# Ovarian Cancer

# METHODS IN MOLECULAR MEDICINE™

## *John M. Walker,* SERIES EDITOR

METHODS IN MOLECULAR MEDICINE™

# Ovarian Cancer

*Methods and Protocols*

Edited by

## John M. S. Bartlett, MD

*Department of Surgery, University of Glasgow, Glasgow, Scotland*

Springer Science+Business Media, LLC

2000 Humana Press Inc.

© Springer Science+Business Media New York 2000
Originally published by Humana Press Inc. in 2000
Softcover reprint of the hardcover 1st edition 2000

This publication is printed on acid-free paper. ∞
ANSI Z39.48-1984 (American Standards Institute)
Permanence of Paper for Printed Library Materials.

Cover design by Patricia F. Cleary
Cover illustration: Fig. 2B from Chapter 26, "Gene Amplification of c-ermB-2 Detected by FISH" by S. Robert Young, Wei-Hua Liu, and Zong-Ren Wang.

For additional copies, pricing for bulk purchases, and/or information about other Humana titles, contact Humana at the above address or at any of the following numbers: Tel.: 973-256-1699; Fax: 973-256-8341; E-mail: humana@humanapr.com; or visit our Website: http://humanapress.com

**Photocopy Authorization Policy:**

Library of Congress Cataloging in Publication Data

Ovarian cancer : methods and protocols / edited by John M. S. Bartlett.
        p.; cm.--(Methods in molecular medicine; 39)
    Includes bibliographical references and index.

    ISBN 978-1-4899-4396-5          ISBN 978-1-59259-071-1 (eBook)
    DOI 10.1007/978-1-59259-071-1

    1. Ovaries--Cancer--Molecular aspects--Research--Methodology. 2. Tumor markers--Research--Methodology. 3. Ovaries--Cancer--Genetic aspects--Research--Methodology. I. Bartlett, John M.S. II. Series
    [DNLM: 1. Ovarian Neoplasms--genetics. 2. Genetics, Biochemical. 3. Models, Biological. 4. Tumor Markers, Biological. WP 322 O9647 2000]
    RC280.O8 O926 2000
    616.99' 465--dc21

                                                                        00-040718
                                                                        CIP

# Preface

If there is one aspect of current cancer research that represents a major challenge for both novice and experienced researchers, it is the rapid advance in our understanding of the disease. Researchers can be required to switch from analysis of gene expression to kinetics of protein activation, from genetic studies to the analysis of protein funtion. Cancers are highly complex disease systems and researchers aiming to understand the functioning of cancer systems require access to a wide range of laboratory techiques from a broad range of research disciplines. Increasingly, however, published methods are incomplete or refer back to a series of previous publications each containing only a small part of the complete protocol. The aim of *Ovarian Cancer: Methods and Protocols* is to provide for ovarian cancer researchers, in the first instance, a laboratory handbook that will facilitate research into cancer systems by providing a series of expert protocols, with proven efficacy, across a broad range of technical expertise. Thus, there are sections on tumor genetics and cellular signal transduction, as well as sections on apoptosis and RNA analysis.

The value of *Ovarian Cancer: Methods and Protocols* to the ovarian cancer researcher will, I trust, be considerably enhanced by (1) the provision of a series of overviews relating to the biology, diagnosis, and treatment of this important neoplasm, and (2) the provision of a series of technical overviews introducing each part that provides an expert review of the applications and pitfalls of the various techniques included.

*Ovarian Cancer: Methods and Protocols* aims to provide a resource for both the novice scientist/clinician coming to grips with laboratory-based research for the first time, as well as for those more experienced investigators seeking to diversify their technological base. Often, we are constrained less by our ideas than by our abilities to carry forward those ideas using different technologies.

No volume can exhaustively cover every aspect of biological research, and there will be gaps that one or another research group will identify. Each section could readily be expanded (and in some cases has been) into a book in its own right. However, I have sought to include a spectrum of techniques that will allow the acquisition of key skills in each area covered. The aim is to give the researcher an understanding of the technical issues covered in each section such that they can then extrapolate their expertise into salient techniques in these areas.

As with all volumes in the *Methods in Molecular Medicine* series, clear instructions in the perfomance of the various protocols is supplemented by additional technical notes that provide valuable insights into the working of the technique in question. Though often brief, these notes provide essential details that allow a successful outcome.

I would like to express my gratitude to all those who have contributed to this volume, who have been patient over the period required to collate their contributions. I am also grateful to Professor John Walker for his encouragement and guidance as series editor. Finally, I would like to thank my wife, Dorothy for patiently proof reading manuscripts and for being understanding on the many occasions when I arrived home late during the preparation of this volume.

*John M. S. Bartlett,* MD

# Contents

# Contributors

EDWIN C. A. ABELN • *Centraal Bureau voor Schimmelcultures, RNAAS Institute, Baarn, The Netherlands*

MAHMOUD ABU-HADID • *Division of Medicine, Roswell Park Cancer Institute, Buffalo, NY*

GREGORY P. ADAMS • *Department of Medical Oncology, Fox Chase Cancer Center, Philadelphia, PA*

GIRIDHAR R. AKKARAJU • *Department of Molecular Biology and Immunology, University of North Texas Health Science Center, Fort Worth, TX*

UWE ALTENSCHMIDT • *Institute for Experimental Cancer Research, Tumor Biology Center, Freiburg, Germany*

RONALD D. ALVAREZ • *Departments of Obstetrics and Gynecology, University of Alabama, Birmingham, AL*

M. JANE ARBOLEDA • *Division of Haematological Oncology, Department of Medicine, UCLA School of Medicine, University of Califorina, Los Angeles, CA*

NELLY AUERSPERG • *Department of Obstetrics and Gynecology, University of British Columbia, BC Women's Hospital, Vancouver, Canada*

MARC AZÉMAR • *Institute for Experimental Cancer Research, Tumor Biology Center, Freiburg, Germany*

JAN P. A. BAAK • *Department of Quantitative Pathology, Academisch Ziekenhuis VrijeUniversiteit De Boelelaan, Amsterdam, The Netherlands*

EMILY BANKS • *ICRG Cancer Epidemiology Unit, Radcliffe Infirmary, Oxford, UK*

JOHN M. S. BARTLETT • *Department of Surgery, Glasgow Royal Infirmary, Glasgow, UK*

ROBERT C. BAST, JR. • *Department of Obstetrics and Gynecology, Duke University Medical Center, NC*

ALAKANANDA BASU • *Department of Molecular Biology and Immunology, University of North Texas Health Science Center, Fort Worth, TX*

EBERHARD P. BECK • *Leitender Oberarzt, Städtische Frauenklinik Berk, Stuttgart, Germany*

ALF BECKMANN • *Klinisher Chemiker, Institut für Klinische Chemie und Laboratoriumsmedizin, Münster, Germany*

MARIA C. BELL • *Department of Cellular Biology and Anatomy, Louisiana State University Medical Center-Shreveport, Shreveport, LA*

BURKHARD BRANDT • *Klinisher Chemiker, Institut für Klinische Chemie und Laboratoriumsmedizin, Münster, Germany*

MURRAY BRILLIANT • *Department of Pathology, Royal University Hospital Saskatoon, Saskatchawan, Canada*

MASSIMO BROGGINI • *Laboratory of Cancer Pharmacology, Mario Negri Institute for Pharmacological Research, Milan, Italy*

ROBERT BROWN • *CRC Department of Medical Oncology, Beatson Laboratories, Glasgow University, Glasgow, UK*

JANE BRUGGHE • *Department of Quantitative Pathology, Academisch Ziekenhuis VrijeUniversiteit De Boelelaan, Amsterdam, The Netherlands*

EMMA J. BRYAN • *Department of Obstetrics and Gynecology, University of Southampton Princess Anne Hospital, Southampton, UK*

RICHARD E. BULLER • *Department of Pharmacology, University of Iowa Hospitals and Clinics, Iowa City, IA*

DAVID J. BURNS • *Breast Cancer Research Unit, Western General Hospital, Edinburgh, Scotland*

IAN G. CAMPBELL • *Department of Obstetrics and Gynecology, University of Southampton Princess Anne Hospital, Southampton, UK*

JENNIFER L. CARROLL • *Department of Cellular Biology and Anatomy, and Obstetrics and Gynecology, Louisiana State University Medical Center-Shreveport, Shreveport, LA*

SETSUKO K. CHAMBERS • *Department of Obstetrics and Gynecology, Yale School of Medicine, New Haven, MA*

ZHIHONG CHEN • *Laboratory of Biomedical Research, Institute of Molecular and Cellular Bioscience, University of Tokyo, Tokyo, Japan*

DENNIS S. CHI • *Gynecology Academic Office, Gynecology Service, Memorial Sloan-Kettering Cancer Center, New York, NY*

CEES J. CORNELISSE • *Department of Pathology, Leiden University Medical Centre, Leiden, The Netherlands*

WILLEM E. CORVER • *Centraal Bureau voor Schimmelcultures, RNAAS Institute, Baarn, The Netherlands*

LUCY J. CURTIS • *Molecular Medicine Centre, Department of Pathology, Edinburgh University, Edinburgh, Scotland*

G. D'AGOSTINO • *Department of Obstetrics and Gynecology, Laboratory of Antienoplastic Pharmacology Zeneca, Catholic University of the Sacred Heart, Rome, Italy*

DEREK S. DAMRON • *Lerner Research Institute, Department of Cancer Biology, Cleveland Clinic Foundation, Cleveland, OH*

HIRANMOY DAS • *Department of Obstetrics and Gynecology, Hyogo Medical Center for Adults 13–70, Akashi, Japan*

A. DE DILECTIS • *Laboratory of Antienoplastic Pharmacology Zeneca, Department of Obstetrics and Gynecology, Catholic University of the Sacred Heart, Rome, Italy*

JESSY DESHANE • *Departments of Pathology, University of Alabama, Birmingham, AL*

JAYNE DEVLIN • *School of Biomedical Sciences, University of Ulster, Coleraine, Northern Ireland*

KARL DOBIANER • *Department fo Cellular Endocrinology, Ludwig Bolzmann Institute for Experimental Endocrinology, General Hospital of Vienna, Vienna, Austria*

INNA DUMLER • *Charité-Franz Volhard Clinic, and Max-Delbrück Center for Molecular Medicine, Humboldt University at Berlin, Berlin, Germany*

JOANNE EDWARDS • *University Department of Surgery, Glasgow, Scotland*

ZEYAD ELAKAWI • *Division of Medicine, Roswell Park Cancer Institute, Buffalo, NY*

GAMAL H. ELTABBAKH • *Department of Gynecologic Oncology, Fletcher Allen Health Care/University of Vermont, Burlington, VT*

MARC S. ERNSTOFF • *Section of Hematology/Oncology, Dartmoth Hitchcock Medical Center, Lebanon, NH*

ARJANG FATTAHI-MEIBODI • *Department of Obstetrics and Gynecology, University of Gottingen, Gottingen, Germany*

GABRIELLA FERRANDINA • *Laboratory of Antienoplastic Pharmacology Zeneca, Department of Obstetrics and Gynecology, Catholic University of the Sacred Heart, Rome, Italy*

WILLIAM FOULKES • *Department of Medicine, Human Genetics, and Oncology, Montreal General Hospital and Sir M. B. Davis-Jewish General Hospital, McGill University, Montreal, Quebec, Canada*

HANI GABRA • *ICRG Medical Oncology Unit, Western General Hospital, Edinburgh, Scotland*

GÜNTHER GASTL • *Department of Hematology and Oncology, University of Innsbruck, Innsbruck,*

FRANK GEBHARDT • *Klinisher Chemiker, Institut für Klinische Chemie und Laboratoriumsmedizin, Münster, Germany*

CICEK GERCEL-TAYLOR • *Division of Gynecologic Oncology, Department of Obstetrics and Gynecology, University of Louisville, Louisville, KY*

RANDALL K. GIBB • *Division of Gynecologic Oncology, Department of Obstetrics and Gynecology, University of Louisville, Louisville, KY*

ANDERS GOBL • *Department of Internal Medicine, University of Uppsala Hospital, Uppsala, Sweden*

JAMES J. GOING • *Department of Pathology, University of Glasgow, Glasgow, Scotland*

BASEM S. GOUELI • *Department of Obstetrics/Gynecology, Jikei University School of Medicine, Tokyo Japan*

SAID A. GOUELI • *Department of Obstetrics/Gynecology, Jikei University School of Medicine, Tokyo Japan*

CHARLES GOURLEY • *Imperial Cancer Research Fund, Medical Oncology Unit, Western General Hospital, Edinburgh, Scotland*

HENNER GRAEFF • *Klinischer Forschergruppe der Frauenklinik der Technischen Universität München, Muenchen, Germany*

BERND GRONER • *Chemotherapeutisches Forschungsinstitut, Georg Speyer Haus, Frankfurt, Germany*

THOMAS W. GRUNT • *Department of Oncology, University Clinic of Internal Medicine, Vienna, Austria*

FRANCESCA GUALANDI • *Institute of Microbiology, School of Medicine, University of Ferrara, Ferrara, Italy*

XIN-YUAN GUAN • *Laboratory of Cancer Genetics, National Human Genome Research Unit, National Institutes of Health, Betheda, MD*

ANNE W. HAMBURGER • *Division of Cell and Molecular Biology, Greenebaum Center for Cancer Research, University of Maryland, Baltimore, MD*

THOMAS C. HAMILTON • *Department of Medical Oncology, Fox Chase Cancer Center, Philadelphia, PA*

KAZUO HASEGAWA • *Department of Obstetrics and Gynecology, Hyogo Medical Center for Adults 13–70, Akashi, Japan*

RUDI HENRIKSEN • *Department of Women's and Children's Health, Obstetrics and Gynecology, University of Uppsala Hospital, Uppsala, Sweden*

SEIMIYA HIROYUKI • *Cancer Chemotherapy Center, Japanese Foundation for Cancer Research, Tokyo, Japan*

GILLIAN L. HIRST • *CRC Department of Medical Oncology, Beatson Laboratories, Glasgow University, Glasgow, Scotland*

SHINJI HORIBE • *Department of Obstetrics and Gynecology, Gifu University School of Medicine, Gifu, Japan*

WILLIAM J. HOSKINS • *Gynecology Academic Office, Gynecology Service, Memorial Sloan-Kettering Cancer Center, New York, NY*

KEVIN HSAIO • *Signal Transduction Group, Promega, and Department of Pathology and Laboratory Medicine, University School of Medicine, Madison, WI*

MARTIN J. HULME • *Breast Cancer Research Unit , Western General Hospital, Edinburgh, Scotland*

MATJAZ HUMAR • *Institute for Experimental Cancer Research, Tumor Biology Center, Freiburg, Germany*

MIEN-CHIE HUNG • *Department of Cancer Biology, Section of Molecular Cell Biology and Department of Surgical Oncology, The University of Texas, Houston, TX*

ATSUSHI IMAI • *Department of Obstetrics and Gynecology, Gifu University School of Medicine, Gifu, Japan*

SEIJI ISONISHI • *Department of Obstetrics/Gynecology, Jikei University School of Medicine, Minato-ku, Tokyo, Japan*

IAN J. JACOBS • *Gynecology Cancer Research Unit, St. Bartholomew's Hospital, West Smithfield, London, UK*

WOLFRAM JAEGER • *Department of Obstetrics and Gynecology, University of Erlangen-Nurmberg, Universität Straße, Erlangen, Germany*

STEVEN W. JOHNSON • *Department of Medical Oncology, Fox Chase Cancer Centre, Philadelphia, PA*

PETER A. KAUFMAN • *Section of Hematology/Oncology, Dartmouth Hitchcock Medical Center, Lebanon, NH*

ROBERT C. KNAPP • *Division of Gynecologic Oncology, Brigham and Women's Hospital, Boston, MA*

MARGARET A. KNOWLES • *ICRF Cancer Medicine Research Unit, St. James's University Hospital, Leeds, UK*

TAMIO KOIZUMI • *Department of Obstetrics and Gynecology, Hyogo Medical Center for Adults 13–70, Akashi, Japan*

GEORG KRUPITZA • *Department of Haematopathology, Institute of Clinical Pathology, Universtiy of Vienna, Vienna, Austria*

SATORU KYO • *Department of Obstetrics and Gynecology, Kanazawa University, Kanazawa, Japan*

SIMON P. LANGDON • *Imperial Cancer Research Fund, Medical Oncology Unit, Western General Hospital, Edinburgh, Scotland*

SANDRA S. LAWRIE • *Imperial CancerResearch Fund, Medical Oncology Unit, Western General Hospital, Edinburgh, Scotland*

THOMAS M. LEBER • *Imperial Cancer Research Fund, Biological Therapies Laboratory, London, UK*

ERNST LENGYEL • *Klinischer Forschergruppe der Frauenklinik der Technischen Universität München, Muenchen, Germany*

THOMAS LIEHR • *Institut für Humangenetik, Jena, Germany*

WEI-HUA LIU • *Department of Obstetrics and Gynecology, University of South Carolina School of Medicine, Columbia, SC*

GABRIELLA MACCHIA • *Laboratory of Antienoplastic Pharmacology Zeneca, Department of Obstetrics and Gynecology, Catholic University of the Sacred Heart, Rome, Italy*

MELANIE MACKEAN • *Department of Medical Oncology, Western General Hospital NHS Trust, Edinburgh Scotland*

VIKTOR MAGDOLEN • *Klinischer Forschergruppe der Frauenklinik der Technischen Universität München, München, Germany*

ANTHONY MAGLIOCCO • *Department of Pathology, Royal University Hospital Saskatoon, Saskatchawan, Canada*

SARAH L. MAINES-BANDIERA • *Department of Obstetrics and Gynecology, University of British Columbia, BC Women's Hospital, Vancouver, Canada*

SALVATORE MANCUSO • *Laboratory of Antienoplastic Pharmacology Zeneca, Department of Obstetrics and Gynecology, Catholic University of the Sacred Heart, Rome, Italy*

MARIA MARONE • *Laboratory of Antienoplastic Pharmacology Zeneca, Department of Obstetrics and Gynecology, Catholic University of the Sacred Heart, Rome, Italy*

DAGMAR MARX • *Department of Obstetrics and Gynecology, University of Gottingen, Gottingen, Germany*

TETSUO MASHIMA • *Laboratory of Biomedical Research, Institute of Molecular and Cellular Bioscience, University of Tokyo, Tokyo, Japan*

J. MICHAEL MATHIS • *Department of Cellular Biology and Anatomy, and Division of Gynecologic Oncology, Department of Obstetrics and Gynecology, Louisiana State University Medical Center-Shreveport, Shreveport, LA*

MARTINA MAURER-GEBHARD • *Institute for Experimental Cancer Research, Tumor Biology Center, Freiburg, Germany*

AMANDA J. MCILWRATH • *CRC Department of Medical Oncology, Glasgow, Scotland*

HARALD MEDEN • *Department of Obstetrics and Gynecology, University of Gottingen, Gottingen, Germany*

MICHAEL MEDL • *Department of Obstetrics and Gynecology, Lainz Medical Center, Vienna, Austria*

GERRIT A. MEIJER • *Department of Quantitative Pathology, Academisch Ziekenhuis VrijeUniversiteit De Boelelaan, Amsterdam, The Netherlands*

VINCENT A. MEMOLI • *Section of Hematology/Oncology, Dartmouth Hitchcock Medical Center, Lebanon, NH*

GORDON B. MILLS • *Department of Obstetrics and Gynecology, Duke University Medical Center, NC*

BERND MUEHLENWEG • *Klinischer Forschergruppe der Frauenklinik der Technischen Universität München, Muenchen, Germany*

PETER MULLEN • *Imperial Cancer Research Fund, Medical Oncology Unit, Western General Hospital, Edinburgh, Scotland*

TAKASHI MURATA • *First Department of Internal Medicine, School of Medicine, Yokohama City University, Yokohama, Japan*

MIKIHIKO NAITO • *Laboratory of Biomedical Research, Institute of Molecular and Cellular Bioscience, University of Tokyo, Tokyo, Japan*

RUPERT P. M. NEGUS • *Imperial Cancer Research Fund, Biological Therapies Laboratory, London, UK*

SUSANN NEUBAUER • *Klinik und Poliklinik für Strahlentherapie, Universitätsstr, Erlangen, Germany*

RYUICHIRO NISHIMURA • *Department of Obstetrics and Gynecology, Hyogo Medical Center for Adults 13–70, Akashi, Japan*

KAZUNORI OCHIAI • *Department of Obstetrics/Gynecology, Jikei University School of Medicine, Minato-ku, Tokyo, Japan*

AIKO OKAMOTO • *Department of Obstetrics/Gynecology, Jikei University School of Medicine, Minato-ku, Tokyo, Japan*

MICHAEL G. ORMEROD • *Reigate, United Kingdom*

GUISEPPE PANDINI • *Istituto di Medicina Interna, Malattie Endocrine e del Metabolismo, Universita di Catania, Catania, Italy*

LAKSHMI PENDYALA • *Division of Medicine, Roswell Park Cancer Center, Buffalo, NY*

RAYMOND P. PEREZ • *Section of Hematology/Oncology, Department of Medicine, Darthmouth-Hitchcock Medical Center, Lebanon, NH*

VINCENZO PEZZINO • *Istituto di Medicina Interna, Malattie Endocrine e del Metabolismo, Universita di Catania, Catania, Italy*

MARIE PLANTE • *Gynecology Service, L'Hotel-Dieu de Quebec, Quebec City, Canada*

SUSAN M. QUIRK • *Department of Animal Science, Cornell University, Ithaca, NY*

GENEVIEVE J. RABIASZ • *Imperial Cancer Research Fund Medical Oncology Unit, Western General Hospital, Edinburgh, Scotland*

FRANS C. S. RAMAEKERS • *Department of Molecular Cell Biology and Genetics, University of Maastricht, Maastricht, Netherlands*

JONATHAN R. REEVES • *Delaware, Ontario, Canada*

UTE REUNING • *Klinischer Forschergruppe der Frauenklinik der Technischen Universität München, Muenchen, Germany*

CHRIS P. M. REUTELINGSPERGER • *Department of Molecular Cell Biology and Genetics, University of Maastricht, Maastricht, Netherlands*

PAOLA RIMESSI • *Institute of Microbiology, School of Medicine, University of Ferrara, Ferrara, Italy*

ALISON A. RITCHIE • *Imperial Cancer Research Fund, Medical Oncology Unit, Western General Hospital, Edinburgh, Scotland*

ANTJE ROETGER • *Klinisher Chemiker, Institut für Klinische Chemie und*

*Laboratoriumsmedizin, Münster, Germany*

JOSEPH E. ROULSTON • *Department of Reproductive and Developmental Sciences, The University of Edinburgh, The Royal Infirmary, Edinburgh, Scotland*

INGO B. RUNNEBAUM • *Molecular Biology Laboratory, Department of Obstetrics and Gynecology, University of Ulm, Ulm, Germany*

S. E. HILARY RUSSELL • *Department of Oncology, The Queen's University of Belfast, Belfast City Hospital, Belfast, Northern Ireland*

YOSHIO SAITO • *Department of Applied Chemistry, Faculty of Science and Technology, Keio University, Kohoku-ku, Yokohama, Japan*

JOSEPH T. SANTOSO • *Division of Gynecologic Oncology, University of Texas Medical Branch, Galveston, TX*

A. KAY SAVAGE • *Department of Histopathology, Royal Free Hospital School of Medicine, Hampstead, London*

GIOVANNI SCAMBIA • *Laboratory of Antienoplastic Pharmacology Zeneca, Department of Obstetrics and Gynecology, Catholic University of the Sacred Heart, Rome, Italy*

ROBERT SCHIER • *Xerion Pharmaceuticals GmbH, Martinsried, Munich, Germany*

ANDREAS SCHNELZER • *Klinischer Forschergruppe der Frauenklinik der Technischen Universität München, München, Germany*

MANFRED SCHMITT • *Klinischer Forschergruppe der Frauenklinik der Technischen Universität München, München, Germany*

BERT SCHUTTE • *Department of Molecular Cell Biology and Genetics, University of Maastricht, Maastricht, Netherlands*

LAURA SCIACCA • *Istituto di Medicina Interna, Malattie Endocrine e del Metabolismo, Universita di Catania, Catania, Italy*

GRANT C. SELLAR • *Imperial Cancer Research Fund Medical Oncology Unit, Western General Hospital, Edinburgh, Scotland*

ANDREW N. SHELLING • *Department of Obstetrics and Gynecology, Research Centre in Reproductive Medicine, National Women's Hospital, Auckland, New Zealand*

GENE P. SIEGAL • *Departments of Pathology and Biology, University of Alabama, Birmingham, AL*

STEVEN J. SKATES • *General Medicine Division, Massachusetts General Hospital and Harvard Medical School, Boston, MA*

DENNIS J. SLAMON • *Division of Haematological Oncology, Department of Medicine, UCLA School of Medicine, University of Califorina, Los Angeles, CA*

BARBARA SMITH • *Jack Birch Unit of Molecular Carcinogenesis, Department of Biology, University of York, York, UK*

ANIL K. SOOD • *Division of Gynecologic Oncology, Department of Obstetrics and Gynecology, University of Iowa Hospitals and Clinics, Iowa City, IA*

JENNIFER SOUTHGATE • *Jack Birch Unit of Molecular Carcinogenesis, Department of Biology, University of York, York, UK*

DANIEL M. SPINNER • *Abteilung Frauenheilkunde und Geburtshilfe I, Universitats Klinik Freiburg, Freiburg, Germany*

JÜRGEN SPONA • *Department of Cellular Endocrinology, Ludwig Boltzmann Institute for Experimental Endocrinology, General Hospital of Vienna, and Department of Obstetrics and Gynecology, University of Vienna, Vienna, Austria*

ATSUSHI TAKAGI • *Department of Obstetrics and Gynecology, Gifu University School of Medicine, Gifu, Japan*

HIROSHI TAKAGI • *Department of Obstetrics and Gynecology, Gifu University School of Medicine, Gifu, Japan*

MASAYUKI TAKEMORI • *Department of Obstetrics and Gynecology, Hyogo Medical Center for Adults 13–70, Akashi, Japan*

TERUHIKO TAMAYA • *Department of Obstetrics and Gynecology, Gifu University School of Medicine, Gifu, Japan*

JEFFREY M. TRENT • *Laboratory of Cancer Genetics, National Human Genome Research Unit, National Institutes of Health, Betheda, MD*

TAKASHI TSURUO • *Laboratory of Biomedical Research, Institute of Molecular and Cellular Bioscience, University of Tokyo, and Cancer Chemotherapy Center, Japanese Foundation for Cancer Research, Tokyo, Japan*

JOHN J. TURCHI • *Department of Biochemistry and Molecular Biology, School of Medicine, Wright State University, Dayton, Ohio*

BEYHAN TÜRKMEN • *Klinischer Forschergruppe der Frauenklinik der Technischen Universität München, Muenchen, Germany*

KAZUO UMEZAWA • *Department of Applied Chemistry, Faculty of Science and Technology, Keio University, Kohoku-ku, Yokohama, Japan*

FRANK H. VALONE • *Section of Hematology/Oncology, Dartmouth Hitchcock Medical Center, Lebanon, NH*

THIJS VAN AKEN • *Department of Molecular Cell Biology and Genetics, University of Maastricht, Maastricht, Netherlands*

PAUL J. VAN DIEST • *Department of Quantitative Pathology, Academisch Ziekenhuis Vrije Universiteit De Boelelaan, Amsterdam, The Netherlands*

STEFAN M. VAN DEN EIJNDE • *Department of Molecular Cell Biology and Genetics, University of Maastricht, Maastricht, Netherlands*

MANON VAN ENGELAND • *Department of Molecular Cell Biology and Genetics, University of Maastricht, Maastricht, Netherlands*

GOPALRAO V. N. VELAGALETI • *Division of Medical Genetics, Department of Pediatrics, Univeristy of Tennessee, Memphis, TN*

CHRISTL VERMEIJ-KEERS • *Department of Molecular Cell Biology and Genetics, University of Maastricht, Maastricht, Netherlands*

FAINA VIKHANSKAYA • *Laboratory of CancerPharmacology, Mario Negri Institute for Pharmacological Research, Milan, Italy*

PAUL K. WALLACE • *Section of Hematology/Oncology, Dartmouth Hitchcock Medical Center, Lebanon, NH*

H. ANNE WALLER • *Imperial College School of Medicine at St. Mary's, Sussex Gardens, London*

ZONG-REN WANG • *Department of Obstetrics and Gynecology, University of South Carolina School of Medicine, Columbia, SC*

SHAN WANG-GOHRKE • *Molecular Biology Laboratory, Department of Obstetrics* and Gynecology, University of Ulm, Ulm, Germany

AMANDA D. WATTERS • *Department of Surgery, Glasgow Royal Infirmary, Glasgow, UK*

WENDY A. WELLS • *Section of Hematology/Oncology, Dartmouth Hitchcock Medical Center, Lebanon, NH*

KAI WIECHEN • *Institute of Pathology, University Clinic Charitie Faculty of Medicine, Humboldt University of Berlin, Berlin, Germany*

ALISTAIR R. W. WILLIAMS • *Department of Pathology, Edinbrugh University, Edinburgh, Scotland*

YAN XU • *Lerner Research Institute, Department of Cancer Biology, Cleveland Clinic Foundation, Cleveland, OH*

DUEN-HWA YAN • *Department of Cancer Biology, Section of Molecular Cell Biology and Department of Surgical Oncology, The University of Texas, Houston, TX*

S. ROBERT YOUNG • *Department of Obstetrics and Gynecology, University of South Carolina School of Medicine, Columbia, SC*

SU ZHANG • *Department of Cancer Biology, Section of Molecular Cell Biology and Department of Surgical Oncology, The University of Texas, Houston, TX*

RONALD P. ZWEEMER • *Department of Obstetrics and Gynecology, University Hospital Vrije Universiteit, Amsterdam, Netherlands*

# I

## INTRODUCTION TO OVARIAN CANCER

# 1

## The Epidemiology of Ovarian Cancer

### Emily Banks

### 1. Introduction

Ovarian cancer is the most common fatal cancer of the female reproductive tract in industrialized countries. At the time of writing, it is the fourth most common cause of cancer death in women in the U.K., after breast, lung, and colorectal cancer, with a lifetime risk of approximately 2% (1). It tends to present at an advanced stage, with limited prospects for treatment and generally poor survival.

The histological classification of ovarian cancer is complex, with a large number of histological subtypes. Because of the rarity of each type, tumor studies have tended to group the types into broader categories of "epithelial" and "nonepithelial" tumors. "Borderline" tumors are distinguished by the absence of stromal invasion. They are considered to be an earlier or less malignant form of ovarian cancer and have similar epidemiological characteristics to epithelial tumors, with a better prognosis.

Generally speaking, ovarian cancer incidence increases with age and is more common in women with a family history of the disease. Reproductive and hormonal factors appear to be the other main determinants of risk, with a decline in risk associated with increasing parity, oral contraceptive use, hysterectomy, and sterilization by tubal ligation. For other factors, such as the use of hormone replacement therapy, fertility drug treatment, breast feeding, and infertility, the evidence remains equivocal. This chapter will discuss the epidemiology of ovarian cancer, starting with a brief outline of patterns of incidence and time trends, before reviewing the evidence to date regarding risk factors for nonepithelial and epithelial tumors. In view of the sparsity of data regarding risk factors for nonepithelial tumors, the bulk of the chapter relates to epithelial ovarian cancer. This chapter presents a general summary; those requiring a more detailed review are directed to an earlier publication (2).

### 2. International and National Variations and Time Trends

National incidence and registry data usually combine all histological types of ovarian cancer, although epithelial types tend to dominate the findings as they represent 80 to 90% of tumors (3). **Figure 1** presents the age-adjusted annual incidence rates of ovarian cancer from a range of cancer registries (1). Ovarian cancer rates vary enormously from country to country and appear to relate to their respective reproductive patterns. Incidence rates are high in most of the industrialized countries of Europe,

From: *Methods in Molecular Medicine, Vol. 39: Ovarian Cancer: Methods and Protocols*
Edited by: J. M. S. Bartlett © Humana Press, Inc., Totowa, NJ

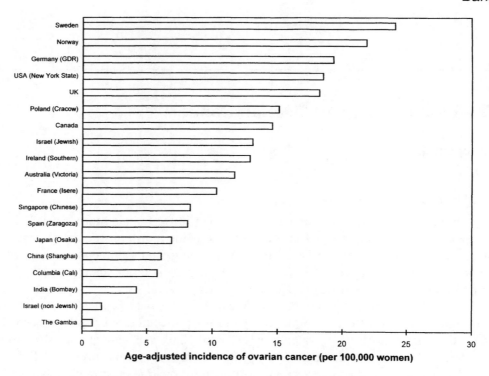

Fig. 1. Age-adjusted annual incidence of ovarian cancer at selected cancer registries.

North America, and Oceania, where women have relatively few children (with the exception of rates in Italy, Japan, and Spain). Ovarian cancer is less common in Asian and African countries with higher fertility rates. Rates of ovarian cancer also vary among different ethnic groups within a particular country. Migration studies have shown that ovarian cancer rates tend to approach those of the country of adoption rather than the country of origin. This suggests that variations within countries are unlikely to be fully explained by racial or genetic differences.

The changing reproductive patterns of Western women are thought to be behind the increases in ovarian cancer witnessed in these countries for most of this century. Changes in incidence are likely to reflect trends in family size (and other factors) from some decades previously. For instance, women who were of reproductive age during the 1930s Depression had a relatively small average family size and consequently higher ovarian cancer risk in later life. Many Western countries have seen recent decreases in ovarian cancer incidence, in the face of continuing declines in fertility. Some authors have proposed that this phenomenon relates to increasing oral contraceptive pill use *(4)*. In contrast, most of the poorer, lower-incidence countries have seen recent increases in ovarian cancer rates.

## 3. Nonepithelial Ovarian Cancer

Nonepithelial tumors account for around 7–10% of all malignant ovarian tumors and are divided into germ cell and sex-cord stromal tumors. They are rare, with an incidence of approximately six per million women per year, and little is known about their risk factor profiles *(5)*.

Fig. 2. Annual incidence of ovarian cancer by age in England and Wales, 1983–1987.

Malignant germ cell tumors are most common in adolescents and young women, with a peak in incidence at around 15–19 years of age. They may be associated with *in utero* exposure to hormones, young maternal age, and high body mass in the woman's mother *(6)*. There are suggestions that parity, recent birth, incomplete pregnancy (miscarriage and abortion), oral contraceptive use, alcohol consumption, and a family history of the disease may influence risk, but findings to date are generally nonsignificant and based on very small numbers of cases *(5,7)*.

Malignant sex-cord stromal tumors have more in common with epithelial ovarian cancer in that they are more frequent in older women and the oral contraceptive pill appears to have a protective effect. However, in contrast to epithelial tumors, findings (once again, based on small numbers) suggest that increasing parity does not appear to protect against these tumors *(5,7)*.

## 4. Epithelial Ovarian Cancer

### 4.1. Personal Characteristics

#### 4.1.1. Age

**Figure 2** shows the log incidence of ovarian cancer by age. Epithelial ovarian cancer is rare among girls and young women and increases exponentially with age *(8)*, until reaching a plateau in incidence around age 50 to 55. Rates increase more slowly in later life *(9,10)*.

#### 4.1.2. Socioeconomic Status

Some studies have found higher risks of epithelial ovarian cancer in women of higher socioeconomic status *(11)*, although this finding is believed to be the result of these women having fewer children *(12–14)*.

### 4.1.3. Weight/Body Mass Index

Results regarding the relationship between body mass index (BMI=weight(kg)/height(m)$^2$) or weight and ovarian cancer are conflicting and inconclusive, and may depend on aspects of study design, such as choice of control group *(15)*. Most studies find no association between weight or BMI and epithelial ovarian cancer *(16–18)*, although some find increasing risk of disease with increasing obesity *(14,19)*. Because the disease process itself can affect body size, study design must address this issue.

### 4.1.4. Genetic/Familial Factors

For more than a century, researchers have reported on rare families with multiple cases of ovarian cancer. In addition, a relationship between breast cancer and ovarian cancer has been reported, both within families and within individuals *(20)*. Clarification of these findings has come with the discovery of the oncogenes *BRCA1* and *BRCA2*, which have been shown to be related to inherited breast and ovarian cancer, through germline mutations in these genes *(21–23)*. Although these rare mutations confer extremely high risks of disease, women reporting a general family history of ovarian cancer are only three to four times more likely to develop ovarian cancer than those without such a family history *(20)*. Whereas these findings are of scientific and aetiological interest, inherited ovarian cancer accounts for only a small proportion of those contracting the disease (less than 5%), and the vast majority of cases are sporadic, occurring among women with no family history of ovarian cancer *(21)*.

### 4.2. Reproductive Factors

### 4.2.1. Menarche and Menopause

The majority of studies have not found any effect of age at first menstrual period (menarche) on epithelial ovarian cancer risk, with one notable exception. Rodriguez et al. *(24)* found a statistically significant decrease in fatal ovarian cancer (all histological types combined) with menarche after age 12, compared with menarche at a younger age.

The age-specific incidence curve (**Fig. 2**) suggests a lessening of the rate of increase in ovarian cancer around the age of menopause, but direct evidence of an effect of menopause on risk has proved somewhat elusive. A study pooling a number of European studies *(25)* reports a doubling in the relative risk of ovarian cancer associated with an age at menopause of 53 or greater compared with menopause under 45 years old, and notes a significant trend of increasing risk of ovarian cancer with later age at menopause. However, the pooled U.S. case-control studies found no trend in ovarian cancer risk with increasing time since last menses *(15)* and Purdie et al. *(14)* found no significant effect of age at menopause on ovarian cancer risk in Australia.

### 4.2.2. Parity and Gravidity

Early classic studies observed high rates of epithelial ovarian cancer among nuns and low rates among groups with generally high parity, including Mormons and Seventh-Day Adventists. The association of increasing parity with decreasing ovarian cancer risk is now well established *(12)* and applies to populations in North America *(13,15)*, Europe *(26,27)*, and Asia *(28)*. Overall, published results show a 40% reduction in ovarian cancer risk associated with the first term pregnancy and trends consistent with a 10–15% average reduction in risk with each term pregnancy *(15)*. A Swedish study found that the risk of ovarian cancer is reduced soon after childbirth and this protective effect appears to diminish with time *(26)*. The effects of incomplete pregnancy (induced abortion and miscarriage) and the effects of the timing of childbirth (such as age at birth of first and/or last child, and birth spacing) require further investigation.

### 4.2.3. Breast Feeding

The effect of breast feeding on ovarian cancer incidence is disputed, and further research is needed on this subject. An analysis based on six U.S. case-control studies *(15)* found a reduced risk of ovarian cancer in women who breast fed compared to those who had not, after controling for parity and oral contraceptive use. Other studies are inconsistent and generally do not support these findings *(2)*.

### 4.2.4. Oral Contraceptive Use

One of the most interesting and striking findings in the epidemiology of epithelial ovarian cancer over the last 20 years is that of the protective effect of the oral contraceptive pill. Studies show consistent results of an approximately 40% reduction in the risk of ovarian cancer with any use of the oral contraceptive pill, and a 5–10% decrease in risk with every year of use *(15,29)*. This protective effect appears to last for at least 15–20 yr after cessation of use and applies to parous as well as nulliparous women. The use of the oral contraceptive pill has been widespread in many countries and the incidence of ovarian cancer has been decreasing, in parallel with increases in oral contraceptive pill use.

### 4.2.5. Hormone Replacement Therapy

Because the age-specific incidence of ovarian cancer suggests that the rate of incidence slows around the time of the menopause, exposure to exogenous hormones in the postmenopausal period could plausibly offset this apparent beneficial effect. Earlier studies of hormone replacement therapy (HRT) tended to compare women who had ever used HRT with never users, and findings are generally consistent with no effect *(2,15)*. However, as more is understood about the effect of oestrogenic and progestagenic hormones on cancer, emphasis has shifted to looking at the effect of current HRT use on ovarian cancer. A pooled analysis of case-control data from the United States found a protective effect of current HRT use in one subgroup, although findings were generally negative *(15)*. In 1995, Rodriguez et al. *(24)* reported on the findings of the only prospective study in this area, which found a 70% increase in risk of ovarian cancer in long-term current HRT users, compared to never users.

Women who use HRT are known to differ from nonusers in a number of ways that may affect their background risk of ovarian cancer. In particular, they are more likely to have had a hysterectomy and to have used the oral contraceptive pill in the past, compared to never users *(30)* and many previous studies have not accounted for these preexisting differences. Further research is needed into the effects of current HRT use, past use, and use of combined oestrogen and progestagen preparations. Other hormonal preparations, such as diethylstilboestrol and depot-medroxyprogesterone acetate do not appear to affect epithelial ovarian cancer risk.

### 4.2.6. Infertility

Women with fertility problems tend to have few children, and because low parity confers an increased risk of epithelial ovarian cancer, investigating the effect of infertility independent of parity has proved problematic. In addition, some researchers have found an increased risk of ovarian cancer in women who have been treated with fertility drugs (*see* **Subheading 4.2.7.**) and that once this drug-treated subgroup is excluded, infertility itself does not affect ovarian cancer risk *(15)*.

Bearing this in mind, there appears to be a fairly consistent relationship between various measures of infertility and an increased risk of ovarian cancer, although this increased risk seems to be confined to women who have never succeeded in becoming pregnant or having a child *(2)*.

### 4.2.7. Fertility Treatment

All of the studies of ovarian cancer and fertility drug treatment are based on very small numbers and findings must be interpreted with caution. In addition, disentangling the effects of fertility drugs from the effects of infertility and low parity has been extremely difficult, if not impossible, with the current data.

Case reports in the late 1980s raised concerns that use of drugs that stimulate ovulation, such as clomiphene citrate, may increase a woman's risk of ovarian cancer. Anxiety was further heightened by the U.S. pooled case-control studies, which showed a 2.8-fold increase in ovarian cancer risk in infertile women who had been treated with fertility drugs compared to women without a history of infertility. The risk was particularly high (more than 20-fold) among women who had been treated with these drugs, but had never become pregnant, compared with never-pregnant women without fertility problems *(15)*. Other studies have shown more moderate increases in risk, and a grouped meta-analysis of the published data in this area shows that at least part of the purported effect of fertility drugs results from the relative infertility of the women taking them *(2)*.

### 4.2.8. Oophorectomy, Hysterectomy, and Sterilization

Previous unilateral oophorectomy has been associated with a decrease in risk of ovarian cancer *(9)*. The majority of studies also show a 30–40% reduction in the risk of ovarian cancer with simple hysterectomy (without removal of the ovaries), which is present after controling for parity and oral contraceptive use. There is evidence to suggest that this protective effect is lasting, with no apparent trend in risk with time since hysterectomy *(15)*, although some authors dispute this. Tubal ligation has been noted to protect against ovarian cancer in a number of studies *(11)* with reported reductions in risk ranging from 40% to 80% *(2,11)*, although some studies have not found this to be the case.

It has been suggested that the apparent protective effect of simple hysterectomy may be the result of misclassification bias, where women reporting hysterectomy only may have had an accompanying oophorectomy that they were not aware of *(11)*. Other researchers have hypothesized that hysterectomy and tubal ligation allow visualization and removal of ovaries noted to have a diseased appearance at surgery *(15)*. This argument is to some extent countered by the finding of a sustained benefit of simple hysterectomy for many years following the operation. Hysterectomy and tubal ligation may also act by impairing ovarian blood supply and inducing anovulation or by preventing passage of carcinogens from the vagina to the ovary, via the uterus *(31)*.

### 4.2.9. Ovulation: Lifetime Frequency

Many of the reproductive findings with respect to epithelial ovarian cancer are consistent with Fathalla's "incessant ovulation" hypothesis *(32)*. This hypothesis relates a woman's risk of ovarian cancer to her lifetime frequency of ovulation, and proposes that ovulation causes trauma to the ovarian epithelium and stimulation of mitoses through exposure to oestrogen-rich follicular fluid, which can result in neoplastic transformation (or promotion of initiated cells).

Pregnancy, oral contraceptive use, breast feeding, late menarche, and early menopause all cause a decrease in a woman's frequency of ovulation, whereas ovarian stimulation with fertility drugs causes increased ovulation. Some studies have used figures relating to these to estimate and evaluate the effect of total duration of ovulation (or "ovulatory age") on ovarian cancer incidence. These studies have generally found an increasing risk of ovarian cancer with increasing duration of ovulation, but find that the degree of protection against ovarian cancer conferred by factors such as the oral contraceptive pill and pregnancy is greater than would be expected based on the duration of anovulation caused *(33)*.

## 4.3. Environmental Factors

### 4.3.1. Diet

Many dietary factors have been investigated in relation to epithelial ovarian cancer; although, only a high intake of saturated fat and a low intake of vegetables have been consistently associated with an increased risk. Earlier findings of associations between milk and lactose intakes, galactose and ovarian cancer have been refuted and evidence to date suggests that neither coffee nor alcohol intake is consistently related to risk *(2)*. The effect of meat and fish consumption is unclear.

### 4.3.2. Smoking

Smoking is known to affect a woman's hormonal milieu and two studies have found increases in ovarian cancer among cigarette smokers, compared to nonsmokers *(14,34)*. However, the majority of studies investigating this issue have shown no association and the effect of smoking on ovarian cancer is likely to be small in comparison with its important effects on lung cancer and cardiovascular disease.

### 4.3.3. Talc

A number of studies have found a significant association between the use of talcum powder on the perineum and ovarian cancer *(2,14)*. This coupled with the chemical similarity of talc and asbestos (a known carcinogen) and the finding of talc particles in normal and cancerous ovaries *(35)* has lead to concerns that this relationship is causal. Other studies have not found an association between talc use and ovarian cancer.

### 4.3.4. Viruses

Earlier claims of a relationship between low rates of mumps virus (and other childhood diseases) and ovarian cancers have not generally been sustained *(28,36,37)*, and have been confused by conflicting serology findings.

### 4.3.5. Ionizing Radiation

Women receiving pelvic irradiation for treatment of metropathia hemorrhagica or for inducing menopause are at an increased risk of pelvic cancer in general, but not of ovarian cancer in particular *(38,39)*. No elevation in risk of ovarian cancer has been found in case-control studies looking at both diagnostic and therapeutic irradiation *(11,18,40)*.

### 4.4. Conclusions

The main established factors influencing epithelial ovarian cancer risk, such as age, parity, oral contraceptive use, and hysterectomy have limited potential for modification or public health intervention. For this reason, factors such as HRT, fertility drugs, and breast feeding are of particular interest. Larger studies and further pooled analyses are likely to clarify their effects.

## References

1. Parkin, D. M., Muir, C. S., Whelan, S. F., et al., (eds.) (1992) *Cancer Incidence in Five Continents.* IARC Scientif. Lyon, France.
2. Banks, E., Beral, V., and Reeves, G. (1997) The epidemiology of epithelial ovarian cancer: a review. *Int. J. Gynecol. Cancer* **7,** 425–438.
3. Mant, J. W. F. and Vessey, M. P. (1994) Ovarian and Endometrial Cancers in *Trends in Cancer Incidence and Mortality* (Doll, R., Fraumeni, Jr. J. F., and Muir, C. S., eds.), Cold Spring Harbor Laboratory, Plainview, NY, pp. 287–307.
4. Beral, V., Hannaford, P., and Kay, C. (1988) Oral contraceptive use and malignancies of the genital tract. Results from the Royal College of General Practitioners' oral contraceptive study. *Lancet* **ii,** 1331–1334.
5. Horn Ross, P. L., Whittemore, A. S., Harris, R., and Itnyre, J. (1992) Characteristics relating to ovarian cancer risk: collaborative analysis of 12 U.S. case-control studies. VI. Non-epithelial cancers among adults. Collaborative Ovarian Cancer Group. *Epidemiol.* **3,** 490–495.
6. Walker, A. H., Ross, R. K., Haile, R. W. C., and Henderson, B. E. (1988) Hormonal factors and risk of ovarian germ cell cancer in young women. *Brit. J. Cancer* **57,** 418–422.
7. Albrektsen, G., Heuch, I., and Kvale, G. (1997) Full-term pregnancies and incidence of ovarian cancer of stromal and germ cell origin: a Norwegian prospective study. *Brit. J. Cancer* **75,** 767–770.
8. Adami, H. O., Bergstrom, R., Persson, I., and Sparen, P. (1990) The incidence of ovarian cancer in Sweden, 1960–1984. *Amer. J. Epidemiol.* **132,** 446–452.
9. Booth, M. and Beral, V. (1985) The epidemiology of ovarian cancer in *Ovarian Cancer* (Hudson, C. N., ed). Oxford University Press, New York, pp. 22–44.
10. Ewertz, M. and Kjaer, S. K. (1988) Ovarian cancer incidence and mortality in Denmark 1943–1982. *Int. J. Cancer* **42,** 690–696.
11. Booth, M., Beral, V., and Smith, P. (1989) Risk factors for ovarian cancer: a case control study. *Brit. J. Cancer* **60,** 592–598.
12. Beral, V., Fraser, P., and Chilvers, C. (1978) Does pregnancy protect against ovarian cancer? *Lancet* **i,** 1083–1087.
13. Risch, H. A., Marrett, L. D., and Howe, G. R. (1994) Parity, contraception, infertility, and the risk of epithelial ovarian cancer. *Amer. J. Epidemiol.* **140,** 585–597.
14. Purdie, D., Green, A., Bain, C., Siskind, V., Ward, B., Hacker, N., et al. (1995) Reproductive and other factors and risk of epithelial ovarian cancer: an Australian case-control study. *Int. J. Cancer* **62,** 678–684.
15. Whittemore, A. S., Harris, R., and Itnyre, J. (1992) Characteristics relating to ovarian cancer risk: collaborative analysis of 12 US case-control studies. II. Invasive epithelial ovarian cancers in white women. Collaborative Ovarian Cancer Group. *Amer. J. Epidemiol.* **136,** 1184–1203.
16. Franceschi, S., La Vecchia, C., Helmrich, S. P., Mangioni, C., and Tognoni, G. (1982) Risk factors for epithelial ovarian cancer in Italy. *Amer. J. Epidemiol.* **115,** 714–719.
17. Hildreth, N. G., Kelsey, J. L., LiVolsi, V. A., Fischer, D. B., Holford, T. R., Mostow, E. D., et al. (1981) An epidemiologic study of epithelial carcinoma of the ovary. *Amer. J. Epidemiol.* **114,** 398–405.
18. Koch, M., Jenkins, H., and Gaedke, H. (1988) Risk factors of ovarian cancer of epithelial origin: a case control study. *Cancer Detect. Prev.* **13,** 131–136.

19. The Centers for Disease Control Cancer and Steroid Hormone Study. (1983) Oral contraceptive use and the risk of ovarian cancer. *JAMA* **249,** 1596–1599.

20. Amos, C. I. and Struewing, J. P. (1993) Genetic epidemiology of epithelial ovarian cancer. *Cancer* **71,** 566–572.

21. Friedman, L. S., Ostermeyer, E. A., Lynch, E. D., Szabo, C. I., Anderson, L. A., Dowd, P., et al. (1994) The search for BRCA1. *Cancer Res.* **54,** 6374–6382.

22. Jacobs, I. and Lancaster, J. (1996) The molecular genetics of sporadic and familial epithelial ovarian cancer. *Int. J. Gynecol. Cancer* **6,** 337–355.

23. Gayther, S. A., Mangion, J., Russell, P., Seal, S., Barfoot, R., Ponder, B. A., et al. (1997) Variation of risks of breast and ovarian cancer associated with different germline mutations of the BRCA2 gene. *Nat. Genet.* **15,** 103–105.

24. Rodriguez, C., Calle, E. E., Coates, R. J., Miracle McMahill, H. L., Thun, M. J., and Heath, C. W., Jr. (1995) Estrogen replacement therapy and fatal ovarian cancer. *Amer. J. Epidemiol.* **141,** 828–835.

25. Franceschi, S., La Vecchia, C., Booth, M., Tzonou, A., Negri, E., Parazzini, F., et al. (1991) Pooled analysis of 3 European case-control studies of ovarian cancer: II. Age at menarche and at menopause. *Int. J. Cancer* **49,** 57–60.

26. Adami, H. O., Hsieh, C. C., Lambe, M., Trichopoulos, D., Leon, D., Persson, I., Ekbom, A., and Janson, P. O. (1994) Parity, age at first childbirth, and risk of ovarian cancer. *Lancet* **344,** 1250–1254.

27. Negri, E., Franceschi, S., Tzonou, A., Booth, M., La Vecchia, C., Parazzini, F., et al. (1991) Pooled analysis of 3 European case-control studies: I. Reproductive factors and risk of epithelial ovarian cancer. *Int. J. Cancer* **49,** 50–56.

28. Chen, Y., Wu, P. C., Lang, J. H., Ge, W. J., Hartge, P., and Brinton, L. A. (1992) Risk factors for epithelial ovarian cancer in Beijing, China. *Int. J. Epidemiol.* **21,** 23–29.

29. Franceschi, S., Parazzini, F., Negri, E., Booth, M., La Vecchia, C., Beral, V., et al. (1991) Pooled analysis of 3 European case-control studies of epithelial ovarian cancer: III. Oral contraceptive use. *Int. J. Cancer* **49,** 61–65.

30. Lancaster, T., Surman, G., Lawrence, M., Mant, D., Vessey, M., Thorogood, M., et al. (1995) Hormone replacement therapy: characteristics of users and non-users in a British general practice cohort identified through computerised prescribing records. *J. Epidemiol. Community Health* **49,** 389–394.

31. Cramer, D. W., Welch, W. R., Scully, R. E., and Wojciechowski, C. A. (1982) Ovarian cancer and talc: a case-control study. *Cancer* **50,** 372–376.

32. Fathalla, M. F. (1971) Incessant ovulation—A factor in ovarian neoplasia? *Lancet* **ii,** 163.

33. Risch, H. A., Weiss, N. S., Lyon, J. L., Daling, J. R., and Liff, J. M. (1983) Events of reproductive life and the incidence of epithelial ovarian cancer. *Amer. J. Epidemiol.* **117,** 128–139.

34. Doll, R., Gray, R., Hafner, B., and Peto, R. (1980) Mortality in relation to smoking: 22 years' observations on female British doctors. *Brit. Med. J.* **280,** 967–971.

35. Henderson, W. J., Joslin, C. A. F., Turnbull, A. C., and Griffiths, K. (1971) Talc and carcinoma of the ovary and cervix. *J. Obstet. Gynaecol. Brit. Comm.* **78,** 266–272.

36. West, R. O. (1966) Epidemiologic study of malignancies of the ovaries. *Cancer* **19,** 1001–1007.

37. McGowan, L., Parent, L., Lednar, W., and Norris, H. J. (1979) The woman at risk for developing ovarian cancer. *Gynecol. Oncol.* **7,** 325–344.

38. Brinkley, D. and Haybrittle, J. L. (1969) The late effects of artificial menopause by X-radiation. *Brit. J. Radiol.* **42,** 519–521.

39. Darby, S. C., Reeves, G., Key, T., Doll, R., and Stovall, M. (1994) Mortality in a cohort of women given X-ray therapy for metropathia haemorrhagica. *Int. J. Cancer* **56,** 793–801.

40. Newhouse, M. L., Pearson, R. M., Fullerton, J. M., Boesen, E. A. M., and Shannon, H. S. (1977) A case control study of carcinoma of the ovary. *Brit. J. Prev. Soc. Med.* **31,** 148–153.

# 2

# Familial Ovarian Cancer

## Ronald P. Zweemer and Ian J. Jacobs

## 1. Introduction

Ovarian cancer represents the fifth most significant cause of cancer-related death for women and is the most frequent cause of death from gynecological neoplasia in the Western world. The incidence of ovarian cancer in the United Kingdom (U.K.) is over 5000 new cases every year, accounting for 4275 deaths per year *(1)*. The lifetime risk of ovarian cancer for women in the U.K. is approximately 1 in 80. Most (80–90%) ovarian tumors are epithelial in origin and arise from the coelomic epithelium. The remainder arise from germ-cell or sex cord/stromal cells. A hereditary component in the latter group is rare, but includes granulosa-cell tumors in patients with Peutz–Jeghers syndrome *(2)* and autosomal dominant inheritance of small-cell carcinoma of the ovary *(3,4)*. Because of their limited contribution to familial ovarian cancer, these nonepithelial tumors will not be considered further in this chapter.

Epithelial ovarian cancer has the highest case fatality rate of all gynecological malignancies, and an overall five-year survival rate of only 30%. This poor prognosis is largely because of the fact that 75% of cases present with extra-ovarian disease, which in turn, reflects the absence of symptoms in early-stage disease. Advanced stage ovarian cancer (stage IV) has a five-year survival rate of approximately 10% whereas early stage (stage I) ovarian cancer has a five-year survival rate of at least 85%. These figures suggest that there may be a survival benefit from the detection of ovarian cancer at an early stage. To be able to develop appropriate screening strategies for ovarian cancer, there is a need to understand the processes of carcinogenesis and tumor progression. For ovarian cancer, there are no recognizable precancerous lesions that could be targeted for screening purposes; this contrasts with other types of cancer (e.g., colorectal or cervical cancer) where many of the critical histological alterations in the development of cancer have been identified. In these cancer types, the precancerous lesions have subsequently been linked to specific molecular genetic events *(5)*. Because very little is still known about the morphological and molecular genetic steps involved in initiation and progression of epithelial ovarian cancer, detection and treatment of premalignant lesions is not yet feasible.

Three large randomized controlled trials of screening for ovarian cancer in the general population are currently underway. Because of the potential survival benefit from

From: *Methods in Molecular Medicine, Vol. 39: Ovarian Cancer: Methods and Protocols*
Edited by: J. M. S. Bartlett © Humana Press, Inc., Totowa, NJ

the detection and treatment of early-stage disease, these studies aim to detect early-stage cancer, rather than premalignant disease. However, none of the current studies have yet reached the stage at which information about the impact on mortality is available. To optimize the efficacy of screening, it may be desirable to target women at the highest risk of developing the disease. Most of the established risk factors for ovarian cancer are associated with the theory of "incessant ovulation" *(6,7)* and include nulliparity, an increased number of ovulatory cycles, early menarche (age at first menstruation), and late menopause (age of last menstruation). Oral contraceptive use and multiparity as well as breast feeding reduce the risk of ovarian cancer. It has long been recognized, however, that the most important risk factor for ovarian cancer besides age, is a positive family history for the disease. In recent years, two genes associated with a genetic predisposition for breast and ovarian cancer, the *BRCA1* and *BRCA2* genes, have been identified. This has led to a growing awareness among the public as well as the medical profession that cancer may be hereditary and the demand for risk counseling and molecular testing has increased dramatically. This chapter aims to provide an integrated overview of both the clinical and molecular genetic background of familial and hereditary ovarian cancer.

## 2. Familial and Hereditary Contribution to the Ovarian Cancer Burden

As ovarian cancer affects approximately 1% of women some families will have a history of ovarian cancer in two or more family members or in combination with a common cancer diagnosed at a young age, just by chance. About 15% of all ovarian cancer patients report a positive family history for the disease and can be included in a working definition of "familial ovarian cancer." Such examples of familial ovarian cancer could be explained by chance, common lifestyle, or exposure to carcinogenic factors or a shared genetic susceptibility. However, an estimated 5–10% of all ovarian cancer cases are thought to be the result of an autosomal-dominant susceptibility factor with high penetrance. These cases can be defined as "hereditary ovarian cancer."

## 3. Clinical Diagnosis

The initial evidence for a hereditary component in ovarian cancer was derived from three observations. First, a family history of ovarian cancer was found to confer the greatest risk of all known factors for developing the disease *(8,9)*. This effect is especially strong in families with more than one relative affected. Analysis of population-based series of ovarian cancer cases has shown that the risk of ovarian cancer in a woman who has a first-degree relative (mother or sister) with the disease is 1 in 30 by the age of 70. This risk is around one in four when two first-degree relatives are affected *(10,11)*. Second, population-based epidemiological studies have shown that there is a significant excess of specific types of cancer in the relatives of ovarian cancer patients. These include additional ovarian cancer cases, breast cancer, colorectal, and stomach cancer *(12)*. Finally, many case reports have identified families with multiple cases of ovarian cancer. The first of these describes ovarian cancer in twins *(13)*. Others have described families with multiple cases of ovarian cancer, often in combination with other types of cancer *(14)*. The occurrence of ovarian cancer in these families is best explained by an autosomal-dominant inheritance factor.

### 3.1. Clinical Syndromes

In families where there is insufficient evidence to diagnose autosomal-dominant disease, ovarian cancer can occur alone or in combination with other types of cancer. These familial cancers are to be distinguished from families where autosomal-dominant inheritance of ovarian cancer is likely. In the latter families, epidemiological studies have provided evidence for three distinct clinical, autosomal-dominant cancer syndromes.

1. Hereditary breast-ovarian cancer (HBOC). Families with a pattern of autosomal-dominant inheritance of ovarian and (usually early-onset) breast cancer.
2. Hereditary ovarian cancer (HOC). Families with clear autosomal-dominant inheritance of ovarian cancer, but without apparent excess of breast cancer.
3. Hereditary nonpolyposis colorectal cancer (HNPCC). Families with an autosomal-dominant pattern of early-onset colorectal cancer often in combination with endometrial cancer and sometimes ovarian cancer.

## 4. Molecular Genetic Diagnosis

The final proof that a genetic predisposition is responsible for familial clustering of a disease was initiated by extensive genetic linkage analysis of several large families. Hall et al. *(15)* identified a susceptibility locus on chromosome *17q21* in several families with autosomal-dominant breast cancer. Narod et al. *(16)* confirmed linkage to the same marker in breast–ovarian cancer families. The putative gene was named *BRCA1* (BReast CAncer1). Subsequent analyses showed this gene to be responsible for over 80% of families with cases of breast and ovarian cancer or ovarian cancer alone *(17)*. The discovery of a candidate gene by Miki et al. *(18)* was confirmed by several studies describing the segregation of inactivating germline mutations in this gene with the breast and ovarian cancer cases in these families. In accordance with the notion that the *BRCA1* gene acts as a tumor suppressor gene, allelic deletions affecting the *17q21* locus have invariably been shown to involve the wild-type allele *(19)*.

### 4.1. BRCA1

The *BRCA1* gene consists of 22 coding exons distributed over 100 kb of genomic DNA. It has 5592 bp of coding sequence and encodes a protein of 1863 amino acids. To date, more than 300 distinct mutations have been described and scattered throughout the gene. Although there are some well-defined founder mutations *(20,21)*, there are no specific hot-spots in the gene and only a minority of mutations are recurrent. Approximately 80% of all mutations are nonsense or frameshift mutations causing a truncation of the protein. Some have suggested a relation between the position of the mutation and penetrance as well as tissue specificity. Gayther et al. *(22)* found a significant correlation between the localization of the mutation in the gene and the ratio of breast and ovarian cancer cases within a family. They found that mutations on the three prime third of the gene conveyed a lower risk of ovarian cancer. Apart from this study, genotype–phenotype correlations within *BRCA1* have not been confirmed. Another possibility is that environmental circumstances and/or modifier genes may influence the penetrance of a specific type of cancer in germline mutation carriers. Phelan et al. *(23)* suggested that the risk of ovarian cancer may be increased in women with a *BRCA1* mutation who carried one of two rare variants of the *HRAS* variable number of tandem repeats (VNTRs) compared to women with the common allele.

It has become clear that mutations in the *BRCA1* gene are responsible for the majority of HBOC and HOC families and, therefore, the clinical distinction between these two syndromes may have become obsolete. Initially it was anticipated that somatic mutations in *BRCA1* would be as important in sporadic ovarian cancer as germline mutations are in hereditary cases. This seemed likely as loss of heterozygosity analysis of unselected ovarian cancers has constantly revealed a very high frequency of LOH on chromosome *17q (24,25)*. However, thus far only a few somatic mutations have been detected in sporadic ovarian cancer cases *(26)*. The explanation for the high frequency of LOH of the *17q* locus in these cases remains unclear and may be because of another tumor suppressor gene in the vicinity of *BRCA1* as suggested by the LOH-results of Jacobs et al. *(27)*.

### 4.2. BRCA2

Localization and cloning of the *BRCA2* gene followed soon after the identification of *BRCA1*. In 1994, Wooster et al. *(28)* localized the gene at chromosome *13q12–13*. Only months later, the same group identified the gene by showing segregation of inactivating mutations of mostly breast cancer in families linked with the *13q* locus *(29)*. The *BRCA2* gene consists of 26 coding exons distributed over approximately 70 kb of genomic DNA. It has 10.254 bp of coding sequence and encodes a 3418 amino acid protein which has little homology to previously identified proteins *(30)*. To date, some 100 distinct mutations have been described and as is the case for *BRCA1* these are scattered throughout the coding sequence and apart from several distinct founder mutations *(31,32)* there are no specific hot-spots. The most frequent type of *BRCA2* mutations are frameshifts, most commonly deletions. It appears that missense mutations are rarer than in *BRCA1*. The contribution of *BRCA2* to hereditary breast cancer (HBC) appears to be similar to the contribution of *BRCA1* whereas only a minority of cases of HBOC and HOC are caused by *BRCA2* germline mutations. Although the overall penetrance for ovarian cancer in *BRCA2* germline mutation carriers is estimated at approximately 25% *(17)*, Gayther et al. *(33)* found evidence for an "ovarian cancer cluster-region" in exon 11. Mutations in this OCCR were suggested to confer a higher risk of ovarian cancer. To a lesser extent than is the case for *BRCA1*, LOH at the *BRCA2* locus is frequent in sporadic ovarian cancer *(34)* and somatic mutations of *BRCA2* are rare in ovarian cancer.

### 4.3. Function of BRCA1 and BRCA2

The 7.8 kb mRNA *BRCA1*-transcript is expressed most abundantly in the testis and thymus and at lower levels in the breast and ovary. The mRNA *BRCA2*-transcript shows a similar tissue-specific expression *(30,35)*. Although *BRCA1* and *BRCA2* are unrelated at the sequence level, there are some intriguing similarities. Both have a large exon 11, which contains more than half of the coding sequence. In both genes, translation site starts at codon 2 and both are relatively A-T rich. Defining the biochemical and biological functions that are responsible for tumorigenesis in large genes such as *BRCA1* and *BRCA2* has proven to be difficult. Both genes probably have several functional domains. The presence of a "zinc-finger" motif suggests a role as a transcription factor for the *BRCA1* protein. *BRCA2* has homology with known transcription factors

*(36)*. Similar motifs have been found in genes directly controlling cellular proliferation and in that respect it is important that *BRCA1* has been found to inhibit cell growth *(37)*. The similarity between *BRCA1* and *BRCA2* also includes their ability to bind and complex with Rad51, a protein involved in the repair of double-strand DNA breaks *(38,39)*. For both *BRCA1* and *BRCA2*, a similar "granin" motif has been described, suggesting that the proteins are secreted in secretory vesicles *(40)*. The localization of the *BRCA1* protein, however, is unclear, conflicting reports have localized the protein in the nucleus as well as the cytoplasm *(41,42)*. Explaining the function of both *BRCA1* and *BRCA2* in tumorigenesis remains a major challenge and will be the subject of research activity for some time.

## 4.4. BRCA1 *and* BRCA2 *Mutation Testing*

The risk of a mutation and the penetrance of this mutation determine an individuals risk of (hereditary) cancer. The level of cancer-risk at which to offer a woman testing for germline mutations in *BRCA1* or *BRCA2* is arbitrary and the decision of whether or not a test should be considered is also depend on the purpose it serves for patients or healthy family members.

The chance that cancer in a given family is because of a *BRCA*-germline mutation can be estimated from data collected by the Breast Cancer Linkage Consortium *(17)*. In summary, the risk of detecting a mutation increases with the following: a) an increasing number of affected relatives; b) a young age at diagnosis; and c) occurrence of related cancers in successive generations.

Furthermore, the chance of detecting a *BRCA1* mutation in a given family increases when ovarian cancer is frequent, when patients with both breast and ovarian cancer are present, and when bilateral breast cancer cases occur. The risk of a *BRCA2* mutation increases when male breast cancer occurs in a family. In specific populations, mutations may also be detected in far less remarkable families especially in populations with a high population frequency of founder mutations, such as the Ashkenazi Jewish population. In this population, up to 39% of ovarian cancer patients with a minimal or negative family history have been found to be caused by *BRCA1* or *BRCA2* germline mutations *(31)*.

DNA testing for cancer predisposition may serve several purposes. Especially for breast cancer patients, the treatment modality and follow-up strategies may be modified if the disease is resulting from a genetic predisposition. For ovarian cancer, there is currently no evidence that treatment should differ if the disease is hereditary in nature. Healthy carriers of predisposing mutations may benefit from screening or preventative surgery. The clearest advantage of testing is obtained in at-risk family members who test negative after a mutation has been identified in the family. For this group preventative measures are no longer indicated. Finally, patients and at-risk relatives may wish to be tested on behalf of their children.

Nondirective counseling and education based on prior risk assessment is aimed at reaching a decision whether or not an individual would like to pursue genetic testing. For the initial mutation testing, the cooperation and consent of live affected relatives will usually be required. It is important to test all available affected family members because coincidental cases of either breast or ovarian cancer (phenocopies) may occur. When a mutation is identified in a family, carrier status for individual unaffected family members can be determined. When a mutation cannot be found, the false–negative rate of the test should be considered. A large variety of methods is currently available for the detection of mutations. There is no one technique that is ideally suited to a complete analysis of *BRCA1* and/or *BRCA2*. Some techniques are simple to perform, but not very sensitive whereas others may be very sensitive but laborious and, therefore, usually expensive. The most commonly used techniques include:

- Direct (semiautomated) sequencing (DS)
  Generally considered the gold standard for mutation detection because of its high sensitivity. Disadvantages are the time-consuming and laborious procedures involved, although the availability of semiautomated, fluorescent sequencing systems has increased the feasibility of this method for large-scale (clinical) use.
- Allele-Specific Oligonucleotide Analysis (ASO)
- Single-Strand Conformation Polymorphism Analysis (SSCP/SSCA) and Heteroduplex Analysis (HA)
  Both techniques are easy to perform and relatively quick. Compared to DS, the sensitivity is much lower at a reputed 60–80%.
- Conformational Sensitive Gel Electrophoresis (CSGE)
  This method has an increased sensitivity compared to HA and SSCP, but is more labor intensive.
- (Constant) Denaturing Gradient Gel Electrophoresis (DGGE/CDGE)
  This techniques, which is based on the melting behavior of the DNA double helix is more sensitive than SSCP, however, the technique only detects differences between both alleles, therefore additional techniques are required to identify the precise nature of the mutation. Another disadvantage of all techniques mentioned thus far is that it may be difficult to distinguish between benign polymorphisms and pathogenic mutations. This problem is overcome by the
- Protein Truncation Test (PTT)
  This method detects nonsense and frameshift mutations that result in a stop codon by visualizing a truncated protein in an in vitro transcription–translation assay.
- Southern Analysis (for genomic deletions)
  Recently, specific founder mutations have been identified that consist of the loss of large fragments of coding sequence. Such genomic alterations can be detected by southern analysis in specific populations, which have a high-expected frequency of such alterations.

Detailed, frequently updated protocols for each of the aforementioned techniques are available from the Breast Cancer Information Core database @http://www.nhgri. nih.gov/Intramural_research/Lab_transfer/Bic/

## 4.5. HNPCC-Related Ovarian Cancer

Hereditary nonpolyposis colorectal cancer (HNPCC) is characterized by the autosomal dominant inheritance of early onset colorectal cancer, without the multiple (usually >100) adenomas that constitute familial adenomatous polyposis (FAP). Endometrial cancer is often seen in HNPCC families and should be considered part of the clinical syndrome. Other cancers, including ovarian cancer are encountered in HNPCC families, but are infrequent. Germline mutations in one of five mismatch repair genes are responsible for the syndrome. *hMSH2* (chromosome *2p*), *hMLH1* (chromosome *3p*), *hPMS1* (chromosome *2q*), *hPMS2* (chromosome *7p*), and *hMSH6* (chromosome *2p*) are all part of a family of genes involved in the repair of DNA-replication errors. Tumors arising in patients with germline mutations in one of these genes are in the vast majority of cases genetically unstable and have an RER (replication error) phenotype, which can most easily be detected by studying somatic length alterations in simple nucleotide repeat sequences. Although mutations in all five genes have been detected in HNPCC-related colorectal cancers, 90% of mutations occur in either the *hMSH2* or *hMLH1* gene. Mutation detection of these genes is particularly arduous because they, too, are large—2.2 to 2.8 kb of coding sequence—and as for *BRCA1* and *BRCA2* mutations, are not confined to specific hot spots. The contribution of germline mutations in one of these five mismatch-repair (*MMR*) genes to the total burden of hereditary ovarian cancer is limited, as the penetrance for ovarian cancer is low at approximately 5%.

## 5. Are There Clinicopathological Differences Between Hereditary and Sporadic Ovarian Cancer?

Because family history of ovarian cancer is not a definitive indicator of an underlying germline mutation, other characteristics of ovarian cancer patients have been suggested to be indicative of hereditary disease. In contrast with HNPCC-related cancers of which the vast majority exhibits the *RER*-phenotype, there are no definitive criteria that allow distinction between hereditary and sporadic ovarian cancer. Differences in histopathological characteristics and clinical presentation, as well as prognosis have, however, been reported. The mean age of hereditary ovarian cancer appears to be on average some eight years younger than in sporadic disease *(43–45)*. Hereditary ovarian cancers are more often of the serous type and are more frequently advanced stage with, according to some authors, higher grade than sporadic ovarian cancer. It has been suggested that despite these unfavorable prognostic factors, hereditary ovarian cancer patients have a better prognosis compared to age and stage-matched controls *(44)*. Survival analyses of patients with hereditary cancer are prone to selection bias and other studies could not confirm this favorable prognosis for hereditary ovarian cancer patients *(46,47)*.

Apart from clinical differences, there are intriguing differences between hereditary and sporadic ovarian cancer at the molecular level. Somatic mutations in *BRCA1* and *BRCA2* are infrequent in sporadic ovarian cancer. Knowledge of the somatic molecular events involved in the pathway of carcinogenesis in both hereditary and sporadic ovarian cancer is emerging. The *p53* tumor suppressor gene has been studied in relation to *BRCA*-associated ovarian cancer and was found to play an important, but probably not essential role *(48,49)*. Limited analysis of HER-2/*neu*, K-*ras*, *C-MYC*, and *AKT2* suggests that these genes may be less important in hereditary than in sporadic ovarian cancer *(49)*. Although a number of somatic genetic events have been identified, their role in tumor development and progression in hereditary ovarian cancer remains largely unknown.

## 6. Integration of Clinical and Molecular Information

Mutation detection in *BRCA1* and *BRCA2* has until recently been performed in a research setting and been restricted to families that either showed linkage to the *BRCA1* or *BRCA2* locus or had a clear pattern of autosomal dominant inheritance. From these families, the lifetime risks (LTR) of breast and ovarian cancer have been estimated

*(17,50,51)*. For *BRCA1*, the LTR of either breast or ovarian cancer was calculated at 95% at age 70. The LTR of breast cancer at 85% and of ovarian cancer 40–60%. For *BRCA2*, the risk of breast cancer is similar to the risk in *BRCA1* mutation carriers whereas the risk of ovarian cancer is lower (approximately 25%). It is likely that these estimates are artificially high because of ascertainment bias in which families with high-penetrant mutations have been preferentially included and, especially for *BRCA2*, are based on the analysis of a relatively small number of families. Now that germline mutation detection for *BRCA1* and *BRCA2* is available for individual patients several studies have been performed to identify mutations in unselected ovarian cancer cases (not based on family history). Mutations in *BRCA1* and/or *BRCA2* are consistently detected in approximately 5% of such cases *(52,53)*. There is evidence of varying penetrance between families. Germline mutations have been detected in families with a weak or moderate history of breast or ovarian cancer and even in apparently sporadic cases. This particularly seems to be the case for *BRCA2* germline mutations. Translation of molecular test results to clinical management and individual risk estimation is therefore difficult outside families with clinically recognisable autosomal dominant disease.

## 7. Multidisciplinary Approach to Ovarian Cancer Families

The recent progress of research into the molecular basis of cancer in general and hereditary cancer in particular, has provided more insight into the aetiology of hereditary cancer. At the same time, publicity about research progress has raised the awareness in the medical profession and lay public that cancer may be hereditary in nature. In the case of ovarian cancer, a disease with a dismal prognosis, many women with a positive family history have come forward to request risk assessment and advice regarding screening and prevention. To provide such families with adequate advice requires expertise in the fields of genetics, screening, oncology, and surgery and, consequently, requires the input of several clinical specialities. Furthermore, genetic testing may have far-reaching emotional and social implications and require psychological support *(54)*. A multidisciplinary approach using protocols established by clinical geneticists for other inherited disorders *(55)* may be beneficial for the management of such families.

### 7.1. Pedigree Analysis

Risk assessment is still primarily based on the family history. An extensive pedigree analysis is required to establish whether an autosomal dominant pattern of inherited susceptibility is likely to be present in a family. Confirmation of reported diagnoses by medical reports, death certificates, or histopathological reevaluation is essential because, especially for gynaecological malignancies, the family history data alone may be unreliable because of recall bias *(56)*.

### 7.2. Genetic Testing

To initiate genetic testing, the cooperation of a live affected relative is usually required. Only when a pathogenic mutation has been detected in an affected family member is testing of healthy at-risk individuals informative. The implications of *BRCA1* and *BRCA2* mutation testing and the available techniques are discussed in **Subheading 4.4.**

## 7.3. Risk Assessment

Analysis of pedigree data in combination with the results of genetic testing should lead to the most accurate individual risk assessment. Often, a level of uncertainty will remain and families will need education on how to interpret their risk to be able to take decisions regarding screening and prevention in their own hands. Psychological support throughout this whole process is essential.

## 7.4. Screening and Prevention

The major aim of individual risk assessment for ovarian cancer is to identify women at the highest risk of developing the disease in the hope that mortality can be reduced for these women by screening and/or prevention. There is currently no evidence about the impact of screening for ovarian cancer on mortality. Many of the problems that occur in screening for the general population (*57*) may be overcome by directing efforts at a high-risk population, but prospective studies are still required to determine the value of specific screening strategies. The most commonly used screening strategy, which is currently the subject of a large U.K.-based prospective study, involves annual transvaginal ultrasonography and serum CA 125 from age 35 (or 5 yr before the youngest cases of ovarian cancer was diagnosed in the family, whichever comes first). Owing to the lack of evidence that screening for ovarian cancer and the subsequent early intervention reduces mortality and the absence of a detectable premalignant stage, some women at the highest level of risk may opt for a prophylactic oophorectomy to prevent ovarian cancer. Unfortunately, even this procedure may not entirely prevent "ovarian" cancer because several studies have reported the occurrence of intraperitoneal carcinomatosis, resembling primary ovarian cancer (*58–60*) and women should therefore be counseled that prophylactic oophorectomy does not provide absolute protection.

Use of the oral contraceptive pill has consistently been shown to reduce the risk of ovarian cancer in the general population. This risk reduction may be as high as 50%. A recent case-control study by Narod et al. (*61*) suggested that this protective effect also applies to women with hereditary ovarian cancer. There is some concern that use of oral contraceptives to prevent ovarian cancer or the use of hormonal replacement therapy after prophylactic oophorectomy may increase the already high risk of breast cancer in these women. Further research is needed to address the issue of whether or not these risks outweigh their obvious benefits.

## References

1. Office of Population Censuses, and Surveys: Cancer Statistics Registrations 1989. London, MB1, Her Majesty's Stationery Office, 1994.
2. Ferry, J. A., Young, R. H., Engel, G., and Scully, R. E. (1994) Oxyphilic Sertoli cell tumor of the ovary: a report of three cases, two in patients with the Peutz-Jeghers syndrome. *Int. J. Gynecol. Pathol.* **13**, 259–266.
3. Lamovec, J., Bracko, M., and Cerar, O. (1995) Familial occurrence of small-cell carcinoma of the ovary. *Arch. Pathol. Lab. Med.* **119**, 523–527.
4. Longy, M., Toulouse, C., Mage, P., Chauvergne, J., and Trojani, M. (1996) Familial cluster of ovarian small cell carcinoma: a new mendelian entity? *J. Med. Genet.* **33**, 333–335.
5. Vogelstein, B., Fearon, E. R., Hamilton, S. R., Kern, S. E., Preisinger, A. C., Leppert, M., et al. (1988) Genetic alterations during colorectal-tumor development. *N. Eng. J. Med.* **319**, 525–532.
6. Fathalla, M. F. (1971) Inscessant ovulation-a factor in ovarian neoplasia? *Lancet* **2**, 163.
7. Casagrande, J. T., Louie, E. W., Pike, M. C., Roy, S., Ross, R. K., and Henderson, B. E. (1979) "Incessant ovulation" and ovarian cancer. *Lancet* **2**, 170–173.

8. Lurain, J. R. and Piver, M. S. (1979) Familial ovarian cancer. *Gynecol. Oncol.* **8,** 185–192.
9. Boyd, J. and Rubin, S. C. (1997) Hereditary ovarian cancer: molecular genetics and clinical implications. *Gynecol. Oncol.* **64,** 196–206.
10. Schildkraut, J. M. and Thompson, W. D. (1988) Familial ovarian cancer: a population-based control study. *Am. J. Epidemiol.* **128,** 456–466.
11. Ponder, B. A. J., Easton, D., and Peto, J. (1990) Risk of ovarian cancer associated with a family history, in *Ovarian Cancer* (Sharp, F., Mason, W. D., and Leake, R. E., eds.), Chapman & Hall, London, pp. 3–6.
12. Ponder, B. A. J. (1996) Familial ovarian cancer, in *Genetic Predisposition to Cancer* (Eeles, R. A., Ponder, B. A. J., Easton, D. F., and Horwich, A., eds.), Chapman & Hall Medical, London, pp. 290–296.
13. Kimbrough, R. A. (1929) Coincidental carcinoma of the ovary in twins. *J. Obstset. Gynecol.* **18,** 148–149.
14. Lynch, H. T., Albano, W., Black, L., Lynch, J. F., Recabaren, J., and Pierson, R. (1981) Familial excess of cancer of the ovary and other anatomic sites. *JAMA* **245,** 261–264.
15. Hall, J. M., Lee, M. K., Newman, B., Morrow, J. E., Anderson, L. A., Huey, B., and King, M. C. (1990) Linkage of early-onset familial breast cancer to chromosome 17q21. *Science* **250,** 1684–1689.
16. Narod, S. A., Feunteun, J., Lynch, H. T., Watson, P., Conway, T., Lynch, J., and Lenoir, G. M. (1991) Familial breast-ovarian cancer locus on chromosome 17q12-q23. *Lancet* **338,** 82,83.
17. Ford, D., Easton, D. F., Stratton, M., Narod, S., Goldgar, D., Devilee, P., et al. (1998) Genetic heterogeneity and penetrance analysis of the *BRCA1* and *BRCA2* genes in breast cancer families. The Breast Cancer Linkage Consortium. *Am. J. Hum. Genet.* **62,** 676–689.
18. Miki, Y., Swensen, J., Shattuck-Eidens, D., Futreal, P. A., Harshman, K., Tavtigian, S., et al. (1994) A strong candidate for the breast and ovarian cancer susceptibility gene *BRCA1*. *Science* **266,** 66–71.
19. Smith, S. A., Easton, D. F., Evans, D. G., and Ponder, B. A. (1992) Allele losses in the region 17q12-21 in familial breast and ovarian cancer involve the wild-type chromosome. *Nat. Genet.* **2,** 128–131.
20. Struewing, J. P., Abeliovich, D., Peretz, T., Avishai, N., Kaback, M. M., Collins, F. S., and Brody, L. C. (1995) The carrier frequency of the *BRCA1* 185delAG mutation is approximately 1 percent in Ashkenazi Jewish individuals. *Nat. Genet.* **11,** 198–200.
21. Peelen, T., van Vliet, V. M., Petrij-Bosch, A., Mieremet, R., Szabo, C., van den Ouweland, A. M., et al. (1997) High proportion of novel mutations in BRCA1 with strong founder effects among Dutch and Belgian hereditary breast and ovarian cancer families. *Am. J. Hum. Genet.* **60,** 1041–1049.
22. Gayther, S. A., Warren, W., Mazoyer, S., Russell, P. A., Harrington, P. A., Chiano, M., et al. (1995) Germline mutations of the *BRCA1* gene in breast and ovarian cancer families provide evidence for a genotype-phenotype correlation. *Nat. Genet.* **11,** 428–433.
23. Phelan, C. M., Rebbeck, T. R., Weber, B. L., Devilee, P., Ruttledge, M. H., Lynch, H. T., et al. (1996) Ovarian cancer risk in BRCA1 carriers is modified by the HRAS1 variable number of tandem repeat (VNTR) locus. *Nat. Genet.* **12,** 309–311.
24. Foulkes, W., Black, D., Solomon, E., and Trowsdale, J. (1991) Allele loss on chromosome 17q in sporadic ovarian cancer. *Lancet* **338,** 444,445.
25. Eccles, D. M., Russell, S. E., Haites, N. E., Atkinson, R., Bell, D. W., Gruber, L., et al. (1992) Early loss of heterozygosity on 17q in ovarian cancer. The Abe Ovarian Cancer Genetics Group. *Oncogene* **7,** 2069–2072.
26. Merajver, S. D., Pham, T. M., Caduff, R. F., Chen, M., Poy, E. L, Cooney, K. A., et al. (1995) Somatic mutations in the BRCA1 gene in sporadic ovarian tumors. *Nat. Genet.* **9,** 439–443.
27. Jacobs, I. J., Smith, S. A., Wiseman, R. W., Futreal, P. A., Harrington, T., Osborne, R. J., et al. (1993) A deletion unit on chromosome 17q in epithelial ovarian tumors distal to the familial breast/ovarian cancer locus. *Cancer Res.* **53,** 1218–1221.
28. Wooster, R., Neuhausen, S. L., Mangion, J., Quirk, Y., Ford, D., Collins, N., et al. (1994) Localization of a breast cancer susceptibility gene, *BRCA2*, to chromosome 13q12-13. *Science* **265,** 2088–2090.
29. Wooster, R., Bignell, G., Lancaster, J., Swift, S., Seal, S., Mangion, J., et al. (1995) Identification of the breast cancer susceptibility gene BRCA2. *Nature* **378,** 789–792.
30. Tavtigian, S. V., Simard, J., Rommens, J., Couch, F., Shattuck-Eidens, D., Neuhausen, S., et al. (1996) The complete BRCA2 gene and mutations in chromosome 13q-linked kindreds. *Nat. Genet.* **12,** 333–337.
31. Levy-Lahad, E., Catane, R., Eisenberg, S., Kaufman, B., Hornreich, G., Lishinsky, E., et al. (1997) Founder *BRCA1* and BRCA2 mutations in Ashkenazi Jews in Israel: frequency and differential penetrance in ovarian cancer and in breast-ovarian cancer families. *Am. J. Hum. Genet.* **60,** 1059–1067.
32. Thorlacius, S., Sigurdsson, S., Bjarnadottir, H., Olafsdottir, G., Jonasson, J. G., Tryggvadottir, L., et al. (1997) Study of a single *BRCA2* mutation with high carrier frequency in a small population. *Am. J. Hum. Genet.* **60,** 1079–1084.

33. Gayther, S. A., Mangion, J., Russell, P., Seal, S., Barfoot, R., Ponder, B. A., et al. (1997) Variation of risks of breast and ovarian cancer associated with different germline mutations of the *BRCA2* gene. *Nat. Genet.* **15,** 103–105.
34. Foster, K. A., Harrington, P., Kerr, J., Russell, P., DiCioccio, R. A., Scott, I. V., et al. (1996) Somatic and germline mutations of the BRCA2 gene in sporadic ovarian cancer. *Cancer Res.* **56,** 3622–3625.
35. Sharan, S. K. and Bradley, A. (1997) Murine BRCA2: sequence, map position, and expression pattern. *Genomics* **40,** 234–241.
36. Milner, J., Ponder, B., Hughes-Davies, L., Seltmann, M., and Kouzarides, T. (1997) Transcriptional activation functions in *BRCA2*. *Nature* **386,** 772,773.
37. Holt, J. T., Thompson, M. E., Szabo, C., Robinson-Benion, C., Arteaga, C. L., King, M. C., and Jensen, R. A. (1996) Growth retardation and tumor inhibition by *BRCA1*. *Nat. Genet.* **12,** 298–302.
38. Scully, R., Chen, J., Plug, A., Xiao, Y. W., Weaver, D., Feunteun, J., et al. (1997) Association of *BRCA1* with Rad51 in mitotic and meiotic cells. *Cell* **88,** 265–275.
39. Sharan, S. K., Morimatsu, M., Albrecht, U., Lim, D. S., Regel, E., Dinh, C., et al. (1997) Embryonic lethality and radiation hypersensitivity mediated by Rad51 in mice lacking BRCA2. *Nature* **386,** 804–810.
40. Jensen, R. A., Thompson, M. E., Jetton, T. L., Szabo, C. I., et al. (1996) BRCA1 is secreted and exhibits properties of a granin. *Nat. Genet.* **12,** 303–308.
41. Chen, Y., Chen, C. F., Riley, D. J., Allred, D. C., Chen, P. L., Von Hoff, D., et al. (1995) Aberrant subcellular localization of BRCA1 in breast cancer. *Science* **3,** 789–791.
42. Sully, R., Ganesan, S., Brown, M., De Caprio, J. A., Cannistra, S. A., Feunteun, J., et al. (1996) Location of BRCA1 in human breast and ovarian cancer cells. *Science* **272,** 123–126.
43. Bewtra, C., Watson, P., Conway, T., Read-Hippee, C., and Lynch, H. T. (1992) Hereditary ovarian cancer: a clinicopathological study. *Int. J. Gynecol. Pathol.* **11,** 180–187.
44. Rubin, S. C., Benjamin, I., Behbakht, K., Takahashi, H., Morgan, M. A., LiVolsi, V. A., et al. (1996) Clinical and pathological features of ovarian cancer in women with germ-line mutations of *BRCA1*. *N. Eng. J. Med.* **335,** 1413–1416.
45. Zweemer, R. P., Verheijen, R. H., Gille, J. J., van Diest, P. J., Pals, G., and Menko, F. H. (1998) Clinical and genetic evaluation of thirty ovarian cancer families. *Am. J. Obstet. Gynecol.* **178,** 85–90.
46. Brunet, J. B., Narod, S. A., and Tonin, P. (1997) *BRCA1* mutations and survival in ovarian cancer. *N. Eng. J. Med.* **336,** 1256.
47. Johannsson, O., Ranstam, J., Borg, A., and Olsson, H. (1997) BRCA1 mutations and survival in ovarian cancer. *N. Eng. J. Med.* **336,** 1256.
48. Zweemer, R. P., Shaw, P. A., Verheijen, R. H. M., Ryan, A., Berchuck, A., Ponder, B. A. J., et al. *p53* overexpression is frequent in ovarian cancers associated with *BRCA1* and *BRCA2* germline mutations, in press.
49. Rhei, E., Bogomolniy, F., Federici, M. G., Maresco, D. L., Offit, K., Robson, M. E., et al. (1998) Molecular genetic characterisation of *BRCA1* and *BRCA2*-linked hereditary ovarian cancers. *Cancer Res.* **58,** 3193–3196.
50. Ford, D., Easton, D. F., Bishop, D. T., Narod, S. A., and Goldgar, D. E. (1994) Risks of cancer in BRCA1-mutation carriers. Breast Cancer Linkage Consortium. *Lancet* **343,** 692–695.
51. Easton, D. F., Ford, D., and Bishop, D. T. (1995) Breast and ovarian cancer incidence in BRCA1-mutation carriers. Breast Cancer Linkage Consortium. *Am. J. Hum. Genet.* **56,** 265–271.
52. Takahashi, H., Behbakht, K., McGovern, P. E., Chiu, H. C., Couch, F. J., Weber, B. L., et al. (1995) Mutation analysis of the BRCA1 gene in ovarian cancers. *Cancer Res.* **55,** 2998–3002.
53. Stratton, J. F., Gayther, S. A., Russell, P., Dearden, J., Gore, M., Blake, P., et al. (1997) Contribution of BRCA1 mutations to ovarian cancer. *N. Eng. J. Med.* **336,** 1125–1130.
54. DudokdeWit, A. C., Tibben, A., Frets, P. G., Meijers-Heijboer, E. J., Devilee, P., Klijn, J. G., et al. (1997) *BRCA1* in the family: a case description of the psychological implications. *Am. J. Med. Genet.* **71,** 63–71.
55. Berchuck, A., Cirisano, F., Lancaster, J. M., Schildkraut, J. M., Wiseman, R. W., Futreal, A., and Marks, J. R. (1996) Role of BRCA1 mutation screening in the management of familial ovarian cancer. *Am. J. Obstet. Gynecol.* **175,** 738–746.
56. Kerber, R. A. and Slattery, M. L. (1997) Comparison of self-reported and database-linked family history of cancer data in a case-control study. *Am. J. Epidemiol.* **146,** 244–248.
57. Rosenthal, A. and Jacobs, I. (1998) Ovarian cancer screening. *Semin. Oncol.* **25,** 315–325.
58. Tobacman, J. K., Greene, M. H., Tucker, M. A., Costa, J., Kase, R., Fraumeni, J. F., Jr. (1982) Intraabdominal carcinomatosis after prophylactic oophorectomy in ovarian-cancer-prone families. *Lancet* **2,** 795–797.
59. Piver, M. S., Jishi, M. F., Tsukada, Y., and Nava, G. (1993) Primary peritoneal carcinoma after prophylactic oophorectomy in women with a family history of ovarian cancer. A report of the Gilda Radner Familial Ovarian Cancer Registry. *Cancer* **71,** 2751–2755.

60. Struewing, J. P., Watson, P., Easton, D. F., Ponder, B. A., Lynch, H. T., and Tucker, M. A. (1995b) Prophylactic oophorectomy in inherited breast/ovarian cancer families. *J. Natl. Cancer Inst. Monogr.* **17,** 33–35.

61. Narod, S. A., Risch, H., Moslehi, R., Dorum, A., Neuhausen, S., Olsson, H., et al. (1998) Oral contraceptives and the risk of hereditary ovarian cancer. Hereditary Ovarian Cancer Clinical Study Group. *N. Engl. J. Med.* **339,** 424–428.

# 3

## The Molecular Pathogenesis of Ovarian Cancer

### S. E. Hilary Russell

## 1. The Genetic Basis of Cancer

In recent years, there has been considerable progress in understanding the molecular events that give rise to clonal tumor development. This is best described by the steps in the development of colorectal tumors in which the activation of cellular protooncogenes and inactivation of several tumor suppressor genes has been elucidated (*1*). The well-defined steps in the development of these tumors from normal epithelium through adenomas or benign tumors to carcinomas has now been paralleled by identification of several genetic loci which are mutated as the tumor develops.

A considerable amount of evidence is available regarding the role of protooncogenes in cellular growth control. In general, they code for proteins involved in signal transduction, i.e., the transmission of regulatory messages from outside the cell to the nucleus. Their role in tumorigenesis is dominant and, as protooncogenes, they are activated to oncogenes by "gain of function" mutations. The involvement of a number of oncogenes in ovarian cancer has been demonstrated and has been reviewed in Chapter 4.

In addition to the activation of protooncogenes, uncontrolled cell growth also requires the inactivation of negative regulatory pathways or the genes that encode them. This was inferred initially by the results of cell-fusion experiments in which malignant and normal cells were fused resulting in loss of the malignant phenotype, suggesting that genes from the normal cell could suppress malignancy (*2*). This concept was developed further by Knudson's "two-hit" hypothesis, which sought to explain by statistical analysis, the differences between the inherited and sporadic forms of the rare childhood cancer, retinoblastoma (*3*). Knudson proposed that retinoblastoma developed from genetic defects of two alleles in a cell. In the inherited form of the disease, one defect was passed down through the germline, as the second was acquired somatically. In sporadic retinoblastoma, both mutations must occur somatically in the same retinal cell. The class of genes that act recessively in tumorigenesis, and are inactivated by Knudson's "two hits," are the tumor suppressor genes. It is now generally accepted that the first allele of a tumor suppressor gene is inactivated by mutation. Various mechanisms for inactivation of the second allele have been proposed and include mitotic nondisjunction resulting in loss of the wild type chromosome, mitotic nondis-

From: *Methods in Molecular Medicine, Vol. 39: Ovarian Cancer: Methods and Protocols*
Edited by: J. M. S. Bartlett © Humana Press, Inc., Totowa, NJ

junction with reduplication of the mutant chromosome, mitotic recombination, deletion of part of the wild type chromosome, or point mutation *(4)*.

Based on an understanding of these mechanisms of inactivation, the mapping of tumor suppressor genes has made use of both cytogenetic and molecular analyses. One particularly useful approach has been loss of heterozygosity analysis in which patterns of loss of alleles in matched control/tumor DNA are determined using polymorphic markers. Originally, this employed minisatellite markers and Southern blotting, but now makes use of the highly polymorphic microsatellite repeat sequences and the polymerase chain reaction (PCR).

## 2. Cytogenetic Analysis of Ovarian Cancer Cells

There have been numerous cytogenetic studies of ovarian cancer *(5–7)* but they have failed to identify consistent chromosomal breakpoints as is observed, for example, in the leukaemias and lymphomas. However, it is clear that the majority of tumors are aneuploid *(8)* with complex karyotypic changes. Abnormalities involving chromosome *1* would seem to be the most common *(5,7,9)*. Low-grade ovarian tumors were characterized by simple specific numeric and structural abnormalities of this chromosome *(10)*. Such abnormalities were also present in high-grade tumors whether the karyotypes were more complex or near diploid *(11)*. In a study of 128 ovarian carcinomas, 89 had breaks involving chromosome *1*. In 42% of these, the breaks involved band *1p36 (12)*. A specific translocation involving chromosomes *6* and *14* was reported in 8 of 14 cases of papillary serous adenocarcinoma of the ovary *(13)*. Additional reports have also suggested a role for aberrations of chromosome 6, mainly involving deletions from *6q (6,14)*. Recurrent alterations of chromosome *9p* have been reported in several studies *(5,9,15)*. A variety of rearrangements were observed but all were in keeping with loss of a distal region of *9p*: *9p13*-ter and *9p22* or *9p23-pter*. Abnormalities involving chromosome *11* were reported in 83% of 23 untreated ovarian tumors *(7)*. Additional studies have also described aberrations of chromosome 11, e.g., loss of a distal region of the short arm *(16)*, but in a much smaller percentage of cases.

Trisomy 12 has been reported as a common abnormality of both benign tumors *(17)* and borderline lesions *(18)* and trisomy 17 was specific for invasive disease *(18)*.

## 3. Loss of Heterozygosity

One of the most useful approaches in locating tumor suppressor genes is through studying patterns of loss of alleles in tumors with polymorphic markers otherwise known as loss of heterozygosity (LOH). A high frequency of allele loss in a specific region of a chromosome in a tumor type indicates the presence of a tumor suppressor gene or genes, the loss of whose function is implicated in the progression of that particular tumor. Ovarian tumors have been analyzed for LOH across the genome and a number of hotspots for allele loss identified on different chromosomes. However, when reviewing these results with a view to producing a consensus allelotype for ovarian tumors, a number of problems are encountered. First of all, many of the studies have analyzed only small numbers of tumors *(20–30)* and these may or may not have included some benign or borderline lesions. Second, because some authors have used microdissected tumor tissue for LOH analysis, many have not. Therefore, if a sample contains a high percentage of contaminating stromal tissue, any LOH in the tumor cells will be masked. Third, there is often considerable variation in the composition of the tumor bank with respect to histological subtype, tumor stage and grade, all of which might be expected to influence the outcome of any LOH analysis. Finally, many studies use only one or two polymorphic markers per chromosome arm and there is often great variation between studies in the marker used. Direct comparisons between studies are therefore very difficult and often lead to conflicting and confusing results. However, in a recent review *(19)*, an attempt has been made to provide a consensus allelotype. Results of chromosome arm loss from several LOH studies were pooled without duplication of data from different studies and using data from mainly malignant tumors. The highest rates of LOH were described for chromosome arms *17p* and *17q* (62 and 56%, respectively). LOH of 40–46% were reported for chromosomes *13q*, *6q*, *18q*, and *22q*. As there is general genetic instability within tumor cell genomes, low levels of LOH would be expected across every chromosomal arm. A background level of 35% in ovarian tumors has been suggested *(20)*. Thus, a percentage LOH greater than this would be considered significant. The pooled data described, therefore, provide a good indication of the chromosomal locations of several tumor suppressor genes involved in the aetiology of ovarian tumors. Each of these regions and additional chromosomal arms indicated from other studies will be discussed in more detail.

### 3.1. Chromosome 6q

Among the earliest LOH studies in ovarian tumors were those employing markers from chromosome 6. Much of this interest was stimulated by cytogenetic reports of aberrations involving this chromosome particularly in serous adenocarcinoma *(13)*. Allelic loss was reported at the oestrogen receptor locus on *6q* in 9/14 informative tumors, i.e., 64% *(21)*. The frequency of LOH was similar in both primary and metastatic lesions. It was also demonstrated that the losses were confined to the more distal regions of *6q*. Further analysis of LOH from chromosome *6q* in a variety of small studies, have confirmed the high rates of LOH initially reported *(22–24)*. Three more extensive studies have concentrated on the terminal region of *6q*. In an analysis of 29 tumors, LOH ranging from 59 to 73% was reported for 5 markers at 6q27 *(25)*. In another study of 70 tumors with nine markers mapping to *6q24–27*, a 1.9-cm common region of deletion at *6q27* was identified from eight serous tumors flanked by the markers D6S193 and D6S149 *(26)*. A second region of deletion at *6q12–23* has also been reported *(20)*. In a large study of 40 tumors with 12 markers from *6q*, a more complex pattern of deletions was described for different histological subtypes *(27)*. For serous tumors, LOH at the distal site was confirmed (70% at D6S193). Evidence was provided for three sites of LOH on proximal *6q*; one at *6q21–23.3* showing LOH at high frequency in benign and endometrioid tumors, one at *6q14–12* also involved in endometrioid lesions, and a small region at 6q16.3-21 involved in early stage tumors. There is, therefore, good evidence that several potentially important genes on chromosome *6q* play a role in the aetiology of ovarian tumors, particularly serous and endometrioid, but not the mucinous subtype.

### 3.2. Chromosome 7

For ovarian carcinoma, the initial studies using chromosome *7* microsatellite polymorphisms reported only very low rates of LOH; 13–19% with the marker D7S23 *(24,28)*, 13% with D7S125 *(29)* and 21% with D7S396 *(30)*. More recent reports of LOH from this chromosome are much higher, e.g., 59% *(31)* and 73% (14/19 informative tumors) with D7S522 at *7q31 (32)*. Two of three Stage I tumors showed LOH with this marker suggesting that this may be an early event in ovarian tumorigenesis. Deletions from *7q* have been demonstrated in a wide variety of tumor types including breast *(33)*, colon *(34)*, and prostate *(35)* and indicate *7q31* as the critical region. Microcell mediated monochromosome transfer of chromosome *7* into two immortalized cell lines, indicates that this may be a senescence gene *(36)*.

### 3.3. Chromosome 11

Evidence for the involvement of a tumor suppressor gene on chromosome *11p* comes from several reports of LOH with markers from this chromosome particularly at the HRAS1 gene locus on *11p15.5 (21,22,37,38)*. On average, the LOH reported was approx 50%. Some reports have suggested that the LOH at *11p15.5* was associated with high-grade ovarian tumors and therefore might be associated with late steps in ovarian tumorigenesis *(23,39,40)*. However, in a more recent report, no significant association between tumor grade or stage and LOH at *11p15.5* was found *(41)*. A second region of deletion at *11p13* has been reported *(42)*, but the target gene would not appear to be WT1 since no abnormalities were found in this gene. LOH from *11p* is rare in mucinous tumors and is strongly associated with high-grade nonmucinous epithelial lesions *(43)*. In this study of 48 tumors, two regions on *11p* were identified; an *11cM* region at *11p15.5–15.3* and a *4cM* region at *11p15.1*.

Two regions of deletion on chromosome *11q* were detected using five polymorphic microsatellite markers *(41)*. LOH was observed in 39/60 (65%) informative tumors at minimally one locus. Significant associations were shown between LOH at two distant loci on both arms of the chromosome whereas intervening loci were not involved. It was, therefore, hypothesized that the pairs of loci may harbor genes which are cooperatively inactivated as part of a multistep process. High rates of LOH, up to 67%, have been reported for distal *11q (44)*. Refinement of the region of LOH at *11q23-ter* has identified two distinct regions of deletion. The proximal region, between D11S925 and D11S1336, is less than 2 megabases while the second more distal region, between D11S912 and D11S439, is approx 8 megabases *(45)*. The LOH on distal *11q* was detected in 50% of grade 1 and 47% of Stage 1 tumors and would therefore seem to be an early event in ovarian tumorigenesis. Interestingly, a large proportion of tumors had small confined deletions from distal *11q*, unlike the situation with many other chromosomes where large deletions and sometimes whole chromosome loss are detected.

### 3.4. Chromosome 13q

Allelic loss from chromosome *13q* has been reported by several groups. Cystadenomas did not show LOH from this chromosome and only low rates of LOH were reported for borderline tumors. But LOH of more than 50% was reported in 35 high-grade tumors *(46)*. This study supported earlier reports of LOH from this chromosome in which loss in only serous tumors was described (6/27 tumors) *(30)* and in 5/19 informative tumors at the *Rb* locus. Two of these tumors were undifferentiated and three were serous. In an analysis of 18 informative tumors, either all or none of the loci examined were lost. If the only target of LOH on *13q* was the *Rb* gene, it would be expected that some tumors would have small deletions confined to the region of the *Rb* locus. LOH at the *Rb* locus was reported in 25/48 informative tumors, but in 23 of the 25 tumors, immunohistochemical staining demonstrated normal *Rb* protein product

*(47)*. The majority of the 25 tumors (22/25) had LOH at all 17 loci evaluated on chromosome 13. Of the remaining three tumors, two retained markers distal to the Rb locus and one retained markers proximal to *Rb*. In a large study of 77 ovarian tumors, benign, borderline, and low- and high-grade malignant tumors were considered separately for LOH at 3 chromosome *13q* loci. Fifteen out of 29 high-grade tumors had LOH at minimally one marker, but no such loss was detected in 15 low-grade tumors *(48)*. Once again, normal *Rb* protein was demonstrated by immunohistochemical staining. This would suggest that because LOH from *13q* may be associated with increased biological aggressiveness in ovarian tumors, the target gene is not the *Rb* locus.

The incidence of ovarian cancer in BRCA2-linked families is much lower than in *BRCA1* families. Nonetheless, the mapping of BRCA2 to *13q12–13 (49)* and its subsequent cloning *(50)* raised the possibility of its involvement in somatic ovarian disease. The entire 10.2kB coding region of BRCA2 was screened for mutations in a series of 130 ovarian tumors. LOH at markers flanking BRCA2 was observed in 56% of tumors. Four germline mutations and two somatic mutations were described and it would, therefore, appear that mutations in *BRCA2* are rare in sporadic ovarian tumors *(51)*.

### 3.5. Chromosome 17

Abnormalities involving loci on chromosome *17* have, to date, been shown as the most frequent in ovarian tumor aetiology. Several regions of this chromosome have been identified as having a fundamental role. Among the earliest reports of LOH analysis of ovarian tumors were those using polymorphisms from *17p* and *17q*. In the late 1980s, the rationale for using *17p* markers was the demonstration that the *p53* gene on *17p13* had tumor-suppressor function and that this gene was inactivated in the development of most tumor types. It was, therefore, not unexpected that the rates of LOH detected in banks of ovarian tumors were significant at approximately 50% in malignant tumors *(21,52,53)*. However, these same studies also demonstrated that the greatest LOH from chromosome *17* (70%) was observed with markers from the long arm, in particular, the marker *pTHH59* at *17q23*-ter. In a combined follow-up study of 146 tumors, which included 22 borderline and 30 benign tumors, LOH was confirmed at 70% on distal *17q* and was even detected in some benign and borderline lesions *(54)*. Allele loss occurred with a significantly greater frequency on *17q* than *17p* and loss on *17q* increased in more advanced stage disease. Other studies have confirmed the high rates of LOH from *17q (24,55)* and the concomitant loss of all informative markers in a high percentage of tumors suggests that there is often loss of one chromosome 17 homolog *(56)*. As tumors with partial deletions are rare, detailed deletion mapping of the putative tumor suppressor gene on *17q* has been more difficult. One such study identified two distinct, commonly deleted regions on *17q*; one between *17q12* and *17q21.3*, which overlaps with the *BRCA1* locus, and a second region between *17q25.1* and *17q25.3 (57)*. Two additional studies have also demonstrated a deletion unit distal of *BRCA1 (58,59)*. In both cases the numbers of tumors are small and there are relatively few markers mapping to the *q23–25* region, but the results are still consistent with a deletion unit in this distal part of the chromosome. More recently, fine-scale deletion mapping has identified a 3-cm common region of deletion at *17q25 (60)*.

The establishment of linkage to chromosome *17q21* in families with an inherited predisposition to early onset breast and ovarian cancer in 1990 *(61)*, suggested initially that the high rates of LOH from *17q* in sporadic tumors may reflect the inactivation of this hereditary gene, *BRCA1*. However, with more detailed linkage analysis in families and extensive deletion mapping in sporadic tumors, it has become clear that two distinct regions were involved. Following the cloning of *BRCA1*, mutation studies have shown that somatic mutations of BRCA1 are rare in sporadic tumors *(62)*.

LOH from the short arm of chromosome *17* has often been assumed to represent inactivation of the *p53* gene at *17p13.1*. However, losses at *17p13.3* were demonstrated in Stage 1 carcinomas and borderline tumors *(55)*. In the latter case, the LOH at *17p13.3* were not accompanied by LOH at *p53*. A common region of deletion of approximately 15 kB was identified between the markers D17S28 and D17S30. Two novel genes have now been identified from this critical region of the chromosome at *17p13.3 (63)*. OVCA1 and OVCA2 are expressed in normal surface epithelial cells of the ovary, but the level of this transcript is reduced or undetectable in 92% of ovarian tumors and tumor cell lines. DNA sequence analysis identified no known functional domains. However, *OVCA1* showed significant sequence identity and similarity to a yeast and nematode sequence.

Another candidate tumor suppressor gene on the short arm of chromosome *17* is *HIC-1* (*17p13.3*), which was isolated from a region undergoing allelic loss and with a hypermethylated CpG island on the remaining allele *(64)*. Hypermethylation is regarded as an indication of a region of DNA, which is transcriptionally repressed *(65)* and thus may be another mechanism for inactivation of tumor suppressor genes. HIC-1 contains a consensus *p53* binding site and, therefore, is a potential downstream target of *p53*. Hypermethylation at *D17S5* (*17p13.3*) was shown to be a frequent event in epithelial ovarian tumors and was specific for that region and not the result of generalized hypermethylation across the genome *(66)*. Hypermethylation at *D17S5* correlated inversely with LOH for chromosome *17* and was found predominantly in tumors of low histological grade.

### 3.5.1. The p53 Gene

The *p53* gene on chromosome *17p13.1* is central to the control and regulation of DNA repair in cells. Deletions and mutations of this gene are observed in around 50% of all human tumors *(67)*. The protein causes arrest of the cell cycle after DNA damage, hence preventing the cell progressing into mitosis, and triggers apoptosis if the damage is too great to be repaired by normal cellular mechanisms *(68)*. There have been many studies to determine the incidence of *p53* alterations in ovarian tumors. In many cases, only small numbers of tumors were examined and often, *p53* protein overexpression was used as an indirect indicator of mutation. Some caution must be used in interpreting such analyses because immunohistochemical and mutation analysis do not always concur *(69)*.

There has been little evidence of *p53* mutation or overexpression in benign epithelial ovarian tumors *(70,71)*. Indeed, such mutations were also rare in borderline tumors. Only one *p53* mutation was observed in a series of 48 borderline tumors *(72)* and *p53* overexpression was detected in 2/49 cases *(71)*. In contrast, mutation and/or overexpression is commonly found in invasive epithelial ovarian tumors. The incidence of mutation ranged from 29 to 74% *(70,72,73)*. Results indicate that *p53* function is lost in 15% of early-stage carcinomas and 50% of late-stage carcinomas, suggesting that *p53* alterations may be a late event in the development of ovarian tumors *(71,74)*.

The fundamental role of the *p53* gene in recognition of DNA damage has led to the hypothesis that primary tumors with *p53* mutation may not recognise DNA damage and thus may not induce the normal apoptotic pathway for self-destruction. A number of studies have looked at the prognostic significance of the *p53* status of a tumor, although the results to date have been inconclusive. In one report, *p53* overexpression was associated with a higher risk of relapse and death in a subset of patients with well or moderately differentiated ovarian carcinoma, but not in patients with high grade or advanced stage tumors *(75)*. In contrast, two studies could find no correlation between *p53* status and survival *(76,77)*. Decreased survival was reported in patients whose tumors overexpressed the *p53* protein, but no significant association was found between response to chemotherapy and *p53* in the 70 patients analyzed.

More recent analysis has examined the response to platinum-based chemotherapy and *p53* mutation. In a study of 33 patients with Stage III/IV disease receiving high-dose cisplatin, mutational status did not predict responsiveness to chemotherapy *(78)*. However, treatment resistance was significantly associated with missense mutation and positive immunostaining. In another study, a strong correlation was reported between *p53* alterations and response to cisplatin chemotherapy *(79)*. In 33 patients receiving a cisplatin-based treatment, 14% of those responding to the drug had a *p53* mutation whereas 82% of nonresponders or patients with only a partial response had a *p53* abnormality. Patients with p53 mutations had a significantly shorter progression-free survival than patients with tumors containing wild type *p53*.

### 3.6. Chromosome 18q

Consideration of the pooled results for allelic losses from chromosome *18 (19)* suggest that LOH from *18q* is approximately 42% and, therefore, above the background level proposed as 35% *(20)*. LOH at *18p* was only 14% indicating a specific role for the long arm of this chromosome. LOH analysis with eight markers from *18q* detected loss in 31 of 52 (60%) informative tumors *(80)*. The most frequent loss was at *D18S11* at *18q23* (21/35 informative tumors). Partial deletions were detected in 11 tumors. In five cases, this excluded the region of the DCC gene with the smallest common region of deletion between *D18S5* and *D18S11*. This suggests that another locus on chromosome *18q* may be involved. Although the results were not statistically significant, loss on chromosome *18*, as judged by the different rate of loss at different clinical stages, appeared to be a late event in ovarian carcinogenesis. No association with histological type or grade was noted.

### 3.7. Chromosome 22q

Reports of LOH from this chromosome in ovarian tumors have shown considerable variation between studies and ranged from only approximately 25%, i.e., background levels *(29,30)* to 71% *(20,24)* which would have considerable significance. The tumor suppressor gene NF2 is on *22q12* and was therefore considered a possible target for loss. In an analysis of 67 ovarian tumors, 23/32 of informative tumors (72%) showed LOH but in the three tumors with partial losses, the common region of deletion was distal of NF2 *(81)*. Furthermore, mutation analysis of 9 of 17 exons of NF2 by single-strand conformational polymorphism (SSCP) did not detect any somatic mutations in this gene. This study has now been extended to include 110 tumors and eight polymorphic markers from *22q (82)*. LOH was detected in 58 tumors (53%) and six tumors had partial deletions. Two separate common regions of deletion were identified. One region, less than 0.5 cM flanked by the markers *D22S284* and *CYP2D*, and a second region that is distal of *D22S276*. An increasing frequency of LOH was observed in higher grade and later-stage tumors suggesting that *22q* LOH is a late event in ovarian tumorigenesis. Moreover, the loss was common in serous and endometrioid tumors and observed only rarely in the mucinous subtype.

## 4. Conclusion

The molecular analysis of epithelial ovarian tumors has identified at least three tumor suppressor genes that play a role in the aetiology of this disease. As with other tumor types, the involvement of the *p53* gene is mainly a late stage event. One *p53* allele is lost as a consequence of loss of one chromosome 17 homolog *(56)* whereas mutations in the second allele are prevalent in late stage disease *(71)*. However, the role of this gene in the important question of response to chemotherapy and its prognostic significance, have yet to be determined. Also, on chromosome *17* are the recently identified tumor suppressors, *OVCA1* and *OVCA2 (63)*. Although there is as yet no information regarding their function, initial evidence would suggest their fundamental role in the majority of malignant ovarian tumors. LOH studies have highlighted some key areas commonly deleted in ovarian tumor aetiology. In many cases, fine deletion mapping has been carried out and positional cloning strategies are under way. Soon, it is to be expected that some of these important genes will be cloned. At least one tumor suppressor on chromosome *6q27* has been identified *(26)* as part of a complex pattern of deletion from this chromosome in mainly serous and endometrioid tumors. A senescence gene on chromosome *7q31* is involved in early stages of tumor development in a high percentage of cases *(32)*. There is evidence for at least one tumor suppressor on chromosome *11p15*, probably inactivated in the development of late-stage nonmucinous tumors. On the long arm of this chromosome, there are at least two tumor suppressor genes at *11q23*-ter which are inactivated in early-stage disease *(45)*. As with chromosome *17*, there appear to be several important genes on chromosome *11*. However, their inactivation is by several smaller regions of deletion rather than loss of one chromosome 11 homolog. A tumor suppressor on chromosome *13q*, in the region of the *Rb* gene, but excluding *Rb*, may play a role in the development of more aggressive disease, but is not involved in benign or borderline lesions *(46)*. In addition to the genes on *17p* already described, there is clear evidence for at least one tumor suppressor on *17q* playing a fundamental role in benign, borderline, and malignant disease of all histological types *(54)*. The deletions at *18q23* are indicative of a late-stage tumor suppressor gene, which is not the *DCC* gene. There are two tumor suppressor genes at *22q12* involved in the development of late stage nonmucinous tumors.

Evidence is emerging that there may be a number of genetic pathways involved in the development of the various epithelial ovarian tumors. The molecular data so far reported, indicates that serous and endometrioid tumors share many genetic alterations and that mucinous tumors are quite distinct. Thus, in serous and endometrioid tumors, loss of a chromosome *17* homolog, LOH from *6q27*, *11p15*, and *22q12* are important, but are not observed in mucinous tumors. However, the *17q25* gene is deleted in mucinous lesions *(83)*. One fundamental question that remains in ovarian tumor biology is the relationship of benign, borderline, and malignant tumors, and if these represent a continuum or are independent lesions. Histological analysis of invasive tumors has shown adjacent benign areas *(84)*, but this still remains controversial. Relatively little LOH has been reported in benign tumors. Recently, by using microdissected tissue, higher rates of LOH have been detected at loci also involved in malignant disease *(85)*. This would support the hypothesis that benign tumors represent a premalignant lesion. Similarly, with borderline tumors, few genetic abnormalities have been identified and it remains to be seen if these tumors represent a precursor to real invasive disease or are a distinct entity. The elucidation of the molecular changes in ovarian tumor aetiology will answer many of these questions. Hopefully, they will also have applicability to the clinical situation. The ability to genetically define a premalignant lesion may lead to earlier detection and indicate those tumors likely to progress to malignancy. Genetic changes associated with the more aggressive forms of disease may also suggest a more appropriate form of treatment. Finally, new forms of treatment may emerge in which the underlying cause of malignancy, i.e., the genetic abnormality, may be the target.

## References

1. Vogelstein, B., Fearon, E. R., Hamilton, S. R., Kerns, S. E., Preisinger, A. C., Leppert, M., et al. (1988) Genetic alterations during colorectal tumor development. *N Engl J. Med.* **319,** 525–532.
2. Harris, H., Miller, O. J., Klein, G., Worst, P., and Tachibana, T. (1969) Suppression of malignancy by cell fusion. *Nature* **223,** 363–368.
3. Knudson, A. G. (1971) Mutation and cancer: statistical study of retinoblastoma. *Proc. Nat. Acad. Sci. USA* **68,** 820–823.
4. Cavenee, W. K., Dryja, T. P., Phillips, R. A., Benedict, W. F., Godbout, R., Gallie, B. L., et al. (1983). Expression of recessive alleles by chromosomal mechanisms in retinoblastoma. *Nature* **305,** 779–784.
5. Whang-Peng, J., Knutsen, T., Douglass, E. C., Chu, E., Ozols, R. F., Hogan, W. M., and Young, R. C. (1984) Cytogenetic studies in ovarian cancer. *Cancer Genet.Cytogenet.* **11,** 91–106.
6. Trent, J. M. and Salmon, S. E. (1981) Karyotypic analysis of human ovarian carcinoma cell lines cloned in short term agar. *Cancer Genet. Cytogenet.* **3,** 279–291.
7. Gallion, H. H., Powell, D. E., Smith, L. W., Morrow, J. K., Martin, A. W., van Nagell, J. R., and Donaldson, E. S. (1990) Chromosome abnormalities in human epithelial ovarian malignancies. *Gynaecol. Oncol.* **38,** 473–477.
8. Berchuk, A., Boente, M. P., and Kerns, B. J. (1992) Ploidy analysis of epithelial ovarian cancers using image cytometry. *Gynecol. Oncol.* **44,** 61–65.
9. Van der Riet-Fox, M. F., Retief, A. E., and Van Niekerk, W. A. (1979) Chromosome changes in 17 human neoplasms studied with banding. *Cancer* **44,** 2108–2119.
10. Thompson, F. H., Liu, Y., Emerson, J., Weinstein, R., Makar, R., Trent, J. M., et al. (1994) Simple numeric abnormalities as primary karyotype changes in ovarian carcinoma. *Genes Chromo. Cancer* **10,** 262–266.
11. Thompson, F. H., Emerson, J., Alberts, D., Liu, Y., Guan, X-Y., Burgess, A., et al. (1994) Clonal chromosome abnormalities in 54 cases of ovarian carcinoma. *Cancer Genet. Cytogenet.* **73,** 33–45.
12. Thompson, F. H., Taetle, R., Trent, J. M., Liu, Y., Massey-Brown, K., Scott, K. M., et al. (1997) Band 1p36 abnormalities and t(1;17) in ovarian carcinoma. *Cancer Genet Cytogenet.* **96,** 106–110.
13. Wake, N., Hreshchyshyn, M. M., Piver, S. M., Matsui, S., and Sandberg, A. (1980) Specific cytogenetic changes in ovarian cancer involving chromosomes 6 and 14. *Cancer Res.* **40,** 4512–4518.
14. Trent, J. M., Thompson, F. H., and Buick, R. N. (1985) Generation of clonal variants in human ovarian carcinoma studied by chromosome banding analysis. *Cancer Genet. Cytogenet.* **14,** 153–161.
15. Bello, M. J., Moreno, S., and Rey, J. A. (1990) Involvement of 9p in metastatic ovarian adenocarcinomas. *Cancer Genet. Cytogenet.* **45,** 223–229.
16. Bello, M. J. and Rey, J. A. (1990) Chromosome aberrations in metastatic ovarian cancer: relationship with abnormalities in primary tumors. *Int. J. Cancer* **45,** 50–54.
17. Yang-Feng, T. L., Li, S., Leung, W-Y., Carcangiu, M. L., and Schwartz, P. E. (1991) Trisomy 12 and K-ras 2 amplification in human ovarian tumors. *Int. J. Cancer* **48,** 678–681.
18. Kohlberger, P. D., Kieback, D. G., Mian, C., Wiener, H., Kainz, C., Gitsch, G., and Breitenecker, G. (1997) Numerical chromosomal aberrations in borderline,benign and malignant epithelial tumors

of the ovary: correlation with p53 protein overexpression and Ki-67. *J. Soc. Gynecol. Invest.* **4,** 262–264.

19. Shelling, A. N., Cooke, I. E., and Ganesan, T. S. (1995) The genetic analysis of ovarian cancer. *Brit. J. Cancer* **72,** 521–527.

20. Cliby, W., Ritland, S., Hartmann, L., Dodson, M., Halling, K. C., Keeny, G., et al. (1993) Human epithelial ovarian cancer allelotype. *Cancer Res.* **53,** 2393–2398.

21. Lee, J. H., Kavanagh, D. M., Wildrick, D. M., Wharton, J. T., and Blick, M. (1990) Frequent loss of heterozygosity on chromosomes 6q,11 and 17 in human ovarian carcinomas. *Cancer Res.* **50,** 2724–2728.

22. Ehlen, T. and Dubeau, L. (1990) Loss of heterozygosity on chromosomal segments 3p, 6q and 11p in human ovarian carcinomas. *Oncogene* **5,** 219–223.

23. Zheng, J., Robinson, W. R., Ehlen, T., Yu, M. C., and Dubeau, L. (1991) Distinction of low grade from high grade human ovarian carcinomas on the basis of loss of heterozygosity on chromosomes 3, 6 and 11 and HER-2/neu gene amplification. *Cancer Res.* **51,** 4045–4051.

24. Dodson, M. K., Hartmann, L. C., Cliby, W. A., Delacey, K. A., Keeney, G. L., Ritland, S. R., et al. (1993) Comparison of loss of heterozygosity patterns in low grade and high grade epithelial ovarian carcinomas. *Cancer Res.* **53,** 4456–4460.

25. Foulkes, W. D., Ragoussis, J., Stamp, G. W. H., Allan, G. J., and Trowsdale, J. (1993) Frequent loss of heterozygosity on chromosome 6 in human ovarian carcinoma. *Brit. J. Cancer* **67,** 551–559.

26. Saito, S., Saito, H., Kooi, S., Sagae, S., Kudo, R., Saito, J., et al. (1992) Fine scale deletion mapping of the distal long arm of chromosome 6 in 70 human ovarian cancers. *Cancer Res.* **52,** 5815–5817.

27. Orphanos, V., McGown, G., Hey, Y., Thorncroft, M., Santibanez-Koref, M., Russell, S. E. H., et al. (1995). Allelic imbalance of chromosome 6q in ovarian tumors. *Brit. J. Cancer* **71,** 666–669.

28. Osborne, R. J. and Leech, V. (1994) Polymerase chain reaction allelotyping of human ovarian cancer. *Brit. J. Cancer* **69,** 429–438.

29. Yang-Feng, T. L., Hong, H., Chen, K. C., Li, S. B., Claus, E. B., Carcangiu, M. L., et al. (1993) Allelic loss in ovarian cancer. *Int. J. Cancer* **54,** 546–551.

30. Sato, T., Saito, H., Motita, R., Koi, S., Lee, J. E., and Nakamura, Y. (1991) Allelotype of human ovarian cancer. *Cancer Res.* **51,** 5118–5122.

31. Edelson, M. I., Scherer, S. W., Tsui, L. C., Welch, W. R., Bell, D. A., Berkowitz, R. S., and Mok, S. C. (1997) Identification of a 1300 kilobase deletion unit on chromosome 7q31.3 in invasive epithelial ovarian carcinomas. *Oncogene* **14,** 2979–2984.

32. Zenklusen, J. C., Weitzel, J. N., Ball, H. G., and Conti, C. J. (1995) Allelic loss at 7q31.1 in human primary ovarian carcinomas suggests the existence of a tumor suppressor gene. *Oncogene* **11,** 359–363.

33. Zenklusen, J. C., Bieche, I., Lidereau, R., and Conti, C. J. (1994) (C-A)n microsatellite repeat D7S522 is the most commonly deleted region in human primary breast cancer. *Proc. Nat. Acad. Sci. USA* **91,** 12,155–12,158.

34. Zenklusen, J. C., Thompson, J. C., Klein-Szanto, A. J., and Conti, C. J. (1995) Frequent loss of heterozygosity in human primary squamous cell and colon carcinomas at 7q31.1: evidence for a broad range tumor suppressor gene. *Cancer Res.* **55,** 1347–1350.

35. Zenklusen, J. C., Thompson, J. C., Troncoso, P., Kagan, J., and Conti, C. J. (1994) Loss of heterozygosity in human prostate carcinomas: A possible tumor suppressor gene at 7q31.1. *Cancer Res.* **54,** 6370–6373.

36. Ogata, T., Ayusawa, D., Namba, M., Takahashi, E., Oshimura, M., and Oishi, M. (1993) Chromosome 7 suppresses indefinite division of nontumorigenic immortalized human fibroblast cell lines KMST-6 and SUSM-1. *Molec. Cell. Biol.* **13,** 6036–6043.

37. Lee, J. H., Kavanagh, J. J., Wharton, J. T., Wildrick, D. M., and Blick, M. (1989) Allele loss at the c-Ha-ras1 locus in human ovarian cancer. *Cancer Res.* **49,** 1229–1222.

38. Viel, A., De Pascale, L., Toffoli, G., Tumiotti, L., Miotto, E., and Boiocchi, M. (1991) Frequent occurrence of Ha-ras1 allelic deletion in human ovarian adenocarcinomas. *Tumorigenesis* **77,** 16–21.

39. Zheng, J., Wan, M., Zweizig, S., Velicescu, M., Yu, M. C., and Dubeau, L. (1993) Histologically benign or low grade malignant tumors adjacent to high grade ovarian carcinomas contain molecular characteristics of high grade carcinomas. *Cancer Res.* **53,** 4138–4142.

40. Gallion, H. H., Powell, D., Morrow, J. K., Pieretti, M., Case, E., Turker, M. S., et al. (1992) Molecular genetic changes in human epithelial ovarian malignancies. *Gynecol. Oncol.* **47,** 137–142.

41. Gabra, H., Taylor, L., Cohen, B. B., Lessels, A., Eccles, D. M., Leonard, R. C., et al. (1995) Chromosome 11 allele imbalance and clinicopathological correlates in ovarian tumors. *Brit. J. Cancer* **72,** 367–375.

42. Viel, A., Giannini, F., Capozzi, E., Canonieri, V., and Scarabelli, C. (1994) Molecular mechanisms possibly affecting WT1 function in human ovarian tumors. *Int. J. Cancer* **57,** 515–521.

43. Lu, K. H., Weitzel, J. N., Kodali, S., Welch, W. R., Berkowitz, R. S., and Mok, S. C. (1997) A novel 4-cM minimally deleted region on chromosome 11p15.1 associated with high grade nonmucinous epithelial ovarian carcinomas. *Cancer Res.* **57,** 387–390.

44. Foulkes, W. D., Campbell, I. G., Stamp, G. W. H., and Trowsdale, J. (1993) Loss of heterozygosity and amplification on chromosome 11q in human ovarian cancer. *Brit. J Cancer* **67,** 268–73.

45. Davis, M., Hitchcock, A., Foulkes, W. D., and Campbell, I. G. (1996) Refinement of two chromosome 11q regions of loss of heterozygosity in ovarian cancer. *Cancer Res.* **56,** 741–744.

46. Cheng, P. C., Gosewehr, J. A., Kim, T. M., Velicescu, M., Wan, M., Zheng, J., et al. (1996) Potential role of the inactive X chromosome in ovarian epithelial tumor development. *J. Nat. Cancer Inst.* **88,** 510–518.

47. Dodson, M. K., Cliby, W. A., Xu, H. J., Delacey, K. A., Hu, S. X., Keeney, G. L., et al. (1994) Evidence of functional RB protein in epithelial ovarian carcinomas despite loss of heterozygosity at the Rb locus. *Cancer Res.* **54,** 610–613.

48. Kim, T. M., Benedict, W. F., Xu, H-J., Hu, S., Gosewehr, J., Velicescu, M., et al. (1994) Loss of heterozygosity on chromosome 13 is common only in the biologically agressive subtypes of ovarian epithelial tumors and is associated with normal retinoblastoma gene expression. *Cancer Res.* **54,** 605–609.

49. Wooster, R., Neuhausen, S. L., Mangion, J., Quirk, Y., Ford, D., Collins, N., et al. (1994) Localisation of a breast cancer susceptibility gene, BRCA2, to chromosome 13q12-13. *Science.* **265,** 2088–2090.

50. Wooster, R., Bignell, G., Lancaster, J., Swift, S., Mangion, J., Collins, N., et al. (1995) Identification of the breast cancer susceptibility gene, BRCA2. *Nature* **378,** 789–792.

51. Takahashi, H., Chiu, H-C., Bandera, C. A., Behbakt, K., Liu, P. C., Couch, F. J., et al. (1996) Mutations of the BRCA2 gene in ovarian carcinomas. *Cancer Res.* **56,** 2738–2741.

52. Eccles, D. M., Cranston, G., Steel, C. M., Nakamura, Y., and Leonard, R. C. F. (1990) Allele loss on chromosome 17 in human epithelial ovarian carcinoma. *Oncogene* **5,** 1599–1601.

53. Russell, S. E. H., Hickey, G. I., Lowry, W. S., White, P., and Atkinson, R. J. (1990). Allele loss from chromosome 17 in ovarian cancer. *Oncogene* **5,** 1581–1582.

54. Eccles, D. M., Russell, S. E. H., Haites, N. E., and the ABE Ovarian Cancer Genetics Group. (1992) Early loss of heterozygosity on 17q in ovarian cancer. *Oncogene* **7,** 2069–2072.

55. Phillips, N. J., Ziegler, M., Saha, B., and Xynos, F. (1993) Allelic loss on chromosome 17 in ovarian cancer. *Int. J. Cancer* **54,** 85–91.

56. Foulkes, W. D., Black, D. M., Stamp, G. W. H., Solomon, E., and Trowsdale, J. (1993) Very frequent loss of heterozygosity throughout chromosome 17 in sporadic ovarian carcinoma. *Int. J. Cancer* **54,** 220–225.

57. Saito, H., Inazawa, J., Saito, S., Kasumi, F., Koi, S., Sagae, S., et al. (1993) Detailed deletion mapping of chromosome 17q in breast and ovarian cancer: 2cM region on 17q21.3 often and commonly deleted in tumors. *Cancer Res.* **53,** 3382–3385.

58. Jacobs, I. J., Smith, S. A., Wiseman, P. A., Futreal, A., Harrington, T., Osborne, R. J., et al. (1993) A deletion unit on chromosome 17q in epithelial ovarian tumours distal to the familial breast/ovarian cancer locus. *Cancer Res.* **53,** 1218–1221.

59. Godwin, A. K., Vanderveer, L., Schultz, D. C., Lynch, H. T., Altomare, D. A., Buetow, K. H., et al. (1994) A common region of deletion fon chromosome 17q in both sporadic and familial epithelial ovarian tumors distal to BRCA1. *Am. J. Hum. Genet.* **55,** 666–677.

60. Kalikin, L. M., Frank, T. S., Svoboda, S. M., Wetzel, J. C., Cooney, K. A., and Petty, E. M. (1997) A region of interstitial 17q25 allelic loss in ovarian tumors coincides with a defined region of loss in breast tumors. *Oncogene* **14,** 1991–1994.

61. Hall, J. M., Lee, M. K., Newman, B., Morrow, J. E., Anderson, L. A., Huey, B., and King, M-C. (1990) Linkage of early-onset familial breast cancer to chromosome 17q21. *Science* **250,** 1684–1689.

62. Futreal, P. A., Liu, Q., Shattuck-Eidens, D., Cochran, C., Harshman, K., Tavtigian, S., et al. (1994) BRCA1 mutations in primary breast and ovarian cancers. *Science* **266,** 120–122.

63. Schultz, D. C., Vanderveer, L., Berman, D. B., Hamilton, T. C., Wong, A. J., and Godwin, A. K. (1996). Identification of two candidate tumor suppressor genes on chromosome 17p13.3. *Cancer Res.* **56,** 1997–2002.

64. Makos-Wales, M., Biel, M. A., El-Deiry, W., Nelkin, B. D., Issa, J-P., Cavanee, W. K., et al. (1995) p53 activates expression of HIC-1, a new candidate tumor suppressor gene on 17p13.3. *Nature Med.* **1,** 570–577.

65. Razin, A. and Riggs, A. D. (1980) DNA methylation and gene function. *Science* **210,** 604–610.

66. Pieretti, M., Powell, D. E., Gallion, H. H., Conway, P. S., Case, E. A., and Turker, M. S. (1995) Hypermethylation at a chromosome 17 'hot spot' is a common event in ovarian cancer. *Human Pathol.* **26,** 398–401.

67. Carson, D. A. and Lois, A. (1995) Cancer progression and p53. *Lancet* **346,** 1009–1011.

68. Lane, D. P. (1992) p53, guardian of the genome. *Nature* **358,** 15–16.
69. Wynford-Thomas, D. (1992) p53 in tumor pathology: can we trust immunocytochemistry? *J. Pathol.* **166,** 329–330.
70. Mazars, R., Pijol, P., Maudelonde, T., Jeanteur, P., and Theillet, C. (1991) p53 mutations in ovarian cancer: a late event? *Oncogene* **6,** 1685–1690.
71. Berchuk, A., Kohler, M. F., Hopkins, M. P., Humphrey, P. A., Robboy, S. J., Rodriguez, G. C., et al. (1994) Overexpression of p53 is not a feature of benign and early-stage borderline ovarian tumors. *Gynecol. Oncol.* **53,** 232–236.
72. Wertheim, I., Muto, M. G., Welsh, W. R., Bell, D. A., Berkowitz, R. S., and Mok, S. C. (1994). p53 gene mutation in human borderline epithelial ovarian tumors. *J. Natl. Cancer. Inst.* **86,** 1549–1551.
73. Okamoto, A., Sameshima, Y., Yokoyama, S., Terashima, Y., Sugimura, T., Terada, M., and Yokata, J. (1991) Frequent allelic losses and mutations of the p53 gene in human ovarian cancer. *Cancer Res.* **51,** 5171–5176.
74. McManus, D. T., Murphy, M., Arthur, K., Hamilton, P. W., Russell, S. E. H., and Toner, P. G. (1996) p53 mutation, allele loss on chromosome 17p and DNA content in ovarian carcinoma. *J. Pathol.* **179,** 177–182.
75. Levesque, M. A., Katsaros, D., and Yu, H. (1995). Mutant p53 protein overexpression is associated with poor outcome in patients with well or moderately differentiated ovarian carcinoma. *Cancer* **75,** 1327–1338.
76. Sheridan, E., Silcocks, P., Smith, J., Hancock, B. W., and Goyns, M. H. (1994) p53 mutation in a series of epithelial ovarian cancers from the UK and it's prognostic significance. *Euro. J. Cancer* **30,** 1701–1704.
77. Niwa, K., Itoh, M., and Murase, T. (1994) Alterations of p53 gene in ovarian carcinoma: Clinico-pathological correlation and prognostic significance. *Brit. J. Cancer* **70,** 1191–1197.
78. Righetti, S. C., Della Torre, G., Pilotti, S., Menard, S., Ottone, F., Colnaghi, M. I., et al. (1996) A comparative study of p53 gene mutations, protein accumulation, and response to cisplatin-based chemotherapy in advanced ovarian carcinoma. *Cancer Res.* **56,** 689–693.
79. Buttitta, F., Marchetti, A., Gadducci, A., Pellegrini, S., Morganti, M., Carcinelli, V., et al. (1997) p53 alterations are predictive of chemoresistance and aggressiveness in ovarian carcinomas: a molecular and immunohistochemical study. *Brit. J. Cancer* **75,** 230–235.
80. Chenevix-Trench, G., Leary, J., Kerr, J., Miche, J., Kefford, R., Hurst, T., et al. (1992) Frequent loss of heterozygosity on chromosome 18 in ovarian carcinoma which does not always include the DCC locus. *Oncogene* **7,** 1039–1065.
81. Engelfield, P., Foulkes, W. D., and Campbell, I. G. (1994) Loss of heterozygosity on chromosome 22 in ovarian carcinoma is distal to and not accompanied by mutations in NF2 at 22q12. *Brit. J. Cancer* **70,** 905–907.
82. Bryan, E. J., Watson, R. H., Davis, M., Hitchcock, A., Foulkes, W., and Campbell, I. G. (1996) Localisation of an ovarian cancer tumor suppressor gene to a 0.5cM region between D22S284 and CYP2D, on chromosome 22q. *Cancer Res.* **56,** 719–721.
83. Pieretti, M., Cavalieri, C., Conway, P. S., Gallion, H. H., Powell, D. E., and Turker, M. S. (1995). Genetic alterations distinguish different types of ovarian tumors. *Int. J. Cancer* **64,** 434–440.
84. Puls, L. E., Powell, D. E., Depriest, P. D., Gallion, H. H., Hunter, J. E., Kryscio, R. J., and Vannagell, J. R. (1992) Transition from benign to malignant epithelium in mucinous and serous ovarian cysta-denocarcinoma. *Gynaecol. Oncol.* **47,** 53–57.
85. Roy, W. J., Watson, R. H., Hitchcock, A., and Campbell, I. G. (1997) Frequent loss of heterozygosity on chromosomes 7 and 9 in benign epithelial ovarian tumors. *Oncogene* **15,** 2031–2035.

# 4

## Alterations in Oncogenes, Tumor Suppressor Genes, and Growth Factors Associated with Epithelial Ovarian Cancers

### Robert C. Bast, Jr. and Gordon B. Mills

### 1. Introduction

More than 90% of epithelial ovarian cancers are clonal neoplasms that arise from the progeny of a single cell *(1–3)*. Comparison of primary and metastatic sites from the same patient has detected similar patterns of loss of heterozygosity (LOH) on different chromosomes, inactivation of the same X chromosome, and identical mutations in the *p53* gene in primary and secondary tumors. Given the clonality of most ovarian cancers, multiple genetic alterations must occur in the progeny of a single cell to permit progression from a normal epithelial phenotype to that of a malignant cell capable of uncontrolled proliferation, invasion, and metastasis. Approximately 10% of ovarian cancers are familial and have been associated with germ-line mutations in *BRCA1*, *BRCA2*, mismatch repair genes, or *p53* (detailed in **Subheading 2.2.**). Somatic mutations have been found in sporadic ovarian cancers that activate oncogenes or that result in loss of tumor suppressor gene function. Different ovarian cancers can also exhibit aberrant autocrine and/or paracrine growth regulation with alteration in the expression of growth factors and their receptors. No single abnormality has been detected in all ovarian cancers and most of the alterations are observed in cancers that arise at other sites. Certain changes in oncogenes, tumor suppressor genes, growth factors, and their receptors occur in a significant fraction of epithelial ovarian cancers, whereas others are uncommon. Consequently, progress has been made in defining the spectrum and profile of genetic and epigenetic changes that occur during transformation of the ovarian epithelium. A better understanding of the genotypic and phenotypic alterations that are associated with different epithelial ovarian cancers may impact on more effective management of the disease through chemoprevention, early detection, precise prognostication, treatment directed toward molecular targets, and individualization of therapy.

### 2. Tumor Suppressor Genes

A number of tumor suppressor genes have been identified in cancers that arise at other sites and subsequently evaluated in ovarian cancers, including *RB*, *VHL*, *WT*, and

From: *Methods in Molecular Medicine, Vol. 39: Ovarian Cancer: Methods and Protocols*
Edited by: J. M. S. Bartlett © Humana Press, Inc., Totowa, NJ

*p53*. In recent years, abnormalities in novel tumor suppressor genes such as *NOEY2* (*ARHI*) have been discovered in ovarian cancers and then found relevant to other tumor types. Candidate genes have been discovered both by positional cloning and by differential display. Different putative suppressor genes encode proteins that extend from the cell matrix to intracellular signaling molecules and transcription factors (**Table 1**).

### 2.1. Tumor Suppresor Genes Identified at Other Sites

Among the tumor suppressor genes first described in other cancers, abnormalities have been detected in *RB*, *WT*, and *VHL*, but loss of function rarely occurs. LOH has been observed at *RB* in more than 50% of high-grade ovarian cancers, but homozygous deletion is uncommon and protein expression is lost in less than 5% of cases *(5–6)*. Reduced expression of *RB* is, however, associated with a poor prognosis when it is encountered in stage I disease *(7)*.

### 2.2. p53

Loss of *p53* function is observed in more than 50% of advanced ovarian cancers, but in only 15% of stage I lesions *(8)*. Mutation of *p53* is only occasionally observed in ovarian cancers with low malignant potential and is rarely detected in benign ovarian tumors. Consequently, abnormalities of *p53* have been considered a "late change" in tumor progression, associated with the acquisition of metastatic potential. Observation of *p53* overexpression in apparently benign inclusion cysts *(9)* suggests that mutation of *p53* might, in fact, be an "early change" in a fraction of cases and might mark a subset of cancers that metastasize when a tumor is still of relatively small volume.

Mutations are observed at multiple sites in the *p53* gene, but there is no single site or codon that is distinctive or unique to ovarian cancer. When *p53* mutations were sequenced in a series of ovarian cancers, the fraction of transitions, transversions, and deletions in *p53* was similar to the fraction of these alterations in the Factor IX gene within the germ line of patients who had inherited Hemophilia B *(10)*. The mutations observed in Factor IX deficiency are thought to be related to spontaneous deamination of nucleotides during DNA replication, rather than to the action of exogenous carcinogens. In this regard, *p53* mutations in ovarian cancer differ from the excess of G–T transversions observed in lung cancer and the excess of transitions at CG pairs found in colon cancer. Molecular alterations in *p53* among ovarian cancers are consistent with epidemiologic observations that have generally failed to identify carcinogens and that point to the importance of ovulation in promoting tumor progression at this site. Ovarian surface epithelial cells are generally quiescent, but can proliferate to heal the wound produced by rupture of a follicle to release an oocyte. Proliferation provides an opportunity for mutations to occur and to be expressed. Factors that increase ovulation—nulliparity, early menarche, late menopause, and use of fertility stimulating drugs—are associated with an increased incidence of ovarian cancer. Conversely, multiple pregnancies, prolonged lactation, or use of oral contraceptives that suppress ovulation are associated with a decreased incidence of the disease. Consistent with a possible link between genetic alteration and ovulation, mutations of *p53* in ovarian cancers have been correlated with the total number of ovulatory cycles in one population based study *(11)*.

In addition to insights regarding the biology of the disease, mutation of *p53* signals a poor prognosis in stage I disease *(12)*, predicts resistance to platinum-based chemo-

**Table 1**
**Putative Tumor Suppressor Genes**
**in Epithelial Ovarian Cancer (modified from ref. *4*)**

| Gene | Chromosome | Function |
|---|---|---|
| *SPARC* | *5q31* | Matrix |
| *DOC2* | *5p13* | Binds GRB2 |
| *MMAC-1 (PTEN)* | *10q23* | Phosphatase |
| *NOEY2* | *1p31* | Induces *p21* |
| | | Inhibits Cyclin D1 |
| *p53* | *17p13* | DNA Stability |
| | | Apoptosis |
| *LOT-1* | *6q25* | Zinc Finger |
| *OVCA1* | *17p13* | Unknown |

therapy *(13)* and may provide a target for gene therapy *(14)*. In this regard, studies of *p53* may provide a model for characterizing the biological and clinical characteristics of other oncogenes whose expression is lost in ovarian cancers. To the extent that information regarding *p53* is utilized in clinical practice, it is important to recognize that immunohistochemical staining of mutant Tp53 may underestimate the incidence of mutation. The TP53 protein is present at low concentrations in normal cells and is generally not detected by immunohistochemical techniques. Missense mutations produce TP53 that accumulates in cells and that can be stained with anti-TP53 antibodies. Loss of *p53* function can also occur in 10–20% of ovarian cancers through loss of both alleles (*p53* null) or through nonsense mutations that produce truncated protein.

## 2.3. Tumor Suppressor Genes Identified in Ovarian Cancers

Several tumor suppressor genes were first recognized in ovarian cancer either by positional cloning or by comparison of gene expression in normal and malignant epithelial cells. SPARC encodes a calcium binding matrix protein that contributes to cell adhesion *(15)*. DOC-2 *(16)* binds to GRB-2 upstream of RAS. Although RAS is not frequently mutated in serous carcinomas, it is physiologically activated in a majority of ovarian cancer cell lines *(17)*. NOEY2 (ARHI) is a RAS/RAP homolog whose expression is downregulated in a majority of ovarian and breast cancers *(18)*. Unlike RAS or RAP, introduction of the ARHI gene induces p21[WAF1/CIP1], downregulates expression of cyclin D1, truncates signaling through RAS/MAP and inhibits the growth of cancer cells that lack its expression. MMAC1/PTEN is a phosphatase that is mutated in a significant fraction of endometrioid ovarian carcinomas *(19)*. Recent studies point to the products of PI3 kinase as important substrates. LOT-1 exhibits a zinc finger motif and may serve as a transcription factor *(20)*. The function of OVCA1 is not known *(21)*. Taken together, it is apparent that putative tumor suppressor genes may be lost at all levels of important signaling pathways such as those regulated through RAS/MAP and PI3 kinase.

Loss of tumor suppressor gene function generally involves inactivation of two alleles through deletion and/or mutation. In the case of *p53*, the mutant protein product may serve as a dominant negative, precluding the necessity for "two hits." The *ARHI* gene is inactivated through maternal imprinting that silences one allele from conception and subsequent deletion of the contralateral allele in 30–40% of breast and ovarian cancers. In addition, expression of the *ARHI* gene is transcriptionally regulated accounting for loss of expression in an even higher fraction of cancers at these sites. To date, there have been no more than 20 imprinted genes described, with some appearing to be clustered. Consequently, areas adjacent to ARHI on chromosome *1p31* might encode additional growth regulatory genes that could play a role in ovarian oncogenesis. Putative tumor suppressor genes have been identified at many, but not all sites of LOH in sporadic ovarian cancers. Additional tumor suppressor genes are likely to be discovered that will map to at least some of these areas. Current development of expression arrays with some $5 \times 10^4$ gene fragments should facilitate studies of differential expression in normal and cancer tissues, identifying potential candidates that can regulate growth. Rapid progress of the human genome project and compilation of more complete EST chromosome maps should facilitate the identification of additional genes that map to sites of LOH.

## 3. Oncogenes

Activation of several oncogenes has been reported in subsets of ovarian cancers. Abnormalities in receptor tyrosine kinases, nonreceptor tyrosine kinases, G proteins, and transcription factors have been observed (**Table 2**).

### 3.1. HER-2/neu

Among the receptor tyrosine kinases, wild type HER-2/neu (HER-2) has been overexpressed in 20–30% of ovarian cancers, associated with a poor prognosis in several, but not all, studies *(22,23)*. Whether a poor prognosis relates to more aggressive growth or to drug resistance has not been resolved. To date, a ligand has not been found that binds to HER-2 alone. Heregulin (HRG) or neu differentiation factor (NDF) binds to homodimers of HER-3 or HER-4 and to heterodimers containing HER-2/HER-3 or HER-2/HER-4. When all three receptors are present, as is the case in ovarian cancers, heterodimers are formed preferentially and have higher affinity for heregulin than do homodimers. Most ovarian cancer cell lines express low levels of HER-3 ($10^4$/cell) and HER-4 ($10^4$/cell), whereas levels of HER-2 vary widely among different cell lines ($10^3$–$10^6$/cell) *(24)*. When high levels of HER-2 are expressed relative to HER-3, the ligand HRG inhibits anchorage independent growth of cancer cells. When low levels of HER-2 and HER-3 (or all three receptors) are present, HRG stimulates clonogenic growth *(24)*. Consequently, the relative expression of HER-2 and HER-3 may be important in determining the response of ovarian cancers to ligand and high levels of HER-2 may be associated with decreased clonogenic growth in the presence of HRG. In contrast to the effect of HRG on clonogenic growth, the ligand enhances the invasiveness of cancer cells that express high levels of HER-2 *(25)*. Thus, an increased capacity for invasion and metastasis, rather than an increased rate of growth, may contribute to the clinical correlation of HER-2 overexpression with a poor prognosis.

In addition to its possible impact on prognosis, overexpression of HER-2 may contribute to taxane resistance *(26)*. HER-2 can also serve as a target for gene- and antibody-based therapy. Introduction of the viral E1A gene downregulates HER-2 expression and inhibits growth of ovarian cancers that overexpress the receptor *(27)*. Treatment with E1A in liposomes has inhibited growth of human ovarian cancer

**Table 2**
**Oncogenes in Epithelial Ovarian Cancer**
**(modified from ref. *4*)**

Receptor Kinases
 Overexpression of HER-2
 Mutation of EGFR
 Novel Expression of FMS
Overexpression of MYC
Nonreceptor Kinases
 Amplification of PI3 Kinase
 Amplification of AKT Kinase
 SRC Kinase Activated Physiologically
Ras Rarely Mutated but Frequently Activated Physiologically

xenografts in nude mice *(27)* and has downregulated HER-2 expression in ascites and pleural effusions of ovarian and breast cancer patients in a phase I clinical trial *(28)*. Preliminary data suggest that introduction of viral E1A can also increase sensitivity to the cytotoxic effect of paclitaxel.

Antibodies against some, but not all, epitopes on the extracellular domain of HER-2 can inhibit clonogenic growth of cancer cells that overexpress the receptor *(29)*. Treatment with anti-HER-2 antibody is associated with modulation of diacylglycerol levels *(30)*, inhibition of phospholipase C gamma, and the induction of apoptosis *(31)*. HRG does not affect these parameters, but activates RAS/MAP and PI3 kinase *(32)*. Incubation with an anti-HER-2 antibody, blocks the ability of HRG to stimulate PI3 kinase *(33)*. A humanized murine anti-HER-2 antibody, designated Herceptin, has induced regression in 12–15% of breast cancers that overexpress HER-2 *(34)*. Anti-HER-2 antibodies can enhance the cytotoxic activity of paclitaxel and doxorubicin against ovarian cancer xenografts *(35)*. In a concurrently controlled clinical trial with breast cancer patients, treatment with Herceptin enhanced the response to paclitaxel and to cyclophosphamide-doxorubicin *(36)*. Clinical studies with Herceptin in patients with ovarian cancer have not yet been reported. If treatment with anti-HER-2 antibodies becomes clinically useful, standardization may be required for quantitating levels of the HER-2 protein in ovarian cancers. Amplification of the HER-2 gene is observed in many, but not all cases where mRNA and protein are overexpressed. The extracellular domain of HER-2 has been detected in serum and correlates with overexpression of the receptor in tumor cells, but has not been elevated in enough patients to provide a useful diagnostic marker *(37)*.

### 3.2. Epidermal Growth Factor Receptor (EGFR)

The fourth member of the HER family of tyrosine kinase receptors is the epidermal growth factor receptor (EGFR). Phosphorylation of certain tyrosine residues of the intracellular domain is required for activation of kinase activity. Among the HER family members, heterodimerization and cross phosphorylation has been observed after binding of relevant ligands, many of which are expressed in ovarian cancers. Normal ovarian surface epithelium expresses EGFR detected by immunohistochemical techniques and this expression is lost in approximately 30% of ovarian cancers, associated with a slightly better prognosis *(38)*. Activation of EGFR can occur through truncation of its extracellular domain and this variant has been observed in some ovarian cancers *(39,40)*.

### 3.3. fms

Normal ovarian surface epithelial cells secrete small amounts of M-CSF (CSF-1) *(41)*, whereas 70% of ovarian cancers secrete sufficient amounts of the ligand to elevate serum levels *(42)*. The CSF-1 receptor *fms* cannot be detected by immunohistochemical techniques in normal ovarian surface epithelial cells, but is expressed in approximately 50% of ovarian cancers providing potential autocrine regulation of tumor cell growth and function *(43)*. Coexpression of CSF-1 and *fms* has been associated with increased invasive potential in ovarian and endometrial cancers.

### 3.4. src

Expression of the intracellular tyrosine kinase *src* is increased in a fraction of ovarian cancer cell lines *(44)* and enhanced *src* activity has been detected in the absence of mutation *(45)*. Stable transfectants bearing antisense to src have exhibited decreased anchorage independent growth and decreased tumorigenicity in nude mice, associated with reduced expression of the angiogenic factor VEGF/VPF *(44)*.

### 3.5. PI3 Kinase and AKT Kinase

The alpha 110 Kd subunit of phosphatidyl inositol 3 kinase (PI3 kinase) is amplified in at least 80% of ovarian cancers, associated with increased kinase activity *(46)*. Inhibition of kinase activity can slow growth of ovarian cancer cell lines, consistent with the possibility that signaling through this pathway is important for regulation of cell proliferation, and/or apoptosis. Elevated levels of membrane phosphatidyl inositol 3,4,5 triphosphate and other products of kinase activity can accumulate either through increased PI3 kinase activity or through inactivation of the MMAC1/PTEN phosphatase.

The AKT serine-threonine kinases are activated by the products of PI3 kinase and can inhibit apoptosis by phosphorylating BAD and/or caspase 9. AKT2 is amplified in 12% of ovarian cancers, associated with poorly differentiated histology *(47)*. Other components of the PI3K pathway are also upregulated in ovarian cancer, possibly related to colocalization with *p110* alpha and AKT2. Strikingly, whereas amplification of *p110* alpha at *3q26* and AKT2 at *19p* are frequently observed in ovarian cancer, these genes are rarely amplified in breast cancer or epithelial malignancies from other sites. Consequently, the PI3K pathway may be particularly important in ovarian cancer.

### 3.6. ras

The GTP-binding protein encoded by *ras* integrates signals from tyrosine kinases and from seven-times across the membrane receptors. Mutation of the *ras* gene activates the protein in 90% of pancreatic cancers and in a majority of lung and colon cancers, but in less than 20% of serous ovarian cancers *(48)*. More frequent *ras* mutations are found in mucinous and borderline tumors *(49)*. Interestingly, activation of the RAS protein has been observed in the absence of mutation in a majority of ovarian cancer cell lines *(17)*, consistent with activation of upstream receptors or with dysregulation of signal transduction through loss of DOC-2. Consequently, ovarian cancers may be a target for farnesyl transferase inhibitors despite the relatively low incidence of *ras* mutation.

### 3.7. myc

Expression of MYC protein is increased in 30% of ovarian cancer *(50)*. In contrast to observations with several other oncogenes, MYC expression does not appear to correlate with prognosis.

## 4. Growth Factors

### 4.1. Autocrine and Paracrine Growth Stimulation

Growth of ovarian cancers can be stimulated by several peptide and lipid growth factors. Peptide ligands that bind to the EGFR are produced by ovarian cancers including EGF, transforming growth factor alpha (TGF-α), and amphiregulin *(51)*. Loss of EGFR expression is associated with a slightly, but significantly better prognosis *(38)*. Antibodies against TGF-α can inhibit the growth of ovarian cancer cell lines that continue to express EGFR, consistent with autocrine growth stimulation *(52)*. Paradoxically, it has been difficult to document activation of the EGFR in ovarian cancer cell lines, challenging the functional importance of this particular receptor for autocrine growth stimulation *(53)*.

Approximately half of ovarian cancers express CSF-1 and have upregulation of the *fms* receptor *(43)*. Expression of *fms* is associated with a poor prognosis. Signaling through this receptor stimulates anchorage independent growth and enhances invasiveness by increasing expression of uPA *(54)*.

In addition to the peptide growth factors that signal through tyrosine kinase growth factor receptors, other ligands, such as lysophosphatidic acid (LPA) and endothelin, signal through G protein-linked seven times across the membrane receptors. A distinctive sn2 form of LPA has 100-fold greater activity in stimulating tumor cells than in stimulating platelets *(55)*. LPA can be produced by tumor cells as well as by platelets and fibroblasts. Sufficient levels are found in plasma and ascites fluid to alter calcium flux, activate EGFR, signal through *ras*/MAP, stimulate proliferation, block apoptosis, increase uPA secretion, and enhance secretion of VEGF/VPF. LPA levels in plasma have the potential to provide a marker for the presence of ovarian cancer, possibly complementing CA125 for detection of early-stage disease.

### 4.2. Autocrine and Paracrine Growth Inhibition

In normal ovarian surface epithelial (OSE) cells, appropriately activated TGF-β inhibits proliferation *(56)*. Normal OSE cells can express the TGF-β1, 2, and 3 isoforms, as well as type I and type II TGF-β receptors *(57)*. During malignant transformation, expression of TGF-β is lost in 40% of cases, interrupting potential autocrine growth inhibition *(58)*. In different cancer cell lines that have been established in culture, exogenous TGF-β can inhibit, fail to affect or even stimulate growth *(59)*. When ovarian cancer cells are isolated directly from ascites fluid, growth can still be inhibited with TGF-β in more than 90% of specimens *(56)*. When explants of solid ovarian cancers were treated with TGF-β, phosphorylation of TGF-β R1 was observed in 3 of 5 cancers, consistent with abnormal signaling downstream *(60)*. Abnormalities of SMADs, commonly found in other tumor types, have yet to be reported in ovarian cancers. Interestingly, TGF-β produces growth arrest in normal OSE, but does not induce apoptosis. With cancer cells, both growth arrest and apoptosis are observed *(56)*. TGF-β induced apoptosis can be inhibited by N-acetylcysteine or by transfection of bcl-2 that would otherwise be downregulated by the growth factor *(61)*. Differential effects on normal OSE and ovarian cancers are also seen with regard to invasiveness, where TGF-β has little effect on normal cells, but increases the invasiveness of ovarian cancer cells *(62)*.

Mullerian inhibitory substance (MIS) bears homology with TGF-β and binds to a receptor with a structure similar to that of the TGF-β receptors. During fetal development MIS is secreted by Sertoli cells and produces regression of the Mullerian duct in male animals *(63)*. Treatment with MIS has inhibited growth of ovarian cancers in cell culture and xenograft models *(64)*.

### 4.3. Factors that can Both Stimulate and Inhibit Growth of Different Cancers

Tumor necrosis factor alpha (TNF-α) can inhibit, fail to affect or stimulate the growth of different ovarian cancers *(65)*. In some ovarian cancer cell lines, TNF-α can induce apoptosis and this is enhanced by treatment with inhibitors of protein synthesis *(66)*. In other cell lines and in 10–25% of ovarian cancers isolated directly from patients, treatment with TNF-α can stimulate anchorage dependent or anchorage-independent growth *(65)*. Incubation with exogenous IL-1 or TNF-α can induce the endogenous expression of TNF-α that, in turn, stimulates proliferation *(65)*. TNF-α expression and function are regulated both transcriptionally and translationally through NF-κB. Most ovarian cancer cell lines have lost expression of TNF-α, but the cytokine can be detected in 80% of ovarian cancers obtained directly from patients *(68)*. TNF-α can also stimulate the nodular and invasive growth of ovarian cancers within the abdominal cavity, associated with increased expression of protease activity *(69)*.

As detailed above, heregulin can either inhibit or stimulate growth of ovarian and breast cancers depending upon the relative expression of HER-2 and HER-3 *(24)*. In addition, like TGF-β and TNF-α, heregulin can increase the invasiveness of ovarian and breast cancers that overexpress HER-2 *(25)*.

### 5. Conclusion

Research over the last two decades has begun to define the profile of alterations in oncogenes, tumor suppressor genes, and growth factors that occur in the ovarian surface epithelium during malignant transformation. Among the tumor suppressor genes, loss of functional *p53* and loss of NOEY2 (ARHI) expression appear to be most prevalent. Among the oncogenes, aberrant expression and/or activation of receptor tyrosine kinases (HER-2/neu, *fms*), cytoplasmic kinases (src, PI3 kinase, and AKT2), G proteins (ras), and transcription factors (myc) have been documented in different subsets of ovarian cancers. Different receptors are involved in stimulation (EGFR, *fms*, LPA), inhibition (TGF-β, MIS) or both (TNF-α, heregulin), depending upon the cellular context. Several growth factors (M-CSF, LPA, TGF-β, TNF-α) can increase invasiveness of ovarian cancers related to the induction of protease activity. Aberrant signaling through the ras/MAP or PI3 kinase pathways has been best studied. Several targets have been identified that may prove useful for more effective diagnosis, prognostication, choice of drugs, or therapy.

Future progress in ovarian cancer research will continue to depend upon the acquisition of ovarian cancer tissue before and after treatment. Prompt freezing of tissues will be all the more critical to assure preservation of RNA as well as DNA and protein. The availability of intact RNA will permit effective analysis of gene expression using conventional and genomic technologies. Comparison of gene expression in normal and malignant ovarian epithelial cells should identify new targets for molecular therapeutics and gene therapy. Correlation with clinical outcomes may permit the identification of patterns of gene expression that predict sensitivity or resistance both to conventional drugs and to agents that target well-defined molecular abnormalities in ovarian cancer cells. In normal tissues, studies of gene expression and of polymorphisms in genes, which encode drug metabolizing enzymes, may aid in identifying patients who would experience severe side effects from cytotoxic agents. Choice of the most effective and least toxic drugs could provide more effective management of the disease. To obtain the data required to permit individualization of therapy will require the study of a substantial number of patients in appropriate protocols that permit sampling of tissue to study the impact of conventional and novel agents. Further development of molecular technologies, which permit study of gene expression in small numbers of cells will be important, as will the close collaboration of laboratory and clinical investigators.

## References

1. Jacobs, I. J., Kohler, M. F., Wiseman, R., et al. (1992) Clonal origin of epithelial ovarian cancer: Analysis by loss of heterozygosity, p53 mutation and X chromosome inactivation. *J. Natl. Cancer Ins.* **84,** 1793–1798.
2. Mok, C. H., Tsao, W. W., Knapp, R. C., et al. (1992) Unifocal origin of advanced human epithelial ovarian cancer. *Cancer Res.* **52,** 5119–5122.
3. Li, S., Han H., Resnik, E., et al. (1993) Advanced ovarian carcinoma: molecular evidence of unifocal origin. *Gyn. Onc.* **51,** 21–25.
4. Bast, R. C. Jr. and Mills, G. B. The molecular pathogenesis of ovarian cancer, in *The Molecular Basis of Cancer,* 2nd ed., Mendelsohn, J., Howley, P., Israel, M., and Liotta, L., in press.
5. Kim, T. M., Benedict, W. F., Xu, H. J., et al. (1994) Loss of heterozygosity on chromosome 13 is common only in the biologically more aggressive subtypes of ovarian epithelial tumors and is associated with normal retinoblastoma gene expression. *Cancer Res.* **54,** 605–609.
6. Dodson, M. K., Cliby, W. A., Xu, H. J., et al. (1994) Evidence of functional RB protein in epithelial ovarian carcinomas despite loss of heterozygosity at the RB locus. *Cancer Res.* **54,** 610–613.
7. Dong, Y., Walsh, M. D., McGuckin, M. A., et al. (1997) Reduced expression of retinoblastoma gene product (pRB) and high expression of p53 are associated with poor prognosis in ovarian cancer. *Int. J. Cancer* **74,** 407–415.
8. Marks, J. R., Davidoff, A. M., Kerns, B. J. M., et al. (1991) Overexpression and mutation of p53 in epithelial ovarian cancer. *Cancer Res.* **51,** 2979–2984.
9. Hutson, R., Ramsdale, J., and Wells, M. (1995) p53 protein expression in putative precursor lesions of epithelial ovarian cancer. *Histopathol.* **27,** 367–371.
10. Kohler, M. F., Marks, J. R., Wiseman, R. W., et al. (1993) Spectrum of mutation and frequency of allelic deletion of the p53 gene in ovarian cancer. *J. Natl. Cancer Inst.* **85,** 1513–1519.
11. Schildkraut, J., Bastos, E., and Berchuck, A. (1997) Relationship between lifetime ovulatory cycles and overexpression of mutant p53 in epithelial ovarian cancer. *J. Nat. Cancer Inst.* **89,** 932–938.
12. Henriksen, R., Strang, P., Wilander, E., Backstrom, T., Tribukait, B., and Oberg, K. (1994) p 53 expression in epithelial ovarian neoplasms: relationship to clinical and pathological parameters, Ki-67 expression and flow cytometry, *Gynecol. Oncol.* **53,** 301–306.
13. Righetti, S. C., Della Torre, G., Pilotti, S., et al. (1996) A comparative study of p53 gene mutations, protein accumulation, and response to cisplatin-based chemotherapy in advanced ovarian carcinoma. *Cancer Res.* **56,** 689–693.
14. Mujoo, K., Maneval, D. C., Anderson, S. C., and Gutterman, J. U. (1996) Adenoviral-mediated p53 tumor suppressor gene therapy of human ovarian carcinoma. *Oncogene* **12,** 1617–1623.
15. Mok, S. C., Chan, W. Y., Wong, K. K., et al. (1996) SPARC, an extracellular matrix protein with tumor-suppressing activity in human ovarian epithelial cells. *Oncogene* **12,** 1895–1901.

16. Mok, S. C., Wong, K. K., Chan, R. K., et al. (1994) Molecular cloning of differentially expressed genes in human epithelial ovarian cancer. *Gynecol. Oncol.* **52,** 247–252.

17. Patton, S. E., Martin, M. L., Nelson, L. L., et al. (1998) Activation of the Ras-MAP pathway and phosphorylation of ets-2 at position threonine 72 in human ovarian cancer cell lines. *Cancer Res.* **58,** 2253–2259.

18. Yu, Y., Xu, F., Fang, X., Zhao, S., Li, Y., Cuevas, B., et al. (1999) NOEY2 (ARHI), an imprinted putative tumor suppressor gene in ovarian and breast carcinomas. *Proc. Nat. Acad. Sci. USA* **96,** 214–219.

19. Steck, P. A., Pershouse, M. A., Jasser, S. A. et al. (1997) Identification of a candidate tumor suppressor gene, MMAC1, at chromosome 10q23.3 that is mutated in multiple advanced cancers. *Nature Gen.* **15,** 356–362.

20. Abdollahi, A., Godwin, A. K., Miller, P. D., et al. (1997) Indentification of a gene containing zinc finger motifs based on lost expression in malignantly transformed rat ovarian surface epithelial cells. *Cancer Res.* **57,** 2029–2034.

21. Schultz, D. C., Vandeweer, L., Berman, D. B., et al. (1996) Identification of two candidate tumor suppressor genes on chromosome 17p13.3. *Cancer Res.* **56,** 1997–2002.

22. Slamon, D. J., Godolphin, W., Jones, L. A., et al. (1989) Studies of the HER-2/neu protooncogene in human breast and ovarian cancer. *Science* **244,** 707–712.

23. Berchuck, A., Kamel, A., Whitaker, R., et al. (1990) Overexpression of HER-2/*neu* is associated with poor survival in advanced epithelial ovarian cancer. *Cancer Res.* **50,** 4087–4091.

24. Xu, F. J., Yu, Y. H., Boyer, C. M., et al. (1996) Stimulation or inhibition of ovarian cancer cell proliferation by heregulin is dependent on the ratio of HER2 to HER3 or HER4 expression. *Proc. Amer. Assoc. Cancer Res.* **37,** 191 (A#1305).

25. Xu, F. J., Stack, S., Boyer, C., et al. (1997) Heregulin and agonistic anti-p185$^{c-erbB2}$ antibodies inhibit proliferation but increase invasiveness of breast cancer cells that overexpress p185$^{c-erbB2}$: Increased invasiveness may contribute to poor prognosis. *Clin. Cancer Res.* **3,** 1629–1634.

26. Yu, D., Wu, B., Jing, T., et al. (1998) Overexpression of both p185 c-erbB2 and p170 MDR render breast cancer cells highly resistant to taxol. *Oncogene* **16,** 2087–2094.

27. Yu, D., Matin, A., and Xia, W. (1995) Liposome-mediated in vivo E1A gene transfer suppressed dissemination of ovarian cancer cells that overexpress HER-2/neu. *Oncogene* **11,** 1383–1388.

28. Ueno, N. T., Hung, M. C., and Zhang, S. (1998) Phase I E1A gene therapy in patents with advanced breast and ovarian cancers. *Proc. Amer. Soc. Clin. Oncol.* **17,** 432a (A#1663).

29. Xu, F. J., Lupu, R., Rodriguez, G., et al. (1993) Antibody induced growth inhibition is mediated through immunochemically and functionally distinct epitopes on the extracellular domain of c-erbB-2 (HER-2/neu). *Int. J. Cancer* **53,** 401–408.

30. Boente, M. P., Berchuck, A., Whitaker, R. S., Kalén, A., Xu, F. J., Clarke-Pearson, D. L., et al. (1998) Suppression of diacylglycerol levels by antibodies reactive with the c-*erb*B-2 (HER-2/neu) gene product p185$^{erbB-2}$ in breast and ovarian cancer cell lines. *Gynecol. Oncol.* **70,** 49–55.

31. Bae, D. S., Xu, F-J., Mills, G., and Bast, R. C. Jr. (1995) Heregulin and antibodies against p185c-erbB-2 (p185) activate distinct signaling pathways. *Proc. Amer. Assoc. Cancer Res.* **36,** 55 (A#328).

32. Le, L., Vadlamudi, R., McWatters, A., Kumar, R., and Bast, R. C. Contrasting effects of heregulin and a tumor-inhibitory monoclonal antibody to HER-2 receptor on mitogen-activated protein kinases and phosphoinositide-3-kinase pathways. *Proc. Amer. Assoc. Cancer Res.*, in press.

33. Adam, L., Vadlamudi, R., Kandapaka, S. B., Chernoff, J., Mendelsohn, J., and Kumar, R. (1998) Heregulin regulates cytoskeletal reorganization and cell migration through the p21-activated kinase-1 via phosphatidyl-inositol-3 kinase. *J. Biol. Chem.* **273,** 28,238–28,246.

34. Baselga, J., Tripathy, D., Mendelsohn, J., et al. (1996) Phase II study of weekly intravenous recombinant humanized anti-p185HER2 monoclonal antibody in patients with HER2/neu-overexpressing metastatic breast cancer. *J. Clin. Onc.* **14,** 737–744.

35. Baselga, J., Norton, L., Albanell, J., et al. (1998) Recombinant humanized anti-HER2 antibody (Herceptin) enhances the antitumor activity of paclitaxel and doxorubicin against HER2/neu overexpressing human breast cancer xenografts. *Cancer Res.* **58,** 2825–2831.

36. Slamon, D., Leyland-Jones, B., Shak, S., et al. (1998) Addition of herceptin (humanized anti-HER2 antibody) to first line chemotherapy for HER2 overexpressing metastatic breast cancer markedly increases anticancer activity: A randomized multinational controlled phase II trial. *Proc. Amer. Soc. Clin. Oncol.* **17,** 98 (A#377).

37. McKenzie, S. J., DeSombre, K. A., Bast, B. S., Hollis, D. R., Whitaker, R. S., Berchuck, A., et al. (1993) Serum levels of HER-2/*neu* (c-*erb*B-2) correlate with overexpression of p185$^{neu}$ in human ovarian cancer. *Cancer* **71,** 3942–3946.

38. Berchuck, A., Rodriguez, G. C., Kamel, A., et al. (1991) Epidermal growth factor receptor expression in normal ovarian epithelium and ovarian cancer. I. Correlation of receptor expression with prognostic factors in patients with ovarian cancer. *Amer. J. Ob. Gynecol.* **164,** 669–674.

39. Huang, H. J. S., Nagane, M., Klingbiel, C. K., et al. (1997) The enhanced tumorigenic activity of a mutant epidermal growth factor receptor common in human cancers is mediated by threshold levels of constitutive tyrosine phosphorylation and unattenuated signaling. *J. Bio. Chem.* **272**, 2927–2935.

40. Ilekis, J. V., Gariti, J., Niederberger, C., et al. (1997) Expression of a truncated epidermal growth factor receptor-like protein (TEGFR) in ovarian cancer. *Gynecol. Oncol.* **65**, 36–41.

41. Lidor, Y. J., Xu, F. J., Martinez-Maza, O., et al. (1993) Constitutive production of macrophage colony stimulating factor and interleukin-6 by human ovarian surface epithelial cells. *Exp. Cell Res.* **207**, 332–339.

42. Xu, F. J., Ramakrishnan, S., Daly, L., Soper, J. T., Berchuck, A., Clarke-Pearson, D., et al. (1991) Increased serum levels of macrophage colony-stimulating factor in ovarian cancer. *Amer. J. Obstet. Gynecol.* **165**, 1356–1362.

43. Kacinski, B. M., Carter, D., Mittal, K., et al. (1990) Ovarian adenocarcinomas express fms-complementary transcripts and fms antigen, often with coexpression of CSF-1. *Amer. J. Path.* **137**, 135–147.

44. Wiener, J., Nakano, K., Kruzelock, R. P., Bucana, C. D., Bast, R. C., Jr., and Gallick, G. E. Reduction of c-src kinase activity abrogates malignant human ovarian cancer tumor growth in a xenograft mouse model. *Submitted for publication.*

45. Budde, R. J., Ke, S., and Levin, V. A. (1994) Activity of pp60c-src in 60 different cell lines derived from human tumors. *Cancer Biochem. Biophys.* **14**, 171–175.

46. Shayesteh, L., Lu, Y., Ku, W. L., et al. (1999) PIK3CA is implicated as an oncogene in ovarian cancer. *Nature Genetics* **21**, 99–102.

47. Bellacosa, A., de Feo, D., Godwin, A. K., et al. (1995) Molecular alterations of the AKT2 oncogene in ovarian and breast carcinomas. *Int. J. Cancer* **64**, 280–285.

48. Enomoto, T., Inoue, M., Perantoni, A. O., et al. (1990) K-ras activation in neoplasms of the human female reproductive tract. *Cancer Res.* **50**, 6139–6145.

49. Mok, S. C., Bell, D. A., Knapp, R. C., et al. (1993) Mutation of K-ras protooncogene in human ovarian epithelial tumors of borderline malignancy. *Cancer Res.* **53**, 1489–1492.

50. Baker, V. V., Borst, M. P., Dixon, D., et al. (1990) c-myc amplification in ovarian cancer. *Gynecol. Onc.* **38**, 340–342.

51. Stromberg, K., Johnson, G. R., O'Connor, D. M., et al. (1994) Frequent immunohistochemical detection of EGF supergene family members in ovarian carcinogenesis. *Int. J. Gynecol. Pathol.* **13**, 342–347.

52. Stromberg, K., Collins, T. J., Gordon, A. W., et al. (1992) Transforming growth factor-alpha acts as an autocrine growth factor in ovarian cancer cell lines. *Cancer Res.* **52**, 341–347.

53. Ottensmeier, C., Swanson, L., Strobel, T., et al. (1996) Absence of constitutive EGF receptor activation in ovarian cancer cell lines. *Brit. J. Cancer* **74**, 446–452.

54. Chambers, S. K., Ivins, C. M., and Carcangiu, M. L. (1997) Expression of plasminogen activator inhibitor-2 in epithelial ovarian cancer: a favorable prognostic factor related to the actions of CSF-1. *Int. J. Cancer* **74**, 571–575.

55. Xu, Y., Gaudette, D. C., Boynton, J., et al. (1994) Characterization of an ovarian cancer activating factor (OCAF) in ascites from ovarian cancer patients. *Clin. Cancer Res.* **1**, 1223–1232.

56. Havrilesky, L. J., Hurteau, J. A., Whitaker, R. S., et al. (1995) Regulation of apoptosis in normal and malignant epithelial cells by transforming growth factor beta. *Cancer Res.* **55**, 944–948.

57. Henriksen, R., Gobl, A., Wilander, E., et al. (1995) Expression and prognostic significance of TGF-beta isotypes, latent TGF-beta 1 binding protein, TGF-beta type I and type II receptors, and endoglin in normal ovary and ovarian neoplasms. *Lab. Invest.* **73**, 213–220.

58. Hurteau, J., Rodriguez, G. C., Whitaker, R. S., et al. (1994) Transforming growth factor-beta inhibits proliferation of human ovarian cancer cells obtained from ascites. *Cancer* **74**, 93–99.

59. Berchuck, A., Rodriguez, G., Olt, G. J., et al. (1992) Regulation of growth of normal ovarian epithelial cells and ovarian cancer cell lines by transforming growth factor-β. *Amer. J. Ob. Gynecol.* **166**, 676–684.

60. Baldwin, R. L., Yamada, D., Bristow, R. E., Chen, L-M., and Karlan, B. Y. (1998) Ovarian epithelial growth regulation, in *Ovarian Cancer 5*, Sharp, F., Blackett, T., Berek, J., Bast, R., eds. Isis Medical Media, Oxford, U.K. pp. 99–107.

61. Lafon, C., Mathieu, C., Guerrin, M., et al. (1996) Transforming growth factor beta 1-induced apoptosis in human ovarian carcinoma cells: protection by the antioxidant N-acetylcysteine and bcl-2. *Cell Growth Differ.* **7**, 1095–1104.

62. Rodriguez, G. C., Berchuck, A., Whitaker, R., et al. (1994) Regulation of invasion in ovarian cancer cell lines by transforming growth factor-beta. *26th Annu. Meeting Soc. Gynecol. Oncol.* **40**.

63. Lee, M. M., Donahoe, P. K., Hasegawa, T., et al. (1996) Mullerian inhibiting substance in humans: normal levels from infancy to adulthood. *J. Clin. Endo. Metabol.* **81**, 571–576.

64. Fuller, A. F., Jr., Guy, S., Budzik, G. P., and Donahoe, P. K. (1982) Mullerian inhibiting substance inhibits colony growth of a human ovarian carcinoma cell line. *J. Clin. Endo. Metabol.* **54,** 1051–1055.

65. Wu, S., Boyer, C. M., Whitaker, R. S., et al. (1993) Tumor necrosis factor alpha as an autocrine and paracrine growth factor for ovarian cancer: monokine induction of tumor cell proliferation and tumor necrosis factor alpha expression. *Cancer Res.* **53,** 1939–1944.

66. Mutch, D. G., Powell, C. B., Kao, M. S., et al. (1992) Resistance to cytolysis by tumor necrosis factor alpha in malignant gynecological cell lines is associated with the expression of protein(s) that prevent the activation of phospholipase A2 by tumor necrosis factor alpha. *Cancer Res.* **52,** 866–872.

67. Wu, S., Xu, F. J., Boyer, C. M., and Bast, R. C., Jr. (1994) Proliferation and induction of NF-kappa B by tumor necrosis factor-a can be mediated through two distinct receptors in human ovarian cancer cells. *Proc. Amer. Assoc. Cancer Res.* **35,** 486 (A#2899).

68. Takeyama, H., Wakamiya, N., O'Hara, C., et al. (1991) Tumor necrosis factor expression by human ovarian carcinoma in vivo. *Cancer Res.* **51,** 4476–4480.

69. Boyer, C. M., Wu, S., Xu, F-J., et al. (1995) Stimulation of human ovarian cancer cell growth *in vivo* with TNFa or IL-1 in immunodeficient scid mice. *Proc. Amer. Assoc. Cancer Res.* **36,** 71(A#422).

# 5

# Pathological Assessment of Ovarian Cancer

## Alistair R. W. Williams

## 1. Introduction

Ovarian neoplasms are notoriously heterogeneous—the World Health Organization classification (*1*) includes 46 different epithelial tumor types, 24 sex cord stromal types, 29 germ cell types, and 13 other categories, not including 17 other tumor-like conditions (**Table 1**). Many of these lesions are very rare, but there is tremendous variation in the biological behavior of different tumor types, and it is very important that histopathological assessment is performed accurately. This is not only crucial to the patient, whose treatment depends on it, but also in investigative work on ovarian cancer. Uniform terminology must be used to allow comparisons between different studies and any research that involves analysis of the biological or clinical features of ovarian tumors must include expert histopathological review of cases.

Over 90% of all malignant ovarian tumors are epithelial in type and most of these are believed to take origin from invaginations of the ovarian surface epithelium (OSE). This is a modified pelvic mesothelium that embryologically derives from the coelomic epithelium. The OSE retains an ability to undergo metaplasia to form a range of müllerian and nonmüllerian epithelia. The reexpression of this capacity in neoplasia explains the genesis of the wide variety of epithelial tumor types that occur. These not only include müllerian tissues—Fallopian tubal epithelium (serous tumors), endometrium (endometrioid tumors), and endocervix (mucinous tumors of endocervical type), but also other forms of nonmüllerian epithelium such as intestine (mucinous tumors of intestinal type) and transitional epithelium (transitional cell tumors and Brenner tumors).

Ovarian sex cord-stromal tumors make up less than 5% of all ovarian malignancies. Their rarity, diverse histology, and variable terminology make sex cord-stromal tumors a confusing and difficult group to study. There is a wide diversity of histological differentiation associated with similar variation in endocrine activity and clinical behavior.

Tumors of germ cell origin make up the third major category of ovarian neoplasms. Totipotential germ cells give rise to a further broad range of benign and malignant neoplasms, the histological types of which recapitulate the capacity of the germ cell to differentiate along somatic and extraembryonic lines.

From: *Methods in Molecular Medicine, Vol. 39: Ovarian Cancer: Methods and Protocols*
Edited by: J. M. S. Bartlett © Humana Press, Inc., Totowa, NJ

**Table 1**
**WHO-Revised Classification of Ovarian Tumors *(1)***

1. Surface epithelial-stromal tumors
Serous tumors
  Benign
    1. Cystadenoma and papillary cystadenoma
    2. Surface papilloma
    3. Adenofibroma and cystadenofibroma
  Of borderline malignancy (of low-malignant potential)
    1. Cystic tumor and papillary cystic tumor
    2. Surface papillary tumor
    3. Adenofibroma and cystadenofibroma
  Malignant
    1. Adenocarcinoma, papillary adenocarcinoma, and papillary cystadenocarcinoma
    2. Surface papillary adenocarcinoma
    3. Adenocarcinofibroma and cystadenocarcinofibroma
Mucinous Tumors: endocervical-like and intestinal type
  Benign
    1. Cystadenoma
    2. Adenofibroma and cystadenofibroma
  Of borderline malignancy (of low-malignant potential)
    1. Cystic tumor
    2. Adenofibroma and cystadenofibroma
  Malignant
    1. Adenocarcinoma and cystadenocarcinoma
    2. Adenocarcinofibroma and cystadenocarcinofibroma
Endometrioid tumors
  Benign
    1. Cystadenoma
    2. Cystadenoma with squamous differentiation
    3. Adenofibroma and cystadenofibroma
    4. Adenofibroma and cystadenofibroma with squamous differentiation
  Of borderline malignancy (of low-malignant potential)
    1. Cystic tumor
    2. Cystic tumor with squamous differentiation
    3. Adenofibroma and cystadenofibroma
    4. Adenofibroma and cystadenofibroma with squamous differentiation
  Malignant
    1. Adenocarcinoma and cystadenocarcinoma
    2. Adenocarcinoma and cystadenocarcinoma with squamous differentiation
    3. Adenocarcinofibroma and cystadenocarcinofibroma
    4. Adenocarcinofibroma and cystadenocarcinofibroma with squamous differentiation
  Epithelial-(endometrioid) stromal and (endometrioid) stromal
    1. Adenosarcoma, homologous and heterologous
    2. Mesodermal (müllerian) mixed tumor (carcinosarcoma), homologous and heterologous
    3. Stromal sarcoma
Clear cell tumors
  Benign
    1. Cystadenoma
    2. Adenofibroma and cystadenofibroma
  Of borderline malignancy (of low-malignant potential)
    3. Cystic tumor
    4. Adenofibroma *and cystadenofibroma*
  Malignant
    1. Adenocarcinoma
    2. Adenocarcinofibroma and cystadenocarcinofibroma
Transitional cell tumors
  Brenner tumor
  Brenner tumor of borderline malignancy (proliferating)

**Table 1** *(continued)*

Malignant Brenner tumor
Transitional cell carcinoma (non-Brenner type)
Squamous cell tumors
Mixed epithelial tumors (specify types)
Benign
Of borderline malignancy (of low-malignant potential)
Malignant
Undifferentiated carcinoma
Unclassified

2. Sex cord-stromal cell tumors
Granulosa-stromal cell tumors
Granulosa cell tumors
1. Juvenile
2. Adult
Tumors of the thecoma-fibroma group
1. Thecoma
a. Typical
b. Luteinized
2. Fibroma
3. Cellular fibroma
4. Fibrosarcoma
5. Stromal tumor with minor sex cord elements
6. Sclerosing stromal tumor
7. Stromal luteoma
8. Unclassified (fibrothecoma)
9. Others
Sertoli-stromal cell tumors; androblastomas
Well differentiated
1. Sertoli cell tumor; tubular androblastoma
2. Sertoli-Leydig cell tumor
3. Leydig cell tumor
Of intermediate differentiation
1. Variant—with heterologous elements (specify types)
Poorly differentiated (sarcomatoid)
1. Variant—with heterologous elements (specify types)
Retiform
Mixed (specify types)
Sex cord tumor with annular tubules
Gynandroblastoma
Steroid (lipid) cell tumor
Stromal luteoma
Leydig cell tumor (hilus cell tumor)
Unclassified
3. Germ cell tumors
Dysgerminoma
Variant—with syncytiotrophoblastic cells
Yolk sac tumor (endodermal sinus tumor)
Variants
Polyvesicular vitelline tumor
Hepatoid
Glandular
Embryonal carcinoma
Polyembryoma
Choriocarcinoma
Teratomas
Immature
Mature

*(continued)*

**Table 1** *(continued)*

 1. Solid
 2. Cystic (dermoid cyst)
 3. With secondary tumor formation (specify type)
 4. Fetiform (homunculus)
Monodermal and highly specialized
 1. Struma ovarii
  a. Variant—with thyroid tumor (specify type)
 2. Carcinoid
  a. Insular
  b. Trabecular
 3. Strumal carcinoid
 4. Mucinous carcinoid
 5. Neuroectodermal tumors
 6. Sebaceous tumors
 7. Others
  Mixed (specify types)
 Mixed (specify types)
4. Gonadoblastoma
  Variant—with dysgerminoma or other germ cell tumor
5. Germ cell-sex cord stromal tumor
  Variant—with dysgerminoma or other germ cell tumor
6. Tumors of rete ovarii
  Adenoma and cystadenoma
  Carcinoma
7. Mesothelial tumors
  Adenomatoid tumor
  Others
8. Tumors of uncertain origin
  Small cell carcinoma
  Tumor of probable Wolffian origin
  Hepatoid carcinoma
  Oncocytoma
9.  Gestational trophoblastic diseases
10. Soft tissue tumors not specific to ovary
11. Malignant lymphomas
12. Unclassified tumors
13. Secondary (metastatic) tumors
14. Tumor-like lesions
  Solitary follicle cyst
  Multiple follicle cysts (polycystic disease) (sclerocystic ovaries)
  Large solitary luteinized follicle cyst of pregnancy and puerperium
  Hyperreactio luteinalis (multiple luteinized follicle cysts)
 1. Variant—with corpora lutea
  Corpus luteum cyst
  Pregnancy luteoma
  Ectopic pregnancy
  Hyperplasia of stroma
  Stromal hyperthecosis
  Massive oedema
  Fibromatosis
  Endometriosis
  Cyst, unclassified (simple cyst)
  Inflammatory lesions
 1. Xanthogranuloma
 2. Malacoplakia
 3. Others

Current areas of particular research interest in the pathology of ovarian cancer are as follows:

1. Biology and pathology of OSE, and its role in the development of epithelial tumors.
2. Molecular pathology of ovarian carcinoma.
3. Early ovarian carcinoma.

## 2. The Ovarian Surface Epithelium (OSE)

The OSE is inconspicuous histologically, but is far more complex and versatile than its appearance would suggest. It is intimately involved in the processes of ovulation, and in the subsequent reconstitution of the ovarian surface. It is believed to give origin to around 90% of adult human ovarian malignancies, including those varieties that contribute most to mortality (2). The OSE has unique features, which are absent from the immediately adjacent pelvic mesothelium, suggesting that local factors in the ovarian cortex may play an important part in modifying the growth and morphology of this cell type. There are close embryological relationships between the OSE and the epithelium lining the Fallopian tubes, endometrium, and endocervix. The surface epithelial cells are a modified peritoneal mesothelium originating from coelomic epithelium, which forms the müllerian duct system, from which derive the uterus, cervix, and Fallopian tubes. There is a pressing need for a greater understanding of this elusive tissue, and the role it plays in ovarian carcinogenesis.

OSE has been poorly studied over the years for several reasons. It is a difficult tissue to handle, which consists of a single layer of cuboidal cells that is easily damaged, often absent from surgical specimens, having been removed during handling. It makes up a minute proportion of the overall ovarian mass, and early attempts to culture OSE in vitro were confused by contamination by various other cell types from ovarian cortex, whose morphology is similar. Recently, reliable methods have been described for establishing OSE in culture, and equally importantly, of characterizing the cell type by immunohistochemical markers, and of distinguishing it from potential contaminants in vitro (3,4). Several studies have employed OSE cells immortalized by viral transforming genes (5,6). The cells show great plasticity of phenotype, and it is clear that culture conditions have an important effect on morphology, migration, proliferation, and differentiation (7). Interactions with the extracellular matrix (ECM) seem fundamental in determining a range of phenotypic and cell kinetic features. Proliferation is dependent on the substratum—when cultured on collagen or fibrin, proliferation is low or absent, but when cultured on plastic alone, there is a high rate of proliferation (3). When cultured on Matrigel, OSE cells are able to show invasion in multicellular aggregates (7). Cell shape, growth, protease production, and integrin expression were also shown to be influenced by the ECM.

Interactions with the ECM are not entirely "one-way traffic," as OSE cells have been shown to have the capacity not only to produce ECM components, but also to induce changes in its composition. In a well-known culture model for wound repair, when plated onto collagen gel and ECM preparations, OSE cells were able to remodel collagen lattice gel inducing its contraction (8). OSE has also been shown to produce proteolytic enzymes, including serine proteases and metalloproteases (7). Although constitutively produced, levels of protease expression are determined by the ECM, and inversely related to cell growth. Low levels of protease expression are seen when OSE is grown on plastic, but high levels when grown on Matrigel. Protease production, and the ability to invade Matrigel, appears to be part of the normal phenotype of OSE and not acquired *de novo* during the process of neoplastic transformation.

It is well known that frequency of ovulation is associated with an increased risk of developing ovarian carcinoma, and it is speculated that carcinogenic effects occur during the proliferative process involved in reconstituting the ovulation-associated wound. Locally produced growth factors and cytokines influence growth and differentiation of OSE during this process and may drive the sequence of events leading to neoplastic change. Expression of cytokines, growth factors, and their receptors has been studied to a limited extent in OSE in culture, as well as in SV40 transformed immortalized OSE cell lines, and in cell lines derived from ovarian carcinomas. In one immunohistochemical study using a monoclonal antibody to the extracellular domain, unmanipulated OSE expressed epidermal growth factor receptor (EGFR) in vitro *(9)*. Other investigators found normal OSE to be weakly positive by immunohistochemistry for EGFR, as well as c-erbB2 protein (homologous with EGFR), while benign epithelial tumors were positive for c-erbB2 and negative for EGFR. Carcinomas showed variable immunohistochemical staining for both proteins *(10)*.

OSE in vitro has been shown to produce transforming growth factor β (TGFβ) protein and mRNA *(11)*. In this study, OSE cells in culture responded to TGFβ by inhibition of proliferation. This has been confirmed by demonstration of inhibition of thymidine incorporation by OSE in response to TGFβ *(12)*. Apoptosis was not seen in normal OSE with TGFβ, but it did occur in an ovarian cancer-derived cell line.

TGFα has also been localized by immunohistochemistry to OSE and mRNA demonstrated in a cell line *(13)*. It is believed that TGFα and TGFβ may act as reciprocal autocrine growth regulators of OSE, producing growth promotion and growth inhibition, respectively.

The effect of interferon γ (IFNγ) on proliferation and expression of EGFR has been examined in OSE and ovarian carcinoma cell lines *(14)*. Normal OSE was unaffected by IFNγ, either in terms of proliferation or EGFR expression, but in cell lines, there was a 30–40% decrease in proliferation despite strikingly increased EGFR expression.

Other cytokines have been examined in OSE by less rigorous techniques than demonstration of mRNA. Bioassay and antibody-neutralization experiments have shown that OSE secretes IL-1, IL-6, and CSF-1, whereas IL-2, IL-3, and IL-4 were absent *(14)*. Similar methods showed constitutive production of M-CSF and IL-6 by OSE *(15)*.

## 3. Molecular Pathology of Ovarian Carcinoma

Ovarian carcinoma usually presents late in its clinical course, and precursor lesions are infrequently encountered and poorly studied. As a consequence, molecular genetic studies have often been limited to analyses of late-stage tumors or ovarian carcinoma cell lines. A variety of techniques have been used. Karyotypic analyses have defined frequent areas of chromosomal disruption, and in an effort to identify potential tumor suppressor genes, areas of deletion have been mapped using polymorphic DNA probes. Alternatively, researchers have studied expression of previously defined candidate molecules at the protein or mRNA levels.

Karyotypic abnormalities are common in ovarian carcinoma, and may be simple aberrations such as trisomy 12 (commonly found in well-differentiated ovarian carcinomas, but also occurring in completely benign ovarian neoplasms) to very complex abnormalities, which mainly comprise chromosome losses, deletions, and unbalanced translocations. These are found frequently in poorly differentiated ovarian carcinomas. It should be noted that in interpreting such changes, it is often uncertain whether the abnormality is involved in causation of the neoplastic process, or whether it is an end result of genetic instability. The bands and regions most commonly involved in such structural rearrangements have been, in decreasing order of frequency: *19p13, 1p36, 1q21, 1q23–25, 3p11–13, 6q21, 19q13, 11p13–15, 11q13, 11q23, 12q24, 12p11–13,* and *7p13–22 (16)*. Analysis of this type may also shed light on other aspects of the disease process. For example, comparative karyotypic and other genetic analyses of primary ovarian tumors and their intraabdominal deposits, indicate ovarian carcinoma usually to be unifocal in origin, sharing distinctive chromosomal and genetic abnormalities. However, there is also evidence that primary serous carcinoma of the peritoneum, which is histologically indistinguishable, and clinically very similar to ovarian serous carcinoma, is of multifocal origin, at least in a significant proportion of cases *(17)*. It has also been recently suggested that "recurrent" ovarian cancer may actually be new primary cancer of the peritoneum. Clonal analysis (involving X chromosome inactivation, *p53* mutations, LOH, and microsatellite instability at multiple loci on multiple chromosomes) has revealed significantly different genetic "fingerprints" in primary and recurrent carcinoma, suggesting the formation of new tumors in the majority of cases *(18,19)*.

DNA aneuploidy (usually measured by integrated DNA densitometry in a flow cytometer) is present in a high proportion of ovarian carcinomas, and there is generally a correlation between aneuploidy and poor prognosis *(20,21)*. DNA aneuploidy is uncommon in early-stage well-differentiated tumors, and similarly is usually absent in borderline tumors. However, it has been shown that DNA aneuploidy may be a marker for the small minority of borderline ovarian tumors that show an aggressive clinical behavior *(22)*.

There have been a large number of "allelotyping" studies in which the presence of putative tumor suppressor genes has been adduced from the occurrence of high levels of allele loss at particular loci. Such studies are often limited by small numbers of tumors for analysis (especially of the rarer histological subtypes), and from inadequate numbers of informative loci examined. However, it has emerged that chromosomes *17p* and *q*, *6q* and *11p* figure regularly among the regions with high rates of allele imbalance, with as yet inconsistent findings of between 0 and 52% for *11q (23–25)*. There is a high rate of whole chromosome 17 loss—LOH at all informative chromosome 17 loci has been found in at least half the cases. This contrasts with chromosomes *6q* and *18q* where the rates of deletion obtained depend on their precise map locations. However, there may be over-representation in these results of chromosomal regions that can be deleted without compromising tumor cell growth. Where the relevant information is given, the frequency of allele imbalance at most loci correlates with histological grade and/or FIGO stage, much of the data being derived from advanced tumors.

By pooling data from several studies on chromosomes *11* and *17*, differences were observed amongst the common epithelial cancers. On chromosome *11*, allele imbalance was similar in serous, mucinous, and endometrioid cancers, but on chromosome *17*, imbalance, particularly on the short arm, is much more frequent in serous than in endometrioid or mucinous carcinomas *(26)*.

The PTEN/MMAC gene on *10q23* is a tumor suppressor gene implicated in the pathogenesis of a wide range of human malignancies. PTEN mutations appear to be relatively frequent in the endometrioid histological subtype of ovarian carcinoma (21%) accompanied by loss of the wild-type allele, but none were found in serous or clear cell types, and only one instance in an atypical mucinous tumor *(27)*.

Positive results in ovarian cancer have been obtained by studying well-established oncogenes and tumor suppressor genes that are known to be significant in other cancers. For example, activated or amplified *ras* has been identified in a minority (around 15%) of mainly advanced tumors, but activated Ki-*ras* has been detected in about one third of mucinous tumors, including some borderline tumors. *c-myc* is overexpressed in around 30% of ovarian carcinomas, especially serous carcinomas. *C-erbB-2* (HER-2/*neu*) has been found to be overexpressed, mainly in poor prognosis tumors, whereas its homologue *c-erbB-3* appears to be more strongly expressed in borderline and early invasive tumors.

The *p53* gene is altered in approximately 50% of human cancers of all types, and its role in ovarian carcinogenesis is not in doubt. Its protein product regulates transition from the G1 to S phases of the cell cycle, controlling entry into DNA repair pathways. Mutations, allele loss and altered protein expression are detectable in up to 50% of ovarian carcinomas, but not in benign tumors, very infrequently in borderline tumors, and apparently not in micropapillary serous carcinoma, a recently described low-grade variant. There is a significant association between *p53* mutation in ovarian carcinoma, and DNA aneuploidy. In carcinomas, missense mutations are the commonest abnormality of *p53*, rather than deletions or insertions (deletions being seven times commoner than insertions) *(28)*. Most *p53* mutations in ovarian carcinomas are transitions, suggesting that they arise spontaneously rather than due to exogenous carcinogens. *p53* mutation is found in a high proportion (82%) of malignant mixed mesodermal tumors (MMMT), and interestingly, monoclonal origin of both the malignant epithelial and mesenchymal components has been shown *(29,30)*. Mutations in *p53* have been found to occur less frequently in mucinous and endometrioid carcinomas than in the other epithelial types, and more often in moderately and poorly differentiated tumors *(31)*. A frequent histological finding in ovarian cancer is that of histologically "benign" cysts adjacent to carcinomas. *p53* mutation analysis of the tumor and the "benign" cyst epithelium has shown the same mutation to be present in both *(32)*. However, the absence of *p53* abnormalities in benign cystadenomas argues against this indicating transition from a preexisting benign tumor, but rather suggests that differentiation towards benign-appearing epithelium may occur in the carcinoma.

Downstream effector proteins of *p53* are potential sites of somatic alterations, and in a variety of human cancers, abnormalities have been found in expression of the *p21* protein product of the WAF1/Cip1 gene, which acts as a universal inhibitor of cyclins. In ovarian cancer, *p21* expression has been found to be significantly higher in the stroma surrounding the tumor than in the tumor itself *(33)*. There seems to be no consistent correlation of *p21*WAF1/Cip1 expression with *p53* expression or *p53* mutation *(34,35)*.

Alterations of retinoblastoma protein appear to be very uncommon in ovarian carcinoma. Similarly, microsatellite instability, present in a variety of other human tumor types, appears to be very infrequent in ovarian carcinoma, and there is also no evidence of its occurrence in benign or borderline ovarian tumors *(36)*.

Study of familial cancers has shown that up to around 10% of epithelial ovarian cancers are associated with inheritance of an autosomal dominant genetic mutation conferring a predisposition to cancer with variable penetrance. It was found that germline mutations in the *BRCA1* gene, located on *17q12–21*, accounted for the majority of breast/ovarian cancer families, with a smaller proportion associated with *BRCA2*. It has been estimated that women harboring *BRCA1* mutations carry up to a 63% lifetime risk of developing ovarian cancer, and an 85% risk of breast cancer. Most *BRCA1* mutations are predicted to result in truncated protein products. *BRCA1* and *BRCA2* are almost certainly tumor suppressor genes, but at least in the case of *BRCA1*, it has also been shown to be essential for the growth and development of embryonic cells. *BRCA1* is large, and its function essentially unknown, but it is probably involved in DNA damage and repair, in cell-cycle regulation and in control of cellular differentiation. In *BRCA1*-associated ovarian carcinomas, somatic mutation of *p53* is common (approximately 80% of cases), but is not an essential requirement for tumorigenesis. Perhaps surprisingly, only a small proportion (around 5%) of patients with sporadic ovarian cancer carry germline mutations in *BRCA1*, and mutations in *BRCA2* are rare. However, levels of *BRCA1* mRNA and protein are decreased in the majority of tumors. The significance of this is as yet unknown, but it has already raised the possibility of therapeutic strategies aimed at increasing expression of wild-type *BRCA1*, which in vitro has also been shown to suppress the growth of ovarian carcinoma cells *(37)*. Cancers associated with the *BRCA1* mutation appear to have a significantly more favorable clinical course compared with sporadic cancers matched for stage, grade and histological subtype *(38)*. *BRCA1* inactivation appears not to be involved in the genesis of borderline ovarian tumors—in a series of 26 cases, only one tumor showed loss of heterozygosity at one of eight polymorphic markers on *17q21 (39)*.

## 4. Early Ovarian Cancer

In the majority of cases, ovarian carcinoma has spread beyond the ovary by the time of presentation. As current treatment has made only a limited impact on survival, attention has increasingly turned to early detection of precursor lesions, in the hope that survival may be improved. There is surprisingly little known of the nature of the precursor lesion, and the sequence of events in development of disseminated ovarian malignancy. It has been recognized for some time that early malignant changes occur in the OSE-lined clefts and inclusion cysts in ovarian cortex, more frequently than on the surface of the ovary itself. Frequently, direct continuity can be demonstrated between apparently nonmalignant epithelia of this type and frank carcinomas. In a study examining the presence of nonmalignant epithelium in ovarian carcinomas *(40)*, benign-appearing epithelial components were identified in 74% of mucinous carcinomas, 46% of endometrioid carcinomas and 39% of clear-cell carcinomas. In contrast, benign epithelium was identified in only 15% of serous carcinomas. It was suggested that the great majority of serous carcinomas arise *de novo* from surface epithelium and its inclusions, but that a significant proportion of mucinous carcinomas arise in a background of mucinous cystadenoma. One study examined the histopathological features of "incidental" ovarian cancers—defined as early ovarian cancers, which were not recognized preoperatively, intraoperatively, or pathologically on gross examination, but discovered only microscopically *(41)*. It is significant that the study, using cases retrieved from the consultation files of a most eminent gynecological pathologist, reported only 14 cases. From the small number of cases available, it seems likely that ovarian cancer may be disseminated at a very early stage—of the 10 patients for whom follow-up data were available in this study, only five were alive and well without recurrence. An alternative explanation is multifocal origin of malignancy, in the ovary and at disseminated sites throughout the peritoneum—a "field effect." However, the evidence is rather against this in the majority of tumors—studies have shown that identical patterns of genetic markers of clonality are found in ovarian and extraovarian deposits, indicating a monoclonal origin *(42)*.

Epithelial inclusion cysts adjacent to and contralateral to serous carcinoma of ovary were examined immunohistochemically for *p53* protein expression *(43)*. In those showing cellular atypicality, immunoreactivity for *p53* was detected in the majority, consistent with the suggestion that such areas of epithelial atypia in inclusion cysts are the precursors of ovarian malignancy.

Endometriosis has long been suspected as another precursor to ovarian carcinomas of endometrioid and clear-cell types, but it is clear that other histological subtypes may be associated with it also. Atypical hyperplasia has been reported in endometriotic foci associated with the development of ovarian carcinomas *(44,45)*. Endometrioid carcinomas are the most frequent tumors associated with endometriosis, followed by clear-cell carcinomas and malignant mixed müllerian tumors. Serous and mucinous carcinomas are less frequently found *(46)*. It is noteworthy that unopposed estrogen stimulation may act on endometriosis leading to premalignant or malignant transformation *(47)*. In a series of cases of endometriosis synchronous with ovarian carcinoma, common genetic lesions were detected in carcinoma and endometriosis in the majority of cases, suggesting a common lineage, and consistent with the notion that carcinoma had arisen by malignant transformation of endometriosis *(48)*.

In conclusion, further progress in elucidating the molecular pathogenesis of ovarian cancer will rely on a fuller understanding of the physiology of the ovarian surface epithelium and a better knowledge of the earliest precursors of ovarian carcinoma. Only then will the molecular techniques that have already contributed so much to our knowledge of advanced ovarian carcinoma begin to unravel the mysteries of the early precursor lesions.

## References

1. Scully, R. E., Fox, H., Russell, P., et al. *International Histological Classification of Ovaria Tumors.* Springer Verlag, Berlin, Germany (in press).
2. Yancik, R. (1993) Ovarian cancer:age contrasts in incidence, histology, disease stage at diagnosis, and mortality. *Cancer* **71,** 517–523.
3. Auersperg, N., Maines-Bandiera, S. L., and Kruk, P. A. (1995) Human ovarian surface epithelium: growth patterns and differentiation, in *Ovarian Cancer 3*, (Sharp, F., Mason, P., Blackett, T., and Berek, J., eds.), Chapman & Hall Medical, London, U.K., pp. 157–170.
4. Salazar, H., Godwin, A. K., Getts, L. A., Testa, J. R., Daly, M., Rosenblum, N., et al. Spontaneous transformation of the ovarian surface epithelium and the biology of ovarian cancer, in Ovarian Cancer 3 (Sharp, F., Mason, P., Blackett, T., and Berek, J., eds.), Chapman & Hall Medical, London, U.K., pp. 145–156.
5. Auersperg, N., Maines-Bandiera, S. L., Dyck, H. G., and Kruk, P. A. (1994) Characterisation of cultured human ovarian surface epithelial cells: phenotypic plasticity and premalignant changes. *Lab. Invest.* **71,** 510–518.
6. Tsao, S. W., Mok, S. C., Fey, E. G., Fletcher, J. A., Wan, T. S., Chew, E. C., et al. Characterisation of human ovarian surface epithelial cells immortalised by human papilloma virus oncogenes (HPV-E6E7 ORFs). *Exp. Cell Res.* **218,** 499–507.

7. Kruk, P. A., Uitto, V. J., Firth, J. D., Dedhar, S., and Auersperg, N. (1994) Reciprocal interactions between human ovarian surface epithelial cells and adjacent extracellular matrix. *Exp. Cell Res.* **215,** 97–108.

8. Kruk, P. A. and Auersperg, N. (1992) Human ovarian surface epithelial cells are capable of physically restructuring extracellular matrix. *Amer. J. Obstet. Gynecol.* **167,** 1437–1443.

9. Berchuck, A., Rodriguez, G. C., Kamel, A., Dodge, R. K., Soper, J. T., Clarke-Pearson, D. L., and Bast, R. C. (1991) Epidermal growth factor receptor expression in normal ovarian epithelium and ovarian cancer I. Correlation of receptor expression with prognostic factors in patients with ovarian cancer. *Amer. J Obstet. Gynecol.* **164,** 669–674.

10. Wang, D. P., Konishi, I., Koshiyama, M., Nanbu, Y., Iwai, T., Nonogaki, H., et al. (1992) Immunohistochemical localisation of c-erb-B2 protein and epidermal growth factor receptor in normal surface epithelium, surface inclusion cysts, and common epithelial tumors of the ovary. *Virchows Archiv. A* **421,** 393–400.

11. Berchuck, A., Rodriguez, G., Olt, G., Whitaker, R., Boente, M. P., Arrick, B. A., et al. (1992) Regulation of growth of normal ovarian epithelial cells and ovarian cancer cell lines by transforming growth factor beta. *Amer. J. Obstet. Gynecol.* **166,** 676–684.

12. Havrilesky, L. J., Hurteau, J. A., Whitaker, R. S., Elbendary, A., Wu, S., Rodriguez, G. C., et al. (1995) Regulation of apoptosis in normal and malignant ovarian epithelial cells by transforming growth factor beta. *Cancer Res.* **55,** 944–948.

13. Jindal, S. K., Snoey, D. M., Lobb, D. K., and Dorrington, J. H. (1994) Transforming growth factor alpha localisation and role in surface epithelium of normal human ovaries and in ovarian carcinoma cells. *Gynecol. Oncol.* **53,** 17–23.

14. Boente, M. P., Berchuck, A., Rodriguez, G. C., Davidoff, A., Whitaker, R., Xu, F. J., et al. (1992) The effect of interferon gamma on epidermal growth factor receptor expression in normal and malignant ovarian epithelial cells. *Amer. J. Obstet. Gynecol.* **167,** 1877–1882.

15. Lidor, Y. J., Xu, F. J., Martinez-Maza, O., Olt, G. J., Marks, J. R., Berchuck, A., et al. (1993) Constitutive production of macrophage colony-stimulating factor and interleukin-6 by human ovarian surface epithelial cells. *Exp. Cell Res.* **207,** 332–339.

16. Pejovic, T. (1995) Genetic changes in ovarian cancer. *Ann. Med.* **27,** 73–78.

17. Muto, M. G., Welch, W. R., Mok, S. C., Bandera, C. A., Fishbaugh, P. M., Tsao, S. W., et al. (1995). Evidence for a multifocal origin of papillary serous carcinoma of the peritoneum. *Cancer Res.* **55,** 490–492.

18. Buller, R. E. Skilling, J. S., Sood, A. K., Plaxe, S., Baergen, R. N., and Lager, D. J. (1998) Field cancerization: why late "recurrent" ovarian cancer is not recurrent. *Amer. J. Obstet. Gynecol.* **178,** 641–649.

19. Provencher, D. M., Lounis, H., Fink, D., Drouin, P., and Mes-Masson, A. M. (1997) Discordance in p53 mutations when comparing ascites and solid tumors from patients with serous ovarian cancer. *Tumor Biol.* **18,** 167–174.

20. Brescia, R. J., Barakat, R. A., Beller, U., Frederickson, G., Suhrland, M. J., et al. (1990) The prognostic significance of nuclear DNA content in malignant epithelial tumors of the ovary. *Cancer* **65,** 141–147.

21. Friedlander, M. L., Hedley, D. H., Taylor, I., Russell, P., and Tattersall, M. H. N. (1984) Influence of cellular DNA content on survival in advanced ovarian cancer. *Cancer Res.* **44,** 397–400.

22. Kaern, J., Trope, C. G., Abeler, V., and Petterson, E. O. (1995) Cellular DNA content: the most important prognostic factor in patients with borderline tumors of the ovary. Can it prevent overtreatment? in *Ovarian Cancer 3* (Sharp, F., Mason, P., Blackett, T., and Berek, J., eds.), Chapman and Hall, London, U.K., pp. 181–188.

23. Foulkes, W. D. and Trowsdale, J. (1995) Isolating tumor suppressor genes relevant to ovarian carcinoma—the role of loss of heterozygosity, in *Ovarian Cancer 3* (Sharp, F., Mason, P., Blackett, T., and Berek, J., eds.), Chapman and Hall, London, U.K., pp. 23–38.

24. Sato, T., Saito, H., Morita, R., Koi, S., Lee, J. H., and Nakamura, Y. (1991) Allelotype of human ovarian cancer. *Cancer Res.* **51,** 5118–5122.

25. Yang-Feng, T. L., Han, H., Chen, K-C., Li, S., Claus, E., Carcangui, M. L., et al. (1993) Allelic loss in ovarian cancer. *Int. J. Cancer* **54,** 546–551.

26. Steel, C. M., Cohen, B. B., Lessels, A., Williams, A. R. W., and Gabra, H. (1997). Other gene aberrations in ovarian cancer, in *Ovarian Cancer 4*, (Sharp, F., Mason, P., Blackett, T., and Berek, J., eds.), Chapman and Hall, London, U.K.

27. Obata, K., Morland, S. J. Watson, R. H., Hitchcock, A., Chenevix-Trench, G., Thomas, E. J., et al. (1998) Frequent PTEN/MMAC mutations in endometrioid but not serous or mucinous epithelial ovarian tumors. *Cancer Res.* **58,** 2095–2097.

28. Skilling, J. S., Sood, A., Niemann, T., Lager, D. J., and Buller, R. E. (1996) An abundance of p53 null mutations in ovarian carcinoma. *Oncogene* **13,** 117–123.

29. Kounelis, S., Jones, M. W., Papadaki, H., Bakker, A., Swalsky, P., and Finkelstein, S. D. (1998) Carcinosarcomas (malignant mixed mullerian tumors) of the female genital tract: comparative molecular analysis of epithelial and mesenchymal components. *Human Pathol.* **29,** 82–87.

30. Abeln, E. C., Smit, V. T., Wessels, J. W., de Leeuw, W. J., Cornelisse, C. J., and Fleuren, G. J. (1997) Molecular genetic evidence for the conversion hypothesis of the origin of malignant mixed müllerian tumors. *J. Pathol.* **183,** 424–431.

31. Skomedal, H., Kristensen, G. B., Abeler, V. M., Borresen-Dale, A. L., Trope, C., and Holm, R. (1997) TP53 protein accumulation and gene mutation in relation to overexpression of MDM2 protein in ovarian borderline tumors and stage I carcinomas. *J. Pathol.* **181,** 158–165.

32. Zheng, J., Benedict, W. F., Xu, S. X., Kim, T. M., Velicescu, M., Wan, M., et al. (1995) Genetic disparity between morphologically benign cysts contiguous to ovarian carcinomas and solitary cystadenomas. *J. Nat. Cancer Inst.* **87,** 1146–1153.

33. Lukas, J., Groshen, S., Saffari, B., Niu, N., Reles, A., Wen, W. H., et al. (1997) WAF1/Cip1 gene polymorphism and expression in carcinomas of the breast, ovary, and endometrium. *Amer. J. Pathol.* **150,** 167–175.

34. Werness, B. A., Jobe, J. S., DiCioccio, R. A., and Piver, M. S. (1997) Expression of the p53 induced tumor suppressor p21waf1/cip1 in ovarian carcinomas: correlation with p53 and Ki-67 immunohistochemistry. *Int. J. Gynecol. Pathol.* **16,** 149–155.

35. Milner, B. J., Hosking, L., Sun, S., Haites, N. E., and Foulkes, W. D. (1996) Polymorphisms in p21CIP1/WAF1 are not correlated with Tp53 status in sporadic ovarian tumors. *Eur. J. Cancer* **32A,** 2360–2363.

36. Shih, Y. C., Kerr, J., Hurst, T. G., Khoo, S. K., Ward, B. G., and Chevenix-Trench, G. (1998) No evidence for microsatellite instability from allelotype analysis of benign and low malignant potential ovarian neoplasms. *Gynecol. Oncol.* **69,** 210–213.

37. Holt, J. T. (1997) Breast cancer genes: therapeutic strategies. *Ann. New York Acad. Sci.* **833,** 34–41.

38. Rubin, S. C., Benjamin, I., Behbakht, K., Takahashi, H., Morgan, M. A., LiVolsi, V. A., et al. (1996) Clinical and pathological features of ovarian cancer in women with germ-line mutations of BRCA1. *New England J. Med.* **335,** 1413–1416.

39. Tangir, J., Muto, M. G., Berkowitz, R. S., Welch, W. R., Bell, D. A., and Mok, S. C. (1996) A 400 kb novel deletion unit centromeric to the BRCA1 gene in sporadic epithelial ovarian cancer. *Oncogene* **12,** 735–740.

40. Scully, R. E., Bell, D. A., and Abu-Jawdeh, G. M. (1995) Update on early ovarian cancer and cancer developing in benign ovarian tumors, in *Ovarian Cancer 3* (Sharp, F., Mason, P., Blackett, T., and Berek, J., eds.), Chapman & Hall Medical, London, U.K., pp. 139–144.

41. Bell, D. A. and Scully, R. E. (1994) Early de novo ovarian carcinoma: a study of 14 cases. *Cancer* **73,** 1859–1864.

42. Park, T. W., Felix, J. C., and Wright, T. C. (1995) X chromosome inactivation and microsatellite instability in early and advanced bilateral ovarian carcinomas. *Cancer Res.* **55,** 4793–4796.

43. Hutson, R., Ramsdale, J., and Wells, M. (1995) P53 protein expression in putative precursor lesions of epithelial ovarian cancer. *Histopathol.* **27,** 367–371.

44. La Grenade, A. and Silverberg, S. G. (1988) Ovarian tumors associated with atypical endometriosis. *Human Pathol.* **19,** 1080–1084.

45. Sainz de la Cuesta, R., Eichhorn, J. H., Rice, L. W., Fuller, A. F., Nikrui, N., and Goff, B. A. (1996) Histologic transformation of benign endometriosis to early epithelial ovarian cancer. *Gynecol. Oncol.* **60,** 238–244.

46. Mostoufizadeh, M. and Scully, R. E. (1980) Malignant tumors arising in endometriosis. *Clin. Obstet. Gynecol.* **23,** 951–963.

47. Gucer, F., Pieber, D., and Arikan, M. G. (1998) Malignancy arising in extraovarian endometriosis during estrogen stimulation. *Eur. J. Gynecol. Oncol.* **19,** 39–41.

48. Jiang, X., Morland, S. J., Hitchcock, A., Thomas, E. J., and Campbell, I. G. (1998) Allelotyping of endometriosis with adjacent ovarian carcinoma reveals evidence of a common lineage. *Cancer Res.* **58,** 1707–1712.

# 6

# Tumor Markers in Screening for Ovarian Cancer

## Steven J. Skates, Ian J. Jacobs, and Robert C. Knapp

## 1. Introduction

Tumor markers are used for multiple purposes in clinical care, including screening asymptomatic subjects, differential diagnosis of symptomatic patients, treatment planning, prognosis during and immediately following treatment, and monitoring for recurrence. Generally, tumor markers have found most clinical utility in monitoring for recurrence of disease *(1)*. Bast and coinvestigators discovered CA125 in 1979 using monoclonal antibody techniques *(2)*, and subsequently demonstrated its utility in monitoring treatment and recurrence of ovarian cancer *(3)*. CA125 is the most widely used ovarian tumor marker, and is currently approved in the United States for monitoring of disease to determine if second-look surgery is required. Tumor markers have not gained wide acceptance for early detection of disease with the one exception of PSA for prostate cancer in the U.S. The lack of acceptance is mainly because of the difficult hurdles a screening strategy must overcome, and few tumor markers have shown sufficient promise in overcoming these hurdles to put them to the test in a randomized controlled trial. Because of the low incidence of most cancers, sample sizes for prospective randomized screening trials are huge, so that sufficient numbers of disease specific events occur by the end of the trial. The significant costs entailed in clinical trials of this size imply that only very promising approaches to screening warrant prospective investigation. For ovarian cancer, three large trials are underway, two trials are planning to randomize 120,000 women followed for 7–8 yr *(4,5)*, and an NCI trial will randomize 74,000 women followed for 16 yr *(6)*.

Screening for ovarian cancer is an appealing approach to reducing mortality from this disease. Ovarian cancer is frequently (75%) detected at late stage when it is often incurable *(7)*. However, when it is detected in early stage, survival rates are high, exceeding 90% five-year survival for well differentiated stage I disease *(8)*. Screening strategies may detect a substantial proportion of ovarian cancers in early stage that would have been clinically detected in late-stage disease. In this case, it is reasonable, but not certain, to expect a significant reduction in disease specific mortality.

Approaches to ovarian cancer screening in the general population can be classified on the basis of the first line test. One approach uses tumor markers *(9,10)*, another approach uses ultrasound, (typically transvaginal ultrasound) *(4,11,12)*, and the third approach uses both modalities *(13)* as the first line test applied to all subjects in the

From: *Methods in Molecular Medicine, Vol. 39: Ovarian Cancer: Methods and Protocols*
Edited by: J. M. S. Bartlett © Humana Press, Inc., Totowa, NJ

target population. Secondary tests are then applied to the much smaller subset of subjects with positive or suspicious results on the first-line test. In the trials using tumor markers as the first-line test, the secondary test is usually ultrasound. Following ultrasound as a first-line test, are color Doppler ultrasound and/or tumor markers. Tumor markers are advocated as a first-line test on the basis of comparatively lower cost, objectivity, easier access for subjects to phlebotomy, and high specificity. Ultrasound is advocated as a first-line test because of high sensitivity for early-stage disease. Costs for ultrasound in a large screening program could be substantially reduced because of volume and efficiencies compared to current charges *(14)*. Objectivity and ease of access remain issues for ultrasound. Bimanual pelvic exam has been shown to be of no value in the early detection of ovarian cancer *(15)*. This chapter examines the first approach to ovarian cancer screening. In particular, we examine the problem of designing a screening strategy based on serial tumor marker levels. This approach has not received much attention in the literature. Using serial tumor marker levels may overcome some of the significant hurdles facing tumor markers in the context of screening. Because this is an introductory chapter, the rationale and the reasons for the power of this approach are discussed in depth. We hope this may encourage investigation of screening for other cancers with known markers that were thought not to have sufficient sensitivity or specificity when using the strategy of a fixed reference level for all subjects. The approach could also be applied to markers yet to be discovered. However, only an overview of the methods and principles underlying this approach can be given, as exact details on the statistical implementation are beyond the scope and space constraints of this chapter.

Whereas many tumor markers IAP, LDH, SA, TGF-$\alpha$, and M-CSF *(16)*, PLAP, CA 15-3 and TAG 72 *(17)*, LASA, DM-70K, UGP, and HER-2 *(18)*, and OVX1 and OVX2 *(19)* have been studied in relation to ovarian cancer, only one marker, CA125, has consistently withstood the test of time. CA125 is the only marker that has been used in three of four large-scale prospective marker based screening studies *(6,9,10)*.

The main concern in using CA125 as a first-line test for ovarian cancer is its apparent lack of sensitivity for early-stage disease *(20)*. Only 50% of stage I ovarian cancer patients have elevated CA125 preoperative serum levels. The traditional cutoff level for a positive CA125 test is 30 or 35 U/mL. It is important to note that this level was established for patients with clinically established disease *(3)*, and was not advocated for as the appropriate cutoff level for screening asymptomatic populations. Furthermore, screening aims to detect ovarian cancers in early stage that would have been detected in late-stage disease. It is not aimed at detecting ovarian cancers that are currently clinically detected in early stages. Therefore, the relevance of CA125 sensitivity in clinically detected ovarian cancer is questionable with regard to early detection. Most late-stage ovarian cancers (> 90%) have serum CA125 levels elevated above 35 U/mL, and in these cases the CA125 level during early-stage asymptomatic disease is simply not known. Zurawski *(21)* discovered elevated CA125 levels up to 60 mo prior to clinical detection of ovarian cancer through analysis of banked serum samples, although the stage of the disease at the time of the blood draw is again unknown. Nevertheless, the low sensitivity for clinically detected early-stage disease is still cause for concern. A further concern is that CA125 is elevated by ovulation so that screening with CA125 as a first-line test would only be applicable to postmenopausal women.

However, the great majority of ovarian cancer cases occur in postmenopausal women, the most well-defined risk group for ovarian cancer. This group has been the target population for tumor marker-based screening tests.

A number of methods have been suggested for circumventing the apparent low sensitivity of CA125 to early-stage disease. The first method is to lower the cutoff level for a positive test, for example, 20 U/mL *(22)*, followed by a specific test such as color Doppler flow. Another method is to use multiple markers. The two markers that appear to complement CA125 are OVX1 *(23)* in recurrence of ovarian cancer, and MCS-F *(24)* in preoperative levels of stage I ovarian cancers. MCS-F improved performance with CA125 slightly better than OVX1 with CA125. Both screening with CA125 and OVX1 *(25)*, and screening with CA125 and either MCS-F or OVX1 have been advocated *(24)*, but neither approach has been tested prospectively.

The third method for improving CA125 sensitivity uses serial levels of CA125 to simultaneously improve the specificity and sensitivity of the screening strategy *(26,27)*. This chapter explains the potential for serial CA125 to improve the performance of an ovarian cancer screening strategy. Statistical analyses of serial CA125 levels from two large screening trials have demonstrated that many women with initially elevated CA125 levels have relatively stable CA125 levels over time, and at the end of the study do not have a diagnosis of ovarian cancer. In contrast, women subsequently diagnosed with ovarian cancer generally have steeply rising CA125 levels, presumably reflecting the rapidly increasing volume of the tumor.

**Figure 1** displays serial CA125 levels in two cases with ovarian cancer *(1,3)*, and in two women without ovarian cancer *(2,4)* at the end of the London study (see below). Women without ovarian cancer have a relatively stable CA125 level over a long period of time, whereas women subsequently diagnosed with ovarian cancer have rapidly increasing CA125 levels.

If basic cell kinetics apply to the unregulated growth of ovarian cancer, then an exponential increase in the volume is to be expected because of a constant tumor volume doubling time. Serial CA125 levels likely reflect the volume of the tumor and will correspondingly increase exponentially over time. A remarkable case is illustrated by the first phase of the Stockholm trial, where five successive CA125 levels increased exponentially before clinical diagnosis occurred *(26)*. By incorporating the extra information in the serial behavior of CA125 into the screening strategy, the sensitivity can be substantially improved, at the same time maintaining or even increasing the already high level of specificity. Another simplified interpretation of this idea, which nevertheless captures its essence, is that each woman serves as her own control. A baseline CA125 level is established for each woman, and only when statistically significant elevations above the individualized baseline occur does the screening strategy indicate a positive result. The method section gives details on the systematic and efficient approach to utilizing the serial information in a first-line CA125-based screening program for ovarian cancer.

It should be emphasized that no researcher currently advocates screening the general public for ovarian cancer. Many researchers have positive outlooks on the prospect for a successful approach to early detection of ovarian cancer *(5,27–30)*, others see substantial difficulties *(16,31–33)*, whereas other authors *(34–37)* have a neutral assessment. However, researchers are unanimous that screening for ovarian cancer is

Fig. 1. CA125 values over time for 2 women with subsequent diagnosis of ovarian cancer (1,3) and two women without a diagnosis (2,4) as of December 1997. The CA125 scale is logarithmic so that exponential rises appear as straight lines. The women with ovarian cancer have exponential rises (1) or have relatively level CA125 profiles followed by an exponential rise (3). In contrast, women without ovarian cancer (2,4) have relatively stable CA125 profiles, even over periods of time exceeding five years.

unproven and advocacy of screening the general public awaits the results of further research, such as refinement of screening tests and outcomes of randomized trials. In fact, it is considered unethical *(38)* to advocate screening for a disease until proof exists that it results in substantial benefits and cost is reasonable. If an unproven strategy, even though promising, is implemented as a public health measure, it may unethically diminish available resources for programs with proven health benefit.

## 2. Materials

Two large-scale CA125 first-line screening trials provide the data for the methods discussed below. Between 1986–1989, 5550 women over the age of 40 were screened with CA125 in Sweden *(9)*. If the CA125 exceeded 35 U/mL (30 U/mL in the second half) the woman was referred for bimanual pelvic exam, ultrasound, and three monthly CA125 tests for one year. An age-matched control subject, with CA125 under the cut-off was also referred and the examining physicians were not told which woman had an elevated CA125. Women were screened at least twice approximately one year apart. Follow-up screenings occurred in 1990 through the Swedish tumor registry and Stockholm hospital registries for cancer outcomes. Further details on the data have been described elsewhere *(27)*.

The second screening trial was centered at the Royal London Hospital, and enrolled 22,000 postmenopausal U.K. women over the age of 45 in a prevalence screen using CA125 between 1986–1990 *(10)*. If elevated above 30 U/mL, women were referred for ultrasound and three monthly CA125 tests. A further three annual CA125 screens were performed on approximately half the women randomized to a screening arm, with the trial ending in mid-1995 and providing more than 50,000 CA125 values. National cancer registries were utilized for follow-up of cancers at the end of 1997.

The data from both trials for each woman consisted of the date of birth, the dates of CA125 measurements, ovarian cancer status (yes/no), and date of ovarian cancer detection.

## 3. Methods

The development of the multi-modal strategy that uses serial CA125 values as a first-line screening test has two steps.

1. Derivation of a method that calculates the probability of having ovarian cancer given one or more CA125 levels, the dates on which the samples were drawn, and the age of the woman.
2. Development of a triaging system that efficiently identifies women with a high enough risk (i.e., probability) of having ovarian cancer to warrant referral to ultrasound.

### 3.1. The Risk of Ovarian Cancer Calculation (ROCC)

The difficulty with using any tumor marker for screening is the variability in the CA125 measurements because of natural biological variation in the CA125 level over time, and assay measurement error. For serial CA125 levels to be useful in screening, it is necessary to distinguish changes over time in CA125 levels because of an increase in ovarian cancer volume from CA125 variability. Statistical analyses quantify the level of noise, which is then used to weigh the evidence between changes due to variation and to ovarian cancer.

**Figure 2** displays hypothetical preclinical CA125 levels over time in two women in the presence of CA125 variability. For the first woman, ovarian cancer inception occurs at year one, with clinical detection after year three. The second woman has relatively stable CA125 levels that are approximately at the same level as the first woman's CA125 levels before tumor inception. The second woman does not have ovarian cancer, yet the CA125 values are the same between the two women at the two time points at which measurements are taken (indicated by the dots). This example illustrates the difficulty with interpreting rising levels of CA125, and the necessity of developing a systematic method for weighing the evidence between the presence and absence of ovarian cancer.

Another hurdle in screening is the low incidence of ovarian cancer, with one case in 2000 postmenopausal women per year. Therefore, it is absolutely imperative that the screening strategy be as efficient as possible. Otherwise, too many false positives will be identified for each true positive case, resulting in the screening program becoming too costly and not being clinically acceptable. Thus, more screening resources, such as extra CA125 tests, and referral to ultrasound, should be devoted to groups of women at higher risk. It is simply inefficient to devote more resources to a group of women with fewer true cases (lower risk) than to another same-sized group of women that has a larger number of true cases (higher risk). More resources should be devoted to detecting the larger number of cases. Any screening strategy that does not base its decisions on the risk of having ovarian cancer is therefore inefficient. That is, an *ad hoc* rule such

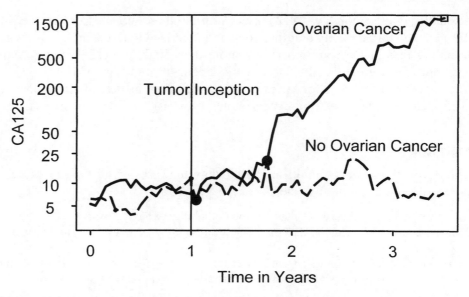

Fig. 2. Hypothetical CA125 profiles of two women, one with ovarian cancer with rising CA125 levels between years 1 and 3, and the other with no ovarian cancer, if CA125 could be measured continuously such as every day. The CA125 fluctuations can obscure whether rises—indicated by two filled circles common to both profiles—are due to presence of ovarian cancer or background fluctuations. Systematic statistical modelling of background fluctuations and expected CA125 profiles in known cases and controls enable accurate weighing of CA125 evidence for new subjects.

as referring women to ultrasound if the CA125 doubles within six months and the initial measurement exceeded 20 U/mL, is inefficient in comparison to a rule based on the risk of having ovarian cancer.

To calculate the risk given the CA125 levels, the dates of the serum samples, and the age of the woman, requires two statistical models. The first model describes the stochastic behavior of CA125 over time in women with ovarian cancer, and the second describes it in women without ovarian cancer. The estimates of the parameters in these models from analyses of the Stockholm and London trials data provide the basis for calculating the risk for a new woman with single of multiple CA125 levels. Examples of the parameters are the baseline CA125 level for a given woman, the age at tumor inception for a woman with ovarian cancer, the rate or CA125 increase after tumor inception, and the variation about the expected CA125 value. The distribution of these parameters over the women with ovarian cancer, for example, describes the stochastic behavior of CA125 over time in this subgroup.

The risk of having ovarian cancer for a new woman is calculated by evaluating the relative closeness of her CA125 data (over time if multiple values are available) to the following:

1.  the CA125 behavior in cases prior to clinical detection in the two trials;
2.  the CA125 behavior over time in women without ovarian cancer (noncases).

If the CA125 values over time in the new woman behave more like the CA125 values in the women with ovarian cancer (cases), then the new woman has a high risk of having undetected ovarian cancer. If on the other hand, the CA125 values behave more like the CA125 levels in the women without ovarian cancer, then the new woman has a low risk. The next two subsections describe the expected behavior in detail. To calculate the exact risk, Bayes' Theorem is used to properly weigh the evidence between the new woman having ovarian cancer and not having ovarian cancer based on her CA125 levels. This procedure accounts for the variability of the CA125 measurements in the new woman, the uncertainty in the parameter estimates of the women with known status (ovarian cancer: yes/no) in the two studies, and the variability of the parameters between the women. The prior odds of having ovarian cancer, derived from cancer registries using the age of the woman, is then multiplied by the correct weight of evidence to determine the final odds of having ovarian cancer. The final risk is calculated from the odds by the simple formula: risk = odds/(odds+1). The weight of evidence is often referred to as the Bayes factor.

### 3.2. The Expected Behavior of CA125 in Women Without Ovarian Cancer (Noncases)

From graphical analyses of the CA125 levels in women without ovarian cancer at the end of the studies (noncases), it is clear that in most noncases CA125 remains relatively level over time. For each noncase, a linear regression with a zero slope, and a standard deviation about the regression line, adequately represents the statistical behavior of CA125 over time. The parameters of the model are the intercept (average CA125 value or level of the regression line) and the standard deviation. Across the population of noncases these parameters have a distribution, and this distribution is estimated simultaneously with the individual linear regressions. (Such a model is referred to as a hierarchical linear model). Because the average CA125 value varies by orders of magnitude across women (from less than five to more than 500 U/mL), it is natural to model the distribution of intercepts across the population on the logarithmic scale. Because of measurement error and biological variation, the actual log(CA125) measurements will vary about the expected values. The variation about the expected values (regression line) is described by the standard deviation.

### 3.3. The Expected Behavior of CA125 in Women with Ovarian Cancer (Cases)

Before an ovarian tumor begins in a (subsequently detected) case, the behavior of CA125 over time is expected to be like the behavior in the noncases; that is, relatively stable over time. However, when the tumor begins and proceeds to double in volume over time, most tumors cause the CA125 levels to rise proportionately. On the original CA125 scale, the proportionate rise results in exponentially increasing levels. Corresponding to the exponential rise on the CA125 scale, the expected log(CA125) values rise linearly. Thus, a change point occurs at the time of tumor inception, with a flat expected value before this point in time, and a linear increasing expected value afterwards. The parameters summarizing this model for the expected log(CA125) values are the initial stable level, the time of tumor inception, the slope of the line after tumor inception, and the standard deviation about the expected line. This type of model is referred to as a change-point model. As before, these parameters have a distribution across the population of cases, which is simultaneously estimated with the parameters for each individual change-point model (referred to as a hierarchical change-point model).

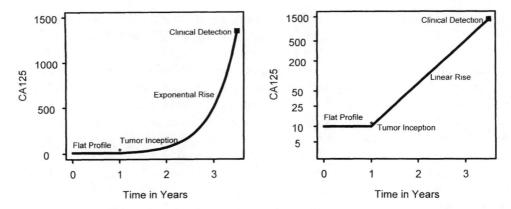

Fig. 3. Expected CA125 profiles in a hypothetical case prior to clinical detection on the original CA125 scale (left) and on the logarithmic scale (right), showing a flat profile followed by a linear rise, similar to profile (4) in **Fig. 1**.

**Figure 3** displays the expected CA125 levels (in the absence of CA125 variability) on the original CA125 scale, and on a logarithmic scale. Tumor inception occurs at year one, after which CA125 values rise exponentially until the tumor is clinically detected in after year three. On the logarithmic scale, the change-point is more clearly delineated, and the CA125 values rise linearly. Statistical analyses estimate the level before tumor inception, the time of tumor inception, and the slope after tumor inception. The analyses also quantify the uncertainty in these estimates. The uncertainty derives from two sources, the first is that CA125 is measured at only a few points in time, and the second is the CA125 variability, both of which obscure the true value of each parameter. The parameters and their uncertainty are used in weighing the evidence (serial CA125 values) from a new woman to determine her risk of having ovarian cancer.

### 3.4. Examples of the ROCC

It is important to note that the risk of ovarian cancer calculation cannot simply be replaced by a general cutoff level for all subjects (standard rule), nor by the slope of the CA125 levels (often called the velocity in PSA literature), nor by the number of standard deviations the last CA125 value is above the average of the previous CA125 values, nor by *ad hoc* CA125 doubling rules such as doubling within 6 months following a level above 15 U/mL. Examples are given of the ROCC that show intuitively the correct behavior in contrast to some of these simpler rules.

**Figure 4** shows serial CA125 levels that display a change-point, indicating possible presence of ovarian cancer. The last level is 22 U/mL, well under the standard level of 35 U/mL, which would therefore have missed the case at this point in time. The risk of ovarian cancer calculation (ROCC) results in a sufficiently high risk for referral to ultrasound, at which point the occult cancer may be discovered well before being discovered by the standard 35 U/mL rule.

**Figure 5** shows two women with rising CA125 values, which have the same slopes, but the second woman has a much higher CA125 value for the last measurement. While the slope does not differentiate between these two women, it is intuitively obvious that

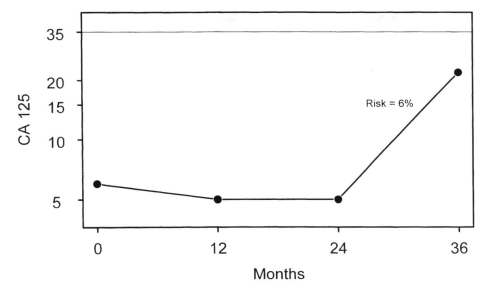

Fig. 4. The risk of having ovarian cancer given the above sequence of CA125 values is 6% or approximately 1 in 16, which would trigger referal to ultrasound and possible detection of ovarian cancer well before detection by the standard 35 U/mL rule.

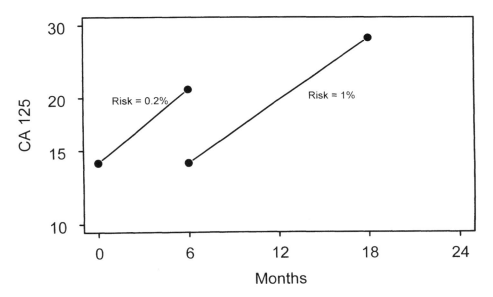

Fig. 5. Two CA125 profiles with the same slope (or CA125 velocity) yet five fold difference in the risk of having ovarian cancer. Intuitively, the second profile has a higher risk due to the larger CA125 result at the second time point which the slope parameter alone does not capture, but the systematic calculation of risk does capture.

the second woman is at much higher risk of having ovarian cancer due to a larger CA125 value. The ROCC indicates a much higher risk for the second woman.

**Figure 6** shows two women, where the first woman has an initial level greater than 15 U/mL, and the final level doubles within six months. For the second women, the

Fig. 6. Ad hoc rules, such as doubling within six months following a CA125 level above 15 U/mL, are not as efficient as systematically calculating the risk. Under the ad-hoc rule the first profile would be referred to ultrasound and not the second. In contrast, systematically calculating the risk results in the second profile having greater risk, and both women would be referred to ultrasound.

initial level is less than 15 U/mL, and the final CA125 level is greater than the final CA125 level for the first woman. The *ad hoc* doubling rule would send the first woman onto ultrasound, and not the second woman, because for the second woman, the initial level was less than 15 U/mL. The ROCC correctly indicates that the second woman is at higher risk than the first, and refers both to ultrasound.

### 3.5. Triaging by Risk of Ovarian Cancer

Having derived a method to convert any number of CA125 levels to a risk, an efficient screening strategy is now developed centered on the ROCC. Screening for ovarian cancer with the tumor marker CA125 is envisaged to start for postmenopausal women (operationally defined as amenorrhea for at least one year), and to measure CA125 annually. The choice of the regular measurement at one year intervals is based on practical and biological grounds. It is unlikely that more frequent testing, such as every 6 months for all women in the target population, would be generally acceptable, nor covered by insurance schemes (private or public). Biologically, ovarian cancer is known to be a rapidly growing tumor, and leaving two-year or greater gaps between CA125 measurements would result in many cases of ovarian cancer not being measured in early-stage disease *(39)*. Therefore, an annual CA125 measurement is proposed for the general postmenopausal population, and refinement of this strategy with the ROCC is discussed next.

All the information about ovarian cancer contained in the CA125 values, their timing, and the age of the woman, are summarized in one number, the risk of ovarian cancer. On the basis of the risk, the screening strategy triaging is designed as follows.

1. A CA125 measurement is made, and the risk calculated based on the current CA125 value, and any previous CA125 values, and the woman's age.
2. For women with low risk (less than baseline level of 1 in 2000), the women return in one year for their next CA125 measurement (**step 1**).
3. For women with intermediate risk (between 1 in 2000 and 1 in 100), the women returns in 6 wk to 6 mo time for another CA125 measurement (**step 1**). The time interval is close to 6 wk for women with risk just below 1 in 100, and in 6 mo for women with risk just above 1 in 2000, and smoothly interpolated for risks in between.
4. For women with high risk (greater than 1 in 100), the woman is referred to ultrasound. If the ultrasound is abnormal, the woman is referred to surgery. For normal ultrasound, the woman returns in 6 wk for another CA125 (**step 1**).

Using this system only 1–2% of the population of screened women are referred to ultrasound, conserving the higher end resources for women at highest risk. Extra CA125 tests are made available to women at intermediate risk, proportionately more rapidly for women with higher levels of intermediate risk. All resource decisions are made on the basis of risk, so that the screening strategy is as efficient as possible given constraints on the number of CA125 tests and ultrasound tests per woman per year.

Step 1 utilizes all the information in serial CA125 levels, and so this screening strategy can be simultaneously more sensitive and more specific than a strategy based on a single cutoff applied uniformly across the screened population. All other steps return to step 1 in a feedback loop, enabling the strategy to identify high-risk women very rapidly. The serial CA125 levels will rule out (indicate low risk) for women with initially high CA125 levels that remain stable, increasing the specificity. For women with initially very low levels of CA125, and whose levels begin to exponentially increase, but not enough to exceed the single cutoff level, the ROCC will identify them as intermediate or high risk long before the standard rule, thereby increasing the sensitivity simultaneously with the specificity. With this approach, a study of serial CA125 levels collected from the London study showed the sensitivity for preclinical detection has increased from 70 to 86% at the same time maintaining the required high level of specificity for a clinically acceptable method. However, only a prospective implementation of the ROCC strategy as a component of a multimodel screening trial will ultimately confirm or deny the impact on ovarian cancer mortality.

### 3.6. Future Directions

The proposed tumor marker screening strategy may still miss cancers that do not shed significant amount of OC125, the antibody to CA125. Information about the behavior over time of a complementary marker, such as OVX1 or MCS-F, would provide the basis for developing a ROCC from serial multiple markers that would be more broadly sensitive at the same time retaining all the specificity of the ROCC based on serial CA125 values. Statistical methods that can accommodate two or more markers, describing their joint behavior over time in both cases and noncases, and translating the behavior into a risk for a new woman with new CA125 levels and other marker levels, need to be developed. Then the next step is to implement and obtain support for a large clinical randomized trial. No treatment strategy has had a significant impact on the long-term mortality rate of ovarian cancer cases in the past three decades (*35*), and given the high specificity and sensitivity achievable with serial CA125 testing, it is time to focus more attention and resources on early detection.

## Acknowledgments

This work was supported by grants from the Women's Cancer Program at Dana Farber/Partners CancerCare, and from the National Cancer Institute (R29-CA57693).

## References

1. Bates, S. E. (1991) Clinical applications of serum tumor markers. *Ann Intern Med.* **115,** 623–638.
2. Bast, R.·C., Jr., Feeney, M., Lazarus, H., et al. (1981) Reactivity of a monoclonal antibody with human ovarian carcinoma. *J Clin Invest.* **68,** 1331–1337.
3. Bast, R. C. Jr., Klug, T. L., St John, E., et al. (1983) A radioimmunoassay using a monoclonal antibody to monitor the course of epithelial ovarian cancer. *New England J. Med.* **309,** 883–887.
4. Parkes, C. A., Smith, D., Wald, N. J., et al. (1994) Feasibility study of a randomised trial of ovarian cancer screening among the general population. *J. Med. Screen.* **1,** 209–214.
5. Rosenthal, A. and Jacobs, I. (1998) Ovarian cancer screening. *Semin. Oncol.* **25,** 315–325.
6. Kramer, B. S., Gohagan, J., Prorok, P. C., et al. (1993) A National Cancer Institute sponsored screening trial for prostatic, lung, colorectal, and ovarian cancers. *Cancer* **71,** 589–593.
7. Wingo, P. A., Ries, L. A., Rosenberg, H. M., et al. (1998) Cancer incidence and mortality, 1973–1995: a report card for the U.S. *Cancer* **82,** 1197–1207.
8. Young, R. C., Walton, L. A., Ellenberg, S. S., et al. (1990) Adjuvant therapy in stage I and stage II epithelial ovarian cancer. Results of two prospective randomized trials [see comments]. *New England J. Med.* **322,** 1021–1027.
9. Einhorn, N., Sjovall, K., Knapp, R. C., et al. (1992) Prospective evaluation of serum CA 125 levels for early detection of ovarian cancer. *Obstet. Gynecol.* **80,** 14–18.
10. Jacobs, I., Davies, A. P., Bridges, J., et al. (1993) Prevalence screening for ovarian cancer in post-menopausal women by CA 125 measurement and ultrasonography [see comments]. *Brit. Med. J.* **306,** 1030–1034.
11. Van Nagell, J. R. Jr., DePriest, P. D., Puls, L. E., et al. (1991) Ovarian cancer screening in asymptomatic postmenopausal women by transvaginal sonography. *Cancer* **68,** 458–462.
12. Kurjak, A., Shalan, H., Kupesic, S., et al. (1994) An attempt to screen asymptomatic women for ovarian and endometrial cancer with transvaginal color and pulsed Doppler sonography. *J. Ultrasound Med.* **13,** 295–301.
13. Prorok, P. (1994) The National Cancer Institute Multi-Screening Trial. *Canadian J. Oncol.* **4,** 98,99; discussion 100,101.
14. Pavlik, E. J., van Nagell, J. R. Jr., DePriest, P. D., et al. (1995) Participation in transvaginal ovarian cancer screening: compliance, correlation factors, and costs. *Gynecol. Oncol.* **57,** 395–400.
15. Grover, S. R. and Quinn, M. A. (1995) Is there any value in bimanual pelvic examination as a screening test [see comments]. *Med. J. Aust.* **162,** 408–410.
16. Chow, S. N., Chien, C. H., and Chen, C. T. (1996) Molecular biology of human ovarian cancer. *Int. Surg.* **81,** 152–157.
17. Gargano, G., Correale, M., Abbate, I., et al. (1990) The role of tumor markers in ovarian cancer. *Clin. Exp. Obstet. Gynecol.* **17,** 23–29.
18. Cane, P., Azen, C., Lopez, E., et al. (1995) Tumor marker trends in asymptomatic women at risk for ovarian cancer: relevance for ovarian cancer screening. *Gynecol. Oncol.* **57,** 240–245.
19. Xu, F. J., Yu, Y. H., Li, B. Y., et al. (1991) Development of two new monoclonal antibodies reactive to a surface antigen present on human ovarian epithelial cancer cells. *Cancer Res.* **51,** 4012–4019.
20. Helzlsouer, K. J., Bush, T. L., Alberg, A. J., et al. (1993) Prospective study of serum CA125 levels as markers of ovarian cancer [see comments]. *JAMA* **269,** 1123–1126.
21. Zurawski, V. R. Jr., Orjaseter, H., Andersen, A., et al. (1988) Elevated serum CA125 levels prior to diagnosis of ovarian neoplasia: relevance for early detection of ovarian cancer. *Int. J. Cancer* **42,** 677–680.
22. Bourne, T. H., Campbell, S., Reynolds, K., et al. (1994) The potential role of serum CA125 in an ultrasound-based screening program for familial ovarian cancer. *Gynecol. Oncol.* **52,** 379–385.
23. Xu, F. J., Yu, Y. H., Daly, L., et al. (1993) OVX1 radioimmunoassay complements CA125 for predicting the presence of residual ovarian carcinoma at second-look surgical surveillance procedures. *J. Clin. Oncol.* **11,** 1506–1510.
24. Woolas, R. P., Xu, F. J., Jacobs, I. J., et al. (1993) Elevation of multiple serum markers in patients with stage I ovarian cancer. *J. Nat. Cancer Inst.* **85,** 1748–1751.
25. Berek, J. S. and Bast, R. C. Jr. (1995) Ovarian cancer screening. The use of serial complementary tumor markers to improve sensitivity and specificity for early detection. *Cancer* **76,** 2092–2096.
26. Zurawski, V. R. Jr., Sjovall, K., Schoenfeld, D. A., et al. (1990) Prospective evaluation of serum CA125 levels in a normal population, phase I: the specificities of single and serial determinations in testing for ovarian cancer. *Gynecol. Oncol.* **36,** 299–305.

27. Skates, S. J., Xu, F. J., Yu, Y. H., et al. (1995) Toward an optimal algorithm for ovarian cancer screening with longitudinal tumor markers. *Cancer* **76**, 2004–2010.

28. DePriest, P. D., van Nagell, J. R. Jr., Gallion, H. H., et al. (1993) Ovarian cancer screening in asymptomatic postmenopausal women. *Gynecol. Oncol.* **51**, 205–209.

29. Bourne, T. H., Hampson, J., Reynolds, K., et al. (1992) Screening for early ovarian cancer. *Brit. J. Hosp. Med.* **48**, 454–459.

30. Wald, N. and Parkes, C. (1993) Screening for ovarian cancer. Still controversial, but encouraging [letter; comment]. *Brit. Med. J.* **306**, 1684.

31. Schwartz, P. E. and Taylor, K. J. (1995) Is early detection of ovarian cancer possible? *Ann. Med.* **27**, 519–528.

32. Wong, J. G. and Feussner, J. R. (1993) Screening for ovarian cancer: not worthwhile for most patients. *N. C. Med. J.* **54**, 438–440.

33. Schapira, M. M., Matchar, D. B., and Young, M. J. (1993) The effectiveness of ovarian cancer screening. A decision analysis model [see comments]. *Ann. Intern. Med.* **118**, 838–843.

34. Ozols, R. F. (1994) Research directions in epithelial ovarian cancer. *Gynecol. Oncol.* **55**, S168–S173.

35. Karlan, B. Y. and Platt, L. D. (1994) The current status of ultrasound and color Doppler imaging in screening for ovarian cancer. *Gynecol. Oncol.* **55**, S28–S33.

36. Einhorn, N. (1992) Ovarian cancer. Early diagnosis and screening. *Hematol. Oncol. Clin. North Amer.* **6**, 843–850.

37. Runowicz, C. D., Goldberg, G. L., and Smith, H. O. (1993) Cancer screening for women older than 40 years of age. *Obstet. Gynecol. Clin. North Amer.* **20**, 391–408.

38. Austoker, J. (1994) Screening for ovarian, prostatic, and testicular cancers [see comments]. *Brit. Med. J.* **309**, 315–320.

39. Bourne, T. H., Campbell, S., Reynolds, K. M., et al. (1993) Screening for early familial ovarian cancer with transvaginal ultrasonography and colour blood flow imaging [see comments]. *Brit. Med. J.* **306**, 1025–1029.

# 7

# Primary Surgical Management of Ovarian Cancer

## Dennis S. Chi and William J. Hoskins

## 1. Introduction

In the United States, ovarian cancer is the fifth most common cause of female cancer death behind lung, breast, colorectal, and pancreatic cancers. It is estimated that 14,500 women in the United States will die of ovarian cancer in 1999 *(1)*. Epithelial ovarian carcinoma accounts for 90% of all ovarian cancers and an even greater percentage of ovarian cancer mortality *(2)*. In this chapter, we will review the role of primary surgery in the management of epithelial ovarian carcinoma. A brief discussion of interval cytoreduction is also included.

Although the management of ovarian cancer generally requires a multimodal approach, surgery is the cornerstone, playing an essential role in both diagnosis and treatment. In cases of apparent early-stage disease, proper surgical management involves comprehensive surgical staging. Advanced-stage disease frequently requires aggressive surgical debulking.

In 1993, Averette et al. *(3)* reported the results of a national survey of care patterns for patients with ovarian carcinoma performed by the American College of Surgeons (ACOS). They collected data on over 12,000 patients, and found that in only 21% of cases was the primary surgeon a gynecologic oncologist. In 45% of cases, the primary surgeon was a general obstetrician-gynecologist; in 21%, it was a general surgeon; and in 13% of cases, the primary surgeon was listed as "other," which included urologists, family practitioners, and resident trainees. Other studies have elucidated the ACOS data, which showed that when a gynecologic oncologist is not present at the initial operation, surgical staging is more often inadequate, tumor cytoreduction is more frequently suboptimal, and long-term survival is significantly shorter *(4,5)*. These poorer results are less a reflection of surgical ability than a representation of the primary surgeon's knowledge about the disease process. In order to provide optimal surgical management, the surgeon must understand the natural history and patterns of spread of ovarian carcinoma.

## 2. Natural History and Patterns of Spread

It is believed that epithelial ovarian carcinomas arise from invaginated surface epithelium within the ovarian stroma *(2)*. By an unidentified mechanism, the invaginated

From: *Methods in Molecular Medicine, Vol. 39: Ovarian Cancer: Methods and Protocols*
Edited by: J. M. S. Bartlett © Humana Press, Inc., Totowa, NJ

epithelium undergoes malignant transformation and forms an epithelial tumor. As the malignant tumor grows, it can spread by one or more of three primary methods:

1. direct extension to adjacent organs;
2. exfoliation of tumor cells from the ovary, followed by their intraperitoneal dissemination; and /or
3. lymphatic embolization to regional and distant lymph nodes.

Blood-borne metastases are rare.

Direct extension occurs after the tumor enlarges to the point that it penetrates the ovarian capsule and invades adjacent pelvic organs by direct contact. The most frequently involved structures are the fallopian tubes, uterus, and contralateral adnexa *(6)*. The peritoneal lining of the bladder, rectum, and cul-de-sac are also frequently involved pelvic structures.

The most significant method of tumor spread occurs via exfoliation of clonogenic malignant cells from the ovary, followed by their dissemination throughout the peritoneal cavity. Although this dissemination is frequently assumed to occur after the ovarian capsule has been penetrated by tumor, the existence of malignant cells within the peritoneal cavity in the presence of an intact ovarian capsule has been documented *(7)*. Once the malignant cells enter the peritoneal cavity, they follow the normal clockwise flow of peritoneal fluid that results from the peristaltic movements of the intestines and the respiratory motions of the diaphragm *(8)*. These cells may implant on any of the peritoneal surfaces and grow to form metastatic tumor nodules. The omentum is a frequent site of metastasis, with omental metastases seen in up to 11% of patients thought at exploration to have localized disease and found in nearly all patients who die of ovarian cancer *(9,10)*. Malignant cells that reach the diaphragm may lead to diaphragmatic metastases, and can be transported by lymphatic channels within the diaphragm to the pleural space *(11)*.

The third method of ovarian cancer spread is via the lymphatics that drain the ovaries. Tumor cells metastasize to lymph nodes by three main routes:

1. they can travel in the lymphatics that accompany the ovarian vessels to the para-aortic lymph nodes;
2. they can follow the drainage in the broad ligament to the external and internal iliac lymph nodes; or
3. they can travel in the lymphatics in the round ligament to the inguinal lymph nodes.

The incidence of lymph node involvement appears to range from 5 to 20% in apparently local disease, and up to 70% in more advanced stages *(8)*.

## 3. Surgical Staging of Early Ovarian Carcinoma

Based on its known patterns of spread, the surgical staging of apparently early-stage ovarian carcinoma requires a meticulous search of the peritoneal cavity for metastatic disease. Accurate surgical staging of early-stage ovarian carcinoma is imperative to the decision-making process regarding adjuvant therapy. **Table 1** summarizes the International Federation of Gynecology and Obstetrics (FIGO) staging system for ovarian cancer *(12)*. The distribution by FIGO stage of over 10,000 ovarian cancer patients is given in **Table 2** *(13)*.

**Table 1**
**International Federation of Gynecology**
**and Obstetrics (FIGO) Staging System for Ovarian Cancer**

| Stage | Characteristics |
|---|---|
| I | Growth limited to the ovaries. |
| A | Growth limited to one ovary; no ascites; no tumor on the external surface; capsule intact. |
| B | Growth limited to both ovaries; no ascites; no tumor on the external surfaces; capsule intact. |
| C | Tumor either Stage IA or IB, but with tumor on the surface of one or both ovaries; or with capsule ruptured; or with malignant cells in ascites or peritoneal washings. |
| II | Growth involving one or both ovaries with pelvic extension. |
| A | Extension and/or metastases to the uterus and/or tubes. |
| B | Extension to other pelvic tissues. |
| C | Tumor either Stage IIA or IIB, but with tumor on the surface of one or both ovaries; or capsule ruptured; or with malignant cells in ascites or peritoneal washings. |
| III | Tumor involving one or both ovaries with peritoneal implants outside the pelvis and/or positive retroperitoneal or inguinal lymph nodes. Superficial liver metastasis equals Stage III. Tumor is limited to the true pelvis but with histologically verified malignant extension small bowel or omentum. |
| A | Tumor grossly limited to the true pelvis but with histologically confirmed microscopic of abdominal peritoneal surfaces. |
| B | Tumor involving one or both ovaries with histologically confirmed implants of abdominal peritoneal surfaces, none exceeding 2 cm in diameter. Nodes are negative. |
| C | Abdominal implants greater than 2 cm in diameter and/or positive retroperitoneal or inguinal nodes. |
| IV | Growth involving one or both ovaries with distant metastases. If pleural effusion is present there must be positive cytology to allot a case to Stage IV. Parenchymal liver metastases equals Stage IV. |

**Table 2**
**Distribution by FIGO Stage of Ovarian**
**Carcinoma Patients *(13)***

| Stage | Number of patients | Percent |
|---|---|---|
| I | 2549 | 23.3 |
| II | 1409 | 13.0 |
| III | 5170 | 47.4 |
| IV | 1784 | 16.3 |
| Total | 10,912 | 100 |

Prior to 1980, the five-year survival for patients with apparently localized ovarian carcinoma was approximately 60%. However, it is now believed that a substantial number of these early-stage patients were "understaged" and actually harbored occult metastatic sites of disease before initiation of postoperative therapy. In 1983, Young et al. *(9)* reported the results of a prospective study performed by the multi-institutional Ovarian Cancer Study Group. This report included 100 patients with a diagnosis of "early" ovarian cancer who underwent surgical restaging. After restaging, 31 of the 100

**Table 3**
**Recommended Primary Surgical Staging Procedure**
**for Patients with Apparently Early Ovarian Carcinoma**

Vertical incision
Multiple peritoneal washings
Total abdominal hysterectomy and bilateral salpingo-oophorectomy
    (Unilateral salpingo-oophorectomy may be appropriate for selected patients with Stage IA
    disease who desire to defer definitive surgery until completion of childbearing)
Infracolic omentectomy
Pelvic and para-aortic lymph node sampling
Peritoneal biopsies from: the cul-de-sac
        rectal and bladder serosa
        right and left pelvic sidewalls
        right and left paracolic gutters
        right and left diaphragm
        any adhesions

patients (31%) were found to have a more advanced stage of disease. Sites of occult
disease included omentum, diaphragm, various peritoneal surfaces, and para-aortic and
pelvic lymph nodes.

**Table 3** outlines the recommended surgical staging procedure for ovarian carcinoma that appears confined to the pelvis. An adequate vertical incision should be used
and the procedures and biopsies performed as listed. Microscopic tumor implants
tend to cause the formation of adhesions; therefore, biopsy of all intraperitoneal
adhesions is recommended. Although complete laparoscopic surgical staging for
ovarian cancer has been reported, its efficacy remains unproven and its role strictly
investigational *(14)*.

A recent study by the Gynecologic Oncology Group (GOG) *(15)* demonstrated that
patients with localized ovarian cancer who undergo comprehensive surgical staging as
described above have a five-year survival rate of over 80%. For patients with well- and
moderately differentiated Stage IA and IB tumors, the five-year survival is over 90%.
Five-year survival rates by FIGO stage are given in **Table 4** *(2,16)*.

## 4. Surgical Cytoreduction of Advanced Ovarian Carcinoma

Despite decades of effort aimed at improving the early detection and diagnosis of
epithelial ovarian carcinoma, the majority of patients present with advanced FIGO
Stage III or IV disease (**Table 2**). Frequently, these patients have an abdomen dis-
tended with ascites along with large tumor masses in the abdomen and pelvis. At
exploration, complete resection of all grossly visible tumor is usually impossible, and
such patients cannot be cured by surgery alone. In these cases, the surgeon must decide
what level of surgical aggressiveness is appropriate.

Primary surgical cytoreduction refers to the removal of as much tumor as possible at
the initial operative procedure. For most human solid tumors, aggressive surgical
resection is justified only if all known tumor can be removed, rendering the operation
potentially curative. However, for epithelial ovarian carcinoma, both theoretical and
clinical benefits have been demonstrated for primary cytoreductive, or debulking, surgery even when all known tumor cannot be resected.

**Table 4**
**Five-Year Survival by Stage**
**for Epithelial Ovarian Carcinoma**

| Stage | Five-year survival |
|---|---|
| I | 80–90% |
| II | 80% |
| III | 15–40% |
| IV | 5–20% |

## 4.1. Theoretical Benefits of Primary Surgical Cytoreduction

Griffiths (*17*) summarized the theoretical benefits of primary surgical cytoreduction. These benefits are based on tumor growth kinetics and the mechanisms of tumor cell destruction by cytotoxic chemotherapy. Initial tumor models suggested that cancers have exponential growth curves. However, subsequent studies have shown that the actual growth of human solid tumors is marked by an increase in cancer cell doubling time as the tumor becomes larger. This increase in doubling time causes a flattening of the growth curve, which has been described as the Gompertzian model of tumor growth and regression (*18*). The growth rate is thought to decrease as the tumor enlarges because of a relative lack of blood supply and nutrients. Additionally, larger tumors are postulated to contain a higher proportion of cells in the resting, or nonproliferating, phase of the cell cycle.

The most important theoretical effect of primary cytoreductive surgery is its impact on the chemosensitivity of the residual tumor nodules. The resection of large bulky masses removes the portion of tumors with poor blood supply that would otherwise receive inadequate doses of chemotherapy. Furthermore, the Gompertzian model suggests that cytoreduction causes a high percentage of resting tumor cells to migrate into the pool of actively dividing cells, with a consequent increase in chemotherapy sensitivity. Small tumor implants between 0.1 and 0.5 cm have virtually 100% of their cells in the dividing pool (*17*).

According to the mathematical model of Goldie and Coldman (*19*), the development of chemotherapy resistance is a function of the spontaneous mutation rate of tumor cells toward drug-resistant phenotypes. As tumor size and cell number increase, the probability of mutations and drug-resistant clones also increases. Therefore, another theoretical benefit to primary cytoreductive surgery is that it may remove existing resistant tumor clones while decreasing the spontaneous development of new resistant phenotypes (*8*).

Some have suggested that the main benefit of surgical cytoreduction is that the removal of large tumor masses leaves fewer cancer cells to be eradicated by postoperative chemotherapy. Surgical cytoreduction of 1 kg of tumor to 1 g represents a decrease in the total number of cancer cells from $10^{12}$ to $10^9$. This amount of cytoreduction is rarely attained. However, even if this amount of debulking was achieved, considering tumor growth that occurs between chemotherapy cycles, an additional seven 3-log cell kills would be required to eradicate the last cancer cell (*17*). The benefit of cytoreduction derived from this mechanism is probably of significance only in patients who undergo resection of all grossly visible disease, leaving only microscopic residual cancer *(20)*.

## 4.2. Clinical Benefits of Primary Surgical Cytoreduction

Surgical removal of bulky disease in a patient with advanced ovarian cancer is believed to not only improve the patient's level of comfort, but also to reduce the adverse metabolic effects of the tumor while helping the patient maintain her nutritional status *(21)*. Overall, debulking surgery appears to measurably improve the quality of life in these patients *(22)*.

However, all of the literature that supports the clinical benefits of primary cytoreductive surgery is based on indirect analyses. To date, no prospective trial has ever randomized patients to aggressive surgical cytoreduction versus less aggressive surgery. The GOG attempted such a trial but was unable to accrue enough patients, reflecting the very strong indirect evidence for the benefits of cytoreductive surgery *(23)*.

In 1968, Munnell *(24)* introduced the concept of the "maximum surgical effort" for patients with ovarian cancer. He reported improved survival in patients who underwent "definitive surgery" compared to those who had "partial removal" or "only biopsy." Similar results were reported by Declos and Quinlan *(25)* who noted a 25% four-year survival rate for patients with Stage III ovarian cancer who had surgical cytoreduction to "nonpalpable" tumor, compared to 9% for those left with "palpable" residual tumor.

It was not until 1975 that residual tumor after primary cytoreduction was accurately quantified and correlated with survival. Griffiths *(26)* reported on 102 patients who received single-agent melphalan following primary surgical cytoreduction. The patients were divided into four groups based on the diameter of the largest residual tumor nodule after surgery. Patients with no residual tumor had a median survival of 39 mo, with median survival progressively decreasing (as residual tumor size increased) down to 11 mo for the group of patients who had residual tumor nodules of >1.5 cm.

Since Griffiths's seminal report, numerous studies have evaluated the effect of residual disease after primary surgical cytoreduction on response rate to chemotherapy (**Table 5**) and survival (**Table 6**). All of these reports use the diameter of the largest remaining tumor nodule as the measurement of residual disease. Most of them divide the patients into "optimal" and "suboptimal" groups, using 2 cm as a cutoff point. Some use other cutoff points, such as 1.0, 1.5, or 3 cm. Overall, a clear clinical benefit can be seen for cytoreductive surgery, with patients in the "optimal" category having a higher complete response rate to chemotherapy (43 vs 24%) and an improved median survival (37 vs 17 mo).

More recently, Hoskins et al. *(38)* reported the results of two studies performed by the GOG that further clarified the role of primary cytoreductive surgery in patients with advanced ovarian cancer. In the first study, they compared the survival of patients with Stage III disease who were found at surgery to have abdominal disease of ≤1 cm, to the survival of those who were found to have abdominal disease of >1 cm, but were then surgically cytoreduced to ≤1 cm. If surgery was the only important factor, then the survival should have been the same in the two groups. However, patients found to have small-volume disease survived longer than patients who were cytoreduced to small-volume disease. Further analysis showed that the age of the patient, the grade of the tumor, and the number of residual tumor nodules were independent prognostic factors.

**Table 5**
**The Effect of Residual Disease After Primary Cytoreductive Surgery**
**on Response Rate in Advanced Ovarian Cancer**

| Author (ref.) | Year | Rx | No. | Residual (cm) | Response (%) Complete | Total |
|---|---|---|---|---|---|---|
| Young et al. *(27)* | 1978 | HexaCAF vs. $_L$-PAM | 19 | <2 | | 84 |
| | | | 58 | >2 | | 53 |
| Ehrlich et al. *(28)* | 1979 | PAC | 14 | <3 | 46 | 78 |
| | | | 25 | >3 | 32 | 54 |
| Wharton and Herson et al. *(29)* | 1981 | $_L$-PAM | 45 | <2 | 12 | 29 |
| | | | 59 | >2 | 8 | 24 |
| Conte et al. *(30)* | 1986 | CAP vs. CP | 37 | <2 | 70 | 76 |
| | | | 38 | >2 | 32 | 82 |
| Total/Mean | | | 115 | Optimal | 42.7 | 66.8 |
| | | | 180 | Suboptimal | 24.0 | 53.3 |

HexaCAF, hexamethylmelamine, cyclophosphamide, amethopterin, 5-fluorouracil; PAC, cisplatin, adriamycin, cyclophosphamide; $_L$-PAM, melphalan; CAP vs. CP, cisplatin, adriamycin, cyclophosphamide versus cisplatin, cyclophosphamide. Used with permission from **ref. 20**.

Although this study in no way showed a lack of effectiveness of primary cytoreductive surgery, it did show that other factors, including the biology of the tumor, were also important.

The second study demonstrated that surgical cytoreduction to ≤2 cm residual disease resulted in a significant survival benefit, but all residual diameters >2 cm had equivalent survival *(39)*. Therefore, unless the tumor could be cytoreduced to a maximum residual tumor diameter of ≤2 cm, aggressive surgical cytoreduction did not affect survival.

**Figure 1** is a composite graph of the survival curves for the two GOG studies. It appears that three distinct groups emerge:

1. those with no grossly visible residual disease;
2. those with optimal residual disease (≤2 cm);
3. those with suboptimal disease (>2 cm in diameter).

Four-year survivals are approximately 60, 35, and less than 20%, respectively *(40)*.

The results of the two GOG studies, as well as the other reports in the literature, were presented in 1994 at the National Institutes of Health Consensus Development Conference on Ovarian Cancer. The consensus statement on the issue of the appropriate management of advanced epithelial ovarian cancer was that "aggressive efforts at maximal cytoreduction are important because minimal residual tumor is associated with improved survival" *(41)*.

## 4.3. Surgical Cytoreduction of Stage IV Disease

Although the role of aggressive surgical cytoreduction in patients with Stage III ovarian carcinoma is well defined, its benefit in Stage IV disease is less clear. Most of

**Table 6**
**The Effect of Residual Disease at the Conclusion**
**of Primary Cytoreductive Surgery on Survival**

| Author (ref.) | Year | Rx | Residual (cm) | No. | Survival (mo) |
|---|---|---|---|---|---|
| Griffiths *(26)* | 1975 | ₗ-PAM | 0 | 29 | 39 |
| | | | 0–0.5 | 28 | 29 |
| | | | 0.6–1.5 | 16 | 18 |
| | | | >1.5 | 29 | 11 |
| Hacker et al. *(31)* | 1983 | varied | <0.5 | 7 | 40 |
| | | | 0.6–1.5 | 24 | 18 |
| | | | >1.5 | 16 | 6 |
| Vogel et al. *(32)* | 1983 | CHAP | <2 | 32 | >40 |
| | | | >2 | 58 | 16 |
| Pohl et al. *(33)* | 1984 | varied | <2 | 37 | 45 |
| | | | >2 | 57 | 16 |
| Delgado et al. *(34)* | 1984 | varied | <2 | 21 | 45 |
| | | | >2 | 54 | 16 |
| Redman et al. *(35)* | 1986 | CAP | <3 | 34 | 38 |
| | | | >3 | 51 | 26 |
| Conte et al. *(30)* | 1986 | CAP vs. CP | <2 | 37 | >40 |
| | | | >2 | 38 | 16 |
| Neijt et al. *(36)* | 1987 | CHAP vs. CP | <1 | 88 | 40 |
| | | | >1 | 219 | 21 |
| Piver et al. *(37)* | 1988 | PAC | <2 | 35 | 48 |
| | | | >2 | 5 | 21 |
| Total/Mean | | | Optimal | 388 | 36.7 |
| | | | Suboptimal | 537 | 16.6 |

ₗ-PAM, melphalan; CHAP, cyclophosphamide, hexamethylmelamine, adriamycin, cisplatin; CAP, cisplatin, adriamycin, cyclophosphamide; CP, cisplatin, cyclophosphamide; PAC, cisplatin, adriamycin, cyclophosphamide. Used with permission from **ref. 20**.

the studies supporting cytoreductive surgery have evaluated Stage III patients alone, or have analyzed Stage III and Stage IV patients collectively. Because patients with Stage IV ovarian carcinoma have, by definition, extraperitoneal and/or intrahepatic metastases, some have questioned the benefit of intraperitoneal surgical cytoreduction in these cases *(42)*. In a series of 35 women with Stage IV ovarian cancer, Goodman et al. *(43)* found no significant survival benefit attributable to optimal versus suboptimal surgical cytoreduction.

However, in a more recent review of Stage IV ovarian carcinoma patients, Curtin et al. *(16)* demonstrated a median survival of 40 mo for 41 patients who underwent optimal surgical cytoreduction compared to 18 mo for 51 patients who had suboptimal debulking. Other reports have confirmed the significant survival benefit associated with optimal surgical cytoreduction in patients with Stage IV ovarian cancer (**Table 7**). Overall, these recent series support the NIH Consensus Statement regarding the importance of aggressive surgical cytoreduction for advanced ovarian carcinoma, even in

Fig. 1. Survival by residual disease, Gynecologic Oncology Group protocols (*PR*) 52 and 97. Used with permission from **ref. *39***.

**Table 7**
**The Effect of Residual Disease at the Conclusion**
**of Primary Cytoreductive Surgery on Survival in Stage IV Ovarian Cancer**

| Author (ref.) | Year | Rx | Residual (cm) | Number Median | Survival (mo) |
|---|---|---|---|---|---|
| Goodman et al. *(43)** | 1992 | platinum-based** | <2 | 23 | 28 |
| | | | >2 | 12 | 22 |
| Curtin et al. *(16)* | 1997 | platinum-based | <2 | 41 | 40 |
| | | | >2 | 51 | 18 |
| Liu et al. *(44)* | 1997 | platinum-based*** | <2 | 14 | 37 |
| | | | >2 | 33 | 17 |
| Munkarah et al. *(45)* | 1997 | platinum-based | <2 | 31 | 25 |
| | | | >2 | 61 | 15 |
| Total/Mean | | | Optimal | 109 | 33 |
| | | | Suboptimal | 157 | 17 |

* includes 11 patients who also underwent interval cytoreduction.
** four patients did not receive platinum-based chemotherapy.
*** three patients did not receive platinum-based chemotherapy

cases where the preoperative findings are compatible with Stage IV disease. **Table 8** lists aggressive surgical procedures that would be considered in patients with advanced ovarian carcinoma should such procedures help achieve optimal cytoreduction *(46)*. However, if optimal cytoreduction is not attainable, then these aggressive procedures would not improve survival and therefore should not be attempted.

**Table 8**
**Aggressive Surgical Procedures That Would
be Considered to Obtain Optimal Tumor Cytoreduction**

Multiple or extensive bowel resection
Rectosigmoid resection
Resection of ureteral/bladder segment
Extensive pelvic/aortic node dissection
Diaphragm stripping
Resection of liver, spleen, kidney, diaphragm

Used with permission from **ref. *46***.

## 4.4. Interval Cytoreduction

The actual percentage of patients with advanced ovarian cancer who can be successfully cytoreduced to optimal residual disease status ranges in the literature from 17 to 87%, with a mean of approximately 35% *(2)*. Because these patients with suboptimal residual disease carry such a poor prognosis, their further management is especially challenging. Some investigators have evaluated the benefit of a brief course of chemotherapy, followed by a second attempt at "interval" cytoreduction before completing a prescribed chemotherapy regimen *(47,48)*. The European Organization for Research on Treatment of Cancer (EORTC) *(49)* recently reported a large, prospective randomized trial that evaluated interval cytoreduction in patients with suboptimally cytoreduced, advanced ovarian cancer. After three cycles of cyclophosphamide and cisplatin, patients without disease progression were randomly assigned to undergo either interval debulking surgery or no surgery, followed by three more cycles of the same chemotherapy. Patients who underwent interval cytoreduction demonstrated a significant improvement in both progression-free survival (18 vs 13 mo) and overall survival (26 vs 20 mo) (**Figs. 2** and **3**).

Based on the results of the EORTC trial and those that have shown the superiority of cisplatin and paclitaxel as first-line chemotherapy in patients with suboptimally cytoreduced, advanced ovarian carcinoma *(50)*, the GOG is currently performing another prospective, randomized trial to evaluate the benefit of interval cytoreduction. The schema of GOG protocol #152 is similar to that of the EORTC trial, except that patients will receive paclitaxel and cisplatin instead of cyclophosphamide and cisplatin.

Because the benefits of aggressive primary surgical cytoreduction for advanced ovarian cancer are well accepted, the role of interval cytoreduction is yet to be established. Until the results of confirmatory studies such as GOG protocol #152 become available, interval cytoreduction should be attempted only in a clinical trial setting.

## 5. Conclusion

The treatment of ovarian carcinoma requires a multidisciplinary approach. Proper primary surgical management should include involvement of a gynecologic oncologist who understands the natural history and patterns of spread of the disease. Apparent early-stage disease requires comprehensive surgical staging, while aggressive surgical cytoreduction is frequently indicated for bulky, advanced-stage disease. Although preliminary results are promising, the role of interval cytoreduction in patients who are suboptimally cytoreduced at primary surgery is yet to be established.

Fig. 2. Survival of patients with advanced epithelial ovarian cancer according to whether they underwent debulking surgery. P = 0.012 for the comparison between the groups by the log-rank test. Used with permission from **ref. 49**.

Fig. 3. Progression-free survival of patients with advanced epithelial ovarian cancer according to whether they underwent debulking surgery. P = 0.013 for the comparison between the groups by log-rank test. Used with permission from **ref. 49**.

## References

1. Landis, S. M., Murray, T., Bolden, S., and Wingo, P. A. (1999) Cancer Statistics, 1999. *Cancer J. Clin.* **49,** 8–31.
2. Ozols, R. F., Rubin, S. C., Thomas, G., and Robboy, S. (1997) Epithelial ovarian cancer, in *Principles and Practice of Gynecologic Oncology, Second Edition.* (Hoskins, W. J., Perez, C. A., and Young, R. C., eds.), Lippincott-Raven, Philadelphia, PA, pp. 919–986.
3. Averette, H. E., Hoskins, W., Nguyen, H. N., et al. (1993) National survey of ovarian carcinoma. I. A patient care evaluation study of the American College of Surgeons. *Cancer* **71,** 1629–1638.
4. McGowan, L., Lesher, L. P., Norris, H. J., and Barnett, M. (1985) Misstaging of ovarian cancer. *Obstet. Gynecol.* **65,** 568–572.
5. Eisenkop, S. M., Spirtos, N. M., Montag, T. W., Nalick, R. N., and Wang, H. J. (1992) The impact of subspecialty training on the management of advanced ovarian cancer. *Gynecol. Oncol.* **47,** 203–209.
6. Fuks, Z. (1980) Patterns of spread of ovarian carcinoma: Relation to therapeutic strategies. *Adv. Biosci.* **26,** 39–57.
7. Keetel, W. C. and Pixley, E. (1958) Diagnostic value of peritoneal washings. *Clin. Obstet. Gynecol.* **1,** 592–606.
8. Rubin, S. C. and Hoskins, W. J. (1993) Primary surgery for ovarian carcinoma, in *Gynecology and Obstetrics* (Sciarra, J. J. and Droegemueller, W., eds), J.B. Lippincott, Philadelphia, PA, pp. 1–11.
9. Young, R. C., Decker, D. G., Wharton, J. T., et al. (1983) Staging laparotomy in early ovarian cancer. *JAMA* **250,** 3072–3076.
10. Hoskins, W. J. (1993) Surgical staging and cytoreductive surgery of epithelial ovarian cancer. *Cancer* **71,** 1534–1540.
11. Feldman, G. B. and Knapp, R. C. (1974) Lymphatic drainage of the peritoneal cavity and its significance in ovarian cancer. *Am. J. Obstet. Gynecol.* **119,** 991–994.
12. Staging Announcement: FIGO Cancer Committee (1986) *Gynecol. Oncol.* **25,** 383–385.
13. Pettersson, F. (1991) Int. Fed. Gynecol. Obstet.: Ann. rep. on the results and treatment in gynecological cancer. Stockholm, Panorama Press AB, vol 21.
14. Childers, J. M., Lang, J., Surwit, E. A., and Hatch, K. D. (1995) Laparoscopic surgical staging of ovarian cancer. *Gynecol. Oncol.* **59,** 25–35.
15. Young, R. C., Walton, L. A., Ellenberg, S. S., et al. (1990) Adjuvant therapy in stage I and stage II epithelial ovarian cancer. Results of two prospective trials. *N. Engl. J. Med.* **322,** 1021–1027.
16. Curtin, J. P., Malik, R., Venkatraman, E. S., et al. (1997) Stage IV ovarian cancer: Impact of surgical debulking. *Gynecol. Oncol.* **64,** 9–12.
17. Griffiths, C. T. (1986) Surgery at the time of diagnosis in ovarian cancer, in *Management of Ovarian Cancer* (Blackledge, G. and Chan, K. K., eds.), Butterworth, London, pp. 60–75.
18. DeVita, V. T. (1993) Principles of chemotherapy, in *Cancer: Principles and Practice of Oncology, Fourth Edition* (Devita, V. T., Hellman, S., and Rosenberg, S. A., eds.), J.B. Lippincott, Philadelphia, PA, pp. 276–292.
19. Goldie, J. H. and Coldman, J. A. (1979) A mathematic model for relating the drug sensitivity of tumors to their spontaneous mutation rate. *Cancer Treat. Rep.* **63,** 1727–1733.
20. Hoskins, W. J. (1993) Primary cytoreduction, in *Cancer of the Ovary* (Markman, M. and Hoskins, W. J., eds.), Raven, New York, pp. 163–173.
21. Hoskins, W. J. and Rubin, S. C. (1991) Surgery in the treatment of patients with advanced ovarian cancer. *Semin. Oncol.* **18,** 213–221.
22. Blythe, J. G. and Wahl, T. P. (1982) Debulking surgery: Does it increase the quality of survival? *Gynecol. Oncol.* **14,** 396–408.
23. Hoskins, W. J. (1993) Primary surgical management of advanced epithelial ovarian cancer, in *Ovarian Cancer.* (Rubin, S. C. and Sutton, G. P., eds), McGraw-Hill, New York, NY, pp. 241–253.
24. Munnell, E. Q. (1968) The changing prognosis and treatment in cancer of the ovary. A report of 235 patients with primary ovarian carcinoma 1952–1961. *Am. J. Obstet. Gynecol.* **100,** 790–805.
25. Declos, L. and Quinlan, E. J. (1969) Malignant tumors of the ovary managed with post operative megavolt irradiation. *Radiology* **93,** 659–663.
26. Griffiths, C. T. (1975) Surgical resection of tumor bulk in the primary treatment of ovarian carcinoma. *Natl. Cancer Inst. Monogr.* **42,** 101–104.
27. Young, R. C., Chabner, B. A., Hubbard, S. P., et al. (1978) Advanced ovarian adenocarcinoma: A prospective clinical trial of melphalan (L-PAM) versus combination chemotherapy. *N. Engl. J. Med.* **299,** 1261–1266.
28. Ehrlich, C. E., Einhorn, L., Williams, S. D., et al. (1979) Chemotherapy for stage II-IV epithelial ovarian cancer with cisdichlorodiammineplatinum (II), adriamycin and cyclophosphamide: A preliminary report. *Cancer Treat. Rep.* **63,** 281–288.
29. Wharton, J. T. and Herson, J. (1981) Surgery for common epithelial tumors of the ovary. *Cancer* **48,** 582–589.

30. Conte, P. F., Bruzzone, M., Chiaro, S., et al. (1986) A randomized trial comparing cisplatin plus cyclophosphamide versus cisplatin, doxorubicin and cyclophosphamide in advanced ovarian cancer. *J. Clin. Oncol.* **4,** 965–971.

31. Hacker, N. F., Berek, J. S., Lagasse, L. D., et al. (1983) Primary cytoreductive surgery for epithelial ovarian cancer. *Obstet. Gynecol.* **61,** 413–420.

32. Vogl, S. E., Pagano, M., Kaplan, B. H., et al. (1983) Cisplatin based combination chemotherapy for advanced ovarian cancer: High overall response rate with curative potential only in women with small tumor burdens. *Cancer* **51,** 2024–2030.

33. Pohl, R., Dallenback-Hellweg, G., Plugge, T., et al. (1984) Prognostic parameters in patients with advanced malignant tumors. *Eur. J. Gynaecol. Oncol.* **3,** 160–169.

34. Delgado, G., Oram, D. H., and Petrilli, E. S. (1984) Stage III epithelial ovarian cancer: The role of maximal surgical reduction. *Gynecol. Oncol.* **18,** 293–298.

35. Redman, J. R., Petroni, G. R., Saigo, P. E., et al. (1986) Prognostic factors in advanced ovarian carcinoma. *J. Clin. Oncol.* **4,** 515–523.

36. Neijt, J. P., ten Bokkel Huinink, W. W., van der Burg, M. E. L., et al. (1987) Randomized trial comparing two combination chemotherapy regimens (CHAP-5 vs CP) in advanced ovarian carcinoma. *J. Clin. Oncol.* **5** 1157–1168.

37. Piver, M. S., Lele, S. B., Marchetti, D. L., et al. (1988) The impact of aggressive debulking surgery and cisplatin based chemotherapy on progression-free survival in stage III and IV ovarian carcinoma. *J. Clin. Oncol.* **6,** 983–989.

38. Hoskins, W. J., Bundy, B. N., Thigpen, J. T., and Omura, G. A. (1992) The influence of cytoreductive surgery on recurrence-free interval and survival in small-volume stage III epithelial ovarian cancer: A Gynecologic Oncology Group study. *Gynecol. Oncol.* **47,** 159–166.

39. Hoskins, W. J., McGuire, W. J., Brady, M. F., et al. (1994) The effect of diameter of largest residual disease on survival after primary cytoreductive surgery in patients with suboptimal residual epithelial ovarian carcinoma. *Am. J. Obstet. Gynecol.* **170,** 974–980.

40. Hoskins, W. J. (1994) Epithelial ovarian carcinoma: Principles of primary surgery. *Gynecol. Oncol.* **55,** S91–S96.

41. National Institutes of Health Consensus Development Conference Statement (1994) Ovarian cancer: screening, treatment, and follow-up. April 5–7, 1994. *Gynecol. Oncol.* **55,** S4–S14.

42. Schwartz, P. E. (1997) Cytoreductive surgery for the management of stage IV ovarian cancer. *Gynecol. Oncol.* **64,** 1–3, (editorial).

43. Goodman, H. M., Harlow, B. L., Sheets, E. E., et al. (1992) The role of cytoreductive surgery in the management of stage IV epithelial ovarian carcinoma. *Gynecol. Oncol.* **46,** 367–371.

44. Liu, P. C., Benjamin, I., Morgan, M. A., et al. (1997) Effect of surgical debulking on survival in stage IV ovarian cancer. *Gynecol. Oncol.* **64,** 4–8.

45. Munkarah, A. R., Hallum, A. V. III, Morris, M., et al. (1997) Prognostic significance of residual disease in patients with stage IV epithelial ovarian cancer. *Gynecol. Oncol.* **64,** 13–17.

46. Morrow, C. P. and Curtin, J. P. (1996) Surgery for ovarian neoplasia, in *Gynecologic Cancer Surgery* (Morrow, C. P. and Curtin, J. P., eds), Churchill Livingstone, New York, NY, pp. 627–716.

47. Lawton, F. G., Redman, C. W. E., Luesley, D. M., et al. (1989) Neoadjuvant (cytoreductive) chemotherapy combined with intervention debulking surgery in advanced, unresected epithelial ovarian cancer. *Obstet. Gynecol.* **73,** 61–65.

48. Ng, L. W., Rubin, S. C., Hoskins, W. J., et al. (1990) Aggressive chemosurgical debulking in patients with advanced ovarian cancer. *Gynecol. Oncol.* **38,** 358–363.

49. van der Burg, M. E. L., van Lent, M., Buyse, M., et al. (1995) The effect of debulking surgery after induction chemotherapy on the prognosis in advanced epithelial ovarian cancer. *N. Engl. J. Med.* **332,** 629–634.

50. McGuire, W. P., Hoskins, W. J., Brady, M. F., et al. (1996) Cyclophosphamide and cisplatin compared with paclitaxel and cisplatin in patients with stage III and stage IV ovarian cancer. *N. Engl. J. Med.* **334,** 1–6.

# 8

## Recent Insights into Drug Resistance in Ovarian Cancer

### Thomas C. Hamilton and Steven W. Johnson

### 1. Introduction

Ovarian cancer, as used in this review on drug resistance, applies to the study of the problem in those malignant tumors which arise from the modified peritoneal mesothelial cells, which cover the ovarian surface. These tumors are, by far, the most common malignancies of the ovary and display a remarkable range of histological features, which generally recapitulate those of the endocervix, endometrium, or Fallopian tube to which the ovarian surface epithelium is embryologically related. Of direct relevance to the issue of chemotherapeutic responsiveness is the fact that, stage for stage, some of these tumor subtypes carry a worse prognosis. The need for chemotherapy in ovarian cancer arises because this disease produces vague symptoms that occur only after it has spread from the confines of the ovary to the surfaces of the peritoneal cavity. At this stage, surgery rarely can eliminate all apparent disease, and even in those cases, experience shows that the disease will recur with high probability. This makes it obvious that residual microscopic disease remained after surgery. Hence, the majority of ovarian cancer patients require chemotherapy and its effective use has proved a tremendous challenge as evidenced by the approximately 14,000 deaths from this disease in the United States in 1997.

The standard of care for advanced-stage ovarian cancer in the United States and most, if not all, of the world is a platinum drug and paclitaxel (1). An example of the impact of paclitaxel on ovarian cancer treatment is the 18-mo progression-free interval and 37.5-mo median survival seen with a cisplatin and paclitaxel combination compared to a 12.9-mo progression-free interval and 24.4-mo median survival seen with cisplatin and cyclophosphamide in stage III and IV patients that had >1-cm residual disease after surgery. Issues that remain to be resolved with this drug combination relate to scheduling, route of administration, dose intensity, and which platinum analog (cisplatin or carboplatin) should be incorporated into the regimen. With regard to this latter point, most clinical trials have shown carboplatin to be equivalent to cisplatin in ovarian cancer. Therefore, carboplatin is generally the preferred platinum analog both because of its better spectrum of toxicity and the ability to deliver the paclitaxel as a 3-h infusion, rather than 24 h, as is required when used with cisplatin to avoid excessive neurotoxicity. It is important to note that additional clinical trials since the arrival of paclitaxel in the clinical arena have confirmed that platinum is the cornerstone for

From: Methods in Molecular Medicine, Vol. 39: Ovarian Cancer: Methods and Protocols
Edited by: J. M. S. Bartlett © Humana Press, Inc., Totowa, NJ

chemotherapy of ovarian cancer, i.e., paclitaxel alone is inferior to platinum alone or a combination of platinum and paclitaxel. Of more direct relevance to this review is the fact that although the addition of paclitaxel to the armamentarium for ovarian cancer treatment has improved the survival of ovarian cancer patients, the majority still die of their disease. This results because when disease recurs it has become resistant to further therapy. It is reasoned that if the basis for this resistance to chemotherapy could be understood, then ways to prevent or reverse this problem could be developed and further improve the prognosis for advanced-stage ovarian cancer patients.

## 2. Basis for Cytotoxicity

There is little controversy that the mechanism by which platinum kills cells is by binding to DNA and paclitaxel by stabilizing microtubules. There is somewhat less certainty as to exactly why cell death occurs. It is clear that platinum DNA binding results in inhibition of DNA replication and transcription, but whether these effects at clinically achievable platinum doses are sufficient to cause cell death through DNA damage and depletion of homeostatic enzymes is uncertain. In the case of taxanes, the stabilization of tubulin results in aberrant mitosis, which is also destructive to DNA. It is currently popular to consider that cell death results because there is sufficient DNA damage to activate programmed cell death pathways, but that this degree of damage is not necessarily sufficient to mandate cell death in the absence of the function of these pathways. Although data with cisplatin are emerging to support this concept (*2*), some caution is warranted considering that the level of cytotoxicity produced by adriamycin and irradiation does not correlate with death by apoptosis (*3*). There is additional uncertainty as to which of the various DNA adducts produced by the aquated forms of cisplatin and carboplatin are critical to cytotoxicity, but it is probably inadvisable to exclude DNA interstrand crosslinks as a major factor. Even though these adducts are not of high abundance, it seems intuitive that such lesions would markedly perturb DNA replication. Also of interest is the fact that when cells (as opposed to naked DNA) are treated with cisplatin or carboplatin, the spectrum of DNA adducts produced is different even though the active form of both drugs is identical (*4*).

## 3. Mechanisms of Drug Resistance

Since its initial descriptions in cell lines exposed to chemotherapeutic agents over two decades ago, considerable effort has been expended to characterize the genetic and biochemical basis for multidrug resistance (MDR). MDR can occur through various cellular changes and studies in cells that have developed MDR by exposure to cisplatin often contain more than one change to account for their resistance to diverse drugs. These multiple mechanisms include those which prevent cytotoxic drugs from reaching their targets and mechanisms which control cellular responses downstream of the drug/target interaction. The first group of resistance mechanisms includes decreased drug accumulation, increased drug inactivation, mutation or altered expression of drug targets, and increased intracellular sequestration by vault proteins. These mechanisms are often drug-specific, that is, a change in the quantity or activity of a particular protein may circumvent the cytotoxic effect of a specific class of drugs (e.g., mutations in β-tubulin for taxanes, increased P-glycoprotein for natural product drugs, or increased glutathione levels for alkylating agents). The second group, which may be characterized as mechanisms that allow a cell to tolerate increased levels of drug-induced damage, consists of enhanced DNA repair, alterations in the types of DNA lesions formed by some drugs, and alterations in the cell cycle and cell death pathways. Some of these mechanisms may confer a more general MDR phenotype which may be more typical of drug refractory recurrent ovarian cancer.

## 3.1. Altered Drug Transport

Increased expression of the human *MDR1* gene product, P-glycoprotein, is the most well-studied MDR mechanism. This 170 kDa plasma membrane glycoprotein is an ATP-dependent drug efflux pump that confers resistance to a wide variety of natural product drugs such as anthracyclines, vinca alkaloids, epipidophylotoxins, and taxanes, but not alkylating agents or platinum drugs. P-glycoprotein is a member of a superfamily of ATP-binding cassette (ABC) transporters which are expressed in diverse prokaryotic and eukaryotic organisms. Expression of the *MDR1* gene messenger RNA or protein product (P-glycoprotein) has been observed in a variety of untreated tumors and tumors from patients treated with chemotherapy. Overexpression of *MDR1* mRNA and/or P-glycoprotein has also been found to be an indicator of poor prognosis in patients treated with chemotherapy. In ovarian cancer, the role of *MDR1* gene expression is presently unclear. In a study by Goldstein et al. *(5)*, no *MDR1* mRNA was observed in ovarian tumors from 16 untreated patients. A similar result was obtained by Bourhis et al. *(6)* who observed no *MDR1* expression in 40 ovarian tumor biopsies from patients who were either untreated or treated with non-MDR chemotherapeutic regimens. In contrast, Holzmayer et al. *(7)* observed 30 of 46 *MDR1* mRNA positive tumors in untreated ovarian cancer patients and 10 of 10 positive tumors in ovarian cancer patients treated with natural product containing chemotherapy regimens. In recent reports, Kavallaris et al. *(8)* observed 19 of 53 *MDR1* positive ovarian tumors by RT-PCR and Izquierdo et al. *(9)* found 9 of 57 (16%) P-glycoprotein positive ovarian tumors by immunostaining. However, no association was found between Pgp expression and either response to chemotherapy or survival. Considering the recent incorporation of paclitaxel into ovarian cancer chemotherapy regimens and that it is a potent substrate for P-glycoprotein, future studies should revisit the significance of P-glycoprotein to the failure of chemotherapy in ovarian cancer.

Reversal of P-glycoprotein-mediated MDR was first described by Tsuruo et al. *(10)*. He showed that verapamil and trifluoperazine increased the steady-state accumulation of vincristine in a multidrug resistant murine leukemia cell line. Although toxicities associated with verapamil precluded its thorough clinical testing as an MDR reversing agent *(11)*, the possibility of modulating clinical resistance fueled the search for other MDR reversing agents. The spectrum of compounds that have subsequently been discovered is broad and includes calcium channel blockers, calmodulin antagonists, protein kinase C inhibitors, cyclic peptides, and steroidal drugs. Most of these agents modulate P-glycoprotein function through direct inhibition of P-glycoprotein-mediated drug efflux. Photoaffinity analogs of several of these compounds have been used to demonstrate their direct interaction with P-glycoprotein. The results of ongoing clinical trials employing second- and third-generation P-glycoprotein inhibitors may determine whether targeting this transporter is a practical approach to reversing clinical MDR, and may have special relevance in ovarian cancer where taxanes have become an important component to therapy.

Following the discovery and characterization of the P-glycoprotein natural product drug transporter, there were several reports describing cell lines which exhibited the MDR phenotype in the absence of P-glycoprotein expression. Evidence for a second transporter was provided by Marquardt et al. *(12)* who showed that an antibody raised against a synthetic peptide of P-glycoprotein recognized a 190 kDa protein in P-glycoprotein expressing and nonexpressing cell lines. Subsequently, an ATP-dependent multidrug transport protein known as MRP was discovered by Cole et al. *(13)* in a non-P-glycoprotein multidrug resistant small cell lung carcinoma cell line (H69AR) developed by step-wise doxorubicin selection. MRP shares little sequence homology with P-glycoprotein except in the nucleotide binding domain, however, the two transporters surprisingly exhibit a similar substrate specificity *(13)*. Transfection of the full-length *MRP* cDNA into drug-sensitive cells confers resistance to doxorubicin, daunorubicin, vincristine, etoposide, rhodamine 123, arsenite, arsenate, and antimonial compounds. Unlike P-glycoprotein-mediated resistance, MRP confers only low levels of resistance to paclitaxel and colchicine and cannot be photolabeled by the classic P-glycoprotein photoaffinity analogs. Concurrent with the discovery of MRP, several investigators were characterizing an efflux system for glutathione S-conjugates known as the GS-X pump (14). This transport activity was associated with the export of a variety of glutathione S-conjugated anions, cations and lipophilic compounds. A number of studies have suggested that the GS-X pump and MRP are the same transport protein. For example, Leier et al. *(15)* and Muller et al. *(16)* demonstrated that plasma membrane vesicles prepared from MRP transfected cells could transport the glutathione S-conjugates $LTC_4$ and DNP-SG. Leier et al. also successfully photolabeled a 190 kDa glycoprotein with $[^3H]$-$LTC_4$, which is consistent with the molecular weight of MRP. Furthermore, depletion of cellular GSH levels using buthionine sulfoximine (BSO) sensitized MRP transfectants to doxorubicin, daunorubicin, vincristine, and etoposide. A reduction in doxorubicin efflux from the transfected cells was also observed relative to the control transfectants. The mechanism by which MRP modulates chemotherapeutic drug resistance is not completely understood and it remains unclear whether conjugation to glutathione is a requirement of MRP substrates or whether glutathione acts as a cofactor for drug transport.

*MRP* is expressed at low levels in a variety of human tissues. The highest levels of expression occur in testes, skeletal muscle, heart, kidney, and lung. Two recent studies have addressed the issue of *MRP* gene expression in tumor biopsies from untreated ovarian cancer patients. Izquierdo et al. *(9)* reported 39 of 57 (68%) samples positive for MRP by immunostaining and Kavallaris et al. *(8)* detected *MRP* mRNA in 23 of 53 (43%) ovarian tumor specimens. Although the frequency of *MRP* expression appears higher than that of *MDR1*, the significance of these results awaits further study. Like P-glycoprotein-mediated MDR, identifying specific MRP inhibitors is important not only to study the biochemistry and pharmacology of this transporter, but also to have compounds available for circumventing clinical MDR resulting from increased MRP activity. Verapamil, which is an effective inhibitor of P-glycoprotein function, has little effect on reversing MDR in cell lines transfected with the *MRP* cDNA. In non-P-glycoprotein expressing MDR cell lines, verapamil and cyclosporin A have shown a low to modest drug-potentiating effect. Other chemosensitizers [reviewed in *(17)*] have been shown to exert varying effects, probably resulting from the drug-selected cell model systems used for study. These cell lines, which express high levels of MRP, may contain other MDR pathways which may be abrogated by these compounds.

Unlike the natural product drugs, no active drug efflux pathway has been described for unconjugated alkylating agents or platinum drugs. However, reduced cellular amounts of these agents is a phenotype often observed in drug-resistant cells, particularly those selected for resistance in vitro. Alkylating agents and platinum drugs may enter cells by passive diffusion or carrier-mediated transport. Decreased expression of certain amino acid transport systems has been shown to be associated with resistance to melphalan and nitrogen mustard *(18,19)*. In a panel of twelve cell lines derived from tumors of ovarian cancer patients who were either untreated or treated with platinum-based chemotherapy, cisplatin accumulation varied fivefold, but was not associated in any direct way with cisplatin sensitivity *(20)*. Evidence for cisplatin uptake by passive diffusion has been provided by studies in which cisplatin uptake was shown to be nonsaturable, even up to its solubility limit, and not inhibited by structural analogs. Cisplatin accumulation has also been shown to be partially energy dependent, ouabain inhibitable, sodium dependent, and affected by membrane potential and cAMP levels which indicate that a carrier-mediated transport protein may have some role in accumulation. Several approaches have been utilized in vitro to circumvent these passive and facilitated transport processes in order to enhance cellular drug accumulation. For example, amphotericin B, a membrane channel forming antibiotic, has been shown to selectively enhance cisplatin uptake in human ovarian cancer cell lines *(21)*. Two calmodulin antagonists have also been shown to increase cisplatin uptake in cisplatin-resistant ovarian cancer cell lines, restoring their intracellular platinum levels to that of the drug-sensitive parental cell line from which they were derived.

### 3.2. Drug Inactivation

A wide variety of detoxication pathways exist that enable a cell to inactivate cytotoxic drugs. The mechanisms that have received the most attention in mediating drug resistance in ovarian cancer include increased levels of glutathione, glutathione S-transferases, and metallothioneins. Glutathione (GSH), the most abundant cellular non-protein thiol, may be present at concentrations as high as 10 m$M$. The spontaneous conjugation of glutathione with melphalan, chlorambucil, and cisplatin has been demonstrated in vitro *(22)* and elevated levels of GSH have been found to be associated with resistance to alkylating agents and platinum drugs *(23)*. Based on these results, several investigators have studied the effects of GSH depletion on drug sensitivity using buthionine sulfoximine (BSO), an inhibitor of γ-glutamylcysteine synthetase which catalyzes the rate-limiting step in GSH synthesis. BSO has been shown to clearly modulate melphalan sensitivity in vitro and in vivo *(24)*. The results demonstrating an effect of GSH depletion on cisplatin sensitivity, however, have been less convincing. Hamilton et al. *(25)* reported a 4.3-fold enhancement of cisplatin cytotoxicity in a cisplatin-resistant ovarian cancer cell line following BSO treatment. In contrast, Andrews et al. *(26)* reported an enhancement of iproplatin cytotoxicity, but not cisplatin or carboplatin cytotoxicity in cells treated with BSO. A differential effect of BSO on sensitization by platinum (II) and platinum (IV) compounds has also been shown. Other studies, however, have shown minimal potentiation of cisplatin and other platinum drug sensitivities in cell lines pretreated with BSO. Overall, the effect of BSO on drug sensitivity has been unpredictable with respect to the various cell lines and platinum drugs examined.

The glutathione-S-transferases (GSTs), are a multigene family whose members catalyze the conjugation of glutathione with electrophilic drugs. They have been implicated in resistance to alkylating agents, anthracyclines, and platinum drugs. Direct evidence favoring this concept comes from transfection studies, which have demonstrated that overexpression of the GSTπ isoform confers resistance to etoposide, ethacrynic acid, cisplatin, and adriamycin *(27)*. Furthermore, transfection of an antisense GSTπ cDNA was shown to sensitize cells two- to threefold to adriamycin, cisplatin, melphalan, and etoposide *(28)*. In vitro studies have also shown that GSTs can catalyze the conjugation of a variety of drugs with GSH. Conflicting data, however, have been reported regarding the relationship between drug resistance and increased levels of activity of GSTs in ovarian cancer cell lines. In clinical material, the role of GSTs in predicting patient response to chemotherapy has been examined using a variety of techniques. The results of five recently published studies indicate that neither tumor GST activity nor expression level is predictive of response to chemotherapy in ovarian cancer patients *(29–33)*.

Owing to their high cysteine content, the metallothionein (MT) proteins have also been suggested to inactivate electrophilic anticancer drugs. Compelling evidence for a role of MTs in drug resistance has been provided by Kelley et al. *(34)* who demonstrated that overexpression of MT-II$_A$ in mouse C127 cells resulted in resistance to cisplatin, melphalan, and chlorambucil. In addition, embryonic fibroblasts isolated from MT-null mice were shown to be hypersensitive to a variety of chemotherapeutic drugs *(35)*. The contribution of MTs to drug resistance, however, is presently unknown. In in vitro models, increased MT levels have been found to be associated with anticancer drug resistance in some cell lines *(34,36)*, but not others *(37,38)*. In an immunohistochemical analysis of ovarian tumor specimens, Germain et al. *(39)* found no correlation between MT expression and patient response to chemotherapy.

### 3.3. Altered Drug Target

Decreased expression or alteration of a gene or its product may enable a cell to escape the cytotoxic effect of certain chemotherapeutic agents. This is of relevance to ovarian cancer in the context of β-tubulin. Paclitaxel binds to and stabilizes polymerized microtubules causing cell cycle arrest prior to mitosis (G$_2$/M). This can either prevent the cell from undergoing mitosis or may result in an aberrant mitosis that leads to cell death. Therefore, alterations in β-tubulin can prevent paclitaxel binding and enable a cell to circumvent the cytotoxic effects of this drug. Several reports have described such alterations in β-tubulin in paclitaxel resistant cells. For example, differential expression of the various isotypes of β-tubulin have been observed and recently, specific mutations in the M40 isotype of β-tubulin were found to be associated with paclitaxel resistance in a human ovarian cancer cell line *(40)*. There have been no reports thus far, however, describing β-tubulin mutations in tumor specimens from ovarian cancer patients.

### 3.4. Drug Sequestration

Trapping or sequestering drugs into cellular compartments is another MDR mechanism that a cell can utilize to prevent active drugs from reaching their cytotoxic targets.

LRP, a protein originally found to be overexpressed in a non-P-glycoprotein MDR lung cancer cell line, was identified as the human major vault protein *(41)*. Transfection of the *LRP* cDNA into the drug-sensitive A2780 human ovarian cancer cell line failed to confer resistance to doxorubicin, vincristine, or etoposide. This result is not surprising because in rat liver cells, vaults are known to be complex ribonucleoprotein complexes containing at least four proteins and an RNA component. Overexpression of multiple vault proteins may be required in order to observe an increased functional effect. The cytoplasm contains the majority of the vault complexes, while a small fraction is localized to the nuclear membrane and nuclear pore complexes *(42)*.

A direct role for LRP in MDR is circumstantial and most of the evidence implicating this protein are offered by *LRP* expression studies. Many cell lines selected for resistance using a variety of drugs express *LRP* mRNA in the absence of *MDR1* gene expression. *MRP*, but not *MDR1*, is often found to be expressed concomitantly with *LRP*. In ovarian cancer, LRP was found to be present in 15 of 20 (75%) untreated ovarian tumors *(43)* and in biopsies from patients treated with chemotherapy, 44 of 57 (77%) specimens immunostained positive using an LRP monoclonal antibody *(9)*. In this study, LRP-positive patients had poorer responses to chemotherapy and shorter overall survival as compared to LRP-negative patients. An understanding of the proteins that interact with LRP will aid in elucidating the function of this putative MDR mechanism. Perhaps antisense or gene "knock-out" strategies will solidify a functional role for this vault protein in MDR.

### 3.5. Increased DNA Repair

Once platinum drugs form cytotoxic DNA adducts, cells must either repair or tolerate the damage in order to survive. Removal of platinum-DNA lesions is believed to occur primarily by the process of nucleotide excision repair (NER). NER involves the activity of a large number of proteins that function to remove bulky and helix-distorting DNA lesions. The study of cell lines defective in NER has been critical in understanding this complex system. Such cell lines include those derived from patients with the repair-deficient syndrome xeroderma pigmentosum (XP) and a rodent model of the syndrome. All of these mutant cells are sensitive to DNA damaging agents that form bulky DNA adducts such as UV light and cisplatin. Many of the nucleotide excision repair proteins have now been purified, characterized, and their corresponding genes have been cloned. Furthermore, human nucleotide excision repair has been reconstituted in an in vitro system using highly purified protein components *(44)*.

Mammalian NER removes DNA damage as part of an oligonucleotide 24–32 residues long. DNA damage is thought to be recognized by the zinc-finger protein XPA in association with the heterotrimeric replication protein RPA. The XPA-RPA complex is then thought to recruit the basal transcription factor TFIIH, which contains eight subunits, to the site of damage. Two of TFIIH's subunits, XPB and XPD, have helicase activities, which are believed to function in opening up the DNA around the damage thus enabling structure-specific nucleases to incise the DNA. The ERCC1-XPF heterodimer is thought to cut the strand on the 5′ side of the damage and the XPG protein incises on the 3′ side. Principal sites of cleavage flanking a d(GpTpG)Pt 1,3-*intrastrand* crosslink in a closed-circular duplex DNA substrate were identified as the ninth phosphodiester bond 3′ to the lesion and the 16th phosphodiester bond 5′ to the lesion *(44)*. DNA polymerase $\delta$ or $\epsilon$ and two accessory proteins, replication factor

C (RFC) and proliferating-cell nuclear antigen (PCNA), participate in the DNA synthesis regard to fill the gap left by removal of the damaged DNA. The DNA is joined by the action of DNA ligase. In addition to the proteins described above, the incision stage of the reaction requires the protein XPC, which may form a heterodimer with the protein hHR23B and may participate in the recognition of damage, as well as stabilizing an incision-reaction intermediate.

Among the types of DNA lesions formed by cisplatin, the interstrand crosslink poses a distinct problem in that both DNA strands are damaged. Although this lesion represents only a small percentage of the platinum-DNA adducts formed, some research supports the idea that they are the most cytotoxic. Repair of interstrand crosslinks in eukaryotic cells is not well understood, but genetic studies in *Escherichia coli* suggest that it may involve both NER and recombination processes *(45)*. It should be mentioned that although other NER defective cell lines are sensitive to DNA crosslinking agents, ERCC1 and XPF(ERCC4) mutants are hypersensitive to these compounds suggesting that these proteins play a unique role in interstrand crosslink repair in addition to their role in the normal NER process. Furthermore, these proteins have yeast homologs [Rad10 (*ERCC1*) and Rad1 (*XPF*)] that are clearly involved in recombination. Recently, a hamster *ERCC1*-knockout cell line was found to be defective in the processing of heteroduplex structures that form during recombination *(46)*.

Another process that should also be mentioned when discussing platinum-DNA adduct repair is transcription-coupled repair. NER can occur preferentially in actively transcribed genes relative to the overall genome. This enhanced repair, termed transcription-coupled repair, is limited to genes that are transcribed by RNA polymerase II and is now thought to involve CSA and CSB, proteins which are defective in Cockayne's syndrome patients *(47)*. Although transcription-coupled repair, like overall genome repair, has been studied most extensively with UV-damaged DNA, there is evidence that platinum-DNA lesions are repaired at higher rates in actively transcribed genes relative to silent genes and noncoding DNA.

The capacity to rapidly and efficiently repair DNA damage clearly plays a role in determining a tumor cell's sensitivity to platinum drugs and other DNA damaging agents. There is recent evidence that suggests that cell lines derived from tumors, which are unusually sensitive to cisplatin, such as testicular nonseminomatous germ cell tumors, are deficient in their ability to repair platinum-DNA adducts *(48)*. Similarly, the relative unresponsiveness of nonsmall cell lung cancer as compared to small cell lung cancer has been associated with an elevated DNA repair capacity *(49)*. Increased repair of platinum-DNA lesions in cisplatin-resistant cell lines as compared to their sensitive counterparts has been shown in several human cancer cell lines including ovarian *(50,51)*, breast *(52)*, and glioma *(53)*, as well as murine leukemia cell lines *(54)*. Evidence for increased repair of cisplatin interstrand crosslinks in specific gene and nongene regions in cisplatin-resistant cell lines has also been demonstrated *(50,51)*. These studies have been done using a variety of in vivo methods including unscheduled DNA synthesis, host cell reactivation of cisplatin-damaged plasmid DNA, atomic absorption spectrometry, quantitative PCR, and renaturing agarose gel electrophoresis. The recent development of highly specific assays for nucleotide excision repair should make it possible to both confirm the hypothesized increase in nucleotide excision repair capacity in resistant cell lines and to isolate the molecular determinants of this resistance mechanism *(44)*.

The molecular basis for the increased platinum-DNA adduct repair capacity of cisplatin resistant cell lines is largely unknown. In contrast, the molecular cause of increased DNA repair is known in some cell lines resistant to other DNA damaging agents such as the chloroethylnitrosoureas (CENUs), where there exists a clear association between increased expression of $0^6$-methylguanine-DNA methyltransferase and decreased drug sensitivity *(55)*. Unlike the direct repair mechanism involved in the correction of adducts caused by the CENU's, the repair of platinum-DNA adducts is complex and involves several proteins. Expression levels of the *ERCC1* and *XPA* genes have been shown to be higher in malignant tissue from ovarian cancer patients resistant to platinum-based therapy compared with those responsive to treatment *(56)*. It is not clear, however, whether *XPA* or *ERCC1* are involved in the rate-limiting step of the NER process. While *XPA* expression was shown to correct the NER deficiency in a mutant cell line, overexpression of the same construct had little effect on repair activity *(57)*. In addition, expression of *ERCC1* has been shown to correct NER deficiencies in *ERCC1* mutant cell lines, whereas overexpression of the ERCC1 protein appears to sensitize cells to cisplatin and inhibit the repair of interstrand crosslinks. Increased levels of XPE, a putative DNA repair protein that recognizes many DNA lesions including platinum-DNA adducts, has been observed in tumor cell lines resistant to cisplatin. It should be noted, however, that XPE is not a necessary component for the in vitro reconstitution of NER *(44)*. Increased expression of DNA polymerases α and β have been observed in cisplatin resistant cell lines and increased expression of these polymerases, as well as DNA ligase, has recently been described in human tumors following cisplatin exposure in vivo *(53)*. The possible significance of these findings is unclear since the primary polymerases involved in NER are thought to be DNA polymerases δ or ε. Although it is probably not involved in NER, DNA polymerase β may be involved in translesion DNA synthesis.

Another active area of research addressing the relationship between DNA repair and platinum drug sensitivity involves the study of platinum-DNA damage-recognition proteins. Binding of proteins to platinum-DNA lesions may serve to recruit the NER machinery to the site of damage or, alternatively, may shield the adduct from recognition by the excision nuclease. In addition to the putative repair proteins XPA and XPE, which were aforementioned, there are several proteins that are known to bind cisplatin-damaged DNA. Included in this group are the nonhistone chromatin proteins HMG1 and HMG2, human upstream binding factor (hUBF), human structure specific recognition factor (SSRP1), and yeast intrastrand crosslink recognition protein (Ixr1). These proteins are all HMG-domain proteins containing one or more HMG1 DNA binding motifs. These structures bind selectively to DNA modified with cisplatin but not its inactive isomer transplatin. Interestingly, two HMG-domain proteins have been shown to inhibit the repair of cisplatin-DNA adducts in an in vitro system *(58)*. Furthermore, a yeast strain with inactivated Ixr1 exhibited significantly less sensitivity to cisplatin than its parental, wild-type strain *(59)*. Recently, the very abundant chromatin protein histone H1 was shown to bind preferentially to cisplatin-modified DNA with an affinity much higher than that of HMG1. In another recent paper, the TATA box binding protein (TBP) was found to bind to cisplatin and UV-damaged DNA with high affinity *(60)*. Despite the abundance of candidates, a correlation between the expression of a platinum-DNA adduct binding protein and cytotoxicity or platinum-DNA adduct repair has not been observed in human tumor cell lines. Therefore, the significance of these findings remains unclear.

There is an abundance of evidence to support a role for increased repair of platinum-DNA adducts in resistance to platinum-based chemotherapy, but which protein alterations are critical remains to be determined. Nonetheless, it should be possible to enhance the efficacy of platinum drugs and classical alkylating agents by inhibiting the repair process. Agents that have been employed in this pursuit to date include nucleoside analogs such as gemcitabine, fludarabine, and cytarabine, the ribonucleotide reductase inhibitor, hydroxyurea, and the inhibitor of DNA polymerases α and γ, and aphidicolin. All of these agents interfere with the repair synthesis stage of various repair processes including nucleotide excision repair. It should be noted that these compounds are also likely to effect DNA replication and as such should not be strictly characterized as repair inhibitors. The potentiation of cisplatin cytotoxicity by treatment with aphidicolin has been studied extensively in human ovarian cancer cell lines. Whereas some studies have demonstrated a clear synergism with this drug combination *(61)*, others have not *(62)*. In an in vivo mouse model of human ovarian cancer, the combined treatment of cisplatin and aphidicolin glycinate, a water soluble form of aphidicolin, was found to be significantly more effective than cisplatin alone *(63)*. The combination of cytarabine and hydroxyurea was found synergistic with cisplatin in a human colon cancer cell line *(64)* and in rat mammary-carcinoma cell lines *(65)*. Moreover, the modulatory effect of cytarabine and hydroxyurea on cisplatin was associated with an increase in DNA interstrand crosslinks in both cellular systems. Similarly, the drugs gemcitabine and fludarabine have both shown synergistic cytotoxicity with cisplatin in in vitro systems. Both of these drugs have been shown to interfere with the removal of cisplatin-DNA adducts. A clinical trial of cisplatin and gemcitabine in relapsed breast and ovarian cancer patients is currently underway. The likelihood of a significant improvement in the therapeutic index of cisplatin in refractory patients by the coadministration of a repair inhibitor, however, is limited by the multifactorial nature typical of resistant tumor cells.

### 3.6. Increased DNA Damage Tolerance

Platinum-DNA damage tolerance is a phenotype that has been observed in both cisplatin-resistant cells derived from chemotherapy-refractory ovarian cancer patients and cells selected for primary cisplatin resistance in vitro. The contribution of this mechanism to resistance is significant and it has been shown to correlate strongly with cisplatin resistance, as well as resistance to other drugs in two ovarian cancer model systems. Like other cisplatin resistance mechanisms, this phenotype may result from alterations in a variety of cellular pathways. One apparently involves the ability of some cisplatin resistant cells to acquire a different spectrum of cisplatin-DNA lesions than sensitive cells *(50)*. An additional component of DNA damage tolerance which has been observed in cisplatin-resistant cells involves dysfunction of the DNA mismatch repair (MMR) system. The main function of the MMR system is to scan newly synthesized DNA and remove mismatches that result from nucleotide incorporation errors made by the DNA polymerases. In addition to causing genomic instability, it has been reported that loss of MMR is associated with low-level cisplatin resistance, and that the selection of cells in culture for resistance to this drug often yields cell lines that have lost a functional MMR system *(66)*. The human colon carcinoma cell line HCT116 is MMR-deficient because of a deletion in one allele of *hMLH1* and a mutation in the other copy of the gene. The HCT116+ch3 subline was rendered MMR-proficient by transfer of a complete chromosome 3, which contains a functional copy of the *hMLH1* gene. The HCT116+ch2 cell line was created by transferring chromosome 2 into the parental HCT116 cell line; this cell line serves as a control for the microcell-mediated chromosome transfer process since chromosome 2 does not contain the *hMLH1* gene. The HCT116+ch2 cells are 2.1-fold resistant to cisplatin and 1.3-fold resistant to carboplatin relative to the HCT116+ch3 cells *(67)*. Hence, the MMR-deficient subline exhibits low-level cisplatin resistance relative to the MMR-proficient subline. A similar system has allowed the impact of hMSH2 function on platinum drug sensitivity to be determined. HEC59 is a human endometrial carcinoma cell line, which is MMR-deficient because of mutations in both alleles of *hMSH2*. In HEC59+ch2 cells, the MMR-deficiency has been corrected by transferring a full-length chromosome 2, which contains the *hMSH2* gene. The MMR-deficient HEC59 cells are 1.8-fold resistant to cisplatin and 1.5-fold resistant to carboplatin relative to the MMR-proficient subline HEC59+ch2 cells. In contrast, neither of the pairs of MMR-proficient and -deficient cells differed with respect to their sensitivity to the cisplatin analog oxaliplatin *(67)*. Although the level of resistance that accompanies loss of mismatch repair is relatively small, loss of MMR has been shown to be sufficient to account for the failure of treatment in model systems *(68)*.

These data are consistent with the hypothesis that the MMR system serves as a detector of cisplatin and carboplatin DNA adducts but not of oxaliplatin adducts. MSH2 alone, and in combination with hMSH6, has been shown to bind to cisplatin 1,2-d(GpG) intrastrand adducts with high efficiency *(69)*. Additionally, hMSH2 and hMLH1-containing protein-DNA complexes were observed using mobility shift assays when nuclear extracts of the MMR-proficient cell lines were incubated with DNA preincubated with cisplatin, but not with oxaliplatin, confirming a difference in the capacity of MMR-deficient and -proficient cell lines to detect the lesions produced by cisplatin vs oxaliplatin. These data suggest that MMR recognition of damage may trigger a programmed cell death pathway rendering cells with intact MMR more sensitive to DNA damage *(67)*. In addition to the data suggesting that MMR may function as a DNA damage sensor, MMR deficiency may also create an environment that promotes the accumulation of mutations in drug sensitivity genes.

The putative basis for the cytotoxicity of *N*-methyl-*N*'-nitro-*N*-nitrosoguanidine (MNNG) and 6-thioguanine involves repeated rounds of synthesis past DNA lesions followed by recognition and subsequent removal of the newly synthesized strand by the MMR system. This futile cycling is believed to generate DNA strand gaps and breaks which can lead to cell death *(70)*. If platinum lesions are also recognized by the MMR system, this same futile cycling may occur within MMR-proficient cells. Loss of MMR would then increase the cell's ability to tolerate platinum-DNA lesions. Replicative bypass, defined as the ability of the replication complex to synthesize DNA past an adduct, has been demonstrated to occur for cisplatin damage *(71)*. Furthermore, this process of translesion DNA synthesis appears to be enhanced in human ovarian cancer cell lines resistant to cisplatin *(71)*. However, a correlation between increased replicative bypass and MMR deficiency has not been demonstrated. Enhanced replicative bypass can be viewed independently as a component of DNA damage tolerance and may occur by a variety of mechanisms. DNA polymerase $\beta$, the most inaccurate of the

DNA polymerases, may function in this process. Interestingly, the activity of this enzyme was found to be significantly increased in cells derived from a human malignant glioma resistant to cisplatin as compared to its drug sensitive counterpart *(53)*.

The tolerance mechanisms described above are related primarily to cisplatin resistance. Because the platinum-DNA damage-tolerance phenotype is often associated with cross-resistance to other unrelated chemotherapeutic drugs, the existence of a more general resistance mechanism must be considered *(20)*. One possible explanation is that the platinum-DNA damage tolerance phenotype is the result of decreased expression or inactivation of one or more components of the programmed cell death pathway. The sequence of events that occur following platinum-DNA adduct formation that lead to cell death are unknown. Cells exposed to cytotoxic levels of cisplatin display the phenotypic and biochemical characteristics of apoptosis. These characteristics, which include chromatin condensation, membrane blebbing, oligonucleosomal DNA fragmentation, and caspase-mediated poly (ADP-ribose) polymerase (PARP) cleavage, have been documented in both cisplatin-sensitive and -resistant cell lines *(72)*. The presence of these apoptotic features following drug-induced cell death suggests that a pathway is present in cells that is responsible for detecting DNA damage and transmitting a signal to the apoptotic machinery. The process of signaling cell death may depend on a variety of factors including 1) cell cycle phase; 2) the influence of mitogenic signaling pathways; and 3) the relative expression of members of the *bcl-2* gene family.

Following exposure to cisplatin, tumor cells arrest in the $G_1$, S, and $G_2$/M phases of the cell cycle *(73,74)*. During this time, cells attempt to repair DNA damage and they also sort through a cascade of signals that determine their fate. This dynamic process is not currently understood, however, several studies have begun to elucidate the proteins that participate in these events. For example, the arrest of cells at the G1 checkpoint following DNA damage is associated with elevated levels and activity of *p53 (75)*. Several downstream events subsequently occur including increased expression of the cdk inhibitor *p21*[WAF1/Cip1] and the growth and DNA damage-inducible protein GADD45. Inhibition of the cell cycle by *p21*[WAF1/Cip1] may be important in allowing cells time to repair DNA damage. This is supported by recent evidence showing that *p21*-deficient cells are hypersensitive to DNA damaging agents *(76)*. The function of the GADD proteins is unknown, however, GADD45 may interact with PCNA to prevent it from assisting DNA polymerases in replicating the damaged DNA template *(77)*. It should be noted that these genes may also be upregulated in the absence of functional *p53*. This may be a factor in the variable results that have been reported from studies attempting to associate platinum drug sensitivity with *p53* status. For example, some cell lines containing mutant *p53* exhibit decreased sensitivity to cisplatin and other chemotherapeutic drugs. Transfection studies, however, have yielded conflicting results. Fan et al. *(78)* showed that transfection of a dominant-negative *p53* mutant gene sensitized MCF-7 breast cancer cells to cisplatin, whereas Eliopoulos and colleagues *(79)* reported that overexpression of a temperature-sensitive *p53* mutant conferred protection from cisplatin-induced apoptosis. Another study showed that adenovirus-mediated transfer of a wild-type *p53* gene into a variety of cancer cell lines resulted in increased cisplatin sensitivity, regardless of *p53* status *(80)*. Thus, the failure of the *p53*-dependent $G_1$ checkpoint in arresting the cell cycle following DNA damage may not be paramount for determining cell survival.

In the absence of functional *p53*, tumor cells will progress through the $G_1/S$ boundary and subsequently arrest in S or $G_2/M$ following cisplatin exposure. This has been shown to occur in CHO cells lacking functional *p53* *(81)*. Evidence for arrest in $G_2/M$ has been provided by Demarq et al. *(74)* using DNA repair deficient CHO/UV41 cells in which a prominent $G_2$ arrest was observed following cisplatin treatment. After a protracted delay, these cells experienced an aberrant mitosis and eventually exhibited apoptotic features. One area of investigation that has not been thoroughly examined is whether the cell cycle profiles of platinum-drug sensitive and -resistant cells are similar following drug exposure. In one study, Vaisman et al. *(73)* showed that cisplatin exposure resulted in similar cell cycle alterations in cisplatin-sensitive and -resistant human ovarian cancer cells. This suggests that if platinum drug-sensitive and -resistant cells exhibit similar cell cycle profiles following platinum-DNA damage, then the platinum-DNA damage-tolerance phenotype may reside in the response of sensitive and resistant cells to other intra- and extracellular signals. A clue to the mechanism(s) by which cells activate programmed cell death in the presence of DNA damage is offered by studies involving cell-cycle checkpoint abrogators. It has been known for many years that caffeine, pentoxyfilline, and staurosporine enhance cellular sensitivity to DNA damaging agents. Some recent insight into the basis for this effect was provided by Bunch et al. *(81)*. In their study, the incubation of cells with 7-hydroxystaurosporine (UCN-01) following cisplatin treatment resulted in rapid progression of the cells through S phase and into $G_2/M$ at which time they subsequently died. This effect was shown to be even more pronounced in cells lacking functional *p53*, perhaps resulting from a larger fraction of the cells being available for S and $G_2/M$ arrest. Based on these data, it is conceivable that drug-sensitive cells may self-abrogate their own checkpoints in response to DNA damage, whereas resistant cells may not receive or may ignore such signals. If these signals are common to most chemotherapeutic drugs, this could explain the broad cross-resistance phenotype that is frequently observed. At this time, it is not clear what signaling pathways influence the response of cells to platinum drugs, however, it has been shown that activators or inhibitors of known signal transduction pathways can influence platinum drug sensitivity. For example, treatment of various cell lines with tamoxifen, EGF, IL-1a, TNF-a bombesin, and rapamycin enhance cisplatin cytotoxicity. Also, the expression of certain proto-oncogenes including Ha-*Ras*, v-*abl*, and Her2/*neu* has been shown in some instances to promote cell survival following cisplatin exposure.

The sensitivity of tumor cells to platinum drugs and other anticancer agents may also occur if the commitment step of apoptosis is attenuated. An example of this is provided by the *bcl-2* gene family, which encodes a group of pro- and antiapoptotic proteins that regulate mitochondrial function and intracellular calcium concentration. These proteins function as a cell survival/cell death rheostat by forming homo- and heterodimers with one another. The antiapoptotic bcl-2 and bcl-XL proteins are localized in the outer mitochondrial membrane and may be involved in the formation or regulation of transmembrane channels. Overexpression of *bcl-2* or *bcl-$X_L$* has been shown to prevent disruption of the mitochondrial transmembrane potential and to prolong cell survival in some cells following exposure to cisplatin and other anticancer drugs *(82)*. The function of these proteins is negated, however, in the presence of high levels of pro-apoptotic proteins such as BAX, another *bcl-2* family member. BAX, which forms homodimers when the ratio of pro- to antiapoptotic proteins is high, is believed to contribute to the formation of a pore or channel in the outer mitochondrial membrane that enables cytochrome C and APAF1 (apoptotic protease activating factor-1) to flow into the cytoplasm *(83)*. This leads to the activation of caspases that specifically cleave vital cellular proteins. Incubating cells with conventional apoptosis inducers in the presence of the broad caspase inhibitor z-VADfmk prevents PARP cleavage and oligonucleosomal DNA fragmentation which indicates that caspase activation is a relatively late event in the apoptotic pathway *(84)*. Thus, inhibiting the late stages of programmed cell death does not confer a resistance phenotype, it may only change the mode of cell death.

## 4. Conclusion

It is apparent that in model systems of cisplatin resistance may mechanisms appear to participate. Presently, it would be helpful to have at least two additional pieces of information. First, it would be helpful to know if the changes observed in model systems are of clinical relevance. This may be facilitated as the various comprehensive gene scanning technologies are applied to clinical samples from cisplatin and paclitaxel responding and nonresponding patients. The second relates to a more obvious indication of how significant observed correlative changes associated with resistance actually contribute to resistance. Hopefully, the future will hold the answers to these questions as these should improve our ability to treat ovarian cancer.

## Acknowledgment

Thomas C. Hamilton was supported by CA51228 and CA56916 from the National Cancer Institute.

## References

1. Ozols, R., Rubin, S., Thomas, G., and Robboy, S. (1997) Epithelial ovarian cancer, in *Principles and Practice of Gynecologic Ocology* (Hoskins, W., Perez, C., and Young, R., eds.), 2nd edition, Lippincott, Philadelphia, PA, pp. 919–986.
2. Barry, M., Behnke, C., and Eastman, A. (1990) Activation of programmed cell death (apoptosis) by cisplatin, other anticancer drugs, toxins and hyperthermia. *Biochem. Pharmacol.* **40,** 2353–2362.
3. Algan, O., Stobbe, C., Helt, A., Hanks, G., and Chapman, J. (1996) Radiation inactivation of human prostate cancer cells: the role of apoptosis. *Radiat. Res.* **146,** 267–275.
4. Blommaert, F., van Kijk-Knijnenburg, H., Dijt, F., den Engelse, L., Baan, R., Berends, F., and Fichtinger-Schepman, A. (1995) Formation of DNA adducts by the anticancer drug carboplatin: different nucleotide sequence preferences in vitro and in cells. *Biochemistry* **34,** 8474–8480.
5. Goldstein, L. J., Galski, H., Fojo, A., Willingham, M., Lai, S. L., Gazdar, A., and Pirker, R.(1989) Expression of a multidrug resistance gene in human cancers. *J. Natl. Cancer Inst.* **81,** 116–124.
6. Bourhis, J., Goldstein, L. J., Riou, G., Pastan, I., Gottesman, M. M., and Benard, J. (1989) Expression of a human multidrug resistance gene in ovarian carcinomas. *Cancer Res.* **49,** 5062–5065.
7. Holzmayer, T. A., Hilsenbeck, S., Von Hoff, D. D., and Roninson, I. B. (1992) Clinical correlates of MDR1 (P-glycoprotein) gene expression in ovarian and small-cell lung carcinomas. *J. Natl. Cancer Inst.* **84,** 1458–1460.
8. Kavallaris, M., Leary, J., Barrett, J., and Friedlander, M. (1996) MDR1 and multidrug resistance-associated protein (MRP) gene expression in epithelial ovarian tumors. *Cancer Lett.* **102,** 7–16.
9. Izquierdo, M., Zee, A. v. d., Vermorken, J., Valk, P. v. d., Belien, J., Giaccone, G., et al. (1995) Drug resistance-associated marker LRP for prediction of response to chemotherapy and prognoses in advanced ovarian carcinoma. *J. Natl. Cancer Inst.* **87,** 1230–1237.
10. Tsuruo, T., Iida, H., Tsukagoshi, S., and Sakurai, Y. (1981) Overcoming of vincristine resistance in P388 leukemia in vivo and in vitro through enhanced cytotoxicity of vincristine and vinblastine by verapamil. *Cancer Res.* **41,** 1967–1972.

11. Ozols, R., Cunnion, R., Klecker Jr., R., Hamilton, T., Y, O., Parrillo, J., and Young, R. (1987) Verapamil and adriamycin in the treatment of drug resistant ovarian cancer patients. *J. Clin. Oncol.* **5,** 641–647.

12. Marquardt, D., McCrone, S., and Center, M. S. (1990) Mechansims of multidrug resistance in HL60 cells: detection of resistance-associated proteins with antibodies against synthetic peptides that correspond to the deduced sequence of P-glycoprotein. *Cancer Res.* **50,** 1426–1430.

13. Cole, S., Bhardwaj, G., Gerlach, J., Mackie, J., Grant, C., Almquist, K., et al. (1992) Overexpression of a transporter gene in a multidrug-resistant human lung cancer cell line. *Science* **258,** 1650–1654.

14. Ishikawa, T. (1992) The ATP-dependent glutathione S-conjugate export pump. *Trends Biochem. Sci.* **17,** 164–166.

15. Leier, I., Jedlitschky, G., Buchholz, U., Cole, S., Deeley, R., and Keppler, D. (1994) The MPR gene encodes an ATP-dependent export pump for leukotriene C4 and structurally related conjugates. *J. Biol. Chem.* **45,** 27,807–27,810.

16. Muller, M., Meijer, C., Zaman, G., Borst, P., Scheper, R., Mulder, N., et al. (1994) Overexpression of the gene encoding the multidrug resistance-associated protein results in increased ATP-dependent glutathione S-conjugate transport. *Proc. Natl. Acad. Sci. USA* **91,** 13,033–13,037.

17. Twentyman, P. and Versantvoort, C. (1996) Experimental modulation of MRP (multidrug resistance-associated protein)-mediated resistance. *Eur. J. Cancer* **32A,** 1002–1009.

18. Wolpert, M. K. and Ruddon, R. W. (1969) A study on the mechanisms of resistance to nitrogen mustard (HN2) in Ehrlich ascites tumor cells: comparison of uptake of HN2-14C into sensitive and resistant cells. *Cancer Res.* **29,** 873–879.

19. Redwood, W. R. and Colvin, M. (1980) Transport of melphalan by sensitive and resistant L1210 cells. *Cancer Res.* **40,** 1144–1149.

20. Johnson, S., Laub, P., Beesley, J., Ozols, R., and Hamilton, T. (1997) Increased platinum-DNA damage tolerance is associated with cisplatin resistance and cross-resistance to various chemotherapeutic agents in unrelated human ovarian cancer cell lines. *Cancer Res.* **57,** 850–856.

21. Sharp, S. Y., Mistry, P., Valenti, M. R., Bryant, A. P., and Kelland, L. R. (1994) Selective potentiation of platinum drug cytotoxicity in cisplatin-sensitive and -resistant human ovarian carcinoma cell lines by amphotericin B. *Cancer Chemother. Pharmacol.* **35,** 137–143.

22. Ishikawa, T. and Ali-Osman, F. (1993) Glutathione-associated cis-diamminedichloroplatinum (II) metabolism and ATP-dependent efflux from leukemia cells. *J. Biol. Chem.* **268,** 20,116–20,125.

23. Godwin, A., Meister, A., O'Dwyer, P., Huang, C., Hamilton, T., and Anderson, M. (1992) High resistance to cisplatin in human ovarian cancer cell lines is associated with marked increase in glutathione synthesis. *Proc. Natl. Acad. Sci. USA* **89,** 3070–3074.

24. O'Dwyer, P., Hamilton, T., Young, R., LaCreta, F., Carp, N., Tew, K., et al. (1992) Depletion of glutathione in normal and malignant human cells in vivo by buthionine sulfoximine: clinical and biochemical results. *J. Natl. Cancer Inst.* **84,** 264–267.

25. Hamilton, T., Winker, M., Louie, K., Batist, G., Behrens, B., Tsuruo, T., et al. (1985) Augmentation of adriamycin, melphalan and cisplatin cytotoxicity in drug-resistant and -sensitive human ovarian cancer cell lines by buthionine sulfoximine mediated glutathione depletion. *Biochem. Pharmacol.* **34,** 2583–2586.

26. Andrews, P. A., Murphy, M. P., and Howell, S. B. (1985) Differential potentiation of alkylating and platinating agent cytotoxicity in human ovarian carcinoma cells by glutathione depletion. *Cancer Res.* **45,** 6250–6253.

27. Nakagawa, K., Saijo, N., Tsuchida, S., Sakai, M., Tsunokawa, Y., Yokota, J., et al. (1990) Glutathione S-transferase p as a determinant of drug resistance in transfectant cell lines. *J. Biol. Chem.* **265,** 4296–4301.

28. Ban, N., Takahashi, Y., Takayama, T., Kura, T., Katahira, T., Sakamaki, S., and Niitsu, Y. (1996) Transfection of glutathione S-transferase (GST)-p antisense complementary DNA increases the sensitivity of a colon cancer cell line to adriamycin, cisplatin, melphalan, and etoposide. *Cancer Res.* **56,** 3577–3582.

29. Ghazal-Aswad, S., Hogarth, L., Hall, A. G., George, M., Sinha, D. P., Lind, M., et al. (1996) The relationship between tumor glutathione concentration, glutathione S-transferase isoenzyme expression and response to single agent carboplatin in epithelial ovarian cancer patients. *Br. J. Cancer* **74,** 468–473.

30. Wrigley, E. C., McGown, A. T., Buckley, H., Hall, A., and Crowther, D. (1996) Glutathione-S-transferase activity and isoenzyme levels measured by two methods in ovarian cancer, and their value as markers of disease outcome. *Br. J. Cancer* **73,** 763–769.

31. Tanner, B., Hengstler, J. G., Dietrich, B., Henrich, M., Steinberg, P., Weikel, W., et al. (1997) Glutathione, glutathione S-transferase a and p, and aldehyde dehydrogenase content in relationship to drug resistance in ovarian cancer. *Gynecol. Oncol.* **65,** 54–62.

32. Ferrandina, G., Scambia, G., Damia, G., Tagliabue, G., Fagotti, A., Benedetti Panici, P., et al. (1997) Glutathione S-transferase activity in epithelial ovarian cancer: association with response to chemotherapy and disease outcome. *Annals Oncol.* **8,** 343–350.

33. Codegoni, A. M., Broggini, M., Pitelli, M. R., Pantarotto, M., Torri, V., Mangioni, C., and D'Incalci, M. (1997) Expression of genes of potential importance in the response to chemotherapy and DNA repair in patients with ovarian cancer. *Gynecol. Oncol.* **65,** 130–137.

34. Kelley, S., Basu, A., Teicher, B., Hacker, M., Hamer, D., and Lazo, J. (1988) Overexpression of metallothionein confers resistance to anticancer drugs. *Science* **241,** 1813–1815.

35. Kondo, Y., Woo, E. S., Michalska, A. E., Choo, K. H. A., and Lazo, J. S. (1995) Metallothionein null cells have increased sensitivity to anticancer drugs. *Cancer Res.* **55,** 2021–2023.

36. Kasahara, K., Fujiwara, Y., Nishio, K., Ohmori, T., Sugimoto, Y., Komiya, K., et al. (1991) Metallothionein content correlates with the sensitivity of human small cell lung cancer cell lines to cisplatin. *Cancer Res.* **51,** 3237–3242.

37. Schilder, R., Hall, L., Monks, A., Handel, L., Fornace, A., Ozols, R., et al. (1990) Metallothionein gene expression and resistance to cisplatin in human ovarian cancer. *Int. J. Cancer* **45,** 416–422.

38. Robson, T., Hall, A., and Lohrer, H. (1992) Increased sensitivity of a Chinese hamster ovary cell line to alkylating agents after overexpression of the human metallothionein II-A gene. *Mutat. Res.* **274,** 177–185.

39. Germain, I., Tetu, B., Brisson, J., Mondor, M., and Cherian, M. G. (1996) Markers of chemoresistance in ovarian carcinomas: an immunohistochemical study of 86 cases. *Int. J. Gynecol. Path.* **15,** 54–62.

40. Giannakakou, P., Sackett, D. L., Kang, Y.-K., Zhan, Z., Buters, J. T. M., Fojo, T., and Poruchynsky, M. S. (1997) Paclitaxel-resistant human ovarian cancer cells have mutant b-tubulins that exhibit impaired paclitaxel-driven polymerization. *J. Biol. Chem.* **272,** 17,118–17,125.

41. Scheper, R., Broxterman, H., Scheffer, G., Kaaijk, P., Dalton, W., van Heijningen, T., et al. (1993) Overexpression of a Mr 110,000 vesicular protein in non-P-glycoprotein-mediated multidrug resistance. *Cancer Res.* **53,** 1475–1479.

42. Chugani, D., Rome, L., and Kedersha, N. (1993) Evidence that vault ribonucleoprotein particles localize to the nuclear pore complex. *J. Cell Sci.* **106,** 23–29.

43. Izquierdo, M., Scheffer, G., Flens, M., Giaccone, G., Broxterman, H., Meijer, C., et al. (1996) Broad distribution of the multidrug resistance-related vault lung resistance protein in nomal human tissues and tumors. *Am. J. Pathol.* **148,** 877–887.

44. Moggs, J., Yarema, K., Essigmann, J., and Wood, R. (1996) Analysis of incision sites produced by human cell extracts and purified proteins during nucleotide excision repair of a 1,3-intrastrand d(GpTpG)-cisplatin adduct. *J. Biol. Chem.* **271,** 7177–7186.

45. Cole, R. (1973) Repair of DNA containing interstrand crosslinks in *Escherichia coli*: sequential excision and recombination. *Proc. Natl. Acad. Sci. USA* **70,** 1064–1068.

46. Sargent, R., Rolig, R., Kilburn, A., Adair, G., Wilson, J., and Nairn, R. (1997) Recombination-dependent deletion formation in mammalian cells deficient in the nucleotide excision repair gene *ERCC1. Proc. Natl. Acad. Sci. USA* **94,** 13,122–13,127.

47. Tantin, D., Kansal, A., and Carey, M. (1997) Recruitment of the putative transcription-repair coupling factor CSB/ERCC6 to RNA polymerase II elongation complexes. *Mol. Cell Biol.* **17,** 6803–6814.

48. Koberle, B., Grimaldi, K., Sunters, A., Hartley, J., Kelland, L., and Masters, J. (1997) DNA repair capacity and cisplatin sensitivity of human testis tumor cells. *Int. J. Cancer* **70,** 551–555.

49. Zeng-Rong, N., Paterson, J., Alpert, L., Tsao, M.-S., Viallet, J., and Alaoui-Jamali, M. (1995) Elevated DNA repair capacity is associated with intrinsic resistance of lung cancer to chemotherapy. *Cancer Res.* **55,** 4760–4764.

50. Johnson, S. W., Swiggard, P. A., Handel, L. M., Brennan, J. M., Godwin, A. K., Ozols, R. F., and Hamilton, T. C. (1994) Relationship between platinum-DNA adduct formation, removal, and cytotoxicity in cisplatin sensitive and resistant human ovarian cancer cells. *Cancer Res.* **54,** 5911–5916.

51. Johnson, S., Perez, R., Godwin, A., Yeung, A., Handel, L., Ozols, R., and Hamilton, T. (1994) Role of platinum-DNA adduct formation and removal in cisplatin resistance in human ovarian cancer cell lines. *Biochem. Pharmacol.* **47,** 689–697.

52. Yen, L., Woo, A., Christopoulopoulos, G., Batist, G., Panasci, L., Roy, R., et al. (1995) Enhanced host cell reactivation capacity and expression of DNA repair genes in human breast cancer cells resistant to bi-functional alkylating agents. *Mutat. Res.* **337,** 179–189.

53. Ali-Osman, F., Berger, M., Rairkar, A., and Stein, D. (1994) Enhanced repair of a cisplatin-damaged reporter chloramphenicol-O-acetyltransferase gene and altered activities of DNA polymerases a and b, and DNA ligase in cells of a human malignant glioma following in vivo cisplatin therapy. *J. Cell. Biochem.* **54,** 11–19.

54. Eastman, A. and Schulte, N. (1988) Enhanced DNA Repair as a Mechanism of Resistance to *cis*-diamminedichloroplatinum(II). *Biochemistry* **27,** 4730–4734.

55. Chaney, S. and Sancar, A. (1996) DNA Repair: enzymatic mechanisms and relevance to drug response. *J. Natl. Cancer Inst.* **88,** 1346–1360.
56. Dabholkar, M., Vionnet, J., Bostick-Bruton, F., Yu, J., and Reed, E. (1994) Messenger RNA levels of XPAC and ERCC1 in ovarian cancer tissue correlate with response to platinum-based chemotherapy. *J. Clin. Invest.* **94,** 703–708.
57. Cleaver, J., Charles, W., McDowell, M., Sadinski, W., and Mitchell, D. (1995) Overexpression of the XPA repair gene increases resistance to ultraviolet radiation in human cells by selective repair of DNA damage. *Cancer Res.* **55,** 6152–6160.
58. Huang, J.-C., Zamble, D., Reardon, J., Lippard, S., and Sancar, A. (1994) HMG-domain proteins specifically inhibit the repair of the major DNA adduct of the anticancer drug cisplatin by human excision nuclease. *Proc. Natl. Acad. Sci. USA* **91,** 10,394–10,398.
59. McA'Nulty, M. and Lippard, S. (1996) The HMG-domain protein Ixr1 blocks excision repair of cisplatin-DNA adducts in yeast. *Mutat. Res.* **362,** 75–86.
60. Vichi, P., Coin, F., Renaud, J., Vermeulen, W., Hoeijmakers, J., Moras, D., and Egly, J. (1997) Cisplatin- and UV-damaged DNA lure the basal transcription factor TFIID/TBP. *EMBO J.* **16,** 7444–7456.
61. Katz, E., Andrews, P., and Howell, S. (1990) The effect of DNA polymerase inhibitors on the cytotoxicity of cisplatin in human ovarian carcinoma cells. *Cancer Comm.* **2,** 159–164.
62. Dempke, W. C. M., Shellard, S. A., Fichtinger-Schepman, A. M. J., and Hill, B. T. (1991) Lack of significant modulation of the formation and removal of platinum-DNA adducts by aphidicolin glycinate in two logarithmically-growing ovarian tumor cell lines in vitro. *Carcinogenesis* **12,** 525–528.
63. O'Dwyer, P., Moyer, J., Suffness, M., Harrison, S., Cysyk, R., Hamilton, T., and Plowman, J. (1994) Antitumor activity and biochemical effects of aphidicolin glycinate (NSC 303812) alone and in combination with cisplatin in vivo. *Cancer Res.* **54,** 724–729.
64. Albain, K., Swinnen, L., Erickson, L., Stiff, P., Fisher, S., and Fisher, R. (1992) Cytotoxic synergy of cisplatin with concurrent hydroxyurea and cytarabine: summary of an in vitro model and initial clinical pilot experience. *Semin. Oncol.* **19,** 102–109.
65. Alaoui-Jamali, M., Loubaba, B.-B., Robyn, S., Tapiero, H., and Batist, G. (1994) Effect of DNA-repair-enzyme modulators on cytotoxicity of L-phenylalanine mustard and cis-diamminedichloroplatinum (II) in mammary carcinoma cells resistant to alkylating agents. *Cancer Chemother. Pharmacol.* **34,** 153–158.
66. Aebi, S., Kurdi-Haidar, B., Gordon, R., Cenni, B., Zheng, H., Fink, D., et al. (1996) Loss of DNA mismatch repair in acquired resistance to cisplatin. *Cancer Res.* **56,** 3087–3090.
67. Fink, D., Nebel, S., Aebi, S., Zheng, H., Cenni, B., Nehme, A., et al. (1996) The role of DNA mismatch repair in platinum drug resistance. *Cancer Res.* **56,** 4881–4886.
68. Fink, D., Zheng, H., Nebel, S., Norris, P., Aebi, S., Lin, T.-P., et al. (1997) *In vitro* and *in vivo* resistance to cisplatin in cells that have lost DNA mismatch repair. *Cancer Res.* **57,** 1841–1845.
69. Duckett, D., Drummond, J., Murchie, A., Reardon, J., Sancar, A., Lilley, D., and Modrich, P. (1996) Human MutSa recognizes damaged DNA base pairs containing 06-methylguanine, O4-methylthymine, or the cisplatin-d(GpG)adduct. *Proc. Natl. Acad. Sci. USA* **93,** 6443–6447.
70. Karran, P. and Bignami, M. (1994) DNA damage tolerance, mismatch repair and genome instability. *BioEssays* **16,** 833–839.
71. Mamenta, E., Poma, E., Kaufmann, W., Delmastro, D., Grady, H., and Chaney, S. (1994) Enhanced replicative bypass of platinum-DNA adducts in cisplatin-resistant human ovarian carcinoma cell lines. *Cancer Res.* **54,** 3500–3505.
72. Henkels, K. and Turchi, J. (1997) Induction of apoptosis in cisplatin-sensitive and -resistant human ovarian cancer cell lines. *Cancer Res.* **57,** 4488–4492.
73. Vaisman, A., Varchenko, M., Said, I., and Chaney, S. (1997) Cell cycle changes associated with formation of Pt-DNA adducts in human ovarian carcinoma cells with different cisplatin sensitivity. *Cytometry* **27,** 54–64.
74. Demarcq, C., Bunch, R., Creswell, D., and Eastman, A. (1994) The role of cell cycle progresson in cisplatin-induced apoptosis in chinese hamster ovary cells. *Cell Growth Differ.* **5,** 983–993.
75. El-Deiry, W., Tokino, T., Velculescu, V., Levy, D., Parsons, R., Trent, J., et al. (1993) WAF1, a potential mediator of p53 tumor suppression. *Cell* **75,** 817–825.
76. McDonald, E. I., Wu, G., Waldman, T., and El-Deiry, W. (1996) Repair defect in p21 WAF1/CIP1 –/– human cancer cells. *Cancer Res.* **56,** 2250–2255.
77. Chen, I., Smith, M., O'Connor, P., and Fornace, A. J. (1995) Direct interaction of Gadd45 with PCNA and evidence for competitive interaction of Gadd45 and p21Waf1/Cip1 with PCNA. *Oncogene* **11,** 1931–1937.
78. Fan, S., Smith, M. L., Rivet, D. J. I., Duba, D., Zhan, Q., Kohn, K. W., et al. (1995) Disruption of p53 function sensitizes breast cancer MCF-7 cells to cisplatin and pentoxyfylline. *Cancer Res.* **55,** 1649–1654.

79. Eliopoulos, A., Kerr, D., Herod, J., Hodgkins, L., Krajewski, S., Reed, J., and Young, L. (1995) The control of apoptosis and drug resistance in ovarian cancer: influence of p53 and Bcl-2. *Oncogene* **11,** 1217–1228.

80. Blagosklonny, M. and Eldeiry, W. (1998) Acute overexpression of WT p53 facilitates anticancer drug-induced death of cancer and normal cells. *Int. J. Cancer* **75,** 933–940.

81. Bunch, R. and Eastman, A. (1997) 7-Hydroxystaurosporine (UCN-01) causes redistribution of proliferating cell nuclear antigen and abrogates cisplatin-induced S-phase arrest in Chinese hamster ovary cells. *Cell Growth Differ.* **8,** 779–788.

82. Miyashita, T. and Reed, J. C. (1993) Bcl-2 oncoprotein blocks chemotherapy-induced apoptosis in a human leukemia cell line. *Blood* **81,** 151–157.

83. Zou, H., Henzel, W., Liu, X., Lutschg, A., and Wang, X. (1997) Apaf-1, a human protein homolgous to C. elegans CED-4, participates in cytochrome c-dependent activation of caspase-3. *Cell* **90,** 405–413.

84. Hirsch, T., Marchetti, P., Susin, S., Dallaporta, B., Zamzami, N., Marzo, I., et al. (1997) The apoptosis-necrosis paradox. Apoptogenic proteases activated after mitochondrial permeability transition determine the mode of cell death. *Oncogene* **15,** 1573–1581.

# II

## TUMOR MARKERS

# 9

## Markers of Tumor Burden

*An Overview*

### Joseph E. Roulston

### 1. Introduction

Since ancient times, cancer has been known to humankind. The ancient Greeks and Romans have left us with writings in which various treatment options are discussed *(1)*. Disease processes and causes were not well understood, however; the humoral pathology established by the ancient Greeks of the school of Galen in the second century AD was to survive virtually intact until the mid-nineteenth century. It is perhaps all the more remarkable then, that the first tumor marker—Bence Jones' protein in multiple myeloma—should come to light in what was still by and large the prescientific medical culture prevailing in 1845.

Multiple myeloma was fully described and named by von Rustizky *(2)* in 1873, but it was Kahler *(3)* who related the disease to Bence Jones' proteinuria and thereby brought a specific tumor marker to medical attention, a marker that is still used to this day to assist in diagnosis.

Despite the lesson of Bence Jones' protein, in which a marker specific for a particular cancer was discovered, many researchers still sought a general test for early diagnosis of all cancer. Homberger *(4)* reviewed more than 60 tests, which had been suggested in the previous 20 (1930–1950) years. Many of these tests were based upon the physicochemical properties of serum proteins and sought to show a difference between precipitation of serum proteins from normal subjects and cancer patients.

With the benefit of hindsight, it is easy to write off such efforts as misplaced; the biochemical techniques available were crude and not always applied with logic. Bodansky *(5)* points out the problems with many early studies. Technically, the tests were deficient because they were based upon a gross and nonspecific measurement—the change in a large fraction of the serum protein pool. Second, these investigations were usually carried out in samples from patients with advanced disease, whereas control groups of similarly aged patients with serious nonmalignant diseases were not studied. When these controls were looked at later, the false positive rate was as high as the true positive rate in the neoplastic group.

From: *Methods in Molecular Medicine, Vol. 39: Ovarian Cancer: Methods and Protocols*
Edited by: J. M. S. Bartlett © Humana Press, Inc., Totowa, NJ

Apart from technical shortcomings, there is also a major assumption in the presupposition that cancers will produce some unique feature that nonneoplastic diseases will not, and for this there is not a shred of evidence *(6)*.

As the biochemical tools and techniques available have grown ever more sophisticated, it has enabled more precisely focused studies to be conducted. The advent of immunoassay techniques in the 1960s and their refinement during the following decades with nonisotopic labels and, especially, the development of monoclonal ("hybridoma") technology has brought levels of analytical sensitivity and specificity, which were orders of magnitude better than those available to previous generations of researchers.

## 2. Theoretical Considerations

In order to assess and apply tests in an appropriate and discerning manner, it is necessary to consider what the aims and objectives are and how one monitors and assesses one's efforts.

At first thought, it appears very simple. First it is intended to apply a test to discriminate between the normal and the diseased subject, that is to assist in diagnosis and possibly to screen populations for occult disease. Second, one may wish to apply a test to monitor the course of the disease in a noninvasive way in order to assess the efficiency of therapy, to watch for drug-resistance, and to predict outcome. Third, one may wish to monitor patients in remission to ensure that they remain disease-free and to get a valuable lead-time to relapse.

In order to achieve these aims, several points must be made clear. First, one must have confidence in the analytical accuracy and precision of the test(s). However, in order to translate the analytical data into clinically meaningful information, it is essential to be aware of what the objectives are. "Is this result normal?" is a question often asked by a requesting clinician and it is worth considering, at the outset, what the word "normal" may or may not mean.

### 2.1. What is "Normal"?

The first problem presenting to workers in clinical medicine is the statistical definition of normal because it is widely misunderstood and even more widely misapplied. Gauss' law of errors applies to repeated measurements on the *same* subject or object, not a series of measurements of the same analyte in different subjects. Gauss' law proposes that if the same measurement were repeated over and over again in the same subject the results' spread would fit a bell-shaped distribution symmetrical about the mean. Abnormal results may then be defined as those outside the 95% confidence limit; in other words, the 2.5% of values at the top and bottom end of the range. There is however no *a priori* reason why this law of distribution should apply to measurements in more than one subject; it was never derived to describe the distribution of a variable (disease-related or otherwise) in a population of subjects. Although it is common practice in laboratories to define a reference range for an analyte as being the limit within which 95% of the healthy population's results fall, these limits *per se* give no indication of morbidity or mortality. Indeed, by definition, 5% of this population will be "abnormal" although disease-free if we assume a 95% (i.e., mean value plus or minus two standard deviations) reference range. It also follows that the more tests performed on each specimen, then the greater the likelihood of at least one of its results being "abnormal"; from 5% for 1 test, to 40% for 10 tests (the chance of 10 tests on a sample all being "normal" is $0.95^{10}$, which is 0.6 or 60%; leaving a 40% chance for an "abnormal"). The percentage error figure rises to 99% ($[1-0.95^{90}] \times 100\%$) for 90 tests.

It is for this reason that most laboratories today eschew the phrase "normal range" and prefer the alternative "reference range," or "referent value;" in order to make clear that the range or cutoff cited is not of necessity a range or cutoff that encompasses or defines the limit of the values of the analyte in all disease-free and excludes all diseased subjects. Often, 95% reference ranges, based upon the mean value plus or minus two standard deviations, are employed as the reference limits because they have been found empirically to provide cutoffs at clinically useful and discriminant values. For tumor markers, however, there is less concern whether a reference range based upon a symmetric distribution is ideal; in practice the optimal cut-off value is sought; a point which discriminates "normal" from "elevated"—there is no lower limit to the "reference range."

In order to establish this cut-off value empirically, it is necessary to discover the value that discriminates the best between disease and nondisease; in other words, produces the fewest misclassifications. In order to do this, large numbers of measurements in the disease group under study and a *suitably matched* control population must be made. Inevitably, there is an overlap between the range of results produced by the control group and the range produced by the diseased group. There will, therefore, be some false positive results (elevated analyte in control subject) and some false negative ("normal" result in diseased subject), and just how many depend upon the test and population in question. In order to proceed further, therefore, it is vital to determine how good the test is in an objective manner.

## 2.2. How Good is The Test?

### 2.2.1. Sensitivity and Specificity

The two most usually applied criteria in order to assess a test are those of sensitivity and specificity. Sensitivity is a measure of how good a test is at picking up the disease in question by giving a positive result. It is expressed in a population with the disease as the number giving a true positive result divided by the sum of true positive and false negative; in other words, what percentage of the diseased cohort were identified correctly by the test.

It is obvious that a test that is 100% sensitive will score perfectly. A test that is 90% sensitive, however, will generate 10 false negatives in each 100 positives.

As well as correctly identifying the presence of disease, a good test must also correctly classify the disease-free subject by giving a negative result. The measure of a test to so discriminate is called the specificity. This is established by measurements in a disease-free population and specificity is defined as the number of true negatives divided by the sum of true negatives plus false positives.

It can be seen that sensitivity and specificity are entirely "test-based" parameters; they take no account of the prevalence of the disease in the population, the sensitivity is calculated by study of a group who are all disease positive, and specificity from a group who are all disease free. This, as will become apparent, is a serious limitation to the application of these parameters because disease prevalence has serious effects upon the clinical usefulness of tests in certain circumstances.

Furthermore, the choice of cutoff, which effectively determines the sensitivity and specificity, cannot improve both sensitivity and specificity simultaneously; moving the chosen cut-off point to a higher referent value will increase specificity, but correspondingly reduce sensitivity. The optimal choice of cutoff, therefore, depends upon whether it is deemed more desirable to optimize sensitivity at the expense of specificity or vice versa, and this consideration, in turn, is influenced by the disease prevalence in the population under study.

### 2.2.2. Incidence and Prevalence

By definition, incidence relates to the frequency of occurrence of an event and is therefore a rate per unit time. For a disease, the incidence rate is the number of new cases per 100,000 of the population per year. The prevalence, by contrast, is the number of patients, per 100,000 of the population who have the given disease at the time of the study; prevalence, therefore, is a snapshot of the status quo.

The incidence of epithelial carcinoma of the ovary is of the order of 15 per 100,000 per year. If the average duration of the disease is 5 yr, it follows that the prevalence, assuming a steady-state situation in the population, must be 75 per 100,000. As a general rule, therefore:

$$\text{Prevalence} = \text{Incidence} \times \text{Duration}$$

The clinical usefulness of a test *in a given situation* will depend upon the prevalence of the disease in the cohort under study; high sensitivity and specificity, although vital, are not enough of themselves to guarantee "usefulness." For example, a test that was 100% specific and 99% sensitive seems to have impressive credentials, but it would fail dismally as a screening test for ovarian cancer. Screening 100,000 women would yield 99% out of the positives, i.e., 74 or 75 women, which is an acceptable "pick-up rate," but it would also generate 1% false positives, i.e., 1000 nondiseased women. Therefore, a positive test result would correctly identify disease presence in less than 7% (75/[1000+75] = 6.98%) of the subjects studied.

It is necessary therefore to use assessment procedures that take into account the prevalence of the disease in the population under study.

### 2.2.3. Bayes' Theorem and the Predictive Value Model

In 1975, Galen and Gambino *(7)* introduced the Predictive Value Model to clinical laboratories. The theoretical basis was hardly new *(8)*. What Bayes' theorem allows is the calculation of the *a posteriori* probability of disease being present in an individual given that the patient has a positive test result. By definition, the *a priori* probability that a patient will have the disease (i.e., before the test), is equal to the prevalence of the disease. From prevalence, sensitivity, and specificity, Bayes calculated the *a posteriori* probability—the so-called predictive value of a positive result or positive predictive value.

Let sensitivity = $a$, specificity = $b$, and prevalence = $p$, then one can describe the positive predictive value (PPV) as follows:

$$\text{PPV} = pa/[pa + (1-b)(1-p)] \tag{1}$$

This simplifies to PPV = true positives/[true positives + false positives].

Since $pa$ = the prevalence of the disease multiplied by the sensitivity of the test for the disease, i.e., the true positive.

**Table 1**
**Positive Predictive Values as a Function of Prevalence**

| Disease Prevalence (%) | Test Sensitivity and Specificity = 95% Positive Predictive Value | Test Sensitivity and Specificity = 99% Positive Predictive Value |
|---|---|---|
| 0.02 | 0 | 2.0 |
| 0.1 | 1.9 | 9.0 |
| 1.0 | 16.1 | 50.0 |
| 2.0 | 27.9 | 66.9 |
| 5.0 | 50.0 | 83.9 |
| 50.0 | 95.0 | 99.0 |

Similarly, *(1–b)(1–p)* = the prevalence of nondisease multiplied by the probability of a positive result in such a disease free person. *1–b*, which is *1–specificity*, is sometimes, albeit incorrectly, referred to as the false positive rate.

The benefit of the predictive value model is apparent immediately; if a test has a 95% PPV in a given area of use, then the clinician may assume that in a patient with a positive result there is a 95% chance that the patient has the disease. The same conclusion cannot be made from sensitivity and specificity values as they take no account of disease prevalence. **Table 1** shows how the predictive value of a positive test varies from virtually 0 to 100% as a result of changing disease prevalence *even when sensitivity and specificity are high*. This gives an important insight to screening procedures; where disease prevalence is low, it is necessary to have tests with greater than 99% sensitivity and specificity to achieve an acceptable positive predictive value.

## 3. Screening for Disease

Screening has been defined as "the presumptive identification of unrecognized disease or defect by the application of tests, examinations, or other procedures that can be applied rapidly" *(9)*. By definition, therefore, a screening test is applied to asymptomatic subjects and is not diagnostic *per se*; confirmatory tests being required. The idea that early warning leads to a better outcome is not easily translated into a practical program. The economic difficulties of testing large numbers of apparently healthy individuals in order to pick up a small number with the disease are enormous. Second, there are difficult ethical considerations when one is investigating healthy subjects without symptoms or any substantive probability of finding disease.

### 3.1. Population Screening

The oncology literature contains many reports of apparently promising markers that fail subsequently to claim a routine clinical role. There are many reasons that contribute to this, but most common is overextrapolating or illogically applying the results. Consider a study in which an investigator tests a novel tumor marker for a particular cancer that has a prevalence of 100/100,000 in the general population and finds that in 100 patients with the tumor under investigation, 99 have a positive test result, that is, the test has a sensitivity of 99%. Equally, when tested on 100 disease-free subjects, only one is test-positive—a specificity of 99%. Owing to this excellent discrimination, it is decided to introduce the test as a screen in the general population in order to detect this tumor at an earlier stage to improve therapeutic efficacy and patient outcome. The results are disastrous; the test appears to have lost its earlier discrimination and is generating many false positives—why?

In the pilot study, the disease prevalence was 50% *by design*; there were 100 patients and 100 controls and the positive predictive value was 99%. In the screening exercise, the prevalence would be 100/100,000, which is 0.1%. Therefore, as well as correctly identifying 99 out of the 100 true positives the test will also *under these circumstances* misclassify 1000 as false positive giving us a positive predictive value of 99/[99 + 1,000], that is 9.0%. In other words, a test that in the pilot investigation yielded 99% correct results, gives, in a screening situation a 91% *a posteriori* probability that elevated results are *not* associated with the disease. The marker sensitivity and specificity remain unchanged, the fall in positive predictive value from 99 to 9% was *entirely* caused by the change in prevalence in the cohort under study from 50 to 0.1%.

If a test is genuinely and completely useless, that is to say it yields positive and negative results in a truly random manner, then the positive predictive value will be the same as the prevalence: the *a priori* probability of disease in the patient equals the *a posteriori* probability of disease. Furthermore, for a test to be random, it is not necessary for sensitivity and specificity each to equal 50%; a test may have 90% sensitivity and still give random results if the specificity is only 10%.

Randomness requires only that: $\Sigma[sensitivity + specificity] = 100\%$. These findings can be derived simply from **Eq. 1**: PPV = $pa/[pa + (1-p)(1-b)]$.

In a random test, the percentage of true positives in the diseased group will equal the percentage of false positives in the well group—by definition. That is: $pa/p = [(1-p)(1-b)]/(1-p)$. Also by definition, $pa/p$ is the sensitivity of the test and $[(1-p)(1-b)]/(1-p) = (1-b) = (1-specificity)$. Therefore, in a random test, sensitivity equals (1 – specificity) which is to say the sum of sensitivity and specificity equals unity (or 100%).

This relationship is of value in the graphical representation of marker performance. When sensitivity is plotted as a function of (1 – specificity) an immediate visual impression of the marker's discrimination is obtained. This graph is termed the Receiver Operating Characteristic or "ROC" plot. A random test will give a straight line graph at 45° to the axes, whereas a good, highly discriminatory test will give a curve of steep slope from the origin, showing a high sensitivity even at high specificity. Therefore, the greater the area under the curve the better the test. ROC plots are particularly useful in that they remove the influence of the "cut-off" point from the marker evaluation.

### 3.2. Optimization

If screening is to be considered, it is necessary to know the disease prevalence, therefore, and to have tests with high sensitivity and specificity in order to calculate whether an acceptable positive predictive value can be achieved. But, it is impossible to optimize simultaneously both sensitivity and specificity; increasing the one automatically decreases the other. Considerations regarding optimization strategies will vary with the natural history of the disease under study (*vide infra*).

The simplest case will be considered; the situation where there is a screening procedure to be optimized and a false negative result carries an equivalent penalty to a false positive result. Under these circumstances we may define our "Index of Mis-classification," $f$, as the sum of the false negative and false positive results.

$$f = FN + FP \qquad (2)$$

False negatives, $FN$, can be calculated as the lack of sensitivity $(1–a)$ multiplied by disease prevalence $p$. Similarly, false positives, $FP$, can be calculated by multiplying lack of disease specificity $(1–b)$ by the prevalence of nondisease in the population under study. Therefore,

$$f = p(1–a) + (1–b)(1–p) \qquad (3)$$

For most cancers, prevalence of disease in a general population screen will be tend to zero. Therefore,

$$f = (1–b) \qquad (4)$$

It follows, therefore, that under the conditions and assumptions outlined—very low prevalence and equality of penalty for false negatives and false positives—one should increase specificity at the expense of sensitivity to minimize misclassifications.

### 3.3. Targeted Screening

The most frequently cited example of successful screening using a tumor marker is the use of human chorionic gonadotropin (hCG) in choriocarcinoma, and it is instructive to consider briefly why hCG has worked so wonderfully well when no other tumor markers are as competent.

Choriocarcinoma is rare; it accounts for 0.02% of all cancer deaths and is almost exclusively confined to women who have had a hydatidiform mole of whom about 8% go on to develop choriocarcinoma. The single key fact that makes the screening program workable is the application of the test to a predetermined group in which the disease is present at a high prevalence.

If we assume that hCG has a sensitivity $(a)$ of 99% and a specificity $(b)$ of 99%, and choriocarcinoma has a prevalence $(p)$ of 8% in our screening group, then we can calculate the positive predictive value of hCG in this context: $PPV = pa/[pa + (1–b)(1–p)]$

$$PPV = (0.08 \times 0.99)/[(0.08 \times 0.99)+(1 - 0.99)(1 - 0.08)] = 89.6\%$$

By contrast, if one attempted to screen for choriocarcinoma, all women whose pregnancies had achieved full term (prevalence 0.01%), the positive predictive value would be vanishingly small:

$$PPV = (0.0001 \times 0.99)/[(0.0001 \times 0.99)+(1 - 0.99)(1 - 0.0001)] = 0.98\%$$

It is therefore apparent that for screening to be effective, a high prevalence group must be identified in order to keep the number of false positives to an acceptable level.

### 4. Clinical Utility

Clinical effectiveness demands that the early intervention afforded by a successful screen is translated into an increased rate of cure or improved survival time. Objective quantification of improvement in survival time is not quite as simple as it first might appear, as studies are subject to various forms of methodological bias.

### 4.1. Lead-Time Bias

Survival is measured from the date of diagnosis to death, rather than from the date of inception to death. The date of diagnosis may therefore vary considerably, depending on the methods of detection used, without altering the true length of survival from the date of inception. Lead time generated by screening, or the period from detection while the woman is still asymptomatic until the appearance of clinical symptoms, which would permit conventional diagnosis, may increase the apparent survival without in fact the individual having benefited from screening. In such circumstances, the patient has to live with the knowledge of their disease longer.

### 4.2. Length Bias

A series of cases diagnosed at screening will be atypical of those arising clinically, because it will contain a disproportionate number of patients with slowly developing tumors with probably a better prognosis. Patients with rapidly progressing tumors are more likely to present with symptoms before the initiation of, or in the interval between, screening tests. This bias is more likely to be manifest at the initiation of screening and is therefore especially important in studies of short duration.

### 4.3. Selection Bias

Selection bias results from entry of a cohort into a screening trial who have a different probability of developing and dying from the disease than the population at large. In self-selected populations, it is common to find a higher-than-normal proportion of individuals presenting for screening because of a positive family history. These individuals are more motivated to present for screening because they are more educated in this respect and are more likely to benefit from it. This has been well demonstrated in breast and cervical screening programmes.

## 5. Optimization Strategies

It was demonstrated earlier that, when prevalence was very low (tending to zero), if false negatives and false positives carried equal penalty, then to minimize misclassifications one should maximize *specificity*. In addition, one should maximize specificity in situations where the disease is serious, but cannot be treated or cured and where, therefore, any false positive result would lead to psychological trauma. Some occult cancers would clearly fall into this group, as well as diseases such as multiple sclerosis. Such incurable diseases should not be subject to population screening as there is usually no benefit to patient or society at large in early diagnosis. In this section, the other options available will be considered and under which circumstances it would be appropriate to use them.

### 5.1. Sensitivity

Sensitivity should be maximized in situations where, although the disease is serious and should not be missed, it *is* treatable and, therefore, false positives are less psychologically damaging. Most treatable infectious diseases would fall into this category, as do phaeochromocytoma and phenylketonuria. Cervical cancer, where the screening program is effective and confirmatory tests are available prior to an effective therapeutic intervention program, is an example of a malignancy, which may fall into this category. Furthermore, the concern caused by the presence of abnormal cells upon a cervical smear can, in large measure, be offset by the patient being aware of the success of early treatment.

## 5.2. Positive Predictive Value

Positive predictive value (PPV) should be maximized in any situation where treatment of a false positive could be seriously damaging. Where the treatment indicated involves major surgery and radiotherapy, such as certain occult carcinomas, instigating treatment in someone who did not have the disease would be a major catastrophe.

## 5.3. Accuracy (or "Efficiency")

Accuracy of a very high order is required when a disease is both serious *and* treatable and false positive and false negative results carry equal penalty. Myocardial infarction has usually been cited as the classical example of where the tests should be optimized for accuracy $[(TP+TN)/(TP+TN+FP+FN)]$, however, a case for optimizing accuracy could be made in testing for certain leukæmias and lymphomas.

## 6. The Use of Multiple Markers

The idea of using a group of markers in order to complement the sensitivity and specificity of each other seems logical enough and can be extremely beneficial. There are certain rules that can be defined and applied, and certain pitfalls to avoid.

There are two distinct approaches to multiple testing. The first, as described in the example above, is so-called *series* testing; the various tests are performed one after the other depending upon the result of the previous test. In series testing, therefore, a "test-positive" patient is one who has scored positive in all the tests. A secondary consideration here is defining the order in which the tests are to be performed to maximise efficacy; although considerations of cost and patient compliance also need to be included in any trial design. In *parallel* testing, all tests are performed upon all patients, a "test-positive" patient in these circumstances is one who is positive on any one (or more) of the tests.

It is usual in a screening exercise that series testing is to be preferred as it maximizes specificity at the expense of sensitivity which, as discussed earlier, is a rational approach where disease prevalence is low. Calculation of the positive predictive value for parallel and series regimes bear this out *(10)*.

For series testing, as not all tests are performed on all samples, there is the option of the order in which the tests are to be performed. There are many considerations; the relative cost of the tests involved, the degree of invasiveness, and the relative sensitivities and specificity's of the tests involved. If variables such as cost are set aside it can be shown that the sensible option is to test in series rather than parallel as the positive predictive value is far higher and the total number of tests performed is a lot less. Also, although positive predictive value is independent of the order of testing, the number of analyses that have to be performed varies considerably, being minimized by application first of the test with the higher (or highest) specificity of those in the panel.

## 6.1. Series Testing

In an abstract *(11)*, a research group reported the results of screening 1010 postmenopausal women for epithelial ovarian cancer using the serum marker *CA125* fol-

**Table 2**
**Data from 1010 Postmenopausal Women Screened**
**for Epithelial Ovarian Cancer (EOC) Using CA125**

|                | EOC Positive | EOC Negative | Totals |
|----------------|--------------|--------------|--------|
| CA125 Positive | 1 (TP)       | 31 (FP)      | 32 (TP+FP) |
| CA125 Negative | 0 (FN)       | 978 (TN)     | 978 (TN+FN) |
| Totals         | 1 (TP+FN)    | 1009(TN+FP)  | 1010 (ALL) |

Sensitivity = TP/(TP+FN) = 1/1 = 100%.
Specificity = TN/(TN+FP) = 978/1009 = 97%.
Prevalence = (TP+FN)/(TP+TN+FP+FN) = 1/1010 = 0.1%.
Accuracy = (TP+TN)/(TP+TN+FP+FN) = 979/1010 = 97%.
Positive Predictive Value = TP/(TP+FP) = 1/32 = 3.1%.
TP = True Positive.
FP = False Positive.
TN = True Negative.
FN = False Negative.

lowed up by ultrasonography. They found a level of greater than 30 units per milliliter (their cut-off level) in 31 women. These 31 were then given ultrasonography; three were deemed abnormal and sent for surgery. One had an early-stage ovarian cancer. The authors concluded that *CA125* had a high specificity for ovarian cancer, that they could increase the sensitivity by lowering the cutoff from 30 to 23 units per milliliter (the widely accepted cut-off value is, in fact, 35 U/mL) and that *CA125* warranted further investigation for early diagnosis.

Their data are shown in **Table 2**. It is apparent that, from these data, there is no good reason to lower the cutoff from 30 to 23 as the sensitivity is already 100%. How reliable that figure is, however, is open to question as there is only one true positive in the study. Furthermore, false negatives—here reported as 0—invariably take longer to emerge from any study and tend to be the most difficult to follow up; for these reasons then, the reported sensitivity may be an overestimate. The one true positive patient had a *CA125* level of 32 U/mL. If, therefore, these workers had followed the axiom of optimizing specificity at the expense of sensitivity, they would, in all probability, have missed the one patient who was to benefit directly from the trial. Their reason for opting for a higher sensitivity in this case was that they had a highly efficient second test (ultrasonography) to filter out the majority of the false positives generated by the *CA125* alone and did not wish to miss any cases. It can be seen from **Table 2** that, despite a sensitivity of 100% a specificity of 97% and an overall accuracy of 97%, the positive predictive value was only 3.1% for *CA125*, hopelessly inadequate as a single selector for exploratory surgery. When, however, ultrasonography is added in as a second-line test the positive predictive value improves by an order of magnitude to 33% (1/3) which is perhaps an acceptable pick-up rate, considering the high mortality rate of the disease if not diagnosed early. In effect, the use of *CA125* in this and other studies generates a subgroup of the population under study who are at higher risk than the population at large; it defines a high-prevalence group, thereby enabling a second line test of similar sensitivity and specificity to produce a positive predictive value that is far higher.

## 6.2. Panel Testing

Evaluation of a panel of tests is, of course, subject to all the same provisions as for the assessment of a single test; particularly the prevalence of the disease in the study group must be typical of the prevalence in the population to which it is intended to apply the test(s).

In a study of ovarian cancer by Ward et al. *(12)* in 1987, it was reported that, by using three markers, the sensitivity in samples from pretreatment patients with Stage I and II disease had increased from 18% using *CA125* alone to 64% using human milk-fat globulin II *(HMFG2)* as the second assay and placental alkaline phosphatase *(PLAP)* as a third marker. That is to say *CA125* had picked up 2/11 of the diseased group, *HMFG2* and *PLAP* had picked up a further 5 of the *CA125* negative group taking the total to 7/11. However, as all the subjects under study were disease positive, it can be seen that neither *CA125* nor *HMFG2* nor *PLAP* performed significantly differently from random chance. They also studied the marker panel in patients with advanced disease. In the 26 patients with advanced (Stage III and IV) disease, 25 had elevated *CA125* (96%) and the 26th had an elevated PLAP. Therefore, all patients with advanced carcinoma of the ovary were positive for at least one of these three markers. These results are not quite as promising as one might at first believe: using such a group of patients where prevalence is 100%, (whether early stage or advanced disease) one could achieve apparently excellent sensitivity by four consecutive coin flips at considerably less cost! (Each flip will have a 50% sensitivity; therefore, in series, the cumulative sensitivity will become 50, 75, 87.5, and 93.75%).

## 7. Conclusions

Disease prevalence is of fundamental importance in the rational application of tumor marker assays. By and large, cancer prevalence is too low in the population to permit effective screening even if the financial and ethical constraints could be overcome. In ovarian cancer, there is therefore a large amount of current research directed at the identification of possible high risk groups—the so-called cancer families—in which prevalence is significantly higher than in the population at large because of genetic predisposition.

The use of tumor markers to monitor disease progress or remission, to track therapeutic efficacy or to give a lead time to relapse are much more successful. Here the markers either are being applied to a group in order to quantify a disease which is known to be present or to pick up a relapse in a group where relapse and, therefore, disease prevalence will be high.

## Acknowledgment

The author is grateful to Churchill Livingstone for permission to use excerpts from his textbook: *Serological Tumour Markers: An Introduction*, Roulston, J. E. and Leonard, R. C. F., 1993.

## References

1. Baum, M. (1988) *Breast Cancer: The facts.* Oxford University Press, New York, NY, pp. 1–6.
2. von Rustizky, J. (1873) Multiple Myeloma. Zentralblatt fur Chirugie (Leipzig) **3,** 102–111.
3. Kahler, O. (1889) Zur symptomatologie des multiplen Myelomas. Wiener Medizinische Presse **30,** 209–253.

4. Homburger, F. (1950) Evaluation of diagnostic tests for cancer. 1: Methodology of evaluation and review of suggested diagnostic procedures. *Cancer* **3,** 143–172.
5. Bodansky, O. (1974) Reflections on biochemical aspects of human cancer. *Cancer* **33,** 364–370.
6. Woodruff, M. (1990) Cellular variation and adaptation in cancer, in *Biological Basis and Therapeutic Consequences*, Oxford University Press, New York, NY, pp. 1–7.
7. Galen, R. S. and Gambino S. R. (1975) *Beyond Normality: The Predictive Value and Efficiency of Medical Diagnoses,* Wiley Medical, New York.
8. Bayes, Rev. T. (1763) An essay toward solving a problem in the doctrine of chance. *Phil. Trans. Roy. Soc.* **53,** 370–418.
9. Miller, A. B. (1985) Principles of screening and of the evaluation of screening programs, in *Screening for Cancer,* Miller, A. B. (ed.), Academic, New York, pp. 3–24.
10. Roulston, J. E. and Leonard, R. C. F. (1993) *Serological Tumor Markers: An Introduction*, Churchill Livingstone, Edinburgh, U.K., pp. 15–34.
11. Jacobs, I. J., Bridges, J., Stabile, I., Kemsley, P., Reynolds, C., and Oram, D. H. (1987) CA-125 and screening for ovarian cancer: serum levels in 1010 apparently healthy postmenopausal women. *Brit. J. Cancer* **55,** 515.
12. Ward, B. G., Cruickshank, D. J., Tucker, D. F., and Love, S. (1987) Independent expression in serum of three tumor-associated antigens: CA125, placental alkaline phosphatase and $HMFG_2$ in human ovarian carcinoma. *Brit. J. Obstet. Gynæcol.* **94,** 696–698.

# 10

## Bioactive Interleukin-6 Levels in Serum and Ascites as a Prognostic Factor in Patients with Epithelial Ovarian Cancer

### Günther Gastl and Marie Plante

## 1. Introduction

Interleukin-6 (IL-6) is a multifunctional cytokine displaying diverse biologic functions that can be produced by a broad variety of normal and malignant cell types (*1*). In vivo, high levels of bioactive IL-6 have been detected in the ascites of patients with epithelial ovarian cancer, suggesting abundant local production of this cytokine at the tumor site (*2–6*). We found IL-6 levels in ascites to correlate significantly with the volume of ascites and nearly so with the size of tumor found at initial surgery (*2*). Notably, IL-6 levels in malignant ascites also correlated with reactive thrombocytosis, and maximum IL-6 bioactivity in ascites and highest platelet counts occurred in patients with undifferentiated ovarian adenocarcinoma or advanced disease (*7*). Patients who responded to chemotherapy tended to have lower ascites IL-6 levels compared with patients who failed to respond to chemotherapy (*4*). Berek et al. concluded that bioactive IL-6 in serum may be a useful tumor marker for ovarian cancer, because in their study it correlated with tumor burden, clinical disease status, and survival time (*3*). Performing a multivariate analysis, Scambia et al. (*6*) found serum IL-6 to have an independent prognostic value, but appeared to be less sensitive than CA-125. In conclusion, most investigators found serum and ascitic IL-6 to be of prognostic value in ovarian cancer. In the following section, the B9-bioassay for the detection of IL-6 in body fluids is described in detail.

## 2. Materials

1. Cell culture medium: RPMI-1640 medium with 5% heat-inactivated fetal bovine serum (FBS), 100 U/mL penicillin, 100 U/mL streptomycin, 50 m$M$ 2-mercaptoethanol, 2 m$M$ L-glutamine. Store at 4°C.
2. Cell culture medium containing 0.25 ng/mL human recombinant IL-6 (*rhu* IL-6; Boehringer Mannheim, Indianapolis, IN).
3. Murine hybridoma cell line B9 (ATCC).
4. [$^3$H]thymidine (specific activity, 185 kBq/mmol).
5. Phosphate-buffered saline (PBS) (pH 7.2).

From: *Methods in Molecular Medicine, Vol. 39: Ovarian Cancer: Methods and Protocols*
Edited by: J. M. S. Bartlett © Humana Press, Inc., Totowa, NJ

6. MTT [3-(4,5-dimethylthiazol-2-ys)-2,5-diphenyl tetrazolium bromide] 6 mg/mL in PBS (filter sterilize and store in darkness).
7. Acidified isopropanol (35 μL of 0.04*N* HCl in 500 mL of 2-propanol).
8. Human recombinant IL-6 (100 pg/mL) in cell culture medium.
9. Goat antihuman IL-6 antibody (R&D Systems, Minneapolis, MN).

## 3. Methods

### 3.1. Sample Collection

1. Collect fresh ascites specimens sterilely. Centrifuge samples at 800*g* for 20 min.
2. Draw blood samples by venipuncture in siliconized glass tubes without anticoagulant and centrifuge at 400*g* for 10 min.
3. Freeze the separated cell-free ascitic fluid and serum samples in aliquots at –20°C (*see* **Note 1**).

### 3.2. B9 Bioassay for the Determination of IL-6 Concentrations

To determine the IL-6 bioactivity in ascitic fluid and/or serum, a standard proliferation assay using the IL-6 dependent murine B9 cell line is used *(8)* (*see* **Note 2**). B9 cells are grown in suspension using T-25 tissue culture flasks (Falcon Labware, Lincoln Park, NJ) and maintained in cell culture medium supplemented *rhu* IL-6. Cultures are split 1:5 to 1:10 every 2–3 d, and refed with fresh medium when the cell density reaches approximately $5 \times 10^5$ cells/mL (*see* **Note 3**). Cultures are maintained at 37°C/ 5% $CO_2$ in a humidified incubator.

1. Dilute each ascitic fluid and serum sample serially in culture medium (1:10, 1:20, 1:40; 1:80, 1:160, 1:320) in flat-bottomed 96-well plates. Test all samples in triplicate in 100 μL volumes (*see* **Note 4**).
2. Prepare an IL-6 standard (*rhu* IL-6) as a serial twofold dilution series in triplicate in 100 μL volume in 96-well microtiter plates. Start the titration of the standard at 100 pg/mL and dilute down to 0.1 pg/mL. As a negative control include culture medium without IL-6.
3. Harvest B9 cells two days after feeding by centrifuging the cells at 250*g* for 10 min.
4. Resuspend in IL-6 free medium and recentrifuging the cells at 250*g* for 10 min. Repeat once.
5. Check the viability of the washed cells by trypan-blue-dye exclusion using a counting chamber. Resuspend cells at a concentration of $5 \times 10^4$ cells/mL in cell culture medium without IL-6.
6. Add 100 μL of cell suspension to each well (standard, test samples, and negative control) and incubate the plates for approximately 72 h in a humidified incubator.
7. To each well, add 37 kBq of [$^3$H]thymidine (specific activity: 185 kBq/mmol).
8. Incubate for 6 h and harvest the cells onto glass filter paper (Printed Filtermat A; Pharmacia Diagnostics, Columbus, OH) using a cell harvester.
9. After drying the filter paper in a microwave oven for 4 min, the filtermat should be put into a sample bag (Pharmacia), soaked in 20 mL scintillation fluid, and sealed. Incorporated radioactivity is determined with a β-scintillation counter.

### 3.3. MTT Procedure

As an alternative for radioactive labeling, cell viability can be measured. In this case, proceed as in **Subheading 3.2., step 6** and continue as below:

1. Add 10 μL of MTT solution. and return the plates to the incubator for another 4 h.
2. Centrifuge plates at 400*g* for 7 min to pellet the cells.

3. Tilt the plate and remove medium carefully (this may be done with a 26-gage needle using vacuum suction).

4. Add 100 µL of acidified isopropanol (35 µL of 0.04*N* HCl/500 mL of 2-propanolol) to each well to extract the dye from the cells (positive cells will be blue). Let stand for 5–10 min.

5. Add 100 µL of distilled water. Read adsorption at a wavelength of 570/690 nm using a microplate reader (Bio-Rad, Richmond, CA).

## *3.4. Calculation of Results*

Plot a standard curve of [$^3$H]uptake (or absorbance) versus concentration of IL-6. For determination of IL-6 bioactivity in unknown samples, compare test results with the standard curve.

## 4. Notes

1. Ascitic fluid and serum samples can be kept frozen at –20°C for >12 mo without significant loss of IL-6 bioactivity. A single freeze-thaw cycle does not affect IL-6 levels either.

2. The B9 bioassay is considered to be specific for IL-6 and not affected by the presence of other interleukins, tumor necrosis factor, interferons, or colony-stimulating factors (*8*). Because after several passages B9 cells tend to become IL-6 independent, aliquots of the original IL-6 dependent B9 clone should be kept frozen until assaying.

3. The proliferative response of B9 cells to increasing concentrations of IL-6 (e.g., *rhu* IL-6) eventually reaches a plateau and declines thereafter. Thus, it is important to serially dilute test samples and to calculate IL-6 concentrations from the linear part of the dose-response curve. Half-maximal [$^3$H]thymidine uptake (or cell viability) can usually be achieved with approximately 5 pg/mL of *rhu* IL-6.

4. To verify that the measured bioactivity is indeed owing to IL-6, a neutralizing polyclonal goat antihuman IL-6 antibody (final dilution, 5 µg/mL) should be tested along with test samples. In the presence of this antibody, B9 cell proliferation should be completely blocked. Use a control antibody (e.g., a neutralizing antibody specific for human GM-CSF) to demonstrate specificity in blocking experiments. The detection limit of the B9 bioassay is approximately 1 pg/mL.

## References

1. Kishimoto, T. (1989) The biology of interleukin-6. *Blood* **74**, 1–10.
2. Plante, M., Rubin, S. C., Wong, G. Y., Federici, M. G., Finstad, C. L., and Gastl, G. A. (1994) Interleukin-6 level in serum and ascites as a prognostic factor in patients with epithelial ovarian cancer. *Cancer* **73**, 1882–1888.
3. Berek, J. S., Chung, C., Kaldi, K., Watson, J. S., Knox, R. M., and Martinez-Maza, O. (1991) Serum interleukin-6 levels correlate with disease status in patients with epithelial ovarian cancer. *Am. J. Obstet. Gynecol.* **164**, 1038–1043.
4. Kutteh, W. H. and Kutteh, C. C. (1992) Quantitation of tumor necrosis factor-alpha, interleukin-1 beta, and interleukin-6 in the effusions of ovarian epithelial neoplasms. *Am. J. Obstet. Gynecol.* **167**, 1864–1869.
5. Scambia, G., Testa, U., Panici, P. B., Martucci, R., Foti, E., Petrini, M., et al. (1994) Interleukin-6 serum levels in patients with gynecological tumors. *Int. J. Cancer* **57**, 318–323.
6. Scambia, G., Testa, U., Benedetti-Panici, P., Foti, E., Martucci, R., Gadducci, A., et al. (1995) Prognostic significance of interleukin-6 serum levels in patients with ovarian cancer. *Br. J. Cancer* **71**, 354–356.
7. Gastl, G., Plante, M., Finstad, C. L., Wong, G. Y., Federici, M. G., Bander, N. H., and Rubin, S. C. (1993) High IL-6 levels in ascitic fluid correlate with reactive thrombocytosis in patients with epithelial ovarian cancer. *Br. J. Haematol.* **83**, 433–441.
8. Aarden, L. A., van DeGroot, E. R., Schaap, O. L., and Lansdorp, P. M. (1987) Production of hybridoma growth factor by human monocytes. *Eur. J. Immunol.* **17**, 1411–1416.

# 11

## ELISA-Based Quantification of *p105* (c-*erbB-2*, *HER2/neu*) in Serum of Ovarian Carcinoma

**Harald Meden, Arjang Fattahi-Meibodi, and Dagmar Marx**

### 1. Introduction

The most important prognostic parameters for gynecologic malignancies are tumor stage, residual tumor after surgical treatment, histological subtype, and degree of malignancy *(1–2)*. However, these factors present an incomplete picture of the tumor biology. Therefore, investigation of other prognostic factors is of special clinical relevance, particularly in view of the unexpectedly progressive course of the disease and frequent relapses in some cases.

In recent years, reports have described the prognostic significance of the amplification and overexpression of the oncogene c-*erbB-2* (*HER2/neu*) in various human cancers. The oncogene c-*erbB-2* characterises a group with unfavourable tumor biology and a significantly worse prognosis *(3–4)*.

The c-*erbB-2* oncogene expression product p185 (**Fig. 1**), a transmembrane protein with intrinsic tyrosine kinase activity, is detectable by immunohistochemical methods. Slamon et al. *(5)* examined 189 breast carcinomas and reported on an amplification of the c-*erbB-2* oncogene in 30% of the cases. Amplification of the c-*erbB-2* oncogene proved to be a significant prognostic parameter for survival times and relapse rates. The association between amplification of the c-*erbB-2* oncogene and the overexpression of the protein (p185) encoded by the c-*erbB-2* oncogene has been confirmed in breast cancer by other several studies *(6–8)*. In addition to studies on breast cancer, Berchuck et al. *(9)* described a rate of 32% overexpression of the oncogene c-*erbB-2* in a study of 73 patients with ovarian carcinoma. Our group reported on a study of 275 ovarian cancer patients, and recorded a rate of 19% for p185-positive cases *(10)*. Analyzing the published data, the percentage of immunohistochemical c-*erbB-2* positive cases in ovarian cancer varies from 9 *(11)* to 32% (**Table 1**).

Because of proteolytic activity, the extracelluar domain of the p185 transmembrane growth factor receptor, a fragment of 105 kD (p105, **Fig. 2**), is released from the surface of human cancer cells that overexpress p185. It is detectable in the extracellular environment in vitro *(12)*. Elevated serum levels of the c-*erbB-2* oncoprotein fragment p105 have been identified in patients with various cancers. In addition, the quantitative detection of p105 in the sera of ovarian cancer patients was published by using a mono-

From: *Methods in Molecular Medicine, Vol. 39: Ovarian Cancer: Methods and Protocols*
Edited by: J. M. S. Bartlett © Humana Press, Inc., Totowa, NJ

Fig. 1. Structure of the transmembrane protein p105.

**Table 1**
**c-*erbB-2* Positivity in Ovarian Cancer**

| Author (ref.) | c-*erbB-2* positive | *n* |
|---|---|---|
| Slamon et al. *(4)* | 25% | 120 |
| Berchuck et al. *(9)* | 32% | 73 |
| Haldane et al. *(11)* | 8,7% | 104 |
| Meden et al. *(10)* | 19% | 275 |

clonal antibody (moAb) ELISA *(13)*. Another study demonstrated that elevated p105 serum levels in patients with newly diagnosed and previously untreated primary ovarian cancer correlate with poor prognosis *(14)*, **Table 2**. Screening for increased c-*erbB-2* oncoprotein fragment levels in ovarian cancer patients could make it possible to identify a subset of high risk patients.

Elevated p105 serum levels can be regarded as a result of increased proteolytic activity in the tumor tissue. Parallel to this, the serum results would support the hypothesis that patients with elevated p105 levels are a subset of immunohistochemical c-*erbB-2*-positive tumors indicating a very aggressive tumor biology in the group of high risk patients *(14)*.

In a previously published study, evaluation of p105 ovarian cancer patients was performed by using a new polyclonal detector antibody-based ELISA (**Table 3**). Elevated p105 serum levels were not related to tumor stage, grade, histology, or residual tumor after primary surgery and age, but on the other hand, these evaluations are comparable to results using the monoclonal-based ELISA in previous studies *(15)*.

## 2. Materials

1. Human Neu (c-*erbB-2*) ELISA (e.g., test kit by Oncogene Science). The test kit contains most of the necessary reagents except distilled/deionized water.

Fig. 2. Structure of the protein p105.

**Table 2**
**Prognostic Value of Pretreatment Serum p105 (ELISA) and Tumor p185 (ICH)**

|  | Positive | | Median survival time (mo) | | |
|---|---|---|---|---|---|
|  | *n* | *%* | positive | negative | *P* value |
| Serum p105 | 6/57 | 11 | 7 | 29 | 0,02 |
| Immunohistochemistry | 8/57 | 14 | 23,5 | 29 | 0,64 |
| Serum p105, stage III | 3/29 | 10 | 6 | 26 | 0,05 |
| Immunohistochemistry, stage III | 2/29 | 7 | 12 | 29 | 0,08 |

2. Manual or automatic microplate washer.
3. Sample material: Serum or plasma treated with heparin, citrate, EDTA, fluoride, oxalate, or tissue.

## 3. Methods

### 3.1. Sample Preparation

Serum and plasma samples should be diluted at 1:50 in sample diluent which contains 2% normal mouse serum (nms) prior to assay. Greater dilutions may be necessary for samples that generate signals exceeding the dynamic range of the standards. This diluent minimizes false positive samples, which may result from autologous antimouse antibodies, rheumatoid factors, and heterophilic antibodies in some samples.

1. Prepare a 5-mL solution of sample diluent containing 4% normal mouse serum by adding 0.2 mL of nms to 4.8 mL of sample diluent.
2. Dilute specimens to 1:25 in untreated sample diluent.
3. Combine 0.125 mL of diluted serum with an equivalent volume of 4% nms sample diluent to provide 0.25 mL of 1:50 sample in 2% nms/sample diluent.
4. Transfer two 100 μL aliquots of each diluted sample to microtiter wells (*see* **Subheading 3.2.1.**, step **2**).

**Table 3**
**Correlation of Immunohistochemical**
**and Serological Findings of the Oncogene c-erbB-2 (n = 53)**

|           | p105 pos. | p105 neg. | Total |
|-----------|-----------|-----------|-------|
| IHC pos.  | 6         | 11        | 17    |
| IHC neg.  | 7         | 29        | 36    |
| total     | 13        | 40        | 53    |

Cutoff level for serum p105 positively: 150 fmol/mL.
IHC: immunohistochemistry.

### 3.2. Eliza Method

Addition of reagents must be in the order specified. All six standards and the test specimens should run in duplicate.

#### 3.2.1. Day 1

1. Before addition of the detector antibody, equilibrate all reagents to room temperature (15–25°C, *see* **Note 1**).
2. Remove the microplate supplied with the kit from the bag. From the number of specimens to be tested, calculate the number of strips required (remember that each specimen dilution or standard requires two wells, and four wells are needed for background determinations. The standard curve, run in duplicate, requires 12 wells). Store unused strips in the zip-lock bag with desiccant at 2–8°C (*see* **Note 2**).
3. Add 100 μL of each diluted sample to duplicate wells.
4. Vortex the standard or specimen dilution thoroughly and add 100 μL to duplicate wells. Set up four wells with untreated sample diluent, two to measure the background absorbance and two to be used as the substrate blank well.
5. Cover the microplate with a piece of plastic wrap and incubate for 12–18 h at room temperature (15–30°C).

#### 3.2.2. Day 2

1. Prepare plate wash. 1 vol of plate wash concentrate should be diluted with 19 vol of distilled or deionized water. Mix well (*see* **Note 2**).
2. Remove the plastic wrap and wash the microplate with plate wash (*see* **Note 3**).
   a. Automatic microplate washer—set the fill volume to 300 μL/well. Prime the instrument with 1X plate wash. Use two 3-cycle washes, rotate the plate 180° and repeat.
   b. Manual microplate washer—wash six times, using 300 μL per well per wash. Fill the entire plate, then aspirate in the same order.
   c. Hand-held syringe-wash six times, using 300 μL per well per wash. Blot the plate upside-down between washes.
3. After the final wash, invert the microplate and firmly strike it on an absorbent surface. Visually check that all wells are empty.
4. Add 100 μL of detector antibody to all wells except the substrate blank well. Incubate at room temperature for 60 min.
5. During the incubation with detector antibody, prepare working conjugate by diluting the conjugate concentrate at 1:50 in conjugate diluent in a clean reagent reservoir.
6. Wash the microplate with plate wash.
7. Add 100 μL of working conjugate to all wells except the substrate blank well. Incubate at room temperature for 30 min.

8. During the incubation with working conjugate, prepare working substrate by dissolving one substrate tablet per 4 mL of substrate diluent. Vortex vigorously to assure complete dissolution. Once prepared, working substrate should be used within 30 min. Avoid exposure to light.

9. Wash the microplate with plate wash.

10. Including the substrate blank well, add 100 μL of working substrate to all wells. Incubate the microplate in the dark at room temperature for 45 min.

11. Add 100 μL of stop solution to each well to stop the reaction.

12. Read the absorbance at 490 nm (with a 620-nm reference filter if possible) within 30 min, using the substrate blank well to zero the reader.

13. Compare absorbances of unknown samples with those of the standard curve to determine quantity of neu (p105) protein. Correct for dilution factor for all samples.

## 4. Notes

1. Preparation of plate wash: If the plate wash concentrate is cold, it is allowed to reach room temperature before use. All crystals must be dissolved. If necessary, warm at 37°C and mix or shake.

2. The protein p105 seems to stable enough to be stored for a longer time at −20°C, but it has to be taken into account that serum samples should only be frozen once.

3. Microplate washing may be automated, semi-automated, or manual, but must be carried out with care to ensure optimal performance of the assay. Plate washing equipment must be properly adjusted, cleaned, and maintained. Whichever method is used, the solution used to wash plates is plate wash. The total volume required will depend on the washing method/instrument used. Approximately 1 L of this solution is required to prime an automated washer and run one microplate. About 700 μL are required for each microplate well when manual washing is performed. Plate wash must be freshly prepared each day. Do not store plate wash.

4. **Caution:** When inverting the microplate to decant or blot, the side tabs of the frame should be pressed inward to prevent the strips from falling out. Uncoated blank strips can be used to fill the unused portion of the holder for mechanical washers.

## 5. Summary

Elevated serum levels of the fragment of the c-*erbB-2* oncoprotein have been identified in patients with various cancers known to overexpress the c-*erbB-2* oncogene. For research purposes, screening for an increased p105 level could make it possible to identify a subset of high-risk patients. Furthermore, the test could be potentially useful for detecting recurrent disease. Systematic detection of c-*erbB-2* gene activation in cancer patients would require ELISAs, which are sensitive and reliable enough to differentiate between healthy normal controls and inapparent carcinoma patients, so it is supposition that serum or plasma samples have to exceed the cut-off level which is set at 150 fmol/mL.

From the methodical point of view, double determinations of plasma or serum specimens are recommended in this polyclonal antibody-based ELISA. In our own observations, remarkable differences in the results of the double determinations have not been found. One major problem are patients with very small inapparent cancers: even if these tumors would show an intensive membrane staining of p185 in immunohistochemical analysis and proteolytic activity would shed the extracellular domain (p105) into circulation, an extensive dilution of the tiny amount of p105 would minimize the chance to discriminate these patients from healthy individuals.

Supporting this theory, in a recently published study *(15)* elevated levels of the p185 oncoprotein fragment (p105) were only found in a small group of ovarian carcinoma patients who had overexpression in their tumors. This may indicate that the aforementioned polyclonal ELISA is yet not of sufficient sensitivity. Slamon et al. *(4)* indicated that fixation of the tumor decreases the sensitivity of the immunohistochemical detection of p185 as compared to fresh frozen specimens. Therefore, the lack of immunohistochemical staining may underestimate the level of expression in these tumors.

In addition, nonspecific proteolytic activities because of invasive growth cause a shedding of the extracellular epitope of p185 in the tumor tissue, so immunohistochemical detector antibodies, e.g. 9G6, cannot bind to the extracellular domain and membrane staining is not detectable. In breast cancer, c-*erbB-2* overexpression is usually homogenously distributed in tumor tissue. In contrast to this, in ovarian tumor cell conglomerates commonly and only a focal membrane staining is detectable. Thus, false negative immunohistochemical results cannot be excluded. In healthy women, the effects of interfering and influencing factors of the analysis of p105 (c-*erbB-2*) oncoprotein fragment in serum are still unclear. In individual analyses, changes of p105 concentrations depending from the menstrual cycle have not been found. Concerning the menstrual status of women, postmenopausal women show significantly higher p105 levels than premenopausal women. Furthermore, in tests, there was found no influence on the reproducibility of results by changing transporting and storing conditions *(16)*. In conclusion, clinical interpretation of female p105 serum values require comparison with normal ranges when considering the menopause as an influencing factor.

Women with hormonal contraception have significant lower serum levels than premenopausal controls. In postmenopausal women with hormone replacement therapy (HRT), serum levels are significant lower than in postmenopausal controls. Furthermore, the activity of the oncogene c-*erbB-2* seems to be influenced by endocrine factors, resulting in decreased p105 serum levels after treatment with sex steroids. Regarding the widespread use of sex steroids for hormonal contraception and HRT, the knowledge of these influencing parameters is important for the interpretation of p185 and p105 levels in clinical studies *(17)*.

Numerous genes activated during human ontogenesis, which by means of growth and regulation factors exercise influence on cell proliferation and differentiation, become deactivated at the end of development. Normal fetal development is associated with activation of cellular oncogenes during pregnancy.

Because the oncogene expression product of c-*erbB-1*, EGFR, has been described as a marker of proliferation, p185 seems to play an important part for specific cell differentiation during organogenesis. Initial serum analyses during pregnancy yielded elevated p105 values compared with a group of nonpregnant women *(16)* (**Table 4**).

At the beginning of the third trimester, and then with increasing gestational age, p105 serum levels increase. This trend was revealed both interindividually and intraindividually, and further analyses of the maternal sera show the highest p105 levels prior delivery *(18)*. Growth factors and oncogenes are of central importance to organogenesis. Protooncogenes are activated to a different extent during fetal and embryonal development. Normal intrauterine embryogenesis has several features in common with the growth of malignant tumors. This includes interalia the invasive and controlled growth of trophoblast compared to invasive uncontrolled tumor growth. One

**Table 4**
**Normal Ranges of p105 Serum Concentrations**
**in 71 Healthy, Nonpregnant Women**

| Control group | *n* | 2.5% to 97.5-quantile |
|---|---|---|
| Premenopausal without hormonal contraception | 47 | 108–181 fmol/mL |
| Premenopausal without hormonal replacement therapy | 24 | 104–256 fmol/mL |

possible reason for increased serum levels in the third trimester is the deactivation of p185 by proteolytic cleavage of its 105 kD extracellular domain, followed by increased appearance in the serum. Moreover, changing filtration conditions in the maternal kidney or in the feto-maternal circulatory system could be responsible for these findings.

Concerning the p105 levels during pregnancy, there is no significant difference between healthy women and patients with *superimposed* preeclampsia. Compared to normal pregnancies of the third trimester, patients with *pure* preeclampsia have significantly higher p105 serum levels. Women with a HELLP syndrome show a significant decrease of p105 in the first and second trimester. The highest values were measured in the third trimester. In comparison to normal pregnant women of the third trimester, patients with pure preeclampsia and HELLP syndrome had significantly higher levels of p105.

In abnormal pregnancies of the first trimester with damage to or modification of the structure of known foci of p185 overexpression there was, unlike in nonpregnant women, no significantly diminished p105 serum level. This result indicates that there may be no relationship between the degree of p185 expression in the tissue and maternal serum level.

Investigating of the cause of the elevated p105 serum levels in instances of preeclampsia and HELLP syndrome, the modifications in the vascular endothelium may play a crucial role: endothelial cells have complex functions in the mediation of immunological reactions, preserve the integrity of the vascular structure, prevent intravascular blood coagulation, and modulate the contractile reaction of the smooth vascular muscle cell on which the endothelial cell rests. These characteristics are relevant to preeclampsia. Endothelial cells may loose these properties and release coagulant, vasoconstrictive, and mitogenetic substances *(19)*.

The differences between the results of pure and superimposed preeclampsia are possibly because of differences in the pathogenesis of these two forms of preeclampsia. The results of our study addressing this issue concur with those of Roberts and Redman who discovered an increased activity of growth factors in the blood of patients with eclampsia compared to a control group *(19)*. These changes normalized after pregnancy, like the p105 serum levels in our series of analyses. Another marker that was significantly elevated in patients with preeclampsia compared to a control group is cellular fibronectin. Furthermore, in the context of the altered function of the endothelial cells, patients with preeclampsia are described as featuring an enhanced release of prostacyclin, an elevated expression of the B-chain of the platelet-derived growth factor, and a reduced release of endothelin *(19)*.

In view of these findings, it is conceivable that the significantly elevated p105 serum levels associated with preeclampsia and HELLP syndrome occur as a result of the endothelial modifications detected for these pregnancy-specific disorder and the expression of an alteration in cell dedifferentiation. Another possible cause of the elevated p105 serum levels in patients with preeclampsia and HELLP syndrome could be the disturbance in the differentiation of the spiral arterioles in the course of implantation.

Because elevated p105 serum levels are detectable in various oncological disorders, during the third trimester of normal pregnancy, in pure preeclampsia, and in cases of HELLP syndrome it would make sense to search for common features among these various entities to establish causalities. The implantation of the trophoblast, the ageing of the placenta before delivery, and the invasive growth of tumor cells are founded in proteolytic processes. In the case of the oncogene c-erbB-2, it has been demonstrated that the extracellular domain (p105) of the p185 expressed by tumor cells is liberated due to proteolytic breakdown, which might explain the elevated p105 serum concentrations in cancer patients.

Because preeclampsia and eclampsia have figured as the principal cause of maternal fatalities in most countries for the last 40 yr, predictive markers for these disorders are of central importance. To what extent elevated p105 serum levels can be specifically employed for prospective diagnostics in the case of clinically asymptomatic women who later develop preeclampsia or HELLP syndrome is unclear at present.

Further studies must take these influencing factors into account, especially in control groups, before one can estimate whether the analysis of p105 concentration is a valuable diagnostic tool for cancer patients.

## References

1. Hacker, N. F., Berek, J. S., Lagasse, L. D., Nieberg, R. K., and Elashoff, R. M. (1983) Primary cytoreductive surgery for epithelial ovarian cancer. *Obstet. Gynecol.* **61,** 413–420.
2. Malkasian, G. D. Jr., Melton, L. J., O'Brien, P. C., and Greene, M. H. (1984) Prognostic significance of histologic classification and grading of epithelial malignancies of the ovary. *Am. J. Obstet. Gynecol.* **149,** 274–284.
3. Bishop, J. M. (1987) The molecular genetics of cancer. *Science* **235,** 305–310.
4. Slamon, D. J., Godolphin, W., Jones, L. A., et al. (1989) Studies of the HER-2/neu proto-oncogene in human breast and ovarian cancer. *Science* **244,** 707–712.
5. Slamon, D. J., Clark, G. M., Wong, S. G., Levin, W. J., Ullrich, A., and McGuire, W. L. (1987) Human breast cancer correlation of relapse and survival with amplification of the HER-2/neu oncogene. *Science* **235,** 177–182.
6. Venter, D. J., Tuzi, N. L., Kumar, S., and Gullick, W. J. (1987) Overexpression of the c-erbB-2 oncoprotein in human breast carcinomas: immunohistological assessment correlation with gene amplification. *Lancet* **2,** 68–72.
7. Berger, M. S., Locher, G. W., Saurer, S., Gullick, W. J., Waterfield, M. D., Groner, B., et al. (1988) Correlation of c-erbB-2 gene amplification and protein expression in human breast carcinoma with nodal status und nuclear grading. *Cancer Res.* **48,** 1238–1243.
8. Marx, D., Schauer, A., Reiche, C., et al. (1990) C-erbB-2 expression in correlation to other biological parameters of breast cancer. *J. Cancer Res. Clin. Oncol.* **116,** 15–20.
9. Berchuck, A., Kamel, A., and Whitaker, R. (1990) Overexpression of HER-2/neu is associated with poor survival in advanced epithelial ovarian cancer. *Cancer Res.* **50,** 4087–4091.
10. Meden, H., Marx, D., Rath, W., Kron, M., Fattahi-Meibodi, A., Hinney, B., et al. (1994) Overexpression of the oncogene c-erbB-2 in primary ovarian cancer. Evaluation of the prognostic value in a Cox proportional hazards multiple regression. *Int. J. Gynecol. Pathol.* **13,** 45–53.
11. Haldane, J. S., Hird, V., Hughes, C. M., and Gullick, W. J. (1990) C-erbB-2 oncogene expression in ovarian cancer. *H. Pathol.* **162,** 231–237.
12. Zabrecky, J. R., Lam, T., McKenzie, S. J., and Carney, W. (1991) The extracellular domain of p185/neu is released from the surface of human breast carcinoma cells. SK-BR-3. *J. Biol. Chem.* **266,** 1716–1720.

13. Meden, H., Marx, D., Fattahi, A., Rath, W., Kron, M., Wuttke, W., et al. (1997) Elevated serum levels of a c-erbB-2 oncogene product in ovarian cancer patients and in pregnancy. *J. Cancer Res. Clin. Oncol.* **129,** 378–381.

14. Meden, H., Marx, D., Wuttke, W., Schauer, A., and Kuhn, W. (1997) Prognostic significance of p105 (c-erbB-2, HER2/neu) serum levels in patients with ovarian carcinoma. *Anticancer Res.* **17,** 757–760.

15. Marx, D., Fattahi-Meibodi, A., Kudelka, R., Uebel, T., Kuhn, W., and Meden, H. (1998) p105 (c-erbB-2, HER2/neu) serum levels, detected by a new polyclonal antibody-based ELISA, in patients with ovarian carcinoma—correlation to patho-morphological results. *Anticancer Res.* **18,** 2891–2894.

16. Mielke, S., Meden, H., Raab, T., Wuttke, W., and Kuhn, W. (1997) Effects of interfering and influencing factors of the analysis of p105 (c-erbB-2) oncoprotein fragment in serum. *Anticancer Res.* **17,** 3125–3128.

17. Meden, H., Mielke, S., Marx, D., Wuttke, W., and Kuhn, W. (1997) Hormonal treatment with sex steroids in women is associated with lower p105 serum concentrations. *Anticancer Res.* **17,** 757–760.

18. Meden, H., Mielke, S., Wuttke, W., and Kuhn, W. (1997) Elevated serum levels of the c-erbB-2 encoded oncoprotein fragment in cases of pure preeclampsia and HELLP syndrome. *J. Obstet. Gynaecol. Res.* **23,** 213–217.

19. Roberts, J. M. and Redman, C. W. (1993) Pre-eclampsia: more than pregnancy-induced hypertension. *Lancet* **341,** 1447–1451.

# 12

# Enzyme Immunoassay of Urinary β-Core Fragment of Human Chorionic Gonadotropin as a Tumor Marker for Ovarian Cancer

**Ryuichiro Nishimura, Tamio Koizumi, Hiranmoy Das, Masayuki Takemori, and Kazuo Hasegawa**

## 1. Introduction

Human chorionic gonadotropin (hCG), a glycoprotein hormone composed of two nonidentical α- and β-subunits, is normally produced by trophoblasts. Serum and urine from some patients with nontrophoblastic tumors are found to contain similar immunoactivity to the β-subunit of hCG and this phenomenon has been recognized as an ectopic hCGβ production *(1)*. Elevated levels of ectopic hCGβ are detected more frequently in urine than in serum. Recent studies have shown that urinary ectopic hCGβ mainly represents hCGβ-core fragment (β-CF) *(2)*. Urinary β-CF consists of residues 6–40 disulfide bridged to residues 55–92 of the β-subunit of hCG *(3,4)*, suggesting that it may be a degradative product of hCGβ. Such partial identity of the amino acid sequence between intact hCG, free hCGβ, and β-CF makes their specific measurements difficult. The existence of two more antigenic sites unique to hCGβ has been demonstrated. The one domain locates in the β-core portion and the other in COOH-terminal region of the β-subunit of hCG (**Fig. 1**). By selecting appropriate pairs of antibodies to construct sandwich enzyme immunoassays (EIAs), it is possible to design methods that measure either intact hCG, free hCGβ, or β-CF (**Table 1**). By using this EIA, the authors assessed the clinical usefulness of urinary β-CF as a tumor marker for nontrophoblastic tumors *(5,6)*. Here, the authors describe the methods to measure urinary β-CF in patients with ovarian cancer.

## 2. Materials

Urine was collected from patients on admission. After centrifuging the urine at 2000*g*, the supernatant was collected and then frozen at –20°C until assayed.

### 2.1. Purification of hCG Subunits

1. 8*M* guanidine hydrochloride.
2. High-performance gel permeation chromatography (GPC) system (e.g., Gilson Model 302 pump, Gilson Model 802 monometric module, M & S Model 311 UV-detector, and Pantos U-228 recoder with 2.5 × 60 cm TSK G3000 SW column.
3. GPC elution buffer: 6*M* guanidine hydrochloride.

From: *Methods in Molecular Medicine, Vol. 39: Ovarian Cancer: Methods and Protocols*
Edited by: J. M. S. Bartlett © Humana Press, Inc., Totowa, NJ

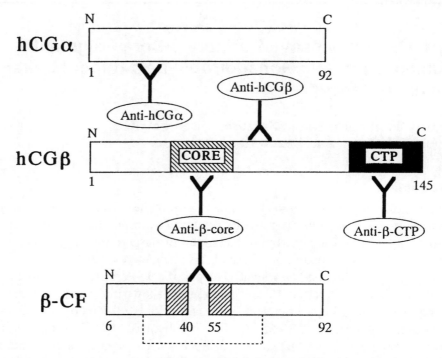

Fig. 1. Two antigenic sites: the first domain is located in the β-core portion and the second domain is located in the COOH-terminal region of the β-subunit of hCG.

## 2.2. Purification of Antibodies

1. Protein-A cellulofine (Seikagaku Kogyo, Tokyo, Japan) in 0.1*M* NaHCO3 containing 0.5*M* NaCl (pH 8.3) packed in a column (0.6 × 8cm).
2. Column prewash: 0.1*M* acetate buffer-0.5 *M* NaCl (pH 4.0).
3. Protein A column loading buffer: 0.01*M* phosphate buffered saline (pH 7.4).
4. Protein A column elution buffer: 0.2*M* Glycine-HCl (pH 2.8).
5. hCGβ-coupled Sepharose (Pharmacia LKB Biotechnology, Uppsala, Sweden) in 0.1*M* NaHCO₃ containing 0.5*M* NaCl (pH 8.3) packed in a column (0.6 × 8cm).
6. hCGβ-Sepharose column loading buffer: 0.5*M* NaCl followed by distilled water.
7. 0.5 *M* NaCl.
8. hCGβ-Sepharose column elution buffer: 1*N* acetic acid.

## 2.3. EIA Systems

1. Polystyrene beads (6.35 mm in diameter, Sekisui Chemical, Osaka, Japan).
2. 0.1*M* sodium bicarbonate, pH 9.5.
3. BSA solution: 1% bovine serum albumin.
4. PBS-BSA: 0.02*M* phosphate buffer, 0.1% bovine serum albumin, pH 7.5.
5. Citrate buffer: Phosphate citrate buffer, 0.02% hydrogen peroxide, 2 mg/mL of o-phenylene diamine, pH 4.65.
6. 1*N* sulfuric acid.

**Table 1**
**Specificities and Sensitivities of Enzyme-Immunoassays Specific for Intact hCG(EIA-1), Free hCGβ(EIA-2), and β-CF(EIA-3)**

| | First antibody | | Second antibody | | | Sensitivity (ng/ml) | Cross-reactivity (%) | | |
| | | | | | | | Intact hCG | Free hCGβ | β-CF |
| Assay | Code | Epitope | Code | Epitope | Specificity | | | | |
|---|---|---|---|---|---|---|---|---|---|
| EIA-1 | No.277(MoAb) | β-CTP | No.224(MoAb) | hcGα | Intact hCG | 0.01 | 100 | 15 | <1.0 |
| EIA-2 | No.209(MoAb) | hCGβ | No.115(PoAb) | β-core | Free hCGβ | 0.01 | 1.9 | 100 | 1.9 |
| EIA-3 | No.229(MoAb) | β-core | No.105(PoAb) | β-core | β-CF | 0.01 | 3.3 | 100 | 100 |

MoAb: monoclonal antibody.
PoAb: polyclonal antibody.

137

## 3. Methods

### 3.1. Production of hCG Subunits

1. Highly purified hCG (4 mg) was dissolved in 0.3 mL of $8M$ guanidine hydrochloride and incubated at 37°C for 2 h.
2. 0.1 mL of distilled water was added before application to a column of high-performance gel permeation chromatography (GPC). In one course of GPC, several aliquots of 0.1-mL hCG solution were injected into the GPC system.
3. hCG subunits were eluted in $6M$ guanidine hydrochloride solution at room temperature. The effluent was collected into 0.5 mL fractions with a flow rate of 0.5 mL/min. Aliquots were removed for identification of immunoactivities of the $\alpha$- and $\beta$-subunits by their respective immunoassays. The fractions comprising each subunit were pooled, exhaustively dialysed against distilled water and lyophilized on a freeze dryer.
4. The resultant purified $\alpha$- and $\beta$-subunits were used as antigens to raise antibodies in animals. To prepare monoclonal antibodies immunization of BALB/c mice was performed as previously described *(7,8)*. After two immunizations of 10 µg subunits, spleen cells were fused with mouse myeloma cells. After 2 wk culture supernatents were tested for production of antibodies against hCG, hCGα, and hCGβ radioimmunoassays.

### 3.2. Enzyme Immunoassay (EIA)

Three types of enzyme immunoassay (EIA) systems for intact hCG, free hCGβ, and β-CF were established as EIA-1, -2, and -3, respectively, by the sandwich method using two different monoclonal and polyclonal antibodies (**Table 1**).

#### 3.2.1. Protein—A Purification of Monoclonal Antibodies

Monoclonal antibodies were purified with the use of protein-A cellulofine (Seikagaku Kogyo, Tokyo, Japan).

1. Protein-A cellulofine is packed in a column and washed with 10 mL of $0.1M$ NaHCO$_3$-$0.5M$ NaCl (pH 8.3).
2. The column is washed with 10 mL of column prewash buffer.
3. The sample is applied to the column.
4. Wash column with ten column volumes of $0.01M$ phosphate buffered saline (pH 7.4).
5. Bound antibody is eluted with $0.2M$ Glycine-HCl (pH 2.8).
6. The eluate is immediately neutralized with ammonium hydroxide.

#### 3.2.2. Purification of Polyclonal Antibodies

The polyclonal antibody was purified by affinity chromatography with an hCGβ-coupled Sepharose column (Pharmacia LKB Biotechnology, Tokyo, Japan).

1. Coupled sepharose is packed in a column and washed with 10 mL of $0.1M$ NaHCO$_3$-$0.5M$ NaCl (pH 8.3).
2. The column is washed with 10 mL of column prewash buffer.
3. The sample is applied to the column.
4. Wash column in 10 vol $0.5M$ NaCl and 10 vol distilled water.
5. Antibody was eluted in $1N$ acetic acid and the eluate immediately neutralized with ammonium hydroxide.

### 3.3. EIA Systems

1. Polystyrene beads were incubated with 50 µg/mL of the purified first monoclonal antibody in $0.1M$ sodium bicarbonate, pH 9.5, overnight at 4°C.

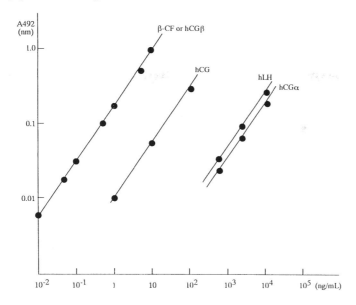

Fig. 2. Standard curve for the enzyme Immunoassays (EIA) of β-CF.

2. After the incubation, the remaining antibody solution was aspirated and the beads were incubated with 1% BSA solution for 1 h at room temperature to block the residual binding sites.
3. The BSA solution was then removed, and the beads were washed with distilled water.
4. The beads coated with the first antibody were incubated with 100 μL of the sample and 200 μL of 0.02$M$ phosphate buffer containing BSA 7.5 for 3 h at 37°C.
5. The beads were washed three times with deionized water and transferred to new assay tubes.
6. 500 μL of citrate buffer (pH 4.65), was added for the color development at room temperature.
7. After 30 min, the reaction was stopped by the addition of 1$N$ sulfuric acid and immediately measured at 492 nm absorbance.
8. The standard curve for EIA of β-CF is shown in **Fig. 2**. Intra-assay and interassay variances were within 10% and the sensitivity was 0.01 ng/mL. The cross-reactivities of pituitary glycoprotein hormones (hLH, hFSH and hTSH) were less than 0.5%.

### 3.4. Assay Specifications

### 3.4.1. Specificity of EIA for β-CF

In our EIA systems, EIA-1 and EIA-2 are essentially specific for intact hCG and free hCGb, respectively, but the assay value of EIA-3 does not always indicate the concentration of β-CF, since EIA-3 recognizes β-CF as well as free hCGβ (**Table 1**). Therefore, the actual amount of β-CF is calculated after subtracting the assay

### 3.4.2. Adjustment of Urinary Concentration of β-CF by Urinary Creatinine Level

Urinary concentration of β-CF is influenced by the urine volume. Therefore, urinary concentration of β-CF should be adjusted by the creatinine level contained in the same

| Stage | Positive rate(%) | Urinary β-CF(ng/mgCr) |
|-------|------------------|------------------------|
| 1 | 66.7%<br>(8/12) | |
| 2 | 100%<br>(5/5) | |
| 3 | 91.3%<br>(21/23) | |
| 4 | 80.0%<br>(4/5) | |

Fig. 3. Levels of urinary β-CF increase as disease progresses.

urine for the evaluation as a tumor marker. Thus, urinary level of β-CF is expressed as nanograms per milligram of creatinine (ng/mgCr).

### 3.4.3. Cutoff Value of Urinary β-CF

The mean level plus or minus standard deviation of β-CF in the urine of nonpregnant healthy women was 0.079 ± 0.052 ng/mgCr. The cutoff value, set at M+2SD, of β-CF in the urine was 0.2 ng/mgCr. Based on this cutoff value, 5.4% of the urine samples from nonpregnant, healthy women were found to contain elevated levels of β-CF. Specificity of urinary β-CF as a tumor marker was investigated by examining urine of patients with gynecologic benign diseases, indicating that the false positive rate was less than 10%.

## 4. Note

The authors studied patients with common epithelial nongerm cell ovarian cancer referred to the Department of Obstetrics and Gynecology of Hyogo Medical Center for Adults. From the 45 patients with ovarian cancer, 38 (84.4%) patients had elevated levels of urinary β-CF, and the incidence increased with disease progression (**Fig. 3**). The positive rates of urinary β-CF classified by histologic types of ovarian cancer were 87.1% (27 of 31) for serous, 75% (6 of 8) for mucinous, and 83.3% (5 of 6) for others. There was no significant correlation between the concentrations of urinary β-CF and serum CA125 and all the patients so far examined were detected by the combination assay of these tumor markers.

## References

1. Braunstein, G. D., Vaitukaitis, J. L., Carbone, P. P., and Ross, G. T. (1973) Ectopic production of human chorinic gonadotropin by neoplasms. *Ann. Intern. Med.* **78,** 39–45.
2. Nishimura, R., Kitajima, T., Hasegawa, K., Takeuchi, K., and Mochizuki, M. (1989) Molecular forms of human chorionic gonadotropin in choriocarcinoma serum and urine. *Jpn. J. Cancer Res.* **80,** 968–974.
3. Birken, S., Armstrong, E. G., Gawinowicz-Kolks, M. A., Cole, L. A., Agosto, G. M., Krichevski, A., et al. (1988) Structure of human chorionic gonadotropin β-subunit fragment from pregnancy urine. *Endocrinol.* **123,** 572–583.

4. Endo, T., Nishimura, R., Saito, S., Kanazawa, K., Nomura, K., Katsuno, M., et al. (1992) Carbohydrate structures of β-core fragment of human chorinoic gonadotropin isolated from a pregnant individual. *Endocrinol.* **130,** 2052–2058.

5. Kinugasa, M., Nishimura, R., Koizumi, T., Morisue, K., Higashida, T., Natazuka, T., et al. (1995) Combination assay of urinary β-core fragment of human chorionic gonadotropin with serum tumor markers in gynecologic cancers. *Jpn. J. Cancer Res.* **86,** 783–789.

6. Yoshimura, M., Nishimura, R., Murotani, A., Miyamoto, Y., Nakagawa, T., Hasegawa, K., et al. (1994) Assessment of urinary β-core fragment of human chorionic gonadotropin as a new tumor marker of lung cancer. *Cancer* **73,** 2745–2752.

# III

## MODEL SYSTEMS

# 13

## Ovarian Cancer Models

*Technical Review*

## Simon P. Langdon, Joanne Edwards, and John M. S. Bartlett

## 1. Introduction

Perhaps the most fundamental question that faces the laboratory scientist is, "Which model system should I use to investigate the problem?" Failure to adequately address this issue can compromise even the most meticulous and inspired research program. If this is such a thorny issue, why use model systems at all? As with most biological systems, ovarian cancer is a complex disorder comprising tumor cells, stromal tissues, neovascularization, inflammatory responses, and other host responses to the tumor. Experimental science best progresses by controling all but a single variable and observing what occurs when that variable is modulated. Almost by definition, this requires a homogenous group of samples to work with. Using human cancer patients for research, it becomes rapidly apparent that the diverse nature of the tumors and the hosts greatly complicates such an approach, hence the development of various model systems. The problem with model systems is simple, they are models—not the true disease states, by their very nature they are less than perfect reflections of the way in which the system under investigation performs in vivo in the normal host. Model systems are essential research tools, but have to be used appropriately.

The choice of model largely depends on the question being asked. It is only within the last 40 years that experimental approaches in the study of cancer have progressed to the use of tissue dispersion techniques. These techniques are used to isolate fully differentiated primary-cell populations for subsequent experimental use. In some cases, these primary cells can be grown or maintained in culture for a number of passages before eventually losing their differentiated characteristics (*1*). These cells can also be used to establish secondary cell lines where tumor characteristics can be studied in vitro or if used within an animal model in vivo. Prior to the development of these techniques, experiments were limited to studies which used either intact organs, tissue extracted from induced animal tumors, or sections of human tumor. Currently, however, a broad range of models systems are available to investigate characteristics of ovarian cancer cells both in vitro and in vivo. Models of malignant and normal ovarian epithelium obtained from the human, rat, and mouse, have been described and their use has extended our knowledge of the properties of ovarian cancer cells (*2*). This over-

From: *Methods in Molecular Medicine, Vol. 39: Ovarian Cancer: Methods and Protocols*
Edited by: J. M. S. Bartlett © Humana Press, Inc., Totowa, NJ

view will briefly outline some of the model systems that are in use and their relative strengths and limitations.

## 2. Clinical Models

Collections of tumors and patients series are the ultimate "clinical model," however, although clinical studies offer valuable information into the nature of ovarian cancer, the great complexity of these systems precludes any control of many of the factors that may affect the system under study. Tumors, as they arise in patients, comprise a genetically, nutritionally, and physiologically highly heterogeneous host group suffering from a broad range of disease pathologies, even within a single tumor group such as ovarian cancer, which is managed by diverse therapies. Nonetheless, at all times the researcher should have in mind the true pathophysiological system, and work toward an understanding of this system with the recognition that ultimately his or her work must be relevant to the behavior of tumors in the patient.

Tumor banks and observational studies have provided significant information relating to the expression and distribution of biological phenotypes within the tumor population. They provide valuable insights into potential mechanisms for in vitro study and also test beds for the analysis of hypotheses developed in vitro.

### 2.1. In Vitro Models

In essence, in vitro systems are divided into three major categories:

1. Primary cell culture.
2. Secondary cell culture.
3. Dual or co-culture systems.

In the first two systems, the objective is to isolate a single cell type, usually the tumor cells, and to investigate their function in isolation from the complex interactions that surround them. Co-culture systems begin to approximate the in vivo system by "rebuilding" the interactions between, for example, stromal and tumor cells and allowing the investigation of interactions between multiple cell systems. Each system has potential benefits and drawbacks. The major advantage of culture systems is their simplicity. Tissue-culture systems allow control of the environment within which the cells are growing, e.g., amount of growth hormones available to the culture and also monitoring of the reaction of a culture to a particular treatment.

### 2.1.1. Primary Cell Culture

#### 2.1.1.1. What is a Primary Culture?

A primary culture is one initiated from cells, tissues, or organs taken directly from an organism. Cells freshly isolated from a particular tissue may survive for days or months either dividing or nondividing before eventually dying, or may divide repeatedly requiring subculturing or passaging (3). If the primary cell culture, once established, continues to grow and divide, it is termed a primary cell line which may die after several passages or may become an established cell line with the apparent potential to be subcultured indefinitely. Refer to Chapter 14 for protocols that describe how to establish ovarian cancer primary cell cultures from ascites, solid primary tumor, or metastatic deposits.

### 2.1.1.2. How are Primary Cultures Derived?

There are several methods for establishing primary cultures, and this varies depending on the composition of the tissue (*see* Chapter 14) *(3)*. Most tissue, however, can be desegregated by one of three techniques or a combination of these; physical disruption, enzymatic digestion, and treatment with chelating agents. Physical disruption is not often used alone, mainly because it is difficult to obtain a uniformed suspension without cell damage. It is, however, usually combined with enzymatic digestion or chelating agents. The most successful enzymes used to desegregate tissues are collagenase and trypsin. Trypsin is usually the enzyme of choice for separation of cells in established cultures, however, for initial isolation of cells, collagenase is more effective as some tissues, especially from adult animals, are refractory to trypsin treatment because of their collagen content *(1)*. Certain tissues, especially epithelial tissues, seem to require divalent cations, particularly calcium and magnesium for their integrity. If these ions are removed by substances that bind them (chelating agents) the tissues may be desegregated very easily. Chelating agents most commonly used are EDTA and EGTA. These agents are rarely used alone for tissue dispersion, however, their use in combination with enzymatic digestion is more common.

The ways in which enzymes and chelating agents are used to form a cell suspension are similar. The tissue (which is usually sliced or chopped) is placed in a solution containing an enzyme or chelating agent or both and rocked or stirred for various lengths of times. It is also common practice to treat a tissue with a chelating agent before the use of an enzyme for further digestion. Once a single cell solution has been obtained, the cells are maintained in sterile culture flasks that contain cell-culture medium. Cell-culture medium is a synthetic replacement for the normal extracellular fluid in the animal. This media needs to be maintained at the correct pH and osmolality, it also requires the correct concentrations of essential inorganic salts, vitamins, amino acids, and growth factors. In most cases, antibiotics such as penicillin, streptomycin, and/or kanamycin are added to the growth media. Other environmental factors also need to be taken into consideration, for example, temperature (37°C) and the culture substrata (tumor cells are less dependent on the substrate).

### 2.1.1.3. What are the Experimental Advantages of Primary Cultures?

Primary cultures, as their name suggests and as described above, represent the first step in ex vivo culture of biological systems. Cancer cells are naturally adaptive. As soon as they are removed from the body and cultured for any length of time, they modify their behavior in ways which may not reflect the behavior in vivo. Simply placed to grow on plastic presents different challenges to growing in vivo! Primary cultures are particularly useful because in studying tumors in the hours and perhaps days since removal from the patient, one is studying the tumor cell in the absence of any culture-induced changes.

The major disadvantage of primary culture systems is that they are short lived and rarely transported from one laboratory to another, thus preventing reproduction of results and confirmation by different groups. In addition, the short-lived nature of these models precludes sequential study of different systems in the same model system. The use of multiple primary cultures allows study of the diversity observed in in vivo tumor studies.

Ovarian carcinoma primary cell-culture models may perhaps best be used to study clinical response to chemotherapy. The level of thymidine uptake by the cultured cells (measurement of cell division) is recorded in response to different chemotherapy regimes. Full agreement has been observed between the degree of thymidine uptake inhibition induced by drugs administered to the cultured cells and the degree of clinical response *(9)*. The predictive accuracy of the in vitro drug sensitivity test has been reported to be in the region of 80% *(10,11)*. This screening test may also provide the choice of the next best drug(s), once the tumor has become resistant to a particular drug. Thus, the overall prognosis of patients at an advanced stage of malignancy could be improved with the help of in vitro predicative tests *(11)*. This method for matching therapies accurately to tumors has, sadly, proven too expensive to be widely utilized, despite the potential patient benefit.

### 2.1.2. Secondary Cell Culture

#### 2.1.2.1. What is a Secondary Cell Culture?

A secondary cell-culture line is a cell line obtained from a primary culture which can be subcultured almost *ad infinitum* *(3)*. It is a general observation that if a primary culture is maintained for a period of time, the cells will enter a period of statis, where cell division or growth slows dramatically or even appears to stop. Many cell lines will die back at this point, however, after maintaining these quiescent cells for periods of weeks, or even months, a proportion will regrow such that they now grow relatively readily on plastic and are amenable to subculturing for an almost indefinite period *(3)*. Once this transition has occurred, the cell line can be readily transported between laboratories and regrown and represents a novel "secondary" cell culture.

#### 2.1.2.2. Development of Secondary Cell Cultures (*see* Chapter 15)

This transition between the primary and established state may occur gradually or suddenly as a result of a transformation (either spontaneous or induced) which can usually be monitored by the identification of a few colonies of rapidly dividing cells. These cells tend to differ from the primary cell line in several ways, e.g., abnormal chromosome number, loss of contact inhibition, shorter population doubling times, and occasionally a loss of specialized function(s) *(4)*. The majority of primary cell lines established from tumors will behave as an established cell line. Many of these cell lines show better retention of specialized function than those derived from normal tissue *(3)*, making tumor material the ideal source of cells for establishment of a secondary cell line *(15)*. Chapter 14 discusses how a primary ovarian cancer cell line can be maintained and develop into an established cell line and also the removal of contaminating cell types, e.g., fibroblasts and mesothelial cells. A large number of ovarian cancer cell lines have now been established and are in widespread use (refer to Table 1 in Chapters 2, 5, 9, 10, 11, 12, and 14). Many of these have been selected to reflect specific situations, e.g., pre- and postchemotherapy models or pathological subtypes. The majority of ovarian cancer patients will develop ascites. Most ovarian lines have been developed from ascitic cells, as this is the most convenient source for sampling *(5)*. Ascitic fluid contains clusters of malignant cells, which are readily obtained by centrifugation. Other cell-line models derived from sites within the patient include the primary tumor, omental metastases, and pleural effusions. Selection of cells according to the source, for example, primary or secondary tumor material, is likely to predetermine certain features of the model system. Ascitic cells reflect features of cells capable of surviving in the peritoneal cavity and are likely to be metastatic; these cells may or may not differ from properties of cells found within the primary tumor. Cell lines derived from these cells may be very appropriate for chemosensitivity testing, however, cell lines obtained directly from primary tumors may be more suitable for investigating early events in ovarian carcinogenesis (6).

### 2.1.2.3. WHAT ARE THE EXPERIMENTAL ADVANTAGES OF SECONDARY CULTURES?

The main advantage of secondary culture over primary culture is avoiding the technical difficulties associated within studying primary cell cultures, particularly in obtaining an initially "pure" population of malignant cells, which is devoid of stromal components such as fibroblasts and mesothelial cells. Secondary cultures, therefore, provide a renewable source of material, which is generally more homogeneous to provide the opportunity for continuous experimentation (1). These systems are the most widely used in current in vitro cancer research. The main disadvantage associated with secondary culture is that clones more suited to culture conditions or which grow more rapidly will dominate, thus resulting in the model becoming less representative of the original tumor (1). Long-term culture may also provide an opportunity for further mutations to occur and it is important to ensure that properties observed in the model truly reflect those found in the original tumor.

However, the problem of dominant clones may, in some cases, be an advantage depending on the question being asked. In some cases, it may be desirable to select clones of cells that exhibit a specific feature of interest, e.g., drug resistance. Clones can be readily obtained by growth of a single-cell suspension in semisolid agar and can be picked out very easily from the matrix by use of a syringe needle or obtained by limiting dilution culture (Chapter 15). Many drug-resistant cell lines, particular those that exhibit this particular feature, have been developed and these have shown that cisplatin-resistance can be generated via multiple mechanisms (7). Other features such as the role of *p53* (Chapter 19) and estrogen regulation (Chapter 20) have also been modeled (26,31). In general, ovarian carcinoma cell cultures are important tools for studying second messenger systems and hormonal regulation of ovarian cancer. The information gained from studying these cell lines can then be utilized in the development of novel therapies, e.g., tyrosine kinase inhibitors (8). Cell cultures are also used in the initial screening phase of newly developed drugs such as tyrosine kinase inhibitors, before such compounds are considered for in vivo investigation (8). The invasiveness of tumor cells can also be measured in vitro using an invasion assay. Chapter 18 discusses an assay that measures invasiveness of relatively low-level invasive ovarian cancer cell lines. The assay involves visual counting of stained cells, which have invaded through a membrane filter.

### 2.1.2.4. CO-CULTURE SYSTEMS

These are essentially a method for combining two or more cell lines (for example, tumor and fibroblast) to investigate interactions between them. Also within this head could be included culturing of cell lines with extracellular matrix (e.g., matrigel). The obvious advantage of such systems is that a closer approximation to the original tumor architecture is achieved. The disadvantage is that modulations may not only affect interactions between cell types, but independently affect each component of the co-culture systems. These systems are thus relatively underused in the study of ovarian cancer.

### 2.2. In Vitro Models Summary

In summary, human tumor cell lines provide valuable model systems to study a wide variety of tumor characteristics including the cell biology, genetic, and chemosensitivity profiles of diseases. Advantages of immortal cell lines are that homogenous cell populations are established without contamination from other cells, which results in better reproducibility of cell cultures. The main disadvantages involved with the use of an immortal cell line are the loss of specialized characteristics, which are retained in primary cultures.

### 3. In Vivo Models

Although murine *(12,13)* and rat *(14)* tumor models of ovarian cancer are available, there has been a much greater interest in studying human ovarian cancer growing in immunodeficient animals. The use of chemoinduced animal models *(14)* reduces, but does not exclude, the tumor heterogeneity seen in clinical samples. Furthermore, there is valid concern that chemoinduced tumors may not reflect the behavior of human systems. The use of immonodeficient mice as surrogate hosts for human tumors has provided a valuable and reproducible system for the investigation of ovarian cancer. Often used in conjunction or subsequent to in vitro systems, these in vivo models represent perhaps the closest approximation to the "normal" tumor.

These models vary depending of the site of implantation. The most commonly used sites are:

1. Subcutaneous (sc).
2. Intraperitoneal (ip).
3. Under the capsule of the ovary.

This overview will discuss when each site should be used as the experimental model and the advantages and disadvantages associated with it.

### 3.1. Subcutaneous Xenografts

The first description of sc xenographs of ovarian cancer tissue into the nude mouse was made by Davy et al. in 1977 *(15)*. Xenografts into nude mice can either be from human ovarian cancer material or from established human tumor cell lines. The most convenient site from the point of view of monitoring features such as tumor growth or recovering the implanted material is sc implantation under the skin in the flank of the animal. Such models have been extensively used in the antitumor testing of experimental agents [e.g., *(16)*] and in the assessment of tumorigenicity where it is important to obtain the best estimates of changes in tumor volume (changes in tumor volume are easily noted by means of calliper measurements). Whereas sc xenograft tumors have been used extensively in the study of cell biology *(17)* and chemotherapy *(18)*, their anatomical localization bears little relation to the natural history of human ovarian cancer.

### 3.2. Intraperitoneal Xenografts

For certain experiments, e.g., pharmacokinetic distribution studies of an antitumor drug, the use of an ovarian xenograft in a site other than the ovary or the peritoneal cavity is of debatable value. In order to solve this problem, Cobb et al. established a human clear-cell carcinoma of the ovary ip in an immunomodulated hamster *(19)*. However, the ip model is now most commonly used in nude mice *(20–23)*. Cells are injected ip and mimic the dissemination process demonstrated by ascitic cell spread. This model is of particular interest for testing the role of therapies administered ip, e.g., cytokines such as gamma-interferon *(24)* and is currently being used to explore the potential of gene therapy *(25–27)*.

### 3.3. Implantation of Tumor Fragments Under the Capsule of the Ovary

A technically more challenging, but more complete, model has recently been reported, which involves the implantation of tumor fragments under the capsule of the ovary *(28)*. These fragments grow locally and then metastasize giving rise to a realistic pattern of metastases involving spread into the peritoneum, colon, and omentum and the production of ascites. A large animal model in cyclosporin-immunosuppressed sheep has also been developed *(29)*.

The above models can either be maintained in vivo or re-established from cell cultures in each experiment. With the primary establishment of the tumor into the immunodeficient mouse either directly from a patient or from a cell line, there is often marked variation in growth rates of individual tumors in different mice even though all are derived from the same source. If these tumors are passaged through several animals, more reproducible growth rates are achieved. Not all cell lines and primary tumor fragments grow readily in immunosuppressed animals. Where difficulty is experienced in establishing xenografts from either cell lines or primary tumors, then use of the extracellular matrix component Matrigel may help (Chapter 21) *(30)*. This appears to be particularly helpful in the initial establishment of the tumor, but unnecessary for subsequent passage. For most ovarian cancer xenografts, the nature of the immunodeficient host does not appear to be overly critical and both nude (T-cell dysfunctional) and SCID mice (T- and B-cell dysfunctional) can be used.

### 3.4. Summary

In summary, the use of human tumor xenografts in immunodeficient animals as a model for human cancers is well established. Their value depends on the extent to which their characteristics reflect the properties of a particular cancer in the clinical situation. Intraperitoneal xenografts seem to be no more difficult to establish than sc xenografts, however, implantation of tumor fragments under the capsule of the ovary is associated with technical difficulties. In experiments where the end point is sacrifice of the animals and measurement of the tumors, ip models mimic the clinical situation more closely than sc xenografts. However, sc xenograft models are more suitable for continuous measurement of tumor parameters, eg dimensions for growth curves, because this is not possible with ip xenografts. At present, the most complete model available involves implantation of tumor material into the ovary, however, ip xenografts or sc xenografts are often sufficient for experimental needs.

## 4. Summary

Many in vitro and in vivo models systems are currently available to investigate characteristics of ovarian cancer cells. The model of choice depends on the aspect of ovarian cancer under investigation. Tissue-culture systems are often sufficient for preliminary studies that involve drug screening and have been responsible for providing much of the information known about hormonal mechanisms, signal transduction, apoptosis, chemoresistance, and other molecular characteristics of this disease. It can, however, be necessary to use an in vivo model where cell cultures have failed to provide a comparable environment to an in vivo human tumor. Whole animal studies may also be required for more extensive metabolic, pharmacokinetic, and toxicological investigations. In summary, many ovarian cancer models are available, however, careful consideration is required before deciding which model is suitable for any one study. It is important to select the most appropriate model to answer the question being posed. The main aims to consider are:

1. the model is simple enough to allow extraction of the information required without complication from irrelevant external parameters,
2. the model is not so simple that it is so far removed from the natural tumor environment that the information obtained is irrelevant.

Deciding on a suitable experimental model is therefore a balance between being simple enough to understand without to many irrelevant complications. This overview has described many of the models available to study ovarian cancer and has highlighted the advantages and disadvantages associated with each of these models.

## References

1. Barnes, K. L., Sirbasku, Z., and Sato, C. (1984) *Cell Culture Methods for Molecular and Cell Biology* (Barnes, ed.), vol. 1.
2. Tsao, S. W., Mok, S. C., Fey, E. G., Fletcher, J. A., Wan, T. S., Chew, E. C., et al. (1995) Characterization of human ovarian surface epithelial cells immortalized by human papilloma viral oncogenes (HPV-E6E7 ORFs). *Exp. Cell Res.* **218,** 499–507.
3. Paul, K. (1970) *Cell and Tissue Culture.* 4th ed. (Paul, ed.), Livingstone.
4. Taub, M. (1985) *Tissue Culture of Epithelial Cells.* 1st ed. (Taub, ed.).
5. Langdon, S. P., Lawrie, S. S., Hay, F. G., Hawkes, M. M., McDonald, A., Hayward, I. P., et al. (1988) Characterization and properties of nine human ovarian adenocarcinoma cell lines. *Cancer Res.* **48,** 6166–6172.
6. Wolf, C. R., Hayward, I. P., Lawrie, S. S., Buckton, K., McIntyre, M. A., Adams, D. J., et al. (1987) Cellular heterogeneity and drug resistance in two ovarian adenocarcinoma cell lines derived from a single patient. *Int. J. Cancer* **39,** 695–702.
7. Kido, M. and Shibuya, M. (1998) Isolation and characterization of mouse ovarian surface epithelial cell lines. *Pathol. Res. Pract.* **194,** 725–730.
8. Trinks, U., Buchdunger, E., Furet, P., Kump, W., Mett, H., Meyer, T., et al. (1994) Dianilinophthalimides: Potent and selective, ATP competitive inhibitors of the EGF receptor protein tyrosine kinase. *J. Med. Chem.* **37,** 1015–1027.
9. Morasca, L., Erba, E., Vaghi, M., et al. (1983) Clinical correlates of in vitro drug sensitivites of ovarian cancer cells. *Br. J. Cancer* **48,** 61–68.
10. Trope, C. and Sigurdsson, K. (1982) Use of tissue culture in predictive testing of drug sensitivity in human ovarian cancer. Correlation between in vitro results and the response in vivo. *Neoplasma* **29,** 309–314.
11. Buckshee, D., Roy, P. K., and Chapekar, T. N. (198) Use of in vitro method to predict response of human ovarian carcinoma cells to chemotherapeutic agents. *Int. J. Gyn. Obst.* **22,** 371–374.
12. Langdon, S. P., Gescher, A., Hickman, J. A., and Stevens, M. F. G. (1984) The chemosensitivity of a new experimental model—the M5076 reticulum cell sarcoma. *Eur. J. Cancer Clin. Oncol.* **20,** 699–705.

13. Ozols, R. F., Locker, G. Y., Doroshow, J. H., Grotzinger, K. R., Myers, C. E., Fisher, R. I., and Young, R. C. (1979) Chemotherapy for murine ovarian cancer: a rationale for i.p. therapy with adriamycin. *Cancer Treat. Rep.* **63**, 269–273.

14. Rose, G. S., Tocco, L. M., Granger, G. A., DiSaia, P. J., Hamilton, T. C., Santin, A. D., and Hiserodt, J. C. (1996) Development and characterization of a clinically useful animal model of epithelial ovarian cancer in the Fischer 344 rat. *Am. J. Obstet. Gynecol.* **175**, 593–599.

15. Davy, M., Mossige, J., and Johannessen, J. V. (1977) Heterologous growth of human ovarian cancer *Acta. Obstet. Gynecol. Scand.* **56**, 55–59.

16. Boven, E., Van der Vijgh, W. J. F., Nauta, M. M., Schluper, H. M. M., and Pinedo, H. M. (1985) Comparative activity and distribution studies of five platinum analogues in nude mice bearing human ovarian carcinoma xenografts. *Cancer Res.* **45**, 86–90.

17. Friendlander, N. L., Russell, P., Taylor, I. W., and Tattersall, M. H. N. (1985) Ovarian tumor xenografts in the study of the biology of human epithelial cancer. *Br. J. Cancer* **51**, 391–333.

18. Jones, A. C., Wilson, P. A., and Steel, G. G. (1984) Cell survival in four ovarian carcinoma xenografts following in vitro exposure to melphalan, cisplatin, and cis-diamline-1,1-cyclobutane dicarbosylate platinum II. *Cancer Chemother. Pharmacol.* **13**, 109–113.

19. Cobb, L. M., Boesen, E. A. M., and Neville, A. (1981) Clear cell carcinoma of the human ovary transplanted to the peritoneal cavity of the hamster. *Transplantation (Baltimore)* **16**, 76–78.

20. Baumal, R., Law, J., Buick, R. N., Kahn, H., Yeger, H., and Sheldon, K. (1986) Monoclonal antibodies to an epithelial ovarian adenocarcinom: distincitve reactivity with xenografts of the original tumor and a culture cell line. *Cancer Res.* **46**, 3994–4000

21. Wahl, R. and Piko, C. (1985) Intraperitoneal delivery of radiolabelled monoclonal antibody to IP induced xenografts of ovarian cancer *Proc. Am. Assoc.* **26**, 29.

22. Ward, B. G., Wallace, K., Shepherd, J. H., and Balkwill, F. R. (1987) Intraperitoneal xenografts of human epithelial ovarian cancer in nude mice. *Cancer Res.* **47**, 2662–2667.

23. Malik, S. T. A., East, N., Boraschi, D., and Balkwill, R. R. (1992) Effects of intraperitoneal recombinant interleukin-1B in intraperitoneal human ovarian cancer xenograft models: comparison with the effects of tumor necrosis factor. *Br. J. Cancer* **65**, 661–666.

24. Malik, S. T., Knowles, R. G., East, N., Lando, D., Stamp, G., and Balkwill, F. R. (1991) Antitumor activity of gamma-interferon in ascitic and solid tumor models of human ovarian cancer. *Cancer Res.* **51**, 6643–6649.

25. Tong, X. W., Block, A., Chen, S. H., Contant, C. F., Agoulnick, I., Blankenburg, K., et al. (1996) In vivo gene therapy of ovarian cancer by adenovirus-mediated thymidine kinase gene transduction and ganciclovir administration. *Gynecol. Oncol.* **61**, 175–179.

26. von Gruenigen, V. E., Santoso, J. T., Coleman, R. L., Muller, C. Y., Miller, D. S., and Mathis, J. M. (1998) In vivo studies of adenovirus-based p53 gene therapy for ovarian cancer. *Gynecol. Oncol.* **69**, 197–204.

27. Mujoo, K., Maneval, D. C., Anderson, S. C., and Gutterman, J. U. (1996) Adenoviral-mediated p53 tumor suppressor gene therapy of human ovarian carcinoma. *Oncogene* **12**, 1617–1623.

28. Fu, X. and Hoffman, R. M. (1993) Human ovarian carcinoma metastatic models constructed in nude mice by orthotopic transplantation of histologically-intact patient pecimens. *Anticancer Res.* **13**, 283–286.

29. Turner, J. H., Rose, A. H., Glancy, R. J., and Penhale, W. J. (1998) Orthotopic xenografts of human melanoma and colonic and ovarian carcinoma in sheep to evaluate radioimmunotherapy. *Br. J. Cancer* **78**, 486–494.

30. Mullen, P., Ritchie, A., Langdon, S. P., and Miller, W. R. (1996) Effect of matrigel on the tumorigenicity of human breast and ovarian cancer cell lines. *Int. J. Cancer* **67**, 816–820.

31. Simpson, B. J. B., Langdon, S. P., Rabiaz., G. J., et al. (1998) *J. Steroid. Biochem. Mol. Biol.* **64**, 137–145.

# 14

## Establishment of Ovarian Cancer Cell Lines

### Simon P. Langdon and Sandra S. Lawrie

### 1. Introduction

Human tumor cell lines have provided valuable model systems to study a wide variety of tumor characteristics including the cell biology, genetics, and chemosensitivity profiles of disease. A large number of ovarian cancer cell lines have now been established and are in widespread use (**Table 1** ) *(1–15)*. Many of these have been selected to reflect specific situations, e.g., pre- and postchemotherapy models or different histological subtypes.

Although ovarian cancer cell lines have been obtained from primary tumors, solid metastatic deposits and pleural effusions (**Table 1**), most have been derived from the peritoneal ascites of ovarian cancer patients because this provides a very convenient source of tumor cells and may be more readily available than primary or metastatic material as it is routinely drained for the alleviation of discomfort. The tumor cells within this fluid are found as single cells or small clusters and this avoids the need for mechanical or enzymatic desegregation. The cells consist not only of malignant carcinoma cells, but also lymphocytes, macrophages, red blood cells, mesothelial cells, and fibroblasts. By use of differential centrifugation and trypsinization techniques, pure populations of carcinoma cells can be selected within several passages. These can then be characterized to verify epithelial origin and the degree of contamination by nonepithelial cells assessed by the use of antibodies targeted to lymphocytes and fibroblasts.

Once established, many ovarian cancer cell lines can be grown in fully defined media, which allows detailed analysis of the influences of regulatory molecules, e.g., the effects of hormones, growth factors, and cytokines or the impact of therapeutic molecules, e.g., cytotoxic drugs such as cisplatin.

### 2. Materials

1. RPMI-1640 medium (Life Technologies Ltd., Paisley, Scotland) + 10% fetal calf serum (Life Technologies) + 100 IU/mL penicillin/100 µg/mL streptomycin (Gibco-BRL, Gaithersburg, MD, Life Technologies Ltd.).
2. 2 m$M$ sodium pyruvate (Sigma, St. Louis, MO).
3. 2.5 µg/mL insulin (Sigma).
4. Phosphate-buffered saline (PBS) (pH 7.4).
5. Histopaque (Sigma).
6. Trypsin (0.05% w/v) / EDTA (0.02% w/v) in PBS.

From: *Methods in Molecular Medicine, Vol. 39: Ovarian Cancer: Methods and Protocols*
Edited by: J. M. S. Bartlett © Humana Press, Inc., Totowa, NJ

**Table 1**
**Properties of Established Ovarian Carcinoma Cell Lines**

| Cell Line | Histology | Source | Prior Treatment | Ref. |
|-----------|-----------|--------|-----------------|------|
| PE01 | P.D. Serous adenoca | Ascites | P/FU/CHL | *1* |
| PE04 | P.D. Serous adenoca | Ascites | P/FU/CHL | *1* |
| PE06 | P.D. Serous adenoca | Ascites | P/FU/CHL | *2* |
| PEA1 | P.D. Adenoca | Pleural | None | *2* |
| PEA2 | P.D. Adenoca | Ascites | P/Pred | *2* |
| PEO16 | P.D. Serous adenoca | Ascites | Radioth | *2* |
| PEO14 | W.D.Serous adenoca | Ascites | None | *2* |
| T014 | W.D.Serous adenoca | Sol. Met | None | *2* |
| PE023 | W.D.Serous adenoca | Ascites | P/CHL | *2* |
| SKOV-3 | Adenoca | Ascites | T | *3* |
| SW626 | Adenoca | — | — | *3* |
| OVCAR-2 | Adenoca | Ascites | P/Cy | *4* |
| OVCAR-3 | P.D. papillary adenoca | Ascites | P/Cy/Adr | *5* |
| OVCAR-4 | Adenoca | Ascites | P/Cy/Adr | *6* |
| OVCAR-5 | Adenoca | Ascites | None | *7* |
| OAW 28 | Adenoca | Ascites | P / Mel | *8* |
| OAW 42 | Serous adenoca | Ascites | P | *8* |
| 41M | Adenoca | Ascites | None | *9* |
| 59M | Endometr adenoca | Ascites | None | *8* |
| CH1 | Papillary adenoca | Ascites | P/ JM8 | *8* |
| 138D | Serous adenoca | Ascites | Carb | *9* |
| 180D | Adenoca | Ascites | P | *9* |
| 200D | Serous adenoca | Solid | None | *9* |
| 253D | Serous adenoca | Ascites | Cy/MPA | *9* |
| HOC-1 | W.D. Serous adenoca | Ascites | None | *10* |
| HOC-7 | W.D. Serous adenoca | Ascites | None | *10* |
| CAOV-3 | Adenoca | Tumour | Cy/Adr/FU | *10* |
| COLO 110 | Serous adenoca | Sol. Met | None | *11* |
| COLO 316 | Serous adenoca | Pleural | None | *11* |
| COLO 319 | Serous adenoca | Ascites | None | *11* |
| COLO 330 | Serous adenoca | Ascites | Mel/Radiother | *11* |
| IGROV1 | Adenoca | Primary | None | *12* |
| HTOA | W.D. serous adenoca | Primary | None | *13* |
| OV-1063 | Papillary adenoca | Ascites | Cy/Adr/P/HMM | *14* |
| DO-s | W.D. mucinous adenoca | Ascites | — | *15* |

P.D. = Poorly differentiated; W.D. = Well differentiated; adenoca = adenocarcinoma; pleural = pleural effusion; Sol.met. = solid metastasis; P = cisplatin; FU = 5-fluorouracil; CHL = chlorambucil; Pred = prednimustine; Radioth = radiotherapy; T = thiotepa; Cy = cyclophosphamide; Adr = adriamycin; Mel = melphalan; Carb = carboplatin; MPA = medroxyprogesterone actetate; HMM = hexamethylmelamine.

## 3. Methods

### 3.1. Initial Culturing from Ascites

1. Freshly obtained ascitic fluid drained from the peritoneum of an ovarian cancer patient at the time of paracentesis or staging laparotomy is transferred to a sterile environment, e.g.,

class II hood (*see* **Notes 1** and **2**). The volume collected from any individual patient is variable, but typically of the order of 1 L.

2. The fluid is centrifuged for 20 min at 3000*g* and 4°C to produce a cell pellet.

3. The fluid is discarded and the cell pellet is resuspended in PBS (20 mL).

4. Red blood cells are removed by use of Histopaque (Sigma). The tumor cell suspension (10 mL) is placed carefully onto Histopaque (10 mL) in a Universal container and centrifuged at 2000*g* for 30 min at room temperature. The tumor cells remain at the interface of the Histopaque and are removed by pastette and transferred to a new Universal container.

5. The cell pellet is resuspended in PBS (10 mL) and centrifuged at 1000*g* for 10 min. The supernatant is discarded. This wash is repeated once.

6. Cells are resuspended in tissue-culture medium (*see* **Notes 3–6**).

7. A cell count is taken. Aliquots of $10^5$ cells/mL (10 mL/25 cm² tissue-culture flask) are then cultured at 37°C, 100% humidity, and 5% $CO_2$ in a tissue-culture incubator. Attachment of cells to the plastic substrate occurs and eventually a monolayer will form.

8. At this initial phase of establishment, cells require careful monitoring (by microscope) because growth is variable. For example, during the establishment of the PE01 and PE04 cell lines, subculturing took place after 21 and 4 wk, respectively (*1*). Tissue-culture medium should be replaced 2–3 times/wk.

## 3.2. Initial Culturing from Solid Primary Tumor or Metastatic Deposit

1. Primary or secondary tumor material is obtained at the time of surgery. Fragments of the tumor are transferred as rapidly as possible into a sterile Universal container containing RPMI-1640 and placed on ice to maintain viability.

2. The Universal container is transferred to a sterile environment (e.g., class II hood). Tumor fragments are then dissociated either mechanically using crossed scalpel blades or enzymatically (*see* **Note 7**). After either mechanical or enzymatic disassociation, cell suspensions can ideally be filtered through a sterile gauze to remove clumps.

3. The cell suspension is then processed according to **Subheading 3.1., steps 6–8**.

## 3.3. Maintenance and Development of Cell Line

After initial culturing, careful monitoring is needed to establish the level of contamination by fibroblasts. Although fibroblasts will cease proliferating after a number of generations, they may outgrow the carcinoma cells if the initial percentage of fibroblasts is too high.

### 3.3.1. Removal of Fibroblasts

1. Selective trypsinization can remove most of the fibroblast population. Fibroblasts tend to detach rapidly from plastic after trypsinization and a short treatment (<2 min) with trypsin/EDTA will remove many of the fibroblasts before the carcinoma cells detach. Fresh media containing serum will then rapidly inactivate remaining trypsin.

2. Fibroblasts attach to plastic more rapidly than the epithelial cells and those cells that attach within the first 2–3 h are predominantly fibroblasts. If the cell suspension is transferred to a new flask after this period, many of the fibroblasts will remain in the original flask which can be discarded.

3. Monoclonal antibodies targeted to fibroblast-specific antigens (e.g., *Thy-1*) can allow selective removal of the fibroblasts when in cell suspension.

### 3.3.2. Removal of Mesothelial Cells

Mesothelial cells may also be present and these can be removed as follows. Mesothelial cells, but not epithelial cells, attach to fibrin meshes, which are produced on initial culturing. A short exposure to trypsin-EDTA (2 min) produces complete detachment of the mesothelial cell sheet attached to the fibrin mesh without removing epithelial islands.

### 3.4. Subculturing and Characterization of Culture

1. When the cell culture approaches confluence, it should be subcultured. Tissue-culture medium is first removed and cells are washed with PBS (20 mL).
2. Trypsin/EDTA is added to the flask for 5–15 min to detach cells.
3. Once cells are in suspension, they are placed into fresh serum / medium and transferred to another flask (*see* **Note 8**).
4. After several passages, the fibroblasts, lymphocytes, and mesothelial cells should have disappeared and only carcinoma cells remain. At this stage, it is appropriate to confirm the epithelial nature of these cells. A small aliquot of cells is placed onto a multispot slide and stained by standard immunocytochemical methods. There are many monoclonal antibodies that can be used for the purpose of identifying specific cell types and we have found the following antibodies to be useful: E29 (Dako, Cambridge, England) targeting epithelial membrane antigen will identify epithelial cells; 2B11 (Dako) targeting leucocyte common antigen (*CD45*) will identify lymphocytes; 5B5 (Dako) targeting the beta subunit of prolyl-4-hydroxylase and the disulphide isomerase will identify fibroblasts.
5. More-detailed assessments of antigen expression may be valuable. Expression of specific cytokeratins and other epithelial markers including human milk fat globulin-2 (*HMFG2*) and *OC 125* (detected by *CA125*) are often measured.
6. Other useful characterization procedures include karyotyping and ploidy analysis.
7. Regular testing for mycoplasma contamination is also advised, e.g., by staining with Hoechst 33528 dye and viewing under a fluorescent microscope or by standard microbiological techniques.

## 4. Notes

1. All ascitic samples should be treated with care and all procedures carried out within class II containment facilities.
2. Heparin has also been widely used to prevent cell aggregation and can be added directly to the initial ascites fluid (10,000 U/L ascites).
3. The choice of specific medium has varied widely between different laboratories. RPMI-1640, DMEM, Ham's F-12, and α-MEM have all been used as the basic medium and the choice depends mainly on the medium in use within the laboratory establishing the cell line. The use of Ham's F12 has also enabled cell lines to develop which otherwise were destined to die *(9)*.
4. The use of additives has also varied widely between different laboratories. In addition to the presence of serum and medium, antibiotics are routinely added and most popular are penicillin and streptomycin although gentamycin (50 µg/mL) and amphotericin (2.5 µg/mL) have also been used. Other standard additives for early cultures include insulin and pyruvate. Historically, extra glutamine was often added to the media, but formulations in current use are more stable.
5. The percentage of fetal calf serum used has most commonly been 10%. Some cell lines have been recorded as growing initially in 10%, but then deteriorating and this effect was prevented by a reduction to 5% serum *(9)*.
6. The use of autologous human ascitic filtrate may help initial establishment and growth of the cell line. This can be added to the media at a level of 10%.
7. Desegregation of solid tumors can be accomplished either mechanically or enzymatically. The simple use of crossed scalpels is easy and if adequate numbers of small clusters of

cells are produced then this is sufficient to generate a cell line. Enzymatic digestion will typically yield a 2–7-fold greater yield of single viable cells. A number of "enzyme cocktails" have been described and the following have all been applied in the establishment of ovarian carcinoma cell lines: collagenase II (0.8 g/100 mL; EC 3.4.24.3; Sigma), DNase I (0.002 g/100 mL; EC 3.1.21.1; Sigma) and pronase (500 U/mL PBS; Boehringer Mannheim, Mannheim, Germany).

8. Subculture in the early stages should involve a split ratio of 1:2 or 1:3; eventually this can be increased to 1:5 to 1:10.

## References

1. Wolf, C. R., Hayward, I. P., Lawrie, S. S., Buckton, K., McIntyre, M. A., Adams, D. J., et al. (1987) Cellular heterogeneity and drug resistance in two ovarian adenocarcinoma cell lines derived from a single patient. *Int. J. Cancer* **39,** 695–702.
2. Langdon, S. P., Lawrie, S. S., Hay, F. G., Hawkes, M. M., McDonald, A., Hayward, I. P., et al. (1988) Characterization and properties of nine human ovarian adenocarcinoma cell lines. *Cancer Res.* **48,** 6166–6172.
3. Fogh, J., Fogh, J. M., and Orfeo, T. (1977) One hundred and twenty seven cultured tumour cell lines producing tumours in nude mice. *J. Natl. Cancer Inst.* **59,** 221–226
4. Pirker, R., FitzGerald, D. J., Hamilton, T. C., Ozols, R. F., Laird, W., Frankel, A. E., et al. (1985) Characterization of immunotoxins active against ovarian cancer cell lines. *J. Clin. Invest.* **76,** 1261–1267.
5. Hamilton, T. C., Young, R. C., McKoy, W. M., Grotzinger, K. R., Green, J. A., Chu, E. W., et al. (1983) Characterization of a human ovarian carcinoma cell line (NIH:OVCAR-3) with androgen and estrogen receptors. *Cancer Res.* **43,** 5379–5389.
6. Louie, K. G., Behrens, B. C., Kinsella, T. J., Hamilton, T. C., Grotzinger, K. R., McKoy, W. M., et al. (1985) Radiation survival parameters of antineoplastic drug-sensitive and -resistant human ovarian cancer cell lines and their modification by buthionine sulfoximine. *Cancer Res.* **45,** 2110–2115.
7. Louie, K. G., Hamilton, T. C., Winker, M. A., Behrens, B. C., Tsuruo, T., Klecker, R. W., et al. (1986) Adriamycin accumulation and metabolism in adriamycin-sensitive and -resistant human ovarian cancer cell lines. *Biochem. Pharmacol.* **35,** 467–472.
8. Hills, C. A., Kelland, L. R., Abel, G., Siracky, J., Wilson, A. P., and Harrap, K. R. (1989) Biological properties of ten human ovarian carcinoma cell lines: calibration in vitro against four platinum complexes. *Br. J. Cancer* **59,** 527–534.
9. Wilson, A. P., Dent, M., Pelovic, T., Hubbold, L., and Radford, H. (1996) Characterisation of seven human ovarian tumour cell lines. *Br. J. Cancer* **74,** 722–727.
10. Buick, R. N., Pullano, R., and Trent, J. M. (1985) Comparative properties of five human ovarian adenocarcinoma cell lines. *Cancer Res.* **45,** 3668–3676.
11. Woods, L. K., Morgan, R. T., Quinn, L. A., Moore, G. E., Semple, T. U., and Stedman, K. E. (1979) Comparison of four new cell lines from patients with adenocarcinoma of the ovary. *Cancer Res.* **39,** 4449–4459.
12. Benard, J., Da Silva, J., De Bois, M-C., Boyer, P., Duvillard, P., Chiric, E., et al. (1985) Characterization of a human ovarian adenocarcinoma line, IGROV1, in tissue culture and in nude mice. *Cancer Res.* **45,** 4970–4979.
13. Ishiwata, I., Ishiwata, C., Soma, M., Nozawa, S., and Ishikawa, H. (1987) Characterization of newly established human ovarian carcinoma cell line—Special reference of the effects of cis-platinum on cellular proliferation and release of CA125. *Gynecol. Oncol.* **26,** 340–354.
14. Horowitz, A. T., Treves, A. J., Voss, R., Okon, E., Fuks, Z., Davidson, L., et al. (1985) A new human ovarian carcinoma cell line: establishment and analysis of tumor-associated markers. *Oncology* **42,** 332–337.
15. Briers, T. W., Stroobants, P., Vandeputte, T. M., Nouwen, E. J., Conraads, M. V., Eestermans, G., et al. (1989) Establishment and characterization of a human ovarian neoplastic cell line DO-s. *Cancer Res.* **49,** 5153–5161.

# 15

# Subcloning of Ovarian Cancer Cell Lines

## Thomas W. Grunt

## 1. Introduction

Cellular heterogeneity of malignant tissues is a well-known phenomenon *(1)*. Intralineal/intraclonal diversity may be explained in part by proposing the concept of a hierarchically ordered, differentiating and self-renewing stem cell system for transformed cell populations *(2)*. However, in many solid tumors, the stem cells are not easily accessible to phenotypic identification. In the past, density gradient centrifugation was successfully used to separate cells from tumors and from cell lines into distinct subpopulations *(3–5)*. Using Percoll density gradients, we isolated undifferentiated clonogenic tumor stem-cell fractions from *HOC-7* human ovarian adenocarcinoma cells. In addition, we also identified a low-density cell subpopulation formed by large, vacuolated, slowly growing, adenoid differentiated cells with very low clonogenic activity *(6–11)*. Further characterization of these cell fractions in terms of stability of the isolated phenotypes is essential for the assessment of their biological significance. Subcloning of the isolated cell fractions by limiting dilution culture *(12)* followed by long-term culture yielded three permanent monoclonal sublines, which reveal a stable adenoid differentiated phenotype, and three subclones representing undifferentiated, clonogenic tumor stem cells *(13)*. These data demonstrate that the isolated phenotypes represent distinct cell entities reflecting specific stages of ovarian surface epithelial cell differentiation.

This chapter describes the use of discontinuous Percoll density gradient centrifugation of human ovarian adenocarcinoma cells for the separation of cells with different phenotypes and the application of limiting dilution culture of these cells for the establishment of monoclonal sublines with stable, tissue-specific stages of differentiation.

## 2. Materials

### 2.1. Cell Culture and Density Gradient Separation
### of Ovarian Cancer Cells

1. Any adherent polyclonal cell line (e.g., *HOC-7* human ovarian adenocarcinoma cell line; kind gift from Dr. R. N. Buick [Ontario Cancer Institute, Toronto, ON], *(14)*).
2. Percoll® (Pharmacia, Uppsala, Sweden) is a medium for density-gradient centrifugation of cells, viruses, and subcellular particles. Percoll is composed of colloidal silica, coated

From: *Methods in Molecular Medicine, Vol. 39: Ovarian Cancer: Methods and Protocols*
Edited by: J. M. S. Bartlett © Humana Press, Inc., Totowa, NJ

with polyvinylpyrrolidone (PVP), which renders the material nontoxic and ideal for use with biological materials *(15)*. It is free from unbound PVP and it is characterized by physiological ionic strength and pH, by low viscosity and low osmotic pressure enabling iso-osmotic conditions throughout the gradient (*see* **Note 1**). Densities ranging from 1.0–1.3 g/mL are achievable by centrifugation. It is supplied sterile (*see* **Note 2**) and may be stored unopened for up to 2 yr at room temperature. When opened, it should be stored at 4°C or –18°C for up to 6 mo. After thawing, the solution should be inverted several times to ensure uniform colloid distribution. Residual Percoll is easily removed from biological materials by dilution with physiological saline or culture medium, followed by centrifugation to collect cells, viruses, or subcellular particles.

3. Density Marker Beads (Pharmacia).
4. Sterile 100-mL cellulose acetate bottle filter with 0.2 µm pore-size (Costar, Cambridge, MA, Cat. No. 8310).
5. 1.5$M$ NaCl (10× concentrated physiological saline). The 10× concentrated NaCl must be filtered through a sterile 0.2-µm bottle filter.
6. α-MEM (Gibco, Karlsruhe, Germany) containing 10% heat inactivated fetal calf serum (FCSHI, Gibco).
7. 0.25% trypsin in 1 m$M$ EDTA solution (Gibco).
8. Dulbecco's phosphate-buffered saline (PBS - Gibco).
9. Viability stain (e.g., 0.4% trypan blue exclusion dye).
10. Dimethyl sulfoxide (Sigma, Deisenhofen, Germany).

## 2.2. Establishing Monoclonal Sublines by Limiting Dilution Culture

1. Cell-culture medium conditioned by the parental polyclonal cell line; can be stored at 4°C for a maximum period of 2 wk (*see* **Subheading 3.2.**)

## 3. Methods

### 3.1. Cell Culture

The human ovarian adenocarcinoma cell line *HOC-7* is maintained in a humidified 5% $CO_2$ atmosphere at 37°C in α-MEM.

1. Pipet 17 mL of a single cell suspension containing $0.5 \times 10^5$ cells/mL into 75 cm² tissue-culture flasks. These cells usually adhere within a few hours to the plastic growth substrate and then grow as a monolayer.
2. After 4 d, the old growth medium is removed and 17 mL of fresh growth medium are added to each T75 tissue-culture flask (*see* **Note 3**). Under these growth conditions, the number of *HOC-7* cells multiplies within 7 d by a factor of 10 reaching a total number of approximately $9 \times 10^6$ cells per flask, which means that the cell monolayer becomes 100% confluent.
3. The medium is removed and 10 mL of PBS is added to the cells.
4. After 2 min, the PBS is removed and the cells are incubated for 15–20 min (37°C, humidified 5% $CO_2$ atmosphere) in 2 mL of trypsin EDTA solution.
5. Cell detachment is facilitated by gently tapping the flask against the palm and is controled microscopically (the cells should already be rounded-up).
6. The action of trypsin is stopped by adding 4 mL of complete growth medium and the cells are dispersed into a single cell suspension by pipeting the cells a few times up and down using a 2 mL disposable plastic pipet (examine the result microscopically).
7. If desired, a trypan blue dye exclusion test can be performed in order to check the viability of the cells: 50 µL of the cell suspension are incubated for 5 min at room temperature with 50 µL of the viability stain. Ten µL of this mixture are then pipeted into a hemocytometer

and are viewed under the microscope for cell counting and for estimation of cell viability (*see* **Note 4**).

8. Subsequently, the total volume of the cell suspension is made up to 10 mL using fresh growth medium and 1 mL of this 1:10 diluted suspension is added to new T75 tissue-culture flasks, respectively. The final volume within the flasks is then brought up to 17 mL by adding another 16 mL of growth medium to each flask.

## 3.2 Gradient Separation of Ovarian Cancer Cells

Percoll (from the bottle) is diluted directly to make a final working solution of known density by the following procedure. In a measuring cylinder, add 0.1 volume of the final desired volume of 1.5*M* NaCl (e.g., 5 mL for 50 mL of working solution). To this add the desired volume of Percoll (from the bottle) calculated using the formula shown below *(15)*. Make up to the final volume with distilled water and store this solution at 4°C for up to 1 mo.

$$V_0 = V [(\rho - 0.1\rho_{10} - 0.9) / (\rho_0 - 1)]$$

Where $V_0$ = volume of Percoll (from the bottle)                    mL

$V$ = volume of the final working solution                    mL
$\rho$ = desired density of the final solution                    g/mL
$\rho_0$ = density of Percoll (from the bottle; varies from batch to batch and is specified on the label, usually $1.130 \pm 0.005$ gm/mL)
$\rho_{10}$ = density of 1.5*M* NaCl = 1.058                    g/mL

For example, to produce 50 mL of working solution of Percoll of density 1.053 g/mL in 0.15*M* NaCl: To 5 mL of 1.5*M* NaCl add Volume of Percoll required = 50 [(1.053 – 0.1058 – 0.9) / (1.130 – 1)] = 18.15 mL (if Percoll density is 1.130 g/mL) and make up to a final volume of 50 mL by adding 26.85 mL distilled water.

For *HOC-7* ovarian adenocarcinoma cells, a discontinuous Percoll density-gradient covering the density range from 1.037 g/mL to 1.069 g/mL was found to be best suited for sensitive separation of the cells (see **Note 5**). It is formed by nine different Percoll density stock solutions with density steps ($\Delta\rho$) of 0.004 g/mL each (**Table 1**). For checking the shape and range of the generated gradient (*see* **Note 6**).

1. On the day of cell separation, prepare the discontinuous Percoll density gradient in sterile polycarbonate tubes (*see* **Note 2**). Start with 1 mL of stock solution 9 (highest density) and then carefully overlaying 1 mL of stock solution 8 (next lower density) on top of solution 9 and proceed in this manner until stock solution 1 is reached. Use extreme caution not to disturb the interfaces between the individual density steps (*see* **Note 7**). Established gradients can be kept at 4°C for up to 24 h. Longer storage is not recommended, as diffusion between the layers will blur the density steps.
2. Trypsinize monolayer cells grown to confluence in a T75 tissue-culture flask using trypsin EDTA solution (*see* **Subheading 3.1., step 1**).
3. Wash the trypsinized cells once with culture medium: Add 18 mL culture medium to 2 mL of trypsinized cells and centrifuge for 5 min at 450*g* and 4°C. Aspirate the supernatant and resuspend the cell pellet in approximately 500 µL of culture medium.
4. Determine the cell number and cell viability (trypan blue dye exclusion) by using a hemocytometer and with culture medium adjust the cell concentration to $1.0–1.5 \times 10^7$/mL. It is essential to avoid cell clumping in the cell suspension. Separation of cell aggregates can be achieved by repeated passage of the cell suspension through a 20-gage aseptic needle.

**Table 1**
**Preparation of Nine Different Percoll Density Stock Solutions**[a]

| Stock Solution | Density ($\rho$) (g/mL) | Percoll (from Bottle) (mL) | Distilled Water (mL) | 1.5$M$ NaCl (mL) |
|---|---|---|---|---|
| 1 | 1.037 | 12.10 | 32.90 | 5 |
| 2 | 1.041 | 13.65 | 31.35 | 5 |
| 3 | 1.045 | 15.20 | 29.80 | 5 |
| 4 | 1.049 | 16.75 | 28.25 | 5 |
| 5 | 1.053 | 18.30 | 26.70 | 5 |
| 6 | 1.057 | 19.85 | 25.15 | 5 |
| 7 | 1.061 | 21.40 | 23.60 | 5 |
| 8 | 1.065 | 22.90 | 22.05 | 5 |
| 9 | 1.069 | 24.45 | 20.50 | 5 |

[a]Percoll density (from the bottle) is 1.129 and final volume is 50 mL.

5. Slowly pipet 1 mL of cells on top of the gradient using a 1000-µL pipette (e.g., Gilson pipetman P1000). As with layering another density gradient solution, too rapid addition can disturb the gradient.
6. Spin the gradients for 30 min at 4°C in a swing-out rotor at 600$g$. Disengage any internal brake so that the rotor can run out evenly avoiding turbulence in the gradient.
7. In *HOC-7* cells, this centrifugation yields 10 cell fractions located at the interfaces between the Percoll density stock solutions.
8. With a 1000-µL pipet remove and discard the upper 0.5 mL of cell-culture medium.
9. Recover each cell fraction formed at the interfaces by aspirating 1 mL of the gradient stepwise and transfer the fractions to new tubes.
10. Wash the cell fractions 2 × with culture medium: Add 9 mL culture medium to 1 mL of cell fraction and centrifuge for 5 min at 450$g$ and 4°C. Aspirate the supernatant and repeat the procedure once. Subsequently, resuspend the cell pellet in 100–200 µl of culture medium (*see* **Note 8**).
11. Determine cell number and viability of the cell fractions as described in **Subheading 3.1., step 1,** and, **Subheading 3.1., step 6.**
12. Cells can now be introduced into individual experiments.

**Table 2** demonstrates the cell recovery for each cell fraction after density gradient centrifugation. Overall recovery after cell separation was approximately 98% *(6)*. For additional methods to check the purity and resolution of the separation technique, *see* **Note 9.**

### 3.3. Preparation of Conditioned Medium

1. To produce conditioned cell-culture medium, subculture 7-day-old confluent *HOC-7* cell cultures in new tissue-culture flasks using α-MEM containing 10% FCSHI (splitting ratio 1:10) (*see* **Note 10**).
2. After 4 d of culture, remove the conditioned medium from the cells.
3. Add 1% (v/v) penicillin-streptomycin (10 mg/mL, Gibco), 25 m$M$ HEPES (Gibco), and 5% (v/v) FCSHI to the conditioned medium (*see* **Note 10**).

**Table 2**
**Recovery of *HOC-7* Cell Fractions after Density-Gradient Separation[a]**

| | Cell Recovery (% of Submitted Cells) | | | | | | | | | | |
| --- | --- | --- | --- | --- | --- | --- | --- | --- | --- | --- | --- |
| | FR1 | FR2 | FR3 | FR4 | FR5 | FR6 | FR7 | FR8 | FR9 | FR10 | Σ |
| Mean | 0.3 | 0.4 | 0.7 | 2.3 | 11.5 | 28.9 | 27.7 | 14.0 | 7.4 | 4.8 | 97.8 |
| SD | 0.1 | 0.4 | 0.6 | 1.6 | 9.8 | 13.4 | 5.8 | 10.7 | 4.8 | 3.1 | 3.8 |

[a]Mean ± SD of 11 experiments.

4. Centrifuge the medium at 460*g* for 10 min at 4°C.
5. Filter sterilize the medium through a 0.2-μm sterile bottle filter and store at 4°C for a maximum of 2 wk.

### 3.4. Establishing Monoclonal Sublines by Limiting Dilution Culture

1. Subject confluent *HOC-7* cells to discontinuous density gradient centrifugation, as described above.
2. After determination of cell number and viability, dilute each cell fraction to a concentration of 2.5 cells/mL in conditioned medium.
3. Plate 200 μL/well of the cell suspensions in 96-well tissue-culture plates; this gives a statistical density of 0.5 cells/well (*see* **Note 11**). For each fraction use a half plate (48 wells).
4. Examine the plates every other day in the microscope and replace half of the volume of the conditioned media (100 μL/well) every 3 d.
5. After 2–3 wk, established *HOC-7* monoclonal microcultures usually get confluent and must be transferred to larger wells. Aspirate the supernatant from the confluent cultures and add 200 μL PBS/well.
6. Remove the PBS, add 40 μL of trypsin EDTA and incubate the plates in the $CO_2$-incubator until the cells round up (15–20 min).
7. Neutralize the trypsin by adding 160 μL unconditioned growth medium to the well and transfer the cell suspension to new 12-well plates, which are filled already with 800 μL of fresh growth medium (total volume is now 1 mL). This first passage monoclonal subline should be refed every 3–4 d.
8. After 1–2 wk of subculture, the cells should again be confluent and should be transferred to T25 tissue-culture flasks, as described above.
9. Cell stocks should be repeatedly frozen in liquid nitrogen during further expansion. Trypsinize, wash, and count the cells, as described above. Adjust the cell number to approximately $2 \times 10^6$/mL in cold (4°C) growth medium and dilute the single cell suspension with an equal volume of cold growth medium containing 20% dimethyl sulfoxide. Aliquot the cell suspension into 1.8-mL cryotubes (1 mL/vial) and place the samples into a precooled Styrofoam box with approximately 1-cm wall thickness. Close the box tightly using adhesive tape and freeze the samples slowly by placing the box in a deep freezer (−30°C or −80°C). On the next day, transfer the vials into the liquid nitrogen tank.

Overall, it takes approximately 5 wk to obtain one T25 flask of a monoclonal *HOC-7* subline. Expansion of the cloned subcultures and freezing of stocks requires another 4–8 wk of cultivation depending on the density fraction from which the clone was derived. In our hands, the proportion of *HOC-7* human ovarian cancer cells, which are able for clonal outgrowth, lies in the range of 1 in $1.6 \times 10^6$ parental cells. Therefore, using $1 \times 10^7$ cells for density gradient separation and subsequent monoclonal expansion by limiting dilution culture always yields a few distinct subclones.

Cell fractions of human ovarian adenocarcinoma cells separated by the isopycnic density-gradient technique described above reveal distinct morphology, anchorage-dependent and -independent growth activities, different immunophenotypes, and specific stages of differentiation including different activity for monoclonal expansion on solid substrates *(6,13)*. Using limiting dilution culture, we demonstrated that the cell fractions of *HOC-7* cells form monoclonal sublines with distinct and stable phenotypes, which reflect specific stages of differentiation *(6,13)*.

## 4. Notes

1. Percoll has a very low osmolality (<20 mOs/kg $H_2O$) and can therefore form a density gradient without itself producing any significant osmolality gradient. Iso-osmotic conditions are generated by adding 1/10 volume of 10X concentrated physiological saline (1.5*M*) to 9/10 volume of aqueous solutions of Percoll (see above); the resulting osmolality will thus be in the physiological range of 280–320 mOs/kg $H_2O$. This is important for reliable isopycnic density separation as the buoyant density of biological particles is crucially dependent on the osmotic pressure of the separation medium.

2. Polycarbonate tubes should be used with Percoll as the particles do not adhere to the walls of these tubes. Percoll may be autoclaved at 120°C for 30 min without any change in properties. This must be carried out without addition of salts, because these cause gelation of Percoll under the above conditions.

3. If T25 flasks are used for tissue culture, we usually add 7 mL of a cell suspension of $0.5 \times 10^5$ *HOC-7* cells/mL to each flask.

4. Incubation of the cells in the trypsin EDTA solution should generally be performed until the cells start to round up. Shorter treatment will result in excessive cell clumping, whereas longer exposure will deteriorate the cell viability. It is the FCSHI within the growth medium, which has trypsin-inhibitory effects. Therefore, it is important to use serum-supplemented medium in order to stop the enzymatic action.

5. One convenient advantage of Percoll is its ability to form self-generated continuous density gradients after high-speed centrifugation (> 10,000*g*, 15–90 min, 4°C) in a fixed-angle rotor. This is a simple and rapid way to obtain highly reproducible density gradients. However, this method yields gradients with wide density ranges, but with low-density resolution precluding successful separation of ovarian cancer cells, which reveal a rather narrow density distribution *(6)*. Therefore, although preparation of step gradients is more laborious and time-consuming (approx four gradients/h) than generation of continuous gradients, step gradients are strongly recommended for the task described above.

6. If desired, color-coded Density Marker Beads (Pharmacia) can be used as an external standard to monitor the gradient shape and range. To 990 µL of culture medium add 10 µL of each bead type (bead numbers 1–9, bead number 10 should not be used if Percoll is diluted with NaCl) and pipet this solution on top of an identical gradient, which should then be treated in the same way as the gradient containing the cells. The colored beads comprise a density range of 1.017–1.142 g/mL. The precise density of each bead type is specific for each lot and is printed on the label of each box. The beads sediment in the gradient according to their specific density and the shape of the gradient can be traced by plotting the distance from the top of the meniscus to each band vs the density of each band.

7. Pipeting of the density solutions is best done with a manual pipetor fitting to 5 mL plastic pipetes thus you can control the flow rate directly with your thumb. Let the solution slowly trickle (approximately 1 mL/min) into the tube keeping the tip on the wall of the tube just

above the surface of the liquid. It is not recommended to hold the tubes vertically, rather tilt them to an angle of approximately 45°. Gentle tilting of the tubes does not affect the integrity of the gradient.

8. Buoyant density of the cells grossly correlates with their size. Thus, large, slowly proliferating, vacuolated adenoid cells are found in the low density fractions (fractions 1–4), whereas smaller, undifferentiated, rapidly growing cells migrate to higher density regions (fractions 5–10). Cells forming colonies in anchorage-independent growth assays (soft agar) are enriched in medium-density fractions. Fraction 6, for instance, reveals a colony-forming efficiency of approximately 9%, whereas low-density fractions 1–4 are virtually devoid of such colony-forming cells (colony-forming efficiency <<1%) *(6)*. The differentiated, large vacuolated cells from the low-density fractions are extremely fragile and must, therefore, be handled very gently during washing and resuspension steps. Cell debris and nonviable cells have low buoyant densities in Percoll and concentrate in fraction 1. In order to avoid much debris from occurring in fraction 1, it is therefore essential that the parental cell culture is in a good proliferative state.

9. The purity of the cell fractions obtained and the resolution of the discontinuous density-gradient separation can be examined by immediate recentrifugation of the cell fractions in a second, identical step gradient using the same conditions (600 g, 30 min, 4°C, swing-out rotor). In our hands, 97 ± 3% (range 90.1–100%) of the cells of each primary fraction sedimented again to their original density region indicating that the purity of the cell fractions ranged between 90 and 100% *(6)*.

10. Select a batch of FCSHI for cloning experiments, which gives a high plating efficiency during tests *(12)*.

11. In order to reach an exact and reproducible final number of 0.5 cells per 200 µL and well, it is necessary to make serial dilutions of the stock cell suspension using a dilution ratio of approximately 1:5.

## Acknowledgment

This work was supported in part by grants from the "Jubilaeumsfonds der Oesterreichischen Nationalbank," the "Anton-Dreher Gedaechtnisschenkung fuer Medizinische Forschung," and the "Oesterreichische Gesellschaft fuer Chemotherapie."

## References

1. Dexter, D. L. and Calabresi, P. (1982) Intraneoplastic diversity. *Biochim. Biophys. Acta* **695,** 97–112.
2. Buick, R. N. and Pollak, M. N. (1984) Perspectives on clonogenic tumor cells, stem cells, and oncogenes. *Cancer Res.* **44,** 4909–4918.
3. Buick, R. N. and MacKillop, W. J. (1981) Measurement of self-renewal in culture of clonogenic cells from human ovarian carcinoma. *Brit. J. Cancer,* **44,** 349–355.
4. Mackillop, W. J., Stewart, S. S., and Buick, R. N. (1982) Density/volume analysis in the study of cellular heterogeneity in human ovarian carcinoma. *Brit. J. Cancer* **45,** 812–820.
5. Resnicoff, M., Medrano, E. E., Podhajcer, O. L., Bravo, A. I., Bover, L., and Mordoh, J. (1987) Subpopulations of MCF7 cells separated by Percoll gradient centrifugation: a model to analyze the heterogeneity of human breast cancer. *Proc. Natl. Acad. Sci. USA* **84,** 7295–7299.
6. Grunt, T. W., Dittrich, E., Somay, C., Wagner, T., and Dittrich, C. (1991) Separation of clonogenic and differentiated cell phenotypes of ovarian cancer cells (HOC-7) by discontinuous density gradient centrifugation. *Cancer Lett.* **58,** 7–16.
7. Grunt, T. W., Somay, C., Pavelka, M., Ellinger, A., Dittrich, E., and Dittrich, C. (1991) The effects of dimethyl sulfoxide and retinoic acid on the cell growth and the phenotype of ovarian cancer cells. *J. Cell Sci.* **100,** 657–666.
8. Grunt, T. W., Somay, C., Ellinger, A., Pavelka, M., Dittrich, E., and Dittrich, C. (1992) The differential effects of transforming growth factor-β1 and N,N-dimethylformamide on proliferation and differentiation of a human ovarian cancer cell line (HOC-7). *J. Cell Physiol.* **151,** 13–22.

9. Grunt, T. W., Somay, C., Oeller, H., Dittrich, E., and Dittrich, C. (1992) Comparative analysis of the effects of dimethyl sulfoxide and retinoic acid on the antigenic pattern of human ovarian adenocarcinoma cells. *J.Cell Sci.* **103,** 501–509.

10. Somay, C., Grunt, T. W., Mannhalter, C., and Dittrich, C. (1992) Relationship of myc protein expression to the phenotype and to the growth potential of HOC-7 ovarian cancer cells. *Brit. J. Cancer* **66,** 93–98.

11. Grunt, T. W., Oeller, H., Somay, C., Dittrich, E., Mannhalter, C., and Dittrich, C. (1993) Modulation of the immunophenotype of ovarian cancer cells by N,N-dimethylformamide and transforming growth factor-$\beta$1. *J. Cell Physiol.* **156,** 358–366.

12. Freshney, R. I. (1987) *Culture of animal cells. A manual of basic technique.* Alan R. Liss, New York.

13. Grunt, T. W., Oeller, H., Somay, C., and Dittrich, C. (1993) Different propensity for spontaneous differentiation of cell clones isolated from the human ovarian surface epithelial cell line HOC-7. *Differentiation* **53,** 45–50.

14. Buick, R. N., Pullano, R., and Trent, J. M. (1985) Comparative properties of five human ovarian adenocarcinoma cell lines. *Cancer Res.* **45,** 3668–3676.

15. Pharmacia Fine Chemicals. Percoll®. *Methodology and Applications.* Uppsala, Sweden.

# 16

## Culture and Characterization of Human Ovarian Surface Epithelium

### Nelly Auersperg and Sarah L. Maines-Bandiera

## 1. Introduction

The ovarian surface epithelium (OSE) is the part of the pelvic mesothelium that covers the ovary. It comprises only a minute fraction of the ovary—however, it is the source of the epithelial ovarian carcinomas which are the prime cause of death from gynecological malignancies in North American and European women. The implication that OSE is the source of the epithelial ovarian cancers is based mainly on the demonstration of histopathological changes (1). The early stages of epithelial ovarian carcinogenesis are poorly understood because these carcinomas are usually diagnosed in late stages and there are no adequate animal models for their study.

In the past decade, methods were established to grow human OSE in tissue culture (2,3). This chapter summarizes the main properties of OSE in vitro, the methods used to culture OSE from surgical specimens, and some of the markers which characterize these cells.

Normal OSE in culture exhibits considerable phenotypic plasticity. Under standard culture conditions, i.e., on plastic substrata with culture media containing 10–15% fetal bovine serum, the cells form compact, cobblestone epithelial monolayers in primary culture and modulate to flat epithelial and atypical fibroblast-like forms with time and passage in vitro. Colonies characterized by whorls of spindly overlapping cells appear to be derived from metaplastic OSE (4). Cultured OSE is influenced by extracellular matrices (ECM) and, in turn, modifies such matrices by synthesis, physical restructuring, and lysis (5,6). For example, on collagen gel, OSE cells assume a mesenchymal, fibroblast-like phenotype, whereas on Matrigel, an in vitro basement membrane substitute, OSE forms aggregates that invade the matrix. ECM also influences rates of OSE proliferation. Proteolytic enzymes, which are produced by OSE include chymotrypsinlike and elastaselike peptidases and a 30 Kd gelatinase (6). Human OSE also secretes ECM, including laminin and collagen types I, III, and IV (7).

Normal OSE cells secrete, and have receptors for agents with growth- and differentiation regulatory capabilities. They produce TGFβ, which acts as an autocrine growth inhibitor (8), and secrete bioactive cytokines including IL-1 and IL-6, M-CSF, G-CSF, and GM-CSF (9). They have receptors for epidermal growth factor, which is a potent

From: *Methods in Molecular Medicine, Vol. 39: Ovarian Cancer: Methods and Protocols*
Edited by: J. M. S. Bartlett © Humana Press, Inc., Totowa, NJ

mitogen for OSE cells *(10,11)* and for amphiregulin, which controls OSE proliferation in a complex manner *(12)*. They also have receptors for ovarian steroids *(13)* and gonadotrophins *(14)*, but the roles of these hormones in OSE are unknown.

Because of the morphologic variability of cultured OSE cells and the possibility of contamination by other cell types at the time of explantation from surgical specimens, it is important to identify the cells as accurately as possible. The following markers have been defined by immunofluorescence microscopy, histochemistry, and Western blotting to distinguish OSE from other ovarian and extraovarian cell types: keratin, vimentin, factor VIII, laminin, collagens I and IV, Ulex europeus lectin (UEAl), wheat germ agglutinin (WGA), lipid, mucin and 17β-hydroxysteroid dehydrogenase *(7,15)*. OSE, endothelial cells, and fibroblasts can be distinguished in live cultures by the amount and pattern of fluorescent (FITC)UEAl binding. By this means, the cells can be identified nondestructively and used subsequently *(7)*.

In the following section, we describe methods for the culture of OSE, including specimen procurement, materials, and methodology, and recommend means of characterization. It is important to realize that culture conditions suitable for OSE from one species are not necessarily suitable for other species. For example, in Waymouth medium 752/1, which supports proliferation of rat OSE very well, human OSE remains stationary *(10,16)*, perhaps because the requirements for calcium concentrations in the culture medium differ between OSE cells from the two species *(17)*.

## 2. Materials

1. Standard basal medium, "199/105"-Medium 199 with Earle's salts, and Medium MCDB 105 (Sigma, St. Louis, MO) mixed 1:1, stored at 4°C up to 8 wk. Fetal bovine serum (FBS, defined, Hyclone, Logan, UT) is added at 15% to 199/105. The bulk of FBS is stored at –70°C for periods of several months. Aliquots of 10 ml are stored at –20°C for up to 8 weeks and thawed immediately before the preparation of complete media.
2. $CO_2$-independent medium—(Life Technologies, Gaithersburg, MD) with 15% FBS and 50 µg/mL gentamicin or 100 IU penicillin/100 µg/mL streptomycin is used to store or transport OSE fragments after isolation from the ovary, if transit to the laboratory is expected to exceed 1 h. Stored at 4°C up to 6 mo.
3. Reduced-serum medium, "OSEM-1"-PC-1ₛ (Ventrex Labs, Portland, ME) is Pedersen's fetuin and a proprietary compound. Stored as 25X stock and added to 199/105 to a final concentration of 500 µg/mL. Insulin, 15 µg/mL, transferrin, 20 µg/mL, lipoic acid, 0.1 µg/mL, phosphatidyl choline, 0.2 µg/mL and ethanolamine, 33 µg/mL (Sigma), are stored as 100X to 1000X individual stock solutions and added to the medium up to 5 d before use *(18,19)*. Complete medium should be used within 2 wk of preparation.
4. Antibiotics and antifungal agents—all from Life Technologies: 50 mg/mL gentamicin, stored at room temperature; 10,000 IU/mL penicillin /10,000 µg/mL streptomycin, stored at –20°C; 250 µg/mL fungizone, stored at –20°C in aliquots of approximately 1.0 mL (N.B. Fungizone should not be thawed and frozen more than 2–3 times).
5. Cell dissociation medium: Trypsin 0.06% (250:1 grade, Life Technologies) and ethylenediaminetetraacetic acid (EDTA), 0.01% (disodium salt, Sigma) dissolved in Hanks' balanced salt solution (HBSS) without calcium and magnesium (Life Technologies) with the final pH adjusted to 7.2–7.4 using 1N HCL or 1N NaOH. Aliquoted and stored at –20°C.
6. Cell separation reagents: 40% Percoll (Sigma) in HBSS with calcium and magnesium (Life Technologies) is stored at 4°C. It is stable for several months.

7. Dimethyl sulfoxide (DMSO) (reagent grade, BDH Chemicals) is stored at room temperature and should be replaced with fresh stock every 6 mo. Immediately before use, freezing medium is made to contain 45% medium 199/105, 45% FBS and 10% DMSO.

## 3. Methods

### 3.1. Specimen Collection

Specimens are obtained either from ovaries removed during surgery for nonmalignant gynecological disorders (e.g., hysterectomies for fibroids) or at laparoscopies, e.g., for tubal ligation (*see* **Note 1**).

#### 3.1.1. Biopsy Specimens

1. At the time of ovariectomy, cut (or have the surgeon cut) a piece of the ovary that includes ovarian surface, immediately after removal from the body cavity or while the ovary is still *in situ* (*see* **Note 2**).
2. Place specimen into a sterile polypropylene container with approximately 25 mL of $CO_2$-independent culture medium and transport to the laboratory at ambient temperature.
3. If the specimen is very bloody, it may be necessary to rinse it with HBSS or serum-free culture medium. The rinse is kept and cultured (see below) because it often contains OSE fragments.
4. The specimen is held with forceps, surface down, over a 35-mm culture dish containing 2 mL of standard basal medium and the ovarian surface is scraped firmly with a white rubber scraper attached to a glass rod, or gently with a blunt instrument (sharp edges or excess pressure increase the risk of stromal cell contamination). For large specimens, a 60-mm dish with 4 mL of medium may be more convenient.
5. The OSE fragments generated from scraping are incubated in the same culture dish where they are collected. Microscopically, they appear as small pieces of flat or rolled-up epithelial monolayers.
6. Cells in the medium used for transport from surgery are collected by centrifugation for 5 min at 80$g$ and plated into a separate 35-mm dish. All cultures are incubated at 37°C in humidified 5% $CO_2$/air and left undisturbed for at least 4 d. Then, culture medium with antibiotics (*see* **step 2** above) is changed as needed until the monolayers become confluent (*see* **Note 3**).

#### 3.1.2. Laparoscopy Specimens

OSE is scraped from the ovary by the surgeon, using the blunt side of laparoscopic scissors, and the fragments are rinsed off the instrument into a 15-mL centrifuge tube containing 2–3 mL of medium. The tube is then transported to the laboratory where the contents are pipetted into a 35-mm culture dish and incubated as above.

#### 3.1.3. Red Blood Cell Removal

Occasionally, the rinses, transport medium, and even the final scraped preparation from a biopsy specimen contain a lot of blood which interferes with the attachment of the OSE to the culture dishes. To remove the RBCs, the following method may be used.

1. Collect blood and OSE fragments by centrifugation for 5 min at 80$g$.
2. Remove supernatant and resuspend pellet in 1–2 mL of basal culture medium, depending on the size of the pellet.

3. Carefully layer this suspension on top of an equal volume of 40% Percoll in a 15-mL centrifuge tube, making sure not to mix the cell suspension into the Percoll.
4. Centrifuge at 2400$g$ at room temperature for 20 min. Do not use centrifuge brakes.
5. Purified cells will be at the medium/Percoll interface, and red blood cells at the bottom of the tube. Remove the cells of interest with a transfer pipet or a Pasteur pipet to a new centrifuge tube while transferring as little Percoll as possible. Add excess (several mL) of medium and wash the cells by gentle mixing to remove as much Percoll as possible. Centrifuge at 80$g$. Resuspend the cells in 2 mL of medium and incubate in a 35-mm dish (*see* **Note 4**).

### 3.2 Maintenance of Cultures

### 3.2.1. Growth

OSE fragments begin to attach within a few days. The cultures should not be disturbed for the first 4 d. Thereafter, medium is changed once a week while the cells are sparse, twice a week or more when they approach confluence. For morphological evaluation of the cells (*see* **Note 5**).

### 3.2.2. Subculture (see **Note 6**).

1. Rinse confluent culture once with Hanks' calcium, magnesium-free BSS with trypsin/EDTA (at room temperature).
2. Add fresh Hanks/trypsin/EDTA for 2–3 min (1.0 mL per 35-mm dish).
3. Pipet with a transfer pipet or Pasteur pipet until the cells detach.
4. Transfer the cell suspension to a centrifuge tube containing 2.0 mL of medium with 15% FBS to neutralize the trypsin, mix, collect the cells by centrifugation at 80$g$ for 5 min.
5. Resuspend the pellet in complete culture medium and plate the cells into new culture dishes.

### 3.2.3. Freezing

OSE fragments may be frozen in liquid nitrogen for future use immediately after they are obtained from surgery, i.e., before culturing, by centrifuging fragments and resuspending in freezing medium, or cultured cells may be trypsinized and frozen.

1. Use cultured cells in the log phase of growth for best recovery.
2. Dissociate cells with trypsin/EDTA, centrifuge.
3. Remove culture medium, resuspend cells in freshly prepared culture medium with 45% FBS and 10% DMSO. Optimal cell concentrations are $5 \times 10^5$ to $1 \times 10^6$ cells/mL.
4. Transfer cells to freezing vials (1.0 to 1.8 mL/vial) and freeze as per instructions on freezing equipment.
5. Store in liquid nitrogen.

## 4. Notes

1. Eligibility of patients from whom tissue is to be obtained. OSE from patients with leiomyomata, ovarian cysts, pelvic inflammatory disease/adhesions, and endometriosis all yield cultures with high success rates. However, precautions must be taken in the case of endometriosis because lesions on the ovarian surface can be overlooked and erroneously included in the culture. Similarly, in the case of adhesions, the operator must ascertain that the scrapings of OSE are derived from the ovarian surface proper and not from adherent extraovarian mesothelium. Ovaries that have been exposed to radiation therapy or chemotherapy, e.g., for endometrial carcinoma, grow very poorly. Age differences up to 65 yr do not seem to influence the success rate.

2. Conditions in the operating room. It is essential that OSE be obtained rapidly, under sterile conditions, with as little handling of the ovary as possible, and with as little blood as possible associated with the specimen. If the ovarian surface is allowed to dry, even *in situ*, the OSE dies within minutes. OSE is only losely attached to the ovary and, therefore, handling of the specimen results in loss of the epithelium. Removal of blood from the ovarian surface by rinsing also tends to result in epithelial detachment, while blood left with the epithelium prevents the OSE from attaching to the culture dishes.

3. Handling of new cultures. OSE is obtained in the form of epithelial fragments. These attach only slowly to plastic, particularly if they are large, and seem to lose the capacity to attach and die if they are still suspended after a few days. Therefore, newly established cultures should remain undisturbed for at least 4 d (longer may be better, but if there are many cells or if there is much blood in the culture, medium should be changed after 4 d). To facilitate cell attachment, we tried to use an adhesive (Cell - Tak, Collaborative Biomedical Products, Bedford, MA), but found its effect to be inconsistent and not warranting the added expense. Occasionally, no fragments or growth are observed for over 1 wk and then, small colonies of monolayered OSE cells appear.

4. Percoll remnants will remain in the cultures and its microscopic appearance resembles a bacterial contamination. Too much Percoll may interfere with cell attachment to plastic; small amounts are harmless and will disappear after a few medium changes.

5. Identification of cultured OSE cells (*see* **Subheading 1.**). The morphology of the cultured OSE is classified as compact (cobblestone) epithelial, flat epithelial, and atypical or fibroblastic. Cells in primary culture tend to be cobblestone epithelial, becoming flat to atypical with increasing passage. Demonstration of keratin by immunofluorescence proved to be the most convenient means of identifying OSE cells. Concomitant to the change in morphology from an epithelial phenotype to a more fibroblastic phenotype is the loss of keratin. This loss may interfere with cellular identification and interpretation of experimental results.

6. Confluent cultures are split 1:3 when in early passage, but when they are senescing can only be split 1:2. Cells can be cultured for up to 12 population doublings (PD). A confluent 35-mm dish of primary OSE will yield up to $3 \times 10^5$ cells, but this number diminishes as the cells age and become large and flat.

7. For studies of growth requirements and hormone/growth factor responsiveness, a medium with low, more defined serum content may be desirable *(18,19)* (*see* **Subheading 2.3.**). In 199/105 supplemented with 500 µg/ml PC-1$_s$, the growth rate is 50–60% of the rate in medium with 15% FBS. If, in addition, the remaining components listed in **Subheading 2.3.** are added to PC-1$_s$, the growth rate is 70–80% of growth in medium with 15% FBS.

## Acknowledgment

This research was supported by the National Cancer Institute of Canada with funds from the Terry Fox run.

## References

1. Scully, R. E. (1995) Pathology of ovarian cancer precursors. *J. Cell. Biochem.* Suppl. **23**, 208–218.
2. Kruk, P. A., Maines-Bandiera, S. L., and Auersperg, N. (1990) A simplified method to culture human ovarian surface epithelium. *Lab. Invest.* **63**, 132–136.
3. Auersperg, N., Maines-Bandiera, S. L., and Dyck, H. G. (1997) Ovarian carcinogenesis and the biology of ovarian surface epithelium. *J. Cell. Physiol.* **173**, 261–265.
4. Wong, A. T. Z., Maines-Bandiera, S. L., Leung, P. C. K., and Auersperg, N. (1998) Metaplastic changes in cultured human ovarian surface epithelium. *In Vitro Cell. Develop. Biol.* **34**, 668–670.
5. Kruk, P. A. and Auersperg, N. (1992) Human ovarian surface epithelial cells are capable of physically restructuring extracellular matrix. *Am. J. Obs. Gyn.* **167**, 1437–1443.

6. Kruk, P. A., Uitto, V. J., Firth, J. D., Dedhar, S., and Auersperg, N. (1994) Reciprocal interactions between human ovarian surface epithelial cells and adjacent extracellular matrix. *Exp. Cell Res.* **215,** 97–108.

7. Auersperg, N., Maines-Bandiera, S. L., Dyck, H. G., and Kruk, P. A. (1994) Characterization of cultured human ovarian surface epithelial cells: phenotypic plasticity and premalignant changes. *Lab. Invest.* **71,** 510–518.

8. Berchuck, A., Rodriguez, G., Olt, G., Whitaker, R., Boente, M. P., Arrick, B. A., et al. (1992) Regulation of growth of normal ovarian epithelial cells and ovarian cancer cell lines by transforming growth factor-beta. *Am. J. Obs. Gyn.* **166,** 676–684.

9. Ziltener, H. J., Maines-Bandiera, S., Schrader, J. W., and Auersperg, N. (1993) Secretion of bioactive interleukin-1, interleukin-6, and colony-stimulating factors by human ovarian surface epithelium. *Bio. Reprod.* **49,** 635–641.

10. Siemens, C. H. and Auersperg, N. (1988) Serial propagation of human ovarian surface epithelium in tissue culture. *J. Cell. Physiol.* **134,** 347–356.

11. Rodriguez, G. C., Berchuck, A., Whitaker, R. S., Schlossman, D., Clarke-Pearson, D. L., and Bast, Jr, R. C. (1991) Epidermal growth factor receptor expression in normal ovarian epithelium and ovarian cancer. II. Relationship between receptor expression and response to epidermal growth factor. *Am. J. Obs. Gyn.* **164,** 745–750.

12. Gordon, A. W., Pegues, J. C., Johnson, G. R., Kannan, B., Auersperg, N., and Stromberg, K. (1994) mRNA phenotyping of the major ligands and receptors of the EGF supergene family in human epithelial cells. *Cancer Lett.* **89,** 63–71.

13. Karlan, B. Y., Jones, J. L., Greenwald, M., and Lagasse, L. D. (1995) Steroid hormone effects on the proliferation of human ovarian surface epithelium in vitro. *Am. J. Obstet. Gynecol.* **173,** 97–104.

14. Zheng, W., Magid, M. S., Kramer, E. E., and Chen, Y. T. (1996) Follicle-stimulating hormone receptor is expressed in human ovarian surface epithelium and Fallopian tube. *Am. J. Pathol.* **148,** 47–53.

15. Auersperg, N., Siemens C. H., and Myrdal, S. E. (1984) Human ovarian surface epithelium in primary culture. *In Vitro* **20,** 743–755.

16. Adams, A. T. and Auersperg, N. (1985) A cell line, ROSE 199, derived from normal rat ovarian surface epithelium. *Exp. Cell Biol.* **53,** 181–188.

17. McNeil, L., Hobson, S., Nipper, V., and Rodland, K. (1998) Functional calcium-sensing receptor expression in ovarian surface epithelial cells. *Am. J. Obstet. Gynecol.* **178,** 305–313.

18. Elliott, W. M. and Auersperg, N. (1993) Growth of normal human ovarian surface epithelial cells in reduced-serum and serum-free media. *In Vitro Cell. Develop. Biol.* **29A,** 9–18.

19. Brewitt, B. and Clark, J. I. (1990) A new method for the study of lens development *in vitro* using pulsatile delivery of PDGF or EGF in HL-1 serum-free medium. *In Vitro Cell Develop. Biol.* **26,** 305–314.

# 17

# MTT Growth Assays in Ovarian Cancer

## Daniel M. Spinner

## 1. Introduction

The MTT (3-[4,5-dimethylthiazol-2yl]-2,5-diphenyl tetrazolium bromide) growth assay developed by Mosmann *(1)* offers a simple, rapid, and precise measurement of cell viability and proliferation of adherent cell lines *(2)*. The value of this assay is in the screening of large numbers of samples. The MTT assay, a quantitative colorimetric assay is based on the living cell's ability to reduce the tetrazolium salt MTT, a pale yellow substrate to a dark-blue formazan product. The mitochondrial succinate-dehydrogenases *(3)* of viable cells cleave the tetrazolium ring in active mitochondria into formazan crystals. The crystals can be dissolved in acid isopropyl alcohol, mineral oil *(4)*, or dimethyl sulfoxide (DMSO) *(5)*. The resulting blue solution can be measured semiautomatically using a scanning multiwell spectrophotometer. Our laboratory has successfully applied the MTT-based growth assay with some modifications *(6)* to investigate the growth effects of human cytokines on *HOC* cell lines *(7)*, but we have to keep its limitations and pitfalls in mind (*see* **Note 1**). For use in tests of floating cell lines, the MTT assay may be less optimal. Using this assay for screening of primary tumor samples may produce limited results, because cell contaminants may result in high-background values *(4)*. However, accepting the limitations of the MTT assay, the optimum assay conditions have to be selected and adapted to the cell lines that are under investigation. The MTT-based growth assay, as described in this chapter, is a reliable and sensitive test for the determination of cell growth of human ovarian-carcinoma cells.

## 2. Materials

1. Growth medium (GM): The standard GM is a modified RPMI-1640 medium with phenol red supplemented with 17% heat inactivated fetal calf serum (FCS), L-glutamine [200 m$M$], penicillin [5000 U/mL], streptomycin [5000 mg/mL], insulin [0.01 mg/mL]; epidermal growth factor [2 ng/mL], and cholera toxin [100 ng/mL].
2. Serum starved medium (SSM) for MTT reduction assay: RPMI-1640 without phenol red (Gibco, Gaithersburg, MD) (*see* **Note 2**) supplemented with 0.05% heat-inactivated FCS and L-glutamine [200 m$M$], penicillin [5000 U/mL], and streptomycin [5000 mg/mL]. Add HEPES buffer and NaHCO$_3$ to the medium and adjust to pH 7.2.
3. MTT solution: MTT was obtained from Sigma Chemicals (St. Louis, MO). Prepare the MTT solution as a 5 mg/mL stock in phosphate-buffered saline (PBS, Dulbecco and Vogt

From: *Methods in Molecular Medicine, Vol. 39: Ovarian Cancer: Methods and Protocols*
Edited by: J. M. S. Bartlett © Humana Press, Inc., Totowa, NJ

formulation without Mg⁺⁺ or Ca⁺⁺). Store at 4°C, stable at 4°C for up to 2 wk, stable for several weeks when stored frozen. Filter the stock solution for use through a 0.2-μm filter and dilute it in RPMI-1640 w/o phenol red to a concentration of [1 mg/mL].

4. Formazan solvent: Anhydrous isopropyl alcohol containing $0.04N$ hydrochloric acid (*see* **Note 8**).
5. Automatic multiwell reader (Titertek Multiscan plus MKII - Spectrophotometer).
6. Microtiter plate shaker (Microshaker II, Dynatech, Chantilly, VA, speed 7).
7. PBS: Dulbecco's PBS, sterile, store at room temperature (RT) (Quality Biological).
8. Hanks' balanced salt solution (HBSS), sterile, store at RT (Quality Biological).

## 3. Methods

1. In a laminar flow hood, wash cells twice with HBSS (*see* **Note 3**). Resuspend cells in GM (*see* **Note 4**).
2. Aseptically seed single *HOC* cell suspensions in duplicate or triplicate in 96-well culture plates at 10,000 cells/100 μL per well (*see* **Note 5**).
3. Incubate cells for 96 h at 37°C (*see* **Note 6**).
4. Wash cells twice with HBSS, while shaking the plates gently and resuspend cells with 100 μL SSM (*see* **Note 7**) per well.
5. Add 100 μL MTT solution [1 mg/mL] into each well. Shake plates gently. Wear gloves and protective clothing when handling MTT solvent (*see* **Note 8**).
6. Incubate cells at 37°C for a further 4 h while gently shaking the plates (*see* **Note 9**).
7. Add 100 μL of acid isopropyl alcohol (*see* **Note 10**) to all wells and shake well (or use a plate shaker at min speed for 5 min), to dissolve the formazan crystals.
8. After a few minutes at RT, ensure that all the crystals are dissolved and read the plates on an automatic plate reader at a wavelength of 570 nm. Subtract background absorbance measured at 690 nm (*see* **Note 11**).

## 4. Notes

1. There is strong evidence *(8)* that changes in cell-culture environments (cell-culture age >96 h, medium pH <> 7.2, low medium glucose concentration, high medium serum concentration) may affect formazan generation and thus introduce artifacts into the MTT growth assay. This may lead to lower sensitivity or to false negative test results. As observed *(8)*, in some cell lines a decrease in the concentration of D-glucose from culture medium is accompanied by a decrease in formazan products. For that reason a full culture medium (e.g., RPMI-1640 w/o phenol red), containing D-glucose is necessary to obtain optimal formazan production. Furthermore, the medium has to be adjusted to neutral pH. The untreated cells should be in exponential growth phase at the time of harvest. When medium containing serum (>0.05 %) is used in the MTT assay, high background values are observed *(6)*. It should be stressed that with the MTT assay, optimal conditions should be elucidated for each cell line. Using MTT concentrations from 0 to 4 mg/mL, with a constant number of cells per well may be useful to identify optimal MTT concentrations especially for novel cell lines.
2. First, the pH indicator phenol red absorbs at 570 nm. This may affect the results of the MTT assays. Second, the contaminants of this indicator have shown substantial estrogenic activity for estrogen-dependent cells in culture. The phenol red may vary the growth pattern of some estrogen responsive cells. Our solution to these problems was to use SSM lacking phenol red.
3. Exponentially growing cultures of *HOC* cell lines were grown in GM (17% FCS) and were maintained in 75-cm² culture flasks (Nunc, Weisbaden-Biebrich, Germany) in a humidified incubator at 37°C in an atmosphere of 95% air and 5% carbon dioxide. Depen-

dent on cell lines others use GM with FCS concentrations of 5, 7.5, or 10% as cell-culture medium. This may not interfere with the MTT assay, for using SSM (0.05% FCS) as medium in this assay. Single-cell suspensions were obtained by trypsination of the mono-layer cultures (incubation with 500 mL trypsin-EDTA [0.02%/0.05% (v/v)] at 37°C for 5 min). Cells were washed twice with sterile HBSS.

4. Disperse the cells by gentle passages through a Pasteur pipet.

5. Count an aliquot of cells directly in a hemocytometer or with an automated cell counter to estimate cell concentration [cells/mL].

6. This preculture period ensure attachment of the cells. On one hand, this period can be reduced, if necessary to a few hours. On the other hand, an incubation time of 96 h allows sufficient time for assessment of chemosensitivity or for growth stimulation tests with cytokines.

7. The serum reduced SSM (0.5% FCS) was used to perform the MTT based growth assay. As mentioned above, high serum-protein concentrations (> 1%) can interfere with the assay, resulting in high background values. Reduction of the serum-protein concentration may result in improved sensitivity of the MTT assay. Although other working groups *(6)* suspended the cells in serum-free medium, the small amount of serum protein (0.5% FCS in SSM) that we used, did not result in higher background values.

8. **Warnings:** MTT solution is harmful if swallowed, inhaled, or absorbed through skin. MTT may alter genetic material. Formazan solvent is flammable and corrosive.

9. Where high sensitivity is not required, the incubation time can be reduced to 1–2 h *(6)*.

10. We used acid isopropyl alcohol as formazan solvent *(1,6)*, reading at a wavelength of 570 nm. Background subtraction was performed at a reference wavelength of 690 nm to minimize background values. However, other working groups used different solvents to enhance the sensitivity of the MTT-based colorimetric assay: Scudiero et al. *(2)* and Park et al. *(5)* used DMSO to solubilize the MTT-formazan product (wavelength: 540 nm). Carmichael et al. *(4)* achieved optimal results by measuring formazan crystals solubilized in mineral-oil at a test wavelength of 570 nm and with DMSO at 540 nm.

11. Culture plates should be read within 1 h after adding the solvent.

## References

1. Mosmann, T. (1983) Rapid colorimetric assay for cellular growth and survival: application to proliferation and cytotoxicity assays. *J. Immunol. Meth.* **65,** 55–63.
2. Scudiero, D. A., Shoemaker, R. H., Paull, K. D., Monks, A., Tierney, S., Nofziger, T. H., et al. (1988) Evaluation of a soluble tetrazolium/formazan assay for cell growth and drug sensitivity in culture using human and other cell lines. *Cancer Res.* **48,** 4827–4833.
3. Slater, T. F., Sawyer, B., and Strauli, U. (1963) Studies on succinate-tetrazolium reductase system III. Points of coupling of four different tetrazolium salts. *Biochem. Biophys. Acta* **77,** 383–393.
4. Carmichael, J., DeGraff, W. G., Gazdar, A. F., Minna, J. D., and Mitchell, J. B. (1987) Evaluation of a tetrazolium-based semiautomated colorimetric assay: Assessment of chemosensitivity testing. *Cancer Res.* **47,** 936–942.
5. Park, J-G., Kramer, B. S., Steinberg, S. M., Carmichael, J., Collins, J. M., Minna, J. D., et al. (1987) Chemosensitivity testing of human colorectal carcinoma cell lines using a tetrazolium-based colorimetric assay. *Cancer Res.* **447,** 5875–5879.
6. Denizot, F. and Lang, R. (1986) Rapid colorimetric assay for cell growth and survival. Modifications to the tetrazolium dye procedure giving improved sensitivity and reliability. *J. Immunol. Meth.* **89,** 271–277.
7. Spinner, D. M., Brandstetter, T., Kiechle-Schwarz, M., duBois, A., Angel, P., and Bauknecht, T. (1995) C-jun expression and growth stimulation in human ovarian carcinoma cell lines following exposure to cytokines. *Int. J. Cancer* **63,** 423–427.
8. Vistica, D. T., Skehan, P., Scudiero, D., Monks, A., Pittman, A., and Boyd, M. R. (1991) Tetrazolium-based assays for cellular viability: a critical examination of selected parameters affecting formazan production. *Cancer Res.* **51,** 2515–2520.

# 18

## In Vitro Invasion Assays

### Setsuko K. Chambers

### 1. Introduction

Epithelial ovarian cancer cells spread by two major pathways. One is by exfoliation of tumor cells from the ovarian surface, with resulting implants on peritoneal surfaces such as omentum, diaphragm, and bowel serosa. The second pathway of spread of epithelial ovarian cancer is that of invasion into lymphatic channels, with involvement of the retroperitoneal lymph nodes. Invasion of tumor cells appears to result from a deregulation of the normal processes that govern physiologic controlled invasion. An example of physiologic invasion is that of trophoblastic implantation of the endometrium followed by invasion to access the maternal blood supply in the uterus. The normal invasive process is controled by a balance between protease activity and that of their inhibitors at the level of the individual cell. For the large majority of tumors, extracellular matrix degrading proteases have been shown to have an important role in tumor invasion and metastases. In epithelial ovarian cancer, the major focus has been on the activities of the serine protease urokinase plasminogen activator (uPA) *(1–4)*, and the matrix metalloproteinases (MMP) *(5,6)*. The cysteine proteases, such as cathepsin B, and aspartic proteases, such as cathepsin D, also play a role in invasiveness of ovarian cancer cells. Each class of proteases contributes to the process of invasion, and cooperates with each other to further the optimal degradation of the extracellular matrix by ovarian cancer cells *(7)*. Urokinase activates plasminogen to plasmin, which activates both pro-uPA and latent MMPs, and cleaves the MMP inhibitor *TIMP-2*. Moreover, cathepsin B, which is expressed by ovarian cancer cells, appears to facilitate the action of uPA, most likely by activating pro-uPA *(8)*.

The invasiveness of tumor cells, a phenotype which can be measured in vitro, is dependent on the combined properties of adhesion, motility, and proteolysis. Thus, measurement of invasion alone should be taken as reflective of all three characteristics of tumor behavior. It is important that proliferation of tumor cells not be understood to be a requirement for invasiveness. In fact in some cases, an increase in invasiveness is observed concomitantly with a decrease in proliferative capacity.

The following is a basic protocol, which we use for measurement of ovarian cancer cell invasion in vitro. This assay is based on a modification of the original Membrane Invasion Culture System (MICS) *(9)*. Most protocols have focused on measurement of invasiveness of the highly invasive melanoma or prostate cancer cells. In our hands,

From: *Methods in Molecular Medicine, Vol. 39: Ovarian Cancer: Methods and Protocols*
Edited by: J. M. S. Bartlett © Humana Press, Inc., Totowa, NJ

the technique has evolved to optimize measurement of invasiveness of the relatively low-level invasive ovarian cancer cell lines. In this assay, the gold standard of visually counting stained cells, which have invaded through the filter is utilized. An alternative protocol has been described *(10)* that has been successfully used for measurement of ovarian cancer cell invasion, which takes advantage of the colorimetric 3-(4,5-dimethylthiazole-2-yl)-2,5-diphenyltetrazolium bromide (MTT) assay adapted for quantitating tumor cell invasion. Other alternative methods to quantify tumor cell invasion, such as spectrophotometric analysis after extraction of crystal violet staining of tumor cells *(11,12)*, has not proven to be sensitive enough for measurement of ovarian cancer cell invasion in our hands.

## 2. Materials

1. Trypsin-EDTA diluted fourfold with PBS pH 7.4 to a final concentration of 0.125% trypsin and 0.05% EDTA.
2. 1% NuSerum (Collaborative Research, Inc., Bedford, MA).
3. MICS chambers (MJC Hendrix, Department of Anatomy and Cell Biology, University of Iowa, Iowa City, IA).
4. 10 µm pore polycarbonate filters (Nuclepore, available through Corning, Acton, MA). Does not have to be polyvinylpyrrolidone (PVP)-free. Cut to size (7.5 × 11.5 cm) and cold gas-sterilize. Store at room temperature.
5. Human defined matrix: 50 µg/mL human laminin (Sigma, St. Louis, MO), 50 µg/mL human type IV collagen (Collaborative Research), and 2 mg/mL gelatin in 10 m$M$ acetic acid. This is a nonmurine matrix, which does not contain known or unknown growth factors, and whose effect on invasion does not depend on different batches. Store at 4°C.
6. Alternatively, Matrigel (Collaborative Research) diluted to 1–4 mg/mL with serum-free media. To reduce the differences in results of invasion studies found with using different lots of Matrigel, it is recommended to assay the protein content of each lot, and dilute to the same final concentration for each experiment. Alternatively, one could request the same lot number when repurchasing Matrigel, depending on availability, or purchase a large amount of the same lot at once, which could be costly. Store at 4°C.

## 3. Methods

### 3.1. Cell Preparation

Ovarian cancer cells should be harvested while in the exponential phase of growth (70–80% confluent), with strict attention made to keeping the passage numbers as consistent as possible from experiment to experiment (*see* **Note 1**).

1. The media of the untreated cells is changed to 1% NuSerum (*see* **Note 2**) 24 h prior to start of the invasion assay,
2. The cells are detached from plastic with trypsin-EDTA diluted fourfold with PBS. The treatment duration is minimized, and the enzymatic action is neutralized by addition of media with NuSerum as soon as the cells detach (*see* **Note 3**).
3. The cells are then washed free of trypsin by briefly centrifuging at 1000$g$ and resuspending the cell pellet in media containing NuSerum. The cells are pelleted and washed in this manner for a total of three times (*see* **Note 4**).
4. Care is taken to disaggregate all clumps by pipeting with a Pasteur pipet. The cells are then counted, and diluted to a final concentration of $2 \times 10^5$ cells/mL of medium containing NuSerum (*see* **Note 5**).

## 3.2. Invasion Assay

The night before the invasion assay, a brief period of time (20 min per chamber) is spent in the tissue-culture hood setting up the experiment. Sterile gloves are used (*see* **Note 6**).

1. A piece of parafilm slightly larger than the size of the filter is placed so that it sticks onto a glass plate that measures approximately 18 cm × 18 cm.
2. The shiny side of the polycarbonate membrane is placed so that it sticks onto the parafilm (dull side up). Mild pressure is exerted by the gloved fingertips to accomplish this step. All four sides of the filter are then secured to the glass plate with Scotch tape (*see* **Note 7**).
3. The uncoated filter affixed to the glass plate, along with the MICS chamber, is then UV sterilized in the tissue-culture hood overnight (minimum of 8 h).
4. On the day of the assay, the sterilized filter on the glass plate is placed in an approximately 27 cm × 30 cm-size Ziplock bag, and transferred to 4°C to chill prior to the filter being coated.
5. A 1-mL pipet is placed within a bucket filled with ice (tip down) while still in its sterile paper wrapper, and extracellular matrix at the final concentration is placed on ice (*see* **Note 8**).
6. An 8-mm glass rod, approximately 13 cm in length, is cleaned with 70% ethanol, wiped, and chilled in the ice bucket.
7. The chilled filter on the glass plate is returned to the tissue-culture hood, and 0.3 mL of chilled matrix is then applied to one end of the filter in a straight line.
8. The chilled glass rod is used to smoothly spread the matrix to the thickness of the Scotch tape across the entire filter in one even motion. Do not push hard. The matrix is then allowed to dry in the hood with the blower off for 30 min.
9. Meanwhile, the pins used to plug the bottom ports of the lower wells, and the screws used to attach the upper plate to the lower plate of the MICS, are then flame sterilized in the hood. Because these metal components are stored in ethanol, they can be placed in a small pile within the hood, and a very small bonfire can be lit with the Bunsen burner. Watch carefully until the fire has been completely extinguished. Alternatively, the metal pins and screws can be presterilized in the autoclave.
10. The pins are then placed into the ports in the lower plate, and media plus NuSerum pipeted into the lower chamber. Fill the lower wells until almost overflowing to ensure that air bubbles do not become entrapped within the lower chamber when placing the coated filter on top of the lower plate (*see* **Note 9**).
11. Carefully cut the dried matrix-coated membrane with a scalpel along the edges of the Scotch tape, and peel off the parafilm backing, using two forceps at corners diagonally across from each other, to avoid the creation of a cigarette roll, which would likely adversely affect the smooth matrix coating.
12. The matrix-coated filter is then placed coated side up on the lower plate. The upper plate is then carefully placed on the lower plate perfectly, matching edges, so that the upper plate is not slid across the lower plate during subsequent adjustment, disturbing the matrix surface. Using the sterilized screws, the upper plate is then affixed to the lower plate.
13. The matrix is then rehydrated for at least 30 min with 0.5 mL media plus NuSerum.
14. It is at this step that, if treatment with cytokines, hormones, antibodies, or drugs are desired, that the matrix can be exposed to the treatment for 1 h in the tissue-culture hood at 2X the final concentration, in the absence of cells (*see* **Note 10**).
15. 0.5 mL of cells at a concentration of $2 \times 10^5$ cells/mL is added to the upper chamber after the matrix is rehydrated and/or treated (*see* **Note 11**).

16. The MICS is then sandwiched between two covers (UV sterilized 96-well plate covers work well) and carefully placed in a Ziplock bag, partly open, in a 37°C incubator for 48 h (*see* **Note 12**).

## 3.3. Staining and Counting of Cells

1. The entire apparatus is dismantled after removing the upper chamber media (*see* **Note 13**), and the filter is affixed bottom side up (invading cell side up) by pins to a parafilm covered wax plate.
2. The filter is then fixed in 0.5% crystal violet in 25% methanol for 20 min, carefully rinsed with $H_2O$, flipped over using two forceps at diagonally opposed corners, and then repinned. At this point, the cells, which have been seeded on top of the filter, are bright purple and fill the entire circle of the well.
3. The edges of the well are marked at four corners for future reference with a fine felt-tipped pen, and the cells on top of the filter carefully wiped off with a wet Q-tip.
4. A square containing each well is then carefully cut out with a scalpel and flipped onto a glass slide such that the invading cells are on top again. Immersion oil is added, followed by a cover slip.
5. Use a X40 lens without phase contrast to count 10–15 fields per well (*see* **Notes 14** and **15**).

## 3.4. Calculation of Percent Invasion

In order to calculate the total number of cells invading through the filter per well, one needs to make certain preliminary calculations using the specific microscope which will be used to count the cells.

Using a well of which the boundaries of the circle are well delineated, first count the number of X40 fields end to end, which can line up along the diameter of the well. Make this calculation more than once, and take a mean. The diameter squared represents the total number of X40 fields, which can fit in the area of the well. For instance, if the number of X40 fields that fit along the diameter of the well is 16.4, then the total number of X40 fields that can fit in the area of the well is $(16.4)^2$, which equals 269. If the mean number of cells/X40 field is 20, then the total number of invading cells is $20 \times 269 = 5380$ cells. Because we loaded $1 \times 10^5$ cells, the invasion rate is 5.4%. By using 4–6 wells per condition, a small standard of error could be obtained.

## 4. Notes

1. It is recommended that a reference cell line, such as the highly invasive melanoma cell line, Bowes, or the prostate cancer cell line, PC-3, be used to ensure reproducibility of results from one experiment to the next. It is especially important when first learning this assay to include a reference cell line *(13)*.
2. 1% NuSerum is used to limit the presence of protease inhibitors, which are likely to be present in calf serum. In our case, because we are studying the effects of *CSF-1* and *CSF-1* receptor on invasion, and because serum has confounding effects on their expression, we use a low final concentration of 1% NuSerum in our invasion assay. Many others have used up to 10% serum in their invasion assay. If pretreatment of the cells with agents such as cytokines or hormones is desired, these can be performed while the cells are on plastic for the predetermined period of time. An alternative to NuSerum that avoids protease inhibitors completely and enables serum-free conditions for the invasion assay is the use of Mito+ (Collaborative Research), which is a serum-free constituent that contains numerous, but defined, growth factors and hormones.

3. At the time of the invasion assay, it is optimal if the cells can be detached from plastic without trypsin, such as with 2 m$M$ EDTA/PBS, pH 7.4, for 10 min. We have found the ovarian cancer cell lines are very adherent, and will not detach with this approach. On long incubation, visualization of toxic effects are seen with the majority of cells still attached to the plastic.

4. If serum-free conditions or low-serum conditions are used, it is recommended that the media be supplemented with 0.1% BSA.

5. In general, we have found that an 80% confluent T25 flask of ovarian cancer cells contains $3–5 \times 10^6$ cells. This number of cells is more than sufficient for the purposes of the invasion assay, even with multiple conditions, and 4–6 wells per condition, because only $1 \times 10^5$ cells are loaded into each well.

6. The MICS chamber *(9)* consists of two portions: a lower plate with 14 blind end wells (12 of which are accessible through side sampling ports), and an upper plate with 14 matching, but open-ended wells. Each well measures 13 mm in diameter. The 10 µm pore polycarbonate filter measuring 7.5 cm × 11.5 cm is uniformly coated with matrix components and placed between the upper and lower components of the MICS chamber, which are then screwed together. We use the MICS chambers for measurement of ovarian cancer cell invasion, because this approach has some advantages: 1) relative ease in setup of the assay, as the entire polycarbonate filter (7.5 cm 11.5 cm) is coated at once, eliminating paraffin pretreatment of chamber walls to decrease meniscus formation, and separate preparations of each well; 2) enhanced reproducibility and even thickness of the surface containing basement membrane components on the filter; and 3) cost savings, as the MICS chambers are durable for many years.

7. Laboratory colored tape was originally recommended to serve as a guide to uniform thickness of the extracellular matrix components on the filter, which resulted in a uniform Matrigel thickness after rehydration of 0.035 mm after spreading 1 mL of full-strength Matrigel on this filter *(9)*. We have found that optimal invasion of ovarian cancer cells could be attained with the use of the thinner Scotch tape as our guide to uniform thickness.

8. We currently use a human defined matrix, containing type IV collagen, and laminin. Human normal ovarian surface epithelium produces such basement membrane components *(14)*. We found that the difference in invasiveness when comparing different ovarian cancer cell lines is, in fact, enhanced when using the human defined matrix, when compared to Matrigel *(13)*. Care is taken that the stock solutions of both types of extracellular matrices are always kept on ice or at 4°C. The matrices will irreversibly gel at room temperature.

9. We occasionally use chemoattractants (such as 25 µg/mL fibronectin) in our invasion assay, which is added in this step if desired. The argument against its use is that it is believed that chemoattractants promote mainly motility, not invasion, thus its use may be confounding, with differential effects on different cell lines. Recently, the chemoattractant fibronectin was shown to enhance secretion of *MMP-9* by ovarian cancer cells *(15)*, which would support a direct effect of fibronectin on invasiveness of these cells. It is possible that the effects of chemoattractants on motility would be evident only with invasion assays of short duration, but not those of 24 h or longer, where differences in invasion rates may predominate.

10. We have found that in the case of *CSF-1* treatment of ovarian cancer cells, for instance, that exposure of the matrix to this cytokine in this step is valuable *(13)*.

11. Additional agents to which the cells will be exposed for the duration of the invasion assay, such as chemotherapeutic drugs or oligonucleotides can also be included in the upper chamber media at this point. Care should be taken to ensure that each well receives the same amount of media and same final concentration of serum or drugs or their vehicles.

12. Invasion has been measured after a duration of as little as 6 h, to as long as 72 h. The optimal duration for assay of invasiveness is dependent on the cell type. For ovarian cancer cells, measurement of invasion at time periods of less than 24 h will usually yield too few cells to accurately quantitate. Thus, ovarian cancer cell invasion has been measured at periods between 24 to 72 h *(8,10,13)*.

13. The MICS was originally designed to have the advantage of being able to access the bottom chamber without having to dismantle the entire apparatus. This was to enable trypsinization of the invading cells off the bottom of the filter by replacing the media in the lower chamber with trypsin-EDTA, and incubating the entire apparatus in the incubator for 20 min. The cells recovered in this manner, after Pasteur pipeting the contents of the lower chamber, were then loaded onto a dot-blot manifold containing 3 μm pore polycarbonate filters, fixed, stained, and counted. We have counted cells floating in the lower chamber media, and found that in the case of ovarian cancer cells, this number is negligible. When using the trypsin approach to recover the invading cells, we found that cellular debris would not infrequently obscure our ability to count cells accurately, and the flow of the trypsinized cells (rescued in media with serum) through the dot blot manifold at times appeared to be excessively slow, with debris blocking the ability to load all the cells. Although we no longer use this approach for recovering the cells, nevertheless, the separate access to the lower chamber can be useful if one needs to add an agent to the lower chamber later. In this case, the 100-μL glass drummond pipetes are ideal, as they fit easily into the side sampling ports in the lower chamber, through which media could be removed, and an equal amount of concentrated drug replaced.

14. There is little debris with this method of staining and counting cells, and the cells are generally clearly identified. Sometimes the cells are all the way out of the pore and starting to form little colonies, many times they are still coming through the pore. Care should be taken in counting, focussing up and down with the fine focus, in order not to miss invading cells as empty pores in the filter. We have found at times, that the intensity of the purple stain fades with time; for this reason we recommend that the cells are counted within 24 h of staining the filters. The filters can be easily restained if necessary.

15. Note that this protocol for invasion could be easily modified to study adhesion (2-h time frame, count cells that have adhered to the human defined matrix on top of the filter), or directed or random motility (6-h time frame, with or without chemoattractants (25 μg/mL fibronectin works well for ovarian cancer cells) in the lower chamber, count cells on the bottom of the filter). In the case of the directed motility assays of ovarian cancer cells, long pseudopodia can be frequently visualized, attached to cells on the bottom surface of the filter.

## References

1. Chambers, S. K., Ivins, C. M., and Carcangiu, M. L. (1998) Urokinase-type plasminogen activator in epithelial ovarian cancer: a poor prognostic factor, associated with advanced stage. *Int. J. Gynecol. Oncol.* **8,** 242–250.
2. Kuhn, W., Pache, L., Schmalfeldt, P., Dettmar, P., Schmitt, M., Janicke, F., et al. (1994) Urokinase (uPA) and PAI-1 predict survival in advanced ovarian cancer patients (FIGO III) after radical surgery and platinum-based chemotherapy. *Gynecol. Oncol.* **55,** 401–409.
3. Van der Burg, M. E. L., Henzen-Logmans, S. C., Berns, E. M. J. J., van Putten, W. L. J., Klijn. J. G. M., and Foekens, J. A. (1996) Expression of urokinase-type plasminogen activator (uPA) and its inhibitor PAI-1 in benign, borderline, malignant primary and metastatic ovarian tumors. *Int. J. Cancer* **69,** 475–479.
4. Chambers, S. K., Ivins, C. M., and Carcangiu, M. L. (1998) Plasminogen activator inhibitor-1 is an independent poor prognostic factor for survival in epithelial ovarian cancer. *Int. J. Cancer* **79,** 1–6.
5. Fishman, D. A., Bafetti, L. M., and Stack, M. S. (1996) Membrane-type matrix metalloproteinase expression and MMP-2 activation in primary human ovarian epithelial cancer cells. *Inv. Metastasis* **16,** 150–159.

6. Davies, B., Brown, P. D., East, N., Crimmin, M. J., and Balkwill, F. R. (1993) A synthetic matrix metalloproteinase inhibitor decreases tumor burden and prolongs survival of mice bearing human ovarian carcinoma xenografts. *Cancer Res.* **53,** 2087–2091.

7. DeClerck, Y. A. and Laug, W. E. (1996) Cooperation between matrix metalloproteinases and plasminogen activator system in tumor progression. *Enzyme Protein* **49,** 72–84.

8. Kobayashi, H., Ohi, H., Sugimura M., Shinohara, H., Fujii, T., and Terao, T. (1992) Inhibition of in vitro ovarian cancer cell invasion by modulation of urokinase-type plasminogen activator and cathepsin B. *Cancer Res.* **52,** 3610–3614.

9. Hendrix, M. J. C., Seftor, E. A., Seftor, R. E. B., and Fidler, I. J. (1987) A simple quantitative assay for studying the invasive potential of high and low human metastatic variants. *Cancer Lett.* **38,** 137–147.

10. Sieuwerts, A. M., Klijn, J. G., and Foekens, J. A. (1997) Assessment of the invasive potential of human gynecological tumor cell lines with the in vitro Boyden chamber assay: influences of the ability of cells to migrate through the filter membrane. *Clin. Exp. Metastasis* **15,** 53–62.

11. Leyton, J., Manyak, M. J., Mukherjee, A. B., Miele, L., Mantile, G., and Patierno, S. R. (1994) Recombinant human uteroglobin inhibits the in vitro invasiveness of human metastatic prostate tumor cells and the release of arachidonic acid stimulated by fibroblast-conditioned medium. *Cancer Res.* **54,** 3696–3699.

12. Saito, K., Oku, T., Ata, N., Miyashiro, H., Hattori, M., and Saiki, I. (1997) A modified and convenient method for assessing tumor cell invasion and migration and its application to screening for inhibitors. *Biol. Pharm. Bull.* **20,** 345–348.

13. Chambers, S. K., Wang, Y., Gertz, R. E., and Kacinski, B. M. (1995) Macrophage colony stimulating factor mediates invasion of ovarian cancer cells through urokinase. *Cancer Res.* **55,** 1578–1585.

14. Kruk, P. A., Uitto, V-J., Firth, J. D., Dedhar, S., and Auersperg, N. (1994) Reciprocal interactions between human ovarian surface epithelial cells and adjacent extracellular matrix. *Exp. Cell. Res.* **215,** 97–108.

15. Shibata, K., Kikkawa, F., Nawa, A., Thant, A. A., Naruse, K., Mizutani, S., et al. (1998) Both focal adhesion kinase and c-ras are required for the enhanced matrix metalloproteinase 9 secretion by fibronectin in ovarian cancer cells. *Cancer Res.* **58,** 900–903.

# 19

## *p53* Transfectants in Ovarian Cancer

### Faina Vikhanskaya and Massimo Broggini

## 1. Introduction

The tumor suppressor gene *tp53* is mutated, deleted, or rearranged in more than 50% of human tumors *(1)*. Wild-type (wt) *tp53* stops growth and/or induces apoptosis in most transformed cells into which it is introduced, thus restricting research of such cells. One means of studying the effects of both wt and mutant *tp53* is to generate cells in which *tp53* activity can be experimentally manipulated using inducible transcriptional control elements to drive wt *tp53* expression *(2–4)*. Alternatively, temperature-sensitive (ts) *tp53* mutants may be used. Such mutants were first analyzed by Oren *(5)* and possess wt *tp53* activity at 32°C, but behave like other mutants *tp53* molecules at 37°C.

There are, however, some disadvantages associated with the use of both inducible and temperature-sensitive constructs. Inducible constructs may adversely affect expression of basal levels of wt *tp53* in the absence of the inducing agent. Temperature-sensitive constructs require transformation, expansion, and cultivation of clones to be performed at 37°C, but experiments must be carried out at 32°C precluding the use of these systems in vivo.

Ovarian cancer cell lines (A2780, IGROV-1, Pa-1, SKOV-3, and so on) can be transfected with plasmid DNA using the Ca-precipitate formation with the plasmid of interest followed by selection on antibiotics. Western blotting of positive clones can be readily used to identify positive clones. There are no particular difficulties in transfecting *tp53* into ovarian cells other than selection of the appropriate plasmid for the experiment, method of identification of positive clones, and careful cultivation of clones to prevent unexpected loss of *tp53* expression.

## 2. Materials

### 2.1. Cell Culture

1. Medium for cell culture: prepare from concentrated stock of DMEM or RPMI. For 500 mL of medium: add 50 mL of 10X DMEM (or RPMI, Gibco, Gaithersburg, MD), 50 mL of fetal calf serum (FCS, Gibco), 5 mL of nonessential amino acids (NEAA Gibco), 5 mL of glutamine (Gibco) to 390 mL of sterile distilled water.
2. Phosphate-buffered saline (PBS) (pH 7.4).
3. Trypsin (0.05% w/v)/EDTA (0.02% w/v) in PBS.

From: *Methods in Molecular Medicine, Vol. 39: Ovarian Cancer: Methods and Protocols*
Edited by: J. M. S. Bartlett © Humana Press, Inc., Totowa, NJ

## 2.2. Solutions for Cell Transfection (see Note 1)

1. 2X HEBS-buffered saline: 8.2 g NaCl (280 m$M$), 0.037 g KCl (10 m$M$), 0.0135 g Na$_2$HPO4x2H$_2$O (1.5 m$M$), 0.1 g dextrose (12 m$M$), 0.5 g HEPES (50 m$M$) are dissolved in 50 mL of sterile distilled water. Titrate to pH 7.05–7.1 with NaOH, filter sterilize and store in 4 mL aliquots at –20° for up to 2 mo.
2. 2.5$M$ CaCl$_2$: 7.34g CaCl$_2$x2H$_2$O or 10.8 g CaCl$_2$x6H$_2$O are dissolved in 20 mL of distilled water. Filter sterilize and store at –20°C for up to 2 mo.
3. Geneticin (G418) 500 mg/mL in culture medium.

## 2.3. Solutions for Western Blot Analysis

1. 5X Tris-glycine running buffer: 15.1 g of Tris base, 94 g glycine, 50 mL of 10% SDS are added to 950 mL of distilled water. The solution can be stored at room temperature for long periods.
2. 2X transfer buffer: 12.1 g Tris-base, 14.3 g glycine, 2 mL SDS 10%, 400 mL methanol, to 1 L with distilled water. The solution can be stored at room temperature for long periods.
3. 2X loading buffer: 0.4 mL 10% SDS, 0.1 mL 1M Tris-HCl pH 6.8, 0.2 mL 100% glycerol, 0.2 mL of 1$M$ DTT, 0.02 mL bromophenol blue (10% in water) to 1 mL of distilled water. The solution is stable if kept at –20°C.
4. Lysis buffer for protein preparation: 5 mL of 1$M$ Tris-HCl pH 7.4 (50 m$M$), 5 mL of 5$M$ NaCl (250 m$M$), 1 mL 10% NP40 (0.1%), 1 mL 0.5$M$ EDTA (5 m$M$), 0.21 g NaF (50 m$M$), (store at 4°C for up to 3 mo). Just before use, add to 1 mL of lysis buffer 10 µL of 200 mMPMSF , 17 µL of aprotinin (prepared as 1.9 mg/mL in water), 4 µL of leupeptin (prepared as a stock 5 mg/mL in water). PMSF and leupeptin must be stored at –20°C, aprotinin can be stored at 4°C.
5. 5% dried milk in PBS.
6. *p53* antibody (*tp53*: DO1, pAB1801, or pAb421, Santa Cruz Biotechnology or Oncogene Science) diluted 1:200 in PBS containing 5% dried milk.
7. Horse radish peroxidase linked secondary antibody (antimouse or antirabbit, depending of the primary antibody used; Amersham, Arlington Hts., IL) diluted 1:2000 in PBS containing 5% milk.
8. ECL Detection system (Amersham).

## 3. Methods

### 3.1. Cell Maintenance

#### 3.1.1. Thawing and Cultivation of Cells

1. Thaw cells from liquid nitrogen rapidly in a 37°C water bath.
2. Transfer to centrifuge tubes in 10 mL of growth medium, centrifuge 10 min at 1000$g$.
3. Discard supernatent, resuspend cell pellet in 5–10 mL growth medium, and transfer to 75-cm$^2$ tissue-culture flasks.

#### 3.1.2. Preparation of Cells for Freezing

1. Prepare 1 million cells/mL in complete culture medium with 10% DMSO. Aliquot 1 mL cell suspension/vial and freeze 20 min in ethanol at –20°C, then put for 2 d at –80°C and then to liquid nitrogen.

### 3.2. Preparation of Cells for Transfection

1. Plate mycoplasma-free cells (5 × 10$^5$ cells in 6-cm diameter Petri dishes in growth medium) the day before transfection.

2. Next day, change medium (from RPMI to DMEM) using 9 mL DMEM with 5% fetal calf serum. DMEM should be used even if it is not the medium of choice for the cells being used, because components of DMEM medium do not interfere with Ca-precipitate used for transfection, whereas RPMI-1640 interferes with precipitate formation.
3. Equilibrate cells for at least 4 h before transfection.

### 3.3. Preparation of Plasmids for Transfection

Plasmids that contain *tp53* under the control of inducible promoter or ts *tp53*, as mentioned in the introduction, should be sterilized as follows:

1. Precipitate DNA in 2 volumes absolute ethanol in the presence of sodium acetate (final concentration $0.3M$) at $-20°C$ for 30 min.
2. Centrifuge at $4°C$ for 15 min at $12,000g$, discard supernatant.
3. Fill Eppendorf with 70% ethanol and leave overnight at room temperature (*see* **Note 2**). For each flask use 5–10 µg of plasmid containing *tp53*.

### 3.4. Transfection of Cells

1. Before transfection, centrifuge the plasmid again, at $4°C$ for 15 min at $12,000g$, discard supernatant and dry in sterile hood.
2. Dissolve the DNA in 450 µL of sterile $H_2O$ and add this solution to an Eppendorf containing 50 µL of $2.5M$ $CaCl_2$.
3. Put in a separate, transparent tube 500 µL of 2X HEBS. Add drop by drop with constant shaking plasmid dissolved in $H_2O$ and $CaCl_2$ to the HEBS. A fine precipitate will appear. Vortex immediately for 5 s.
4. Leave the tube for complete formation of precipitate for another 20 min at room temperature.
5. Add the entire solution (1 mL) to the flasks with the cells containing 9 mL of medium (*see* **Subheading 3.2., step 2**). Leave overnight at $37°C$ in incubator (*see* **Note 3**).

### 3.5 Selection of Clones

1. The day after transfection, discard medium, wash cells two or three times with 10 mL of PBS until the precipitate has been completely removed, and add complete medium (RPMI-1640) for cell cultivation.
2. Allow the cells to grow for the next 2 d.
3. Detach cells with trypsin-EDTA and split cells 1:6 into selective medium (*see* **Note 4**).

### 3.6. Results

Demonstration of *tp53* presence and activity in clones selected can be done by using several tests.

1. Demonstration of *tp53* insertion in genomic DNA of transfected cells using Southern blotting or PCR. This analysis confirms the stable introduction of plasmid into genomic DNA, but does not give information on the activity of *tp53*.
2. Demonstration of *tp53* expression at the level of transcriptions by Northern blot analysis or RT-PCR. This analysis demonstrates that plasmid after introduction can be transcribed and confirms the *tp53* RNA presence in transfected clones.
3. Demonstrations of *tp53* expression at the level of proteins by Western blot analysis. This analysis demonstrates that *tp53* can be translated by the translational system of the cell. We recommend this approach for analysis of transfectants as the most simple which supports the full production of the gene introduced into the parental cells.

4. Investigations of *tp53*-related genes expression: GADD45, waf/cip1, bax. Analysis can be done at the level of transcription or expression of proteins. Presence of *tp53*-related gene expression confirms that introduced *tp53* is transcriptionally active.
5. Analysis of cell cycle arrest after gamma irradiation. In presence of functional *tp53*, cells should stop in the phase G1 phase of the cell cycle. This test can be recommended as additional.
6. Investigation of apoptosis induced by DNA-damaging agents. This test cannot be recommended as additional because apoptosis is not typical for all kinds of cell.

The tests 2–6, for inducible promoters of *tp53* expression, should be carried out in conditions that allow *tp53* expression (i.e., by addition of the inducer).

In the case of ts *tp53*, DNA analysis, Northern, and Western blot analysis can be performed either at 37°C or 32°C without altering the results. For 4–6, it is important to shift the temperature from 37°C to 32°C for at least 6 h before analysis to allow for *tp53* protein to change conformation from mut to wt. In the case of ts mutants, the use of functional tests (and particularly test 4) is mandatory for confirmation of clones under analysis.

We present in detail a method for Western blot analysis.

### 3.7. Western Blot Analysis

1. Preparation of proteins from clones. Use 1–2 million cells for each sample. Remove the medium by aspiration and wash the cells with 5 mL of PBS.
2. Remove all the PBS and add 200–500 µL of lysis buffer for protein preparation and incubate for approximately 30 min. on ice. Scrape the cells and transfer to 1.5-mL Eppendorf tubes.
3. Spin at 12,000*g* for 5 min, take supernatant, freeze, and keep at –20°C.
4. Electrophoresis of proteins. Prepare a 12% resolving gel. Then overlayer a 5% stacking gel and put them inside the cassette for protein separation.
5. Measure the concentrations of proteins, take 20–30 mg for each sample.
6. Add an equal volume of loading buffer, boil at 90°C 5 min, spin, and load into the gel.
7. Run at 100–150 V for 1–1.5 h. Detach the gel and use it for transferring proteins to nitrocellulose.
8. Electroblotting of proteins. Soak nitrocellulose membrane in $H_2O$, soak 4 sheets of 3 MM paper and 2 sponges in transfer buffer.
9. Remove stacking gel, take plastic transfer cassette, and assemble transfer sandwich: sponge, 2 sheets of 3 MM, gel, membrane, 2 sheets of 3 MM, sponge. Remove any air bubbles between gel and filter papers.
10. Put the cassette inside the apparatus, apply current for 1.5–3 h at 50 V.
11. Stain the protein on the membrane with Ponceau Red, rinse with $H_2O$, and air-dry.
12. Cut membrane according to the molecular weights and block the membrane in 5% dry milk dissolved in PBS for at least 1 h (it can be done overnight) with constant, gentle agitation.
13. Add the primary antibody for 1 h at room temperature with constant, gentle agitation.
14. Wash three times (each time for 5 min) with PBS.
15. Add secondary antibody (antimouse or antirabbit, depending of the primary antibody used) diluted 1:2000 in PBS containing 5% milk for 1 h at room temperature with constant, gentle agitation.
16. Wash three times (each time for 5 min) in PBS.
17. Detect the protein using the enhanced chemiluminescence (ECL, Amersham) method, following the manufacturer's instructions.

## 4. Notes

1. The quality of these two solutions should be checked immediately before use by mixing 2X HEBS and CaCl$_2$ as follows: in one tube, put 450 μL of H$_2$O and 50 μL of 2.5$M$ CaCl$_2$; in another transparent tube, put 500 μL of 2X HEBS. Drop by drop put the mixture of H$_2$O+CaCl$_2$ in the tube with 2X HEBS with constant mixing (which can be done by bubbling air with an automatic pipettor). A fine precipitate should develop that is readily visible under a microscope. It is important to check and adjust the pH of 2X HEBS every time before precipitation. Remake 2X HEBS if no precipitate is seen.

2. Transfection will be optimal if the gene is inserted in a plasmid containing a selective marker. However, it is also possible to do transfection with *tp53* by cotransfection with a separate plasmid containing a selective marker. In this case co-transfection with plasmid containing *tp53* and vector containing selective marker is carried out in the ratio 5–10 : 1 to ensure the presence of both plasmids in selected clones.

3. In the case of ts *tp53* all procedure should be done at 37°C, any drop of temperature during changes of medium, washing and splitting of cells after introduction of plasmid with ts *tp53* could decrease the efficiency of transfection. From two flasks with 10$^6$ cells prepared for transfection with 2–4 mg of vector containing selective marker, you should have about 30–50 colonies resistant to G418.

4. Selective medium contains antibiotic correspondent to the selective marker used in the transfection. From our experience, the most convenient for selection is the resistance to neomycin which allows selection in geneticin G418 (500 mg/mL, concentration which is generally used for many types of cells). It is, however, necessary to check before experiment the toxicity of the antibiotic in the cell line to be used. This can be done by plating the cells in different flasks and treating them with increasing concentrations of G418 (for example, from 10 to 1000 μg/mL). After 1 wk, visualize under microscope the cell remained attached to the plastic. The minimal concentration of G418 that is able to kill all the cells should be used. Feed cells with selective medium every 3–4 d for 14 d. Pick large colonies by using cloning cylinders and sterile vaseline. Cells forming colonies are detached and seeded in 24 wells plates. Following expansion and freezing demonstrate the presence of *tp53* expression and functions. After the procedure of cotransfection you should have 1–2 positive clones from every 10 colonies carrying resistance to antibiotic. It is important to keep and freeze several clones with different level of *tp53* expression.

    Freeze one clone that has been transfected with plasmid containing the neomycin resistance gene only and use this clone as a control in all your experiments. The cultivation at 32°C invariably slows down the growth of cells independently of the transfection. The use of appropriate controls strongly reduces this inconvenience and allows a proper analysis of the results obtained. It is necessary from time to time to check expression of *tp53* in your cells. Freeze some part of cells after this examination to keep constant stocks of cells at –80°C.

## References

1. Hollstein, M., Sidransky, D., Vogelstein, B., and Harris, C. C. (1991) p53 mutations in human cancers. *Science* **253,** 49–53.
2. Shaw, P., Bovey, R., Tardy, S., Sahli, R., Sorda, B. T., and Costa, J. (1992) Induction of apoptosis by wild-type p53 in human colon tumor-derived cell line. *Proc. Natl. Acad. Sci. USA* **89,** 4495–4499.
3. Lin, D., Shields, M. T., Ullrich, S. J., Appella, E., and Mercer, W. E. (1992) Growth arrest induced by wild-type p53 protein block cells prior to or near the restriction point near late G1 phase. *Proc. Natl. Acad. Sci. USA* **89,** 9210–9214.
4. Agawal, M. L., Agawal, A., Taylor, W. R., and Stark, G. R. (1995) p53 controls both the G2/M and G1 cell cycle checkpoints and mediates revesible growth arrest in human fibroblasts. *Proc. Natl. Acad. Sci. USA* **92,** 8493–8497.
5. Michalovitz, D., Halevy, O., and Oren, M. (1990) Conditional inhibition of transformation and of cell proliferation by temperature-sensitive mutant of p53. *Cell,* **62,** 671–680.

# 20 _____

## Estrogen-Responsive Ovarian Cancer Xenografts

### Alison A. Ritchie and Simon P. Langdon

## 1. Introduction

The use of human tumor xenografts grown in immunodeficient animals as a model for human cancers is well established and their value depends on the extent to which their characteristics reflect the properties of a particular cancer in the clinical situation. For endocrine-sensitive tumors, the retention of hormone receptors in xenografts and their responsiveness to hormonal stimuli are essential criteria if they are to serve as appropriate models. Provided these criteria are met, such experimental systems allow detailed studies of the effects of hormones on hormone-sensitive tumor cells and the potential of endocrine therapies in an in vivo system *(1)*.

Interest in the estrogen regulation of ovarian cancer and the possible use of antiestrogen-based therapies has led to the development of estrogen-responsive ovarian carcinoma xenografts as models of estrogen-sensitive disease *(2–7)* (**Table 1**). In contrast to estrogen-responsive breast cancer xenografts, ovarian carcinoma xenografts will grow in intact adult female mice without the need for exogenous hormonal supplementation. However, to provide defined levels of circulating estrogen, the ovaries can be removed and estrogen administered in slow-release pellets *(2,5)*. Alternatively, male mice can be used, because the circulating estrogen levels are similar to those in ovariectomized animals *(2,6)*. Using these models, information on the impact of estrogen on the growth and regulation of certain proteins such as the progesterone receptor and the evaluation of antiestrogen therapies have been obtained, e.g., **Fig. 1** *(2,3,7)*.

## 2. Materials
### 2.1. Animals and Animal Husbandry

1. Female nude (*nu/nu*) mice (Harlan Olac, Oxford, England).
2. Negative pressure isolators (Moredun Isolators, Penicuik, Scotland).
3. Sterile water (Baxter Travenol, Thetford, England).
4. Gold Chip bedding (B.S. and S. (Scotland) Ltd., Edinburgh, Scotland).
5. RM3 (E) animal feed–irradiated with 2.5 mrad (SDS Diet Services, Witham, England).
6. Hibicet (chlorhexidine gluconate/cetrimide solution; Zeneca Ltd., Macclesfield, England).
7. Alcide sterilant (Labcare Precision Ltd., Aldington, England).

From: *Methods in Molecular Medicine, Vol. 39: Ovarian Cancer: Methods and Protocols*
Edited by: J. M. S. Bartlett © Humana Press, Inc., Totowa, NJ

**Table 1**
**Estrogen Sensitive Ovarian Carcinoma Xenograft Models**

| Xenograft | Histology | ER content (fmol/mg) | Reference |
|---|---|---|---|
| PE04 | Poorly differentiated serous adenocarcinoma | 242 | *2,3* |
| BG-1 | Poorly differentiated adenocarcinoma | 23 | *4,5* |
| OVA-5 | Serous cystadenocarcinoma | 22 | *6* |
| OVCAR-3 | Poorly differentiated adenocarcinoma | 28 | *7* |

Fig. 1. Effect of tamoxifen on the growth of the ER-positive PE04 and ER-negative HOX 60 ovarian carcinoma xenografts. Each point represents the mean ± standard error of nine tumors. 2.5 mg tamoxifen; untreated control. * $p < 0.05$, statistically different from control group (Student's t-test).

## 2.2. Culture Medium

1. RPMI-1640 medium (Life Technologies Ltd., Paisley, Scotland) containing 10% fetal calf serum (FCS) (Advanced Protein Products, Brierly Hill, England) with penicillin (100 U/mL) /streptomycin (100 μg/mL), (Gibco-BRL).
2. Dulbecco's phosphate-buffered saline (PBS) (Oxoid, Unipath Ltd., Basingstoke, England).
3. Trypsin (0.05%) - EDTA (0.02%) (Gibco-BRL).

## 2.3. Primary Tissue Implantation

1. 12 gage needle 3″ trochar with 3 1/2″ objurator (International Market Supply, Congleton, Cheshire, England).
2. 10.5-cm small iris scissors (Brookwick, Ward, Glenrothes, Fife, Scotland).
3. 10-cm iris forceps (Brookwick).

## 2.4. Estrogen and Other Hormone Pellet Implantation

1. 0.72 mg 17 β-estradiol 60-d release pellets (Innovative Research of America, Sarasota, FL).
2. Anprolene ethylene oxide ampoules (H.W. Anderson, Clacton-on-Sea, Essex).
3. Ethyl chloride B.P. Fine jet ampoule (Roche, Welwyn Garden City, UK).

### 2.5. Ovariectomy

1. General anaesthetic (injectible or by inhalation).
2. Michel clips (7.5 × 2.5 mm, International Market Supply).

## 3. Methods

### 3.1. Host Maintenance

1. Female nu/nu mice (Harlan Olac) are maintained in negative pressure isolators (Moredun Isolators).
2. All husbandry items are sterilized by autoclave, irradiation, or ethylene oxide gas.
3. Prior to admission into isolator, items are externally sterilized by Alcide spray (Labcare Precision Ltd.) and left in a transfer isolator for 30 min.
4. After arrival, mice are acclimatized for at least 1 wk.
5. All husbandry and experimental procedures are conducted within the isolator.

### 3.2. Xenografting from Cells in Culture

1. The cell line of interest (e.g., the ER-positive PE04 line) is first grown in appropriate medium, e.g., RPMI-1640 as a monolayer in 75-cm$^2$ plastic tissue-culture flasks at 37°C in a tissue-culture incubator.
2. When cells are at near confluence, tissue-culture medium is removed and cells are washed with PBS.
3. Trypsin–EDTA (5 mL) is added to each 75-cm$^2$ flask to detach cells for the minimum period required for cell detachment (typically 5–20 min.).
4. Cell suspension is transferred to a Universal container and 20 mL RPMI-1640 / FCS added to deactivate trypsin.
5. Centrifuge at 1000$g$ for 5 min and discard fluid to leave cell pellet.
6. Cell pellet resuspended in RPMI-1640 and cell number counted on a Coulter Counter or by hemocytometer.
7. Cell number corrected to $5 \times 10^7$–$10^8$ / mL.
8. Universal container containing cell suspension is placed into isolator port container, sprayed with Alcide and left for 30 min.
9. Universal container is then brought into isolator and the cell suspension is loaded into a 1-mL syringe and a 21-gage needle attached.
10. Cell suspension (100 µL; $5 \times 10^6$–$10^7$ cells) is then injected subcutaneously either into just one flank or bilaterally into both flanks.

### 3.3. Xenografting from Primary Tumors

1. Primary tumor is collected at the time of patient surgery and a fragment is placed into RPMI-1640 in a Universal container (Bibby Sterilin, Stone, Staffs, England).
2. The Universal container is transported into isolator as described in **Subheading 3.2.**
3. Once inside the isolator, the tumor fragment in RPMI-1640 is placed into a Petri dish (Bibby Sterilin).
4. The tumor is then cut into small fragments (approx. 1 mm$^3$) using scalpel blades (Swann-Morton Ltd., Sheffield, England) taking care to use only healthy tissue (*see* **Note 3**).
5. The objurator of the implantation trochar (12-gage needle 3″ trochar with 3-1/2″ objurator) (International Market Supply) is drawn back approximately 5 mm below the tip of the trochar and a tumor fragment is picked up from the Petri dish using a 21-gage needle and placed into the tip of the trochar.

6. The trochar is then introduced subcutaneously under the skin of the mouse and the objurator is pushed upwards to deposit the fragment under the skin (*see* **Note 4**). Fragments may either be deposited individually into a single flank or bilaterally into both flanks.

### 3.4. Tumor Maintenance

1. If the tumor is to be maintained as a continuous in vivo cell line, it should be transferred into further animals before it becomes too large (> 1 cm$^3$) and begins to necrose or ulcerate.
2. To transfer the tumor, the host mouse is first killed by cervical dislocation and then laid ventral side uppermost.
3. A midline incision is made with scissors (Brookwick) and skin flaps laid back to expose the tumor.
4. The xenograft is separated from the skin by the use of a scalpel and placed into a Petri dish containing PBS.
5. It is then cut into 1-mm$^3$ fragments and implanted subcutaneously by trochar as described in **Subheading 3.3.**

### 3.5. Implantation of Hormone Pellets

1. Hormone pellets (e.g., 17 β-estradiol; 0.72 mg, 60-d slow release) (Innovative Research of America) are implanted subcutaneously. If implanted at the same time as the tumor fragment, the same incision site can be used for insertion.
2. The area where the incision is to be made is sprayed with ethyl chloride B. P. local anesthetic.
3. After creating a small incision with a trochar or scissors, forceps (Brookwick) are used to create a channel under the skin.
4. The hormone pellet is then pushed along this channel with minimal trauma to surrounding tissue.
5. Care should be taken to avoid placing the pellet too close to the tumor cell or fragment implant.

### 3.6. Ovariectomy

1. To obtain a defined level of circulating estrogen, it may be desirable to remove the ovaries. Female mice of at least 6–8 wk should be used.
2. General anaesthesia (injectible or by inhalation) is first induced either by injection or inhalation.
3. In ventral recumbancy, a midline transverse skin insertion not exceeding 1 cm is made above the lumbar vertebrae.
4. Via this skin incision, two further incisions, not exceeding 0.5 cm, are made on each side of the lumbar vertebrae into the muscular abdominal wall to allow dorsal entry into the abdominal cavity for access into the adjacent ovaries.
5. The ovaries are located and pulled out in turn via the above incisions by forceps and snipped off with fine scissors or cauterized.
6. The skin incision is then closed by Michel clips (7.5 × 2.5 mm) (International Market Supply) and the animal is allowed to recover from the anesthetic with standard postoperative care and supervision.
7. An estrogen pellet of the desired dose may then be implanted subcutaneously (described in **Subheading 3.5.**).

### 3.7. Tumor growth experiments

1. To compare the effects of an endocrine therapy (e.g., tamoxifen) on the growth of the xenograft, the xenograft is placed into a large group (e.g. 30–40) animals.

2. The xenograft is first removed from a host animal (**Subheading 3.4.**) and cut into fragments.
3. For comparison of, e.g., three doses of tamoxifen with a no treatment control group, four groups would be required. For good statistical power, 5–8 animals are needed/group and so a minimum of 32 animals will be implanted with tumor as described in **Subheading 3.3.** (2 fragments/animal).
4. The xenografts are then allowed to grow to reach a measurable volume, typically 4–6 mm in diameter. At this point, measurement of tumor volumes begins and treatment is initiated (defined as day 0).
5. Individual volumes are estimated by the use of vernier calipers. The maximum length ($l$) and maximum perpendicular width ($w$) are first measured. The volume is then estimated based on the formula: volume $= \pi/6 \times l \times w^2$.
6. Animals are randomized / stratified into groups such that the mean tumor volumes of each group are similar. Not all tumors will be appropriate for the study; some tumors may not have grown or be too small, whereas others may be too large. The "useable" range depends on the size of the effect being studied.
7. Tumors are measured at least once weekly, but two or three times weekly if the volume doubling time is < 5 d.
8. Because the range of volumes is normally large (typically a 10-fold range between the largest and the smallest tumor used in an experiment) it is usual to compare relative tumor volumes for individual tumors rather than absolute values. For an individual tumor, the relative tumor volume ($V_t/V_0$) is calculated from its volume at a particular time ($V_t$) divided by its volume at the start of treatment ($V_0$) on day 0. The mean or median relative tumor volume for the group is then plotted against time for each group to compare effects.
9. An example is shown in **Fig. 1**, which demonstrates the growth inhibitory effect of the antiestrogen tamoxifen against the PE04 ovarian carcinoma xenograft, which contains estrogen receptors. The HOX 60 ovarian carcinoma is estrogen receptor-negative and is unresponsive to tamoxifen.

## 4. Notes

1. All experiments using animals should conform to internationally recognized guidelines. These include the UKCCCR Guidelines for the Welfare of Animals in Experimental Neoplasia (UKCCCCR, PO Box 123, Lincoln's Inn Fields, London, England) and the Interdisciplinary Principles and Guidelines for the Use of Animals in Research, Testing and Education issued by the New York Academy of Sciences' Ad Hoc Committee on Animal Research (available from the Marketing Department, New York Academy of Sciences, 2 East 63rd St, New York, NY 10021-7289).
2. Tumor fragments or cells lose viability after 2 h outside the host or cell-culture incubator. Therefore, all procedures should be completed within this time frame.
3. Viable, healthy tumor is generally of a cream coloration and pearlescent, whereas necrotic tissue is often white or brown and fragments easily.
4. A small piece of tissue paper may be pressed onto the injection site as the needle is withdrawn (after injection of cells) to prevent cell leakage. If tumor cells or fragments are being implanted into two different sites of the animal, these should be kept as far apart as possible, otherwise the two implants can conglomerate to form a single tumor.
5. If appropriate husbandry and sterilization techniques are employed, infection should not arise. However, if it is felt that some risk is present at the implantation site, it can be dabbed with a piece of tissue soaked with 15% hibitane solution.
6. Care should be taken when implanting hormone pellets to site them away from the xenograft sites.

7. Slow-release hormone pellets have specified lifetimes, e.g., 30, 60, or 90 d. At the end of this time period, new pellets should be implanted.

## References

1. Van Steenbrugge, G. J. (1991) "Hormones," in *The Nude Mouse in Oncology Research* (Boven, E. and Winograd, B., eds.) CRC, Boca Raton, FL, pp. 21–229.
2. Langdon, S. P., Ritchie, A. A., Young, K., Crew, A. J., Sweeting, V., Bramley, T, et al. (1993) Contrasting effects of 17 β-estradiol on the growth of human ovarian carcinoma cells in vitro and in vivo. *Int. J. Cancer* **55,** 459–464.
3. Langdon, S. P., Crew, A. J., Ritchie, A. A., Muir, M., Wakeling, A., Smyth, J. F., and Miller, W. R. (1994) Growth inhibition of oestrogen receptor-positive human ovarian carcinoma by anti-oestrogens in vitro and in a xenograft model. *Eur. J. Cancer* **30A,** 682–686.
4. Geisinger, K. R., Kute, T. E., Pettenati, M. J., Welander, C. E., Dennard, Y., Collins, L. A., and Berens, M. E. (1989) Characterization of a human ovarian carcinoma cell line with estrogen and progesterone receptors. *Cancer* **63,** 280–288.
5. Zimniski, S. J., Garola, R. E., Fendl, K., and Peterson, C. M. (1989) Endocrine characterization of a human ovarian carcinoma (BG-1) established in nude mice. *Steroids* **54,** 593–606.
6. Sawada, M., Terada, N., Wada, A., Mori, Y., Yamasaki, M., Saga, T., and Endo, K. (1990) Estrogen and androgen-responsive growth of human ovarian adenocarcinoma heterotransplanted into nude mice. *Int. J. Cancer.* **45,** 359–363.
7. Hamilton, T. C., Behrens, B. C., Louie, K. G., and Ozols, R. F. (1984) Induction of progesterone receptor with 17 beta-estradiol in human ovarian cancer. *J. Clin. Endocrinol Metab.* **59,** 561–563.

# 21

# The Use of Matrigel in the Establishment of Ovarian Carcinoma Cell Lines as Xenografts

## Peter Mullen and Simon P. Langdon

## 1. Introduction

The fact that human tumor xenografts grown in immunodeficient mice have proven to be useful models of human cancer is well documented. However, the establishment of such xenografts from cell lines cultured in vitro has proven to be fraught with difficulties—these problems become even more apparent when one tries to establish xenografts from primary clinical material *(1–3)*. Nevertheless, the inclusion of Matrigel has been shown to enhance the tumorigenicity of a number of cell lines in vivo *(4–10)*, including those of ovarian origin *(11)*. There are also reports of Matrigel enhancing the tumorigenic potential of breast primary material *(12)*. Furthermore, it has been shown that xenografts established in the presence of Matrigel can be excised, transferred into recipient animals, and subsequently grown in the absence of Matrigel, which suggests that it is required only for the initial establishment of tumors *(11)*. Matrigel is, therefore, extremely useful for establishing a variety of cell lines as routine xenografts, which could otherwise prove difficult to take, as illustrated in **Table 1** and **Fig. 1** (adapted from *[11]*).

Matrigel is a solubilized tissue basement membrane matrix isolated from the Engelbreth-Holm-Swarm (EHS) mouse tumor, which is known to be rich in extracellular matrix proteins. It is comprised mainly of laminin, together with collagen IV, heparan sulphate proteoglycans, and entactin (nidogen); various growth factors such as transforming growth factor-β, fibroblast growth factor and tissue plasminogen activator are also present. Matrigel polymerizes under normal physiological conditions to produce a reconstituted, biologically active stable matrix, which is effective for the attachment and differentiation of normal and transformed anchorage-dependent cell types *(13,14)*.

## 2. Materials

### 2.1. Preparation of Matrigel

1. Matrigel (Collaborative Biological Research, Bedford, MA).

### 2.2. Animals and Animal Husbandry

1. Female nude (*nu/nu*) mice (Harlan Olac, Oxford, England).
2. Negative-pressure isolator (Moredun Isolators Ltd., Edinburgh, Scotland).

From: *Methods in Molecular Medicine, Vol. 39: Ovarian Cancer: Methods and Protocols*
Edited by: J. M. S. Bartlett © Humana Press, Inc., Totowa, NJ

**Table 1**
**Take Rate of Ovarian Cancer Cell Lines Inoculated**
**in the Absence/Presence of Matrigel[a]**

| Cell line | Take rate (– Matrigel) | Take rate (+ Matrigel) |
|---|---|---|
| PE01 | 0/17 (0%) | 10/10 (100%) |
| PE01cDDPr | 0/11 (0%) | 10/10 (100%) |
| PE04 | 0/6 (0%) | 6/6 (100%) |
| PE014 | 3/10 (30%) | 10/10 (100%) |
| Ov(hyg)CAR3 | 0/6 (0%) | 2/6 (33%) |

[a]Take rate equals the number of tumors established/the number of inoculations carried out.

3. Open filter box cages (North Kent Plastics, Erith, Kent, England).
4. Implant trochar (International Market Supply, Congleton, England).

## 2.3. Cell Culture

1. Cell lines as required; e.g., PE01 ovarian cancer cells *(15)*.
2 Dulbecco's phosphate buffered saline (PBS) (Oxoid, Unipath Ltd., Basingstoke, England).
3. 1X Trypsin-EDTA (Gibco-BRL, Life Technologies Ltd., Paisley, Scotland).
4. RPMI/PS: RPMI-1640 (Gibco-BRL) + 100 iU/mL penicillin/100 μg/mL streptomycin (Gibco-BRL).
5. RPMI/PS/10% FCS: RPMI-1640 + 100 iU/mL penicillin/100 μg/mL streptomycin + 10% FCS (Advanced Protein Products, Brierley Hill, England) (*see* **Note 1**).

# 3. Methods
## 3.1. Preparation of Matrigel

1. Place Matrigel (Collaborative Biological Research) in the refridgerator overnight at 4°C (*see* **Notes 2** and **3**).
2. Transfer Matrigel on *ice* into the tissue-culture hood, along with sterile 1.5 mL microcentrifuge tubes and Gilson 1-mL tips (*see* **Notes 4** and **5**).
3. Leave for 5 min to chill.
4. Wipe top of vial with 70% ethanol and air-dry.
5. Open vial carefully to maintain sterility.
6. Gently swirl vial to evenly disperse Matrigel, but do not allow to warm up.
7. Using a prechilled 1-mL tip, aliquot 250 μL into each of 40 prechilled microcentrifuge tubes (10 mL Matrigel).
8. Matrigel aliquots should then immediately be refrozen at –20°C prior to use, thus minimizing the number of freeze/thaw cycles.
9. Each ampoule can then be removed from the freezer and thawed *on ice* just prior to use.

## 3.2. Animals and Animal Husbandry

1. Upon delivery, female nude (*nu/nu*) mice (Harlan Olac) are transferred into the negative-pressure isolator (Moredun Isolators Ltd.) until ready for use. RM3(E) animal feed irradiated to 2.5 mrad (SDS Diet Services, Witham, England) and sterile water (Baxter Travenol, Thetford, England) are available *ad libitum*. All bedding (BS & S (Scotland) Ltd., Edinburgh, Scotland) is changed twice per week.
2. Prior to experimentation, remove mice from the isolator and transfer to open filter-box cages (North Kent Plastics).

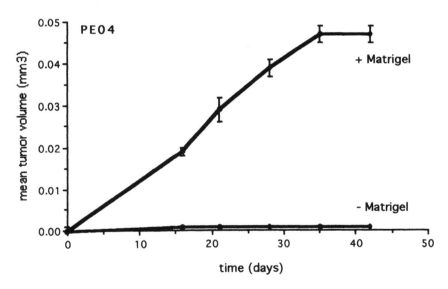

Fig. 1. Growth of PE01 and PE04 ovarian cancer xenografts inoculated in the absence/presence of Matrigel (mean tumor volume +/- standard error).

3. Affix ear identification tags (Brookwick Ward, Glenrothes, Fife, Scotland) to aid identification of individual mice if required.

### 3.3. Cell Culture

1. Suspend $2.5 \times 10^6$ (e.g.) PE01 (*15*) cells in RPMI/PS/10% FCS (25 mL) and transfer to a 75 cm$^2$ tissue-culture flask (Life Technologies Ltd.). Place in a 5% $CO_2$ humidified incubator at 37°C.

2. Allow cells to grow to confluence, feeding twice per week by aspirating the spent media, washing with 20 mL Dulbecco's PBS (Oxoid, Unipath Ltd.) and then adding fresh media (25 mL).

3. When cells become confluent, remove spent tissue-culture media and wash cells in PBS (10 mL). Discard PBS.

4. Add 5 mL trypsin / EDTA (Gibco-BRL, Life Technologies Ltd.) to each 75-cm$^2$ flask and place in incubator until cells have become detached (*see* **Note 6**).

5. Transfer cell suspension to a universal container using a sterile pipet; wash the flask out with 20 mL RPMI/PS/10% FCS (to deactivate the trypsin) and pool with cells in the universal container (total volume = 25 mL).

6. Centrifuge at 600$g$ for 5 min.

7. Resuspend pellet in 5 mL RPMI/PS/10% FCS, syringe with a 21G (green) needle (X3) to break up the pellet, and then make up to 125 mL with RPMI/PS/10% FCS. Aliquot 25 mL into each of five 75-cm$^2$ flasks (1 in 5 split). Replace in incubator.

8. Repeat "splitting" process (**Subheading 3.3., steps 3–7**). until sufficient cells are available to carry out experiment).

### 3.4 Preparation and Delivery of Inoculations

1. Harvest cells as described in **steps 3.3.3.–3.3.6.**

2. Resuspend pellet in 5 mL RPMI/PS (*no FCS from this point on*).

3. Syringe cell suspension with a 10 mL syringe plus 21G (green) needle (×3) to remove clumps—make up to 25 ml with RPMI/PS.

4. Count total number of cells using a haemocytometer, i.e.,

$$\frac{\text{cell count } (n) \times \text{total volume (25 mL)} \times 10{,}000}{\text{number of squares counted}}$$

5. Prepare a suspension of cells at a concentration of $4 \times 10^6$ cells per 250 μL.

6. Allow cells to sit *on ice* for 5 min to chill.

7. Aliquot 250 μL of cell suspension into sterile microcentrifuge vials containing 250 μL of Matrigel (test) or 250 μL RPMI/PS (control).

8. Close all microcentrifuge lids and transfer *on ice* prior to where inoculations are to be carried out.

9. Place all syringes and needles *on ice* to chill for 5 min prior to inoculation (*see* **Note 4**).

10. Gently mix tubes before drawing Matrigel/cell suspension up into the syringe.

11. Inoculate all mice in the flank (*see* **Note 7**), being careful to prevent back-spill when the needle is removed (one inoculation can be made on each side of the mouse, allowing each animal to have its own negative control if required). A preparatory aerosol sealer can be applied if it becomes a problem (*see* **Note 8**).

12. Mice are maintained in the open filter-box cages and measurements made twice a week using callipers.

## 4. Notes

1. Fetal calf serum (FCS) must be heat-inactivated prior to use by heating in a water bath for 30 min at 56°C. It can then be aliquoted out (100 mL) and stored at –20°C.

2. Matrigel is shipped frozen and should be stored at –20°C until ready for use. However, it naturally polymerizes as the temperature rises above 4°C. Because this polymerization is nonreversible, once removed from the freezer *it is imperative that Matrigel is kept on ice at all times prior to the point of inoculation.*

3. Although Matrigel is commercially available from more than one supplier, our experience suggests that some sources are considerably better than others. It is therefore recommended that, in the first instance, Matrigel is obtained from the source cited.

4. Because 1) tissue culture by definition requires sterile technique, and 2) Matrigel must be kept "on ice" at all times, the most practical way of achieving this is to obtain a large, shallow polystyrene box, which can be filled with ice and then placed into the tissue-culture hood. All preparatory manipulations involving Matrigel can then be carried out *on ice* within a sterile environment.

5. In order to prevent Matrigel from polymerizing within the barrel of the syringe during the inoculation, all tubes, tips, syringes, needles, and so on must be chilled on ice prior to use.

6. The time interval for cells to become detached from the plastic is dependent upon the cell line being used, but is usually in the order of 5–10 min.

7. Whereas there is evidence to suggest that better take rates are obtained if the inoculations are made into the mammary fat pad of the mice *(16)*, in our hands this did not prove to be the case, probably because the pad was so small in relation to the volume being introduced. Mice were therefore simply inoculated subcutaneously.

8. It is possible that the cell suspension can "leak" back out of the inoculation site when the needle is removed. This is because of a hole produced in the skin by the trochar. A preparatory aerosol sealer can be applied in order to seal the wound and so retain the cell suspension if this becomes a problem.

## References

1. Bailey, M. J, Gazet, J-C., and Peckham, M. J. (1980) Human breast-cancer xenografts in immune-suppressed mice. *Brit. J. Cancer* **42,** 524–529.
2. Rae-Venter, B. and Reid, L. M. (1980) Growth of human breast carcinomas in nude mice and subsequent establishment in tissue culture. *Cancer Res.* **40,** 95–100.
3. Giovanella, B. C., Vardeman, D. M., Williams, L. J., Taylor, J., de Ipolyi, P. D., Greeff, P. J., et al. (1991) Heterotransplantation of human breast carcinomas in nude mice. Correlation between successful heterotransplants, poor prognosis and amplification of the *HER-2/neu oncogene. Int. J. Cancer* **47,** 66–71.
4. Fridman, R., Giaccone, G., Kanemoto, T., Martin, G. R., Gazdar, A. F., and Mulshine, J. L. (1990) Reconstituted basement membrane (Matrigel) and laminin can enhance the tumorigenicity and the drug resistance of small cell lung cancer cell lines. *Proc. Natl. Acad. Sci. USA* **87,** 6698–6702.
5. Fridman, R., Kibbey, M. C., Royce, L. S., Zain, M., Sweeney, T. M., Jicha, D. L., et al. (1991) Enhanced tumor growth of both primary and established human and murine tumor cells in athymic mice after coinjection with matrigel. *J. Nat. Cancer Inst.* **83,** 769–774.
6. Pretlow, T. G., Delmoro, C. M., Dilley, G. G., Spadafora, C. G., and Pretlow, T. P. (1991) Transplantation of human prostatic carcinoma into nude mice in Matrigel. *Cancer Res.* **51,** 3814–3817.
7. Albini, A., Melchiori, A., Garofalo, A., Noonan, D. M., Basolo, F., Taraboletti, G., et al. (1992) Matrigel promotes retinoblastoma cell-growth in vitro and in-vivo. *Int. J. Cancer* **52,** 234–240.
8. Noel, A., Simon, N., Raus, J., and Foidart, J. M. (1992) Basement-membrane components (Matrigel) promote the tumorigenicity of human breast adenocarcinoma MCF-7 cells and provide an in-vivo model to assess the responsiveness of cells to estrogen. *Biochem. Pharmacol.* **43,** 1263–1267.
9. Vukicevic, S., Somogyi, L., Martinovic, I., Zic, R., Kleinman, H. K., and Marusic, M. (1992) Reconstituted basement membrane (Matrigel) promotes the survival and influences the growth of murine tumours. *Int. J. Cancer* **50,** 791–795.
10. Noel, A., De Pauw-Gillet, M-C., Purnell, G., Nusgens, B., Lapiere, C-M., and Foidart, J-M. (1993) Enhancement of tumorigenicity of human breast adenocarcioma cells in nude-mice by Matrigel and fibroblasts. *Brit. J. Cancer* **68,** 909–915.
11. Mullen, P., Ritchie, A., Langdon, S. P., and Miller, W. R. (1996) Effect of matrigel on the tumorigenicity of human breast and ovarian carcinoma cell lines. *Int. J. Cancer* **67,** 816–820.
12. Mehta, R. R., Graves, J. M., Hart, G. D., Shilkaitis, A., and Dasgupta, T. K. (1993) Growth and metastasis of human breast carcinomas with matrigel in athymic mice. *Breast Cancer Res. Treat.* **25,** 65–71.
13. Kleinman, H. K., McGarvey, M. L., Liotta, L. A., Robey, P. G., Tryggvason, K., and Martin, G. R. (1982) Isolation and characterisation of type IV procollagen, laminin and heparan sulfate proteoglycans from the EHS sarcoma. *Biochemistry* **21,** 6188–6193.
14. Baatout, S. (1997) Endothelial differentiation using Matrigel. *Anticancer Res.* **17,** 451–455.
15. Langdon, S. P., Lawrie, S. S., Hay, F. G., Hawkes, M. M., McDonald, A., Hayward, I. P., et al. (1988) Characterization and properties of nine human ovarian adenocarcinoma cell lines. *Cancer Res.* **48,** 6166–6172.
16. Price, J. E., Polyzos, A., Zhang, R. D., and Daniels, L. M. (1990) Tumorigenicity and metastasis of human breast carcinoma cell lines in nude mice. *Cancer Res.* **50,** 717–721.

# IV

# CYTOGENETICS

# 22

## Cytogenetics of Ovarian Cancer

*Technical Overview*

**Thomas Liehr**

### 1. Introduction

Cytogenetics in ovarian cancer has been restricted to conventional cytogenetic analysis of G-banded metaphase chromosomes up to the early 1980s. The detection of cytogenetic changes in solid tumors was relatively limited, as cytogenetic preparations from solid tumor tissue often have a low yield of metaphases with poor quality chromosomes *(1)*. Following the advent of the fluorescence *in situ* hybridization (FISH) technique *(2,3)* it became possible to obtain huge amounts of additional cytogenetic information from the material available. This fact is demonstrated very clearly by the following comparison: Mitelman summarizes in the 4th edition of *Catalog of Chromosome Aberrations in Cancer* only 185 cases of ovarian cancer, which were characterized by conventional cytogenetic analysis between about 1970 to 1991 *(4)*. On the other hand, 135 cases of ovarian cancer have been analyzed by means of comparative genomic hybridization (CGH) in the shorter time period 1995 to 1997 *(5–8)*.

This overview of current cytogenetic techniques will focus on:

1. Conventional cytogenetic preparations and their use for FISH
2. Interphase cytogenetics
3. Primed *in situ* hybridization (PRINS)
4. Flow cytometry
5. CGH

### 2. Methods

Five percent of all malignant tumors in women are ovarian cancers *(9)*, a tumor type which is treated by surgical removal. Thus, scientific studies on ovarian cancer are normally not restricted by a lack of material, which is the case for other less-frequent or inoperable tumor types.

#### 2.1. Cytogenetic Preparations

##### 2.1.1. Conventional Cytogenetics in Ovarian Cancer Studies

Conventional cytogenetics includes a variety of banding techniques such as C-banding, NOR-technique, Q-banding, and GTG-banding (= G-bands by using Trypsin and Giemsa) *(1)*. All these techniques require tissue cultivation. After several days to weeks,

From: *Methods in Molecular Medicine, Vol. 39: Ovarian Cancer: Methods and Protocols*
Edited by: J. M. S. Bartlett © Humana Press, Inc., Totowa, NJ

if culture succeeds (*see* **Note 1**), the cells are harvested, treated with hypotonic solution, and fixed in methanol/glacial acetic acid (3:1) *(1)*. In most cases, virtually no metaphases will be detectable after this laborious procedure because of the low mitotic index of most primary cell cultures.

A major problem of cytogenetic analysis in ovarian tumor—as in most solid tumors—is that owing to the limited number of available metaphases, less information can be obtained on the quantitative proportions of chromosomally abnormal clones in the overall tumor cell population. Thus, a rather sporadic knowledge of numerical chromosomal changes and, in particular, of specific gains or losses of chromosomes in the type of tumors has been obtained using this approach *(4,10)*. In most cases, human ovarian carcinomas have been characterized as having multiple cytogenetic alterations *(11,12)*. Nevertheless, specific cytogenetic changes were detected for some subclasses of ovarian cancer; e.g., trisomy 12 in granulosa cell tumors *(13)* or monosomy 22 in mixed germ cell-sex cord-stromal tumors *(14)*.

One method proposed to enhance the yield of metaphases was the induction of premature chromosome condensation by fusing the interphase target cells with mitotic cells *(15,16)*. However, this technique is both expensive and technically limited and is not recommended *(10)*.

### 2.1.2. FISH-Studies on Metaphase Chromosomes of Ovarian Cancer

Today, with the multiple possibilities offered by FISH-techniques, it is possible to get much more information from the relatively rare metaphases in cytogenetic preparations using all kinds of probes suitable for FISH-analysis (cosmids, P1-clones, yeast artificial chromosomes, satellite probes, band-specific microdissection libraries, whole chromosome arm libraries, or whole chromosome libraries). Although in most cases it is sufficient to use 1–3-color-FISH *(17)*, the possibilities offered by multicolor-FISH approaches should not be ignored *(18–20)*.

Metaphase FISH is a field where much work could still be done using archived cytogenetic slides *(21,22)*.

### 2.2. Interphase Cytogenetics

FISH techniques using chromosome-specific DNA probes have made feasible new cytogenetics studies in solid tumors *(2,3)*, as for metaphase FISH. Karyotypic analysis by direct demonstration of DNA sequences in interphase nuclei (interphase cytogenetics or interphase FISH) can be applied to a wide variety of cellular material, including cytogenetic preparations, fresh material (touch-preparations), cryofixed, and paraffin-embedded tissue. Contrary to metaphase FISH, only cosmids, P1-clones, YACs, and satellite probes are suitable for interphase FISH. Detection and quantitation of structural chromosome aberrations, oncogene amplification, or deletion of tumor suppressor genes in solid tumors, including ovarian cancer, thus became possible. A two-color-FISH approach seems to be the maximum possible without the use of sophisticated imaging-analysis software.

The major advantage of interphase cytogenetics is that it offers the opportunity to analyze the huge amounts of previously superfluous interphase nuclei in cytogenetic preparations with specific probes and to obtain additional "cytogenetic information." Moreover, completely new classes of material can be used for cytogenetic analysis including touch preparations, cryofixed material, and formalin-fixed and, subsequently, paraffin-embedded tissue. Additionally, as chromosome aberrations can be quantified, interphase FISH can be used to study tumor cell heterogeneity within malignant cell populations *(10)*. However, interphase FISH is limited to the analysis of a few chromosomal segments at a time *(8)*, which is an important restriction.

To date, only fresh tumor material *(10,23,24)* or formalin-fixed and, subsequently, paraffin-embedded and sectioned tissue has been used for interphase cytogenetic studies in ovarian tumors (e.g., *10,24*). No nucleus extraction procedures (e.g., *17,25*), cryofixed tissue *(17)*, or "old" cytogenetic slides *(21,22)* have been used as archival ovarian tumor samples in interphase FISH studies up to now.

Archival material (cryofixed or paraffin-embedded tissue) has the disadvantage that it can be damaged concerning its tissue structure and or its whole genomic DNA. This holds true especially for the DNA quality of formalin-fixed and, subsequently, paraffin-embedded archival tissue. In many cases, no reproducible fixation protocol and unbuffered formalin have been used—two factors often leading to highly degraded DNA in the archival material making it unfit for any kind of molecular or molecular cytogenetic experiment. In fresh material (touch and or fresh cytogenetic preparations) this cannot happen as it can be prepared according to the corresponding research project immediately.

## 2.3. Primed In Situ *Hybridization (PRINS)*

Although FISH remains the principal established method for interphase cytogenetics more recently PRINS has been introduced as an alternative *(26)*. The principle of PRINS is that an unlabeled oligonucleotide probe is hybridized to its complementary target sequence in the chromatin where it serves as primer for a chain elongation reaction *in situ* catalyzed by a suitable thermostable *(Taq-)* DNA polymerase. The chromosomal DNA acts as a template for the chain elongation and, using labeled nucleotides as a substrate for DNA polymerase, the target DNA is labeled and can be visualized under the microscope *(27)*.

Because PRINS is much faster—results can be obtained within 2 to 4 h—and approximately 10 times less expensive than FISH, this method is discussed as a real alternative to FISH *(28)*. Even though methods for double-color PRINS have recently been published *(28)*, up to now reliable and reproducible results with PRINS have mainly been reported for centromeric, highly repetitive target sequences in the human genome. Thus, PRINS interphase studies are still limited to numerical chromosomal changes, whereas interphase FISH studies can focus on numerical, as well as structural, chromosomal aberrations.

## 2.4. Flow Cytometry

Inclusion of interphase nuclei in the cytogenetic studies of solid tumors is not only possible using FISH-techniques or PRINS; flow cytometry for interphase karyotyping is another practicable way *(29)*.

Flow cytometry is performed on interphase nuclei isolated from cultured, cryofixed, or paraffin-embedded cells. Nuclear DNA is stained with a DNA-binding agent like *propidium* iodide and nuclei are analyzed in a flow cytometer. The percentage of fractions of hypodiploid, (near-) diploid, and hyperdiploid cells, as well as the percentages of G1, S, and G2/M fractions in cycling cells can be analyzed *(13,30)*.

Flow cytometry has been shown to be a valuable prognostic parameter in ovarian cancer. Aneuploid DNA content is correlated with more aggressive biological behavior, and, therefore, an adverse prognosis *(31,32)*. However, although quantitating the DNA content of tumor cell populations, flow cytometry yields no information on specific chromosome abnormalities or minor cytogenetic deviations *(10)*. To overcome this problem, a combination of this technique with other cytogenetic or molecular genetic techniques are required, e.g., FISH *(30)* or PCR *(33)*.

## 2.5. Comparative Genomic Hybridization (CGH)

CGH is one of the most recent developments in the field of molecular cytogenetics. The principle of this technique is described best by Kallioniemi and coworkers *(34)* as follows: "CGH produces a map of DNA sequence copy number as a function of chromosomal location throughout the entire genome. Differentially labeled tumor DNA and normal-reference DNA are hybridized simultaneously to normal chromosome spreads. The hybridization is detected with two different fluorochromes. Regions of gain or loss of DNA sequences, such as deletions, duplications, or amplifications, are seen as changes in the ratio of the intensities of the two fluorochromes along the target chromosomes."

CGH proved to be a highly efficient tool to acquire a genome-wide screening of chromosomal copy number changes within a single experiment *(5–8)*. This method does not require mitotic cells, cell culture, or prior knowledge of regions of abnormality, and can be performed with small amounts of DNA *(5)*.

The standard CGH protocol relies on the availability of macroscopic tumor samples, which do not contain high proportions of nontumor normal cells. Most tumor samples are contaminated with such normal tissue and if the ratio of tumor:normal cells is lower than 1:1 *(35)*, CGH-analysis does not provide reliable results. In such cases, a combination of microdissection tumor tissue, DOP-PCR, and CGH can be the solution. As shown by Kuukasjarvi and coworkers *(36)* this approach provides an excellent tool to study genetic aberrations in different histological subpopulations of malignant, as well as, precancerous, lesions. DOP-PCR CGH analysis also improves the success rate of conventional paraffin-block CGH *(36)*, as the poor-quality low-yield DNA can be compensated for by universal DNA amplification using DOP-PCR.

It has been demonstrated, that the technical equipment (CCD-camera, image-analyzing system, or microscope) is not the critical point of the CGH-procedure *(37,38)*. However, the quality of the metaphase chromosomes used for CGH is highly critical. They have to be much "harder" than chromosomes used for normal metaphase FISH analysis and many approaches are suggested to achieve such "steel" chromosomes. Karhu and coworkers *(39)* give an update of the current methods for the preparation of CGH-metaphase spreads and propose a rapid denaturation assay to test the suitability of each batch (*see* **Note 2**).

Whereas the major advantage of CGH is its ability to survey the entire genome starting from just a few nanograms of genomic DNA, the technique is limited by the resolution of the hybridization target, the metaphase chromosomes. Genetic changes are detected only when the size of the chromosomal region affected exceeds 5–10 Mb. Changes that affect regions smaller than this are only detectable in the case of high-level amplifications (e.g., 5–10-fold amplification of 1 Mb) *(35)*.

CGH has proved its ability to resolve complex karyotypes and to provide karyotype information when metaphase chromosomes are not available. But the following limitations must be kept in mind to avoid misinterpretations of the results: 1) for technical reasons the telomeric, pericentromeric, or heterochromatic regions sometimes fall outside the reliably evaluable range, because the signal intensities are low—these regions are excluded from all analysis; 2) CGH only detects genetic aberrations that involve gain or loss of DNA sequences; balanced translocations or inversions are not detectable; 3) CGH cannot distinguish diploid from true triploid or tetraploid tumors—ploidy must be determined independently by flow cytometry or interphase FISH; 4) CGH detects the average copy number of sequences in all cells included in the specimen; thus, intratumoral genetic heterogeneity cannot be detected by CGH *(40)*.

## 3. Conclusion

All techniques aforementioned are molecular cytogenetic methods that provide powerful supplements to classical cancer cytogenetics. But, as discussed, each technique has advantages and limitations. Thus, they should be used in combination, depending on the problem to be addressed by studying the corresponding tumor samples. The choice of prospectively harvested fresh tumor material vs retrospective studies with cryofixed or paraffin-embedded tissue, will critically influence both the ease of analysis and the range of analyses performed. In a prospective study, all kinds of molecular cytogenetic approaches aforementioned may be used as cell culture can be performed and touch-preparations, cryofixation, or paraffin-fixation, as well as DNA-extraction of the tumor sample can be done. Thus, conventional cytogenetics, FISH and/or PRINS on metaphase or interphase, and CGH can be carried out. In a retrospective study with archival material only, no conventional cytogenetics and metaphase FISH is possible. Interphase cytogenetics on sections, old touch preparations or extracted nuclei, flow cytometry, and CGH—most likely to be carried out with DOP-PCR amplified tumor-DNA—are the methods to be combined.

A good example for the combination of three of the cytogenetic methods aforementioned is reported by Becher and coworkers *(41)*. They gained basic information about specific chromosomal aberrations of a testicular germ cell tumor by conventional cytogenetics. FISH analysis allowed further characterization of the specific *i(12p)* marker chromosome, and CGH, finally, identified chromosomal subregions that may harbor genes important for tumorigenesis or progression. Similar approaches in human ovarian tumor samples would be desirable.

## 4. Notes

1. The success of growing ovarian tumors in tissue culture varies strongly depending on tumor subtype, tumor grade, and between different laboratories. In our own experience, a short-term culture of ovarian tumors is possible in at least 50% of the cases.
2. As a quick test for each batch of CGH-slides, Karhu and coworkers *(39)* suggest testing the effects of denaturation (73°C for 3 min) on chromosome morphology, visualized by DAPI staining.

## References

1. Heim, S. and Mitelman, F. (1995) *Cancer Cytogenetics.* 2nd Ed., Wiley-Liss, New York.
2. Langer, P. R., Waldrop, A. A., and Ward, D. C. (1981) Enzymatic synthesis of biotin-labeled polynucleotides: Novel nucleic acid affinity probes. *Proc. Natl. Acad. Sci. USA* **78,** 6633–6637.

3.  Pinkel, D., Straume, T., and Gray, J. W. (1986) Cytogenetic analysis using quantitative, high sensitivity, fluorescence hybridization. *Proc. Natl. Acad. Sci. USA* **83,** 2934–2938.
4.  Mitelman, F. (1991) Catalog of Chromosome Aberrations in Cancer. 4th Ed., Wiley-Liss, New York.
5.  Iwabuchi, H., Sakamoto, M., Sakanaga, H., Ma, Y. Y., Carcangiu, M. L., Pinkel, D., et al. (1995) Genetic analysis of benign, low-grade, and high-grade ovarian tumors. *Cancer Res.* **55,** 6172–6180.
6.  Arnold, N., Hagele, L., Walz, L., Schempp, W., Pfisterer, J., Bauknecht, T., and Kiechle, M. (1996) Overrepresentation of 3q and 8q material and loss of 18q material are recurrent findings in advanced human ovarian cancer. *Genes Chr. Cancer* **16,** 46–54.
7.  Wasenius, V. M., Jekunen, A., Monni, O., Joensuu, H., Aebi, S., Howell, S. B., and Knuutila, S. (1997) Comparative genomic hybridization analysis of chromosomal changes occurring during development of acquired resistance to cisplatin in human ovarian carcinoma cells. *Genes Chr. Cancer* **18,** 286–291.
8.  Wolff, E., Liehr, T., Vorderwülbecke, U., Tulusan, A. H., Husslein, E. M., and Gebhart, E. (1997) Frequent gains and losses of specific chromosome segments in human ovarian carcinomas shown by comparative genomic hybridization. *Int. J. Oncol.* **11,** 19–23.
9.  Alberts, B., Bray, D., Lewis, J., Raff, M., Roberts, K., and Watson, J. D. (1994) Molecular Biology of the Cell. 3rd Ed., Garland, New Garland, New York, London.
10. Liehr, T., Stübinger, A., Thoma, K., Tulusan, H. A., and Gebhart, E. (1994) Comparative interphase cytogenetics using FISH on human ovarian carcinomas. *Anticancer Res.* **14,** 183–188.
11. Augustus, M., Brüderlein, S., and Gebhart, E. (1986) Cytogenetics and cell cycle studies in metastatic cells from ovarian carcinomas. *Anticancer Res.* **6,** 283–290.
12. Di Cicco, R. A. and Piver, M. S. (1992) The genetics of ovarian cancer. *Cancer Invest.* **10,** 135–141.
13. Górski, G. K., McMorrow, L. E., Blumstein, L., Faasse, D., and Donaldson, M. H. (1992) Trisomy 14 in two cases of granulosa cell tumor of the ovary. *Cancer Genet. Cytogenet.* **60,** 202–205.
14. Speleman, F., Dermaut, B., De Potter, C. R., Van Gele, M., Van Roy, N., De Paepe, A., and Laureys, G. (1997) Monosomy 22 in a mixed germ cell-sex cord-stromal tumor of the ovary. *Genes Chr. Cancer* **19,** 192–194.
15. Brüderlein, S., Gebhart, E., Siebert, E., and Augustus, M. (1987) Premature chromosome condensation studies on human metastatic carcinoma cells. *Hum. Genet.* **73,** 44–52.
16. Hittelman, W. N., Petkovic, I., and Agbor, P. (1988) Improvements in the premature chromosome condensation technique for cytogenetic analysis. *Cancer Genet. Cytogenet.* **30,** 301–312.
17. Liehr, T., Grehl, H., and Rautenstrauss, B. (1996) A rapid method for FISH analysis of interphase nuclei extracted from cryofixed tissue. *Trends Genet.* **12,** 505–506.
18. Speicher, M. R., Gwyn Ballard, S., and Ward, D. C. (1996) Karyotyping human chromosomes by combinatorial multi-fluor FISH. *Nat. Genet.* **12,** 368–375.
19. Schröck, E., Veldman, T., Padilla-Nash, H., Ning, Y., Spurbeck, J., Jalal, S., et al. (1997) Spectral karyotyping refines cytogenetic diagnostics of constitutonal chromosomal abnormalities. *Hum. Genet.* **101,** 255–262.
20. Chudoba, I., Plesch, A., Lörch, T., Claussen, U., and Senger, G. (1998) Multi-color-banding for the identification of interstitial deletion of chromosome 5. *Medgen.* **10,** 116 (abstract CT-6).
21. Gebhart, E., Hofbeck, P., Hofmann, Y., Lerch, R., Schmitt, G., and Liehr, T. (1996) Recovering of archival tumor cytogenetic slides for two-color-interphase FISH. *Appl. Cytogenet.* **22,** 146–148.
22. Gerdes, A. M., Pandis, N., Bomme, L., Dietrich, C. U., Teixeira, M. R., Bardi, G., and Heim, S. (1997) Fluorescence in situ hybridization of old G-banded and mounted chromosome preparations. *Cancer Genet. Cytogenet.* **98,** 9–15.
23. Liehr, T., Atanasov, N., Tulusan, H. A., and Gebhart, E. (1993) Amplification of proto-oncogenes in human ovarian carcinomas. *Int. J. Oncol.* **2,** 155–160.
24. Neubauer, S., Liehr, T., Tulusan, H. A., and Gebhart, E. (1994) Interphase cytogenetics by FISH on archival paraffin material and cultured cells of human ovarian tumors. *Int. J. Oncol.* **4,** 317–321.
25. Liehr, T., Grehl, H., and Rautenstrauss, B. (1995) FISH analysis of interphase nuclei extracted from paraffin-embedded tissue. *Trends Genet.* **11,** 377,378.
26. Wolfe, K. Q. and Herrington, C. S. (1997) Interphase cytogenetics and pathology: a tool for diagnostics and research. *J. Pathol.* **181,** 359–361.
27. Koch, J. E., Kolvraa, S., Petersen, K. B., Gregersen, N., and Bolund, L. (1989) Oligonucleotide-priming methods for chromosome-specific labelling of alpha satellite DNA *in situ. Chromosoma* **98,** 259–265.
28. Werner, M., Nasarek, A., Tchinda, J., von Wasielewski, R., Komminoth, P., and Wilkens, L. (1997) Applications of single-color and double-color oligonucleotide primed in situ labelling in cytology. *Mod. Pathol.* **10,** 1164–1171.
29. Barlogie, B., Johnson, D. A., Smallwood, L., Raber, M. N, Maddox, A. M., Latreille, J., et al. (1982) Prognostic implications of ploidy and proliferative activity in human solid tumors. *Cancer Genet. Cytogenet.* **6,** 17–28.

30. Persons, D. L., Hartmann, L. C., Herath, J. F., Borell, T. J., Keeney, G. L., and Jenkins, R. B., (1993) Interphase molecular cytogenetic analysis of epithelial ovarian tumors. *Am. J. Clin. Pathol.* **142,** 733–741.

31. Gajewski, W. H., Fuller, A. F. Jr., Pastel-Ley, C., Flotte, T. J., and Bell, D. A. (1994) Prognostic significance of DNA content in epithelial ovarian cancer. *Gynecol. Oncol.* **53,** 5–12.

32. Schueler, J. A., Trimbos, J. B., V. d. Burg, M., Cornelisse, C. J., Hermans, J., and Fleuren, G. J. (1996) DNA index reflects the biological behavior of ovarian carcinoma stage I-IIa. *Gynecol. Oncol.* **62,** 59–66.

33. Abeln, E. C., Corver, W. E., Kuipers-Dijkshoorn, N. J., Fleuren, G. J., and Cornelisse, C. J. (1994) Molecular genetic analysis of flow-sorted ovarian tumor cells: improved detection of loss of heterozygosity. *Br. J. Cancer* **70,** 255–262.

34. Kallioniemi, A., Kallioniemi, O. P., Sudar, D., Rutovitz, D., Gray, J. W., Waldman, F., and Pinkel, D. (1992) Comparative genomic hybridization for molecular cytogenetic analysis of solid tumors. *Science* **258,** 818–821.

35. Speicher, M. R., du Manoir, S., Schröck, E., Holtgreve-Grez, H., Schoell, B., Lengauer, C., et al. (1993) Molecular cytogenetic analysis of formalin-fixed, paraffin-embedded solid tumors by comparative genomic hybridization after universal DNA-amplification. *Hum. Mol. Genet.* **2,** 1907–1914.

36. Kuukasjarvi, T., Tanner, M., Pennanen, S., Karhu, R., Visakorpi, T., and Isola, J. (1997) Optimizing DOP-PCR for universal amplification of small DNA samples in comparative genomic hybridization. *Genes Chr. Cancer* **18,** 94–101.

37. Tirkkonen, M., Karhu, R., Kallioniemi, O., and Isola, J. (1996) Evaluation of camera requirements for comparative genomic hybridization. *Cytometry* **25,** 394–398.

38. Du Manoir, S., Schröck, E., Bentz, M., Speicher, M. R., Joos, S., Ried, T., et al. (1995) Quantitative analysis of comparative genomic hybridization. *Cytometry* **19,** 27–41.

39. Karhu, R., Kahkonen, M., Kuukasjarvi, T., Pennanen, S., Tirkkonen, M., and Kallioniemi, O. (1997) Quality control of CGH: impact of metaphase chromosomes and the dynamic range of hybridization. *Cytometry* **28,** 198–205.

40. Kallioniemi, O.-P., Kallioniemi, A., Piper, J., Isola, J., Waldman, F. M., Gray, J. W., and Pinkel, D. (1994) Optimizing comparative genomic hybridization for analysis of DNA sequence copy number changes in solid tumors. *Genes Chr. Cancer* **10,** 231–243.

41. Becher, R., Korn, W. M, and Prescher, G. (1997) Use of fluorescence *in situ* hybridization and comparative genomic hybridization in the cytogenetic analysis of testicular germ cell tumors and uveal melanomas. *Cancer Genet Cytogenet.* **93,** 22–28.

# 23

# Interphase Cytogenetics in Frozen Ovarian Tumor Tissue

## Thomas Liehr

## 1. Introduction

Resulting from problems of low yield of metaphases and poor-quality chromosomes, detection of cytogenetic changes in solid tumors has been relatively limited *(1)*. The advent of fluorescence *in situ* hybridization (FISH) rendered it possible to obtain "cytogenetic information" from interphase nuclei *(2,3)*. Since that time, interphase cytogenetics has become a powerful tool to investigate numerical chromosomal aberrations *(4,5)*, amplification of oncogenes *(6)*, or deletion of tumor suppressor genes in solid tumors *(7)*, including ovarian cancer. Both fresh tumor material *(8–10)* or formalin-fixed and, subsequently, paraffin-embedded tissue have been used for interphase cytogenetic studies in ovarian tumors *(4–6,8–10)*.

Formalin-fixed/paraffin-embedded tissue is readily available, as this kind of tissue fixation is the most common standard technique in clinical practice. But there are some disadvantages in connection with this material and an increasing number of laboratories now collect archival formalin-fixed/paraffin-embedded and cryofixed tissue samples. Formalin-fixed/paraffin-embedded tissue is, for example, not suitable for all kinds of immunohistochemical approaches as specific antigens may be destroyed during the fixation procedure. Moreover, if formalin fixation is performed in unbuffered formalin and/or incubation is too long, tissue becomes unsuitable for any kind of FISH studies, because DNA is degraded and washed out of the cells *(11)*.

Nevertheless, most interphase cytogenetic studies on archival tumor material have been performed on formalin-fixed/paraffin-embedded tissue sections *(4,9)*, even though there are some additional problems when using sectioned material. The most important ones arise during evaluation of the slides: 1) there is the problem of not evaluable, overlapping nuclei, because of the presence of several cell layers, one on top of the other; and 2) the problem of cut nuclei, leading to artificial signal loss in interphase cytogenetic studies *(9,12)*.

These problems can be solved using a technique called nuclear extraction, first described in 1983 *(13)*. However, there is only one protocol that concerns nuclear extraction from cryofixed tissues in the literature *(14)* and it can be used for cryofixed ovarian tumor tissue, as well (*see* **Fig. 1**).

From: *Methods in Molecular Medicine, Vol. 39: Ovarian Cancer: Methods and Protocols*
Edited by: J. M. S. Bartlett © Humana Press, Inc., Totowa, NJ

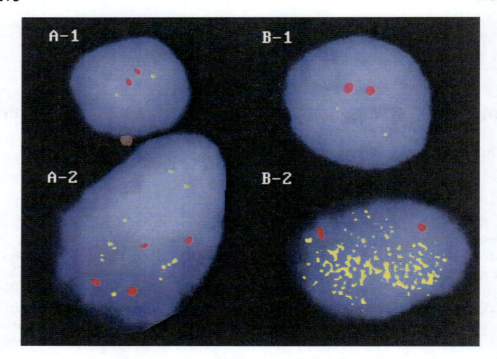

Fig. 1. Four interphase nuclei, extracted from two different cases of cryofixed ovarian tumors are shown. Case A was a dedifferentiated cystadenocarcinoma (GIII) and case B a papillary cystadenocarcinoma (GIII). Both tissues were taken in 1991 and the tumor tissue stored at −20°C up to its use for nucleus extraction in 1997. Both cases have been hybridized with an alphoid, digoxygenated probe for chromosome 8 (ONCOR), detected in red, and a specific, biotinylated probe for the c-*myc* gene (ONCOR), detected in green. Nuclei are blue as a result of DAPI-counterstaining. In **A-1** and **B-1**, one interphase nucleus with two signals each is shown, representing a "normal" cell for these two tissue probes—maybe nuclei of lymphocytes or fibroblasts. In **A-2** and **B-2** nuclei with amplification of the c-*myc* gene are presented. In case B (B-2) two copies of the alphoid region for chromosome 8 and many copies of the c-*myc* gene indicate the presence of double minutes as cytogenetic equivalents of c-*myc* gene amlification; while four copies of the alphoid region for chromosome 8 and 13 copies of the c-*myc* gene, visible in case A (A-2) indicate a c-*myc* "amplification" because of a multiplication of parts of the long arm of chromosome 8, including the c-*myc* gene. Images were captured with the ISIS digital FISH imaging system (MetaSystems, Altlussheim, Germany) using a XC77 CCD camera with on-chip integration (Sony).

The principle of this method is summarized as follows:

1. Cryofixed tissue is cut into small pieces while still frozen, formalin fixed, washed, and treated with proteinase K to digest the cytoplasm and free nuclei. During this treatment, damaged and cut nuclei are eliminated. Interphase nuclei are separated from debris by passing through a nylon mesh. Nuclei are washed in phosphate-buffered saline (PBS) and placed on uncoated, clean slides and fixed. Small tissue pieces (5 mm × 2 mm × 0.5 mm) are sufficient to produce two to five slides with extracted nuclei suitable for interphase FISH analyses.
2. For a FISH approach, these slides are treated with RNase and pepsin prior to denaturation.

3. Denaturation of the slides is performed for about 12 min at 75°C. Biotinylated and digoxigenated alphoid probes are denatured for 5 min and hybridized on the slides for three nights at 37°C in a humid chamber. After a postwashing, series detection of the biotinylated probe is performed with a FITC-avidin system leading to green and of the digoxigenated probe with antidigoxigenin-rhodamine leading to red signals (*see* **Fig. 1**). After counterstaining of the nuclei with DAPI and addition of antifade solution, slides can be evaluated on a fluorescence microscope.

## 2. Materials

### 2.1. Nuclear Extraction

1. Formalin buffer: 3% (v/v) of acid-free formaldehyde (37%; Roth), in 1X PBS pH 7.0; make fresh as required.
2. 10X PBS stock solution: 0.076% (w/v) NaCl, 0.004% (w/v) $NaH_2PO_4$, 0.0013% (w/v) $Na_2HPO_4$, pH 7.0; set up with $ddH_2O$, autoclave, and store at room temperature.
3. PK-solution: 5 mg proteinase K (Boehringer, Mannheim, Germany), 50 µL $1M$ Tris-HCl (pH 7.5), 20 µL $0.5M$ EDTA (pH 7.0), 2 µL $5M$ NaCl, make up to 1 mL with $ddH_2O$; make fresh as required.
4. 55 µm nylon mesh (Nytal 55 SEFAR-AG, Thal, Switzerland).

### 2.2. Slide Pretreatment

1. 20X standard saline citrate (SSC) stock solution: $3.0M$ NaCl, $0.3M$ Na-citrate; set up with $ddH_2O$, adjust to pH 7.0, autoclave, and store at room temperature.
2. RNase stock solution: 5 µg/µL of RNase type A (Boehringer); set up with filtered $ddH_2O$; aliquot and store at –20°C.
3. RNase solution: per slide 100 µL 2X SSC plus 1 µL of RNase stock solution are necessary; make fresh as required.
4. Pepsin stock solution 10% (w/v): dissolve 100 mg pepsin (Serva, Heidelberg, Germany) in 1 mL of filtered $ddH_2O$ at 37°C; aliquot and store at –20°C.
5. Pepsin-buffer: Add 1 mL of $1M$ HCl to 99 mL of distilled water and incubate at 37°C for about 20 min; then add 50 µL of the pepsin stock solution 10% (w/v) and leave the coplin jar at 37°C; make fresh as required.
6. 1X PBS/$MgCl_2$: 5% (v/v) $1M$ $MgCl_2$ in 1X PBS.

### 2.3. Fluorescence In Situ Hybridization (FISH)

#### 2.3.1. Slide Denaturation

1. Denaturation buffer: 70% (v/v) deionized formamide, 10% (v/v) $ddH_2O$, 10% (v/v) 20X SSC, 10% (v/v) phosphate buffer; make fresh as required.
2. Deionized formamide: Add 5 g of ion exchanger Amberlite MB1 (Serva) to 100 mL of formamide (Merck, Darmstadt, Mannheim, Germany), stir for 2 h (room temperature) and filter twice through Whatmann no. 1 filter paper. Aliquot and store at –20°C.
3. Phosphate buffer: prepare $0.5M$ $Na_2HPO_4$ and $0.5M$ $NaH_2PO_4$, mix these two solutions (1 : 1) to get pH 7.0, then aliquot and store at –20°C.

#### 2.3.2. Probe Denaturation

1. Hybridization buffer: Dissolve 2 g dextran sulfate in 10 mL 50% deionized formamide/ 2X SSC/50 m$M$ phosphate buffer for 3 h at 70°C. Aliquot and store at –20°C.

#### 2.3.3. Posthybridization and Detection Washing

1. Solution I: FITC-avidin (CAMON Vector Laboratories) in 4X SSC/0.2% Tween/5% BSA (1 : 300 both Sigma); make fresh as required.

2. Solution II: Biotinylated antiavidin (CAMON Vector Laboratories)/Antidigoxinenin-rhodamine (Boehringer Mannheim)/ in 4X SSC/0.2% Tween/5% BSA (1:20:100); make fresh as required.
3. DAPI-solution: Dissolve 5 μL of DAPI (4,6-diamidino-2-phenylindol.2HCl stock-solution; Serva) in 100 mL 4X SSC/0.2% Tween; make fresh as required.

## 3. Methods

### *3.1. Nuclear Extraction*

This section describes a method for extraction of intact interphase nuclei from cryofixed tissue stored for up to several years at –20 to –80°C. Extracted nuclei are suitable for FISH analysis (*see* **Subheading 3.3.** and **Fig. 1**).

1. Transfer cryofixed tissue from –80°C to –20°C freezer for 1 h.
2. Transfer tissue in a glass dish on ice and cut into small pieces (not larger than 1 mm cubed) using precooled (+4°C) scalpel and forceps (*see* **Note 1**).
3. Add 1 mL of formalin buffer at room temperature (RT) to the cold tissue pieces and transfer them together with the buffer into a 1.5-mL microtube. Tissue should thaw on addition of formalin buffer.
4. Incubate the tissue in formalin buffer for 1 to 3 h at RT without agitation (*see* **Note 2**).
5. Pellet the tissue pieces by centrifugation (3800*g*, 30 s, RT). If necessary, repeat this step.
6. Remove the fluid, add 1 mL of sterile 0.9% NaCl (w/v) and vortex the microtube.
7. Repeat **step 5**.
8. Repeat **steps 6** and **7**.
9. Remove the fluid, add—depending on the amount of tissue—0.2 to 1 mL of PK-solution and vortex the microtube (*see* **Note 3**).
10. Incubate the microtube at 37°C for 30 min. During this time, vortex the microtube every 5 min to promote tissue disaggregation.
11. Transfer the fluid onto 55-μm nylon mesh (*see* **Note 4**). Fluid and nuclei will pass through the mesh by force of gravity and are collected in a 15-mL plastic tube. Nuclei remaining in the mesh are washed out by 4 mL 1X PBS, passed through the mesh, and collected in the 15-mL plastic tube.
12. Pellet the extracted nuclei by centrifugation (850*g*, 8 min); remove the supernatant with the exception of about 300 μL.
13. Resuspend the pellet in 4 mL 1X PBS and repeat **step 12**.
14. Resuspend the cell suspension in the remaining 300 μL of 1X PBS.
15. Distribute the suspension on 2–6 clean and dry slides by pipeting the fluid on the slide surfaces. Place one drop (30–90 μL) of about 1 cm in diameter/slide (*see* **Note 5**).
16. Allow drops to dry out on a 40°C warming plate and afterward at RT overnight.
17. Fix slides in 100 mL formalin buffer in a coplin jar for 10 min (RT).
18 Replace formalin buffer in the coplin jar with 1X PBS. After 5 min of incubation at RT, 1X PBS is replaced by distilled water.
19. Remove the water after 1 min, perform an ethanol series (70, 90, 100%, 3 min each) to dehydrate slides and air-dry. An evaluation of the success of the nuclear extraction can be performed by phase contrast light microscopy (*see* **Note 6**).

### *3.2. Slide Pretreatment*

As in a conventional FISH approach, a pretreatment of the slides with RNase and pepsin followed by a postfixation with formalin buffer is required to reduce background *(15)*.

1. Slides with the extracted nuclei are incubated in 2X SSC for 5 min at RT (in a 100 mL coplin jar on a shaker).
2. Remove slides from the coplin jar, add 100 µL of RNase solution/slide and cover with a 24 × 50 mm coverslip.
3. Incubate the slides in a humid chamber for 15 min at 37°C (*see* **Note 7**).
4. Put slides back into the coplin jar with 100 mL 2X SSC (RT) and remove the coverslips by forceps. Leave slides in 2X SSC solution for 3 min with gentle agitation.
5. Discard 2X SSC and replace it with 100 mL 1X PBS (RT) for 5 min (shaker).
6. Replace 1X PBS with 100 mL prewarmed pepsin buffer (37°C) and incubate the slides for 10 min at 37°C, without agitation (*see* **Note 7**).
7. Replace fluid with 100 mL 1X PBS/MgCl$_2$, incubate at RT for 5 min with gentle agitation. MgCl$_2$ will block the enzymatic activity of pepsin.
8. Postfix nuclei on the slide surfaces by replacing 1X PBS/MgCl$_2$ with 100 mL of formalin buffer for 10 min (RT, with gentle agitation).
9. Formalin buffer is replaced by 100 mL 1X PBS for 2 min (RT, with gentle agitation).
10. Finally, slides are dehydrated by an ethanol series (70, 90, 100%, 3 min each) and air-dried (*see* **Note 8**).

## *3.3. Fluorescence* In Situ *Hybridization (FISH)*

FISH has become a standard technique in cytogenetic laboratories *(15–17)*. For hybridization of archival cryomaterial, however, a prolonged denaturation time and a higher concentration of probes and detection solutions are necessary.

### *3.3.1. Slide Denaturation*

1. Add 100 µL denaturation buffer to the slides and cover with (24 × 50 mm) coverslips.
2. Incubate slides on a warming plate for 12 min at 75°C (*see* **Note 9**).
3. Remove the coverslips immediately by forceps and place slides in a coplin jar filled with 70% ethanol (4°C) to conserve target DNA as single strands.
4. Dehydrate slides in ethanol (70, 90, 100%, 4°C, 3 min each) and air-dry.

### *3.3.2. Probe Denaturation*

1. For each slide to be hybridized, add 1.5 µL each of biotin and digoxigenin labeled chromosome specific probes (ONCOR, Inc.) and 3 µL of 1 µg/µL COT1-DNA (Gibco) to 20 µL of the hybridization buffer in a 1.5-ml microtube, vortex, and spin down (*see* **Note 10**).
2. Denature probe-solution at 75°C for 5 min and cool immediately on ice to conserve probe DNA in single strands (*see* **Note 11**).

### *3.3.3. Hybridization*

1. Add 20 µL of probe-solution onto each denatured slide, put 24 × 50-mm coverslips on the drops and seal with rubber cement (Fixogum; Marabu).
2. Incubate slides for three nights at 37°C in a humid chamber (*see* **Note 12**).

### *3.3.4. Posthybridization and Detection Washing*

1. Take the slides out of 37°C, remove rubber cement with forceps and coverslips by letting them swim off in 4X SSC/0.2%Tween (RT, 100-mL coplin jar) (*see* **Note 13**).
2. Postwash the slides 3 × 5 min in formamide-solution (45°C) followed by 3 × 5 min in 2X SSC (37°C) in a 100-mL coplin jar, with gentle agitation.
3. Put the slides in 4X SSC/0.2% Tween (100 mL, RT), for a few seconds.
4. Add 50 µL of solution I to each slide, cover with 24 × 50-mm coverslips and incubate at 37°C for 30 min in a humid chamber.

5. Remove the coverslips and wash 3 × 3 min in 4X SSC/0.2% Tween (RT, with gentle agitation).
6. Add 50 µL of solution II to each slide, cover with 24 × 50-mm coverslips and incubate at 37°C for 75 min in a humid chamber.
7. Repeat **step 5**.
8. Repeat **step 4**.
9. Repeat **step 5**.
10. Counterstain the slides with DAPI-solution (100 mL in a coplin jar, RT) for 8 min.
11. Wash slides several times in water for a few seconds and air-dry.
12. Add 15 µL of antifade Vectashield (CAMON Vector Laboratories H1000), cover with coverslips, and look at the results in a fluorescence microscope.

## 4. Notes

1. If only small amounts of cryofixed tissue are available, tissue can be cut on a cryostat. About 15 25-µm cryosections (2–5 mm in diameter) are sufficient for about five slides with extracted interphase nuclei.
2. Incubation of the tissue in formalin-buffer can be done by agitation as well, with no difference in the quality or quantity of resulting extracted nuclei.
3. If only small amounts of tissue are to be digested (*see* **Note 1**) 0.2–0.4 mL of PK-solution are sufficient.
4. Nytal 55—the nylon mesh has to be cut in 5 cm × 5 cm squares. Such a square can be formed to a funnel, pinned by a stapler, and used as the required filter.
5. The resulting suspension has a certain turbidity reflecting the number of extracted nuclei. With experience, an assessment of the amount of slides on which the suspension should be distributed will be possible. For the first-time user a distribution of suspension on two slides is suggested.
6. An evaluation of quantity and quality of extracted nuclei is not possible before this step of the protocol, because of crystallization of PBS salts on the slide surface. Now they have been washed away during the **Subheading 3.1., steps 17–19**.
7. RNase and pepsin pretreatment conditions should be tested in each laboratory on a single slide first. Both RNase and pepsin concentrations can be too stringent, resulting in clean slides without any remaining nuclei.
8. The pretreated slides can be hybridized immediately or stored at RT for up to 3 wk. If longer storage is necessary slides are stable at –20°C for several months.
9. Owing to the fact that DNA in archival tissues has undergone some fixation steps and has been stored up to several years, a prolonged denaturation time seems useful. Moreover, in other FISH-protocols with denaturation times of 2–5 min only, the maintenance of available metaphase chromosomes is the main aspect, which is of no significance in the actual protocol.
10. COT1-DNA normally is added to the hybridization mix, when nonrepetitive sequences are to be detected (cosmids, chromosome libraries, or genomic DNA, used in comparative genomic hybridization studies) *(18–20)*. Because of the long hybridization time (72 h) it makes sense to block repetitive sequences, when using repetitive satellite probes, as well. If no COT1-DNA is added, the specific centromeric probes would not only label "their" specific chromosome, but undesired cross hybridization would also occur.
11. In **Fig. 1**, the result of a FISH-experiment using a digoxigenated alphoid probe for chromosome 8 and a biotinylated probe for the c-*myc* oncogene is shown. 1.5 µL of the alphoid probe, 1.5 µL of COT1-DNA (1 µg/µL) and 15 µL hybridization buffer have been denatured at 75°C for 5 min, put on ice, and mixed now with 5 µL of the c-*myc* probe (ONCOR). The latter has been incubated before at 37°C for 20 min—according to manufacturers instructions.

12. Incubation can be stopped—if necessary—after 48 or 96 h, as well. Whereas in the first case, weaker signals are possible, in the second case, some cross hybridization problems may arise.

13. During the washing steps, it is important to prevent the slide surfaces from drying out, otherwise background problems may arise.

## References

1. Heim, S. and Mitelman, F. (1995) Cancer Cytogenetics. 2nd Ed., Wiley-Liss, New York.
2. Langer, P. R., Waldrop, A. A., and Ward, D. C. (1981) Enzymatic synthesis of biotin-labeled polynucleitides: novel nucleic acid affinity probes. *Proc. Natl. Acad. Sci. USA* **78,** 6633–6637.
3. Pinkel, D., Straume, T., and Gray, J. W. (1986) Cytogenetic analysis using quantitative, high sensitivity, fluorescence hybridization. *Proc. Natl. Acad. Sci. USA* **83,** 2934–2938.
4. Persons, D. L., Hartmann, L. C., Herath, J. F., Borell, T. J., Keeney, G. L., and Jenkins, R. B. (1993) Interphase molecular cytogenetic analysis of epithelial ovarian tumors. *Am. J. Clin. Pathol.* **142,** 733–741.
5. Gibas, Z. and Talermann, A. (1993) Analysis of chromosome aneuploidy in ovarian dysgerminoma by flow cytometry and fluorescence *in situ* hybridization. *Diagn. Mol. Pathol.* **2,** 50–56.
6. Young, S. R., Liu, W.-H., Brock, J.-A., and Smith, S. T. (1996) ERBB2 and chromosome 17 centromere studies of ovarian cancer by fluorescence in situ hybridization. *Genes Chr. Cancer* **16,** 130–137.
7. Tsuji, T., Tagawa, Y., Hisamatsu, T., Nakamura, S., Terada, R., Sawai, T., et al. (1997) p53 alterations and chromosome 17 aberrations in non-small cell lung cancer. *Gan To Kagaku Ryoho* **24 Suppl. 2,** 263–268.
8. Liehr, T., Atanasov, N., Tulusan, H. A., and Gebhart, E. (1993) Amplification of proto-oncogenes in human ovarian carcinomas. *Int. J. Oncol.* **2,** 155–160.
9. Neubauer, S., Liehr, T., Tulusan, H. A., and Gebhart, E. (1994) Interphase cytogenetics by FISH on archival paraffin material and cultured cells of human ovarian tumors. *Int. J. Oncol.* **4,** 317–321.
10. Liehr, T., Stübinger, A., Thoma, K., Tulusan, H. A., and Gebhart, E. (1994) Comparative interphase cytogenetics using FISH on human ovarian carcinomas. *Anticancer Res.* **14,** 183–188.
11. Long, A. A., Komminoth, P., Lee, E., and Wolfe, H. J. (1993) Comparison of indirect and direct in-situ polymerase chain reaction in cell preparations and tissue sections. Detection of viral DNA, gene rearrangements and chromosomal translocations. *Histochem.* **99,** 151–162.
12. Dhingra, K., Sahin, A., Supak, J., Kim, S. Y., Hortobagyi, G., and Hittelman, W. N. (1992) Chromosome *in situ* hybridization on formalin-fixed mammary tissue using non-isotopic, non-fluorescent probes: technical considerations and biological implications. *Breast Cancer Res. Treat.* **23,** 201–210.
13. Hedley, D. W., Friedlander, M. L., Taylor, I. W., Rugg, C. A., and Musgrove, E. A. (1983) Method for analysis of cellular DNA content of paraffin-embedded pathological material using flow cytometry. J. Histochem. *Cytochem.* **31,** 1333–1335.
14. Liehr, T., Grehl, H., and Rautenstrauss, B. (1996) A rapid method for FISH analysis on interphase nuclei extracted from cryofixed tissue. *Trends Genet.* **12,** 505,506.
15. Liehr, T., Thoma, K., Kammler, K., Gehring, C., Ekici, A., Bathke, K. D., et al. (1995) Direct preparation of uncultured EDTA-treated or heparinized blood for interphase FISH analysis. *Appl. Cytogenet.* **21,** 185–188.
16. Fox, J. L., Hsu, P. H., Legator, M. S., Morrison, L. E., and Seelig, S. A. (1995) Flourescence *in situ* hybridization: powerful molecular tool for cancer prognosis. *Clin. Chem.* **41,** 1554–1559.
17. Mark, H. F., Jenkins, R., and Miller, W. A. (1997) Current applications of molecular cytogenetic technologies. *Ann. Clin. Lab. Sci.* **27,** 47–56.
18. Wolff, E., Liehr, T., Vorderwülbecke, U., Tulusan, A. H., Husslein, E. M., and Gebhart, E. (1997) Frequent gains and losses of specific chromosome segments in human ovarian carcinomas shown by comparative genomic hybridization. *Int. J. Oncol.* **11,** 19–23.
19. Neubauer, S., Gebhart, E., Schmitt, G., Birkenhake, S., and Dunst, J. (1996) Is chromosome in situ suppression (CISS) hybridization suited as a predictive test for intrinsic radiosensitivity in cancer patients? *Int. J. Oncol.* **8,** 707–712.
20. Kraus, C., Liehr, T., Hülsken, J., Behrens, J., Birchmeier, W., Greschick, K. H., and Ballhausen, W. G. (1994) Localization of the human β-catenin gene (CTNNB1) to 3p21: a region implicated in tumor development. *Genomics* **23,** 272–274.

# 24

# Interphase Cytogenetics
# in Paraffin-Embedded Ovarian Tissue

**Susann Neubauer and Thomas Liehr**

## 1. Introduction

Interphase cytogenetics using formalin-fixed/paraffin-embedded tissue is now a well-established technique, which renders it possible to obtain "cytogenetic information" from interphase nuclei of solid tumors (*1,2*, for ovarian cancer, e.g., *3–8*). It is the only tool to investigate specific numerical chromosomal aberrations (*3–7*), amplification of oncogenes (*8*), deletion of tumor suppressor genes (*9*), or chromosomal translocations (*10*) in formalin-fixed/paraffin-embedded tissue samples on a single-cell level. For numerical chromosomal aberrations using centromeric probes, even automated assessment of the fluorescence *in situ* hybridization (FISH) signals has become possible (*11*).

Interphase FISH studies on formalin-fixed/paraffin-embedded tissue can be done, on the one hand, on sectioned material and, on the other hand, on extracted interphase nuclei (*12*). As concluded in (*13*), both methods are comparable and reliable for detection of chromosomal changes in archival tissue, however, each of them has advantages and disadvantages. The first approach is recommended, when the tissue architecture must be studied intact, e.g., in the case of small and/or invasive tumors, whereas the second technique can be applied successfully when more or less homogenous (tumor)-tissue samples are under study (*12*). During evaluation of tissue sections, there often arise the problem of not evaluable, overlapping nuclei, because of the presence of several cell layers, one on top of the other; and that of cut nuclei, leading to artificial signal loss in interphase cytogenetic studies (*7,14,15*); two problems not present in nuclear extraction techniques (*12,13,16*). However, only sectioned material makes it possible to identify small subclones and their localization within a tumorous tissue, which is impossible after nuclear extraction.

A method for an interphase cytogenetics approach for tissue sections is described (*6*). The three main steps of this technique are as follows:

1. Formalin-fixed/paraffin-embedded tissue, sectioned and mounted on 3-aminopropyltriethoxysilane coated slides, dewaxed, and dehydrated prior to hybridization.
2. Treatment with proteinase K, RNase, pepsin, and formalin prior to denaturation.

From: *Methods in Molecular Medicine, Vol. 39: Ovarian Cancer: Methods and Protocols*
Edited by: J. M. S. Bartlett © Humana Press, Inc., Totowa, NJ

3. Denaturation of slides performed; labeled probes are denatured and hybridized on the slides for 72 h. After a postwashing series, detection of the biotinylated probe is performed with a FITC-avidin system leading to green and of the digoxigenin labeled probe with antidigoxigenin-rhodamine leading to red signals. Counterstaining of the sections and addition of antifade solution finishes the procedure and slides can be evaluated on a fluorescence microscope.

## 2. Materials

### 2.1. Deparaffinization

1. 3-aminopropyltriethoxysilan-coated slides: clean and dry slides are put in a 3% 3-aminopropyltriethoxysilane solution in 100% acetone (room temperature) for 15 s and rinsed two times in acetone and double-distilled water for a few seconds each. Slides are dried overnight at 37°C. Prior to use, slides can be stored at 4°C for about 3 wk.
2. 10X phosphate-buffered saline (PBS) stock solution: 0.076% (w/v) NaCl, 0.004% (w/v) $NaH_2PO_4$, 0.0013% (w/v) $Na_2HPO_4$; pH 7.0; in double-distilled water, autoclave and store at room temperature.

### 2.2. Slide Pretreatment

1. PK-solution: 5 mg proteinase K (Boehringer, Mannheim, Germany), 50 µL $1M$ Tris-HCl (pH 7.5), 20 µL $0.5M$ EDTA (pH 7.0), 2 µL $5M$ NaCl, make up to 1 mL in filtered double-distilled water; make fresh as required.
2. 20X standard saline citrate (SSC) stock solution: $3.0M$ NaCl, $0.3M$ Na-citrate; set up with double-distilled water, adjust to pH 7.0, autoclave, and store at room temperature.
3. RNase stock solution: 5 µg/µL of RNase type A (Boehringer); set up with filtered double-distilled water; aliquot and store at –20°C.
4. RNase solution: per slide 100 µL 2X SSC plus 20 µL of RNase stock solution are necessary; make fresh as required.
5. Pepsin stock solution 10% (w/v): dissolve 100 mg pepsin (Serva, Heidelberg, Germany) in 1 mL of filtered double-distilled water at 37°C; aliquot and store at –20°C.
6. Pepsin buffer: Add 1 mL of $1M$ HCl to 99 mL of distilled water and incubate at 37°C for about 20 min; then add 50 µL of the pepsin stock solution 10% (w/v) and leave the coplin jar at 37°C; make fresh as required.
7. 1X PBS/ $MgCl_2$: 5% (v/v) $1M$ $MgCl_2$ in 1X PBS.
8. Formalin buffer: 3% (v/v) of acid-free formaldehyde (37%; Roth) in 1X PBS; make fresh as required.

### 2.3. Fluorescence In Situ Hybridization (FISH)

#### 2.3.1. Slide Denaturation

1. Denaturation buffer: 70% (v/v) deionized formamide, 10% (v/v) filtered double-distilled water, 10% (v/v) 20X SSC, 10% (v/v) phosphate buffer; make fresh as required.
2. Deionized formamide: Add 5 g of ion exchanger Amberlite MB1 (Serva) to 100 mL of formamide (Merck, Darmstadt, Mannheim, Germany) stir for 2 h (room temperature) and filter twice through Whatmann no. 1 filter paper. Aliquot and store at –20°C.
3. Phosphate buffer: prepare $0.5M$ $Na_2HPO_4$ and $0.5M$ $NaH_2PO_4$, mix these two solutions (1:1) to get pH 7.0, then aliquot and store at –20°C.

#### 2.3.2. Probe Denaturation

1. Hybridization buffer: Dissolve 2 g dextran sulfate in 10 mL 50% deionized formamide/ 2X SSC/50 m$M$ phosphate buffer for 3 h at 70°C. Aliquot and store at –20°C.

### 2.3.3. Posthybridization and Detection Washing

1. Formamide solution: 50% (v/v) formamide (Merck), 10% (v/v) 20X SSC, 40% (v/v) distilled water; make fresh as required.
2. Solution I: FITC-avidin (CAMON Vector Laboratories)/4X SSC/0.2 %Tween/5% BSA (1:300 both Sigma, St. Louis, MO); make fresh as required.
3. Solution II: Biotinylated antiavidin (CAMON Vector Laboratories)/Anti-digoxigenin-rhodamine (Boehringer Mannheim, Germany)/4X SSC/0.2%Tween/5% BSA (1:20:100); make fresh as required.
4. DAPI-solution: Dissolve 5 µL of DAPI (4,6-diamidino-2-phenylindol.2HCl stock-solution; Serva) in 100 mL 4X SSC/0.2% Tween; make fresh as required.

## 3. Methods

### 3.1. Deparaffinization

This section describes the deparaffinization of formalin-fixed/paraffin-embedded tissue mounted on 3-aminopropyltriethoxisilan coated slides (*see* **Subheading 2.1., item 2.**). Tissue sections should be about 5–6 µm (*see* **Note 1**).

1. Place slides with mounted tissue sections in 100% xylene at room temperature (RT) for 5–10 min (*see* **Note 2**).
2. Rehydrate through an ethanol series (100, 100, 95, 70, 50% 2 min each at RT) and 1X PBS (2 min at RT) in a 100-mL coplin jar.
3. Replace PBS by water (for a few seconds) and perform following pretreatment procedure immediately without allowing slides to dry.

### 3.2. Slide Pretreatment

As in a conventional FISH approach, a pretreatment of the slides is necessary. But prior to the usual RNase and pepsin treatment followed by a postfixation with formalin-buffer (*17*), a proteinase K (PK) treatment is necessary (*6*).

1. Transfer slides to a humid chamber at 37°C, add 100–500 µL PK-solution per section to cover the whole tissue. The amount of the PK-solution depends on the diameter of the section. Do not cover the section with a cover slip (*see* **Note 3**).
2. Incubate for 10 min at 37°C.
3. Stop PK treatment by putting the slides in a coplin jar with 100 mL 1X PBS/MgCl$_2$ (RT) for 3 min.
4. Sections can be assessed for completeness of PK digestion in the microscope (*see* **Note 4**). Take care that sections do not dry out. If PK digestion is not completed: repeat **steps 1–3**; if it is: go on with **step 5**.
5. Slides are incubated in 2X SSC for 5 min at RT (in a 100-mL coplin jar).
6. Remove slides from the coplin jar, add 100–500 µL of RNase solution to each section. The amount of the RNase solution depends on the diameter of the section. Do not cover the section with a cover slip (*see* **Note 3**).
7. Incubate the slides in a humid chamber for 10 min at 37°C.
8. Put the slides back into the coplin jar with 100 mL 2X SSC (RT). Leave slides in 2X SSC solution for 3 min without agitation.
9. Discard the 2X SSC and replace by 100 mL 1X PBS (RT) for 5 min.
10. Replace the 1X PBS by 100 mL prewarmed pepsin-buffer (37°C) and incubate the slides for 5 min at 37°C, without agitation (*see* **Note 3**).
11. Replace fluid by 100 mL 1X PBS/ MgCl$_2$ and incubate at RT for 5 min without agitation. MgCl$_2$ will block the enzymatic activity of pepsin.

12. Sections can be assessed for completeness of pepsin digestion in the microscope (*see* **Note 5**). Take care that the sections do not dry out. If pepsin digestion is not completed: repeat **steps 10–12**; if it is: go on with **step 13**.

13. Postfix the sections on the slide surfaces by incubating the slides in 100 mL of formalin buffer for 10 min (RT, without agitation).

14. Replace formalin buffer 100 mL 1X PBS for 2 min (RT, without agitation).

15. Dehydrate slides through an ethanol series (70, 90, 100%, 3 min each) and air-dry (*see* **Note 6**).

### 3.3. Fluorescence In Situ Hybridization (FISH)

FISH is a standard technique in cytogenetic and pathological laboratories (**1,17–19**). For hybridization of archival sections, however, a prolonged slide denaturation time and higher concentration of probes and detection solutions than usual are necessary.

#### 3.3.1. Slide Denaturation

1. Add 200 µL denaturation buffer to the slide surfaces and put cover slips on them ($24 \times 50$ mm).

2. Incubate the slides on a warming plate for 8 min at 75°C (*see* **Note 7**).

3. Remove cover slips immediately by forceps and place slides in a coplin jar filled with 70% ethanol (4°C) to conserve target DNA as single strands.

4. Dehydrate slides in ethanol (70, 90, 100%, 4°C, 3 min each) and air-dry.

#### 3.3.2. Probe Denaturation

1. For each slide to be hybridized, add 1.5 µL each of biotin and digoxigenin labeled chromosome specific probes (ONCOR, Inc.) and 3 µL of 1 µg/µL COT1-DNA (Gibco) to 40 µL of the hybridization buffer in a 1.5-mL microtube, vortex and spin down (*see* **Note 8**).

2. Denature probe-solution at 75°C for 5 min and cool immediately on ice to conserve probe DNA in single strands.

#### 3.3.3. Hybridization

1. Add 40 µL of the denatured probe solution onto each of the denatured slides (from **Subheading 3.3.1., step 4**) put $24 \times 50$ mm cover slips on the drops and seal with rubber cement (Fixogum; Marabu).

2. Incubate slides 72 h at 37°C in a humid chamber.

#### 3.3.4. Posthybridization and Detection Washing

1. Take the slides out of 37°C, remove rubber cement with forceps and cover slips by letting them swim off in 4X SSC/0.2% Tween 20 (RT, 100-mL coplin jar).

2. Postwash the slides $3 \times 5$ min in formamide-solution (45°C) followed by $3 \times 5$ min in 2X SSC (37°C) in a 100-mL coplin jar, with gentle agitation.

3. Put the slides in 4X SSC/0.2% Tween (100 mL, RT), for a few seconds.

4. Add 50 µL of solution I to each slide, cover with $24 \times 50$-mm cover slips and incubate at 37°C for 30 min in a humid chamber.

5. Remove the cover slips and wash $3 \times 3$ min in 4X SSC/0.2% Tween (RT, with gentle agitation).

6. Add 50 µL of solution II to each slide, cover with $24 \times 50$ mm coverslips and incubate at 37°C for 75 min in a humid chamber.

7. Repeat **step 5**.

8. Repeat **step 4**.

9. Repeat **step 5**.

10. Counterstain the slides with DAPI-solution (100 mL in a coplin jar, RT) for 8 min.
11. Wash slides several times in water for a few seconds and air-dry.
12. Add 20 µL of antifade Vectashield (CAMON Vector Laboratories H1000), cover with 20 × 60-mm cover slips and look at the results in a fluorescence microscope.

## 4. Notes

1. Tissue section should be in the range of 5–6 µm to reduce the problem of cut nuclei leading to artificial signal loss.
2. Incubation in xylene for 5–10 min is sufficient to remove the paraffin from the tissue. Longer incubation times at this step do not lead to better FISH results.
3. A cover slip would enhance the possibility of floating or damaging of the section during the pretreatment steps. Performing the pretreatment steps in a humid chamber or a coplin jar reduces this possibility.
4. PK-treatment is sufficient, when the tissue starts to become less compact, because of loss of cytoplasmic components and loss of some (damaged) nuclei. Nevertheless, the assessment of the digestion of a tissue section requires some experience.
5. Pepsin treatment is finished when the section is less compact than in the beginning and nuclei of the section are well visible and more or less free of disturbing plasmatic components. Some experience in the assessment of tissue sections must be learned by trial and error.
6. The pretreated slides must be hybridized immediately, even though air-drying of the slides is now—after the formalin postfixation—required and possible.
7. DNA in archival tissues has undergone some fixation steps and has been stored up to several years, thus, a prolonged denaturation time makes sense. Moreover, in other FISH protocols with denaturation times of 2–5 min only, the maintenance of evaluable metaphase chromosomes is the main aspect, which is of no significance in this approach.
8. COT1-DNA normally is added to the hybridization mix, when nonrepetitive sequences shall be detected (cosmids, chromosome libraries or genomic DNA, used in comparative genomic hybridization studies) *(20–22)*. Owing to the long hybridization time (72 h), blocking of repetitive sequences is necessary to avoid undesired crosshybridization of the specific centromeric probes.

## References

1. Wolfe, K. Q. and Herrington, C. S. (1997) Interphase cytogenetics and pathology: a tool for diagnosis and research. *J. Pathol.* **181,** 359–361.
2. Hackel, C. and VarellaGarcia, M. (1997) Interphase cytogenetics using fluorescence *in situ* hybridization: an overview of its application to diffuse and solid tissue. *Braz. J. Genet.* **20,** 97–106.
3. Wolf, G. N., Abdul-Karim, F. W., Schork, N. J., and Schwartz, S. (1996) Origins of heterogeneous ovarian carcinomas. A molecular cytogenetic analysis of histologically benign, low malignant potential, and fully malignant components. *Am. J. Pathol.* **149,** 511–520.
4. Persons, D. L., Hartmann, L. C., Herath, J. F., Borell, T. J., Keeney, G. L., and Jenkins, R. B. (1993) Interphase molecular cytogenetic analysis of epithelial ovarian tumors. *Am. J. Clin. Pathol.* **142,** 733–741.
5. Liehr, T., Atanasov, N., Tulusan, H. A., and Gebhart, E. (1993) Amplification of proto-oncogenes in human ovarian carcinomas. *Int. J. Oncol.* **2,** 155–160.
6. Neubauer, S., Liehr, T., Tulusan, H. A., and Gebhart, E. (1994) Interphase cytogenetics by FISH on archival paraffin material and cultured cells of human ovarian tumors. *Int. J. Oncol.* **4,** 317–321.
7. Liehr, T., Stübinger, A., Thoma, K., Tulusan, H. A., and Gebhart, E. (1994) Comparative interphase cytogenetics using FISH on human ovarian carcinomas. *Anticancer Res.* **14,** 183–188.
8. Young, S. R., Liu, W.-H., Brock, J.-A., and Smith, S. T. (1996) ERBB2 and chromosome 17 centromere studies of ovarian cancer by fluorescence *in situ* hybridization. *Genes Chr. Cancer* **16,** 130–137.
9. Tsuji, T., Tagawa, Y., Hisamatsu, T., Nakamura, S., Terada, R., Sawai, T., et al. (1997) p53 alterations and chromosome 17 aberrations in non-small cell lung cancer. *Gan To Kagaku Ryoho* **24,** 263–268.

10. Yoshida, H., Nagao, K., Ito, H., Yamamoto, K., and Ushigome, S. (1997) Chromosomal translocations in human soft tissue sarcomas by interphase fluorescence *in situ* hybridization. *Pathol. Internat.* **47,** 222–229.

11. Mesker, W. E., Alers, J. C., Sloos, W. C. R., Vrolijk, H., Raap, A. K., Dekken, H. V., and Tanke, H. J. (1996) Automated assessment of numerical chromosomal aberrations in paraffin embedded prostate tumor cells stained by *in situ* hybridization. *Cytometry* **26,** 298–304.

12. Köpf, I., Hanson, C., Delle, U., Verbiené, I., and Weimarck, A. (1996) A rapid and simplified technique for analysis of archival formalin-fixed, paraffin-embedded tissue by fluorescence *in situ* hybridization (FISH). *Anticancer Res.* **16,** 2533–2536.

13. Qian, J. Q., Bostwick, D. G., Takahashi, S., Borell, T. J., Brown, J. A., Lieber, M. M., and Jenkins, R. B. (1996) Comparison of fluorescence *in situ* hybridization analysis of isolated nuclei and routine histological sections from paraffin-embedded prostatic adenocarcinoma specimens. *Am. J. Pathol.* **149,** 1193–1199.

14. Hopman, A. H. N., Van Hooren, E., Van de Kaa, C. A., Vooijs, P. G. P., and Ramaekers, F. C. S. (1991) Detection of numerical chromosome aberrations using *in situ* hybridization in paraffin sections of routinely processed bladder cancers. *Mod. Pathol.* **4,** 503–513.

15. Dhingra, K., Sahin, A., Supak, J., Kim, S. Y., Hortobagyi, G., and Hittelman, W. N. (1992) Chromosome *in situ* hybridization on formalin-fixed mammary tissue using non-isotopic, nonfluorescent probes: technical considerations and biological implications. *Breast Cancer Res. Treat.* **23,** 201–210.

16. Liehr, T., Grehl, H., and Rautenstrauss, B. (1995) FISH analysis of interphase nuclei extracted from paraffin-embedded tissue. *Trends Genet.* **11,** 377,378.

17. Liehr, T., Thoma, K., Kammler, K., Gehring, C., Ekici, A., Bathke, K. D., et al. (1995) Direct preparation of uncultured EDTA-treated or heparinized blood for interphase FISH analysis. *Appl. Cytogenet.* **21,** 185–188.

18. Fox, J. L., Hsu, P. H., Legator, M. S., Morrison, L. E., and Seelig, S. A. (1995) Fluorescence *in situ* hybridization: powerful molecular tool for cancer prognosis. *Clin. Chem.* **41,** 1554–1559.

19. Mark, H. F., Jenkins, R., and Miller, W. A. (1997) Current applications of molecular cytogenetic technologies. *Ann. Clin. Lab. Sci.* **27,** 47–56.

20. Wolff, E., Liehr, T., Vorderwülbecke, U., Tulusan, A. H., Husslein, E. M., and Gebhart, E. (1997) Frequent gains and losses of specific chromosome segments in human ovarian carcinomas shown by comparative genomic hybridization. *Int. J. Oncol.* **11,** 19–23.

21. Neubauer, S., Gebhart, E., Schmitt, G., Birkenhake, S., and Dunst, J. (1996) Is chromosome *in situ* suppression (CISS) hybridization suited as a predictive test for intrinsic radiosensitivity in cancer patients? *Int. J. Oncol.* **8,** 707–712.

22. Kraus, C., Liehr, T., Hülsken, J., Behrens, J., Birchmeier, W., Greschick, K. H., and Ballhausen, W. G. (1994) Localization of the human β-catenin gene (CTNNB1) to 3p21: a region implicated in tumor development. *Genomics* **23,** 272–274.

# 25

# Rapid Identification of Chromosomes Using Primed *In Situ* Labeling (PRINS)

## GopalRao V. N. Velagaleti

## 1. Introduction

Primed *in situ* labeling (PRINS) was introduced by Koch and colleagues *(1)* for the visualization of chromosome centromeres. The concept is based on the knowledge that the alpha satellite repeat monomers at the human centromeres exhibit variation among chromosomes *(2)*, and by targeting such variation, it is possible to obtain chromosome-specific markers for identification of individual chromosomes *(3)*. PRINS reaction involves annealing of short, unlabeled oligonucleotide primers to specific genomic targets on metaphase chromosomes or interphase nuclei *in situ* and the subsequent extension of the primer sequences in the presence of labeled nucleotides using *Taq* DNA polymerase. The high efficiency with which PRINS can distinguish the alpha satellite sequences of human chromosomes and identify the individual chromosomes is well documented *(4–6)*. PRINS has many advantages compared to fluorescence *in situ* hybridization (FISH), including its specificity and sensitivity; no limitations on probe size; short reaction time; no pretreatment of slides; and minimal cost *(7–10)*. PRINS is used for various clinical applications including identification of marker chromosomes *(11)*. Of all its applications, interphase analysis for detection of aneuploidy is of utmost importance. Interphase analysis permits screening of a large number of cells that are not amenable to analysis through conventional culture methods. PRINS has been used for rapid assessment of aneuploidy in interphase cells of prenatal samples *(12)*, frozen tissue sections *(13)*, and sperm *(14)*. For interphase analysis, PRINS was shown to be more sensitive than chromosome analysis and as sensitive as FISH *(15)*. Thus, PRINS can be a viable and effective alternative to FISH for molecular cytogenetic diagnosis.

## 2. Materials
### 2.1. Preparation of Metaphase Chromosomes from Lymphocytes

1. RPMI-1640 culture media (Gibco-BRL, Grand Island, NY; store at 4°C until expiration date on the bottle). Prepare culture medium by adding 77 mL of RPMI culture media, 20 mL of fetal calf serum (Gibco-BRL; store at –20°C until expiration date), 1 mL of L-glutamine (200 m*M*; aliquot 1–2 mL into small tubes (JRH Biosciences, Lenexa, KS; store at –20°C until expiration date), 1 mL of Gentamycin sulfate (aliquot 1–2 mL into

From: *Methods in Molecular Medicine, Vol. 39: Ovarian Cancer: Methods and Protocols*
Edited by: J. M. S. Bartlett © Humana Press, Inc., Totowa, NJ

small tubes; Irvine Scientific, Santa Ana, CA; store at 15–20°C until expiration date), and 1 mL of penicillin/streptomycin (10,000 U/mL and 10 mG/mL respectively; aliquot 1–2 mL into small tubes [Gibco-BRL]; store at –20°C until expiration date). Store this reconstituted media at 4°C up to 1 mo (*see* **Note 1**).

2. Phytohemagglutinin—reconstitute with 5 mL of distilled water (Murex Diagnostics, Dartford, UK); store at 4°C up to 1 wk (*see* **Note 2**).

3. Thioglycollate medium (Sigma, St. Louis, MO). Prepare the medium by adding 29.8 g of powder media to 1 L of sterile distilled water. Dissolve the media by boiling with occasional stirring. Dispense 10 mL into sterile tubes, and autoclave at 121°C for 15 min. Cool and store at 4°C until expiration date.

4. Colcemid (10 μg/mL in distilled water; Sigma; store at 4°C up to 1 mo).

5. Hypotonic solution (0.075$M$ KCl—prepare in distilled water, store at room temperature up to 1 wk).

6. Fixative (3:1 Methanol: Glacial acetic acid; prepare fresh each day).

## 2.2. Preparation of Slides for PRINS Reaction

1. Deionized Formamide (Sigma) (store at 4°C up to 6 mo). Prepare denaturation solution (70% formamide/2X SSC) by adding 28 mL of deionized formamide; 8 mL of distilled water, and 4 mL of 20X SSC solution. Adjust the pH to 7.0. Prepare once a week and store at room temperature.

2. 20X SSC: 3$M$ NaCl, 0.3$M$ trisodium citrate, pH 7.5 (store at room temperature up to 6 mo).

## 2.3. PRINS Reaction

1. Nucleotide mixture (dNTP mix). Prepare the nucleotide mixture by adding equal volumes (e.g., 10 μL each) of dATP (2′-Deoxyadenosine 5′-triphosphate; 10 m$M$; Perkin-Elmer, Norwalk, CT; store at –20°C), dCTP (2′-Deoxycytidine 5′-triphosphate; 10 m$M$; Perkin-Elmer; store at –20°C), dGTP (2′-Deoxyguanosine 5′-triphosphate; 10 m$M$; Perkin-Elmer; store at –20°C) and dTTP (2′-Deoxythymidine 5′-triphosphate; 10 m$M$; Perkin-Elmer; store at –20°C; dilute 1:10 with distilled water). Mix thoroughly and store at –20°C for up to 2 mo.

2. Reaction mixture (prepare fresh each time). Prepare PRINS reaction mixture by adding the following (numbers in the parenthesis indicate end concentration):
   a. Oligonucleotide primer (100–200 pmol)
      Research Genetics, Huntsville, AL; store at –20°C (*see* **Note 3** and **Table 1**).      1 μL
   b. dNTP mixture (0.2 m$M$ of each dATP, dCTP, dGTP, and 0.02 m$M$ dTTP).      4 μL
   c. dig-11-dUTP (0.02 m$M$) 1 m$M$
      Boehringer-Mannheim, Indianapolis, IN; store at –20°C (*see* **Notes 4** and **5**).      1 μL
   d. PCR Buffer (10 m$M$ Tris-HCl, pH 8.3; 50 m$M$ KCl) 10X
      Perkin-Elmer; store at –20°C.      5 μL
   e. Magnesium chloride (1.5 m$M$) 25 m$M$
      Perkin-Elmer; store at –20°C (*see* **Note 6**).      3 μL
   f. AmpliTaq DNA polymerase (2.5 U) 5 U/ μL
      Perkin-Elmer; store at –20°C.      0.5 μL
   g. Bovine Serum Albumin (0.01%) 0.5% in distilled water
      Sigma (98%) store at –20°C.      1 μL
   h. Distilled water (to make up the volume to 50 μL)      34.5 μL

3. Stop buffer: 500 m$M$ NaCl, 50 m$M$ EDTA, pH 8.0 (store at room temperature up to 6 mo).

**Table 1**
**Primer Sequences and Annealing Temperatures** [a]

| Chromosome | Locus | Sequence | Annealing Temperature (°C) |
|---|---|---|---|
| 1 | α sat | 5′ ATTCCATTAGATGATGACCCCTTTCAT 3′ | 61 |
| 2 | α sat | 5′ CTGTTCAACACTGTGACTTCAATTG 3′ | 71 |
| 3 | α sat | 5′ TGAGTTGAACACACACGTAC 3′ | 68 |
| 5 | α sat | 5′ TTCTGTCTAGCCTTACAGGAAAAAAA 3′ | 70 |
| 7 | α sat | 5′ AGCGATTTGAGGACAATTGC 3′ | 56 |
| 8 | α sat | 5′ CAAACTGCTCTATCAATAGAAATGTTCAGCACACTT 3′ | 67 |
| 9 | α sat | 5′ AATCAACCCGAGTGCAATC 3′ | 56 |
| 10 | α sat | 5′ ACTGGAACGGACAGATGACAAAGC 3′ | 63 |
| 11 | α sat | 5′ GAGGGGTTTCAGAGCTGCTC 3′ | 65 |
| 12 | α sat | 5′ GTTCAATTCACAGAGTAT 3′ | 62 |
| 13 | α sat | 5′ TGATGTGTGTACCCAGCT 3′ | 60 |
| 16 | α sat | 5′ TTCTTTTCATACCGCATTCT 3′ | 53 |
| 17 | α sat | 5′ AATTTCAGCTGACTAAACA 3′ | 50 |
| 18 | α sat | 5′ ATGTGTGTCCTCAACTAAAG 3′ | 65 |
| 21 | α sat | 5′ TGATGTGTGTACCCAGCC 3′ | 61 |
| X | α sat | 5′ GTTCAGCTCTGTGAGTGAAA 3′ | 68 |
| Y | α sat | 5′ TCCATTCGATTCCATTTTTTTCGAGAA 3′ | 60 |

[a] Source of primer sequences: Pellestor et al. (personal communication).

### 2.4. Signal Detection

1. 1,4-diazabicyclo [2.2.2.] octane (DABCO): 2.5 g dissolved in 10 mL of distilled water and add 90 mL of glycerol and mix well (Sigma); store at 4°C up to 1 yr. **Warning: DABCO is fatal if inhaled and harmful on contact. Wearing gloves and goggles prepare reagent in hood.**
2. Wash buffer: 4X SSC, pH 7.0, 0.05% Tween-20 (Boehringer-Mannheim); store at room temperature up to 6 mo.
3. Blocking buffer: 4X SSC, pH 7.0, 0.05% Tween-20 with 5% nonfat dry milk (prepare fresh every time).

## 3. Methods
### 3.1. Preparation of Metaphase Chromosomes from Lymphocytes

1. Set up lymphocyte cultures in graduated centrifuge tubes by adding 1 mL of peripheral blood to 9 mL of reconstituted culture media, 0.15 mL of Phytohemagglutinin in a centrifuge tube. Mix well and incubate in an incubator at 37°C for 72 h.
2. At the end of 72 h, add 0.02 mL of colcemid solution to each tube, mix well and incubate at 37°C for an additional 20 min.
3. Centrifuge the tubes at 170*g* for 10 min.
4. Remove the supernatant, vortex gently to mix the cell pellet, and very slowly add 8–9 mL of hypotonic solution. Invert the tubes 5–6 times to mix well and incubate at 37°C for 20 min.
5. Add 1 mL of fixative very slowly to the tubes and mix well (*see* **Note 7**).
6. Centrifuge the tubes at 170*g* for 10 min.

7. Remove the supernatant, vortex gently to mix the cell pellet and slowly add 8–9 mL of fixative. Invert the tubes 5–6 times to mix well and incubate at room temperature for 10 min.
8. Centrifuge the tubes at 170g for 10 min.
9. Repeat **steps 7** and **8** two more times.
10. After the second centrifugation, remove all but 0.5 mL of supernatant and add 1–2 mL of fresh fixative and tap the tubes gently to mix the cell pellet.
11. Using a glass Pasteur pipet, drop 3–4 drops of the cell pellet solution onto a precleaned and chilled glass microscope slide from a height of about 3–4 ft to obtain better spreading of the metaphase chromosomes . Dry the slides on a hot plate set at 65°C up to 10–15 min.

### 3.2. Preparation of Slides for PRINS Reaction

1. Prepare metaphase chromosomes using the above technique (*see* **Note 8**).
2. Immediately before PRINS reaction, denature the slides in 70% deionized Formamide, 2X SSC at 70°C for 3 min in a water bath.
3. Dehydrate the slides in chilled (4°C) ethanol series (70, 80, 90%, and absolute) for 2 min in each and allow the slides to air-dry.

### 3.3. PRINS Reaction

1. Turn on the PCR machine fitted with a flat plate block (*see* **Note 9**) and set the program for appropriate temperature (*see* **Note 10**). The PRINS reaction consists of two steps:
   a. An initial annealing step of 15 min is specific to each primer, (e.g., for chromosome 18 the annealing temperature is set at 65°C) (**Table 1**).
      During this step, the denatured slide and a glass cover slip are heated to the specific annealing temperature (65°C for chromosome 18) for 5 min. Following the preheating, PRINS reaction mix is placed on the slide and spread evenly by placing a glass cover slip on the slide. Avoid air bubbles when placing the cover slip (22 × 50 mm). The primer in the reaction mix is allowed to anneal to the target DNA sequence on the slide for 10 min at the same temperature.
   b. The second step involves a 30-min primer extension. During this step, the temperature of the hot plate is automatically raised to 72°C to facilitate primer extension. Irrespective of the primer used, the primer extension temperature is always 72°C (*see* **Note 11**).
2. Immediately following the primer extension, transfer the slide into a coplin jar containing 50 mL of stop buffer at 72°C in a water bath for 5 min to stop the reaction.

### 3.4. Signal Detection

1. Wash the slides in wash buffer at room temperature for 5 min (*see* **Note 12**).
2. Drain the slides and apply 60 µL of fluorescein-labeled antidigoxigenin Fab fragment (20 µg/mL; from sheep; Boehringer-Mannheim; store at –20°C) in blocking buffer. Place a plastic cover slip (22 × 60 mm; Oncor, Inc., MD) without air bubbles and incubate at 37°C in a humid chamber for 20 min.
3. Carefully remove the cover slip and wash the slides three times in 50 mL of wash buffer at room temperature for 3 min each time with occasional agitation.
4. Drain the excess fluid without letting the slides dry. Apply 20 µL of counterstain propidium iodide (0.25 µg/mL in DABCO; Sigma). Place a 22 × 60 mm glass cover slip carefully without air bubbles. Place the slide under a paper towel and gently squeeze the paper towel to drain excess counterstain from the slide.
5. Examine the slide under a fluorescence microscope equipped with appropriate filters (e.g., FITC, Propidium Iodide, DAPI, and so on). (*See* **Note 13** and **Figs. 1** and **2**.)

Fig. 1. Metaphase plate from a patient with a marker chromosome. PRINS was carried out with primer for chromosome 13. Arrows point to normal chromosomes 13 and the arrowhead points to marker chromosome.

Fig. 2. Metaphase plate from a patient with a marker chromosome. PRINS was carried out with primer for chromosome 18. Arrows point to normal chromosomes 18 and the arrowhead points to marker chromosome.

## 4. Notes

1. After reconstituting the culture media, check the media for contamination by placing 1 mL of the reconstituted media into Thioglycollate culture tubes. Incubate the tubes at 37°C up to 96 h. Check the tubes for microbial growth periodically every 24 h. If growth is observed, discard the media and reconstitute media fresh.

2. After reconstituting check the phytohemagglutinin solution every day for turbidity. If the solution becomes turbid, discard immediately as it is contaminated.

3. Most of the oligonucleotide primers are targeted at the alpha satellite repeat monomers of the human centromeres and are selected based on the maximum divergence among the human chromosomes *(14)*. Most of these primers are available from Research Genetics, Huntsville, AL, however, one can synthesize the primers. The primers need to be ultra purified for optimum results, hence it is necessary to gel purify the primers after synthesis. The primer sequences and annealing temperatures are given in **Table 1**. All the primer sequences are courtesy of Dr. Franck Pellestor, CNRS, Montepellier, France.

4. Biotin-11-dUTP or Biotin-16-dUTP can also be incorporated into the synthesized product instead of digoxigenin-11-dUTP and can be detected with fluorescein-labeled avidin. One can also use direct-labeled nucleotides such as fluorescein dUTP, etc. Usage of direct labeled nucleotides eliminates the detection steps thereby reducing the time further. However, in our experience, we noticed that the signals are stronger with digoxigenin-11-dUTP in comparison to other labeled nucleotides.

5. If the signals appear too strong, the concentration of the digoxigenin-dUTP can be further reduced.

6. The annealing temperatures and the concentration of magnesium chloride should be optimized for each primer using regular PCR method. The annealing temperature may vary slightly from the regular PCR. In order to measure the accurate concentration of magnesium chloride, an optimization kit such as Opti-Primer PCR Kit (Stratagene, La Jolla, CA) is useful.

7. This step (conditional fix) is very critical in the culture harvest method. Before adding the fixative, make sure the cell pellet is completely dissolved. Add the 1 mL of fix very slowly in order to achieve good fixation and better spreading of the metaphases.

8. In our experience, we noticed that when the slides are prepared fresh, the results are better, with absolutely no background. Even though aged slides also work with this procedure, the background appears to increase with aging. It is better to drop the slides a few hours before starting PRINS reaction. Storage of pellets in fixative is the preferred option in our laboratory.

9. PRINS reactions can be carried out using water baths set at two different temperatures for annealing and extension. However, for optimum results, it is necessary to use a programmable thermocycler equipped with flat plate block. There are several advantages of such a machine, including accurate temperature control with 0.1°C precision, and ease of programming temperature changes.

10. For each of the primers listed in **Table 1**, the annealing temperatures are calculated based on the melting temperatures, but the optimal annealing temperatures are determined empirically, thus resulting in slight variation between the theoretical melting temperatures and the recommended annealing temperatures. Each laboratory should determine the annealing temperatures empirically starting with the recommended temperature. There may be a slight variation of up to +5°C to –5°C from laboratory to laboratory.

11. Depending on the target chromosome, the duration of annealing and extension can be shortened. For example, for chromosomes that are rich in alpha satellite sequences like chromosome 18, the annealing can be as short as 5 min and extension can be as short as 5 min.

12. Slides can be stored in wash buffer up to 1 wk at 4°C, if required. For shorter duration like a few hours, slides can be stored in wash buffer at room temperature.

13. In our experience, we noticed that placing the slides in refrigerator after counterstaining for a few minutes to up to 1 hr improves the overall intensity of counterstain, as well as signal fluorescence.

## Acknowledgments

The author wishes to express his sincere gratitude to Dr. Franck Pellestor for his continued support and assistance without which this manuscript would not have been possible. The author is also thankful to Ms. Paula Martens for help and critical reading, Dr. Avirachan T. Tharapel for continued support, and helpful comments and discussion during the preparation of this manuscript.

## References

1. Koch, J., Kolvarra, S., Gregersen, N., Petersen, K. B., and Bolund, L. (1989) Oligonucleotide priming methods for the chromosome-specific labeling of alpha satellite DNA in situ. *Chromosoma* **98,** 259–265.
2. Bachvarov, D. R., Markov, G. G., and Ivanov, I. G. (1987) Sequence heterogeneity of the human alphoid satellite DNA and thermal stability of mismatched alphoid DNA duplexes. *Int. J. Biochem.* **19,** 963–971.
3. Koch, J., Kolvraa, S., Gregersen, N., Petersen, K. B., and Bolund, L. (1988) PRINS and PAL—two new techniques for the visualization of specific DNA sequences. *Genome* **30,** 446.
4. Koch, J., Hindkjaer, J., Mogensen, J., Kolvraa, S., and Bolund, L. (1991) An improved method for chromosome-specific labelling of satellite DNA in situ by using denatured double-stranded DNA probes as primers in a primed in situ labelling (PRINS) procedure. *GATA* **8,** 171–178.
5. Gosden, J. and Lawson, D. (1994) Rapid chromosome identification by oligonucleotide-primed in situ DNA synthesis (PRINS). *Hum. Molec. Genet.* **3,** 931–936.
6. Pellestor, F., Girardet, A., Lefort, G., Andreo, B., and Charlieu, J. P. (1994) A polymorphic alpha satellite sequence specific for human chromosome 13 detected by oligonucleotide primed *in situ* labelling (PRINS). *Hum. Genet.* **94,** 346–348.
7. Gosden, J. and Hanratty, D. (1993) PCR in situ: A rapid alternative to in situ hybridization for mapping short, low copy number sequences without isotopes. *Biotechniques* **15,** 78–80.
8. Gosden, J. and Lawson, D. (1995) Instant PRINS: A rapid method for chromosome identification by detecting repeated sequences in situ. *Cytogenet. Cell Genet.* **68,** 57–60.
9. Hindkjaer, J., Koch, J., Terkelsen, C., Brandt, C. A., Kolvraa, S., and Bolund, L. (1994) Fast, sensitive multicolor detection of nucleic acids in situ by primed in situ labelling (PRINS). *Cytogenet. Cell Genet.* **66,** 152–154.
10. Velagaleti, G. V. N., Tharapel, S. A., Martens, P. R., and Tharapel, A. T. (1997) Rapid identification of marker chromosomes using primed in situ labelling (PRINS). *Am. J. Med. Genet.* **71,** 130–133.
11. Velagaleti, G. V. N., Carpenter, N. J., and Tharapel, A. T. (1997) Clinical applications of primed in situ labelling (PRINS): rapid identification of a marker chromosomes in a fetus. *Ann. Genet.* **40,** 154–157.
12. Velagaleti, G. V. N., Phillips, O. P., Tharapel, S. A., Tharapel, A. T., and Shulman, L. P. (1998) Rapid assessment of aneuploidy in prenatal samples. *Am. J. Obstet. Gynecol.*, **178,** 1313–1320.
13. Speel, E. J. M., Lawson, D., Ramaekers, F. C. S., Gosden, J. R., and Hopman, A. H. N. (1996) Rapid bright-field detection of oligonucleotide primed in situ (PRINS)-labelled DNA in chromosome preparations and frozen tissue sections. *BioTechniques* **20,** 226–234.
14. Pellestor, F. and Charlieu, J. P. (1996) Analysis of sperm aneuploidy by PRINS, in *Methods in Molecular Biology* (Gosden, J. R., ed.), Humana, Totowa, NJ, pp. 23–29.
15. Velagaleti, G. V. N., Tharapel, S. A., and Tharapel, A. T. (1999) Validation of primed in situ labelling (PRINS) for interphase analysis. Comparative studies with conventional FISH and chromosome analyses. *Cancer Genet. Cyto Genet.*, **108,** 100–106.

# 26

# Gene Amplification of *c-erbB-2* Detected by FISH

**S. Robert Young, Wei-Hua Liu, and Zong-Ren Wang**

## 1. Introduction

In 1981, a novel transforming gene called *neu*, related to, but distinct from, the *c-erbB* protooncogene, was identified *(1–3)*. In 1985, two groups independently isolated identical *erbB*-related genes from human DNA that they called *HER*-2 *(4)* and *c-erbB-2 (5)* located at chromosome band *17q11.2* and encoding a 185,000 Dalton tyrosine kinase *(2,4)*. Studies conducted on human breast cancers showed 28% to have amplified *HER2/neu* present *(7)* and it was suggested that amplification or increased protein expression might confer a selective advantage *(6)*. Over the last ten years, many studies have confirmed the value of using overexpression or amplification of the *HER2/neu* gene as a predictor of poor outcome in cases of breast cancer *(7–9)*. Clinical trials are currently underway using anti-*HER2/neu* in an attempt to destroy malignant breast cells *(10,11)*.

Overexpression of the *HER2/neu* protein is generally studied using immunohistochemical techniques. However, there is considerable variability in the sensitivity of *HER2/neu* antibody preparations *(12,13)*. Amplification of the *HER2/neu* gene is usually studied by Southern blot or quantitative polymerase chain reaction (PCR). Although specific and reproducible, both study the product of many cells at the same time. Because most malignant tissue samples are contaminated with normal cells, and cancer cells are highly heterogeneous, the results are unreliable.

Fluorescence *in situ* hybridization (FISH) makes use of a highly specific interaction between two single strands of denatured DNA: the probe under study and any complementary target sequences within the cell. A variety of cell samples can be studied; cells can be disaggregated, washed, and fixed. This method gives the cleanest, easiest way to score preparations; however, the tissue architecture is lost. Cell preparations can be made by merely touching the tissue to a microscope slide. This method produces a sample with some tissue architecture, but there is an uneven layer of cells on the slide. Tissue sections can be cut from frozen or paraffin-embedded blocks. Because many cells are dissected, these samples are harder to score, but tissue integrity is preserved. The ability to use paraffin-embedded samples allows FISH to be carried out on valuable, archived material. We have successfully studied ovarian cancer tissue blocks that were 15 yr old and had not been stored under any special conditions. The methods described can be used to study virtually any DNA probe and any type of tissue.

From: *Methods in Molecular Medicine, Vol. 39: Ovarian Cancer: Methods and Protocols*
Edited by: J. M. S. Bartlett © Humana Press, Inc., Totowa, NJ

## 2. Materials

Solutions, glassware, and plasticware should be sterile.

### 2.1. Preparation of Samples

#### 2.1.1. Touch Slide Preparation for Interphase Cell Analysis

1. Hanks balanced salt solution (HBSS).
2. Fixative: Methanol:glacial acetic acid (3:1).

#### 2.1.2. Disaggregated Cell Preparation for Metaphase and Interphase Analysis

1. Culture medium: 100 mL RPMI-1640, 20 mL heat inactivated fetal bovine serum (FBS), 1 mL L-glutamine (200 m$M$), 1 mL 10,000 U/mL penicillin, and 10,000 μg/mL streptomycin solution.
2. Collagenase IA (250–300 U/mL in RPMI-1640 medium) (Sigma, St. Louis, MO).
3. Trypsin-EDTA (0.25% Trypsin, 1 m$M$ EDTA): 2.5 g Trypsin, and 0.38 g EDTA.4Na/L in HBBS without Ca$^{++}$ and Mg$^{++}$.
4. 10 μg/mL KaryoMAX Colcemid Solution (Gibco, BRL, Gaithersburg, MD).
5. Hypotonic solution: 0.075$M$ KCl (5.59 g/L of distilled H$_2$O).

#### 2.1.3. Preparation of Paraffin-Embedded Tissue and Pretreating Slides

1. Hemo-De clearing agent (Fisher Scientific, Pittsburgh, PA).
2. 0.2 $N$ hydrochloric acid (HCl).
3. Protease solution: add 160 mg of powdered pepsin in prewarmed 40 mL of 0.9% NaCl, pH 2.0, at 37°C to a final concentration 4 mg/mL or 1200 U/mL (made fresh daily).
4. 1.0$M$ NaSCN solution: 81.07 g sodium thiocyanate in H$_2$O.
5. 2X SSC, pH 7.4 wash buffer: 3$M$ sodium chloride, 1$M$ sodium citrate.

### 2.2. Hybridization Reagents

#### 2.2.1. Denaturing and Hybridization

Probes (either direct or indirect labeled probes maybe used). Obtain from commercial manufacturer such as Vysis, Inc., Downers Grove, IL, or Oncor, Inc., Gaithersburg, MD.

1. *HER2/neu* (ERBB-2) DNA probe (*17q11.2-q12*).
2. Chromosome 17 alpha-satellite probe.
3. 70% Formamide/2X SSC, pH 7.0.
4. Hybridization buffer: 4X SSC, 20% Dextran sulfate.
5. 70, 85, and 100% ice-cold ethanol.

#### 2.2.2. Postwashes and Signal Detection

1. 50% Formamide in 2X SSC, pH 7.0.
2. 2X SSC, pH 7.0.
3. 2X × SSC/0.1% NP-40.
4. Avidin-FITC (Oncor).
5. Antidigoxigenin-rhodamine (Boehringer or Oncor).
6. 4X SSC/0.1% Tween-20, pH 7.0.
7. 4′,6-Diamidino-2 phenylindole dihydrochloride (DAPI)/antifade solution (150 ng/mL or 600 ng/mL).
8. 1X PBD: 120 m$M$ sodium chloride, 2.7 m$M$ potassium chloride, 0.05% Tween-20.

## 3. Methods

### 3.1. Preparation of the Specimen

In the operating room or pathology laboratory, tumor material (15–50 g) is placed in sterile Hanks balanced salt solution (HBSS) or isotonic saline and maintained at room temperature. The tumor is then transported to the cytogenetics laboratory where, in a laminar flow hood, it is transferred to a Petri dish containing a small amount of sterile HBSS or culture medium.

### 3.1.1. Touch Slides

1. With sterile forceps, remove tissue from the Petri dish and cut off a small piece with a sterile blade. With forceps, take the tissue piece, blot off excess solution, and apply gently to areas on treated slides (*see* **Note 1**). Try to roll the tissue so that large clumps of tissue are not deposited onto the slide. The cells transferred to the slide should barely be visible.
2. Air-dry for a few minutes.
3. Fix the cells for 20 min in methanol : glacial acetic acid fixative.
4. Transfer slides to fresh fixative for an additional 20 min.
5. Air-dry slides.

### 3.1.2. Disaggregated Cells

1. Under sterile conditions, mince a portion of the tissue sample in a small Petri dish (35 or 60 mm) into pieces small enough to pass into a Pasteur pipet.
2. The minced tissue pieces are then treated with 1–2 mL of either trypsin/EDTA 1 h, or collagenase Ia for 4–16 h, at 37°C for disaggregation.
3. Transfer the disaggregated cells to a sterile 15-mL plastic centrifuge tube containing about 10 mL of sterile HBSS. Allow any remaining tissue pieces to settle to the bottom for a few minutes and transfer the cell rich upper solution to a fresh sterile centrifuge tube.
4. Wash cells twice in HBSS by centrifugation at 400$g$ for 10 min, discard supernatant each time.
5. Resuspend cells in 2.0 mL HBSS for interphase (**Subheading 3.1.2., step 1**) and/or metaphase (**Subheading 3.1.2., step 2**) studies.

#### 3.1.2.1. INTERPHASE

1. Spin down 1 mL of disaggregated cells at 400$g$ for 10 min.
2. Discard supernatant and resuspend in 10 mL of hypotonic solution for 15 min.
3. Spin down cells, discard supernatant, and resuspend in 5 mL methanol : glacial acetic acid (3:1) fixative.
4. After 15 min repeat **step 3**.
5. After an additional 15 min, spin down the cells, discard the supernatant, and resuspend the cells in about 1 mL of fresh fixative.
6. Place one drop of the suspended cells onto a treated glass slide and allow it to dry.
7. Check the cell density on the slide using phase contrast microscope and adjust cell concentration if needed. The cells should be spread apart, but not so far apart as to make study difficult.

#### 3.1.2.2. METAPHASE

1. Place several drops of the disaggregated cells (from **Subheading 3.1.2.**) into a sterile T25 culture flask and add 5.0 mL of culture medium. Final concentration of cells should be approximately $10^6$ cells/5mL
2. Incubate at 37°C in a humidified, 5% $CO_2$ incubator for 48–96 h.

3. To begin harvest, add Colcemid to a concentration of 0.01 µg/mL. Continue culturing for 1–4 h at 37°C.
4. Take off the culture medium and place in a 15-mL plastic centrifuge tube. Put 1.0 mL of 0.25% trypsin/EDTA into culture flask and incubate at 37°C for 5–10 min.
5. Take off the trypsin/EDTA and detached cells and place in the plastic centrifuge tube.
6. Centrifuge the cells at 400*g* for 5 min and discard the supernatant.
7. Gently resuspend pelleted cells in 5–7 mL of hypotonic solution. After 15 min, the cells are centrifuged at 400*g* for 5 min and the supernatant is discarded.
8. The pelleted cells are slowly resuspended in methanol:glacial acetic acid fixative to a total volume of 10 mL for 20 min.
9. Repeat **step 8**.
10. The cells are then resuspended in about 1.0 mL of fresh fixative and one drop is dropped on cold (4°C) wet slides. Blowing gently on the freshly dropped slides sometimes improves metaphase chromosome spreading.

### 3.1.3. Paraffin Slides

#### 3.1.3.1. SAMPLE PREPARATION

1. Cut 5 µm paraffin sections using a microtome.
2. Float the sections on a protein-free (triple distilled) water bath at 40°C.
3. Mount a tissue section in the center of a treated slide (*see* **Note 1**).
4. Air-dry the slides and bake overnight at 56°C.

#### 3.1.3.2. PRETREATMENT OF PARAFFIN SLIDES

1. Immerse slides in Hemo-De clearing agent (Fisher Scientific) for 10 min at room temperature three times.
2. Dehydrate slides in 100% EtOH for 5 min twice at room temperature.
3. Air-dry slides.
4. Put slides in 0.2 *N* HCl for 20 min.
5. Put slides in distilled water for 3 min.
6. Put slides in 2X SSC for 3 min.
7. Put slides in 1.0*M* sodium thiocyanate solution at 81°C for 20 min.
8. Put slides in distilled water for 1 min.
9. Put slides in 2X SSC for 3 min two times.
10. Put slides in protease solution at 37°C for 10 min.
11. Inactivate pepsin by rinsing slides in 2X SSC for 5 min twice.
12. Dry slides on a 45°C slide warmer for 5 min.
13. Immerse slides in the 10% Formalin for 10 min at room temperature.
14. Rinse slides in 2X SSC for 5 min twice.
15. Dry slides on a 45°C slide warmer for 5 min.

### 3.2. FISH Summary and Principle

FISH involves the precise annealing of a single-stranded DNA probe to a complementary target DNA sequence. The hybridization of the probe with the cellular DNA site is visualized by fluorescence microscopy using a probe either indirectly or directly labeled with a fluorophore.

### 3.2.1. Probe Preparation and Denaturation

Because it is certainly possible to make and label your own probes for FISH studies, we have found it very convenient to purchase commercially prepared probes. High-quality direct- and indirect-labeled probes are available from a number of manufacturers. A direct-labeled probe has the fluorochrome already attached to it. An indirect-labeled probe has a hapten (e.g., biotin or digoxigenin) attached to it. After hybridization has taken place, fluorochrome-labeled antibodies to the hapten are used for probe detection. The amount of probe and hybridization buffer needed depends on the target area to be studied. For studying a 22 × 22-mm coverslip area, you need 10 μL of probe mixture. For a 22 × 40-mm coverslip area, 20 μL of probe mixture is needed.

### 3.2.1.1. INDIRECT LABELING PROBE (SUCH AS THAT FROM ONCOR, INC.)

1. Prewarm vial chromosome 17 α satellite (biotin labeled) probe at 37°C for 5 min.
2. Vortex and centrifuge for 2–3 s.
3. If area to study is 22 × 22 mm, add 0.5 μL of chromosome 17 α satellite probe to 5 μL of hybridization buffer in a microcentrifuge tube. Increase this amount for as many slides as you are going to study.
4. Vortex and centrifuge 2–3 s.
5. Denature the probe at 73°C for 5 min. Immediately put in ice bath until use.
6. The *HER2/neu* (digoxigenin labeled) probe is already denatured. Take 5.0 μL of prewarmed *HER2/neu* probe and 5.5 μL of denatured chromosome 17 α satellite probe and mix well by vortex. Centrifuge for a few seconds. Proceed with hybridization (*see* **Subheading 3.2.3.**).

### 3.2.1.2. DIRECT LABELING PROBE (SUCH AS THAT FROM VYSIS, INC.)

1. Prewarm *HER2/neu* (Spectrum Orange labeled) and chromosome 17 α satellite (Spectrum Green labeled) probes at 37°C for 5 min. These probes can sometimes be purchased premixed.
2. Vortex and centrifuge 2–3 s.
3. If the study area is 22 × 22 mm, add 0.5 μL *HER2/neu* probe, 0.5 μL chromosome #17 α satellite probe, 2 μL purified $H_2O$, and 7 μL LSI hybridization buffer to a microcentrifuge tube and mix (according to Vysis, Inc., directions). Increase this amount for as many slides as you are going to study.
4. Vortex and centrifuge 2–3 s.
5. Denature probe mixture in a 73 ± 1°C waterbath for 5 min.
6. Place tube in a 45°C water bath until ready to apply probe to target DNA (*see* **Subheading 3.2.3.**).

## 3.2.2. Slide Denaturation for FISH

1. Place specimen slides in 70% formamide/2X SSC, pH 7.0, at 73 ± 1°C for 4 min.
2. Dehydrate specimen slides in a series of 1 min ice-cold EtOH washes (70, 85, 100%) to maintain the denatured state in the specimen.
3. Dry slides by touching the bottom edge of the slides to a paper towel and wipe the underside of the slides dry.
4. Place slides on a 45–50°C slide warmer to evaporate remaining EtOH.

## 3.2.3. Hybridizing

1. Apply 10 μL of probe mixture to target area on each slide and cover with a 22 × 22 mm glass coverslip. (Or apply 20 μL of probe mix and cover with a 22 × 40 mm glass coverslip.)
2. Seal coverslip with rubber cement.
3. Incubate slides at 37°C for 12–16 h in a prewarmed humidified chamber. To prevent drying of the slides, it may prove best to support the slides over damp paper towels in a sealed small plastic box placed in an incubator or humidified incubator.

### 3.2.4. Posthybridization Wash

1. Prewarm three glass Coplin jars containing 40 mL of 50% formamide/2X SSC pH7.0, in a 45°C water bath for 30 min.
2. Prewarm 40 mL of 2X SSC and 40 mL of 2X SSC/0.1% NP-40 in two glass Coplin jars in a 37°C water bath for 30 min.
3. Carefully remove the rubber cement from the cover slips and place the slides in the 50% formamide/2X SSC. Agitate lightly for a few seconds and the cover slips should come free from the slides. If the cover slips do not float free, carefully remove cover slip from the slide.
4. After 5 min, pass the slides to the second 50% formamide/2X SSC Coplin jar for an additional 5 min.
5. Pass slides to third Coplin jar for 5 min.
6. Immerse slides in Coplin jar containing warm 2X SSC. Agitate slides for 1–3 s. Remove slides after 2 min.
7. Immerse slides in Coplin jar containing 2X SSC/0.1% NP-40 for 5 min.
8. Put slides in 1X PBD. Slides can be kept in 1X PBD at room temperature for several minutes or in the refrigerator for several days.

### 3.2.5. Detection and Counterstaining

#### 3.2.5.1. DETECTION OF INDIRECT LABELING PROBES

1. Place 15 µL of Fluorescein-labeled Avidin and 15 µL of Rhodamine-labeled Anti-Digoxigenin into a microcentrifuge tube. Mix and vortex.
2. Remove the slide from 1X PBD (*see* **Subheading 3.2.4., steps 1–8**) and blot excess fluid from the edge.
3. Apply the 30 µL mixed detection reagent to the slide and cover with a plastic cover slip. There is no need to attempt to seal this cover slip.
4. Incubate the slide at 37°C for 5–20 min in a prewarmed humidified chamber.
5. Carefully remove the plastic coverslip and immerse the slide in 40 mL of 4X SSC/0.1% Tween-20 for 2 min at room temperature, three times.

#### 3.2.5.2. FLUORESCENCE COUNTERSTAINING

1. Remove slide from the 4X × SSC/0.1% Tween-20 and blot the excess fluid from the edge.
2. Apply 10 µL DAPI/antifade counterstain to the target area of slide and apply a 22 × 22-mm glass cover slip (20 µL if using a 22 × 40-mm cover slip).
3. Carefully press out air bubbles and take off excess DAPI/ antifade with a paper towel.
4. Seal cover slip with rubber cement.
5. It is best to analyze slides immediately, but the slides can be stored at –20°C in the dark. If the signal is strong it may be visible for several months.

## 3.3. Score FISH Results

Slides may be viewed using a epifluorescence ultraviolet (UV)-equipped microscope and a triple bandpass filter unit (*see* **Notes**). There is no single accepted method of scoring FISH studies at the present time. Several investigators *(14,15)* have used the method outlined here. **Figure 1** graphically describes the scoring procedure. **Figure 2** shows examples of *HER2/neu* and chromosome 17 α satellite dual color FISH. Photographs were taken with Kodak Ektachrome 400 film and a Zeiss MC 100 Autoexposure Camera. Exposure times varied from about 30 to 120 s. These photographs were not enhanced in any way.

Do not count these cells with overlapping nuclei, it is difficult to tell which nucleus contains the signal.

In each of the above, score two 17 alpha centromere signals and two HER2/neu signals. A single chromosome signal can often appear as two (presumably when the cell is in G2).

Score these cells as having a decreased HER2/neu signal.

Score as HER2/neu signal amplification; diffuse type(middle) and cluster type(right).

Fig. 1. Schematic representation of *HER2/neu* and chromosome 17 alpha satellite FISH scoring. Large circles represent nucleii, gray dots represent *HER2/neu* gene signals, and black signals are chromosome #17 centromeres.

1. Count 100–200 single, nonoverlapping, well-defined nuclei from different quadrants of the slide. This helps minimize any problem there might be from variation in hybridization efficiency or probe detection. If studying paraffin tissue samples it would be useful to compare a companion hematoxalin/eosin (H&E) stained slide to assist in selecting tumor regions to analyze.

2. Only count cells that have at least one chromosome 17 centromere (green) and/or one *HER2/neu* (red) signal to assure that there was nuclear probe penetration.

3. Record the number of *HER2/neu* and centromeric signals counted in each cell. A 2 × 2 table showing the number of oncogene and centromere copies per cell can easily be constructed.

4. It is common to report the average oncogene amplification ratio *(14,15)*. To calculate this value, the ratio of *HER2/neu* signals to centromere 17 copies was calculated for each cell in a particular sample. Then, the average of these ratios was computed to create the amplification ratio for that particular sample. A sample with an amplification ratio between 1.5 and 2.0 is considered moderately amplified, and a ratio exceeding 2.0 is highly amplified.

Fig. 2. Examples of *HER2/neu* (red) and chromosome 17 α satellite (green) dual-color FISH (Vysis, Inc., Downers Grove, IL). Photographs were taken with Kodak Ektachrome 400 film. (**A**) Normal metaphase spread with 2–#17 centromeres and 2 –*HER2/neu* oncogenes. (**B**) Ovarian cancer cell line (SKOV-3) metaphase spread. Arrow points to chromosome #17 with amplified amount of *HER2/neu*. (Cell line kindly provided by Dr. A. Berchuck, Duke University.) (**C**) Paraffin-embedded ovarian cancer tissue. Lower left cells show amplified *HER2/neu* and polysomy of 17; upper right cells with 2 copies of *HER2/neu* and disomy 17. (**D**) Two ovarian cancer cells with polysomy 17 and multiple copies of *HER2/neu*. One centromere has a small cluster of oncogene nearby.

5. An individual cell is said to be amplified if there are twice as many *HER2/neu* signals as chromosome 17 centromeres. In some samples, cells will have as many as 20–30 copies of the oncogene with the distribution being either "clustered" or "dispersed." The "clustered" pattern is generally ascribed to the presence of an HSR, whereas the "dispersed" pattern is ascribed to the presence of double minutes. The presence of even a small percentage of such cells in a tissue sample may prove to be of clinical importance.

6. Documentary photographs can be made with 400 ASA Ektachrome film.

## 4. Notes

1. You must use treated slides because the harsh solutions strip the cells/tissue away. Slides may be treated by dipping them in a saline solution of 1.0 mL 3-Aminopropyl

triethoxysilane (Sigma A 3648) and 49.0 mL of acetone, rinsing twice in distilled water, and then dried. Alternatively, many kinds of treated slides can be purchased from manufacturers.

2. Because the temperatures of the solutions and the timing are so critical, we have found it best to work with only four slides at a time. Placing more slides in a Coplin jar at one time appears to alter the temperature sufficiently enough to disturb results.

3. Because many FISH studies use propidium iodide as the counterstain, DAPI is best for dual color FISH. It may prove useful to use the more dilute DAPI when studying paraffin samples.

4. If at completion of the procedure you find no signal or a weak signal, 1) check the temperatures and pH of all solutions; 2) the denaturing temperature may be too low; 3) the hybridization temperature may be too low or the length of time too short; 4) if using paraffin samples, and the cell morphology/DAPI stain poor, fix the sample longer; or 5) the filters may be damaged or old.

5. We have found it possible to redenature and use slides that had been FISH studied before. By carefully documenting the location of previously studied cells, we have been able to study the same cells with the same or other probes.

## References

1. Shih, C., Padhy, L. C., Murray, M., and Weinberg, R. A. (1981) Transforming genes of carcinomas and neuroblasts introduced into mouse fibroblasts. *Nature* **290**, 261–264.
2. Schechter, A. L., Stern, D. F., Vaidyanathan, L., Decker, S. J., Drebin, J. A., Greene, M. I., and Weinberg, R. A. (1984) The neu oncogene: an erb-B-related gene encoding a 185,000-Mr tumor antigen. *Nature* **312**, 513–516.
3. Semba, K., Kamata, N., Toyoshima, K., and Yamamoto, T. (1985) A v-erbB-related protooncogene, c-erbB-2, is distinct from the c-erbB-1/epidermal growth factor-receptor gene and is amplified in a human salivary gland adenocarcinoma. *Proc. Natl. Acad. Sci. USA* **82**, 6497–6501.
4. Coussens, L., Yang-Feng, T. L., Liao, Y.-C., Chen, E., Gray, A., McGrath, J., et al. (1985) Tyrosine kinase receptor with extensive homology to EGF receptor shares chromosomal location with neu oncogene. *Science* **230**, 1132–1139.
5. Schechter, A. L., Hung, M-C., Vaidyanathan, L., Weinberg, R. A., Yang-Feng, T. L., Francke, U., et al. (1985) The neu gene: an erbB-homologous gene distinct from and unlinked to the gene encoding the EGF receptor. *Science* **229**, 976–978.
6. King, C. R., Kraus, M. H., and Aaronson, S. A. (1985) Amplification of a novel v-erbB-related gene in a human mammary carcinoma. *Science* **229**, 974–976.
7. Slamon, D. J., Clark, G. M., Wong, S. G., Levin, W. J., Ullrich, A., and McGuire, W. L. (1987) Human breast cancer: correlation of relapse and survival with amplification of the HER-2/neu oncogene. *Science* **235**, 177–182.
8. Paterson, M. C., Dietrich, K. D., Danyluk, J., Paterson, A. H. G., Lees, A. W., Jamil, N., et al. (1991) Correlation between c-erbB-2 amplification and risk of recurrent disease in node-negative breast cancer. *Cancer Res.* **51**, 556–567.
9. Menard, S., Casalini, P., Pilotti, S., Cascinelli, N., Rilke, F., and Colnaghi, M. I. (1996) No additive impact on patient survival of the double alteration of p53 and c-erbB-2 in breast carcinomas. *JNCI* **88**, 1002,1003.
10. Weiner, L. M., Clark, J. I., Davey, M., Li, W. S., Garcia de Palazzo, I., Ring, D. B., and Alpaugh, R. K. (1995) Phase I trial of 2B1, a bispecific monoclonal antibody targeting c-erbB-2 and Fc gamma RIII. *Cancer Res.* **55**, 4586–4593.
11. Baselga, J., Tripathy, D., Mendelsohn, J., Baughman, S., Benz, C. C., Dantis, L., et al. (1996) Phase II study of weekly intravenous recombinant humanized anti-p185HER2 monoclonal antibody in patients with HER2/neu-overexpressing metastatic breast cancer. *J. Clin. Oncol.* **14**, 737–744.
12. Press, M. F., Hung, G., Godolphin, W., and Slamon, D. J. (1994) Sensitivity of HER-2/neu antibodies in archival tissue samples: potential source of error in immunohistochemical studies of oncogene expression. *Cancer Res.* **54**, 2771–2777.
13. Busmanis, I., Feleppa, F., Jones, A., McGrath, K. M., Reed, R., Collins, J., et al. (1994) Analysis of cerbB2 expression using a panel of 6 commercially available antibodies. *Pathology* **26**, 261–267.
14. Sauter, G., Moch, H., Moore, D., Carroll, P., Chew, K., Mihatsch, M. J., et al. (1993) Heterogeneity of erbB-2 gene amplification in bladder cancer. *Cancer Res.* **54**, 2199–2203.
15. Kallioniemi, O.-P., Kallioniemi, A., Kurisu, W., Thor, A., Chen, L.-C., Smith, H. S., et al. (1992) ERBB2 amplification in breast cancer analyzed by fluorescence in situ hybridization. *Proc. Natl. Acad. Sci. USA* **89**, 130–134.

# 27

## Chromosome Microdissection for Detection of Subchromosomal Alterations by FISH

### Xin-yuan Guan and Jeffrey M. Trent

## 1. Introduction

Chromosome microdissection is a recently developed molecular cytogenetic technique that has become increasingly important as a bridge connecting cytogenetics to molecular genetics. After a decade of effort, this approach has been developed into a useful and reproducible approach for several purposes, including 1) the isolation of DNA from any cytogenetically recognizable region which can be used to generate DNA microclone libraries for molecular analysis and positional cloning (1,2); 2) the generation of fluorescence *in situ* hybridization (FISH) probes for whole chromosome painting probes (3), and chromosome arm painting probes (4) for cytogenetic study; 3) combined with FISH, microdissection has been applied to detecte virtually any kind of visible chromosome rearrangements (5,6); and more recently, 4) microdissection combined with hybrid selection has been applied to identify genes associated with homogeneously staining regions (HSRs) in human cancers (7,8).

The process of chromosome microdissection technique includes two parts: microdissection of a target chromosomal region under a microscope using a finely drawn glass needle and subsequent amplification of the dissected DNA fragments with a degerate oligonucleotide primer by polymerase chain reaction (PCR). Briefly, 5–10 copies of target chromosomeal region are microdissected with glass needle and transfered to a PCR tube containing collection solution. Microdissected DNA fragments are then treated with Topoisomerase I and amplified by PCR. FISH with labeled microdissected PCR products is then routinely used in this protocol to evaluate the experimental result.

## 2. Materials
### 2.1. Preparation of Metaphase Chromosome

1. Complete RPMI-1640 medium (100 mL) (store at 4°C): Mix 81 mL RPMI-1640 medium, 15 mL heat inactivated fetal calf serum (FCS), 1 mL glutamine (200 m$M$), 1 mL penicillin/ streptomycin (10,000 U/mL), and 2 mL phytohemagglutinin (PHA) (Murex Biotech Ltd., Dartford, England).
2. Carnoy's fixative solution: 3:1 methanol and glacial acetic acid, freshly prepared.

From: *Methods in Molecular Medicine, Vol. 39: Ovarian Cancer: Methods and Protocols*
Edited by: J. M. S. Bartlett © Humana Press, Inc., Totowa, NJ

3. 22 × 60-mm glass cover slip: The glass cover slip should be washed with detergent and stored in methanol and dried with clean tissue wiper before dropping the metaphase spreads.

4. Trypsin working solution (0.005% trypsin): Dilute 0.05% trypsin (Gibco/BRL, Gaithersburg, MD) with Hank's balanced salt solution (HBSS) without calcium and magnesium (Gibco/BRL), freshly prepared.

5. Giemsa stain working solution: Dilute 1 mL Giemsa stock solution (BDH Chemicals Ltd., Poole, England) in 50 mL 0.01$M$ sodium phosphate balance solution (pH 7.0).

## 2.2. Microdissection and Topoisomerase I Treatment

1. Microdissection glass needle: Prepare glass needle by pipet puller using glass capillary tube (1.2-mm wide and 4-in in length) from World Precision Instruments (WPI, Sarasota FL).

2. Pipet puller: Recommend the Kopf needle/pipet puller, model 750. Use the patch program to prepare fine, closed point needles. The width of the needle's point is about the width of a chromosome. Prior to use, glass needles are irradiated with UV light for 5 min (Straalinker 2400, Strategene, La Jolla CA).

3. Collection solution (50 µL): Mix 5 µL 10X Topo I buffer (40 m$M$ Tris-HCl, pH 7.5, 20 m$M$ MgCl$_2$, 50 m$M$ NaCl), 5 µL 10X dNTP (2 m$M$ each, Pharmacia LKB, Piscataway, NJ), 1 µL UN1 primer (50 µ$M$) (5'-CCGACTCGAGNNNNNNATGTGG), 1 µL Topoisomerase I (10 U/µL, Promega Corp., Madison, WI), and 38 µL dH$_2$O, prepare fresh, aliquot 5 µL each into 0.5-mL tubes and place tubes on ice.

## 2.3. Amplification of Dissected DNA

PCR reaction mixture (50 µL): Mix 5 µL 10X PCR buffer (100 m$M$ Tris-HCl, pH 8.4, 20 m$M$ MgCl$_2$, 500 m$M$ KCl, 0.1 mg/mL gelatin), 5 µL 10X dNTP (2 m$M$ each), 1 µL UN1 primer (50 µ$M$), 0.4 µL AmpliTaq LD (5 U/µL, Perkin Elmer, Norwalk, CT), and 38.6 µL dH$_2$O.

## 2.4. Fluorescent In Situ Hybridization (FISH)

1. Denaturing solution (50 mL): Mix 35 mL formamide, 5 mL 20X SSC, and 10 mL dH$_2$O thoroughly and place in a glass coplin jar. This solution can be repeatly used for several months.

2. Hybridization mixture (10 µL): Mix 7 µL hybridization buffer (70% formamide, 2X SSC, 10% dextran sulfate), 1–2 µL labeled probe (about 100 ng), 1 µL Human Cot I DNA (1 µg/µL) (Gibco/BRL), and 0–1 µL dH$_2$O.

3. PNM buffer (100 mL): Mix 95 mL 0.1$M$ sodium phosphate, 0.1 mL NP40, 20 mg sodium azide, and 5 g nonfat dry milk. Incubate the mixture in a 37°C water bath for 2 h and shake several times during the period to allow all of the milk go into the solution. Leave the solution at room temperature for 1 d, followed by spinning in a table top centrifuge at 2,000$g$ for 20 min to pellet the solids. Transfer the supernatant to another bottle and stored at 4°C until used.

# 3. Methods

## 3.1. Preparation of Metaphase Chromosome

1. Add 0.5 mL peripheral blood to 4.5 mL complete RPMI-1640 medium and culture for 64–68 h at 37°C.

2. Add 25 µL colcemid (10 µg/mL) to the culture medium and incubate at 37°C for 20 min.

3. Transfer the cells to a 15-mL centrifuge tube and centrifuge at 250$g$ for 5 min and then carefully discard the supernatant.

4. Resuspend and incubate the remaining cell pellet in 10 mL of hypotonic solution (0.075$M$ KCl) in a 37°C water bath for 18 min. Centrifuge at 250$g$ for 5 min and then remove the supernatant, leaving 0.2–0.5 mL to resuspend cell pellet.

5. Resuspend the remaining cell pellet thouroghly but gently in 8 mL freshly prepared Carnoy's fixative and place on ice for a minimum of 2 h (*see* **Note 1**). Centrifuge at 250$g$ for 5 min and then remove the supernatant carefully.

6. Wash the cells twice with 5 mL Carnoy's fixative by centrifuging at 250$g$ for 5 min.

7. Resuspend the cell pellet in 0.5–1.5 ml Carnoy's fixative to obtain a lightly opaque cell suspension before preparing slides.

8. Drop 2–3 drops of cell suspension onto a clean cover slip (22 × 60 mm) held at 45° angle, allowing the cell suspension to run down the length of the coverslip. Do not blow the slide to avoid contamination.

9. Keep the prepared coverslips in a sterile container at room temperature for 3–10 d prior to banding.

10. Standard G-banding with trypsin-Giemsa (GTG) was performed prior to microdissection (*9*). Briefly, treat the slide with trypsin working solution at room temperature for 1–2 min. Transfer the slide to Giemsa working solution for 6 min at room temperature, then rinse the slide with distilled water and air-dry (*see* **Note 2**).

All above steps should be performed under sterile conditions.

## 3.2. Microdissection and Topoisomerase I Treatment

1. Find the target chromosome under an inverted microscope fitted with a stage that can be freely rotated to allow positioning of any chromosome perpendicular to the axis along which the glass needle is moved. If possible, the microscope should reside on a massive stand to dampen out vibration.

2. Dissect the target chromosomal region with glass needles controlled by a hydraulic micro-manipulator (Narishige, Japan) attached to the inverted microscope.

3. Pick up the dissected DNA fragment with the needle by positioning the tip of the needle directly above the DNA fragment and then moving the needle down and lightly touching the fragment. The DNA fragment will be held to the tip by electrostatic forces and then is transfered into a 5 µL collection solution by touching the needle tip to the fluid.

4. After the desired number of dissected DNA fragments (5–10 copies) are collected, the collection solution is covered with a drop of mineral oil. Before the amplification of microdissected DNA, the DNA is treated with Topoisomerase I to relax the very tight DNA coiling which has been shown to dramatically enhance the recovery of sequences from dissected DNA (*10*). Incubate the collection solution containing dissected DNA fragments at 37°C for 1 h, and then terminate the reaction by heating to 96°C for 10 min.

## 3.3. Amplification of Dissected DNA

1. An initial 5–8 cycles of PCR (denaturation at 94°C for 1 min, annealing at 30°C for 2 min, and extension at 37°C for 2 min) are conducted by adding approx 0.3 U of Sequenase (US Biochemicals, Cleveland, OH) at 30°C each cycle [Sequenase (13 U/µL) is diluted 1 to 8 in enzyme dilution buffer (US Biochemicals), and 0.2 µL is added to 5 µL reaction mixture].

2. Following this preamplification step, a conventional PCR reaction catalyzed by *Taq* DNA polymerase is performed in the same tube. 50 µL PCR reaction mixture is then added and the reaction is heated to 95°C for 3 min followed by 30 cycles at 94°C for 1 min, 1 min at 56°C, 2 min at 72°C, with a 5 min final extension at 72°C.

3. Add 2 μL of above PCR products into another 50 μL PCR reaction mixture and perform 20 PCR cycles identical to that described above.

4. The success of the process can be judged at this point by agarose gel analysis of 5 μL of the amplified PCR products. The size distribution of PCR products is in the size range of 200 to 600 base pairs (*see* **Note 3**).

## 3.4. FISH

1. Prepare FISH probe by the addition of 2 μL of second round PCR products into a 50 μL PCR reaction mixture identical to that described above except for the addition of 20 μ*M* Biotin-16-dUTP (Boehringer Mannheim GmbH, Germany) for final concentration. The PCR reaction is continued for 15–20 cycles of 1 min at 94°C, 1 min at 56°C, and 2 min at 72°C, with a 5 min final extension at 72°C.

2. Remove unincorporated Biotin-16-dUTP from the product by centrifuging on a Bio-gel P6 filtration column (Bio-Rad, Hercules, CA) following the manufacture's instructions. Briefly, resuspend the settled gel, snap off the tip and place the column in a 2.0-mL microcentrifuge tube, allow the excess packing buffer to drain by gravity and discard the drained buffer, centriguge the column for 2 min at 1000*g* to remove the remaining packing buffer, place the column in a clean 1.5-mL microcentrifuge tube, load sample directly to the center of the column and centrifuge the column for 4 min at 1,000*g*.

3. Recover the probe by precipitation with 1/10 volume of 3*M* sodium acetate (pH 5.2) and 2 volumes of ethanol for 10 min at 4°C and centrifugation at 10,000*g* for 15 min at 4°C. Resuspend the probe in 40 μL TE buffer (10 m*M* Tris·HCl, 1 m*M* EDTA, pH 7.5).

4. Hybridization of the FISH probes is based upon the procedure described previously *(11)*. Briefly, for each hybridization, about 100 ng labeled probe (2 μL) is mixed in 10 μL hybridization mixture, which is denatured at 75°C for 5 min followed by 20 min incubation at 37°C.

5. Denature a slide bearing metaphase spreads for 2 min at 70°C in denaturing solution, then dehydrate the slide through a series of 70, 85, and 100% ethanol.

6. Place the hybridization mixture on the slide previouly denatured and cover with a 22 × 22-mm cover slip, seal with rubber cement, and incubate the slide at 37°C overnight in a humidified container.

7. After hybridization, the cover slip is removed and the slide is processed through a series of three washes in 50% formamide, 2X SSC, 1 wash in 4X SSC, 0.1% NP40 (Calbiochem, La Jolla, CA) and 1 wash at 4X SSC, all at 45°C, for 5–10 minutes each.

8. Hybridization involving only directly labeled probes can be analyzed at this point. Hybridization involving biotin labeled probe is then treated with 40 μL FITC-conjugated avidin (5 μg/mL) (Vector Laboratories, Burlingame, CA) in PNM buffer for 20 min at room temperature. The slide is then washed three times in 4X SSC, 0.1% NP40 and one time in 4X SSC at room temperature 2 min each.

9. The fluorescence signal is then amplified by treating the slide with 40 μL antiavidin antibody (5 μg/mL) (Vector Laboratories) in PNM buffer for 20 min at room temperature. The slide is then washed three times in 4X SSC, 0.1% NP40 and once in 4X SSC at room temperature 2 min each.

10. The slide is usually treated with one more layer of FITC-conjugated avidin identical to that described above.

11. The slide is dehydrated through a series of 70%, 85%, and 100% ethanol washes and air-dried. Counterstain the slide with 40 μL antifade solution (Vector Laboratories) containing DAPI (0.5–1 μg/mL) or propidium iodide (0.5 μg/mL). The slide is then cover slipped and examined with an epi-fluorescence microscope equipped with appropriate filters.

## 4. Notes

1. The cell pellet can be stored in Carnoy's fixative at –20°C for at least a couple of years. No obvious effect of glacial acetic acid in Carnoy's fixative is observed in our microdissection experiments.
2. The cover slip with metaphase chromosomes has to be used within a month if it is kept at room temperature. However, the cover slip with metaphase chromosomes is still good for microdissection after 6 mo if it is stored at –20°C.
3. DNA contamination is a critical problem in the amplification of microdissected DNA. Since the initial amount of dissected material is exceedingly small (in the range of $10^{-13}$ to $10^{-14}$ g/fragment), even minute amounts of contaminating DNA can overwhelm the microdissected DNA leading to useless amplification products. The contaminated DNA may derive from a glass needle which touches DNA other than the target DNA, or from DNA introduced into the collection drop from the air when the tube is repeatedly opened and closed, or frequently from one of the reagents which has been contaminated with extraneous DNA. Therefore, all reagents used for microdissection should be tested for contamination, as well as their efficiency prior to any microdissection experiment. The test is carried out by using the aforementioned PCR reaction using UN1 primer with 0.1 ng total DNA as a positive control with no added DNA as negative control. After 40 cycles (94°C for 1 min, 56°C for 1 min, 72°C for 2 min), the purity of the tested PCR reagents can be checked by agarose gel analysis of PCR products. If the positive control produces extensive products in the size range of 200 to 600 bp, while the negative control produces little or no visible high molecular weight products, the tested reagent is suitable for microdissection. Otherwise, it is necessary systematically to replace each reagent untill a negative blank is obtained. This is critical for success. After all PCR reagents are confirmed suitable for the amplification of microdissected DNA, *Topo I* and Sequenase should also be tested following the protocol described above. To diminish the impact of contamination, all glassware for the preparation of reagents should be washed and autoclaved twice before use. Water with highest purified grade should be filtered through a 0.22-micron filtration unit, then autoclaved twice for 40 min before use. Likewise, salts solutions must be prepared from reagents of the highest available purity, and filtered and autocalved in the same fashion as the water.

## References

1. Lüdecke, H-J., Senger, G., Claussen, U., and Horsthemke, B. (1989) Cloning defined regions of the human genome by microdissection of banded chromosomes and enzymatic amplification. *Nature* **338,** 348–350.
2. Kao, F-T. and Yu, J-W. (1991) Chromosome microdissection and cloning in human genome and genetic disease analysis. *Proc. Natl. Acad. Sci. USA* **88,** 1844–1848.
3. Guan, X-Y., Meltzer, P. S., and Trent, J. M. (1994) Rapid construction of whole chromosome painting probes by chromosome microdissection. *Genomics* **22,** 101–107.
4. Guan, X-Y., Zhang, H., Bittner, M., Jiang, Y., Meltzer, P. S., and Trent, J. M. (1996) Rapid generation of human chromosome arm painting probes (CAPs) by chromosome microdissection. *Nature Genet.* **12,** 10,11.
5. Meltzer, P. S., Guan X-Y., Burgess, A., and Trent, J. M. (1992) Rapid generation of region specific probes by chromosome microdissection and their application. *Nature Genet.* **1,** 24–28.
6. Guan, X-Y., Meltzer, P. S., Dalton, W. S., and Trent, J. M. (1994) Identification of cryptic sites of DNA sequence amplification in human breast cancer by chromosome microdissection. *Nature Genet.* **8,** 155–161.
7. Su, Y., Meltzer, P. S., Guan, X-Y., and Trent, J. M. (1994) Direct isolation of expressed sequences encoded within a homogeneous staining region by chromosome microdissection. *Proc. Natl. Acad. Sci. USA* **91,** 9121–9125.
8. Guan, X-Y., Xu, J., Anzick, S. L., Zhang, H., Trent, J. M., and Meltzer, P. S. (1996) Hybrid selection of transcribed sequences from microdissected DNA: isolation of genes within an amplified region at 20q11-q13.2 in breast cancer. *Cancer Res.* **56,** 3446–3450.

9. Trent, J. M. and Thompson, F. H. (1987) Methods for chromosome banding of human and experimental tumors in vitro. *Methods Enzymol.* **151,** 267–279.
10. Guan, X-Y., Trent, J. M., and Meltzer, P. S. (1993) Generation of band-specific painting probes from a single microdissected chromosome. *Human Mol. Genet.* **2,** 1117–1121.
11. Pinkel, D., Landegent, J., Collins, C., Fuscoe, J., Segraves, R., Lucas, J., and Gray, J. (1988) Fluorescence in situ hybridization with human chromosome-specific libraries: Detection of trisomy 21 and translocation of chromosome 4. *Proc. Natl. Acad. Sci. USA* **85,** 9138–9142.

# 28

## Quantitation of FISH Signals in Archival Tumors

### Amanda D. Watters and John M. S. Bartlett

## 1. Introduction

The term interphase cytogenetics was first used in 1986 by Cremer *(1,2)* to describe detection of chromosomal alterations using *in situ* techniques in interphase nuclei. This was a distinct advantage over conventional analyses as solid tumors could now be studied *(2,3)* and the possibility of applying the technique to specimens received in a diagnostic laboratory realised *(4)*. The nonradioactive *in situ* method, fluorescence *in situ* hybridization (FISH), has been widely applied to study chromosomal rearrangements, malignancies, and chromosome mapping *(4)*.

Despite numerous reports of chromosomal aberrations *(5–12)*, there is wide variation in methods employed to quantify results. Correlation of results between studies and laboratories is hampered by poor application or description of techniques for scoring gene or chromosomal copy number. Without precise and accurate methods for quantifying signals in FISH sections, the diagnostic potential of this technique is unlikely to be fully realized.

There are a number of central principles embodied in current approaches to scoring FISHed tissue sections or touch preparations, which do not apply to extracted nuclear preparations.

It is essential that only nonoverlapping nuclei are scored, and thus for highly dense tissues increasingly thin tissue sections may be required *(1)*. In addition, scoring should be limited to signals with similar intensity of fluorescence. Dual observer scoring is a valuable method of achieving close concordance of results and validation of what is otherwise a purely objective interpretation of results *(5)*. A minimum number of nuclei should be scored to provide an accurate representation of the tissue make up, between 200–500 nuclei per tumor area assess is recommended *(6,8,9,11)*.

Performing FISH in a true *in situ* context, without disruption of tissue, undoubtedly provides a more accurate and relevant interpretation of signal copy number. It must be remembered that tissue sections are limited by the phenomenon of nuclear truncation, making it essential that 1) control genes are used for loss of signals or signal amplification, and 2) that some correction [such as that described by Pahplatz *(13)*] for this artefact is applied.

From: *Methods in Molecular Medicine, Vol. 39: Ovarian Cancer: Methods and Protocols*
Edited by: J. M. S. Bartlett © Humana Press, Inc., Totowa, NJ

Finally, a consensus on the scoring of aneusomic cell populations is required. Whereas some reports reflect only aneusomic populations representing >20% of nuclei scored *(8,9)*, others are less stringent *(6,11)*, resulting in higher frequencies of aneusomies. Wolman et al. *(12)* warned of the problems associated with thin tissue sections and diagnosing a monosomy. Losses, particularly in touch preparations may indicate failed hybridization and large numbers of nuclei need to be scored to be confident of the result. They suggest a cut-off of 45%. A study by Visscher et al. *(14)* compared whole nuclei in suspension with tissue sections and concluded that signal loss was largely a result of nuclear truncation. All such methods employ arbitrary cut-offs and all ignore large proportions of the data set, particularly normal nuclei.

In view of the time-consuming nature of manual scoring, a number of automated systems have been developed; however, apart from specialized applications, these remain developmental *(10,11,15)*. There remains a wide variation in methods for quantifying the results of FISH. In order to apply the technique to a diagnostic setting a clear protocol is required. We have used FISH to assess chromosomal copy number in routine histology sections from solid, archival tumours with probes to repeat sequences around the centromere and have developed a rigorously quality-controled quantitation method *(16)*, which is outlined below using normal tissues as a reference for normosomic signals. We believe this circumvents previous variations in methodology and provides straightforward guidelines.

## 2. Materials

1. Pepsin (Fluka, UK): Prepare a 10% w/v stock solution in 0.2 $N$ HCl, aliquot and store at −20°C for up to 4 mo. Prepare fresh 0.4% pepsin in 0.2 $N$ HCl.
2. 20 × SSC pH 7.0: 175.3 g sodium chloride, 88.2 g sodium citrate, made up to 1 L with distilled water.
3. Hybridization buffer: 50% formamide, 2X SSC, 0.5 mg/mL salmon sperm DNA, 2% dextran sulphate (All Sigma, UK).
4. PNT is 0.1$M$ phosphate buffer, pH 8.0 and 0.05% Tween.
5. PNTB is PNT with 10% blocker (Boehringer, UK).
6. 4,6-diamidino-2 phenylindole-2 hydrochloride (DAPI) (Sigma) 200 ng/mL in Antifade mounting medium (Vectashield) (Vectorlabs, UK).
7. "Streck" Molecular Biology Fixative (MBF) (Alphalabs, UK).
8. Repeat sequence probes (Appligene Oncor, UK), dilute as recommended in hybridization buffer.
9. Sheep anti digoxigenin (Boehringer, UK) 1 µg/mL in PNTB.
10. Rabbit antisheep (Stratech, UK) dilute 18 µg/mL in PNTB.
11. FITC labeled donkey antirabbit (Stratech) dilute 3 µg/mL in PNTB.
12. *In situ* hybridization block (e.g., Misha Unit, Hybaid, UK).
13. 50% Formamide (Fluka) 1X SSC posthybridization wash.
14. 2X SSC posthybridization wash.
15. Epifluorescence microscope.

## 3. Methods

### 3.1. Pretreatment of Slides

1. Prepare tissue sections (5–6 µ$M$ thick) on silane-treated glass slides (Sigma).
2. Dewax slides in two changes of 100% xylene, 10 min each.

3. Rehydrate sections in two changes of 100% methanol, 5 min each. Leave to air-dry (*see* **Note 1**).
4. Prewarm sufficient 0.2 *N* HCl for all sections to 37°C. Immediately prior to use add pepsin to 0.4%.
5. Treat sections with 0.4% pepsin in 0.2 *N* HCl at 37°C for 45 min. Replace pepsin/HCl with fresh prewarmed 0.4% pepsin after 30 min.
6 Rinse 5 × with distilled water.
7. Stain nuclei with 200 ng/mL DAPI (4,6,-diamidino-2 phenylindole-2 hydrochloride, Sigma) in Vectashield (Vector Labs).
8. Assess the extent of the digestion (*see* **Note 2**), extend/curtail digestion as appropriate. If digestion needs to be shortened start digestion again with fresh sections.
9. Dehydrate slides through 70% and 100% alcohol, 2 min each. Leave to air-dry.

## 3.2. In Situ *Hybridization*

1. Rinse slides in 2X SSC, 1 min at room temperature.
2. Postfix in molecular biology fixative (Alphalabs) for 10 min at room temperature.
3. Dehydrate through 70 and 100% alcohol for 2 min each. Leave sections to air-dry.
4. Apply relevant repeat sequence probe (Appligene Oncor) diluted 1 : 10 in hybridization mixture giving a final probe concentration of 10 ng/mL, cover with glass cover slips and seal with rubber cement (Halfords, UK). Tissue and probe are simultaneously denatured on a Misha (Shandon, UK) unit for 5 min at 72°C and hybridized overnight at 37°C (*see* **Note 3**).

## 3.3. Posthybridization Washes

1. Prewarm sufficient 50% formamide/1X SSC and 2X SSC for posthybridization washes to 42°C (or use Misha wash station).
2. Immerse slides in posthybridization wash in 50% formamide, 1X SSC at 42°C for 20 min.
3. Immerse slides in 2X SSC respectively at 42°C for 20 min (*see* **Note 4**).
4. Place slides in PNT at room temperature for 2 min.
5. Block nonspecific tissue binding with PNTB at room temperature for 10 min (*see* **Note 5**).
6. Apply sheep antidigoxigenin (Boehringer) for 45 min at room temperature.
7. Rinse in PNT, for 10 min.
8. Apply rabbit antisheep Fab fragments (Stratech, for 20 min at room temperature.
9. Repeat **step 7** (*see* **Note 6**).
10. Apply FITC donkey antirabbit (Stratech) for 40 min at room temperature.
11. Rinse in PNT, for 20 min.
12. Dehydrate in 70 and 100% alcohol 2 min each.
13. Air-dry slides and mount in antifade with 200 ng/mL DAPI added.
14. Seal with nail varnish and store in the dark. Signals are stable for up to 8 wks.
15. Visualize the signals using an epifluorescence microscope such as the Leica, DMLB (*see* **Notes 7** and **8**).

## 3.4. Quantitation of Hybridization Signals

1. Identify regions for analysis by FISH using adjacent haematoxylin and eosin stained slides and mark areas to be scored on an enlarged photocopy (200%) of the section (*see* **Note 9**).
2. Analyze 1–3 tumor areas, depending on the section size (*see* **Note 11**).
3. Count signals for each chromosome in 200 nonoverlapping nuclei in the control and carcinoma sections using a *multichannel counter* (*see* **Note 10**). The number of signals (0 to ≥4) observed in each individual nucleus are recorded.

**Table 1**
**Scoring Results**

| Chromosome | Observer[a] | Number of signals | | | | | IOV[b] |
|---|---|---|---|---|---|---|---|
| | | 0 | 1 | 2 | 3 | ≥4 | % |
| 10 | A | 5 | 61 | 133 | 0 | 1 | |
| | B | 4 | 48 | 143 | 5 | 0 | 2.79 |
| 11 | A | 7 | 46 | 146 | 1 | 0 | |
| | B | 33 | 45 | 148 | 4 | 0 | 3.46 |
| 9 | A | 18 | 139 | 43 | 0 | 0 | |
| | C | 30 | 109 | 60 | 0 | 0 | 3.06 |
| 9 | A | 12 | 154 | 34 | 0 | 0 | |
| | C | 27 | 117 | 56 | 0 | 0 | 3.10 |
| 17 | A | 1 | 45 | 153 | 1 | 0 | |
| | D | 11 | 47 | 140 | 1 | 0 | 6.52 |
| 17 | A | 4 | 13 | 71 | 12 | 0 | |
| | D | 0 | 21 | 69 | 10 | 0 | 1.39 |
| 17 | A | 4 | 54 | 91 | 43 | 7 | |
| | C | 0 | 21 | 94 | 73 | 12 | 18.35 |
| 17 | A | 2 | 32 | 74 | 48 | 44 | |
| | C | 1 | 4 | 34 | 48 | 63 | 24.86 |

[a]Examples of scoring results as assessed by independent observers (A–D).
[b]IOV= interobserver variation.

4. Enter number of signals/nucleus on a spreadsheet (*see* **Table 1**). Calculate MCCN (mean chromosomal copy number) and percentage of cells with 0,1,2, and so on, signals, and interobserver (*see* **Note 12** and **Table 2**). MCCN is essentially the total number of signals observed divided by total number of nuclei scored.

# 4. Notes

1. Two control sections are included in every FISH run: a positive, which is treated exactly as the test sections and a negative, where the probe is missed out and hybridization mix only applied. This controls for hybridization efficiency and nonspecific staining. The use of control material is further referred to in **Note 9**.

2. When assessing the nuclei for extent of digestion, the staining intensity resulting from the intercalation of DAPI with DNA in the nucleus is a good indicator. Nuclei that stain grey to grey/blue are underdigested and, once the cover slip is removed, can be reintroduced to a fresh batch of pepsin/HCl for up to 15 min. Nuclei that stain blue with clearly visible nuclear borders are suitably digested. Where nuclear borders are lost these sections are over digested and are discarded. The digestion is repeated with different sections for 30 min. It is important to examine areas from different parts of the slide when dealing with thin sections that have been formalin fixed and paraffin processed, as there will inevitably be variations in the fixation effects and therefore in the effect of pepsin digestion. If the digestion of at least two-thirds of the *tumor* is acceptable, then these slides will be suitable for hybridizing.

3. The concentrations of formamide and/or probe may need to be altered if hybridization efficiency is not optimal for example if weak nonspecific hybridization is observed.

4. An alternative is a nontoxic high temperature (72°C) 2X SSC wash for 5 min.

**Table 2**
**Normal Values for 2 Chromosomes** [a]

|  | MCP | TCP/PCP | MCCN |
|---|---|---|---|
| chromosome 7 | 32.3% ± 4.7% | 0.00% | 1.63 ± 0.07 |
| range | 27.2% – 41.0% |  | 1.51 – 1.73 |
| chromosome 17 | 34.1% ± 7.2% | 0.00% | 1.61 ± 0.08 |
| range | 25.0% – 44.7% |  | 1.47 – 1.72 |

[a] This table shows the mean figures for the results of 10 sections of control bladder tissue used to establish disomic values. MCP (monosomic cell population), TCP (trisomic cell population), PCP (polysomic cell population), and MCCN (mean signal to nuclear ratio). Figures are Represented, ± SD.

5. The addition of Tween and blocking agent will reduce nonspecific binding of probe particularly to collagen *(17)*.

6. Use of Fab fragmented antibodies reduces background staining *(17)*.

7. Microscope filters, which are appropriate to the specific fluors, are essential. We use a triple band-pass filter system that allows the combination of FITC and DAPI to be visualized.

8. A 100-W mercury arc lamp and a x40 objective are used to view the sections. Scoring is performed with either a x40 or a x100 objective.

9. Most conventional photocopiers will produce an adequate image of a stained slide for use as a template and permanent record of the area scored.

10. As mentioned in **Note 1**, control sections should always be included, preferably on a section of tissue similar to that being assessed. Where possible, use a morphologically normal block of mucosa, although a carcinoma is perfectly acceptable, providing the tissue has previously been assessed for ploidy and found to be diploid or at least disomic for the probes being used. An additional control for hybridization is inherent in the tumors being assessed, as the cases are observed *in situ* and hybridization of surrounding nontumor areas can clearly be visualized. We have frequently noted that stromal areas in particular hybridize with a greater degree of efficiency than mucosa.

11. The technique of scoring was initially established by two observers using control sections and repeatedly assessing specific fields. The numbers of nuclei per field were between 50 and 100 and a clear baseline for scoring criteria was then confirmed. Nonoverlapping nuclei only were scored. Small nuclei with no signals were ignored, if these were within an area of good hybridization. Split signals, if very close together, were scored as one and if signals with weak intensity were seen together with very bright ones, only the brightest were recorded. *See* **Notes 5** and **6** regarding nonspecific staining. Once established, the technique was then applied to both control and tumor sections. Interobserver variation (IOV) has been low indicating good concordance of scoring, apart from areas of trisomy or polysomy where IOV does tend to be consistently higher. However, as the raw data shows (**Table1**) there are significant numbers of nuclei with three or more signals scored by each observer and these tumors can be said with confidence to be exhibiting trisomy or polysomy, based on the criteria stated in **Note 12**.

12. Chromosome copy number was assessed in two distinct ways. MCCN: The mean chromosomal copy number represented the total number of hybridization signals/total number of nuclei. This was used as a measure of overall chromosome copy number. To define more accurately monosomy, trisomy, and polysomy the percentage of cells with 0–1, ≥3, and ≥4 signals was calculated representing the Monosomic Cell Population (MCP 0-1 signals/

Fig. 1. Photomicrographs of FISH results using repeat sequence probes. Magnification throughout is x1000, hybridization signals show a green fluorescence (FITC) and nuclei a blue fluorescence (DAPI). **(A)** Disomy demonstrated using a classical satellite probe for chromosome 9. **(B)** Monosomy demonstrated using a classical satellite probe for chromosome 9.

Fig. 1. *(continued)* (**C**) Trisomy/tetrasomy demonstrated using an alpha satellite probe for chromosome 17. (**D**) Polysomy demonstrated using an alpha satellite probe for chromosome 8.

cell), Trisomic Cell Population (TCP ≥3 signals/cell), and Polysomic Cell Population (PCP ≥4 signals/per cell). Normal ranges for MCCN and MCP were defined as the mean ≥ 3 × SD (for normal values), tumors outwith these ranges were scored as abnormal. For trisomic or polysomic cell populations, abnormality was defined as ≥10% of cells with at least 3 or 4 hybridization signals per nucleus, respectively. MCCN could never be two for disomic cell populations because of nuclear truncation and this must be taken into account when analyzing the results. This is particularly important when scoring a monosomy, as discussed by Wolman *(12)* and Bartlett et al. *(16)* who addressed this problem in their paper on monosomy of chromosome 9.

## Acknowledgment

This work was supported by a Scottish Office Home and Health Department grant, no. SHHD C2263.

## References

1. Hopman, A. H. N., Ramaekers, F. C. S., Raap, A. K., Beck, J. L. M., Devilee, P., van der Ploeg, M., and Vooijs, G. P. (1988) In situ hybridisation as a tool to study numerical chromosome aberrations in solid bladder tumors. *Histochem.* **89,** 307–316.
2. Wolfe, K. Q. and Herrington, C. S. (1997) Interphase cytogenetics and pathology: a tool for diagnosis and research. Mini review. *J. Pathol.* **181,** 359–361.
3. Mark, H. F. L., Jenkins, R., and Miller, W. A. (1997) Current applications of molecular cytogenetic technologies. Review. *Ann. Clin. Lab. Sci.* **27,** 47–56.
4. Price, C. M. (1993) Fluorescence in situ hybridisation. *Blood Rev.* **7,** 127–134.
5. Hopman, A. H. N., van Hooren, E., van de Kaa, C. A., Vooijs, P. G. P., and Ramaekers, F. C. S. (1991) Detection of numerical chromosome aberrations using *in situ* hybridization in paraffin sections of routinely processed bladder cancers. *Mod. Pathol.* **4,** 503–513.
6. Waldman, F. M., Carroll, P. R., Kerschmann, R., Cohen, M. B., Field, F. G., and Mayall, B. H. (1991) Centromeric copy number of chromosome 7 is strongly correlated with tumour grade and labelling index in human bladder cancer. *Canc. Res.* **51,** 3807–3813.
7. Macoska, J. A., Micale, M. A., Sakr, W. A., Benson, P. D., and Wolman, S. R. (1993) Extensive genetic alterations in prostate cancer revealed by dual PCR and FISH analysis. *Genes, Chromos. Cancer* **8,** 88–97.
8. Sauter, G., Deng, G., Moch, H., Kerschmann, R., Matsumara, K., De Vries, S., et al. (1994) Physical deletion of the p53 gene in bladder cancer. Detection by fluorescence *in situ* hybridization. *Am. J. Pathol.* **144,** 756–766.
9. Sauter, G., Moch, H., Carroll, P., Kerschmann, R., Mihatsch, M. J., and Waldman, F. M. (1995) Chromosome-9 loss detected by fluorescence in situ hybridization in bladder cancer. *Int. J. Cancer* **64,** 99–103.
10. Murphy, D. S., McHardy, P., Coutts, J., Mallon, E. A., George, W. D., Kaye, S. B., et al. (1995) Interphase cytogenetic analysis of *erb*B2 and topoII∝ co-amplification in invasive breast cancer and polysomy of chromosome 17 in ductal carcinoma *in situ. Int. J. Cancer* **64,** 18–26.
11. Pycha, A., Mian, C., Haitel, A., Hofbauer, J., Wiene, H., and Marberger, M. (1997) Fluorescence in situ hybridization identifies more aggressive types of primary non invasive (stage pTa) bladder cancer. *J. Urol.* **157,** 2116–2119.
12. Wolman, S. R. (1994) Fluorescence in situ hybridization; a new tool for the pathologist. *Human Pathol.* **25,** 586–590.
13. Pahphlatz, M. M. M., de Wilde, P. C. M., Poddighe, P., Dekken, H. V., Vooijs, G. P., and Hanselaar, A. G. J. M. (1995) A model for evaluation of in situ hybridisation spot-count distributions in tissue sections. *Cytometry* **20,** 193–202.
14. Visscher, D. W., Wallis, T., and Ritchie, C. A. (1995) Detection of chromosome aneuploidy in breast lesions with fluorescence in situ hybridization: comparison of whole nuclei to thin tissue sections and correlation with flow cytometric DNA analysis. *Cytometry* **21,** 95–100.
15. Coignet, L. J. A., Van de Rijke, F. M., Vrolijk, J., Bertheas, M. F., Raap, A. K., and Tanke, H. J. (1996) Automated spot counting of in situ hybridization dots in interphase cells of leukemia samples. *Leukemia* **10,** 1065–1071.
16. Bartlett, J. M. S., Watters, A. D., Ballantyne, S. A., Going, J. J., Grigor, K. M., and Cooke, T. G. (1998) Quantitative FISH: is chromosome 9 loss a marker of disease recurrence in TCC of the bladder? *Brit. J. Cancer,* **77,** 2193–2198.
17. Warford, T. (1994) An overview of in situ hybridisation, in *A Guide to in situ,* Hybaid Ltd., UK.

# 29

## Comparative Genomic Hybridization for the Analysis of Unbalanced Chromosomal Abnormalities in Ovarian Tumors

Lucy J. Curtis

## 1. Introduction

Comparative genomic hybridization (CGH) is a powerful technique for the quantitative detection of changes in chromosome copy number *(1–3)*. It offers an advantage over conventional cytogenetic techniques in the analysis of tumor karyotypes through its utilization of DNA as the material of study, thus avoiding the problems associated with obtaining good quality metaphases from tumor material. Though CGH is not sensitive to balanced chromosomal rearrangements and changes in DNA ploidy, it can be sensitive to twofold differences in chromosome copy number, making identification of mono- and trisomic karyotype straightforward. Furthermore, deletions and amplifications as small as 2 Mb can be detected, and identification of such regions by CGH analyses of ovarian cancers *(4–6)* have already contributed to the identification of the putative oncogene *PIK3CA (7)*.

The CGH method comprises several steps. First, slides of normal metaphases are made for use as templates. Genomic DNA is extracted from both normal and tumor tissues and whole genome probes are created by labeling DNA with either digoxigenin or biotin, respectively, by nick translation. Normal and test probes are hybridized simultaneously, along with Cot-1 DNA to suppress binding to repetitive sequences, onto denatured metaphases and, after incubation, detection is carried out by the addition of streptavidin-coupled fluorescein and antidigoxigenin-rhodamine. Analysis requires a system comprising an epifluorescence microscope, filter wheel, camera, and appropriate software. The entire procedure is relatively lengthy, and time can be saved by purchasing ready-made items and kits such as metaphase slides, nick translation and hybridization kit, and control DNA. Although an excellent alternative in many ways, they may be prohibitively expensive for many laboratories. The following method is a low-cost procedure that consistently produces results of high quality.

## 2. Materials

Water used in solutions is distilled and deionized.

From: *Methods in Molecular Medicine, Vol. 39: Ovarian Cancer: Methods and Protocols*
Edited by: J. M. S. Bartlett © Humana Press, Inc., Totowa, NJ

## 2.1. Metaphase Preparation from Peripheral Lymphocytes

1. Medium for lymphocyte culture: RPMI medium (Dutch modification, Life Technologies Ltd., Bethesda, MD) supplemented with 10% heat-inactivated fetal bovine serum, 2 m$M$ L-glutamine and 0.5% phytohemagglutinin-M (*see* **Note 1**), (PHA, Life Technologies, Ltd). Filter through a 0.2-μm filter. Medium keeps for 2–3 wk at 4°C once made up. If recurrent problems with bacterial infection are encountered, 1% penicillin (5000 IU/mL)/ streptomycin (5000 μg/mL) solution can be added. Note that both bovine serum and blood represent potential biological hazards must be handled and disposed of accordingly.
2. Hypotonic solution: 2.796 g potassium chloride in 500 mL water (0.075$M$).
3. Fixative: 150 mL methanol and 50 mL glacial acetic acid, made fresh (*see* **Note 2**) and cooled for at least 20 min in a –20°C freezer before use.
4. Clean slides: Prepare good quality microscope slides (e.g., "Select," Chance-Propper, Fisher Scientific) in advance by soaking overnight in a solution of 5% detergent (e.g., Decon 90, Fisher Scientific, Pittsburgh, PA), rinsing for several minutes with tap water and soaking overnight in ethanol containing 0.1% hydrochloric acid. Slides can be stored in ethanol until needed (*see* **Note 3**).

## 2.2. Extraction of Genomic DNA

### 2.2.1. Extraction of Genomic DNA from Blood

1. Lysis buffer: 0.1$M$ Tris-HCl pH 8.0, 20 m$M$ sodium chloride and 1 m$M$ EDTA (ethylene-diaminetetraacetic acid, disodium salt), sterilize by autoclaving, and add 4% sodium dodecyl sulphate (SDS).

### 2.2.2. Extraction of Genomic DNA from Frozen Tissue

1. TE: 10 m$M$ Tris-HCl pH 8.0 and 1 m$M$ EDTA, sterilize by autoclaving.
2. TE-9 SDS/pK: 500 m$M$ Tris-HCl pH 8.0, 20 m$M$ EDTA and 10 m$M$ sodium chloride, sterilize by autoclaving, and add 1% SDS and 0.5 mg/mL proteinase K.

## 2.3. Nick Translation

1. Nick translation buffer: 0.5$M$ Tris-HCl pH 7.5, 0.1$M$ magnesium sulphate, 1 m$M$ dithiothreitol and 500 μg/mL bovine serum albumin fraction V.
2. dNTP mix: 0.5 m$M$ dATP (deoxyadenine triphosphate), 0.5 m$M$ dGTP (deoxyguanine triphosphate), 0.5 m$M$ dCTP (deoxycytosine triphosphate), and 0.4 m$M$ dTTP (deoxythymidine triphosphate).
3. Agarose gel: 1.5 g agarose in 150 mL 1X TBE buffer (10X TBE buffer stock: 107.8 g Tris, 55 g boric acid and 7.44 g EDTA in 1 L water, pH 8.3), boil and add 200 ng/mL ethidium bromide.

## 2.4. Hybridization

Prepare the following stock solutions:

1. 20×SSC: 3$M$ sodium chloride and 0.3$M$ trisodium citrate, pH 7.0; also prepare stock solution of 4X, 2X and 0.1X SSC.
2. Deionised formamide: Add 10 g deionising resin beads (AG501-X8[D] resin, 20–50 mesh, Bio-Rad Laboratories Ltd., Richmond, CA) per 100 mL formamide, mix for 1 h and filter through Whatman No.1 paper to remove the beads. Beads can be used twice. Stored at –20°C.
3. CGH buffer: mix together 200 μL 20X SSC, 40 μL 50% Dextran sulphate and 200 μL water. Store at 4°C.

4. Proteinase K (pK) buffer: 20 m$M$ Tris-HCl pH 7.5 and 2 m$M$ calcium chloride. Prepare the following fresh solutions, in Coplin jars, for processing up to 10 slides:
5. 50 mL RNase A solution: 10 µg/mL RNase A in 50 mL 2X SSC, also 50 mL 2X SSC for rinsing.
6. 50 mL pK solution: 100 ng/mL proteinase K in pK buffer, also 50 mL pK buffer for rinsing.
7. 50 mL 70% formamide solution: 35 mL deionised formamide, 5 mL 20X SSC and 10 mL water.
8. Ethanol series: 100 mL 70% ethanol (50 mL at room temperature and 50 mL on ice), 50 mL 90% ethanol, and 50 mL 100% ethanol at room temperature.

## 2.5. Detection

Prepare the following stock solutions:

1. Tween solution: 0.1% Tween-20 (Fisher Scientific Ltd.) in 4X SSC.
2. DAPI/antifade solution: 0.75 µg/mL 4′-6-diamidino-2-phenylindole (DAPI, Sigma Diagnostics Ltd., St. Louis, MO) in antifade solution (Vectashield, Vector Laboratories Ltd., Burlingame, CA).

Prepare the following fresh solutions, for processing up to 10 slides:

1. Washes: 150 mL 50% deionized formamide/2X SSC, 150 mL 2X SSC and 150 mL 0.1X SSC.
2. Blocking buffer: 0.5 g dried skimmed milk in 10 mL 4X SSC. Warm to dissolve, aliquot into Eppendorf tubes and centrifuge at 8000$g$ for 15 min at 4°C. Carefully remove clean supernatent from precipitate and surface debris and place in a clean tube.
3. Fluorescein/rhodamine solution: 5 µg/mL fluorescein-avidin DN (Vector Laboratories Ltd.) in 1 mL blocking buffer. Centrifuge at 8000$g$ for 15 min at 4°C and remove supernatent to a clean tube. Add 1 µg/mL antidigoxigenin rhodamine (Sigma Diagnostics Ltd.) and place at 4°C protected from light. Make fresh.

## 2.6. Analysis of CGH

Analysis of CGH requires the following equipment: a good quality epifluorescence microscope fitted with a 50- or 100-W mercury lamp (depending on microscope type) and a ×63 or ×100 objective (and also, preferably, a lower power objective for scanning), a filter set comprising single-band exciters for DAPI, FITC, and rhodamine, polychroic mirror and triple bandpass emission filter, a monochrome charged couple device (CCD) camera, and appropriate software. Software must be capable of identifying and segmenting chromosomes, providing a quantitative assessment of fluorescence imbalances, and averaging this over several chromosomes. Such software is commercially available and, furthermore, suppliers are willing to provide all system components. We use the Vysis QUIPS Imaging Software, a Zeiss Axioskop 20 microscope fitted with both ×100 and ×40 Plan Neofluar oil immersion objectives, a Chroma Technology 83000 filter set, and a Photometrics SenSys cooled CCD camera.

## 3. Methods
### 3.1. Metaphase Preparation from Peripheral Lymphocytes (see Note 3)

1. Collect adult blood in an anticoagulant (lithium heparin or sodium heparin) vacutainer and mix well (*see* **Note 4**). Add 0.8 to 10 mL medium, swirl to mix, and incubate in an atmosphere of 5% $CO_2$ at 37°C for 71 h (*see* **Note 5**).

2. Add colcemid to a final concentration of 0.1 µg/mL, swirl to mix and incubate at 37°C for 55 min (*see* **Note 6**). Prewarm hypotonic solution to 37°C and place fixative at –20°C.
3. Transfer the culture to a 15-mL centrifuge tube and spin at 500*g* for 5 min to pellet cells.
4. Remove the supernatent and discard into disinfectant solution (e.g., Presept, Surgikos Ltd.). Loosen the pellet by gentle tapping and resuspend in 10 mL prewarmed hypotonic solution. Invert gently to mix and incubate in a 37°C water bath for 8 min.
5. Centrifuge at 500*g* for 5 min to pellet cells.
6. Carefully remove the supernatent, place the tube onto a vortexer set at a low "shake" speed and add cold fixative one drop at a time (*see* **Note 7**). The pellet should darken immediately. After addition of 20 or so drops the pellet is fixed, and fixative can be added in larger volumes. Make the final volume up to 10 mL.
7. Centrifuge at 500*g* for 5 min, remove the supernatent and resuspend the cells in 10 mL cold fixative. Repeat. The pellet should now be white (*see* **Note 8**).
8. Centrifuge at 500*g* for 5 min and remove the supernatent. For making slides immediately, resuspend the pellet in a few drops of fixative such that a milky solution is produced. For storage, resuspend in 10 mL fixative. Metaphases can be stored indefinitely at –20°C, and are good for CGH for up to two years.
9. Polish slides with a soft lint-free cloth (*see* **Note 9**). Cool slides 2–3 at a time in a –20°C freezer for about 2 min, remove one at a time and immediately use one drop of metaphase solution from a height of 10–60 cm (*see* **Note 10**). Allow to dry and check spreading on a phase contrast microscope at 100× magnification. Adjust the concentration of the metaphase solution such that at least 2–6 metaphases are present in one field of view.
10. Mark the positions of each drop with a diamond pencil. Store at room temperature in a vacuum desiccator for 3–10 d before use (*see* **Note 11**).

## *3.2. Extraction of Genomic DNA*

### *3.2.1. Extraction of Genomic DNA from Blood*

Normal DNA for counterhybridization can be obtained from several sources, but blood is usually the most convenient.

1. Collect 10 mL fresh blood in 1% EDTA to prevent clotting. Lyse in an equal volume of lysis buffer, mix, and leave at room temperature for 30 min.
2. Add an equal volume of water-saturated phenol and mix thoroughly. Centrifuge at 1000*g* for 20 min.
3. Remove the top layer into a clean tube and add a half volume (~10 mL) of 7.5*M* ammonium acetate and twice the volume (~40 mL) of cold isopropanol. Leave this at –20°C for at least 1 h to precipitate the DNA.
4. Centrifuge at 1000*g* for 30 min carefully invert the tube to drain the pellet. Add proteinase K as in **Subheading 3.2.2., step 1** and proceed as for frozen tissue.

### *3.2.2. Extraction of Genomic DNA from Frozen Tissue*

1. Chop frozen tissue into small pieces in 0.5 mL TE-9 SDS/pK and incubate for 48 h at 48°C, mixing occasionally.
2. Add an equal volume of water-saturated phenol, mix by vortexing and centrifuge at 8000*g* for 2 min. Remove the top layer to a clean tube and repeat (*see* **Note 12**).
3. Remove the top layer again and add to it an equal volume of a 24:1 solution of chloroform: isoamyl alcohol, mix by vortexing, and centrifuge again.

4. Remove the top layer once again and add to it 0.5 vol of 7.5$M$ ammonium acetate and 2 vol of ethanol, mix by inversion, and leave $-20°C$ for at least 1 h to precipitate the DNA.

5. Centrifuge at 8000$g$ at 4°C for 20 min, drain the supernatent and either dry the pellet on a vacuum centrifuge or invert the tube and air dry. Once dry, resuspend in 250 µL TE, allow at least 3 h at 4°C for the DNA to dissolve, and measure the optical density (OD) on a spectrophotometer at a wavelength of 260 nm.

### 3.3. Nick Translation of Control and Test DNA

1. Make up DNase solution: Add 1 µL 10 U/µL DNase (RNase-free, Boehringer-Mannheim Ltd. Mannheim, Germany) to 12 mL ice-cold water and mix by gentle inversion (*see* **Note 13**).

2. On ice, mix together: 2 µg normal DNA or 2 µg test DNA (*see* **Note 14**), 8 µL dNTP mix, 4 µL nick translation buffer, 0.8 nmol digoxigenin-11-dUTP (for normal) or biotin-16-dUTP (for test), 1 µL diluted DNase and 10 U DNA polymerase I. Make up to 40 µL with water. Mix gently, pulse-spin to collect the mixture, and incubate for 1 h at 16°C.

3. Replace the reactions on ice. Remove 10 µL and check the fragment size by electrophoresis on a 1% agarose gel against a suitable molecular weight marker such as 1 kb ladder (Life Technologies Ltd.). For optimum results, fragments should appear as a smear of between 300 and 3000 bp. If fragments are larger, add another 1 µL diluted DNase, incubate for a further 10–30 min, and check fragment size again. If fragments are much smaller than 300 bp, the labeled DNA must be discarded. When the fragment size is approximately correct, stop the reactions by addition of 1-2 µL 200 m$M$ EDTA/1% SDS.

4. Clean biotin-labeled DNA through an appropriate spin column, such as Microspin S-200 HR (Pharmacia Biotech Ltd. Uppsala, Sweden), to remove unincorporated nucleotides and small fragments of DNA. Digoxigenin-labeled DNA does not require cleaning prior to use. Store at $-20°C$.

### 3.4. Hybridization

The following protocol is a modification of the method of Kallioniemi et al. (*1*).

1. Prepare labeled probes for hybridization (*see* **Note 15**) by mixing together: 500 ng digoxigenin-labeled normal genomic DNA, 500 ng biotin-labeled test DNA, 15 µL (15 µg) human Cot-1 DNA (Life Technologies Ltd.) and 100 µL ice-cold ethanol (*see* **Note 16**). Place at $-70°C$ for at least 20 min, or at $-20°C$ overnight, and dry on a vacuum centrifuge. Lyophilized probe can be stored at 4°C indefinitely. Approximately 1 h before use, resuspend the probe in 7.5 µL CGH buffer, vortex thoroughly to mix, and leave at room temperature to dissolve. At this point, also prepare a moist hybridization chamber at 37°C (*see* **Note 16**).

2. Place slides into RNase A solution at 37°C for 1 h. Rinse with 2X SSC at 37°C.

3. Rinse slides with pK buffer at 37°C, place into pK solution at 37°C for 2.5 min, and rinse with pK buffer again (*see* **Note 17**).

4. Dehydrate slides by placing sequentially into 70, 90, and 100% ethanol for 2 min each air-dry.

5. Denature probe by adding to it 7.5 µL deionised formamide, vortex thoroughly to mix and pulse-spin to collect. Place at 70°C for 5 min then immediately at 37°C for 30–60 minutes while continuing with the slide denaturation protocol.

6. Prewarm slides to approximately 70°C on a hotplate for about 2 min. To denature chromosomal DNA, place slides in 70°C formamide solution for 3 min (*see* **Note 18**). Plunge them immediately into ice-cold 70% ethanol and leave for 5 min. Meanwhile, clean a sufficient number of small (22 × 22mm) cover slips with ethanol.

7. Dehydrate as in **step 4** and air-dry. Use the denatured slides as soon as possible.
8. Warm the slides and coverslips to 37°C on a hotplate. Add each probe to a metaphase, avoiding bubbles (*see* **Note 19**), and seal a coverslip on top with rubber solution (e.g., Cow Gum). Allow to hybridize at 37°C for 48 h in moist hybridization chamber.

### 3.5. Detection

1. Carefully remove the rubber solution from the slides. Wash three times with 50% formamide solution at 45°C for 3 min, allowing the coverslips to float off in the first wash. Do not allow the slides to dry out until the detection process is complete.
2. Wash slides three times with 2X SSC at 45°C for 3 min, then three times with 0.1X SSC at 45°C for 3 min. Place into 4X SSC/Tween solution for about 2 min at room temperature.
3. Remove slides and drain, but do not allow them to dry. Add 100 µL blocking buffer to each metaphase and leave for 5 min. Add more if necessary to prevent the slide from drying. Meanwhile, clean a sufficient number of large (22 × 40mm) cover slips with ethanol.
4. Place 100 µL fluorescein/rhodamine solution to a large cover slip, drain blocking buffer from slide, and place it carefully onto the cover slip. Gently squeeze the coverslip to remove any bubbles. Note that from now on the slides must be protected from light as far as is reasonably practicable to prevent bleaching of the fluorochromes. Incubate at 37°C for 30 min in the hybridization chamber.
5. Wash with SSC/Tween solution at 37°C for 2 min, allowing the cover slips to float off.
6. Drain, leave to dry, and mount in 35 µL DAPI/antifade solution (Vectashield, Vector Laboratories Ltd.). Seal the edges of the cover slips with nail varnish and store protected from light at 4°C (*see* **Note 20**).

### 3.6. Analysis of CGH

As yet there is no standardized procedure for the analysis of CGH. We use the following guidelines.

1. Check slides by eye first. Good quality slides display even, nongrainy hybridization and blue coloration of centromeres and heterochromatic regions. Briefly check that both the normal/normal and tumor/normal controls and show the expected pattern of chromosomal gains and losses.
2. Analyze the normal control first. Karyotype (*see* **Note 21**) between five and ten metaphase spreads and generate green/red ratios for all undamaged and nonoverlapping chromosomes. Create an average profile and ensure that the observed standard deviation for all euchromatic areas is within the range from 0.85 to 1.15. Do not use any batch of slides where the variation of the normal control is outwith these values. Blocking of probe binding in centromeric and heterochromatic regions by Cot-1 means that even small variations in the proportion green and red signals in these regions can result in large fluctuations of the green : red ratio. These regions must therefore be excluded from analysis.
3. Analyze further samples in the same manner, setting the cutoff point for positive scoring of gains and losses at a ratio which must be greater than the maximum variation of the normal control. We find that this can be as low as 1.125 and 0.875, respectively. Exercise caution in the interpretation of chromosome regions 1p32-pter, 16p, 19, and 22 as repetitive DNA in these areas has been reported to lead to aberrant results (*2*). In our hands, chromosome 19 is the only one of these regions which occasionally presents such problems.

## 4. Notes

1. PHA is added to stimulate lymphocyte growth. The manufacturer is unable to assign weight/volume values for PHA, but the final concentration used here is approximately 10 µg/mL.

2. Acid/alcohol fixation of metaphases both "fixes" the DNA and protein content of the nucleus and dehydrates it. When cells are dropped onto slides, the energy of rehydration allows them to spread. It is particularly important that fixative is made fresh, because it absorbs water during standing and through the process of esterification.

3. Laboratories without ready access to tissue culture facilities may prefer to purchase metaphase slides. Slides of excellent quality can be purchased from Vysis U.K. Ltd., though we currently find them prohibitively expensive for large-scale use.

4. We use male blood for making metaphases for CGH, because the use of female metaphases preclude analysis of the Y chromosome. It is best to use blood on the day of collection, though it can be stored for up to 3 d at 4°C before use if necessary.

5. 25cm$^2$ plastic tissue culture flasks, or glass or plastic universal containers are convenient for this purpose. We find it convenient to set up four flasks at a time for simultaneous harvest, because our bench centrifuge holds four tubes. Larger volumes can be obtained by setting up multiples of four flasks and staggering the harvest. Avoid increasing the volume of blood culture and harvesting in tubes larger than those recommended since this can cause difficulties with fixation. As an alternative to growing cells in an atmosphere of 5% $CO_2$, cultures can be maintained in a normal atmosphere with the lids tightly sealed.

6. Colcemid prevents spindle formation, arresting cells in mitosis and enriching for cells in metaphase. However, longer exposures result in shortening of chromosomes, eventually making them unsuitable for CGH. A balance must be struck between maximizing the number of metaphases and producing chromosomes of suitable length. An incubation of 55 min in colcemid works well in our hands.

7. Constant mixing of the entire cell pellet is essential in order to prevent cells clumping on addition of fixative. Insufficient mixing invariably results in the production of poor quality metaphases, which are unsuitable for CGH. Mixing must, however, be done gently; metaphases are quite delicate at this stage and vigorous agitation results in breakage and scattering of chromosomes. As an alternative to shaking on a vortexer, the cells can be agitated by repeatedly flicking the tip of the tube. This is done by first flicking the tip of the tube to resuspend the pellet and then applying one drop of fixative to the mouth of the tube from a pastette as the tube is held almost horizontal. The tube is brought upright and the pellet flicked repeatedly so that the cells are moving as the fixative comes into contact with them. This is repeated until several drops of fixative have been added, after which larger volumes can be added to bring the final volume up to 10 mL.

8. If the pellet contains a brown residue, then mixing during the fixation step has not been adequate. Metaphases are very unlikely to be of high enough quality for CGH and should be discarded.

9. Slides must be very clean in order to facilitate spreading. Test this by breathing on them; if condensation evaporates evenly then they are clean, but if streaks are apparent return the slides to ethanol and polish them again.

10. Good metaphase spreads should be largely free from cytoplasm and spread sufficiently to eliminate most chromosomal overlaps while maintaining the metaphase intact. There are no hard and fast rules as to how this is achieved; trial and error are often required to determine optimal conditions for obtaining good spreads, and dropping height, slide humidity, slide temperature, and metaphase concentration may need to be altered. Too concentrated a solution of metaphases will impede spreading. In addition, because spreading is partly humidity-dependent, placing slides in the freezer immediately prior to use usually produces enough condensation to spread the metaphases well, but spreading can also be improved by increasing dropping height. Conversely, if metaphases are broken, dropping height should be decreased or slides should be used at room temperature instead of chilled.

11. Although we obtain best CGH results after slide storage for around 1 wk in a desiccator, others successfully store slides in sealed bags at –20°C for many weeks. The latter method allows the production of large batches of slides which can then be batch tested for suitability for CGH. Many investigators advocate batch testing of slides; we find this to be unecessary. Rather, we find batch testing of each blood culture harvest to be necessary because, in our hands, variation between individual harvests appears to be the factor most affecting the quality of CGH results.

12. Occasionally, the phenol and aqueous layer invert. This is easy to see when the phenol used contains a coloring such as hydroxyquinoline. It can be remedied by adding water to the mixture (a volume approximately equal to half that of the aqueous layer is usually sufficient), vortexing, centrifuging, and proceeding as usual.

13. The DNase concentration in this nick translation method is much lower than in protocols where DNA is labeled for purposes other than CGH. This is because, for CGH, maintaining a fragment size of between 300 and 3000 base pairs is critical to obtaining smooth hybridization. Even slight inaccuracies of measurement caused by variations between pipets can result in differences in DNase concentration large enough to significantly affect fragment size. It is therefore essential that each investigator determines their own optimum DNase dilution for nick translation before embarking on large numbers of reactions. Dilution factor must be adjusted such that nick-translated DNA is not less than 300–3000 base pairs in length after a 1 h reaction.

14. We use 2 μg DNA in order to allow for further size checks if necessary. Where only small amounts of DNA are available, the nick-translation reaction can easily be scaled down to utilize 1 μg, which is sufficient for the protocol presented here, or as little as 500 ng. In the latter case, hybridizations can be scaled down to utilize as little as 100 ng of each probe, though we have found this to produce less satisfactory results. Alternatively, probes can be generated from as little as 50 pg by degenerate oligonucleotide PCR (8).

15. Each experiment should include a normal control (digoxigenin-labeled normal DNA vs biotin-labeled normal DNA) and also, if possible, a control sample with known chromosomal abnormalities. Characterised tumor-derived DNA of this type can be purchased from Vysis U.K. Ltd. The sex chromosomes in a hybridization of normal male vs normal female DNA can also serve as a useful control.

16. A moist hybridization chamber can be created from a plastic box with dampened tissues in the bottom, preferably with a sealed lid. Floating the box into a waterbath at 37°C ensures that it will not dry out.

17. Some protocols dispense with proteinase K treatment altogether; we find that it enhances the quality of hybridization when used with care. The 2.5 min incubation is used for slides 7–10 d old and should be reduced to 1 min for 3-d-old slides. Care must be taken not to overdigest, as this leads to loss of chromosome morphology.

18. Formamide temperature is critical to denaturation and should be carefully controlled. Too little denaturation results in poor probe hybridization, whereas too much damages chromosome morphology and precludes adequate DAPI-banding. Formamide must be heated in a fume hood, in which it cools rapidly when uncovered, so it is important to minimize temperature loss by keeping to a minimum the time in which the solution and water bath are uncovered. Addition of slides, even when prewarmed, causes a drop in temperature and it is therefore sensible to denature no more than two at once.

19. The best way to avoid bubbles while adding the probe to the metaphase is to place the probe solution onto a cover slip, invert the slide and gently place it onto the probe. This usually avoids the risk of damaging the metaphase by squeezing out bubbles.

20. Slides can be stored in this way for several months.
21. Current software for automatic karyotyping claims to achieve correct identification of over 90% of chromosomes. In practice, unless DAPI banding is excellent, its efficiency is often significantly less. It is essential that karyotypes are checked by an experienced cytogeneticist to correct errors made by the automated karyotyper.

## Acknowledgment

The author is grateful to Mr. H. Morrison at the Human Genetics Unit, MRC, Edinburgh, Scotland, for help and advice.

## References

1. Kallioniemi, A., Kallioniemi, O. P., Sudar, D., Rutovitz, D., Gray, J. W., Waldman, F., and Pinkel, D. (1992) Comparative genomic hybridization for molecular cytogenetic analysis of solid tumors. *Science* **258,** 818–821.
2. Kallioniemi, O. P., Kallioniemi, A., Piper, J., Isola, J., Waldman, F. M., Gray, J. W., and Pinkel, D. (1994) Optimizing comparative genomic hybridization for analysis of DNA sequence copy number changes in solid tumors. *Genes Chromosom. Cancer* **10,** 231–243.
3. DuManoir, S., Speicher, M. R., Joos, S., Schrock, E., Popp, S., Dohner, H., et al. (1993) Detection of complete and partial chromosome gains and losses by comparative genomic in situ hybridization. *Human Genet.* **90,** 590–610.
4. Arnold, N., Hagele, L., Walz, L., Schempp, W., Pfisterer, J., Bauknecht, T., and Kiechle, M. (1996) Over-representation of 3q and 8q material and loss of 18q material are recurrent findings in advanced human ovarian cancer. *Genes Chromosom. Cancer* **16,** 46–54.
5. Sonoda, G., Palazzo, J., DuManoir, S., Godwin, A. K., Yakushiji, M., and Testa, J. R. (1997) Comparative genomic hybridization detects frequent over-representations of chromosomal material from 3q25, 8q24 and 20q13 in human ovarian carcinomas. *Genes Chromosom. Cancer* **20,** 320–328.
6. Wolff, E., Liehr, T., Vorderwulbecke, U., Tulusan, A. H., Husslein, E. M., and Gebhart, E. (1997) Frequent gains and losses of specific chromosome segments in human ovarian carcinomas shown by comparative genomic hybridisation. *Int. J. Oncol.* **11,** 19–23.
7. Shayesteh, L., Lu, Y. L., Kuo, W. L., Baldocchi, R., Godfrey, T., Collins, C., et al. (1999) PIK3CA is implicated as an oncogene in ovarian cancer. *Nature Genet.* **21,** 99–102.
8. Kuukasjärvi, T., Tanner, M., Pennanen, S., Karhu, R., Visakorpi, T., and Isoa, J. (1997) Optimizing DOP-PCR for universal amplification of small DNA samples in comparative genomic hybridization. *Genes Chromosom. Cancer* **18,** 94–101.

# V

# MOLECULAR GENETIC IMBALANCES IN OVARIAN TUMORS

# 30

## Molecular Genetics of Ovarian Cancer

*A Technical Overview*

**William Foulkes and Andrew N. Shelling**

## 1. Introduction

This chapter is an overview, from a technical perspective, of the approaches that can be used to analyze genetic changes in ovarian cancers. Traditional gene localization methods are discussed, followed by a section on gene identification techniques. Once a putative disease-associated gene has been cloned, mutations have to be identified and analyzed. There are numerous mutation detection methods, and the most common ones are outlined. In the penultimate section, the role of immunohistochemistry as a surrogate method for mutation analysis is considered. Finally, the possible use of functional assays is discussed. The number of techniques used in the molecular analysis of ovarian cancer is immense, and it is beyond the scope of this book to describe all of these methods. However, the most important methods have been outlined in this overview chapter, and many are described in detail in the following chapters.

Molecular genetic abnormalities in ovarian cancer can be broadly divided into changes occurring in three different classes of genes. The most widely investigated class are tumor suppressor genes. The classical example is *RB-1*, the retinoblastoma gene that was found to be altered in hereditary retinoblastoma (*1*), and is also mutated in nonhereditary (sporadic) retinoblastoma. In the latter case, mutations are present only in the retinoblastoma cells, and not in any other cells in the body. Therefore, unlike germ-line mutations, these somatic mutations cannot be transmitted to the offspring of the person with retinoblastoma. This is important not only because the risk of second cancers for affected children is absent, but also because future children will not be at increased risk of retinoblastoma. Other tumor suppressor genes include *APC*, the gene responsible for familial adenomatous polyposis and *VHL*, the gene responsible for von-Hippel Lindau disease. In both of these cases, mutations in the relevant genes in the sporadic counterparts of the hereditary tumors are very common, if not mandatory. This latter rate-limiting role has led to the use of the term "gatekeeper" for these types of tumor suppressor genes. More relevant to ovarian cancer are the breast and ovarian cancer susceptibility genes, *BRCA1* and *BRCA2*, which were identified in 1994 (*2*) and 1995 (*3*), respectively. These two genes illustrate an interesting and novel aspect of tumor suppressor gene function. Despite being the two most important breast and

From: *Methods in Molecular Medicine, Vol. 39: Ovarian Cancer: Methods and Protocols*
Edited by: J. M. S. Bartlett © Humana Press, Inc., Totowa, NJ

ovarian cancer genes thus far identified, somatic mutations in *BRCA1* and *BRCA2* are infrequently in breast *(4,5)* or ovarian cancers *(5–7)*. This suggests they do not act as gatekeepers, but as "caretakers" of the genome, which is supported by evidence that both gene products bind to the human homolog of *Rad51*, a yeast DNA repair gene *(8)*. Interestingly, an inverse relationship between germ-line and somatic mutations exists for ovarian cancer: Li-Fraumeni syndrome, caused by mutations in *TP53*, rarely features ovarian cancer, whereas 50% or more of serous ovarian cancers display mutations in the same gene *(9)*.

Our knowledge about the role of DNA repair genes in human cancer was, for some time, limited to rare inherited recessive disorders such as xeroderma pigmentosa. However, in the last five years it has become clear that mutations in a broad class of genes, the mismatch repair (MMR) genes, are responsible for a much commoner hereditary cancer syndrome, hereditary nonpolyposis colorectal cancer (HNPCC). In this syndrome, colorectal cancer is the most common cancer observed in families. Endometrial adenocarcinoma is the second most frequently observed cancer. Ovarian cancer is seen in a small minority of individuals from HNPCC kindreds: the lifetime risk for a female carrier of a mutation in one of the five genes thus far implicated in HNPCC is not more than 10%. Interestingly, sporadic ovarian cancers do not commonly show microsatellite instability (MSI), a hallmark feature of tumors occurring in HNPCC kindreds. The mismatch repair genes (*MLH1*, *MSH2*, *MSH6*, *PMS1*, and *PMS2*) can be viewed as caretakers rather than gatekeepers of the genomes. It seems that somatic mutations in these genes are not rate-limiting steps in carcinogenesis, but rather lead to genome-wide instability with mutations in numerous genes, particularly in those with runs of monotonous repetitive sequences, such as $A_{(n)}$ or $CA_{(n)}$, where $n > \sim 8$.

The final group of genes to be discussed in this introductory section are the oncogenes. This class of genes was the first to be unequivocally linked to carcinogenesis by assays that transfected DNA from human tumors to mouse 3T3 cells. Following transformation, the resultant cells were capable of causing tumors in nude mice. When the DNA segments responsible for this transformation were cloned, they were found to be cellular homologs of viral oncogenes such as *H* (Harvey) *ras*. The cellular oncogenes that were capable of causing cancer differed from their normal counterparts (so-called proto-oncogenes) either by minor sequence variation, by being overexpressed in the tumor, by gene amplification or by other mechanisms. More than 50 oncogenes have now been identified in human cancers and they possess very diverse functions. Oncogenes are commonly altered in ovarian cancer; *ERBB2* (also known as c-*erbB2* or *neu*), *MYCC* (also known as C-*MYC*), and the *RAS* family of oncogenes have been the most intensively studied and differences have been noted. For example, *ERBB2* is amplified and/or overexpressed in a subset of serous ovarian carcinomas *(10)*, whereas codon 12 *RASK* mutations appear to be more common in mucinous ovarian carcinomas *(11)*.

## 2. Traditional Approaches to Gene Localization

(*See* Chapters 33 and 40.)

### 2.1. Meiotic Linkage

Some genetic mutations that predispose to cancer are directly inherited by children from their parents. These types of mutations (germ-line mutations) in cancer susceptibility genes are important: for example, mutations in *BRCA1* or *BRCA2* account for 5–10% of cases of ovarian cancer. Since 1987, when the locus for familial adenomatous polyposis (FAP) was localized to chromosome 5q, a score of cancer susceptibility loci have been identified using linkage analysis *(12)*. The principle of linkage analysis was developed experimentally by Mendel and later by Morgan and Sturtevant, who constructed the first linkage map in 1913. The first definite evidence of linkage in humans was obtained by studying a pedigree where color blindness and hemophilia were seen in male family members. This occurs because the two responsible loci are sufficiently close together on the X chromosome that random assortment in meiosis does not occur and the loci, along with their resulting diseases, remain together in the next generation. If one of the two diseases here is replaced with an anonymous marker (*see* below) the proximity of the marker to the disease locus can be measured by seeing how often the disease and the marker appear in the same person. The closer the two loci, the less likely they are to be separated by meiosis. The likelihood that the marker is linked to the disease can be expressed as a lod score, (logarithm of odds): the higher the lod score, the more likely that the marker is close to the locus. Traditionally, a lod score of 3 (1000 : 1 in favor of linkage) at a recombination fraction of 0 is accepted as proof that the marker is truly physically close to the locus.

The problem is how to distinguish between different versions of the marker. Proteins are not very polymorphic, which hampered earlier work. It was the identification of restriction fragment length polymorphism's (RFLPs) that permitted the identification of the location of the first cancer susceptibility genes in 1987. Linkage analysis was used by Narod and colleagues *(14)* to demonstrate linkage of markers on chromosome 17 to breast and ovarian cancer occurring in large pedigrees with at least one case of ovarian carcinoma. At that time, Southern blotting followed by radioactively labeled DNA probe hybridization (*see* below) was used to identify the alleles used in linkage analysis. The polymorphisms revealed by these techniques, known as RFLPs are biallelic and in general are not very "informative." That is, it is not possible to distinguish the parent of origin of most alleles, as the two alleles are identical (e.g., 2,2, which is termed homozygous and not 1,2, which is termed heterozygous). For example, an RFLP marker with allele frequencies of 0.35 for allele *a* and 0.65 for allele *b* would result in heterozygosity, *ab* (and therefore be useful as a marker) only 46% of the time. Therefore, over half of the time, the marker would be uninformative for linkage.

These problems were partially overcome in the late 1980s by the utilization of minisatellite markers (also known as variable number of tandem repeats, or VNTRs). These markers are made up of multiple-repeated simple units. The number of repeat units is extremely variable between unrelated individuals, some with >90% heterozygosity. The problem is that most of these types of markers are located at the telomeric ends of chromosomes and this limits their usefulness, as ideally, markers should be equally distributed throughout the genome. Since the early 1990s, linkage analyses have become much easier with the use of highly polymorphic microsatellite markers, utilizing PCR technology. In comparison to previous existing techniques, microsatellite analysis has the following advantages: it is easier and faster to perform, it is more informative, the markers have a more even distribution throughout the genome, the analysis requires less DNA and can be performed using archival tissue such as microscope slides or paraffin blocks (*see* Chapter 31).

The localization of *BRCA1* and *BRCA2* by linkage analysis and their subsequent identification has permitted predictive testing. Now, unaffected individuals who are mutation carriers can be enrolled into risk reduction programs and can be offered screening that might lead to earlier cancer detection and treatment of disease. This is particularly pertinent in ovarian cancer, where the prognosis is poor.

### 2.2. Cytogenetics and Comparative Genomic Hybridization

(*See* Part IV–Cytogenetics, Chapters 22–29.)

### 2.2.1. Background

In common solid tumors, chromosomal abnormalities are complex and it is difficult to identify specific karyotypic changes that are consistently present for a particular type of cancer. It has often been difficult to identify with certainty the chromosomal origins of markers, subtle translocations, or complex chromosomal rearrangements. The majority of ovarian carcinomas appear to be aneuploid and contain a variety of structural chromosomal abnormalities. Various nonrandom alterations have been identified including changes to chromosomes 1, 3, 6, 9, 11, 12, 17, and 19. There is a great deal of speculation as to whether these chromosomal abnormalities play a significant role in tumorigenesis, or whether they are random events related to increased cell division.

### 2.2.2. Flow-Cytometry

It is possible to determine evidence of major cytogenetic changes by measurement of the DNA content of tumor cells using flow cytometry. Polyploidy and/or aneuploid peaks of DNA content are common in ovarian cancer. In general, early stage tumors tend to be diploid, while advanced tumors tend to be aneuploid. Tumor ploidy has been shown in several studies to be an independent prognostic variable and an important predictor of survival.

### 2.2.3. Fluorescence In Situ *Hybridization*

The use of fluorescence *in situ* hybridization (FISH) and other chromosome painting techniques are useful in detecting chromosomal rearrangements. FISH involves hybridization of biotin- or digoxigenin-labeled DNA probes to denatured metaphase chromosomes or interphase nuclei fixed *in situ* to a microscope slide. These probes are visualized by microscopy with fluorochrome-conjugated reagents. Minor variations in hybridization and washing conditions permit the use of a variety of probes, and these can be categorized by their complexity. Whole chromosome paints can be used on metaphase chromosomes, and are useful for the analysis of translocations and particularly of complex cytogenetic rearrangements. Centromere probes consist of chromosome-specific sequences. These sequences, composed of highly repetitive human satellite DNA, provide strong hybridization signals, and are valuable in detecting aneuploidy of specific chromosomes. Locus specific probes are usually cloned DNA sequences covering a specified human chromosomal region. The use of a combination of these types of probes has allowed the mapping of changes on specific chromosomes, and at a finer level, to smaller chromosomal regions *(14)*. The use of FISH in the analysis of ovarian cancers has been hampered by problems associated with the preparation of high-quality cytological specimens. Despite time-consuming karyotype and FISH analysis, some changes are too complex to identify clearly. Furthermore, the identification of chromosomal abnormalities is quite crude, especially at the nucleotide level, and may only serve to identify chromosomal areas that deserve further analysis, for example, by allele loss studies.

### 2.2.4. Comparative Genomic Hybridization

Comparative genomic hybridization (CGH) is a DNA- and FISH-based procedure that enables direct chromosomal visualization of genomic imbalances in tumor DNA. The method involves hybridization of labeled tumor DNA mixed with normal DNA onto normal metaphase cells to identify regions of genomic copy number imbalance in the tumor DNA. Consistent genomic changes have been demonstrated for several different types of primary tumors, and provide opportunities to correlate them with etiologic and clinical features of tumors. CGH findings further provide starting points for positional cloning strategies to isolate unidentified genes involved in tumorigenesis. CGH has confirmed previously identified chromosomal abnormalities, and more significantly, has revealed many previously unsuspected regions of gain, loss or amplification of DNA *(15)*. Limitations of CGH are a reflection of its ability to only detect genetic aberrations that involve loss or gain of DNA sequences. Balanced translocation or inversions are not detectable by CGH, nor are point mutations and small intragenic rearrangements. Small deletions will not be observed, as the lower size limit of detection has been estimated to be approximately 20–30 Mb in primary tumors *(16)*, effectively the size of an average chromosomal band.

### 2.2.5. Multicolor FISH

Multicolor FISH (M-FISH) or spectral karyotyping (SKY) is a newly developed technique allowing the global analysis of human chromosome abnormalities *(17)*. A pool of chromosome painting probes, each differently labeled with fluorescent dye, are hybridized to the tumor cell DNA, and analyzed by spectral imaging that allows the unique display of all human chromosomes in different colors. In combination with conventional karyotype analysis, M-FISH greatly increases the resolution of numerical and structural chromosomal aberrations.

### 2.3. Microcell Fusion and Chromosome Transfer

(*See* Chapter 37.)

Chromosomes that contain putative tumor suppressor genes may be identified by the technique of microcell fusion where a hybrid cell containing a normal chromosome is fused to a malignant cell line. The use of this technique has lead to the suppression of tumorgenicity in several malignant cell lines by the introduction of a specific chromosome containing tumor suppressive information for that tumor type *(18)*. To allow for transfer and selective retention of single specific chromosomes, dominant selectable markers, such as the bacterial *neo* gene are integrated into individual human chromosomes. Most studies have shown that the transfer of a chromosome with an intact tumor suppressor gene has a tumor suppressing effect, whereas the transfer of irrelevant chromosomes has no such effect. However, in some experiments, the irrelevant control chromosome has also lead to tumor cell line growth suppression. Several chromosomes containing putative tumor suppressors (e.g., chromosome 3 and 11) have been identified in ovarian cancer *(19)*.

Attempts have been made to further sublocalize chromosomal regions by selection and transfer of reduced hybrids, however, this is technically very difficult, as each subfragment must contain telomeres, a centromere, and the selectable marker. There is considerable technical difficulty in creating a panel of individual chromosomal subfragments, and even with these panels, gene localization is crude. Nonetheless, the identification of a suppressing chromosomal fragment is valuable functional proof of the presence of a tumor suppressor gene, and may also indicate the relative strength of the gene's suppressive qualities, at least in that particular cell line. Yeast artificial chromosomes (YACs) have also been used effectively as minichromosomes or small chromosomal regions. However, it is has proven to be technically difficult to introduce YACs into human cells. The methods involved are complex, and require carefully maintained cell-culture conditions, as well as highly skilled personnel. The absence of recent publications using this method might suggest that other methods of gene localization, such as allele loss studies, may be technically more feasible.

### 2.4. Loss of Heterozygosity

(*See* Chapters 33, 34, and 40.)

The loss or inactivation (by mutation) of normal growth regulation may lead to tumor progression. Because the loss of these genes results in cancer, they could be said to normally function as "tumor suppressors." The phrase "tumor suppressor gene" was first used in the context of experiments where the introduction of whole chromosomes or chromosomal fragments led to the reversion of a tumorigenic phenotype, or tumor suppression. Later, the work of Cavenee and White showed that loss of heterozygosity (LOH) was an important mechanism in human cancers. LOH does not imply a loss of chromosomal material (although this does often occur), but rather the loss of variation at a locus such that only one parental allele is represented in the tumor. Tumor suppressor genes are recessive at the cellular level: one remaining normal copy is sufficient to suppress tumorigenesis. In this case, the remaining allele is not normal, but contains a mutation of some type, usually at the nucleotide level (such as a point mutation or a small deletion). If only a mutated allele is present in the tumor when heterozygous markers corresponding to this locus are tested, only one parental allele will be observed and heterozygosity will be reduced to homozygosity, hence the name LOH. The absence of the two normal alleles of a tumor suppressor gene may be enough to promote, if not initiate, cancer. The search for LOH is now widely accepted as a means of identifying genes involved in the etiology of hereditary and sporadic tumors. Frequent LOH at specific loci may suggest that these loci normally suppress ovarian tumorigenesis. It is often difficult to decide upon a meaningful level of LOH, but the figure of 35% is generally accepted as representing a level of loss that is worth investigating further with more detailed mapping studies. It appears that for ovarian cancer, loss of heterozygosity for a single marker on a chromosome arm frequently equates with loss of heterozygosity of all informative markers on that arm. LOH studies have shown quite variable results between different groups, often making it difficult to clearly identify regions of interest. Some reasons for these variable results are outlined in **Table 1**.

**Table 1**
**LOH: Some Reasons for Discordant Findings in Different Studies**

Small number of tumors studied

Small number of chromosomal arms evaluated

Different loci on chromosomal arms tested in different studies

Many loci uninformative (where RFLPs have been used)

Different histopathological subtype, stage, grade, and incidence of prior treatment in the tumors

Genetic differences in the study population

Different methods in selecting tumor material away from normal tissue

Over the past five years, microsatellite markers have completely replaced RFLPs as the preferred method of detecting LOH, and now whole genome LOH scans are permissible using multiple, regularly spaced markers. To prevent false negatives with sensitive PCR-based techniques, it may be necessary to microdissect samples carefully (*see* Chapter 31). Microsatellite markers permit the utilization of samples from a variety of sources, such as paraffin-embedded tissues, frozen sections, touch preparations direct from tumors, flow-sorted ovarian tumor cells and cell lines. A blood sample, or normal tissue nearby to the tumor may be required as a source of nontumor DNA. It has been shown that the use of fluorescent primers and automated sequencing machines can give better results and a higher throughput than radioactive-based manual procedures *(20)*. However, misreads of gels is a common problem with automated systems. With all methods, there can be difficulties in interpretation as a result of stutter/shadow bands from polymerase slippage.

Complete loss of one allele should be distinguished from allelic imbalance, which could be artefactual (nonmalignant tissue in specimen, differential amplification of alleles) or real (amplification of one allele, or LOH at the other allele). It is important to note this, as complete LOH can only be caused by LOH itself, whereas allelic imbalance can have several causes.

## 3. Old and New Methods of Gene Identification

### 3.1. Southern Blotting

This widely used technique of transferring DNA from liquid form to a solid support was devised by Ed Southern when he was at Edinburgh University. The generation of large amounts of restriction endonucleases permitted their wide use in molecular biology. Their ability to digest DNA into numerous fragments is based on the multiple occurrence of simple recognition sites (such as GAATTC digested by *EcoRI*) throughout the genome. Once genomic DNA has been digested into small fragments (the majority being <50 kb in size) and loaded into the wells of an agarose gel, it is possible to size fractionate by electrophoresis as DNA is a charged molecule. After depurination with hydrochloric acid, the fractionated DNA can then be transferred and fixed onto a filter (originally nitrocellulose, now nylon) that is then ready to be hybridized with a radioactively labeled DNA probe. The probe is treated thermally or chemically so that the two strands separate and thus can hybridize to the complementary DNA present on the filter. This technique is extremely simple and is the basis of many other techniques such as Northern and Western blotting. Southern analysis has been used to study copy number for amplified oncogenes, it has formed the basis of much of the initial work on loss of heterozygosity (*see* **Subheading 2.4.**), and it can be used to detect small, but crucially important deletions and insertions in cancer susceptibility genes. Southern blotting would have correctly identified *BRCA1* if families with genomic deletions including *BRCA1* (which are known to exist) had been screened with probes close to or within this gene.

### 3.2. Pulsed Field Gel Electrophoresis

This technique is derived from Southern blotting, but instead of using a constant current to fractionate the endonuclease-digested fragments, a pulsed current from a series of geometrically organized multiple electrodes is applied to a low percentage (fragile!) agarose gel. The origin of the current changes from one electrode to another in a set (but variable) spatiotemporal pattern. This results in high molecular weight DNA entering the gel in a snake-like manner *(21)*. The conditions are very flexible, allowing the separation of different sized DNA fragments. Very large fragments of human genomic DNA, suitable for examination by pulsed-field gel electrophoresis (PFGE), can be produced by digesting genomic DNA with restriction endonucleases that are methylation-sensitive and require an eight basepair recognition site. These so-called rare cutters (e.g., *Not*I, *Sac*II, and *Bss*HII) can be used to build up a "long range map" using probes separated by up to 1 Mb that can hybridize to the same fragment. The relevance of the methylation sensitivity of the endonucleases resides in the observation that the 5' end of genes tend to be CG-rich. Genes are often associated with CpG islands, particularly if multiple rather than single rare cutter sites are present at the island in question. These "CpG islands" can be identified by PFGE. The identification of *NF1*, *NF2*, *WT1*, and *VHL* all relied heavily on the use of PFGE, although it is perhaps a less-popular technique now than it was a decade ago.

### 3.3. Representational Difference Analysis (RDA)

The basis of this technique is that small differences between otherwise very similar genomes can be detected by hybridization of one genome against the other *(22)*. Two very similar genomes would be the typical "normal-tumor pair" used in LOH studies (*see* **Subheading 2.4.**), so this technique resembles a genome scan for regions of homozygous deletion.

A brief outline of the technique is as follows:

Step 1: ligation of small restriction endonuclease fragments (such as those produced by *Bgl*II) to oligonucleotide adaptors and subsequent PCR.
Step 2: reiterative hybridization/selection.

The two genomes are called "driver" and "tester." If tumor DNA is used as a driver, then normal DNA "tests" for the presence of sequence. If sequences are missing from the driver, there will be a loss of restriction fragments. When the products are run out on agarose gels, no bands will be seen in the samples with homozygous deletions.

This technique is useful only if the loss of a tumor suppressor gene is by homozygous deletion. Previous techniques such as cosmid hybridization with competition were limited to the investigation of rather small, previously well-mapped intervals, whereas RDA makes no assumptions about where the deletions may lie. In practice, this technique has been used to identify several genes of relevance to ovarian cancer, in particular *BRCA2*, where RDA detected a homozygous deletion on chromosome 13q in an 84-yr-old woman with localized pancreatic cancer *(23)*. Interestingly, *BRCA2* was later found to be located entirely within this deletion. RDA has also been used to identify a somatically deleted gene on chromosome 18q known as *DPC4 (24)*, that was later found to be mutated in the germ-line of patients with the inherited cancer syndrome, juvenile polyposis *(25)*. RDA is one of the most successful new techniques for gene identification.

### 3.4. Differential Display Reverse Transcriptase—Polymerase Chain Reaction (DDRT-PCR)

(*See* Chapter 50.)

DDRT-PCR has been used successfully to identify genes that are differentially expressed in tissues or cell lines. The basis of this method is to amplify the specific mRNA species following reverse transcription-PCR (RT-PCR). It uses combinations of arbitrary primers with anchored cDNA primers and generates fragments that originate mostly from the poly(A) tail and extend upstream. The bands that are found to be differentially expressed are amplified prior to direct use in methods to confirm differential expression by an independent RNA analysis technique (Northern blotting, RNase protection, and/or nuclear run-on). The bands can also be amplified for cloning and sequencing. Under the appropriate conditions, the pattern of fragments derived from one type of cell is reproducible and can be compared with that of another cell type *(26)*. Application of the technique is complicated by the appearance on non-reproducible bands, perhaps as many as 20–40% of the total number. It appears that DDRT-PCR is not a totally quantitative method, as even dramatic differences on DDRT-PCR may not correlate to expression levels. The nonreproducible bands are probably from a variety of sources, including imperfect annealing of primers to mRNA sequences, and contamination of RNA samples with chromosomal DNA. DDRT-PCR offers many advantages over previous techniques such as subtractive or differential hybridization libraries, including the ease of operation, the requirement for only small amounts of RNA, the simultaneous display of more than two RNA populations, and the ability to measure both increased and decreased gene expression.

### 3.5. One-Dimensional Genome Scanning

(*See* Chapter 39.)

This new technique is a comparative one that uses a modification of Southern blotting, followed by hybridization with a probe with <2000 repetitive elements (such as *RTLV-H*) which can then detect amplifications, deletions, and other alterations. Genomic DNA from lymphocyte and tumor sources can be compared lane by lane. Not only is a "whole genome snapshot" provided, but the aberrant fragments can be directly cloned and evaluated. This technique has not yet received wide acceptance, possibly as a result of the special equipment required. However, it certainly could gain importance if technical modifications permitted the use of standard equipment.

## 4. Mutation Screening by Fragment Analysis
### 4.1. Single Strand Conformation Polymorphism (SSCP)

(*See* Chapter 35.)

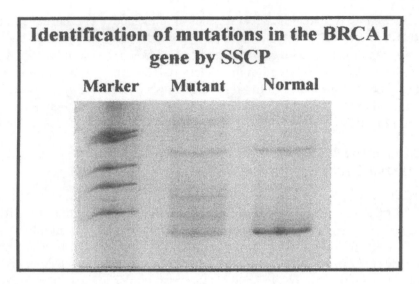

Fig. 1. Example of a SSCP gel showing two bands in the normal lane, and the two extra variant bands in the mutant lane. Gel courtesy of Kirstine Francis-Thickpenny.

This technique has become the most widely used mutation screening test in ovarian cancer genetics (*see* **Fig. 1**) for an example. This is because it is simple, inexpensive, robust, and can detect up to 70–80% of all mutations in a given fragment. Numerous modifications such as differing concentrations of polyacrylamide, glycerol, or TBE and different visualization methods (ethidium bromide, silver-staining) have been made to the original protocol of Orita et al. *(27)*. They all depend upon the principle that single DNA strands of a pair have different mobilities in a nondenaturing gel, even if their sequences do not differ. This permits the visualization of at least two, and sometimes four or more, bands in the wild-type situation. When sequence variants are present, new bands appear on the gel, which indicate the presence of a change in the test DNA. These sequence variants can be easily characterized either by cutting the variant band directly from the dried gel and DNA sequencing, or by direct sequencing with the original primer pairs used for the SSCP. It is often recommended that fragments not larger than 250 bp be analyzed by SSCP. In our laboratory, the addition of 5% glycerol, and 0.5X TBE to the gel mix results in a high detection frequency when the gels are run at room temperature overnight. Every laboratory will develop their own inventory of modifications that seem to slightly improve the detection of potentially important sequence variants.

## 4.2. Protein Truncation Test (PTT)

This test for mutations is also known as IVSP (for in vitro-synthesized protein), which is a more informative name, but the acronym PTT seems to have stuck. It is a particularly useful mutation screening technique for genes such as *APC* and *BRCA1/2* because

1. >80% of all reported mutations result in a truncated protein and are detectable by PTT.
2. These genes all possess one very large exon which permits examination of 50% or more of the total exonic DNA in assays using primers within these large exons. Therefore, they do not require RNA.

In general, however, it is preferable to have RNA as the starting material as other exons cannot be readily examined without this.

The PTT technique relies on the use of a T7 promoter sequence and a consensus sequence for eukaryotic translation initiation, which are both incorporated into a primary or nested PCR amplification. These reactions can be carried out using commercially available in vitro transcription/translation kits, and the products are visualized on a SDS-PAGE gel. The main problems with PTT are the presence of multiple bands because of cryptic translation initiation sequences in the fragment to be analyzed. PTT is an expensive test, and problems arise owing to the difficulty to identify variants because of the instability of the mutant mRNA.

## 4.3. Cleavase Fragment Length Polymorphism (CFLP)

This new method of mutation detection is one of most sensitive enzyme-based techniques and relies upon the fact that the cleavase enzyme recognizes DNA molecules differing by a single base pair. The slow cooling after denaturation encourages the development of DNA hairpins that are recognized by cleavase if they differ from wild-type hairpins by as little as one base pair. Upon electrophoresis, the fragment carrying the mutation, which has been cleaved, will run as two smaller fragments and these can be easily distinguished. A cleavase fingerprint can be detected using fragments as large as one kilobase, and normal and tumor DNA samples can be compared very easily lane by lane. The technique is quick, inexpensive, and detects up to 95% of all mutations.

## 4.4. Heteroduplex Analysis (HA)

Heteroduplex formation is the basis of a number of different techniques discussed here. In its simplest form, HA relies upon the use of different polyacrylamide gel matrices to detect homo- and heteroduplexes in double-stranded normal and tumor DNA fragment pairs (usually <300 base pairs), when run side by side. Alternatively, germ-line DNA from patients who may be carriers of mutations in cancer susceptibility genes could be studied. The main drawback is the lack of sensitivity. Multiplex HA has been used to detect germ-line *BRCA1* mutations in women with ovarian cancer *(28)*, but the results of this study suggest that the method does not detect more than 70% of all possible mutations.

## 4.5. Denaturing Gradient Gel Electrophoresis (DGGE)

This is a nonradioactive technique that separates DNA fragments according to their melting temperature. When electrophoresed through a linearly increasing gradient of denaturants, DNA fragments remain double stranded until they reach a concentration of denaturants equivalent to a melting temperature ($t_m$) that causes the lower-temperature domains of the fragment to melt. This causes the DNA to branch and the mobility of the fragment is markedly decreased. Single basepair changes in the lower $t_m$ domain can result in DNA fragments melting at a slightly different concentration of denaturants, in turn resulting in a band shift. When modified by the addition of a 40–50 base pair GC rich "clamp," using PCR, higher $t_m$ domains become available for analysis, as the GC clamp has a higher $t_m$ than any test fragment. This enables detection of almost 100% of mutations *(27)*. It is therefore an attractive technique, but its wholesale adoption by researchers has been limited by several important drawbacks:

1. Special equipment is required.
2. GC clamps have to be added, results in greater oligonucleotide costs.
3. A melting map has to be plotted for each fragment.
4. The choice of primers is critical, requiring careful design.

Newer techniques based on a mixture of older techniques like SSCP and DGGE, such as conformation sensitive gel electrophoresis (CSGE) *(29)* are more likely to become widely used. In this radioactive technique, heteroduplexes are formed by heating the samples to 98°C for 10 min, after which the temperature is slowly dropped to 65°C and held at 60°C for 15 min before being allowed to slowly return to room temperature (over at least 30 min). Samples are then electrophoresed through 6% polyacrylamide gels overnight at 4 W.

### 4.6. Chemical Cleavage (CCM)

This technique theoretically detects 100% of mutations as it is based on the chemical reaction of hydroxylamine with mismatched cytosine (for CG) and osmium tetroxide with thymidine (for AT). After cleavage of modified mismatch heteroduplexes with piperidine, samples are denatured by heating and loaded onto denaturing urea gels. Mismatches show up as new bands, as the piperidine cleaves at the mismatch and thereby creates a smaller fragment on electrophoresis *(30)*. Large fragments can be analyzed, and newer methods have now been introduced, which obviate the need for toxic chemicals like osmium tetroxide. These two factors make CCM an attractive option, particularly if large fragments can be multiplexed.

## 5. Direct Mutation Identification

### 5.1. Allele-Specific Oligonucleotide Hybridization (ASO)

This method is particularly valuable in identifying common mutations, or for confirming known mutations within a family. Radiolabeled allele-specific oligonucleotide (ASO) probes are hybridized to dot blots containing PCR-amplified DNA products. The "normal" or wild-type oligonucleotide probe is designed to precisely match the normal DNA sequence. It hybridizes only to the wild-type sequence and not to an imperfect complementary sequence in which there are one or more mismatches as a result of a base change. The "mutant" probe will bind only to DNA sequences that differ from the "normal" sequence by a specific base pair changes. Differential washing allows mutations to be detected. Detection by ASO is direct and is less subject to errors or misinterpretations than other methods. Problems encountered are one of two types: the specific hybridization signal is too low or the background hybridization is too high. Adjusting the hybridization and wash temperatures can usually overcome these problems. Its main limitation is that it can only detect a single mutation at a time.

### 5.2. Amplification Refractory Mutation System (ARMS)

This direct mutation identification method is also known as allele-specific amplification. It is ideally suited to detecting mutations where it is very important to include an internal negative control, such as detecting specific *BRCA1* mutations in a family where a mutation has already been identified. The negative control ensures that the absence of a mutation is not incorrectly interpreted as a negative result in situations where the amplification simply did not occur. This method is often favored by service laboratories, often they test only a specific mutation. Furthermore, the technique is suitable for automation.

Briefly, two sets of primers are used. One set to amplify only the mutated allele and the other to amplify only the normal allele. This is achieved by using one primer that mismatches with its wild-type target sequence by only one nucleotide (and therefore anneals to the mutant allele) at the 3' end of the primer. These primers will not amplify the DNA to which they anneal. If they are carefully designed, all four primers can be used in one PCR amplification. It is useful to create a large flanking fragment that should be present in all individuals, whether wild-type or not.

Although this method has been used to detect known mutations in *BRCA1 (31)*, in our hands, we have had problems getting repeatable results when all four primers are added to the same reaction. If two reactions have to be used, the advantage of ARMS is somewhat lost.

## 5.3. DNA Sequencing

DNA sequencing is the technique for determining the exact order of nucleotides in a DNA sequence. The method most widely used is the Sanger dideoxy method, which utilizes the controled interruption of DNA polymerase mediated replication of single stranded template DNA. In addition to the four deoxy-ribonucleoside triphosphates (which are radioactively labeled), the incubation mixture contains a 2'-3'-dideoxy (ddNTPs) analog of one of triphosphates. The incorporation of the ddNTP blocks further growth of the new chain because it lacks the 3'-hydroxyl terminus needed to form the next phosphodiester bond. Fragments of various lengths are produced in which the ddNTP is at the 3' end. Four such sets of chain-terminated fragments (one for each ddNTP) are then separated by electrophoresis in a polyacrylamide gel, and the base sequence is read from the autoradiograph.

DNA sequencing is usually the necessary final step of all mutation detection strategies, as it defines the location and nature of the changes. However, DNA sequencing can also be used as a direct method of mutation detection. Direct sequencing refers to the direct sequence analysis of PCR products without prior subcloning into sequencing vectors and can be the primary method of mutation detection. The use of automation and new fluorescence detection technology will make this method faster and more accurate. However, DNA sequencing tends to be laborious, expensive and generates excessive information. Difficulties are frequently experienced in identifying heterozygotes in automated systems. Fluorescent peaks may be partially hidden, and not identified by sequence recognition programs.

## 5.4. DNA Chip Technology

Techniques are now available for direct analysis of gene mutations by high-density arrays of oligonucleotides. It is possible to synthesize more than 90,000 oligonucleotides *in situ* on silicon chips, to represent all possible nucleotide substitutions and common mutations for each gene. The target gene sequence is fragmented into 50–100 nucleotides, fluor labeled, and hybridized to the chip. Computer assisted comparison of the hybridization pattern of the target sequence vs the wild-type sequences, results in the detection of mutations from two types of signal. First, the gain of signal resulting from new hybridization by the mutant fragment, and second, the loss of signal resulting from the loss of the wild-type signal. Analysis is computer based and uses a confocal scanning microscope fitted with an argon laser to read the data from the chip *(32)*.

Chip technology to scan entire genes for mutations is expected to be the technology of the future, because of its high specificity, speed, and ability to be automated. However, this may be several years away, as many technical limitations still need to be addressed, including sequence-dependent variability in hybridization efficiency. In addition, chips continue to be expensive and are only produced in limited numbers, the equipment and software is expensive, and significant expertise is required. Direct sequencing is still required to confirm the result.

## 6. Somatic and Germ-Line Mutations in Ovarian Cancers that Show Microsatellite Instability

*(See* Chapter 41)

It is well recognized that human neoplasms are the end result of a multistep process, in which accumulation of several genetic alterations can take place. At least three types of cancer-related genes have been recognized; tumor suppressor genes, oncogenes, and mismatch repair genes. The accumulation of mutations within these genes is associated with the development of a variety of cancers. Microsatellite instability (MSI) or replication error (RER) is widely accepted as an indicator of loss of DNA mismatch repair activity in human tumor cells. This is because of mutations in the four mismatch repair genes that result in HNPCC: *hMSH2, hMLH1, hPMS1, hPMS2,* on human chromosomes 2p, 3p, and 7p. The recently identified *hMSH6* on chromosome 2 may not be associated with MSI. It has yet to be determined whether all of these genes confer an increased risk of ovarian cancer.

MSI has been observed in a wide variety of sporadic cancer. However, it has been difficult to accurately assess the contribution of MSI to sporadic cancer, including ovarian cancer *(33)*. This is for several reasons.

1. In some of these studies, it has been difficult to determine whether tumor-associated MSI is in fact owing to the presence of a germ-line mutation in a mismatch repair gene. However, the proportion of familial ovarian cases (<10%) that are a result of HNPCC is low, and thus the percentage of ovarian carcinomas in general that could be attributed to mutations in these genes is less than 1%.
2. There have been considerable experimental differences between different studies, and indeed, there has not been a consensus on how to define MSI. In the past, different groups have not only used different numbers of microsatellites, but have used different microsatellites. The variable use of criteria has been controversial, and if research is to be compared from different laboratories, the definitions need to be standardized. Recent meetings have outlined a set of loci and frequency of MSI. Some consider that genetic instability in ovarian tumors may have previously been underestimated *(34)* and that standard PCR-based assays are not sufficiently sensitive to reproducibly detect instability of polymorphic microsatellites from most sources.
3. MSI seems to be associated with a certain histological type and stage of tumor. Therefore, the results may be quite different from different studies, depending on the particular tumor samples studied.

To avoid these complications, some studies have looked directly at the expression of mismatch repair genes, rather than looking at the observed phenotype (MSI). Gene expression (Northern analysis) and protein expression (Western analysis) can be used. Immunohistochemistry (IHC) is also possible (*see* Chapter 42). As well, functional tests have been reported (*see* **Subheading 8.**).

## 7. Immunohistochemistry as a Surrogate for Mutation Analysis

(*See* Chapter 42.)

Immunohistochemistry (IHC) is used to measure protein expression in both fresh and archival paraffin-embedded tissues, making use of suitable monoclonal antibodies. It is one of a few techniques that can be reliably used with archival tissues, and which is relatively fast. Measurement is subjective, but is sufficient to give an estimation of protein expression. We focus on two genes that have been studied in detail by IHC in ovarian cancer.

### 7.1. TP53

Mutations in the *TP53* tumor suppressor gene are one of the most common genetic alterations in human cancer, and such mutations are frequent in ovarian cancer. The methods most often used to detect mutations in *TP53* include DNA sequencing, SSCA and IHC *(35)*. Point mutations within *TP53* frequently cause conformational changes that stabilize and extend the half-life of the mutant TP53 proteins, causing them to accumulate in the nucleus and effectively leading to relative overexpression. The accumulated mutant protein in the nucleus can be detected immunohistochemically, serving as a rapid and effective means of screening for *TP53* mutations. The small amounts of *TP53* present in normal cells are not detectable. Consequently, IHC-detected TP53 protein has generally been assumed to indicate an underlying *TP53* mutation. Although this has been validated in some earlier studies, not all studies are in agreement, and this has lead to some caution over the simplistic interpretation of TP53 IHC. Detection of overexpression of TP53 protein alone, in the absence of *TP53* mutation may be misleading, as stabilization of TP53 may be a transient phenomenon.

Both methods seem to identify different groups of patients, with approximately 90% overlap. It is interesting that in some studies, IHC has proven to be more effective in defining patients with poor prognosis, whereas in others, the reverse is true. Even if the true mutation status is not revealed by IHC, it has been suggested that this methodological approach may provide information more reflective of the functional status of the TP53 protein than that proved by molecular biological techniques such as complete DNA sequencing.

It is difficult to determine why some DNA sequence-defined *TP53* mutations are not detected by IHC. In some cases, premature truncations and large deletions or insertions could lead to complete absence of protein. Other possible explanations include changes in or loss of antibody epitope, or the presence of mutations that cause reduced stability of the mutated protein.

### 7.2. Mismatch Repair Protein

(*See* Chapter 42.)

Mismatch repair proteins, such as *hMLH1* and *hMSH2* studied by IHC show that loss of protein staining corresponds very closely with loss of function as measured by MSI. This method may offer a more direct approach toward identifying loss of protein expression, however, as shown in *TP53*, this may not always correlate with loss of function or with the presence of a mutation in the gene whose product is under study.

## 8. Functional Assays for Mutated Genes

Mutations can be detected and identified by several methods and several combinations of methods, and usually confirmed by DNA sequencing. However, DNA sequence data will not distinguish whether a variant is a polymorphism or a disease causing mutation. Some biologically relevant mutations are expected to alter gene function, so an assay that detects the functional consequence of a missense mutation would be valuable to help distinguish rare polymorphisms from cancer-causing mutations.

Yeast-based functional assays have been developed, whereby gene PCR products are cloned directly into yeast expression vectors in vivo, used to transform appropriate yeast hosts, and subsequently tested for transcriptional activity in a simple growth assay. Assay systems have been developed for the detection of missense mutations, such as in *TP53* and *BRCA1 (36–38)*. These assays have identified that growth suppression is not observed in neutral polymorphisms, but is abolished or diminished by frameshift, nonsense, or disease-associated missense mutations.

In a variation of this assay, known as the stop codon assay, it is possible to test for truncating mutations. For genes such as *APC* and *BRCA1*, truncating mutations predominate. The PCR-amplified coding sequence is inserted by homologous recombination into the yeast URA fusion protein, and transformants are assayed for growth in the absence of uracil. If the target fragment has a truncation mutation, the fusion protein will not be produced and selection on URA-medium will identify whether URA was expressed.

The advantages of a functional assay are immediately apparent: the absence of gels, toxic or radioactive chemicals, the ability to analyze quite large DNA fragments, and a relatively fast assay time (4–5 d to get an answer). These methods will only work for a limited number of genes that will also function in yeast. It is not always obvious that an abnormality in a yeast assay implies an abnormality in humans, particularly for missense mutations. Work with yeast can prove to be problematic to those not familiar with yeast genetics. In addition, there is a need to construct a new vector for each gene you wish to study.

## 9. Conclusions

In this introductory chapter we have provided a brief overview of the technical aspects of ovarian cancer genetics, without providing too much practical detail as this will be found in the relevant chapters. Molecular genetic techniques have advanced very rapidly, and it is difficult, if not foolish, to predict from where the next advance will come. However, the basic principles of careful collection and recording of specimens, full collaboration with pathology colleagues, and good laboratory practice still form the basis of any successful ovarian cancer genetics project.

A recent significant development in the genetic analysis of ovarian cancer is the rapid emergence of DNA microarray technology in the analysis of gene expression. A recent supplement to *Nature Genetics* (Volume 21, January 1999) was devoted to "microarray" technology. The application of this technology has the potential to make a substantial increase in our understanding of the genes involved in the development of ovarian cancer, and thereby provide new targets for drug design and gene therapy.

## Acknowledgments

We would like to thank Dr. P. Sanséau and Ms. C. Serruya for their contributions to this manuscript.

## References

1. Friend, S. H., Bernards, R., Rogelj, S., et al. (1986) A human DNA segment with properties of the gene that predisposes to retinoblastoma and osteosarcoma. *Nature* **323,** 643–646.
2. Miki, Y., Swensen, J., Shattuck-Eidens, D., et al. (1994) A strong candidate for the breast and ovarian cancer susceptibility gene BRCA1. *Science* **266,** 66–71.
3. Wooster, R., Bignell, G., Lancaster, J., et al. (1995) Identification of the breast cancer susceptibility gene BRCA2. *Nature* **378,** 789–792.
4. Miki, Y., Katagiri, T., Kasumi, F., Yoshimoto, T., and Nakamura, Y. (1996) Mutation analysis in the BRCA2 gene in primary breast cancers. *Nature Genet.* **13,** 245–247.
5. Futreal, P. A., Liu, Q., Shattuck-Eidens, D., et al. (1994) BRCA1 mutations in primary breast and ovarian carcinomas. *Science* **266,** 120–122.
6. Merajver, S. D., Pham, T. M., Caduff, R. F., et al. (1995) Somatic mutations in the BRCA1 gene in sporadic ovarian tumors. *Nature Genet.* **9,** 439–443.
7. Foster, K. A., Harrington, P., Kerr, J., et al. (1996) Somatic and germline mutations of the BRCA2 gene in sporadic ovarian cancer. *Cancer Res.* **56,** 3622–3625.
8. Scully, R., Chen, J., Plug, A., et al. (1997) Association of BRCA1 with Rad51 in mitotic and meiotic cells. *Cell* **88,** 265–275.
9. Kupryjanczyk, J., Thor, A. D., Beauchamp, R., et al. (1993) p53 gene mutations and protein accumulation in human ovarian cancer. *Proc. Natl. Acad. Sci. USA* **90,** 4961–4965.
10. Fajac, A., Benard, J., Lhomme, C., et al. (1995) c-erbB2 gene amplification and protein expression in ovarian epithelial tumors: evaluation of their respective prognostic significance by multivariate analysis. *Int. J. Cancer* **64,** 146–151.
11. Pieretti, M., Cavalieri, C., Conway, P. S., Gallion, H. H., Powell, D. E., and Turker, M. S. (1995) Genetic alterations distinguish different types of ovarian tumors. *Int. J. Cancer* **64,** 434–440.
12. St. Jean, P. and Schork, N. (1988) Genetic epidemiologic approaches to finding genes that influence susceptibility to cancer, in *Inherited susceptibility to cancer: clinical, predictive and ethical perspectives,* Foulkes, W. D. and Hodgson, S. V., eds. Cambridge: CUP, pp. 109–133.
13. Narod, S. A., Feunteun, J., Lynch, H. T., et al. (1991) Familial breast-ovarian cancer locus on chromosome 17q12-q23. *Lancet* **338,** 82,83.
14. Lastowska, M. A., Lillington, D. M., Shelling, A. N., et al. (1994) Fluorescence in situ hybridization analysis using cosmid probes to define chromosome 6q abnormalities in ovarian carcinoma cell lines. *Cancer Genet Cytogenet.* **77,** 99–105.
15. Kallioniemi, A., Kallioniemi, O. P., Sudar, D., et al. (1992) Comparative genomic hybridization for molecular cytogenetic analysis of solid tumors. *Science* **258,** 818–821.
16. Bentz, M., Plesch, A., Stilgenbauer, S., Dohner, H., and Lichter, P. (1998) Minimal sizes of deletions detected by comparative genomic hybridization. *Genes, Chromosomes Cancer* **21,** 172–175.
17. Speicher, M. R., Gwyn, Ballard, S., and Ward, D. C. (1996) Karyotyping human chromosomes by combinatorial multi-fluor FISH. *Nature Genet.* **12,** 368–375.
18. Stanbridge, E. J. (1992) Functional evidence for human tumor suppressor genes: chromosome and molecular genetic studies. *Cancer Surveys* **12,** 5–24.
19. Rimessi, P., Gualandi, F., Morelli, C., et al. (1994) Transfer of human chromosome 3 to an ovarian carcinoma cell line identifies three regions on 3p involved in ovarian cancer. *Oncogene* **9,** 3467–3474.
20. Cooke, I. E., Shelling, A. N., Le Meuth, V. G., Charnock, F. M. L., and Ganesan, T. S. (1996) Allele loss on chromosome arm 6q and fine mapping of the region at 6q27 in epithelial ovarian cancer. *Genes, Chromosomes, Cancer* **14,** 223–233.
21. Bustamante, C., Gurrieri, S., and Smith, S. B. (1993) Towards a molecular description of pulsed-field gel electrophoresis. *Trends In Biotechnol.* **11,** 23–30.
22. Lisitsyn, N. A., Lisitsina, N. M., Dalbagni, G., et al. (1995) Comparative genomic analysis of tumors: detection of DNA losses and amplification. *Proc. Natl. Acad. Sci. USA* **92,** 151–155.
23. Schutte, M., da Costa, L. T., Hahn, S. A., et al. (1995) Identification by representational difference analysis of a homozygous deletion in pancreatic carcinoma that lies within the BRCA2 region. *Proc. Natl. Acad. Sci. USA* **92,** 5950–5954.
24. Hahn, S. A., Schutte, M., Hoque, A. T. M. S., et al. (1996) DPC4, a candidate tumor suppressor gene at human chromosome 18q21.1. *Science* **271,** 350–353.
25. Howe, J. R., Roth, S., Ringold, J. C., et al. (1998) Mutations in the SMAD4/DPC4 gene in juvenile polyposis. *Science* **280,** 1086–1088.
26. Liang, P. and Pardee, A. B. (1992) Differential display of eukaryotic messenger RNA by means of the polymerase chain reaction. *Science* **257,** 967–971.
27. Orita, M., Iwahana, H., Kanazawa, H., Hayashi, K., and Sekiya, T. (1989) Detection of polymorphisms of human DNA by gel electrophoresis as single-strand conformation polymorphisms. *Proc. Natl. Acad. Sci. USA* **86,** 2766–2770.

28. Stratton, J. F., Gayther, S. A., Russell, P., et al. (1997) Contribution of BRCA1 mutations to ovarian cancer. *N. Engl. J. Med.* **336,** 1125–1130.

29. Ganguly, A., Rock, M. J., and Prockop, D. J. (1993) Conformation-sensitive gel electrophoresis for rapid detection of single-base differences in double-stranded PCR products and DNA fragments: evidence for solvent-induced bends in DNA heteroduplexes. *Proc. Natl. Acad. Sci. USA* **90,** 10,325–10,329.

30. Cotton, R. G. and Campbell, R. D. (1989) Chemical reactivity of matched cytosine and thymine bases near mismatched and unmatched bases in a heteroduplex between DNA strands with multiple differences. *Nucleic Acids Res.* **17,** 4223–4233.

31. FitzGerald, M. G., MacDonald, D. J., Krainer, M., et al. (1996) Germ-line BRCA1 mutations in Jewish and non-Jewish women with early-onset breast cancer. *N. Engl. J. Med.* **334,** 143–149.

32. Hacia, J. G., Brody, L. C., Chee, M. S., Fodor, S. P., and Collins, F. S. (1996) Detection of heterozygous mutations in BRCA1 using high density oligonucleotide arrays and two-colour fluorescence analysis. *Nature Genet.* **14,** 441–447.

33. King, B. L., Carcangiu, M. L., Carter, D., et al. (1995) Microsatellite instability in ovarian neoplasms. *Br. J. Cancer* **72,** 376–382.

34. Orth, K., Hung, J., Gazdar, A., Bowcock, A., Mathis, J. M., and Sambrook, J. (1994) Genetic instability in human ovarian cancer cell lines. *Proc. Natl. Acad. Sci. USA* **91,** 9495–9499.

35. Casey, G., Lopez, M. E., Ramos, J. C., et al. (1996) DNA sequence analysis of exons 2 through 11 and immunohistochemical staining are required to detect all known p53 alterations in human malignancies. *Oncogene* **13,** 1971–1981.

36. Ishioka, C., Frebourg, T., Yan, Y. X., et al. (1993) Screening patients for heterozygous p53 mutations using a functional assay in yeast. *Nature Genet.* **5,** 124–129.

37. Ishioka, C., Suzuki, T., FitzGerald, M., et al. (1997) Detection of heterozygous truncating mutations in the BRCA1 and APC genes by using a rapid screening assay in yeast. *Proc. Natl. Acad. Sci. USA* **94,** 2449–2453.

38. Humphrey, J. S., Salim, A., Erdos, M. R., Collins, F. S., Brody, L. C., and Klausner, R. D. (1997) Human BRCA1 inhibits growth in yeast: potential use in diagnostic testing. *Proc. Natl. Acad. Sci. USA* **94,** 5820–5825.

# 31

# Extraction of DNA from Microdissected Archival Tissues

## James J. Going

## 1. Introduction

Many modern analytical methods require little material, which has made feasible biochemical and molecular analyses of small tissue fragments, even individual cells, by microdissection of histological sections *(1,2)*. Polymerase chain reaction (PCR) can potentially be applied to the analysis of single DNA molecules, as in the analysis of single haploid cells, such as spermatozoa *(3)*. This sensitivity requires careful attention to technique and proper controls to avoid false positive or other spurious results.

Microdissection techniques used by different research groups are diverse, and recent papers explore different techniques *(4–7)*. This chapter presents a technique of histological microdissection applicable to a variety of tissues.

Microdissection can be applied to paraffin or frozen sections of human and animal tissues, depending on availability, but in human studies, it may be necessary to work with formalin-fixed paraffin-embedded archival tissues. Although fixed tissues have disadvantages, particularly degradation of nucleic acids after fixation, which may make successful PCR amplification less easy, better preservation of tissue morphology compensates. This may be important, as one purpose of histological microdissection is to bring together molecular and morphological analysis of the same cells. Fixed tissue sections may be easier to handle than unfixed tissues during microdissection. This chapter will concentrate on fixed tissues.

## 2. Materials

All reagents should be of molecular biology quality.

1. Proteinase K from *Tritirachium album* (Sigma, St. Louis, MO), 20 mg/mL stock solution. Store 50-μL aliquots at –20°C; thaw and dilute to 1 mL with digestion buffer containing 1% Tween to give working stock solution of proteinase K, 1 mg/mL for tissue digestion to release DNA.
2. Proteinase K digestion buffer, pH 8.3. (TRIS-HCl, 2.2 g/L; TRIS base 4.4 g/L; EDTA 0.37 g/L; separate batches of the buffer should be prepared detergent-free and containing 1% Tween).
3. Leica model 'M' mechanical micromanipulator (other micromanipulators may be suitable).

From: *Methods in Molecular Medicine, Vol. 39: Ovarian Cancer: Methods and Protocols*
Edited by: J. M. S. Bartlett © Humana Press, Inc., Totowa, NJ

4. 0.5-mm diameter tungsten wire for dissection needles (or ready-made needles); bacteriological loop holders for mounting needles in micromanipulator.
5. Facility for electrolytic sharpening of tungsten needles (*see* **Subheading 3.5.**).

## 3. Methods

### 3.1. Section Cutting

Careful clean techniques should be used when cutting sections for PCR analysis.

1. Use a new part of the microtome blade to cut each section, to avoid possible carryover of DNA from one tissue block to sections of the next.
2. Ribbons of sections should be floated out on a clean water bath and no buildup of section debris permitted.
3. Glass slides upon which sections are mounted should be scrupulously clean. Dry mount sections at 56°C for 2 h (*see* **Note 1**).

### 3.2. Dewaxing and Staining Sections

Dewax sections completely prior to microdissection.

1. Immerse 6–7 $\mu M$ sections in a slide rack for 10 min in xylene. Drain surplus xylene thoroughly from the sections to minimize carryover of dissolved wax and transfer to a second xylene bath for 2 min. Avoid breathing xylene vapor and be aware of the fire hazards of organic solvents.
2. Take sections through two baths of 99% industrial methylated spirits to remove xylene and a third bath of 95% industrial methylated spirits.
3. Transfer sections to distilled or deionised water of a satisfactory standard for preparing PCR reagents. Stain by immersion for 30 s in 0.05% w/v toluidine blue in distilled water (*see* **Note 2**).
4. Wash in distilled water (*see* **Note 3**).
5. After dissection, dehydrate and mount slides with a cover slip to provide a permanent record of the dissection (*see* **Note 4**).

### 3.4. Microdissection Tools

Successful dissection can be carried out freehand using sterile, curved, scalpel blades or sterile hypodermic needles, with or without a dissecting microscope.

1. Take a section for dissection from the water bath immediately before it is needed, drain it, and blot any surplus water from around the section with a disposable, lint-free tissue (do not touch the section).
2. Stroke the edge of the scalpel blade decisively across the section to remove a strip of tissue, the width of which varies with the angle between blade and section (*see* **Note 5**).
3. For more precise dissection with the micromanipulator, an electrolytically sharpened tungsten needle is ideal (**Fig. 1**). This tool consists of 25 mm of tungsten wire, 0.5 mm in diameter, sharpened and polished electrolytically to a fine point (tip radius several microns).
4. Mount the needle in a collet-type bacteriological loop holder.
5. Mount the loop holder in the tool holder of the micromanipulator and angle it downward 25°–30°.

### 3.5. Making and Maintaining Tungsten Microneedles

Tungsten needles can be obtained ready-made as "ohmic probe needles," but are easily fabricated from plain 0.5 mm tungsten wire (obtainable from suppliers of equipment for electron microscopy). This requires an electrolytic cell (*see* **Note 6**).

Fig. 1. Microdissection (stills from a video). **Frame 1:** the needle is placed at the periphery of an island of carcinoma cells (colonic carcinoma, paraffin section, toluidine blue stain).

1. Obtain ~10 cm of platinum wire (e.g., from an old electrophoresis apparatus) and make a circular loop in it, just small enough to fit inside a standard 20-mL universal container, with a "tail" 2–3 cm long.
2. Drill a 1-mm hole in the side of universal container near the base and thread the platinum wire tail through it, with the loop neatly placed at the base of the container. Seal the hole inside and out with an epoxy resin glue, e.g., Araldite.
3. Almost fill the cell with 0.1$M$ potassium hydroxide (KOH; 1.2 g in 20 mL) in water (**caution:** KOH is caustic).
4. Connect the platinum wire cathode to the negative (–) terminal of a standard 9-V radio battery (dry cell), and make the tungsten wire, mounted in its bacteriological loop holder, the anode (+). Ensure that the cell cannot fall over, spilling caustic electrolyte solution.
5. Complete the circuit by dipping 5–10 mm of the tungsten wire vertically into the KOH solution. Hydrogen bubbles appear at the platinum cathode and nascent oxygen removes tungsten from the anode, which sharpens to a fine, polished point. New needles are made this way and damaged needles refurbished. If sharpening does not occur, check polarity.
6. Straighten bent needles by rolling firmly between glass slides, then polish/resharpen.
7. Rinse needles with distilled water from a wash bottle after sharpening or resharpening to remove droplets of KOH electrolyte.

8. Store prepared needles in a covered Petri dish with the blunt end pressed lightly into a ring of modelling clay or similar. Handle with fine forceps.

## 3.6. Performing Microdissection

1. Retrieve the slide to be dissected from distilled water and dry the back of the slide and around the section, using a clean, disposable, laboratory tissue.
2. Place the section on the microscope stage (*see* **Note 7**) and cover with a pool of proteinase K lysis buffer (without detergent) from a disposable sterile Pasteur pipet with a rubber bulb pipet filler. Spread the pool of buffer until it extends 3–4 mm beyond all edges of the section and is as deep as possible without spillage.
3. Center the area of cells in the section to be retrieved for subsequent analysis in the microscope field at an appropriate magnification.
4. Using the coarse motion controls of the micromanipulator, place the needle over the area to be dissected.
5. Lower the needle gently at the edge of the area to be dissected until its tip just touches the slide. Stop lowering the needle when a small lateral deflection of the needle tip occurs (*see* **Note 9**).
6. Microdissection techniques vary for different specimens. In general, attempt by blunt dissection to develop cleavage between groups of cells. Work around the area to be dissected, developing a split between the area to be kept and the area to be removed (**Fig. 2**). Then use the point of the needle gradually to undermine the area to be recovered, pushing and pulling with the tip and side of the needle until the area to be retrieved has been peeled from the slide and floats freely in the buffer pool (**Fig. 3**).
7. If it is not clear whether the fragment is still attached to the section, gently agitate of the slide. Attached fragments do not move freely.
8. Sometimes a tissue fragment remains attached by a few strands of collagen; a second tungsten needle in a bacteriological loop holder, used freehand, will often detach it.

## 3.7. Retrieving Dissected Fragments

1. Bring the tip of the pipet close to the fragment to be retrieved, and capture the fragment by suddenly releasing the pipet plunger, dragging fragment and a fixed volume of buffer into the pipet tip (*see* **Note 8**).
2. Expel the captured specimen into a labeled microcentrifuge tube, ready for further processing (*see* **Note 9**).
3. Check that the microdissected specimen is actually in the tube. It helps if the fragment is easily seen with the naked eye. Use a magnifying lens or the microscope to be certain. Toluidine blue-stained fragments are easy to see; unstained fragments may be practically invisible.

## 3.8. Extracting DNA: Proteinase K Digestion

In a fixed specimen, nucleic acids are present in a dense array of crosslinked proteins. Proteinase K digestion appears effectively to release them and make them available for subsequent PCR.

1. Add an equal volume of proteinase K digestion buffer pH 8.3 containing 1 mg/mL of proteinase K and 1 mg/mL proteinase K to each specimen tube.
2. Digest microdissected specimen in proteinase K (final concentration 500 µg/mL), at 37°C overnight in a water bath or incubator (digestion can continue over a weekend without detriment).

Fig. 2. **Frame 2:** about half of the island of tumor cells has been separated from the glass slide.

3. Heat specimens in a PCR block (95°C for 10'), to inactivate PK.
4. Spin the specimen down by brief centrifugation.
5. Specimens are stable at room temperature for subsequent DNA PCR. Store for longer periods at 4°C or –20°C.
6. Accurate labeling is crucial (*see* **Note 10**).

### *3.9. DNA Purification after PK Digestion*

The 25-µL or 50-µL sample remaining after PK digestion of a microdissected tissue fragment contains only small quantities of nucleic acids (DNA, RNA). One thousand cells contain about 6 ng of DNA, and will contain, at most, 2000 copies of an amplifiable DNA sequence; only 1000 copies of each of two different alleles. An attempt to purify such quantities of DNA or RNA risks losing the specimen, although techniques have been described. Such purification does not obviously improve subsequent PCR amplification. Carefully optimize your PCR using the unpurified digest before you conclude that such purification is essential. Several published microdissection studies using the techniques described here have employed 1-µL aliquots of sample

Fig. 3. **Frame 3:** the whole island is completely detached, shown by slight rotation with respect to the position it occupied in the section. The sample is ready for collection, proteinase K digestion, and further analysis.

as template *(8–11)*. Strategies such as hot start, touchdown, nested, or real-time PCR may to help to obtain good PCR results by decreasing amplification of spurious products.

Techniques exist for whole-genome amplification of DNA from small samples, even single cells *(12–14)*, to expand the template pool available for subsequent PCR analysis. The possibility of introducing artifacts should be considered, but with appropriate controls may be used for projects with scanty material.

### 3.10. Frozen vs Paraffin Sections

Frozen sections are less easy to microdissect than paraffin sections. Unfixed are less robust than fixed tissues, and stand up not as well to the manipulation necessary to detach the specimen.

### 3.11. Analysis of RNA from Microdissected Material

RNA from unfixed tissue may be more suitable for analysis than RNA from fixed tissue; but RNA in unfixed tissue may be more susceptible to degradation, and RT-PCR of RNA from microdissected fixed tissue fragments can be achieved. Rather than performing the microdissection in a guanidinium-containing buffer, which removes toluidine blue from the section, perform microdissection in distilled water and transfer fragments subsequently to RT-PCR buffers.

## 4. Notes

1. Drying influences the firmness with which sections adhere to the slide, and ease of dissection. In general slides coated with poly-L-lysine or treated with silanes should be avoided. It may be difficult to detach tissue from such slides. Conventional 3–4 μm histological sections are a compromise between ease of cutting, depth of staining, and visibility of cytological detail. For histological microdissection, slightly thicker sections (6–8 μm) contain more nucleic acid per unit area, and slightly increased thickness does not usually cause interpretation problems. Over 10 μm poorer visualization of cells is a disadvantage. Cut and dried sections should be stored in dust-free conditions. There appears to be no need to store them in a refrigerator or freezer. Disposable latex gloves should be worn for all manipulations to reduce contamination.

2. Staining reveals tissue structure, but unstained sections may be dissectable, especially if a serial haematoxylin and eosin section is available for reference. Staining often makes dissection easier. Toluidine blue staining is easy and does not appear to interfere with subsequent PCR, although this should be verified for particular applications.

3. Stained sections can be stored in distilled water until dissection. Refrigeration at 4°C in water overnight causes some destaining and sections may lift from the slide. Stained sections can be stored dry, but it is best not to dewax and stain more sections than can be used in a single dissecting session.

4. A serial haematoxylin and eosin section shows what has been removed. A magnified photocopy or digital image of such a serial section can be annotated on hard copy or digitally to record the dissection. Photocopy histological sections through an acetate sheet to avoid scratching the photocopier glass or smearing it with mounting medium.

5. A scalpel blade vertically in contact with the section will remove a narrow strip of tissue. The blade at a flatter angle will remove a wider strip. Tissue so removed can often be rolled into a small ball or "pill," picked up on the tip of the scalpel blade or sterile hypodermic needle, and transferred to a microcentrifuge tube for further processing. Tissue is most easily handled when damp, but without excess water, in which dispersed tissue fragments are hard to retrieve or too dry and brittle. Static electricity may be troublesome.

6. Bacteriological loop holders and tungsten wire are inexpensive. Either prepare enough needles in advance to use a new needle for each microdissection if necessary or briefly repolish the needle between samples, which exposes a new tungsten surface. The risk of DNA carryover on the needle from one specimen to the next appears largely theoretical. In a study of *ras* mutation in colorectal carcinomas *(10)*, no false positives were detected in the analysis of several hundred separate microdissected normal and tumor tissue samples.

7. Any microscope can be used if there is enough space between objective and stage for access to the specimen. Ordinary or inverted standard microscopes can be used, but a stereo dissecting microscope with relatively high maximum magnification (up to ×120) is ideal.

8. 12.5 or 25 μL capture volumes work well. The pipet should be nearly vertical to minimize the risk of damaging the section. Use a Gilson-type pipet with a wide-bore polypropylene tip. Such tips are in many manufacturer's catalogs, or cut the end off an ordinary pipet tip. *Steady your hand, holding the pipet, against your fist resting on the microscope stage.* The fragment may be hard to retrieve if it lies flat on the section or slide. Briskly expelling buffer toward the fragment will usually lift the fragment to a level from which it may

easily be recovered. Retrieval of dissected fragments without damage to the section is easier from a deep pool of buffer. The buffer should not contain detergent such as Triton X-100 which, by reducing surface tension, prevents the formation of a deep standing pool of buffer.

9. If the specimen adheres to the inside of the pipet tip, it can sometimes be dislodged by repeated indrawing and expulsion of buffer. It may be picked out with a needle, or cut off the pipet tip and place that, with the tissue fragment, in the tube for subsequent digestion. Sticking can usually be avoided by coating pipet tips before use with a silicone such as Sigmacote. Draw (e.g., 50 μL) of Sigmacote into the tip, expel it again, shake off any excess, and allow to dry. Coat tips 1 hr or 2 before you need them. Collect microdissected fragments for further processing in 500-μL tubes with screw-on lids sealed with rubber O rings. The O ring prevents loss of specimen volume by evaporation during subsequent processing and 500-μL tubes fit most PCR thermal cycling blocks for heating to inactivate proteinase K after the digestion process is complete.

10. Labeling must survive overnight incubation in the water bath and subsequent heat inactivation in the PCR thermal cycler block, the wells of which often contain oil traces which may dissolve even "permanent" marker pen inks. Write specimen numbers on the lid of the container as well. Typing correction fluid on the lid gives a white surface on which graphite pencil is permanent. If you label the lid you must not transpose lids. Do not open more than one specimen tube at a time, and replace the lid at once.

## References

1. Schriever, F., Freeman, G. and Nadler, L. M. (1991) Follicular dendritic cells contain a unique gene repertoire demonstrated by single-cell polymerase chain reaction. *Blood* **77,** 787–791.
2. Trumper, L. H., Brady, G., Bagg, A., Gray, D., Loke, S. L., Griesser, H., et al. (1993) Single-cell analysis of Hodgkin and Reed-Sternberg cells: molecular heterogeneity of gene expression and p53 mutations. *Blood* **81,** 3097–3115.
3. Hubert, R., Weber, J. L., Schmitt, K., and Arnheim, N. (1992) A new source of polymorphic DNA markers for sperm typing: analysis of microsatellite repeats in single cells. *Am. J. Hum. Genet.* **51,** 985–991.
4. Emmert-Buck, M. R., Bonner, R. F., Smith, P. D., Chuaqui, R. F., Zhuang, Z. P., Goldstein, S. R., et al. (1996) Laser capture microdissection. *Science* **274,** 998–1001.
5. Moskaluk, C. A. and Kern, S. E. (1997) Microdissection and polymerase chain reaction amplification of genomic DNA from histological tissue sections. *Am. J. Pathol.* **150,** 1547–1552.
6. Bohm, M., Wieland, I., Schutze, K., and Rubben, H. (1997) Microbeam MOMeNT - non-contact laser microdissection of membrane-mounted native tissue. *Am. J. Pathol.* **151,** 63–67.
7. Fend, F., Emmert-Buck, M. R., Lee, J., Cole, K., Chaqui, R. F., Liotta, L. A., and Raffeld, M. (1998) Immuno-LCM: laser capture microdissection of immunostained frozen sections for RNA analysis. *Modern Pathol.* **11,** A185.
8. Murphy, D. S., Hoare, S. F., Going, J. J., Mallon, E. A., George, W. D., Kaye, S. B., et al. (1995) Characterisation of extensive genetic alterations in ductal carcinoma in situ by fluorescence in situ hybridisation and molecular analysis. *J. Natl. Cancer Inst.* **87,** 1694–1704.
9. Going, J. J. and Lamb, R. F. (1996) Practical histological dissection for PCR analysis. *J. Pathol.* **179,** 121–124.
10. Lamb, R. F., Going, J. J., Pickford, I., and Birnie, G. D. (1996) Allelic imbalance at the NME1 locus in microdissected primary and metastatic human colorectal carcinomas is frequent, but not associated with metastasis to lymph nodes or liver. *Cancer Res.* **56,** 916–920.
11. Al Mulla, F., Going, J. J., Sowden, E. T. H. H., Winter, A., Pickford, I. R., and Birnie, G. D. (1998) Heterogeneity of mutant versus wild-type Ki-ras in primary and metastatic colorectal carcinomas, and association of codon-12 valine with early mortality. *J. Pathol.* **185,** 130–138.
12. Zhang, L., Cui, X., Schmitt, K., Hubert, R., Navidi, W., and Arnheim, N. (1992) Whole genome amplification from a single cell: implications for genetic analysis. *Proc. Natl. Acad. Sci. USA* **89,** 5847–5851.
13. Telenius, H., Carter, N. P., Bebb, C. E., Nordenskjold, M., Ponder, B. A. J., and Tunnacliffe, A. (1992) Degenerate oligonucleotide-primed PCR: general amplification of target DNA by a single degenerate primer. *Genomics* **13,** 718–725.
14. Grothues, D., Cantor, C. R., and Smith, C. L. (1993) PCR amplification of megabase DNA with tagged random primers (T-PCR). *Nucleic Acids Res.* **5,** 1321,1322.

# 32

# RFLP Molecular Analysis of the Urokinase-Type Plasminogen Activator Gene

**Bernd Muehlenweg, Andreas Schnelzer, Beyhan Türkmen, Ernst Lengyel, Ute Reuning, Henner Graeff, Manfred Schmitt, and Viktor Magdolen**

## 1. Introduction

Several cell biological studies have shown that the invasiveness of a variety of tumors depend on the regulated expression of proteolytic enzymes that degrade the surrounding extracellular matrix and dissociate cell–cell and/or cell–matrix attachments. One such enzyme, the serine protease urokinase-type plasminogen activator (uPA), converts enzymatically inactive plasminogen into the widely acting protease plasmin, which degrades several extracellular matrix components and also activates proenzyme forms of matrix metalloproteases. Thus, uPA is a central molecule in pericellular proteolysis (1–4). uPA (as well as other factors of the plasminogen activator system, the cell surface-associated uPA receptor [uPAR], and the plasminogen activator inhibitor type-1 [PAI-1]) is an important prognostic factor predicting relapse-free and/or survival in patients with a variety of solid malignant tumors including ovarian cancer; in all cases, high levels of uPA are associated with a poor prognosis (4–6).

In view of the important role of uPA, uPAR, and PAI-1 for tumor cell spreading, it is tempting to speculate that alterations in these genes may be a cause for the development or the progression of cancer. Therefore, we analyzed whether the genes encoding these factors are altered in ovarian cancer (7,8). In the case of uPA, a so-far unknown mutation in codon 121 (located in the kringle domain of uPA) has been identified resulting in a proline to leucine exchange. This exchange creates an *Alu* I restriction site thus making restriction fragment length polymorphism (RFLP) analyses possible.

In the present paper, we describe the basic protocols for the handling of tumor tissue, RNA and DNA preparation, polymerase chain reaction (PCR) amplification and RFLP analysis using molecular analysis of the *uPA* gene as an example. These protocols can be used for the analyses of any other given gene.

## 2. Materials

Ovarian cancer tissue specimens from primary tumors or metastases were obtained at surgery (8). In order to obtain undegraded RNA, it is important to freeze the samples as fast as possible in liquid nitrogen or less preferably at –80°C. In most cases, it is not

From: *Methods in Molecular Medicine, Vol. 39: Ovarian Cancer: Methods and Protocols*
Edited by: J. M. S. Bartlett © Humana Press, Inc., Totowa, NJ

possible to freeze the tissue immediately because the tissue specimens are examined by the pathologist after surgery. Under these circumstances the tissue must stay on ice prior to freezing for not longer than 30 min.

### 2.1. Isolation of Genomic DNA

1. QIAamp™ Blood and tissue kit (Qiagen, Chatsworth, CA).
2. Blood collection tube containing citrate solution.

### 2.2. RNA Extraction from Tissue

1. TRIzol Reagent (Gibco, Life Technologies, Bethesda, MI).
2. Chloroform (ultrapure, Merck, Rahway, NJ).
3. Isopropanol (ultrapure, Merck).
4. 75% Ethanol:25% Di-ethyl-pyrocarbonate (DEPC-) treated water (Sigma).
5. RNAse-free water (Sigma).

### 2.3. DNase-I Digestion

1. RNase-Inhibitor, 10 U/μL; Gibco, Life Technologies).
2. DNase-I 100 U/μL; (DNase-I amplification grade, RNase free; Gibco, Life Technologies), with buffer and 25 m$M$ EDTA.
3. Random hexamer primer: p(dN)$_6$, 50 A$_{260}$ U in 200 μL RNase free water (Roche, Mannheim, Germany).

### 2.4. Reverse Transcription

1. Superscript-II RNase H⁻-Reverse transcriptase and buffer (Gibco, Life technologies).
2. dNTP mixture, 10 m$M$ each of dATP, dCTP, dGTP, dTTP (Amersham, Arlington Heights, IL).
3. 5X first strand synthesis buffer (250 m$M$ Tris-HCl, ph 8.3, 375 m$M$ KCl, 15 m$M$ MgCl$_2$, supplied with superscript-II RNase H⁻-Reverse transcriptase.
4. 100 m$M$ DTT.

### 2.5. Polymerase Chain Reaction

1. uPA Primers 10 pmol/μL: uPA-up: 5′-GCC TCA GAG TCT TTT GGC -3′, uPA-down: 5′-CTG ATG CTC TTC AGC TGG -3′.
2. dNTP-PCR mixture, 2.5 m$M$ each of dATP, dCTP, dGTP, dTTP (Amersham).
3. GeneAmp™ PCR Buffer: (100 m$M$ Tris-HCl, pH 8.3, 500 m$M$ KCl, 15 m$M$ MgCl$_2$, 0.01% (w/v) gelatin; Perkin Elmer, Norwalk, CT) and AmpliTaq Gold.

### 2.6. Restriction Fragment Length Polymorphism

1. Phenol:chloroform:isoamylalchohol (P:C:I; 24:1:1; v/v/v).
2. 4$M$ lithium chloride (LiCl).
3. Glycogen: 20 mg/mL in water.
4. *Alu* I restriction enzyme (10 U/μL, Promega, Madison, WI) with Core buffer B.
5. TBE Buffer: Tris-Borate-EDTA Buffer (Sigma, St. Louis, MO).

## 3. Methods

### 3.1. Isolation of Genomic DNA

#### 3.1.1. Extraction from Tissue

Preparation of high molecular weight genomic DNA is performed as described in detail in the handbook of the QIAamp® Blood and Tissue Kit (Qiagen).

Fig. 1. PCR amplification of *uPA* gene probes using genomic DNA or total RNA isolated from ovarian cancer tissue as template. (**A**) Genomic DNA and (**B**) total RNA isolated from three different ovarian cancer tissues (lanes 2,3,4); lane 1, 1 kb ladder (PeqLab). Genomic DNA (**C**) and cDNA obtained by reverse transcription of total RNA (**D**) were used as template for PCR amplification using primers directed to exon 5 (uPA-down) and exon 7 (uPA-up) of the *uPA* gene (lanes 2,3,4); lane 1, 100 bp ladder (PeqLab). The PCR products differ in size because of the presence of intronic sequences in the genomic DNA (for details see **Fig. 2A** and **B**).

1. 25 mg of each ovarian cancer tissue (0.5 cm³) is cut into small pieces and incubated at 55°C in 180 µL buffer ATL (= Tris/HCl-buffer, pH 8.3, containing a detergent) and 20 µL of proteinase K (18 mg/mL) until the tissue is completely lysed.
2. 200 µL of buffer AL (= aqueous solution of guanidine hydrochloride) is added to the sample and the sample is incubated at 70°C for 10 min.
3. After addition of 210 µL ethanol, the sample is mixed thoroughly by vortexing and is then applied to a QIAamp spin column and centrifuged for 1 min at 6000$g$ in a microfuge.
4. The spun column is washed twice by centrifugation (1 min, 6000$g$) with 500 µL of buffer AW (= Tris-buffered saline).
5. The genomic DNA is subsequently eluted by centrifugation (1 min, 6000$g$) with 200 µL of a basic buffer (10 m$M$ Tris-HCl, pH 9.0).
6. The quality and quantity of the purified DNA is determined by measuring the absorbance at 260 and 280 nm (*see* **Note 1**, ratio $A_{260/280}$ should be between 1.7 and 1.9) and by gel electrophoresis using a 0.8–1% (w/v) agarose gel stained with ethidium bromide (**Fig. 1A**).

### 3.1.2. Extraction from Peripheral Blood

In order to analyze, whether detected mutations represent *de novo* tumor-specific *mutations*, the results obtained with genomic DNA derived from tumor tissue have to be compared to those using genomic DNA from normal cells, e.g., from peripheral blood. Therefore, we also routinely isolate DNA from blood samples. For this, we first prepare a so-called buffy coat (which is a leukocyte enriched fraction of whole blood) and then isolate genomic DNA from the buffy coat.

1. 5 mL of venous blood is collected in a tube containing 0.5 mL citrate solution.
2. The sample is centrifuged for 20 min at 4500$g$ at room temperature (RT).
3. After centrifugation, three layers are visible. The intermediate layer representing the buffy coat is isolated.
4. 25 µL proteinase K (18 mg/mL) and 200 µL of buffer AL (= aqueous solution of guanidine hydrochloride) are added to 200 µL of buffy coat and the mixed sample is subsequently incubated at 70°C for 10 min.
5. Further steps are identical as described in **steps 3–6** for isolation of genomic DNA from tumor tissue (**Subheading 3.1.1.**, *see* **Note 1**).

## 3.2. RNA Extraction from Tissue

There are several commercially available kits for total RNA isolation based on the original method of Chomczynski and Sacchi *(9)*, using guanidinium thiocyanate as denaturing agent. The use of reagents such as TRIzol offers several advantages: The brief protocol reduces the risk of contamination and degradation through RNases. Moreover, TRIzol can be used to extract RNA, DNA as well as proteins from the same sample *(10)*.

1. Cool a ceramic mortar and the pestle with liquid nitrogen (always leave some nitrogen in the mortar).
2. Transfer about 100 mg of the frozen tissue sample from the vial to the mortar.
3. After evaporation of the nitrogen, homogenize the tissue sample into a fine powder.
4. Add 1 mL of TRIzol Reagent (4°C; Gibco, Life Technologies) to the frozen powder. Let the TRIzol reagent freeze in the cold mortar without adding any nitrogen.
5. Homogenize and mix the frozen TRIzol reagent with the tissue powder.
6. Allow thawing of the mix. During this process (which can last up to 45–60 min), carefully stir the thawing mixture. Transfer the thawed, viscous solution into a RNase-free 2 mL microfuge tube (the solution can now be stored at –20°C).
7. Incubate the homogenate at RT for 5 min to permit complete dissociation of the nuclear protein complexes.
8. Add 200 µL of chloroform and vortex the tube vigorously for 15 s. Incubate the tube for 3 min at RT.
9. Centrifuge at 12,000$g$ for 10 min at 4°C and transfer the aqueous phase into another RNase-free tube (the organic phase should be saved if isolation of DNA or protein is desired).
10. Add 500 µL of isopropanol and mix by inverting the tube several times (do not vortex).
11. Incubate the sample for 10 min at RT and centrifuge the tube at 12,000$g$ for 10 min at 4°C.
12. Carefully remove the supernatant (the RNA has formed a gel-like pellet which can be hardly seen).
13. Wash the pellet once with 1 mL of 75% EtOH/25% DEPC-treated $H_2O$; vortex briefly and centrifuge the tube again at 7,500$g$ for 5 min at 4°C. Carefully remove the supernatant.
14. Invert the tube to dry the pellet at RT (do not dry the pellet completely as solubility will decrease dramatically).
15. Dissolve the RNA pellet in RNase-free $H_2O$ (30–100 µL).
16. Determine the RNA content by a photometrical measurement at $\lambda = 260$ nm (*see* **Note 1**). If the $A_{260/280}$ ratio is <1.6, the RNA is not resuspended properly or degraded *(11)*.

17. As a control, analyze the RNA preparation by gel electrophoresis (1% w/v agarose; 5–10 µg total RNA per lane) as shown in **Fig. 1B**. The comb and the tray for pouring the gel should be incubated overnight in 0.5 *N* NaOH and subsequently washed in DEPC-treated $H_2O$.

18. RNA dissolved in $H_2O$ can be stored for up to 1 yr at –80°C. For longer storage, keep the RNA ethanol-precipitated at –80°C.

### 3.3. DNase-I Digestion

Without DNase-I digestion, you run the risk of getting false positive results during PCR amplification because of genomic DNA contamination. This is especially true if in the PCR two primers are used, which target sequences within a single exon or if processed pseudogenes of the target gene are present in the genomic DNA *(12)*.

1. For DNase-I digestion of total RNA add: x µL RNA (1 µg), (6-x) µL RNase-free $H_2O$, 1 µL RNase-Inhibitor (10 U/µL; Gibco, Life Technologies), 1 µL DNase-I (100 U/µL; DNase-I amplification grade, RNAse-free; Gibco, Life Technologies), 1 µL 10X DNase-buffer (supplied with DNase I). Incubate the microfuge tube at RT for 15 min.

2. Add 1 µL EDTA (25 m*M*, supplied with DNase I) to stop the reaction, mix by pipetting up and down (total 10 µL).

3. Heat the tube to 70°C for 10 min to denature DNase I.

4. After 4 min, add 1 µL random primer (p(dN)$_6$, 50 $A_{260}$ U in 200 µL RNase-free $H_2O$; Boehringer Mannheim) to the reaction mix, to make sure that all primers are single-stranded. This is important for efficient annealing in the subsequent reverse transcription reaction.

5. After 10 min, place the tube on ice (total volume 11 µL).

### 3.4. Reverse Transcription

The reverse transcriptase Superscript-II-RT, a type of Moloney murine leukemia virus (MMLV) reverse transcriptase, synthesizes high yields of full length cDNAs because of a point mutation in the RNase H-domain (H⁻). After initial RNA-dependent DNA synthesis, the mRNA is, in contrast to other reverse transcriptase reactions, not hydrolyzed and functions more than once as a template. However, amplification of some PCR targets over 1 kbp may require the removal of the mRNA complementary to its cDNA by addition of RNase H.

1. For reverse transcription add to 11 µL reaction mix (*see* **Subheading 3.3., step 5.**): 4 µL of 5X first strand synthesis buffer, 2 µL DTT (100 m*M*), 1 µL dNTP-mix (10 m*M*), 1 µL reverse transcriptase (*see* **Note 2**).

2. Place one drop (30 µL) of mineral oil (Sigma) on top of the reaction mix (19 µL total volume) to minimize evaporation and risk of contamination.

3. Incubate the reaction mix in the thermocycler (e.g., Perkin Elmer GeneAmp® PCR System 2400) performing following steps: 1) 10 min, 25 °C; 2) 10 s, 30°C; 3) 10 s, 35°C; 4) 50 min, 42°C.

4. Cool the microfuge tube on ice (probes may be stored at –20°C).

### 3.5. Polymerase Chain Reaction (PCR)

1. For the PCR-reaction mix: 2 µL template (cDNA or genomic DNA), 5 µL primer uPA-up, 5 µL primer uPA-down, 5 µL dNTP-PCR mixture (2.5 m*M*), 5 µL GeneAmp®PCR buffer, 0.2 µL AmpliTaq Gold™ (5 U/µL), 27.8 µL $H_2O$ (*see* **Note 3**).

2. Briefly vortex the PCR mixture and run the following program on the thermal cycler:

| Activation of *Taq* Polymerase | | 94°C | 9 min |
|---|---|---|---|
| Amplification | 10 cycles | 94°C | 45 s |
| | | 37°C | 45 s |
| | | 72°C | 45 s |
| | 20 cycles | 94°C | 45 s |
| | | 54°C | 45 s |
| | | 72°C | 45 s |
| Extension | | 72°C | 7 min |

3. As a control, visualize 10 µL of the amplified PCR mixture on a 1–2 % (w/v) agarose gel stained with ethidium bromide (*see* **Notes 4–6**). Examples of amplification of genomic DNA and cDNA, respectively, are depicted in **Figs. 1C** and **D**.

### 3.6. Restriction Fragment Length Polymorphism (RFLP)

1. Extract the PCR-amplified DNA with 1 vol phenol:cholorform:isoamylalcohol (P:C:I) (24:1:1) and separate the phases via centrifugation at 12,000*g* for 3 min at RT.
2. Transfer the aqueous phase into a new microfuge tube and precipitate the DNA by adding 10%-vol. 4 *M* LiCl, 1 µL glycogen (20 mg/mL) per 100 µL PCR-mixture (to facilitate DNA precipitation) and 2 vol. EtOH 100%.
3. Leave the mixture on ice for 20 min.
4. Centrifuge the mixture for 20 min (4°C, 12,000*g*), decant EtOH, dry the pellet, and resuspended the pellet in 20 µL $H_2O$.
5. To 17 µL of the DNA solution, add 2 µL *Alu* I digestion buffer and 1 µL (10 U) *Alu* 1. Digest the DNA with *Alu* I overnight at 37°C and repeat **steps 1–3**.
6. After resuspending the pellet in 10–20 µL $H_2O$, the sample is visualized using a 8% TBE-polyacrylamide or by a 1–2% (w/v) agarose gel stained with ethidium bromide (examples are shown in **Fig. 2**, *see* **Note 7**).

## 4. Notes

1. In the present paper, we describe methods for isolating both DNA and RNA from ovarian cancer tissue and peripheral blood. The typical yields from 25 mg ovarian cancer tissue or 250 µL buffy coat, respectively, range between 20 and 40 µg of genomic DNA. The yield of RNA is between 1 and 10 µg/mg tissue, depending on tissue origin and quality.
2. The random hexamers used as primers for reverse transcription are oligodeoxynucleotides (6-mers) exhibiting extended sequence diversity to ensure that at least some oligodeoxynucleotides will anneal to the template and serve as primers for reverse transcription. Different oligodeoxynucleotides will bind randomly to different sequences, leading to high copies of the template. Thus, all parts of the sequence should be copied in equal amounts if each random primer is present at equal concentration.
3. Using primers from different exons (exon 5 and 7 in the case of the analysis of the *Pro/Leu121* polymorphism, which is encoded by exon 6 of the *uPA* gene), an amplification of a processed pseudogene with genomic DNA as template can be ruled out without further controls. However, to exclusively analyze transcribed genes, e.g., by PCR or by Northern blots (qualitatively and quantitatively), the preparation of high-quality mRNA is necessary. For this, it is an absolute requirement that the tissue has been handled appropriately, otherwise the mRNA will be more or less degraded. After reverse transcription, the cDNA

Fig. 2. Detection of the *Pro121Leu* exchange in *uPA* by restriction fragment length poly-morphism (RFLP). Localization of the *Alu* I sites in the exon-6 containing amplicons using primers uPA-down/uPA-up and genomic DNA (**A**) or cDNA obtained by reverse transcription of total RNA (**B**), respectively, as template. *Alu* I digestion of exon6-containing PCR products derived from genomic DNA (**C**) or total RNA (**D**), respectively, of three different ovarian can-cer tissues. Lane 1, sample of a tumor tissue containing both alleles; lane 2, sample of a tumor tissue homozygous for the *Leu121* allel; lane 3, sample of a tumor tissue homozygous for the *Pro121* allel; lane 4, 100 bp ladder (PeqLab). The small DNA fragments appearing after *Alu* I digestion of each PCR-derived DNA fragment (69 bp and 12 bp in the case of genomic DNA-derived PCR products; 12 bp in the case of cDNA-derived PCR products) are not shown.

can be used in an identical manner as the genomic DNA. An aliquot of the DNase-treated RNA sample should be subjected to PCR amplification (without reverse transcription) to control for the absence of DNA-derived products.

4. In some cases, the described PCR protocol does not yield a visible band after PCR amplification (e.g., when mRNA of the target gene is low expressed and, therefore, the yield of cDNA is low). Therefore, a nested PCR with internal primers of the generated (nonvisible) amplification fragment has to be performed *(12)*.

5. If large amounts of so-called primer-dimers are present, DNA fragments should be gel-purified prior to RFLP or sequence analysis. The freeze-squeeze method described by Tautz and Renz *(13)* yields DNA which is an excellent template for DNA sequencing (and RFLP analysis). However, other commercially available kits for gel purification of DNA fragments may also be used.

6. Sequence variants can be easily detected by direct DNA sequencing of the PCR products. In our hands, DNA sequencing reactions are carried out using cycle sequencing (50–200 ng DNA per reaction, depending on fragment size), and the individual reactions are loaded on an ABI Model 377 Sequencer *(8)*.

7. RFLP analysis is a powerful tool for initial screening of a series of probes for genomic mutations. However, new methods and instruments are emerging which allow an extremely high throughput genotyping and PCR product quantification. The LightCycler (developed by Idaho Technology and Roche), for example, is a rapid thermal cycler (performing 30 PCR cycles in less than 20 min) combined with a microvolume fluorimeter allowing genotyping with melting peaks *(14)*.

## References

1. Dano, K., Andreasen, P. A., Grondahl-Hansen, J., Kristensen, P., Nielsen, L. S., and Skriver, L. (1985) Plasminogen activators, tissue degradation, and cancer. *Adv. Cancer Res.* **44,** 139–266.
2. Schmitt, M., Wilhelm, O., Jänicke, F., Magdolen, V., Reuning, U., Ohi, H., et al. (1995) Urokinase-type plasminogen activator (uPA) and its receptor (CD87): a new target in tumor invasion and metastasis. *J. Obstet. Gynaecol.* **21,** 151–165.
3. Blasi, F. (1997) uPA, uPAR, PAI-1: key intersection of proteolytic, adhesive and chemotactic highways? *Immunol. Today* **18,** 415–417.
4. Schmitt, M., Harbeck, N., Thomssen, C., Wilhelm, O., Magdolen, V., Reuning, U., et al. (1997) Clinical impact of the plasminogen activation system in tumor invasion and metastasis: prognostic relevance and target for therapy. *Thromb. Haemost.* **78,** 285–296.
5. Kuhn, W., Pache, L., Schmalfeldt, B., Dettmar, P., Schmitt, M., Jänicke, F., and Graeff, H. (1994) Urokinase (uPA) and PAI-1 predict survival in advanced ovarian cancer patients (FIGO III) after radical surgery and platinum-based chemotherapy. *Gynecol. Oncol.* **55,** 401–409.
6. Schmalfeldt, B., Kuhn, W., Reuning, U., Pache, L., Dettmar, P., Schmitt, M., et al. (1995) Primary tumor and metastasis in ovarian cancer differ in their content of urokinase-type plasminogen activator, its receptor, and inhibitors types 1 and 2. *Cancer Res.* **55,** 3958–3963.
7. Türkmen, B., Magdolen, V., Trommler, P., Creutzburg, S., Graeff, H., and Schmitt, M. (1997) Sequence analysis of cDNAs encoding PAI-1, uPA and uPAR from ovarian cancer cell lines, in *Adv. Exp. Biol.* **425,** 266–267.
8. Türkmen, B., Schmitt, M., Schmalfeldt, B., Trommler, P., Hell, W., Creutzburg, S., et al. (1997) Mutational analysis of the genes encoding urokinase-type plasminogen activator (uPA) and its inhibitor (PAI-1) in advanced ovarian cancer *Electrophoresis* **18,** 686–689.
9. Chomczynski, P. and Sachi, N. (1987) Single step method of RNA isolation by acid guanidinium thiocyanate-phenol-chloroform extraction. *Anal. Biochem.* **162,** 156.
10. Chomczynski, P. (1995) A reagent for the single-step simultaneous isolation of RNA, DNA and proteins from cell and tissue samples. *BioTechniques* **15,** 532–534.
11. Sambrook, J., Fritsch, E. F., and Maniatis, T. (1989) *Molecular Cloning. A Laboratory Manual.* Cold Spring Harbor Laboratory Press, Cold Spring Harbor, New York.
12. Rolfs, A., Schuller, I., Finckh, U., and Weber-Rolfs, I. (1992) *PCR: Clinical Diagnostics and Research.* Springer Laboratory, Springer-Verlag, Berlin, Germany.
13. Tautz, D. and Renz, M. (1993) An optimized freeze-squeeze method for the recovery of DNA fragments from agarose gels. *Anal. Biochem.* **132,** 14–19.
14. Wittwer, C., Ririe, K., Andrew, R., David, D., Gundry, R., and Balis, U. (1997) The LightCycler: a micro-volume multisample fluorimeter with rapid temperature control. *BioTechniques* **22,** 176–181.

# 33

## PCR Microsatellite Analysis of LOH in Ovarian Tumors

### Jayne Devlin and Margaret A. Knowles

### 1. Introduction

The "two-hit" theory of tumor suppressor gene (TSG) inactivation predicts that loss of function is a result of two separate genetic events, one affecting each allele *(1)*. One hit is commonly a deletion of part of, or the entire allele sequence and can be detected by loss of heterozygosity (LOH) analysis in which "normal" DNA is compared with tumor DNA at various loci. At heterozygous loci, the two alleles in normal DNA are observed as separate bands; if an allele has been lost in a tumor, one of the bands is absent in the tumor DNA. Such deletions are termed LOH and indicate a likely site of a TSG. When LOH occurs, it is predicted that the retained allele is nonfunctional either because of a point mutation or a microdeletion. The next step in testing the authenticity of the putative suppressor gene is to look for small genetic alterations in the retained allele.

Mapping genes by LOH relies on normal DNA being heterozygous for alleles under test. Highly polymorphic markers are therefore vital to the success of genetic mapping projects. The most commonly used polymorphic markers in mapping and linkage studies are the microsatellites; the most popular being the (dC-dA)n dinucleotide repeats, which are distributed at high density throughout the genome *(2)*. Microsatellites are relatively short DNA fragments, usually less than 100 basepairs. This together with the fact that they are usually embedded in unique sequence DNA means that they can be readily amplified by PCR using appropriately designed primers and so many samples can be typed very rapidly. It is also possible to amplify sequences from formalin-fixed paraffin-embedded tissue from archival samples; normal DNA can be obtained from tissue adjacent to the tumor when no blood is available.

In order to identify the chromosomes that harbor putative TSGs, allelotypes are constructed. Large numbers of tumors are screened for LOH using a small number of microsatellite markers on each autosomal chromosomal arm. The arms which are most frequently involved in deletions are the likely sites for TSGs. High-density deletion mapping is then performed on specific chromosome arms to build up a deletion profile and further define the regions of loss. Large numbers of tumors often show LOH at all informative loci on a chromosome and this usually represents monosomy. Generally very few tumors have small terminal or interstitial deletions and are therefore very valuable in deletion-mapping studies. Tumors of different histology or differentiation

From: *Methods in Molecular Medicine, Vol. 39: Ovarian Cancer: Methods and Protocols*
Edited by: J. M. S. Bartlett © Humana Press, Inc., Totowa, NJ

states can be compared to see whether the same TSG is inactivated. In addition, deletion maps from a second tumor that recurs can be compared with the original to determine whether it is "genetically similar."

The standard protocol for microsatellite typing tumors using radioactive procedures is detailed below. There are various modifications to this protocol involving nonradioactive methods *(3)*.

## 2. Materials

### 2.1. DNA Extraction

1. Lysis buffer A: 0.32$M$ sucrose, 10 m$M$ Tris-HCl pH 7.5, 5 m$M$ MgCl$_2$, 1% Triton-100, autoclave before use and store at 4°C.
2. Lysis buffer B: 0.075$M$ NaCl, 0.024$M$ EDTA pH 8.0, store at room temperature.
3. Lysis buffer B containing 0.1% SDS and 100 µg/mL proteinase K.
4. Lysis buffer B containing 1% SDS and 170 µg/mL proteinase K.
5. TE Saturated Phenol
6. 1:1 Phenol:chloroform
7. TE: 10 m$M$ Tris, 0.5$M$ EDTA pH 8.0.

### 2.2. End Labeling

1. Oligonucleotide primer (CA or F) strand (Research Genetics), supplied at 200 µ$M$, dilute with water and use at 10 µ$M$. Store at –20°C.
2. γ $^{32}$P -dATP (Amersham, Arlington Hts., IL).
3. T4 polynucleotide kinase (Promega, U.K.). Enzyme is diluted to 1 U/µL in 50 m$M$ Tris-HCl pH 8.0 before use as concentrated enzyme can often result in lower levels of incorporation.

### 2.3. Polymerase Chain Reaction

1. Oligonucleotide primer (GT or R) strand, (working concentration and storage temperature as for CA strand; *see* **Subheading 2.2.**).
2. *Taq* polymerase (supplied with buffers and separate magnesium chloride solution).
3. 2 m$M$ dNTP stock (2 m$M$ each dATP, dCTP, dTTP, dGTP).

### 2.4. Gel Electrophoresis

1. 10% ammonium persulphate, make fresh.
2. Loading buffer: 95% formamide, 10 m$M$ EDTA pH 8.0, 0.05% xylene, 0.05% bromophenol blue, and store at room temperature.
3. 10X TBE: 1$M$ Tris-HCl, 0.9$M$ boric acid, 0.01$M$ EDTA, pH 8.3.
4. Gel fix: 10% methanol, 10% glacial acetic acid in water, make up fresh.

## 3. Methods

### 3.1. DNA Extraction

#### 3.1.1. From Leukocytes

High molecular weight DNA is prepared from blood leukocytes. A 10-mL venous blood sample from each patient is collected in EDTA tubes from which leukocyte DNA is prepared.

1. Lyse red cells in 40 mL lysis buffer A on ice for 10 min.
2. Centrifuge at 1500$g$ for 15 min at 4°C to separate the white cells. Discard supernatant.
3. Resuspend and lyse cell pellet in 2.8 mL lysis buffer B, containing 0.1% SDS and 100 µg/mL Proteinase K, at 55°C for 2–4 h.

4. Add an equal volume of phenol, mix slowly for 15 min and spin at 5000$g$ for 15 min.
5. Use a large bore pipet to transfer the upper aqueous phase to a fresh tube taking care not to disturb the organic layer.
6. Add an equal volume of phenol:chloroform (1:1) mix slowly for 15 min and spin at 5000$g$ for 15 min.
7. Transfer the upper aqueous phase to a fresh tube and add an equal volume of chloroform mix slowly for 15 min and spin at 5000$g$ for 15 min.
8. Transfer the upper aqueous phase to a fresh tube.
9. Adjust to 0.3$M$ with 5$M$ sodium acetate and precipitate with two volumes of ice-cold absolute ethanol.
10. Centrifuge at 15,000$g$ for 30 min to pellet DNA. Carefully discard supernatant.
11. Wash pellet in 70% ice-cold ethanol and recentrifuge. Discard supernatant.
12. Completely dry the pellet and resuspend in TE for 1–2 h at room temperature.
13. Quantitate DNA at OD 260 nm using a spectrophotometer and dilute and aliquot to 5–10 ng/µL.

### 3.1.2. From Tumor Samples

Tumors are collected and stored at −70°C until processing. They are then finely minced with a razor blade and the DNA extracted.

1. Lyse minced tumor tissue in lysis buffer B containing 1% SDS and 170 µg/mL proteinase K.
2. The remainder of the DNA extraction is as the leukocyte method, **Subheading 3.1.1., steps 4–13**.

## 3.2. Radiolabeling of (CA) Strand Primers

$\gamma$ $^{32}$P -dATP is used to end-label one of the primers, generally the CA strand primer. At all stages where radioactivity is involved, screw-top Eppendorf tubes are used. This protocol for microsatellite typing is designed for the large-scale typing of tumors. The volumes of master mixes given are for 96 samples; PCRs are carried out in 96-well plates so that 48 blood-tumor pairs can be typed in one reaction.

1. Prepare a tube containing 5 µL T4 polynucleotide kinase 10x buffer, 20 µL DNA primer, CA strand, 10 µL $\gamma$ $^{32}$P -dATP, 11 µL water, and 4 µL T4 polynucleotide kinase.
2. Incubate at 37°C for 45 min.
3. Place at 68°C for 15 min to inactivate the enzyme. The labeled primer can either be kept on ice until used or at −20°C in a 1-cm thick perspex box for 3–4 d.

## 3.3. Polymerase Chain Reaction

The PCR protocol employs a "hot start" approach. The MgCl$_2$ concentration most often used is 1.5 m$M$. However, sometimes 1 m$M$ or 2 m$M$ are preferred for some primer pairs (*see* **Note 1**). In addition, the melting temperature (*Tm*) of primer pairs varies depending on nucleotide composition. The *Tm* of most primers should be ≥55°C but, this should be calculated and adjusted and the annealing temperature optimized for each pair. It is possible to amplify more than one microsatellite sequence in one reaction mixture. Such duplex or multiplex reactions are useful when resources are limited. The volume of water in the master mix must be adjusted to allow for the increase in primer volume. It is necessary to check that allele sizes of the different microsatellites do not overlap as this leads to confusion in scoring. In addition, some primer combinations do not work so it is best to perform a trial before starting large-scale typing.

1. Mastermix is prepared for 100 reactions to allow for minor losses in pipeting. Prepare a tube containing: 125 μL 10X *Taq* buffer, 100 μL dNTP mix (2 m*M* stock), 20 μL cold primer, GT strand, 37.6 μL 50 m*M* MgCl$_2$, 817.4 μL water. Keep on ice. (If carrying out a duplex reaction reduce the amount of water in the mastermix by the appropriate volume).

2. Add 1 μL (5–10 ng) DNA into wells of a 96-well dish. It is possible to store the plates at –20°C at this stage for later use.

3. Prepare *Taq* polymerase by diluting the enzyme to 1 U/μL with 1×*Taq* buffer. It is best to prepare enough enzyme for 1.5 × number of wells. Prepare a tube containing: 15 μL 10X buffer, 4.5 μL MgCl$_2$, 100.5 μL water, and 30 μL *Taq* polymerase. Keep on ice.

4. Spin down hot primer mix from **Subheading 3.2.** and add to master mix. Vortex briefly, spin down, add 10 μL master mix to each well and then a drop of mineral oil.

5. Transfer plate to PCR machine and denature at 95°C for 10 min. Toward the end of this period begin to add 1 μL of enzyme to each well and mix well by pipetting up and down. It may be necessary to pause the program at 95°C to complete the addition of the enzyme.

6. Then perform 27 cycles of 95°C for 1 min, 55°C (or appropriate annealing temperature) for 1 min, 72°C for 1.5 min followed by a final extension of 72°C for 10 min. At this stage the samples can either be prepared for loading onto the gel (**Subheading 3.4.**) or alternatively the plate can be placed in a 1-cm thick perspex box and stored at –20°C for up to a week before loading.

## 3.4. Gel Electrophoresis

Before pouring the gel, it is necessary to ensure that the plates are thoroughly cleaned and free from grease as this will affect the even running of the gel.

1. Wash both glass plates with detergent and rinse well. Clean the larger back plate with ethanol. Cover the shorter front plate with a thin film of neat 'Silane' (γ Methacryloxypropyltrimethoxysilane), allow to dry. Wash with water and then ethanol.

2. Using 0.4-mm spacers, clamp plates together and seal with tape or rubber casting foot.

3. Prepare a 6% polyacrylamide sequencing gel. Into a 200-mL beaker, add 80 mL SequaGel-6 monomer solution (National Diagnostics), 20 mL SequaGel-6 buffer reagent, and 800 μL 10% ammonium persulphate.

4. Mix and pour using a 50-mL syringe. Insert shark's tooth comb with flat edge toward gel to form a well and secure with bulldog clips.

5. Cover with Saran Wrap and allow to set for 45 min. The gel can be stored 1–2 d at +4°C.

6. Clear any unpolymerized acrylamide from the top of the gel using a scalpel, and gently remove the combs. Untape the plates and transfer to the gel system. Prerun gel at 60 W for 30 min with 1X TBE as running buffer. The plates should be warm to touch (45–50°C).

7. Add 10 μL loading buffer to each sample in the 96-well plate.

8. Denature samples at 80°C for 6 min and place immediately on ice. Fill a large perspex box with hinged lid with ice and place the plate in this. The lid can be used as a shield while loading the samples.

9. Wash top of gel with buffer and insert comb to form wells. Load 3 μL sample and run at 60 W for approximately 2 h depending on the expected size of PCR product. The remainder of the samples can be stored at –20°C for up to a week and rerun if necessary.

10. Remove gel from the gel system and place in a large plastic tray. Carefully prise the upper short plate off the gel. Pour a generous amount of fixative onto the gel and leave for 5 min. Drain off the excess fixative and spread 3MM paper over the gel. Peel back carefully and place on top of two sheets of blotting paper. Cover with Saran Wrap and cut around the gel.

11. Dry at 80°C for 1–1.5 h using a vacuum drier. Place the dried gel in a cassette, expose to X-ray film and place at –70°C overnight. Depending on the intensity of bands, a further exposure may be necessary.

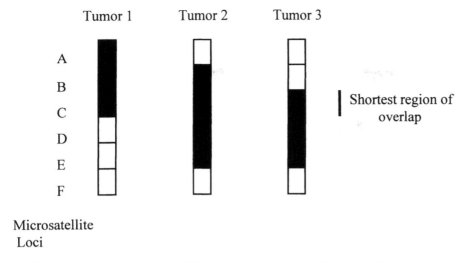

Fig. 1. Typical results of microsatellite typing of tumors. Informative deletion maps can be constructed with the results of LOH analysis using only a small number of markers. □ Retention of heterozygosity, ■ Loss of heterozygosity. *See* text for interpretation.

12. X-ray film can be developed by using either an automatic X-ray film processor or manually. In the latter procedure, developer and fixer are diluted appropriately in deionized water according to the manufacturer's instructions. Place film in developer for 3 min, wash for 1 min in deionized water, transfer to fixer for 3 min, and then rinse in deionized water. Allow film to dry and score (*see* **Notes 2–5**).

The results of LOH analysis of critical tumors, i.e., those with terminal or interstitial deletions are usually presented as deletion maps. These chromosome maps give detailed information of losses and retentions of heterozygosity at each microsatellite locus along a particular chromosome. **Figure 1** shows specimen results from a typical microsatellite typing of a chromosome performed in a series of tumors. Tumor 1 has a large terminal deletion with retention of heterozygosity at locus D and loss of all distal loci. Tumors 2 and 3 have smaller interstitial deletions, with losses between loci A and F and loci B and F respectively. Taking data from all three tumors into account, it is possible to localize a potential TSG to between loci B and D.

## 4. Notes

1. Occasionally, nonspecific bands of various sizes appear in both blood and tumor DNA lanes, indicating that PCR is not optimal. Optimize PCR conditions to yield a specific product by adjusting the concentration of $MgCl_2$, by adding 10% DMSO or altering the annealing temperature of the PCR reaction.
2. Extra shadow bands are often present below the main allele signal even after PCR optimization (*see* **Note 1**). These are artifacts of PCR. These stutter bands or truncated products are thought to be the result of polymerase slippage during the primer elongation step and are less common when amplifying trinucleotide and tetranucleotide repeats.
3. Often the tumor DNA does not show a clear loss at a particular locus, but the relative intensities of the two alleles in the tumor sample differ from those in the blood. This pattern of banding is commonly termed allelic imbalance and results from differences in

Fig. 2. Autoradiographs showing the pattern of LOH in ovarian tumors. Tumor 9 has an interstitial deletion on chromosome 9: retention of IFNA and HXB and LOH of D9S53. In tumor 7, the banding pattern of D9S103 indicates the presence of contaminating normal DNA in the tumor sample.

dosage of the two alleles. This may indicate underrepresentation of one allele (LOH) with signal from the second allele derived from contaminating normal cell DNA in the sample or overrepresentation of one allele (**Fig. 2**, Tumor 7). Overrepresentation may indicate the presence of multiple copies of an entire chromosome or local DNA amplification. Accurate estimation of allele dosage can be made using Southern blotting and RFLP markers followed by phosphoimager analysis.

4.  In some incidences an element of caution is needed in interpreting autoradiographs. A faint retention of heterozygosity signal from tumor template compared with normal DNA may be an indication of a homozygous deletion in tumor DNA. This apparent retention signal can be explained by the presence of small quantities of contaminating normal tissue in a tumor sample that can contribute disproportionately to the PCR product. Therefore, the number of PCR cycles must be restricted when testing for homozygous deletions. At a locus where homozygous deletion is suspected, duplex PCRs are set up using two sets of primers, one for the marker in question and another for an adjacent informative marker

Fig. 3. Autoradiographs showing the pattern of LOH and homozygous deletion in bladder tumors. Duplex PCRs were carried out in tumors 9 and 11 using D9S162 and IFNA and in tumor 15 using D9S171 and D9S126.

that serves as an internal control. The ratio of intensity of signal from blood and tumor lanes is compared for both markers. If the signals from both are similar at the control locus then it is likely that the tumor has a homozygous deletion at the test locus. **Figure 3** illustrates the pattern of homozygous deletion in bladder tumors. In tumor 9, the much weaker signal for IFNA from the tumor template, compared with the blood, indicates homozygous deletion of this locus. Similarly, tumors 11 and 15 have homozygous deletions of IFNA and D9S736, and D9S171, respectively.

5. Amplification of tumor DNA sometimes produces additional bands that are not present in the normal DNA. The difference in size is a result of changes in the number of repeat units in the microsatellite and results from microsatellite instability. This phenomenon was first described in colorectal cancer as a result of deficient mismatch repair (MMR) and has recently been observed in a variety of sporadic cancers (*4*). Mutations in MMR genes

decrease the capacity of the cell to correct errors during DNA replication. Microsatellite instability is much more common in tri- and tetranucleotide repeats than in dinucleotide repeats. This discrepancy may be explained by the underreporting of instances of microsatellite instability in dinucleotides because of masking of novel alleles by "stutters"—strand slippage products common to dinucleotide repeats.

## References

1. Knudson, A. G. (1971) Mutation and cancer: statistical study of retinoblastoma. *Proc. Natl. Acad. Sci. USA* **68,** 820–823.
2. Weber, J. L. and May, P. E. (1989) Abundant class of human DNA polymorphisms which can be typed using the polymerase chain reaction. *Am. J. Hum. Genet.* **44,** 388–396.
3. Hearne, C. M., Ghosh, S., and Todd, J. A. (1992) Microsatellites for linkage analysis of genetic traits. *Trends Genet.* **8,** 288–294.
4. Wooster, R., Cleton-Jansen, A.-M., Collins, N., Mangion, J., Cornelis, R. S., Cooper, C. S., et al. (1994) Instability of short tandem repeats (microsatellites) in human cancers. *Nat. Gen.* **6,** 152–156.

# 34

## Molecular Genetic Analysis of Flow-Sorted and Microdissected Ovarian Tumor Cells

*Improved Detection of Loss of Heterozygosity*

**Edwin C. A. Abeln and Willem E. Corver**

## 1. Introduction

Study of loss of heterozygosity (LOH) is widely used to identify chromosomal locations of putative tumor suppressor genes. In this type of analysis, DNA extracted from tumor tissue is compared with constitutive DNA from the same patient by the use of polymorphic DNA markers (*1*). This approach has two intrinsic limitations. First, tumor specimens with a high fraction of nonneoplastic cells have to be excluded from this analysis because LOH in tumor cells may be undetectable, because of the low concentration of tumor DNA. This may lead to a selection bias, which affects the representativity of the results. A second limitation is that the analysis of DNA extracted from homogenized tumor samples may obscure the presence of intratumor genetic heterogeneity.

In this chapter we describe a method to overcome this limitation: dissociation of tumor specimens followed by specific staining of cellular macromolecules (proteins and/or DNA) and flow-cytometric cell sorting. This approach has several advantages: 1) Over 50% of the ovarian malignancies are DNA aneuploid, which provides a selectable marker for neoplastic cells; 2) different macromolecules can be stained simultaneously—specific tumor markers can be used, which makes it possible to recognize subpopulations of tumor cells; and 3) the speed of the current generation flow-cytometric sorters allows the analysis of large numbers of cells or nuclei. Hereby very small (sub) populations can be isolated from a large number of cells. Disadvantages of the sorting approach are the facts that original histology is lost and that tumors have to be dissociated directly after surgery although sorting of nuclei is possible from paraffin-embedded specimens (*2*) and from frozen specimens (*3*).

We have investigated the possibility to perform molecular genetic (LOH) analysis on flowsorted tumor cells (*4,5*). The specific genetic analysis of specified tumor cell subpopulations may contribute to the understanding of the sequence of molecular-genetic events in the progression of solid tumors.

From: *Methods in Molecular Medicine, Vol. 39: Ovarian Cancer: Methods and Protocols*
Edited by: J. M. S. Bartlett © Humana Press, Inc., Totowa, NJ

## 2. Materials

### 2.1. Isolation of Cells from Solid Ovarian Tumors

1. For DNA-flow-cytometry: Tumor specimens should be fixed in buffered formalin and embedded in paraffin, the usual standard preservation in pathology laboratories (*see* **Note 1**). For multiparameter flow cytometry: fresh tumor tissue is used. Nonneoplastic tissue for isolation of normal DNA, this may be blood or normal tissue adjacent to the tumor.
2. Collagenase Type IA and IV (Sigma, St. Louis, MO), hyaluronidase type V (Sigma), trypsin (GibcoBRL, Gaithersburg, MD), DNase I, type II (Sigma). A mixture of enzymes can be prepared in DMEM, without FCS, and stored in the freezer. Aliquots of 10 mL are suitable. The mixture contains: 0.05% collagenase type IA, 0.1% collagenase type IV, hyaluronidase type V (0.05%), and 0.001% DNase I, type II. Avoid repeatedly freezing and thawing.
3. 2.5% trypsin stock solution (GibcoBRL) stored at –20°C.

### 2.2. Staining of Cellular Proteins

1. mAbs directed against surface antigens [e.g., antiepithelial cell adhesion molecule (Ep-CAM), clone Ber-Ep4 (DAKO, Santa Barbara, CA)], directed against intermediate filaments (e.g., antikeratin or vimentin, DAKO) or directed against nuclear associated proteins [e.g., anti-Ki-67 (clone Ki-67, DAKO), antiproliferating cell nuclear antigen (PCNA, clone PC10, DAKO)].
2. FITC or RPE conjugated goat antimouse IgG or IgG subclass specific secondary reagents (e.g., Southern Biotechnology Associates, Birmingham, AL).
3. Phosphate-buffered (PBS, pH 7.4) paraformaldehyde (PF, E.M. grade, methanol-free, e.g., Merck, Rahway, NJ), freshly prepared from 8X stock solution (8.0% PF).
4. Lysolecithin from egg yolk (Sigma), stock solution 10 mg/mL, dissolved in 100% methanol and stored in the freezer.
5. Phosphate-buffered paraformaldehyde/lysolecithin solution (80–160 µg/mL).
6. PBS containing 0.5% bovine serum albumin (PBA) (BSA fraction V, Sigma), pH 7.4. Store at 4°C.

### 2.3. DNA Staining

1. RNase (Sigma), 10X stock dissolved in PBS, stored at –20°C.
2. 100 m$M$ propidium iodide (Molecular Probes, Eugene, OR), made from 1$M$ 10X stock solution dissolved in PBS, stored at –20°C (*see* **Notes 2** and **3**, about DNA stains).

### 2.4. Special Equipment

1. FACStar flow cytometer flow sorter FACSstar (Becton Dickinson, Mountain View, CA) equipped with an Argon-ion laser (Coherent, Innova 90) giving a light emission of 300 mW at 488 nm and with Lysis 2.0 software (*see* **Note 4**).
2. Sheath fluid (e.g., Becton Dickinson/Pharmingen or Beckmann/Coulter) or (much cheaper) phosphate-buffered saline (PBS): 150 m$M$ NaCl (e.g., Merck), 1.165 m$M$ $Na_2HPO_4.2H_2O$ (Merck), and 0.234 m$M$ $KH_2PO_4$ (Merck). This solution must be prepared in highly purified $H_2O$, filtered over a 0.22-µm filter. A 10X stock solution of 10 L (100 L of sheath fluid) is easily prepared and can be stored at room temperature, pH 7.5 after dilution.

### 2.5. DNA Extraction and PCR

1. DNA extraction buffer: 10 m$M$ Tris-HCl, pH 9.0; 1.5 m$M$ $MgCl_2$; 50 m$M$ KCl; 0.01% gelatin; 0.1% Triton X100, 0.5% proteinase K.

2. 10X nucleotide mix: 2 m*M* each dGTP, dTTP, dATP, and 25 m*M* dCTP (Pharmacia, Uppsala, Sweden).
3. Loading buffer 0.3% xylenecyanol (Sigma); 0.3% bromphenol blue (Sigma); 10 m*M* EDTA pH 8.0; 90% (v/v) formamide.
4. 6.5% polyacrylamide gel containing 7*M* urea (29 : 1 acrylamide:bisacrylamide) and running buffer 0.5 × TBE.

## 3. Methods

Preparation of cells for flow cytometry is essentially as described in Chapter 56 by Corver and Cornelisse to which reference can be made for further details. The tumor sample which is going to be processed for flow-cytometric analysis should be weighed before dissociation to allow monitoring yield and viability of the tumor cells obtained from the specimen using the Trypan blue method.

### 3.1. Isolation of Cells from Solid Ovarian Tumors

1. Fill a flat polystyrene box with ice and put a Petri dish on top of it.
2. Weigh the tumor sample (Petri dish included) and weigh an empty Petri dish. Subtract the results (= sample weight). Put the sample with the Petri dish on ice.
3. Moisture the tissue with 1.0 mL of standard pre-cooled (4°C) culture DMEM-medium, without FCS.
4. Cut the tumor sample into fragments of approximately 1–2 mm$^3$ using scalpel blades. Use a pair of tweezers to fix the tumor sample to Petri dish bottom.
5. Incubate fragments overnight at 4°C with 10 mL of DMEM (GibcoBRL), without FCS, per 1.0 g tissue, containing the enzyme mix.
6. Next day, dissociate tumor chunks at 37°C using an incubator.
7. After 2 h of incubation, add trypsin to a final concentration of 0.25%.
8. After 15 min of incubation at 37°C, gently pass the suspension several times through a 1.5-mm syringe needle and filter over a nylon sieve with a pore size of 100 mm.
9. Put the suspension on ice (4°C) and add FCS to a final concentration of 20% to block proteolytic activity.
10. Spin cells down at 250*g* for 5 min. A centrifuge with cooling facility (4°C) is preferred.
11. Vortex the cell pellet gently and add medium dropwise. The volume can range from about 1 to 10 or more mL, depending on the size of the cell pellet.
12. Count the cells using the Trypan blue method applying a hemocytometer (Bürker) chamber. Adjust the cell concentration to 1 × 10$^6$/mL and store cells on ice (4°C) until further preparation.

### 3.2. Staining of Cellular Proteins

#### 3.2.1. Staining of Surface Proteins (one parameter, no fixation)

1. Use 0.5–1 × 10$^6$ cells per test tube and spin cells down for 5 min at 250*g*. [A cooled centrifuge (4°C) is preferred.]
2. Discard the supernatant or other medium by turning the test tubes upside down in one stroke. Keep the tubes upside down and place the tubes in a tube rack containing a tissue, placed on the bottom of the tube rack. The last drop of supernatant will be taken up by the tissue.
3. Turn the tubes again, add 1.0 mL of cold PBA, vortex gently and spin cells down at 250*g*, for 5 min.
4. Discard the PBA in the same way as described by **step 2**.
5. Add 100 µL of diluted monoclonal antibody (MAb) (e.g., Ber-Ep4, DAKO) to the cells, vortex gently, and incubate for 30 min on ice (4°C) (*see* **Note 5**).

6. Add 1.0 mL of cold PBA to the cells, vortex, and spin cells down (250*g*, 5 min, 4°C).
7. Repeat **step 6** and add 100 µL of diluted secondary reagent, e.g., goat antimouse Ig-FITC (DAKO) (*see* **Note 5**).
8. Vortex gently and put the cells on ice for 30 min (4°C).
9. Repeat **step 6** twice.
10. Add 0.5 mL of ice-cold PBA containing PI at a final concentration of 1.0 µ*M* to the cells, vortex gently and store the cells on ice (4°C). Low concentrations of PI allow good discrimination between dead and viable cells (*see* **Note 2**).
11. Cells are ready for flow-cytometric analysis after 30 min.

Note: **Steps 6–8** can be omitted when direct labeled antibodies are applied.

### 3.3. DNA Staining

1. Add 0.5 mL of 0.1% RNase (in PBA) containing 100 µ*M* of PI.
2. Vortex gently and incubate the cells for 30 min at 37°C using a water-heated incubator.
3. Put the cells on ice (4°C). Cells are ready for flow cytometric analysis after 30 min (*see* **Note 6**).

### 3.4. Flowcytometric Sorting of Cells and Nuclei

1. Cells/nuclei are sorted directly in 1.5-mL microfuge tubes.
2. Electronic doublet discrimination should be used to omit the sorting of cell aggregates. The FL2 pulse area must be plotted against the peak pulsewidth, which enables discrimination of singlets from doublets because the latter have a wider peak pulsewidth *(6,7)*.
3. Two fractions can be sorted simultaneously. A minimum of 1000 cells per fraction should be sorted.
4. DNA should be isolated directly after sorting or the fractions should be stored at –20°C.

### 3.5. DNA Isolation from Sorted Cells or Nuclei

1. Adjust the titer of the sorted cells or nuclei to 50 nuclei or cells per µL by adding DNA extraction buffer.
2. Incubate overnight at 56°C.
3. Incubate 10 minutes at 100°C to inactivate proteinase K.
4. Use directly or store at –20°C.

### 3.6. Detection of LOH

### 3.6.1. Polymerase Chain Reaction (PCR)

1. Make for *n* reactions 1.1*n* times PCR master mix containing 7 µL sterile water, 1.5 µL 10X PCR-buffer (Sphaero Q, HT Biotechnology LTD, Cambridge, UK), 1.5 µL dNTP-mix, 1.5 µL BSA-solution (10%), 1.5 µL primer mix (1 µ*M* of each primer), 0.1 µL $^{32}$P-[γ]-dCTP, and 0.05 µL Super *Taq* DNA polymerase (Sphaero Q) per reaction (*see* **Notes 7 and 8**).
2. Fill out the microtiter plate with 2 µL of the DNA solution. Samples should be arranged in couples of normal-DNA and tumor-DNA next to each other.
3. Add 13 µL of the PCR master mix to each well.
4. Add 1 drop of mineral oil (Sigma-Aldrich, Zwijndrecht, The Netherlands).
5. Run the following PCR program: 5 min 95°C followed by 33 cycles (1 min 94°C, 2 min primer 55°C, 1 min 72°C) and a final extension of 6 min at 72°C.

### 3.6.2. Polyacrylamide Gel Electorphoresis

1. Add 1 drop (≈10 µL) of loading buffer to each well of the microtiter plate.
2. Denature the samples by heating for 5 min at 95°C

3. Snap cool the samples to 0°C on ice to prevent renaturation.
4. Load 2.5 µL on the polyacrylamide gel.
5. Run the samples for 2 h at 90 W.
6. Dry the gel under vacuum at for 2 h at 80°C.
7. Expose an X-ray film. Usually overnight exposure is sufficient (*see* **Notes 9** and **10**).

## 4. Notes

1. Nonbuffered formalin may be acidic and will cause serious random degradation of DNA. Longer fixation times will, in these cases, yield shorter DNA fragments which will decrease the chance at successful amplification during PCR. DNA isolated from archival specimens is known to exist as shorter molecules owing to degradation. Effects of fixative and retention time are reviewed by Greer et al. *(8)*.

2. Paraformaldehyde (PF) is a water-soluble chemical protein crosslinker. An 8% stock can be prepared easily by dissolving 8 g of PF in distilled water heated to 60°C, while stirring. Use a safety cabinet. Avoid evaporation. Add a few drops of 1*M* NaOH dropwise under constant swirling until the solution clears. Cool the solution down using running cold tap water. Filter the solution over a paper filter and store it at 4°C. A 1% PF working solution can be made by diluting the 8% PF stock in PBS. The pH should be between 7.2 and 7.4. The stock solution can be stored for several weeks at 4°C. A short fixation with PF [5 min on ice (4°C)] is sufficient for crosslinking membrane-bound proteins and stabilizing the cells for permeabilization without significant loss of membrane antigen staining. PF is unstable in solution and should be freshly prepared, because formic acid is gradually formed during storage. Discard the stock solution if pH drops below 7.2.

3. Propidium iodide (PI) is the most commonly used DNA stain for flow cytometric analysis of DNA content. This intercalating dye has a relative high affinity to both dsDNA and dsRNA, requiring RNase treatment of the cells before analysis. It has a broad excitation spectrum making it suitable for both UV excitation and visible blue light excitation. The latter is one of the reasons why PI is a very popular DNA stain, because almost all modern bench-top flow cytometers are equipped with the blue 488-nm Argon-ion laser, allowing PI excitation. A disadvantage of the use of PI is the broad orange to red emission spectrum, requiring substantial compensation. This makes the combination of PI with other fluorochromes emitting in the orange range, e.g., RPE, of the spectrum less appropriate. However, proteins which are highly expressed, e.g., intermediate filaments like keratin and vimentin, and stained using RPE conjugated reagents can be easily detected in clinical samples, which were also stained for DNA-ploidy analysis using high concentrations of PI. Also, spectral overlap of RPE/PI positive cells into the green fluorescence channel can not entirely be corrected for using hardware compensation facilities. 7-Amino-actinomycin-D (7-AAD, Molecular Probes) is frequently used as an alternative for PI for measurements of multiple cellular proteins in combination with DNA-ploidy analysis using single laser excitation. This G-C specific DNA dye has a larger "Stokes" shift (difference between excitation wavelength and maximum emission wavelength) than PI, allowing a better discrimination between RPE and 7-AAD fluorescent signals. However, Brockhoff and coworkers clearly demonstrated that 7-AAD also shows considerable spectral overlap with RPE and that PI is still in favor because of the low CV's of the DNA-histogram peaks and good stoichiometry of DNA binding. These findings were confirmed in our laboratory.

4. Flexibility in choice of DNA stain increases using flow cytometers with double (or more) excitation capability. Recently, PARTEC and Becton Dickinson introduced bench-top flow cytometers capable of double excitation using a 488-nm Argon-ion laser line and a Mercury-Arc lamp (UV excitation) or a 488-nm Argon-ion laser line in combination with a red diode laser (approximate excitation: 635 nm.), respectively. The Mercury Arc-lamp

**Table 1**
**Microsatellite Markers for Detection of LOH**

| Marker | Chromosomal Location | Primer 1 5′ → 3′ | Primer 2 5′ → 3′ |
|---|---|---|---|
| D1S103 | 1q32-qter | ACGAACATTCTACAAGTTAC | TTTCAGAGAAACTGACCTGT |
| D3S11 | 3p21-p14 | TTTCAGAGAAACTGACCTGT | GTACACCATCATGAGGAGTCTGG |
| GLUT2 | 3q26-q26.3 | TCCGTCAGCAGCTATTCTAG | CAAATAGTCCTCATGCAGAA |
| D4S230 | 4pter-p15 | TAGGAATAGGAAACAAATGCA | TTAGGATGCTGACTTCACCA |
| D6S105 | 6p22 | GCCCTATAAAATCCTAATTAAC | GAAGGAGAATTGTAATTCCG |
| IGF2R | 6q25-q27 | CTGGTGAATTCAAACAACCT | TTTTCTCTGACACCTCAACT |
| D6S251 | 6q13-q21.1 | TTCCTAACCAGGTTTCAATG | ATATTTTTAAAGTAAGTTGCAC |
| D11S875 | 11pter-p11.2 | ACTGTCCTCTCATCCTACTG | TACAGAGCTGAGTTTGTAGC |
| D11S35 | 11q22 | ACAATTGGATTACTACTAGC | TGTATTTGTATCGATTAACC |
| D17S513 | 17p13 | TTCACTTGTGGGCTGCTGTC | TAAGAAAGGCTCCCACAAGCA |
| D17S579 | 17q12-q21 | CAGTTTCATACCAAGTTCCT | AGTCCTGTAGACAAAACCTG |
| 46E6 | 17q23-q24 | TTCATGGGGCTTACTGTGTTC | TAGCACTCTGCCTTCCAACATAC |
| D17S250 | 17q11.2-q12 | AAAAGGAAGAATCAAATAGAC | ATATATTTAAACCATTTGAAAG |
| D17S520 | 17p12 | GGAGAAAGTGATACAAGGGA | TAGTTAGATTAATACCCACC |
| D18S40 | 18p11.2-p11.3 | CAAGATAGATGCATTTTCCAGT | CATCCAAAGGGTGAATGTGT |
| D18S35 | 18q11-q12 | AGCTAGATTTTTACTTCTCTG | CTGGTTGTACATGCCTGAC |
| D18S34 | 18q11 | CAGAAAATTCTCTCTGGCTA | CTCATGTTCCTGGCAAGAAT |
| MBP | 18q22-qter | GGACCTCGTGAATTACAATC | ATTTACCTACCTGTTCATCC |
| DXS453 | Xp1.23-q21.1 | GCCCCTACCTTGGCTAGTTA | AACCTCAGCTTATACCCAAG |
| XS454 | Xq21.1-q23 | AGAAGACATAAGGATACTGC | GATCCCAACTATTTCTTTCT |

can be used for excitation of DAPI (2,4 diamidino-6-phenylindole, Molecular Probes), allowing analysis of multiple proteins and DNA with minimal spectral crossover problems. DAPI is a DNA specific dye with excellent DNA binding characteristics. The red diode laser can be used for the excitation of TO-PRO-3 Iodide (TP3, Molecular Probes), a recently developed DNA dye. Its usefulness as DNA dye has already been proven in clinical samples stained for two cellular proteins and DNA, analyzed by a double-excitation flowcytometer. Instead of a FACSstar, other sorters may be used as well. The advantage of a droplet sorter is that the volume of the sorted fractions remains relatively small even if very small subpopulations are sorted.

5. One of the major drawbacks of flow cytometry is the lack of visual control of the stained cells being analyzed. mAbs, which are going to be used for flow-cytometric analysis, must be carefully selected, especially mAbs directed against intracellular antigens. Staining for intracellular antigens is sensitive to nonspecific binding of mAbs (e.g., *p53*). Nonetheless, many antibodies suitable for immunohistochemistry can also be used for flow cytometry. However, the MAb must comply with certain criteria. The antibody must be titrated using cells expressing the target protein (positive control) and cells lacking the protein of interest (negative control). Cells must also be cultured on cover slips or spotted on glass sections allowing microscopically examination of protein localization using the same fixation, permeabilization, and staining procedure used for flow cytometry. Results should be compared to data from literature or the signals should at least be localized at the expected site of the cell. Standard immunohistochemistry on tissue section can contribute to verification of the antibody (e.g., antikeratin antibodies should not react with the stromal compartment of a tumor). Western blotting must confirm the expected size of the protein of interest.

6. A prolonged storage of the cells at 4°C in the presence of PI will improve the CV's of the DNA histograms peaks. Stained and PF fixed, lysolecithin permeabilized cells can be stored for several days at 4°C without significant loss of cell surface fluorescence (author's observations).

7. The loading buffer contains some water to help the buffer pass the oil layer on top of the PCR reaction.

8. Some useful microsatellite primers that give easy interpretable banding patterns are listed in **Table 1** (primer sequences were retrieved from Human Genomic Data Bank from the Johns Hopkins University School of Medicine, Baltimore, MD).

9. The use of amplification screens may shorten the needed exposure time. However, it also results in broader bands, which hampers the interpretation. Therefore, longer exposures without screens are preferable.

10. LOH can be scored by visual comparison of the intensity of alleles of constitutional and tumor DNA on autoradiograms *(9–11)*. Owing to the applied enrichment steps, this is usually easy. In some cases, despite the selection of specific cells, heterogeneity may still be present and can cause less easy interpretable bands. In those cases, densitometry is advisable.

## References

1. Lasko, D., Cavenee, W., and Nordenskjöld, M. (1991) Loss of constitutional heterozygosity in human cancer. *Annu. Rev. Genet.* **25,** 281–314.
2. Hedley, D. W., Friedlander, M. L., Taylor, I. W., Rugg, C. A., and Musgrove, E. A. (1983) Method for analysis of cellular DNA content of paraffin-embedded pathological material using flow cytometry. *J. Histochem. Cytochem.* **31,** 1333–1335.
3. Vindelov, L. L., Christensen, I. J., and Nissen, N. I. (1983) A detergent-trypsin method for the preparation of nuclei for flow cytometric DNA analysis. *Cytometry* **3,** 323–327.
4. Abeln, E. C. A., Corver, W. E., Kuipers-Dijkshoorn, N. J., Fleuren, G.-J., and Cornelisse, C. J. (1994) Molecular genetic analysis of flow-sorted ovarian tumor cells: Improved detection of loss of heterozygosity. *Br. J. Cancer* **70,** 255–262.
5. Corver, W. E., Cornelisse, C. J., and Fleuren, G. J. (1994) Simultaneous measurement of two cellular antigens and DNA using fluorescein-isothiocyanate, R-phycoerythrin, and propidium iodide on a standard FACScan. *Cytometry* **15,** 117–128.
6. Sharpless, T., Traganos, F., Darzynkiewicz, Z., and Melamed, M. R. (1975) Flow cytofluorimetry: discrimination between single cell aggregates by direct size measurements. *Acta Cytologica* **19,** 577–581.
7. Göhde, W., Schumann, J., and Früh, J. (1976) Coincidence in eliminating device in pulse cytophotometry in *Pulse Cytophotometry* (Gödhe, W., Schumann, J., and Büchner, T., eds.), European Press Medikon, Ghent. pp. 79–85.
8. Greer, C. E., Peterson, S. L., Kiviat, N. B., and Manos, M. M. (1991) PCR amplification from paraffin-embedded tissues.Effects of XX fixative and fixation time see comments. *Am. J. Clin. Pathol.* **95,** 117–124.
9. Futreal, P. A., Söderkvist, P., Marks, J. R., Iglehart, J. D., Cochran, C., Barrett, J. C., and Wiseman, R. W. (1992) Detection of frequent allelic loss on proximal chromosome XX 17q in sporadic breast carcinoma using microsatellite length XX polymorphisms. *Cancer Res.* **52,** 2624–2627.
10. Jones, M. H. and Nakamura, Y. (1992) Deletion mapping of chromosome 3p in female genital tract malignancies using microsatellite polymorphisms. *Oncogene* **7,** 1631–1634.
11. Weber, J. L. and May, P. E. (1989) Abundant class of human DNA polymorphisms which can be typed using the polymerase chain reaction. *Am. J. Hum. Genet.* **44,** 388–396.

# 35

## SSCP and Sequence Analysis of *p53* Mutations in Ovarian Tumors

**Anil K. Sood and Richard E. Buller**

## 1. Introduction

The *p53* tumor suppressor gene encodes a 53-kD nuclear phosphoprotein and is the most commonly altered gene in human cancers *(1)*. There are a large variety of methods currently employed for detection of alterations in the *p53* gene. The reported abnormalities in *p53* have been detected with a variety of techniques including immunohistochemical staining (IHCS) as a primary screening modality and less frequently single-strand conformation polymorphism (SSCP) screening. However, certain mutations such as frameshift mutations may not be detectable by IHCS, and most studies using SSCP have limited their search to exons 5–8 *(2)*. As shown previously by our lab, this strategy can lead to underreporting of the true frequency of *p53* null mutations *(3)*. We routinely perform a complete evaluation of the *p53* open reading frame (exons 2–11) using SSCP analysis with an estimated sensitivity of over 90% *(3)*. This approach significantly enhances the detection of null mutations, especially insertion/deletion type mutations.

Single-strand conformation polymorphism analysis (SSCP) was introduced in 1989 by Orita et al. and provides rapid analysis of genes of interest *(4)*. The DNA segment of interest is amplified by polymerase chain reaction (PCR), the strands of the PCR product are separated by denaturation, then submitted to gel electrophoresis under nondenaturing conditions. Each individual strand may self-anneal and fold to achieve the most thermodynamically stable conformation. Electrophoretic differences occur with as little as a single base change if the amplimer is not too large. There is no single recipe for SSCP that is adequate for screening various regions of the *p53* gene. Optimally, these parameters are determined for each new pair of amplimers. We present different SSCP methods for different exons to obtain optimal mutation detection.

Direct sequencing is a powerful technique that enables search for mutations in a defined fragment of DNA rapidly. Tumor DNA with suspicious migratory patterns on SSCP analysis can be sequenced to identify the specific mutation. The general approach to sequencing includes: 1) amplification of the desired double-stranded DNA template; 2) purification of the PCR product to remove residual primers, nucleotides, and salts; and 3) use the purified DNA as a template for the sequencing reaction using a single end-labeled forward- or reverse-primer.

From: *Methods in Molecular Medicine, Vol. 39: Ovarian Cancer: Methods and Protocols*
Edited by: J. M. S. Bartlett © Humana Press, Inc., Totowa, NJ

## 2. Materials

### 2.1. Single-Strand Conformation Polymorphism (SSCP)

These reactions can be run on either nondenaturing polyacrylamide gels or Mutation Detection Enhancement (MDE™) gels. The specific types of gels will be specified for each exon under methods.

1. γ-[$^{32}$P] ATP (10 mCi/mL, Amersham, Arlington Heights, IL).
2. *Taq* DNA Polymerase (5 U/µL, with buffers included, Boehringer Mannheim, Germany).
3. dNTP (2 m*M* each dATP, dCTP, dGTP & dTTP).
4. Dilution buffer (0.1% SDS, 10 m*M* EDTA, pH 8.0).
5. SSCP loading dye for polyacrylamide gels: 95% formamide, 20 m*M* EDTA, 0.05% bromophenol blue, and 0.05% xylene cyanol
6. SSCP loading dye for MDE gels: 95% formamide, 10 m*M* NaOH, 0.25% bromophenol blue, and 0.25% xylene cyanol.
7. The polyacrylamide gels are 6% nondenaturing gels with or without 5% glycerol.
8. For MDE, gels the prepared material is provided by FMC Bioproducts (Rockland, ME).
9. The gel buffer for polyacrylamide gels is 1X TBE with or without 5% glycerol. 0.6X TBE buffer is used for the MDE gels. (10X TBE: Dissolve 242 g Tris-base, 123.4 g boric acid, and 14.88 g EDTA in 4 L of dH$_2$O, pH 8.3).

### 2.2. Labeling Reaction for Primers

1. Polynucleotide kinase (PNK) and buffer: 70 m*M* Tris-HCl (pH 7.6), 10 m*M* MgCl$_2$, 5 m*M* dithiothreitol.
2. Fix solution (for polyacrylamide gels): 15% acetic acid/15% methanol (v/v). This solution can be stored at room temperature and reused 5–6 times.

### 2.3. Sequence Analysis

1. Fmol® DNA Sequencing System (Promega Corporation, Madison, WI) which includes: Sequence grade T4 PNK. Sequence grade T4 PNK buffer (10X): 500 m*M* Tris-HCl, pH 7.5 at 25°C, 100 m*M* MgCl$_2$, 50 m*M* dithiothreitol, 1 m*M* spermidine. Sequence grade *Taq* polymerase
2. 5X reaction buffer: 250 m*M* Tris HCl, pH 9.0 at 25°C, 10 m*M* MgCl$_2$.
3. Stop solution: 95% formamide, 10 m*M* NaOH, 0.05% bromophenol blue, 0.05% xylene cyanol.
4. Loading dye for agarose gel: 0.25% bromophenol blue, 0.25% xylene cyanol, and 30% glycerol.
5. Gels: 8*M* urea, 8% polyacrylamide gel.

## 3. Methods

### 3.1. Single-Strand Conformation Polymorphism (SSCP)

1. Labeling Reaction: This mix can be scaled up or down as needed. The mix should be prepared on ice. The primers used for SSCP are listed in **Table 1**. The standard concentration for primers in our lab is 6.7 pmol/µL. Set up, for each primer pair, the following reaction mix: 5 µL γ-[$^{32}$P], 1.5 µL each forward and reverse primers, 1 µL PNK buffer and 1 µL PNK (total 10 µL).
2. Incubate at 37°C for 15 min, 90°C for 2 min, then store at –20°C until used. The labeled oligonucleotide is stable for several weeks at –20°C, and its use is limited only by the half-life of the radioactive substance used.
3. Prepare SSCP reactions (*see* **Notes 1, 3, 4**) for each exon as shown in **Table 2**.

**Table 1**
**Intron-Based *p53* Primer Pairs**

| Exon | Primer pairs | Product size |
|------|--------------|--------------|
| 2 | 5'-AGCGTCTCATGCTGGATCCC-3'<br>5'-CTTCCCACAGGTCTCTGCTA-3' | 204 |
| 3 | 5'-TAGCAGAGACCTGTGGGAAG-3'<br>5'-TCCATTGCTTGGGACGGCAA-3' | 197 |
| 4 | 5'-TGAGGACCTGGTCCTCTGAC-3'<br>5'-CAGGCATTGAAGTCTCATGG-3' | 366 |
| 5 | 5'-TTCAACTCTGTCTCCTTCCT-3'<br>5'-CAGCCCTGTCGTCTCTCCAG-3' | 247 |
| 6 | 5'-ACGACAGGGCTGGTTGCCCA-3'<br>5'-GAGGTCAAATAAGCAGCAGG-3' | 276 |
| 7 | 5'-CTTGCCACAGGTCTCCCCAA-3'<br>5'-AGCAGGCCAGTGTGCAGGGT-3' | 206 |
| 8 | 5'-CTGCCTCTTGCTTCTCTTTT-3'<br>5'-TCTCCTCCACCGCTTCTTGT-3' | 204 |
| 9 | 5'-GCAGTTATGCCTCAGATTCA-3'<br>5'-GGCATTTTGAGTGTTAGACT-3' | 185 |
| 10 | 5'-CAATTGTAACTTGAACCATC-3'<br>5'-ATGAGAATGGAATCCTATGG-3' | 258 |
| 11 | 5'-AGACCCTCTCACTCATGTGA-3'<br>5'-GGGGGAGGGAGGCTGTCAGTG-3' | 158 |

**Table 2**
**SSCP Reaction Mix**

| Item | Exons<br>2–4 & 6–9 | Exon 5 | Exon 10 | Exon 11 |
|------|---------|--------|---------|---------|
| dd $H_2O$ | 5.6 µL | 4.6 µL | 3.6 µL | 4.6 µL |
| 10X reaction buffer | 1 µL | 1 µL[a] | 1 µL | 1 µL |
| dNTP (2 m$M$ each) | 1 µL | 1 µL | 1 µL | 1 µL |
| Labeled primer mix | 1 µL | 2 µL | 3 µL | 2 µL |
| *Taq* polymerase (5 U/µL) | 0.2 µL | 0.2 µL | 0.2 µL | 0.2 µL |
| Total | 8.8 µL | 8.8 µL | 8.8 µL | 8.8 µL |

[a]For exon 5, $MgCl_2$ 2.5 m$M$, pH 9.0 buffer should be used. Add 1.2 µL DNA per reaction and 1 drop of light mineral oil per reaction.

4. Set up PCR conditions as follows: 94°C for 5 min followed by 30 cycles of 94°C for 40 s, 60°C for 60 s, 72°C for 120 s with a final extension time of 8 min at 72°C. Keep the samples at 4°C until ready to use.

5. The PCR product from above is diluted 1:25 with the dilution buffer.

6. The diluted mix is denatured to single-stranded DNA: 5 µL diluted PCR product + 4 µL SSCP dye.

7. Heat the samples at 80°C for 5 mins. Place on ice. Immediately load 6–8 µL in the wells of the gel. The optimal gel type and conditions are listed in **Table 3** (*see* **Notes 2, 5–7**).

8. Run the SSCP gel electrophoresis at 6–14 W for 12–16 h in 1X TBE. The MDE gel should be run in 0.6X TBE at 4 W for 14 h (trailing dye front should be 8–10 cm from the bottom of the gel).

**Table 3**
**Optimal SSCP Gel Type and Conditions**

| Exons | Gel type | Temperature |
|---|---|---|
| 3, 9 | 6% polyacrylamide gel, no glycerol | 4°C |
| 4, 5, 7, 8, 10, 11 | 6% polyacrylamide gel with 5% glycerol | Room temperature |
| 6 | 6% polyacrylamide gel with 5% glycerol | 4°C |
| 2, 4 | MDE | Room temperature |

9. Open the gel plates carefully and place the gel in fix solution for 15 min in a tray followed by water for 15 min. MDE gels do not need to be fixed and can be dried as in the next step.
10. Transfer the gel to a piece of 3 MM Whatman paper (Clifton, NJ) and cover the surface of gel with cling film and dry on a gel dryer for 30 min.
11. Expose to autoradiograph film on intensifying plates for 2–4 h depending on the radioactivity level.

## 3.2. Sequence Analysis

1. Labeling Reaction: This mix volume can be scaled up or down as needed. The mix should be prepared on ice. Set up, for each primer, the following reaction mix: 5 μL γ-[$^{32}$P], 1.5 μL primer, 1.5 μL ddH$_2$O, 1 μL PNK buffer and 1 μL PNK (total 10 μL). Incubate at 37°C for 15 min, 90°C for 2 minutes, then store at –20°C until used. The labeled oligonucleotide is stable for several weeks at –20°C, and its use is limited only by the half-life of the radioactive substance used (*see* **Note 11**).
2. The PCR product to be analyzed is generated in a 50-μL reaction in the proportions described under the section on SSCP.
3. The yield of the PCR product should be checked on a 2% agarose gel prior to proceeding with the sequencing reaction. Mix 6 μL PCR product with 3 μL loading dye and run on a 2% agarose gel stained with ethidium bromide. If an appropriate size band is present, then proceed with sequencing.
4. Purify the PCR product by using the Wizard™ DNA purification system (Promega Biotech, Madison, WI). Adjust elution volume from 20 to 50 μL depending on band intensity detected on the agarose gel to increase the amount of DNA in the sequencing reaction.
5. For each set of sequencing reactions, label four 0.5 mL microcentrifuge tubes (G, A, T, C). Add 2 μL of the appropriate dNTP mix to each tube and store on ice until needed.
6. Prepare the master mix for the sequencing reaction (*see* **Notes 8–10**): 5 μL ddH$_2$O, 4.5 μL Template DNA, 5 μL 5X buffer, 1 μL Sequence *Taq* polymerase and 1.5 μL of labeled primer (total 17 μL).
7. Add 4 μL of the master mix from **step 6** to each tube containing the dNTP.
8. Add 1 drop mineral oil and briefly spin in a microcentrifuge.
9. Place the reaction tubes in a thermal cycler that has been preheated to 95°C and start the cycling program. PCR conditions: 94°C for 5 min, followed by 30 cycles of 94°C for 40 s, 60°C for 60 s, 72°C for 120 s with a final extension of 72°C for 8 min. Keep the samples at 4°C until ready to use.
10. Add 3 μL of sequencing stop solution and spin down all samples in microcentrifuge.
11. Heat samples at 85°C for 5 min prior to loading on gel.
12. Remove the oil from each tube and load 3.5 μL in each well.
13. Run the gel at 35 W for 4–6 h.
14. Open the gel plates carefully and place the gel in fix solution for 15 min in a tray followed by water for 15 min.

Fig. 1. (**A**) SSCP polyacrylamide gel. Lanes 1–2, and 4 show a normal pattern. Lane 3 shows an abnormal pattern which on sequencing revealed a 4-base pair deletion (GAAG) mutation at nucleotide 12108. The codon 72 polymorphism (C*G*C or C*C*C) is not detectable on this gel. (**B**) MDE gel. The abnormal pattern in lane 3 is readily apparent. In addition, the codon 72 polymorphism is easily detectable (lane 1 is homozygous C, lane 2 is G with LOH, and lane 4 reveals a heterozygous C/G individual).

15. Transfer the gel to a piece of 3 MM Whatman paper and cover the surface of gel with cling film and dry.
16. Expose to autoradiograph for 2–4 h depending on the radioactivity level (*see* **Note 11**).

## 4. Notes

1. The sensitivity of SSCP and sequencing techniques may depend upon the amount of tumor cells present in the tissue samples. SSCP can reliably detect band shifts in mixed populations of cells where the mutant cells constitute as little as 25% of the total population while sequencing can detect mutations with only 20% mutant cells (*5*). Thus, it is important to obtain an estimate of tumor composition of the tissue being analyzed.
2. The electrophoretic mobility of the single DNA strands can be influenced by electrophoretic conditions such as concentration of the polyacrylamide gel, buffer concentration, pH, temperature, and presence of additives like glycerol (*6*).
3. Exon 4 is the largest exon in the *p53* gene and contains a clinically useful polymorphism at codon 72 (*7*). Although mutations in exon 4 can be effectively detected using the polyacrylamide gels, the polymorphism is best detected by using the MDE gel (**Fig. 1**). Alternatively, a smaller fragment of exon 4 can be amplified, which readily resolves the polymorphism, but does not allow for complete mutation screening.

4. If the SSCP pattern definitely appears abnormal, but the sequence is normal, then recheck the percentage of tumor cells in the tissue. If the tumor percentage is low (<25%), then the investigator may need to cut out the abnormal band from the SSCP gel, extract the DNA and reamplify (nested primers work best in this setting). If the tumor percentage is adequate, then the investigator needs to use new primers to increase the fragment size because the base change lies too near the primer to detect with the sequencing approach above. Alternatively, the fragment can be cloned with sequence done off an universal site in the vector that is adjacent to the primer sequence.

5. If there are blurred bands on SSCP gels, then add glycerol or lower the electrophoresis temperature.

6. SSCP patterns are highly reproducible. Include a nondenatured sample (occasionally, the nondenatured band will comigrate with one of the amplimers). Also, include a positive control for each SSCP gel. These steps provide quality control, and if the SSCP pattern of the controls does not look right, then the results for the remaining samples may be questionable.

7. High electrophoresis temperatures may result in secondary or tertiary structural changes of amplimers. Long runs at lower wattage may give the best results, unless a temperature-controlled apparatus is used.

8. We routinely sequence all samples in both directions. If a mutation is detected, a separate (independent) PCR reaction is performed to confirm the mutation and avoid mistaking an early cycle PCR error as a mutation.

9. The quality of the sequence can depend on the quality of the DNA and the location of the primer. The same primers used to generate the SSCP product usually will also work well for the sequencing reaction when DNA is prepared from snap-frozen fresh tissue. However, DNA prepared from paraffin-embedded tissue by sonication technique *(8)* can be more difficult to sequence. For sonicated DNA, nested primers often work better. DNA extracted from some paraffin-embedded tissues may not amplify well at all. When this is the case, be careful because these samples will yield different results from different sequencing reactions.

10. A benefit of using intron-based primers is detection of abnormalities at consensus splice sites.

11. Faint or absent bands can result from various reasons such as insufficient template, insufficient enzyme activity, old isotope, contamination of sequence reaction with salt, and insufficient primer labeling.

## References

1. Levine, A. J., Momand, J., and Finlay, C. A. (1991) The p53 tumour suppressor gene. *Nature* **351,** 453–456.
2. Greenblatt, M. S., Grollman, A. P., and Harris, C. C. (1996) Deletions and insertions in the p53 tumor suppressor gene in human cancers: Confirmation of the DNA polymerase slippage/misalignment model. *Cancer Res.* **56,** 2130–2136.
3. Skilling, J. S., Sood, A. K., Niemann, T., Lager, D. J., and Buller, R. E. (1996) An abundance of p53 null mutations in ovarian carcinoma. *Oncogene* **13,** 117–123.
4. Orita, M., Suzuki, Y., Sekiya, T., and Hayashi, K. (1989) Rapid and sensitive detection of point mutations and DNA polymorphisms using the polymerase chain reaction. *Genomics* **5,** 874–879.
5. Smith, T. A., Whelan, J., and Parry, P. J. (1992) Detection of single-base mutations in a mixed population of cells: A comparison of SSCP and direct sequencing. *GATA* **9,** 143–145.
6. Teschauer, W., Mussack, T., Braun, A., Waldner, H., and Fink, E. (1996) Conditions for single strand conformation polymorphism (SSCP) analysis with broad applicability: A study on the effects of acrylamide, buffer and glycerol concentrations in SSCP analysis of exons of the p53 gene. *Eur. J. Clin. Chem. Clin. Biochem.* **34,** 125–131.
7. Buller, R. E., Sood, A., Fullenkamp, C., Sorosky, J., Powills, K., and Anderson, B. (1997) The influence of the p53 codon 72 polymorphism on ovarian carcinogenesis and prognosis. *Cancer Gene Ther.* **4,** 239–245.
8. Heller, M. J., Burgart, L. J., TenEyck, C. J., Anderson, M. E., Greiner, T. C., and Robinson, R. A. (1991) An efficient method for the extraction of DNA from formalin-fixed, paraffin-embedded tissue by sonication. *BioTechniques* **1,** 372–377.

# 36

## Multiplex PCR (MPCR) Screening Can Detect Small Intragenic *p53* Deletion and Insertion Mutations

### Ingo B. Runnebaum and Shan Wang-Gohrke

## 1. Introduction

Mutations of the *p53* tumor suppressor gene are the most common alterations associated with malignancy identified so far. Inactivation of the *p53* gene contributes to loss of a cell-cycle check point at the G1-S boundary and to genetic instability of the cell eventually allowing cells to replicate in an uncontrolled fashion (*1*). Inactivating *p53* mutations have frequently been identified in many different forms of cancer including more than 50% of ovarian cancers (*2,3*). The type and location of *p53* mutations occurring in human tumors are nonrandom. In a compilation of more than 4200 *p53* mutations in human cancers by Soussi et al., 50% of the mutations were missense mutations, 37% frameshift mutations, and 13% nonsense mutations (*4*). Small intragenic deletions and insertions have gained little attention in the analyses of the *p53* gene in human tumors (*5,6*). However, a review that compiled 740 *p53* mutations from a wide variety of cancers showed that 10% of the mutations were either deletions or insertions (*7*). Insertions were mostly flanked by short direct repeats of up to 14 basepairs (bp). Deletions of up to 37 bp often occurred in areas of sequence repeats. Such structural changes may be explained by a slipped mispairing mechanism during DNA replication (*7*).

Deletions or insertions at the *p53* gene locus appear in a variety of human tumor types (*7*). Deletions from 1 to 167 bp have been observed in Li-Frauenmani syndrome and Friend virus-induced erythroleukemia, respectively (*8*). In early studies on *p53* alterations in ovarian cancer, a mutational screening based upon polymerase chain reaction (PCR) with subsequent search for single-strand conformation polymorphisms (SSCP) had been applied. Small intragenic structural aberrations have been detected with an overall frequency of only 4.7% in ovarian cancer (*9–11*). A recent study revealed that a high incidence of p53 deletions/insertions (15.6%) exists in this type of cancer (*12*). In this chapter, we introduce a single step and reliable screening procedure for intragenic deletions or insertions of *p53* using a multiplex PCR (MPCR) strategy. The coding region was amplified by using four sets of oligonucleotides essentially as described previously (*13*). In brief, primer set I amplifies exon 2–4 resulting in a 641-bp fragment; set II exon 5–6 resulting in a 399-bp fragment; set III exon 7–9 resulting in a 810-bp fragment; and set IV exon 10–11 resulting in a 1264-bp fragment.

From: *Methods in Molecular Medicine, Vol. 39: Ovarian Cancer: Methods and Protocols*
Edited by: J. M. S. Bartlett © Humana Press, Inc., Totowa, NJ

A pair of internal control primers was included amplifying a 220-bp fragment of the gene specifying subunit VIII of cytochrome c oxidase (COX VIII) localized on chromosome 11 *(14)*. A high-resolution polymer was used to analyze the *p53* gene for larger, smaller, or missing fragments after PCR amplification *(15)*. Eleven ovarian cancer cell lines were analyzed by this method as well as by cycle sequencing.

## 2. Materials

### 2.1. Multiplex PCR (MPCR)

1. Eleven permanent human tumor cell lines were established from 11 patients with serous adenocarcinoma of the ovary as described previously *(16)*. Genomic DNA was isolated from all 11 cell lines for further analysis. Oligomer sequences (100 pmol/μL stock solution):
2. Exons 2–4: Set I sense 5′AGAATTCGATCCTCTTGCAGCAGCCAGAC3′ and antisense 5′ACCTAGGCTCAGGGCAACTGACCGTGCAA3′.
3. Exons 5–6: Set II sense 5′AGAATTCCTCTTCCTGCAGTACTCCCCTG3′ and antisense 5′CGGAATTCAGGCGGCTCATAGGGC3′.
4. Exons 7–9: Set III sense 5′AGAATTCCTCCTAGGTTGGCTCTGACTGT3′ and antisense 5′ACCTAGGCCAAGACTTAGTACCTGAAGGG3′.
5. Exons 10–11: Set IV sense 5′GGGAATTCAGATCCGTGGGCGTGAG3′ and antisense 5′ACCTAGGGCTGTCAGTGGGGAACAAGAAG3′.
6. Control: Set COX VIII sense 5′GGGCTTACCTCCTGCTTCGTGACCTTCCTC3′ and antisense 5′GAGGTCATGATTGCAGAAGAGGTGACTGGA3′.
7. Reaction mix (per 10 μL): 1.5 m$M$ of each dNTP (Pharmacia, Milwaukee, WI), 10% v/v DMSO, 10 pmol of each of the 10 primers, 1 U of *Taq* polymerase (Perkin Elmer Cetus, Norwalk, CT), 2X reaction buffer.
8. 5X reaction buffer: 335 m$M$ Tris-HCl, pH 8.8, 33.5 m$M$ MgCl$_2$, 83 m$M$ ammonium sulfate, 50 m$M$ beta-mercaptoethanol, 34 μ$M$ EDTA, 850 μg/mL BSA.

### 2.2. Gel Electrophoresis

1. 5X TBE (Tris-borate): 0.45 $M$ Tris-borate, 0.01 $M$ EDTA.
2. 2X MDE (Hydrolink-MDE, AT Biochem, Malvern, PA/Serva, Heidelberg, Germany).
3. Gel-loading dye: 0.25% bromophenol blue, 0.25% xylene cyanol FF, and 40% (w/v) sucrose in distilled water.
4. 10 μg/mL Ethidium bromide in distilled water (shield from light, teratogenic and mutagenic).

### 2.3. Cycle Sequencing

1. Digoxigenin-labeled oligonucleotides of the same sequence for priming as given above.
2. Centricon-100 concentrator (spin column, Amicon, Beverly, MA).
3. Dig *Taq* sequencing kit (# 1449443, Boehringer Mannheim, Mannheim, Germany).
4. Sequencing stop solution: 95% formamide, 20 m$M$ EDTA, 0.05% bromophenol blue, 0.05% xylene cyanol FF, and 20 m$M$ NaOH.
5. 6% (29:1) Acrylamide:Bis-acrylamide with 7.5$M$ Urea, 1X TBE.
6. N-Nylon membrane (Betagen, Waltham, MA).
7. DIG Luminescent Detection Kit (# 1363514, Boehringer Mannheim).

## 3. Methods

### 3.1. MPCR

1. Prepare sufficient reaction mixture for samples to be analyzed (10 μL per reaction).
2. Label tubes for each sample and add 100 ng DNA in 10 μL. Add 10 μL reaction mix to each tube, mix briefly, and pulse spin reagents to bottom of tube.

3. Overlay reaction mix with 20 µL mineral oil (*see* **Note 1**).
4. Perform amplification reaction with an initial denaturation step of 2 min 94°C, followed by 30 cycles consisting of three steps: 94°C for 30 s, 53°C for 30 s, and 65°C for 2 min. The last cycle was followed by an extension step of 5 min at 65°C (*see* **Note 2**).

## 3.2. Gel Electrophoresis

1. Prepare a 42-cm long, 0.6-mm thick, 32-well 1X MDE gel (provided as 2×) hydrolink gel (*see* **Note 3**). Preparation of 1X MDE gel solution (100 mL volume): MDE Gel Solution (2×) 50 mL, 5X TBE 12 mL, deionized water (fill to) 100 mL, mix well; TEMED 40 µL, 10% APS 400 µL, quickly mix well, and carefully pour the gel. If the plates were clean, there should be no trapped air bubbles.
2. Mix 5 µL of the PCR product with 2 µL gel loading dye and load on MDE gel.
3. Electrophorese under nondenaturing conditions in 0.6X TBE buffer for 14 h at 800 V with constant power.
4. Following electrophoresis the gels were stained for 5 min in ethidium bromide.
5. Gels were destained for 10 min in distilled water and photographed on an ultraviolet (UV) light box.

## 3.3. Cycle Sequencing

For sequence analysis of MPCR fragments a cycle sequencing strategy was applied using digoxigenin-labeled oligonucleotides of the same sequence for priming as given above.

### 3.3.1. Template Preparation

1. Bands were excised from the MDE gel under UV fluorescence.
2. MDE gel cannot be redissolved or melted at 37°C in TE buffer overnight usually.
3. PCR products were purified on a Centricon-100 concentrator (spin column, Amicon, Beverly, MA) when using a single primer set or were band-isolated prior to purification when using a multiplex primer set.

### 3.3.2. Cycle Sequencing

1. For each template label tubes A, T, C, G, and add (in a total volume of 6 µL) 1 pmol template DNA, 1 pmol digoxigenin-labeled primer, 50 m$M$ KCl, 10 m$M$ Tris-HCl (pH 8.3), 1.5 m$M$ MgCl$_2$, 0.6 U *Taq* DNA polymerase, 8.3 µ$M$ of each dNTP, and 283 µ$M$ ddATP (A tube), or 133 µ$M$ ddCTP (C Tube) or 25 µ$M$ ddGTP (G tube) or 425 µ$M$ ddTTP (T tube).
2. Overlay reaction mix with 10 µL mineral oil (*see* **Note 1**).
3. Perform cycle sequencing with an initial denaturation step of 3 min at 94°C followed by 30 cycles of 94°C for 30 s, 54°C for 30 s, and 70°C for 1 min (*see* **Note 2**).
4. After thermal cycling 1 µL of the reaction mix was added to 3 µL of sequencing stop solution.
5. The samples were denatured by heating to 95°C for 5 min and chilled on ice.

### 3.3.3. Electrophoresis and Detection

For electrophoresis and blotting an Autotrans 350 Direct transfer electrophoresis system (Betagen, Waltham, MA) was used.

1. A 35-cm long, 0.2-mm thick, 6% polyacrylamide gel containing 7.5$M$ urea was prepared.
2. Sufficient volume of 1X TBE buffer was preheated to 45°C for electrophoresis.

3. Before loading the samples, the gel was prerun in preheated (45°C) 1X TBE buffer at 32 W for 30 min. One µL of each of the sequencing (A, C, T, G) reactions mixes was loaded into separate lanes on the gel.

4. Samples were run into the gel for 60 min, followed by the combined electrophoresis and membrane transfer using a direct transfer electrophoresis system (AutoTrans 350, Betagen) for another 3–4 h at a membrane web speed of 1.8 mm/min. Electrophoresed fragments were directly blotted onto a N-Nylon membrane (Betagen) during the electrophoresis.

5. The transferred sequencing ladder was UV-crosslinked to the membrane under Optimal Crosslink Mode (120 mJ/cm$^2$, Spectrolinker™ XL-1000 UV Crosslinker, Spectronics Corporation, NY).

6. For detection of nucleic acids on the membrane the DIG Luminescent Detection Kit (# 1363514, Boehringer Mannheim) was used. The membrane was washed briefly (5 min) in washing buffer (supplied with the kit) and incubated in blocking buffer (supplied with the kit) for 30 min. Antidigoxigenin-AP FAb fragments were diluted to 75 mU/mL (1 : 10,000) in blocking buffer. The membrane was incubated in diluted antibody conjugate solution for 30 min. After removing unbound conjugate by washing 2× for 15 min in washing buffer and equilibrating the membrane for 5 min, the membrane was incubated in substrate solution (Lumigen PPD) for 5 min. Excess liquid was allowed to drip off, but not complete to dryness. The damp membrane was sealed in a hybridization bag. The sealed membrane was kept at 37°C for 15 min.

7. A Kodak X-omat S film was exposed to the membrane at room temperature for 20 min and developed.

Simultaneous amplification of four genomic *p53* segments comprising the complete coding region separated by intron stretches of 660 bp (intron 4), 760 bp (intron 6), and 2560 bp (intron 9) yielded four bands of expected size without undesirable run-through and spurious extra bands. Sequence analysis of the gel-isolated four bands using the same multiplex oligonucleotides for priming on genomic placental DNA proved their derivation as expected. The included PCR of a COX VIII sequence served as a sensitive internal control to indicate an optimal amplification reaction. Smaller or larger PCR products or missing amplification were observed in 6 out of 11 cell lines tested. Amplification of segment I (exon 2–4, 641 bp) of cell line #6 resulted in a subtle, but reproducible change in electrophoretic mobility indicating a slightly smaller fragment (**Fig. 1**). More distinctly, the PCR products of segment II (exon 5–6, 399 bp) of cell line #3 as well as of segment III (exon 7–9, 810 bp) of cell lines #2 and #5 resulted in a smaller band (**Fig. 1**). In addition to the smaller fragment, no band of expected size was observed in these cases. Larger bands indicating a possible insertional event were seen in segment I (exon 2–4, 641 bp) as the larger band occurred on top of the regular size band of cell lines #4 (**Fig. 1**). No amplification was observed from segment I of cell line #1 (**Fig. 1**). When loaded on a 3% agarose gel, no size differences were observed (data not shown). The consistent results were seen in three different amplifications.

Nucleotide sequence analysis was carried out to determine the exact changes leading to the shifted bands on a nondenaturing high resolution gel. In the fragment of exon 2–4 of cell line #6 a homozygous deletion of two basepairs (TCC to T) in codon 99 was found (**Fig. 2**). In cell line #4, the double bands in segment I were gel-isolated and each used as template for cycle sequencing. The band running at the expected size was shown to be of wild-type sequence, whereas the upper band showed an insertion of 16 bp (GACCTGGAGGGCTGGG) in intron 3 (data not shown).

Fig. 1. Photograph of an ethidium bromide-stained high-resolution polymer gel showing the electrophoresed MPCR products of six ovarian cancer cell lines (lanes 1–6). (P) Placental DNA as wild-type control. (M) Molecular weight marker, phiX HaeIII digest. 1264 bp band, exon 10–11. 810-bp band exon 7–9, 641-bp band, exon 2–4. 399-bp band, exon 5–6. 220-bp band, COX VIII gene as internal control for the fidelity of the reaction mix.

Fig. 2. Autoradiograph of a DIG-labeled sequencing reaction of the genomic segment of exon 2–4 of cell line #6. A deletion of two basepairs in codon 99 is detected (TCC to T). The reaction using the antisense primer is shown (loss of two G).

In six out of seven alterations detected by MPCR, no wild-type allele was visible in the sequence analysis indicating homozygosity for these six cases. Only in cell line #4, we found two bands representing the same segment of the gene amplified from two alleles differing in sequence. The heterozygosity of this aberration was demonstrated by sequence analysis. One band of expected size showed wild-type nucleotide sequence representing the wild-type allele, the larger PCR product revealed an insertion in intron 3 resulting in a slower electrophoretic mobility and representing a second polymorphic allele. In all other cases, it is very likely that a larger deletion leading to LOH eliminated the wild-type allele. Missing amplification of different segments of *p53* as observed in cell line 1 for exon 2–4 could be due to gross deletion in this region or a mutation in the sequence of primer annealing.

Structural *p53* gene aberrations as detected by MPCR have been described for ovarian cancer only rarely. This may be because of the fact that the methodology previously applied concentrated on point mutational changes in the conserved regions (exons 5–8) of the gene. Point mutations have so far been detected with a frequency of more than 50% in ovarian cancer mostly in conjunction with LOH *(9,17–20)*. The relatively higher frequency of LOH, compared to point mutations identified in these studies, suggested that additional genetic alterations such as deletions and insertions of few bases could occur in the remaining allele. In previous studies on *p53* alterations in ovarian cancer, a mutational screening based upon PCR with subsequent search for SSCP has been applied mainly on *p53* exons 5–8. By this procedure, only few such structural alterations have been detected in ovarian cancer: 1/30 primary tumors showed an 18-bp deletion *(9)*, 2/31 with a deletion of 10 and 1 bp, respectively *(19)*, 3/66 with a deletion of 6, 3, and 2 bp, respectively *(10)*. Only in 1/66 ovarian tumors an insertion (of 4 bp) had been detected *(10)*. A recent study revealed that a high incidence of *p53* deletions/insertions (15.6%) exists in this type of cancer when SSCP was performed for the entire ORF of the *p53* gene *(12)*. Similar results (14.3%) were described in a study on 56 ovarian cancer patients *(21)*. These results implicate that intragenic deletions are generally more common than insertions and that they are not rare events in ovarian cancer. The incidence of such alterations has to be ascertained in a large number of primary ovarian carcinomas to determine the overall frequency of this type of *p53* mutations. Systematic analyses should be related to epidemiologic data such as use of oral contraceptives, age of menarche and menopause, length of lactation, length of menstrual cycle (total number of ovulations?), exposure to possible carcinogens (talcum powder), or to irradiation, to identify possible mechanisms leading to certain deletion mutations in *p53*.

## 4. Notes

1. Mineral oil is not required if the PCR block has a heated lid.
2. The amplification reaction was carried out in a Maxicycler and Minicycler (MJ Research, Watertown, MA), different PCR blocks have different cycling parameters (ramp speed, etc.), which may require modification of the conditions described here.
3. In order to improve the degree of gel seperation, we applied Hydrolink MDE polymer gel. On a 3% normal agarose gel, bands can be sensitively separated when the fragment size difference are more than 25 bp. In the current protocol, a difference of 2 bp could readily be observed on a Hydrolink MDE polymer gel. An improved detection of heteroduplices as well as SSCPs using a MDE polymer has been reported *(15)*. Any type of high-resolution

electrophoresis applicable to nucleotide sequencing could be applied to detect minute size aberration in MPCR analysis. Labeling MPCR primers with fluorescent dye should make the use of an semiautomated sequencing equipment feasible and may expedite the detection step.

## Acknowledgment

This work was supported by the Deutsche Forschungsgemeinschaft (Grant no. RU476) and institutional awards granted to I.B.R.

## References

1. Levine, A. J. (1997) p53, the cellular gatekeeper for growth and division. *Cell* **88,** 323–331.
2. Fujita, M., Enomoto, T., Inoue, M., Tanizawa, O., Ozaki, M., Rice, J. M., and Nomura, T. (1994) Alteration of the p53 tumor suppressor gene occurs independently of K-ras activation and more frequently in serous adenocarcinomas than in other common epithelial tumors of the human ovary. *Japanese J. Cancer Res.* **85,** 1247–1256.
3. Kohler, M. F., Kerns, B. J., Humphrey, P. A., Marks, J. R., Bast, R. J., and Berchuck A. (1993) Mutation and overexpression of p53 in early-stage epithelial ovarian cancer. *Obstet. Gynecol.* **81,** 643–650.
4. Beroud, C., Verdier, F., and Soussi, T. (1996) p53 gene mutation: software and database. *Nucleic Acids Res.* **24,** 147–150.
5. Hollstein, M., Sidransky, D., Vogelstein, B., and Harris, C. C. (1991) p53 Mutations in human cancers. *Science* **253,** 49–53.
6. de Frommentel, C. C. and Soussi, T. (1992) TP53 tumor suppressor gene: A model for investigating human mutagenesis. *Genes Chromosomes Cancer* 41–15.
7. Jego, N., Thomas, G., and Hamelin, R. (1993) Short direct repeats flanking deletions, and duplication insertions in p53 gene in human cancers. *Oncogene* **8,** 209–213.
8. Varley, J. M., McGown, G., Thorncroft, M., Santibanez-Koref, M. F., Kelsey, A. M., Tricker, K. J., et al. (1997) Germ-line mutations of TP53 in li-fraumeni families: An extended study of 39 families. *Cancer Res.* **57,** 3245–3252.
9. Mazars, R., Pujol, P., Maudelonde, T., Jeanteur, P., and Theillet, C. (1991) p53 mutations in ovarian cancer: A late event? *Oncogene* **6,** 1685–1690.
10. Milner, B. J., Allan, L. A., Eccles, D. M., Kitchener, H. C., Leonard, R. C. F., Kelly, K. F., et al. (1993) p53 Mutation is a common genetic event in ovarian carcinoma. *Cancer Res.* **53,** 2128–2132.
11. Wang-Gohrke, S., Hees, S., Pochon, A., Wen, W., Reles, A., Press, M. F., Kreienberg, R., and Runnebaum, I. B. (1998) Genomic semi-automated cycle sequencing as a sensitive screening technique for p53 mutations in frozen tumor samples. *Oncol. Rep.* **5,** 65–68.
12. Skilling, J. S., Sood, A., Niemann, T., Lager, D. J., and Buller, R. E. (1996) An abundance of p53 null mutations in ovarian carcinoma. *Oncogene* **13,** 117–123.
13. Runnebaum, I. B., Nagarajan, M., Bowman, M., Soto, D., and Sukumar, S. (1991) Mutations in p53 as potential molecular markers for human breast cancer. *Proc. Natl. Acad. Sci. USA* **88,** 10,657–10,661.
14. Rizzuto, R., Nakase, H., Darras, B., Francke, U., Fabrizi, G. M., Mengel, T., et al. (1989) A gene specifying subunit VIII of human cytochrome c oxidase is localized to chromosome 11 and is expressed in both muscle and non-muscle tissues. *J. Biological Chem.* **264,** 10,595–10,600.
15. Soto, D. and Sukumar, S. (1992) Improved detection of mutations in the p53 gene in human tumors as single-stranded conformation polymorphs and double-stranded heteroduplex DNA. *PCR Methods and Applications* **2,** 96–98.
16. Moebus, V., Gerharz, C. D., Press, U., Moll, R., Beck, T., Mellin, W., et al. (1992) Morphological, immunohistochemical and biochemical characterization of 6 newly established human ovarian carcinoma cell lines. *Int. J. Cancer* **52,** 76–84.
17. Kupryjanczyk, J., Thor, A. D., Beauchamp, R., Merritt, V., Edgerton, S. M., Bell, D. A., Yandell, D. W. (1993) p53 gene mutations and protein accumulation in human ovarian cancer. *Proc. Natl. Acad. Sci. USA* **90,** 4961–4965.
18. Marks, J. R., Davidoff, A. M., Kerns, B. J., Humphrey, P. A., Pence, J. C., and Dodge, R. K. (1991) Overexpression and mutation of p53 in epithelial ovarian cancer. *Cancer Res.* **51,** 2979–2984.
19. Okamoto, A., Sameshima, Y., Yokoyama, S., Terashima, Y., Sugimura, T., Terada, M., and Yokota, J. (1991) Frequent allelic losses and mutations of the p53 gene in human ovarian cancer. *Cancer Res.* **51,** 5171–5176.
20. Teneriello, M. G., Ebina, M., Linnoila, R. I., Henry, M., Nash, J. D., Park, R. C., and Birrer, M. J. (1993) p53 and Ki-ras gene mutations in epithelial ovarian neoplasms. *Cancer Res.* **53,** 3103–3108.
21. Angelopoulou, K., Levesque, M. A., Katsaros, D., Shipman, R., and Diamandis, E. P. (1998) Exon 5 of the p53 gene is a target for deletions in ovarian cancer. *Clin. Chem.* 4472–4477.

# 37

## Transfer of Human Chromosome 3 to an Ovarian Carcinoma Cell Line Identifies Regions Involved in Ovarian Cancer

**Paola Rimessi and Francesca Gualandi**

## 1. Introduction

Earlier studies with somatic cell hybrids had clearly shown that when malignant cells were fused with normal cells, the resulting hybrid cells were nontumorigenic and that reexpression of tumorigenicity was often associated with the loss of specific chromosomes derived from the normal parental cells (1). A more direct approach to identify chromosomes carrying tumor suppressor genes is the introduction of specific chromosomes into tumor cells by microcell monochromosome transfer (MMCT) (2). The key feature of this technique is that the transferred chromosome is retained as a complete structural unit in succeeding generations of recipient cells, unlike the technique of metaphase chromosome transfer, where the transferred chromosome is rapidly degraded. To allow for transfer and selective retention of single specific chromosomes, dominant selectable markers such as the bacterial *neo* gene, which encodes an aminoglycoside 3′phosphotransferase (APH), are integrated into individual human chromosomes via plasmid DNA transfection or retroviral infection. Chromosomes tagged with dominant selectable markers can then be transferred from normal cells into cancer cells previously shown to have deletions in specific chromosome regions (3). The MMCT procedure is schematically outlined in **Fig. 1**. MMCT was used successfully with cell lines from tumors of different histotypes to detect chromosomal regions containing tumor suppressor genes and to identify chromosomes involved in the tumorigenic phenotype.

Several studies report the nonrandom loss of heterozygosity for alleles located at chromosomes 3p, 6q, 11p, 17, and 18q in ovarian carcinoma (4–9). However, no functional proof has been provided of tumor suppressor activity influencing malignant phenotype in ovarian cancer located in these chromosomal regions.

Here we describe the transfer of normal human chromosomes 3 and 11, via MMCT, into an ovarian carcinoma cell line (HEY cell line) to identify regions involved in ovarian cancer. The present study shows that introduction of chromosome 3 by MMCT into HEY cell line produces growth arrest and tumor suppression suggesting the presence on chromosome 3 of tumor suppression functions involved in the development of

From: *Methods in Molecular Medicine, Vol. 39: Ovarian Cancer: Methods and Protocols*
Edited by: J. M. S. Bartlett © Humana Press, Inc., Totowa, NJ

Fig. 1. Microcell fusion technique.

ovarian carcinoma. We also identify two distinct regions on 3p whose loss may represent a critical event in the pathogenesis of ovarian cancer: a proximal region in 3p21 1–21.2 of 3 cM and a distal region in 3p23–24.2 smaller than 13 cM. It is notable that the same regions were found to be deleted in other tumors *(10–12)*. These concordant results strongly support the presence of tumor suppressor genes in the commonly deleted regions and raise the possibility that the same genes may be involved in tumors of different histotypes.

## 2. Materials

### 2.1. Cell Lines and Culture Media

1. Recipient cells: HEY cell line derives from a human ovarian cancer xenograft in nude mice originally grown from a peritoneal deposit of a patient with moderately differentiated papillary cystoadenocarcinoma of the ovary *(13)*.

2. Donor cells: A9-3*neo* and MCH-556 are murine A9 cells containing a pSV2*neo*-tagged normal human chromosome 3 or chromosome 11, respectively.
3. Monochromosomic hybrids: HEY/H3 and HEY/H11 hybrids were grown in DMEM F12 with 400 µg/mL geneticin.

## 2.2. Reagents

1. Colcemid: Demecolcine (Sigma, GIBCO-BRL, Paisley, Scotland) powder is stored desiccated and protected from light at –20°C. Stock solutions of 1 mg/mL in 0.9% (w/v) NaCl are stable for at least 6 mo at –20°C, if protected from light.
2. HEY cells were grown in DMEM/F12 medium supplemented with 10% FCS.
3. Donor cells were grown in DMEM/F12 containing 600 µg/mL geneticin.
4. Cytochalasin B (Sigma): powder is stored desicated and protected from light at –20°C. Stock solutions of 10 mg/mL in dimethyl sulfoxide (DMSO) are stable indefinitely at 4°C, if protected from light.
5. Phytohemagglutinin P (PHA-P) (Cat. No. 3110-57-3; Difco, Detroit, MI): powder is a lyophilized stock consisting of equal parts by weight of PHA-P and salt. PHA-P solutions are always prepared fresh; the powder is stored at 4°C.
6. Polyethylene glycol (PEG) 1500 (Boehringer Mannheim, Indianapolis, IN): 50% PEG 1500 (w/v) in 75 m$M$ HEPES (pH 8.0), ready to use.
7. Geneticin (G418) (Boehringer Mannheim): Stock solution of 100 mg/mL in HEPES 100 m$M$, pH 7.0 stored at –20°C.
8. Enucleation medium, serum-free medium containing 10 µg/mL cytochalasin B (diluted from a 10 mg/mL stock in DMSO).

# 3. Methods
## 3.1. Determination of G418 Killing Curve

Before proceeding to MMCT, it is advisable to clone the recipient cell line and to check for mycoplasma contamination (*see* **Notes 1** and **2**). The amount of drug required for selection varies with the cell type. In practice, one needs to determine the minimal concentration of G418 required to kill all cells in the population over a period of 2–3 wk.

1. The recipient cells are plated in a 6-well (35-mm) tissue-culture plate at approx $3 \times 10^5$ cells/well and incubated at 37°C overnight.
2. A series of increasing concentrations of G418, ranging from 100 µg/mL to 1.2 mg/mL, are prepared in growth medium.
3. Each concentration of selective medium is added to any single well and replaced every 2 d, leaving one well without drug as control.
4. 400 µg/mL of G418 was determined as the lowest drug concentration resulting in 100% kill for HEY cells.

## 3.2. Determination of Colcemid Concentration and Time of Exposure

Efficient micronucleation by prolonged mitotic arrest *(14)* depends on careful determination of the optimal colcemid concentration and time of exposure. Colcemid concentrations in the range 0.01–0.5 µg/mL effectively induce micronucleation of most rodent cells; however, within that range the effective concentration for a given cell line is usually narrow so that each cell line to be employed as a microcell donor should be tested individually (*see* **Note 3**). The kinetics of mitotic arrest and subsequent micronucleation in colcemid depend on the generation times of the donor populations. In general, rapidly growing cells micronucleate faster and more efficiently than slowly growing lines. To reduce cell toxicity, colcemid arrest should be performed in medium supplemented with 20% FCS.

1. Donor cells are seeded at 30–40% confluence in a 6-well (35-mm) tissue-culture plate and incubated overnight.
2. Various concentrations of colcemid, spanning a range of 0.01–0.5 µg/mL, are added to the cells in nonselective medium.
3. Plates are assessed for micronucleation and cell toxicity periodically over the course of 72 h. Visualization under phase contrast is generally sufficient to assess the micronucleation index semiquantitatively.
4. Colcemid at a concentration of 0.2 µg/mL for 48 h resulted as the optimal condition for micronucleating both A9-3*neo* and MCH 556 donor cells.

### 3.3. Microcell-Mediated Chromosome Transfer

The steps involved in MMCT are shown in **Fig. 1**. The procedure can be divided into several parts: micronucleation of donor cells, enucleation in the presence of cytochalasin B, purification of microcells, fusion with intact recipients, and biochemical selection of microcell hybrids.

#### 3.3.1. Micronucleation of Donor Cells

The initial step in microcell fusion is to induce donor cells to become micronucleate. This can be accomplished, among other approaches, by prolonged mitotic arrest *(14)*. In this procedure, exponentially growing cultures are exposed to Colcemid, an inhibitor of microtubule polymerization. Cells are initially blocked in metaphase, but a significant proportion escape the block and enters G1 phase of the cell cycle. However, because there is no mitotic spindle formation, the chromosomes condense as an individual unit, resulting in a multinucleate cell containing large numbers of micronuclei, each of which contains one or several chromosomes.

1. Donor cells are split into six 25-cm$^2$ straight-neck Costar flasks (Costar, Cambridge, MA) resistant to centrifugal force up to 12,500$g$ with 5 mL of growth medium and incubated at 37°C until 70–80% confluent.
2. Colcemid is added to the determined optimal concentration (0.2 µg/mL for A9-3*neo* and MCH 556) and the flasks further incubated for 48 h at 37°C.
3. Micronucleation is visualized under phase contrast to verify the efficiency of the process.

#### 3.3.2. Enucleation of Micronucleate Populations

Enucleation of micronucleate donor cells can be accomplished by centrifugation in the presence of cytochalasin B, a fungal metabolite that interferes with cytokinesis. These conditions result in extrusion of the nucleus or micronuclei, each surrounded by a thin rim of cytoplasm and plasma membrane *(15)*. A convenient method of enucleation involves attachment of the donor cells to a solid surface that can be centrifuged in cytochalasin B-containing medium. In this case, cytoplasts remain attached to the surface while extruded nuclear material is sheared from the cells by centrifugal force and pelleted to the bottom of the surface. Cells can be enucleated directly from T-flasks or other surfaces (*see* **Note 4**).

1. Enucleation medium is prepared and prewarmed at 37°C.
2. The six Costar flasks of donor cells are filled to the neck with enucleation medium and incubated for 30 min at 37°C.
3. The empty rotor and chamber are prewarmed by spinning at 12,500*g* for 10–15 min at 34°C using Beckman J2-21centrifuge (Fullerton, CA; JA-14 rotor).
4. The flasks are placed with the bottoms facing out, in the Beckman JA-14 rotor containing 100 mL of water in each well as a cushion and centrifuged at 12,500*g* for 65 min at 34°C without using the brake.
5. After centrifugation, a small microcell pellet should be apparent in the bottom of each flask. By examination under phase-contrast, illumination is possible to monitor the degree of enucleation; if incomplete, respin the flask. Once enucleation is complete, the cytochalasin-containing medium is collected in a sterile bottle. Enucleation medium can be reused to process a second set of flasks or filter sterilized for future use.
6. Each microcell pellet is carefully resuspended in 2 mL serum-free medium and collected in a 15-mL tube.

### 3.3.3. Purification of Microcell Preparations

The crude microcell pellet is a heterogeneous mixture of particles including microcells, cytoplasmic vesicles, whole nuclei (karyoplasts), and intact cells (*see* **Note 5**). Membrane filtration through polycarbonate filters is the simplest and most widely used method for microcell purification *(16)*. We find sequential filtration through polycarbonate filters of 8-, 5-, and 3-μm pore size (Nuclepore, Pleasanton, CA) to be adequate for excluding whole cells and karyoplasts.

1. Filters are mounted in Swinnex adapters (Millipore, Bedford, MA), wrapped in foil, and autoclaved prior to fusion.
2. For filtration, adapters are mounted on sterile 20-mL syringes from which plungers have been removed (in processing the microcell pellet from six flasks, we used a series of three filters).
3. Microcell suspension in serum-free medium (12 mL/filter set) is poured into the syringe. The suspension will usually flow through the 8-μm membrane by gravity; application of gentle pressure is necessary for the 5 and 3-μm filtration.
4. The final microcell suspension has to be centrifuged at 800*g* for 15 min at room temperature to pellet microcells for fusion. An aliquot of the pooled filtrate should be reserved for particle quantitations.
5. The total number of particles is determined by counting an aliquot of the pellet using a haemocytometer; the number of microcells in the preparation can then be calculated.

### 3.3.4. Suspension/Monolayer Fusion

Use of the chemical fusogen polyethylene glycol (PEG) is the method of choice for most types of somatic cell fusion *(17)*. Polyethylene glycol is widely available and produces rapid, efficient, and reproducible fusion (*see* **Note 6**). Microcells are first allowed to agglutinate with the monolayer of recipient cells in the presence of phytohemagglutinin P (PHA-P). The microcells are then fused with recipient cells by brief exposure to PEG. A fraction of the microcell heterokaryons will subsequently divide to form microcell hybrid clones. We observe efficient microcell fusion with microcell-recipient cell ratios between 1:1 and 5:1. This generally requires $0.5$–$2 \times 10^7$ microcells/25-cm$^2$ recipient flask.

1. Recipient cells are plated into 25-cm² flasks on the day prior to fusion such that the monolayer will be 70–80% confluent at the time of fusion. An extra flask of recipient cells should be prepared to be processed as a self-fused control, without addition of microcells.
2. PHA-P (50 μg/mL in serum-free medium) is prepared fresh and filter sterilized.
3. The microcell pellet is resuspended in 2 mL serum-free medium (D-MEM F12) containing PHA-P (50 μg/mL) and vigorously pipeted to break clumps.
4. The recipient monolayer is rinsed with 5 mL serum-free medium and the microcell suspension then added to the recipient flask. The flask is gently shaken to spread microcells over the monolayer allowing the microcells to settle by gravity and to attach for 15–20 min at 37°C. During PHA, incubation is necessary to check the flask under the microscope to ensure that the microcells have agglutinated to the recipient monolayer and to monitor cell toxicity.
5. The microcells attached to the recipient monolayer are fused as follow: PHA-P containing medium is aspirated, the flask inverted and 1 mL of 50% (w/v) polyethylene glycol (PEG) 1500 added to the cells. The flask is turned over, and, while beginning timing, slowly rocked back and forth to spread the PEG over the monolayer. After 60 s, PEG is aspirated and the cells rinsed rapidly with three changes of serum-free medium.
6. Complete nonselective medium containing antibiotics is added and the cells incubated for 24 h at 37°C.
7. The following day, the flask is split 1:15 into selective medium (400 μg/mL G418).

### 3.3.5. Biochemical Selection of Microcell Hybrids

It is not possible to predict the number of hybrid clones that will be generated in a microcell fusion experiment, as each donor-recipient pair will behave differently. In general, the efficiency of microcell fusion should be on the order of $0.5–5 \times 10^{-5}$ relative to the number of recipient cells fused (*see* **Note 7**).

1. Selective medium has to be periodically replaced (every 2 d). G418-resistant hybrid clones are usually visible in 2–3 wk.
2. After the clones have reached a sufficient size, they are surrounded with glass cylinders fixed to the flask with silicone and collected by trypsinization. The cells are then transferred to 48-well plates in which individual clones can be expanded for further analysis.

### 3.4. Analysis of Microcell Hybrid Clones

Upon transfer of a *neo*-tagged chromosome 3 to HEY cells, in three successive microcell fusion experiments, only four G418-resistant clones were isolated. All the clones, with the exception of clone 5, which could be propagated as a cell line, ceased to grow before 20 population doublings and showed morphological alterations consistent with a slow process of irreversible growth arrest reminiscent of senescence (*see* **Note 8**). The reduced growth rate and the senescence process of HEY/H3 clones precluded the study of their in vitro phenotype. However, tumorigenicity assay was possible for all HEY/H3 clones and genotypic analysis was performed on clones 2, 3, and 5.

In three independent transfer experiments of a normal human chromosome 11 to HEY cells, 15 G418-resistant clones were obtained. All HEY/H11 clones maintained the immortalized phenotype and were propagated as cell lines. No differences were observed in the morphology of HEY/H11 hybrids compared with the HEY recipient cells. Seven among fifteen HEY/H11 clones were analyzed in tumorigenicity and in vitro growth assays and genotyped.

Data obtained from molecular studies, together with the analysis of in vivo and in vitro phenotype of HEY/H3 hybrids, clearly demonstrated that the introduction of chromosome 3 suppresses the tumorigenicity of HEY cells and produces a severe reduction of cellular growth and morphological changes attributable to a process of senescence. In contrast, transfer of chromosome 11 to HEY cells, although influencing the characteristic of growth in vitro, does not consistently control tumorigenicity.

Dinucleotide repeat polymorphisms of microsatellites mapped on chromosome 3 (primer sequences from the Genome Data Base, Baltimore, MD), have been analyzed by PCR amplification and the results allowed the identification of regions on 3p whose loss is involved in ovarian carcinogenesis *(18)*. Our findings confirm microcell fusion as a powerful technique for gene mapping purposes and for genetic analysis of complex cellular phenotype (*see* **Note 9**).

## 4. Notes

1. Before proceeding to chromosome transfer, it is advisable to clone the recipient cell line to rule out that any inherent heterogeneity could account for the phenotypic differences detected in hybrid clones. An advantageous method of cell cloning is growth in soft agar, because it ensures a selection toward a high growth rate often associated with tumorigenicity. Necessary features for a useful recipient cell line are a high tumorigenicity (100%) with a low number of cells per inoculum and a short latency period in tumor development.

2. Mycoplasma infection causes changes in cell genotype and phenotype and can result in poor hybrid yields; periodically screen all cell lines for mycoplasma contamination by fluorescent Hoechst 33258 staining preliminary to any experiments.

3. The reported condition for micronucleation has been optimized for A9-3*neo* and MCH 556 donor cells and needs to be properly modified for other donor cell lines. Optimal conditions are easier to achieve for rapidly growing cells and it is helpful to add colcemid in exponentially growing cultures. For rodent cells, micronucleation indexes of 60–90% are generally attainable. Micronucleation of human cells is more variable, and the micronucleation percentage may be as low as 20–30%, even under optimal conditions.

4. The efficiency of the enucleation phase depends on firm attachment of the cells to the substrate and on generation of sufficient centrifugal force to shear the nuclei from the cells. The optimal speed and time of centrifugation are variables that should be determined empirically for each donor line. In general, centrifugation at 18,000–30,000$g$ for 30–70 min is appropriate. Cytochalasin-induced enucleation does not occur if the temperature of the medium is less than about 25°C *(19)*. Therefore the medium in the flasks must be warm during enucleation. The appropriate temperature settings for each individual centrifuge should be determined empirically. Following each spin the surface of the flask should be examined under phase-contrast illumination to assess the degree of enucleation. Completely enucleated monolayers will contain only cytoplasmic remnants attached to the surface. Incompletely enucleated monolayers will have threads of material, resembling beads on a string, attached to the cytoplasmic remnants. If significant numbers of micronuclei remain attached, longer centrifugation is required, and the flasks may be simply returned to the centrifuge. Even poorly adherent cells or cells that grow in suspension can be enucleated by attaching them to plastic surfaces to which concanavalin A has been covalently linked *(20)*.

5. If the crude preparation of microcell contains more than 10% intact cells and/or karyoplasts, significant numbers of whole-cell hybrids and/or donor cell clones will sur-

vive unless they can be eliminated by biochemical selection. Filtration is a necessary step when using A9 derived donor cells, highly resistant to any selective drugs if compared with human cells. A main cause of failure of MMCT technique is the possibility for A9 cells to escape the purification step through membrane filtration and to overwhelm hybrid clones growth. Filters may fail if set improperly in the adapter or if excessive pressure is used to force the suspension through, so each aliquot should be checked prior to pooling the filtrate. Filtration will result in some loss of microcells due to clogging and nonspecific adherence of particles to plastic, but this can be minimized by diluting the crude enucleation preparation and use of an adequate number of filters.

6. The most important variable at the fusion stage is the concentration of PEG, which is generally 44–50% (w/v) *(16)*. After PHA-P-induced agglutination, it is usually possible to achieve efficient fusion of most cell types with 44–46% PEG, but some relatively nonfusogenic recipients require higher concentrations. For an initial fusion involving a given donor-recipient pair, it is informative to fuse several different recipient flasks, each at a different PEG concentrations. The protocol described, referred to recipient cells growing as monolayer, can be modified when using cells growing in suspension: PHA-P incubation and PEG fusion steps will be performed by mixing microcells and recipient cells in a 50-mL Falcon tube in a total volume of 2 mL for each incubation.

7. If a given fusion does not produce microcell hybrid clones it could be because of a specific effect induced by the transferred chromosome. Nevertheless it is important, to exclude technical inaccuracy, to critically examine the data collected during the experiment regarding micronucleation, enucleation, and composition of the final microcell preparation. Other seemingly minor events such as inappropriate temperature during enucleation, especially high temperature, may also compromise hybrid yield. Several fusion experiments may be required to optimize all of the variables that contribute to efficient microcell transfer.

8. To exclude the possibility that the expression of the bacterial *neo* gene (inserted as selectable marker in the transferred chromosome) can influence cellular growth properties and tumorigenicity, it is advisable to introduce pSV2*neo* plasmid into recipient cells and analyze G418 resistant clones for growth rate and tumorigenicity.

9. During microcell fusion spontaneous chromosome fragmentation can occur and hybrids containing deleted chromosomes can be extremely useful to identify and map specific functions affecting hybrid phenotype. It is also possible to irradiate isolated microcells prior to fusion, thus generating more extensive chromosome fragmentation *(21)*. Fragment-containing hybrids have proved to be useful material for high-resolution mapping, isolation of genomic markers and cloning of expressed genes from defined chromosomal regions.

## References

1. Stanbridge, E. J. (1976) Suppression of malignancy in human cells. *Nature* **260,** 17–20.
2. Fournier, R. E. K. and Ruddle, F. H. (1977) Microcell-mediated transfer of murine chromosomes into mouse, Chinese hamster and human somatic cells. *Proc. Natl. Acad. Sci. USA* **74,** 319–323.
3. Saxon, P. J., Srivatsan, E. S., Leipzig, G. V., et al. (1985) Selective transfer of individual human chromosomes to recipient cells. *Mol. Cell Biol.* **5,** 140.
4. Lee, J. H., Kavanagh, J. J., Wildrick, D. M., et al. (1990) Frequent loss of heterozygosity on chromosome 6q, 11, and 17 in human ovarian carcinomas. *Cancer Res.* **59,** 2724–2728.
5. Eccles, D. M., Cranston, G., Steel, C. M., et al. (1990) Allele losses on chromosome 17 in human epithelial ovarian carcinoma. *Oncogene* **5,** 1599–1601.
6. Ehlen, T. and Dubeau, L. (1990) Loss of heterozygosity on chromosomal segments 3p, 6q and 11p in human ovarian carcinomas. *Oncogene* **5,** 219–223.
7. Chenevix-Trench, G., Leary, J., Kerr, J., et al. (1992) Frequent loss of heterozygosity on chromosome 18 in ovarian adenocarcinoma which does not always include the DCC locus. *Oncogene* **7,** 1059–1065.

8. Kiechle-Schwarz, M., Bauknecht, T., Wienker. T., et al. (1993) Loss of costitutional heterozygosity on chromosome 11p in human ovarian cancer. Positive correlation with grade of differentiation. *Cancer* **72,** 2423–2432.

9. Kohler, M. F., Marks, J. R., Wiseman, R. W., et al. (1993) Spectrum of mutations and frequency of allelic deletion of the p53 gene in ovarian cancer. *J. Natl. Cancer Inst.* **85,** 1513–1519.

10. Hibi, K., Takahashi, T., Yamakawa, K., et al. (1992) Three distinct regions involved in 3p deletion in human lung cancer. *Oncogene* **7,** 445–449.

11. Yamakawa, K., Morita, R., Takahashi, E., et al. (1991) A detailed deletion mapping of the short arm of chromosome 3 in sporadic renal cell carcinoma. *Cancer Res.* **51,** 4707–4711.

12. Kohno, T., Takayama, H., Hamaguchi, M., et al. (1993) Deletion mapping of chromosome 3p in human uterine cervical cancer. *Oncogene* **8,** 1825–1832.

13. Buick, R. N., Pullano, R., and Trent, J. M. (1985) Comparative properties of five human ovarian adenocarcinoma cell lines *Cancer Res.* **45,** 3668–3676.

14. Phillips, S. G. and Phillips, D. M. (1969) Sites of nucleolus production in cultured Chinese hamster cells. *J. Cell Biol.* **40,** 248–268.

15. Ege, T. and Ringertz, N. R. (1974) Preparation of microcells by enucleation of micronucleate cells. *Exp. Cell Res.* **87,** 378–382.

16. Fournier, R. E. K. (1981) A general high-efficiency procedure for production of microcell hybrids. *Proc. Natl. Acad. Sci. USA* **78,** 6349–6353.

17. Pontecorvo, G. (1975) Production of mammalian somatic cell hybrids by means of polyethylene glycol treatment. *Somat. Cell Genet.* **1,** 397–400.

18. Rimessi, P., Gualandi, F., Morelli, C., et al. (1994) Transfer of human chromosome 3 to an ovarian carcinoma cell line identifies three regions on 3p involved in ovarian cancer. *Oncogene* **9,** 3467–3474.

19. McNeill, C. A. and Brown, R. L. (1980) Genetic manipulation by means of microcell-mediated transfer of normal human chromosomes into recipient mouse cells. *Proc. Natl. Acad. Sci. USA* **77,** 5394–5398.

20. Gopalakrishnan, T. V. and Thompson, E. B. (1975) A method for enucleating cultured mammalian cells. *Exp. Cell Res.* **96,** 435–439.

21. Dowdy, S. F., Scanlon, C. L., Fusching, G., et al. (1990) Irradiation microcell-mediated chromosome transfer (XMMCT): the generation of specific chromosomal arm deletions. *Genes Chromo. Cancer* **2,** 318–327.

# 38

## Double- and Competitive-Differential PCR for Gene Dosage Quantitation

**Burkhard Brandt, Alf Beckmann, Antje Roetger, and Frank Gebhardt**

## 1. Introduction

An association of a loss of DNA replication control and the activation of *erbB* oncogenes can be deduced from studies with different cancers *(1–5)*. In the first study on ovarian cancer 26% of the tumors had c-*erbB-2* amplifications *(6)*. The correlation between c-*erbB-2* amplification and expression on mRNA and protein level was perfect. The median survival time of patients with ovarian cancers was negatively correlated to the degree of amplification. The association of *egfr* (c-*erbB-1*) amplification and overexpression with ovarian cancer prognosis has not been investigated as extensively as for c-*erbB-2*. EGF-R is expressed in normal ovarian epithelium and patients whose ovarian cancer continues to express EGF-R have a worse prognosis *(7)*. Rearrangements of the *egfr* gene in ovarian cancer were also described, as identified by Southern blot analysis *(8)*. Bauknecht submitted that a failure of chemotherapy was seen for ovarian cancers with low EGF-R expression *(8)*.

PCR is a universal method for gene dosage estimation. PCR is influenced by reaction conditions, but also by sample preparation, machine performance, and the presence of inhibitors. Approaches to circumvent these difficulties include differential and competitive PCR. We describe a quantitative PCR method, double-differential PCR (ddPCR) for gene dosage estimation of *egfr* and c-*erbB-2*. ddPCR uses comprised of the coamplification of the single-copy gene *HBB* (β-globin), the *erbB-1*, and *erbB-2* oncogenes and the second single-copy reference gene *SOD2* (super-oxide dismutase 2) under identical reaction conditions. The ratio of band intensities of the PCR products in stained electrophoresis gels expresses the average gene copy number (AGCN) per cell of the *erbB* oncogenes. Applying this quantitative PCR method was found to be more sensitive for measuring low-level gene amplification and gene dosage decreases than standard hybridization techniques *(9)*. Low levels of *erbB* amplification appear to have clinical significance in that disease outcome and therapeutic response of the tumor are affected by these genetic changes *(4)*. To control ddPCR sensitivity and reliability, we have recently developed a competitive-differential PCR technique (*cdPCR*) in which target DNA is PCR-amplified along with two internal standards (competitors) using the same primer pairs as in ddPCR (**Fig. 1**). The copy number is determined in this

From: *Methods in Molecular Medicine, Vol. 39: Ovarian Cancer: Methods and Protocols*
Edited by: J. M. S. Bartlett © Humana Press, Inc., Totowa, NJ

Fig. 1. Construction of competitive templates. Primer 1 is the conventional upstream PCR primer corresponding to the target sequence. The recombinant primer A2 comprises segment A corresponding to the target sequence $n$ bp (typically $n = 20$–$30$ bp) upstream from the recognition site of the conventional downstream primer 2 and the primer 2 sequence. PCR with these primers yields a product $n$ bp shorter than the conventional PCR product, which can serve as an internal standard for quantitative PCR, including the recognition sites for primers 1 and 2.

assay by comparing genomic with competing target PCR products on the same gel *(10)*. One of the competing target sequences is based on the genomic target sequences of c-*erbB-1* and c-*erbB-2*, respectively, whereas the other is derived from the single copy reference gene *HBB*. The method combines the advantages of differential and competitive PCR. Using this method, we confirmed *egfr* and *erbB-2* amplification in cancer cell lines and tumor tissue. cdPCR facilitates the detection of both increases and decreases in AGCN with high reproducibility, sensitivity, and accuracy.

## 2. Materials

### 2.1. Isolation of Genomic DNA

1. Nucleon™ II DNA Extraction Kit (Scotlab, Wiesloch, Germany).
2. QiaAmp Tissue Kit (Qiagen, Hilden, Germany).

### 2.2. Double-Differential PCR

1. 5000 U/mL stock of *Taq* DNA Polymerase (Promega, Heidelberg, Germany).
2. 10X ddPCR-Reaction buffer: Add 1200 µL 10X PCR reaction buffer, magnesium-free (Promega, $0.5M$ KCl, $0.1M$ Tris-HCl [pH 9.0], 1% Triton X-100 (w/v)), and 729 µL 25 m$M$ MgCl$_2$ (Promega).
3. 10 m$M$ stocks of dATP, dCTP, dGTP, dTTP in water (Perkin Elmer, Weiterstadt, Germany).

### 2.3. Competitive-Differential PCR

#### 2.3.1. Construction of Competitor Templates

1. TE buffer, pH 8.0 (10 m$M$ Tris-HCl, 1 m$M$ EDTA)
2. TA Cloning™ Kit (Invitrogen, DeSchelp, The Netherlands) containing Vector pCR™ II (25 ng/µL, linearized) TA Cloning( Reagents (T4 DNA Ligase, 10X Ligase buffer), One Shot™ Reagents (0.5 M β-mercaptoethanol, SOC Medium), and One Shot cells (bacteria INV (αF′).

**Table 1**
**Primer Sequences and Recombinant Primer Sequences**
**for Double-Differential and Competitive-Differential PCR**

| Gene and genomic PCR product | Primer Sequences[a] |
|---|---|
| *erbB-1* (144 bp) | Competitor:124 bp |
| Primer 1 | 5′-GCC ATT ATC CGA CGC TGG CTC TAA G-3′ |
| Primer 2 | 5′-**GAC TTG CAG CCC AGC CTA TGT CC**-3′ |
| Recombinant primer | 5′-**GAC TTG CAG CCC AGC CTA TGT C**CC AGG GTC CCC TTC CCC CTT TC-3′ |
| | |
| *erbB-2* (132 bp) | Competitor:107 bp |
| Primer 1 | 5′-GGT GTG ACT GTG TGG GAG CTG ATG-3′ |
| Primer 2 | 5′-**GTA GAC ATC AAT GGT GCA GAT GGG**-3′ |
| Recombinant primer | 5′-**GTA GAC ATC AAT GGT GCA GAT GGG** TCC AGC AGG TCA GGG ATC TC-3′ |
| | |
| *HBB* (252 bp) | Competitor:223 bp |
| Primer 1 | 5′-GCA CTG ACT CTC TCT GCC TAT TGG-3′ |
| Primer 2 | 5′-**GAT CCA CGT GCA GCT TGT CAC AG**-3′ |
| Recombinant primer | 5′-**GAT CCA CGT GCA GCT TGT CAC AG**C TTG AGG TTG TCC AGG TGA GC-3′ |
| | |
| *SOD2* (143 bp) | |
| Primer 1 | 5′-CCTCTGCAGTGATACTTCTGGTAGA-3′ |
| Primer 2 | 5′-GAGATTGGGCTCAAGCATAGCTGC-3′ |

[a]Primer 1 and the recombinant primer were used for construction of competitor templates. Primer 1 and 2 were used for PCR amplification of genomic sequences in double-differential PCR, and genomic and competitor sequences in competitive-differential PCR. Bold letters indicate the identical sequences of primer 2 and the recombinant primer. Primers 1 and 2 were developed previously *(9)*.

3. The cloning and plasmid preparation procedures used throughout this chapter are standard techniques, and the materials and equipment required have been described in detail elsewhere *(11)*. The special reagents for clone selection are as follows: 70 mg/ml Kanamycin (Boehringer, Mannheim, Germany), 100 mg/mL Ampicillin (Serva, Heidelberg, Germany), and 40 mg/mL 5-bromo-4-chloro-3-indolyl-β-D-galactoside (X-Gal) solved in dimethylformamide (DMF).
4. JETSPIN plasmid DNA preparation kit (Genomed, Bad Oeynhausen, Germany).
5. 50 U restriction enzyme *Hind*III and10X buffer E (Promega).

### 2.3.2. Competitive-Differential PCR Assay

1. Oligonucleotide stocks for oncogene and reference gene PCR amplification (HBB) (concentrations as indicated by the manufacturer; Eurogentec); the sequences of the required oligonucleotides are given in **Table 1**.
2. Stock solutions of competitors 0.02 and 0.16 attomoles in 1 m*M* Tris-EDTA buffer.

### 2.4. PCR Product Separation and Evaluation

1. 50X TAE buffer: Add 242 g Tris base, 57.1 mL acetic acid, and 100 mL 0.5*M* EDTA (pH 8.0) to 1 L of distilled water.
2. Gel loading dye: 0.25% bromophenol blue (w/v), 40% sucrose.
3. 1 µg/mL ethidium bromide as gel staining solution.

**Table 2**
**Pipeting Protocol of the ddPCR and cdPCR**

| Steps | | Double-Differential PCR | | Competitive-Differential PCR |
|---|---|---|---|---|
| | | oncogene dosage | reference gene dosage | general assay[a] |
| 1 | DNA | 200 ng | 200 ng | 200 ng |
| 2 | Primer pair reference gene *HBB* | 30 pmol each | 30 pmol each | 50 pmol each |
| 3 | Primer pair reference gene *SOD2* | — | 30 pmol each | — |
| 4 | Primer pair oncogene (*egfr* or c-*erbB-2*) | 30 pmol each | — | 50 pmol each |
| 5 | 10X reaction buffer | 5 µL | 5 µL | 5 µL |
| 6 | 25 m*M* Mgcl$_2$ | 3 µL | 3 µL | 3 µL |
| 7 | 100 µ*M* Nucleotide stocks (dATP, dCTP, dGTP, dTTP) | 4 µL | 4 µL | 4 µL |
| 8 | *Taq* polymerase | 0.3 µL | 0.3 µL | 0.3 µL |
| 9 | Competitors for *HBB* and oncogenes | — | — | 0–0.64 amol |
| 10 | Sterile water | to 50 µL | to 50 µL | to 50 µL |
| 11 | DMSO | — | — | 3.5 µL |
| 12 | Mineral oil for molecular biology | 30 µL | 30 µL | 30 µL |

[a]Standard curve preparation for *egfr* and c-*erbB-2* gene dosage quantitation by cdPCR is described in **Table 3**.

## 3. Methods

### 3.1. Isolation of Genomic DNA

The efficiency of quantitative PCR depends mainly on DNA quality. Therefore, only methods that yield high molecular weight DNA (> 5000 bps) should be used for the isolation of DNA from tissue samples.

1. For the isolation of large DNA amounts from leukocytes and cell lines the authors performed Nucleon II DNA Extraction Kit (Scotlab).
2. For isolation of DNA from small tumor tissue samples the QiaAmp Tissue Kit (Qiagen) was applied by the authors.

Both of the methods for DNA isolation used by the authors were performed according to the manufacturer's instructions.

### 3.2. Double-Differential PCR

The pipeting steps for the reaction mixtures and cycling conditions follow a similar protocol for ddPCR and cdPCR according to standard techniques, which have been described elsewhere *(12)*. Therefore, they are presented in tables.

1. PCR was performed in a total volume of 50 µL in 500 µL thin wall tubes on fixed-temperature thermal cyclers.
2. Double-differential PCR reaction mix: refer to **Table 2**.
3. Double-differential PCR reaction conditions: 3 min at 94°C followed by 32 cycles of 94°C for 1 min, 62°C for 1 min and 72°C for 1 min, with a final extension step of 72°C for 7 min.

### 3.3. Competitive-Differential PCR

#### 3.3.1. Construction of Competitor Templates

The competitive sequences (competitors) for *egfr*, c-*erbB-2*, and *HBB* were synthesized by a PCR method using recombinant oligonucleotide primers (**Fig. 1**) *(13)*. The sequences of the primers are shown in **Table 1** indicated as recombinant primers. The length of the genomic DNA sequences and the competitor sequences are also shown in **Table 1**.

The construction procedure comprises a PCR for the synthesis of the templates for the competitors (template synthesis PCR) for ligation into a plasmid (ligation product PCR), ligation and cloning of the template containing plasmid, plasmid preparation, linearization, and competitor dilution.

1. Template synthesis PCR: Add 200 ng leukocyte DNA, 25 pmol primer 1, 25 pmol recombinant primer, 5 μL 10X PCR reaction buffer, 3 μL MgCl$_2$ (25 m$M$), 4 μL stock of nucleotides (100 μ$M$ each nucleotide), 0.3 μL *Taq* polymerase (1.5 U) add to 50 μL with sterile water and overlay with 30 μL mineral oil.
2. PCR reaction conditions: 3 minutes at 94°C followed by 32 cycles of 94°C for 1 min, 62°C for 1 min and 72°C for 1 min, with a final extension step of 72°C for 7 min.
3. Mix five parts of PCR product with one part of gel loading dye.
4. Load 15 μL in lanes of a 4% agarose gel and electrophorese (5 V/cm in 1X TAE buffer) to separate the PCR products, which are shortened by 20–29 bps and contain the recognition sites for primer 1 and 2 (**Table 1**).
5. Gels are stained after electrophoresis by ethidium bromide (1 μg/mL) for 10 min and destained in water for 30 min.
6. The UV illuminated gels are documented using Polaroid 667 film.
7. The bands of the shortened PCR products are excised with a scalpel. The following steps have to be performed on the same day. The TA Cloning Kit uses 3′-A overhangs which are attached by *Taq* DNA polymerase.
8. Ligation product PCR: Add a 1:10$^4$ dilution of the shortened PCR products from step 7, 50 pmol primer 1, 50 pmol primer 2, 5 μL 10X PCR reaction buffer, 3 μL MgCl$_2$ (25 m$M$), 4 μL stock of nucleotides (100 μ$M$ each nucleotide), 0.3 μL *Taq* polymerase (1.5 U) make up to 50 μL with sterile water and overlay with 30 μL mineral oil.
9. PCR reaction conditions: 3 min at 94°C followed by 32 cycles of 94°C for 1 min, 62°C for 1 min, and 72°C for 1 min, with a final extension step of 72°C for 7 min.
10. Dilute PCR product 5:1 with gel loading buffer and separate 10 μL of the PCR reaction mix on an agarose gel, stain and estimate the amount of PCR product.
11. According to the instructions of the TA Cloning Kit (Invitrogen) add 0.5–1.0 μL freshly prepared PCR product, 1 μL ligase buffer, 2 μL plasmid vector pCR™II, 1 μL T4 DNA ligase and make up to 10 μL with sterile water. Incubate overnight at 14°C. This ligation mix is ready to be used directly in the transformation.
12. For *Escherichia coli* transformation, 2 μL of 0.5$M$ β-mecapto-ethanol are added to 50 μl INV αF' cells on ice and gently mixed. The cells are provided in the kit as One Shot competent cells, which can be transformed without pretreatment. Add 2 μL of the ligation mix from **step 11** and incubate for a further 30 min on ice. Heat to 42°C for 30 s (heat shock) to enhance plasma membrane penetrance for plasmid DNA. Put on ice for 2 min. Add 450 μL SOC medium and shake gently at 37°C for 1 h to induce resistance to antibiotics. Take 100 μL and 400 μL from the suspension and mix rapidly with warm YT-top agar containing 50 μg/mL ampicillin and 20 μg/mL X-Gal and mount on YT-agar dishes

also containing 50 µg/ml ampicillin. Incubate the dishes at 37°C for 18 h. Take white clones (insertion of the PCR product in β-galactosidase gene) for plasmid preparation.

13. Small-scale preparation of plasmid DNA can be performed according to the standard method as described in *Molecular Cloning (11)*.

14. For large-scale preparation of plasmid DNA (50–100 µg) the white colonies of *E. coli* INV αF′ are suspended in 2 mL 2YT medium containing 50 µg/mL kanamycin. Incubate overnight with gentle shaking (225 rpm) at 37°C. Mix culture suspension with 2 mL glycerol and freeze in aliquots at –80°C. One 100-µL aliquot of the glycerol containing *E. coli* culture is resuspended in 25 mL 2YT medium containing 50 mg/mL kanamycin. Incubate overnight at 37°C at 225 rpm. Centrifuge the suspension at 10,000$g$ and 4°C for 10 min. Resuspend the *E. coli* INV αF′ pellet in 1.2 mL F1 buffer and add cell lysis F2 buffer as provided in the absorption column system JETSPIN (Genomed). Mix gently and incubate at room temperature for 5 min. Add 1.6 mL F3 buffer gently and centrifuge at 15,000$g$ and room temperature for 10 min. Apply the supernatant to the JETSPIN column and centrifuge at 5000$g$ for 1 min. Add 3 mL F4 buffer on the top of the column and centrifuge at 5000$g$ for 5 min. Discard the outlet of the column. Add 800 µL TE buffer on the top of the column and centrifuge at 5000$g$ for 2 min.

15. To linearize the plasmids by restriction enzyme digest with *Hind*III (Promega) 0.5–1.0 µg plasmid DNA (10 µl of the TE buffer solution of plasmid DNA from **step 14**) are mixed with 1 µL restriction enzyme (10 U), 2 µL 10X reaction buffer, and 7 µL water. Incubate at 37°C for 1 h. Inactivate enzyme at 65°C for 10 min. Control restriction of plasmid DNA by agarose gel electrophoresis.

16. Measure the concentration of competitor DNA in a UV/VIS spectrometer applying the formula of Warburg and Christian *(14)* as follows: $C_{DNA} = 62.9 \times (E_{260} - E_{320}) - 36.0 \times (E_{280} - E_{320})$ (ng/µL)

17. Prepare 0.02 amol/µL and 0.16 amol/µL stock solutions of competitors in TE buffer (pH 8.0) using the molecular weights of the linearized plasmids as follows: pCR II *erbB-1*, 4072 bps, 2,507,705 (g/mol); pCR II *erbB-2*, 4055 bps, 2,497,238 (g/mol); pCR II β-Globin, 4171 bps, 2,568,683 (g/mol).

### 3.3.2. Competitive-Differential PCR

The general assay procedure is described in **Table 2**. The quantitation assay with 6 standard points is performed as described in **Table 3**. PCR conditions are 3 min at 94°C followed by 32 cycles of 94°C for 1 min, 62°C for 1 min, and 72°C for 1 min, with a final extension step of 72°C for 7 min.

### 3.4. PCR Product Separation and Evaluation

(For alternative methods, see **Note 4**.)

1. Mix five parts of PCR product with one part of gel loading dye.
2. Load 15 µL in lanes of a 4% agarose gel and electrophorese to separate the PCR products.
3. Gels are stained after electrophoresis with ethidium bromide (1 µg/mL) for 10 min and destained in water for 30 min.
4. The UV illuminated gels are documented using Polaroid 667 films.
5. Quantitate the PCR products by scanning the photograph on a four-color scanner (Epson GT 6000) and evaluate the results by the Scan Pack program (Biometra, Güttingen, Germany).
6. Calculate the gene dosages from the ddPCR assay following formula:
   AGCN = area of the oncogene band/area of the reference gene band × length of the reference gene PCR product (bps)/length of the oncogene product (bps). The assay is evaluable if the length-corrected band ratio of the two reference genes HBB and SOD2 ranges from 0.7 to 1.3.

**Table 3**
**Standard Curve Preparation for Quantitation of *egfr***
**and *c-erbB-2* Gene Dosage by cdPCR**

| Sample | DNA | Preparation steps as described in **Table 2** | Stock of competitor 0.02 amol/µL | Stock of competitor 0.16 amol/µL |
|---|---|---|---|---|
| 1 | 200 ng | 2, 4–8, 10–12 | 0 µL | 0 µL |
| 2 | 0 ng | 2, 4–8, 10–12 | 0 µL | 1 µL |
| 3 | 200 ng | 2, 4–8, 10–12 | 2 µL | 0 µL |
| 4 | 200 ng | 2, 4–8, 10–12 | 4 µL | 0 µL |
| 5 | 200 ng | 2, 4–8, 10–12 | 0 µL | 1 µL |
| 6 | 200 ng | 2, 4–8, 10–12 | 0 µL | 2 µL |
| 7 | 200 ng | 2, 4–8, 10–12 | 0 µL | 4 µL |

7. Calculate the gene dosages from the cdPCR assay the following formula:

$$AGCN = \frac{Oncogene}{Oncogene\ competitor} \times \frac{Reference\ gene\ competitor}{Reference\ gene}$$

AGCN = average gene copy number; oncogene = area of the oncogene band; oncogene competitor = area of the competitor band; reference gene = area of the reference gene band; reference gene competitor = area of the reference gene competitor.

## 4. Notes

1. High-quality DNA as defined by the ratio of $E(260nm/280nm) = 1.7 – 2.0$ should be used for gene dosage quantitation.
2. DNA from tissues and blood should be isolated with methods giving high-quality DNA.
3. When creating new primers, their $T_m$ must have nearly the same value (difference: up to 1° and the PCR products should not have big differences in length (difference: up to 150 bp) to guarantee equal amplification efficiencies in ddPCR (**Fig. 2**).
4. The amplification efficiencies are highly influenced by the variation of the $MgCl_2$ concentration and the addition of DMSO.
5. Since DNA destruction during isolation cannot be excluded it is important that DNA concentrations under 200 ng per reaction vial should be avoided to guarantee a correct template amount for all target sequences.
6. All primers have to be of equal concentration in the ddPCR. Our investigations showed an optimal concentration of 50 pmol for each primer per reaction vial.
7. Any gene dosage analysis has to include a DNA free sample for the detection of DNA contamination and positive (recommended cell lines: *erbB-1*: MDA-MB-468, A431; *erbB-2*: SKBR3, BT474) as well as normal control DNA samples (lymphocytes).
8. All PCR components for gene dosage analysis of the same oncogene sequence have to be premixed and added to the different DNA samples.
9. Using *Taq* DNA polymerase, either all dPCR components should be added on ice or a hot start PCR should be preferred to prevent unspecific PCR reactions during preparation. This can be avoided by using Ampli*Taq* Gold™ (Perkin Elmer).
10. Using UV-detection of ethidium bromide staining, a "factor of length" (length$_{comparative\ gene\ sequence\ (bp)}$/ length$_{oncogene\ sequence\ (bp)}$) needs to be included in the calculation of gene dosages (*see* **Subheading 3.4.**).
11. The intra-assay coefficient of variation (CV) of the AGCN has to be determined from at least 10 independent normal samples for each ddPCR assay to determine the degree of

Fig. 2. **(A)** Gene dosage estimation by ddPCR. After PCR 30 cycles the amplification products were separated on a 20% polyacrylamide gel at constant voltage. The gel was silver stained and scanned with a four color scanner (Epson GT 6000). The degree of amplification was determined by comparison of band intensity of the oncogene (2 left gel) and the second reference gene PCR product (2 right gel) with the reference gene gel band (1 in both gels) in the ScanPack-Program (Biometra, Göttingen, Germany), respectively. **(B)** Gene dosage estimation by cdPCR. In 32 PCR cycles, competitor plasmids for c-*erbB-2* and *HBB* from 0.04 to 0.64 attomoles were amplified with 200 ng of genomic DNA from leukocytes.

analytical sensitivity which is defined by the formula: $dk = 2 \times 2 \times SD$ (standard deviation). A sample could be considered to carry an amplification having a gene dosage (AGCN) greater equal $1 + dk$.

12. Any gene dosage analysis must be repeated to eliminate runaways.
13. Mineral oil should be not exposed to UV radiation. PCR inhibitors are produced by UV induced chemical reactions in the mineral oil.
14. For constructing competitor plasmids, it is essential to linearize the vectors containing the competitive inserts before using them for cdPCR. Supercoiled DNA is more resistant to denaturation in the first PCR amplification step than linearized DNA; this results in a false competitor/target ratio after amplification. Thus, linearized plasmids are the preferred competitors for chromosomal linear DNA.
15. Accurate determination of the competitor plasmids' DNA concentration is essential for cdPCR. We recommend the use of a high-quality densitometer to determine the optical density at 260 nm wavelength. Exact dilution of the competitor plasmids is of major importance, because even slight differences in the copy number of oncogene competitor and reference gene competitor before amplification would result in large differences in the PCR products, and therefore in inaccurate gene quantification. For this reason, we suggest making an 1:1 mixture of oncogene competitor and reference gene competitor before dilution of the mixture to 0.04 and 0.16 attomoles, respectively. It is reasonable to

create a large stock of these 1 : 1 mixtures of 0.04 and 0.16 attomoles competitors to obtain constancy for a large number of clinical samples.

16. To avoid problems by dilution errors as aforementioned, it would be ideal to clone reference gene competitor and oncogene competitor into one plasmid. By doing so, the oncogene competitor/reference gene competitor ratio equals 1 in any case.

17. Dilution of competitor plasmids should be done in Tris-EDTA buffer, pH 8.0, and dilutions should be stored at –20°C. Competitor dilutions stored according to these recommendations will be stable for several years. cdPCR works well with up to 8 μL TE buffer in the reaction mixture.

18. If you cannot achieve a gene copy number of 1 by cdPCR in DNA from benign tissues or leukocytes, even if dilution of competitors was very accurate, this can be because of secondary structures of the genomic target sequences. Addition of DMSO or formamide in concentrations of 1% to 10% to the PCR reaction may solve this problem.

19. Analyzing DNA from different sources requires an adaptation of competitor concentrations to obtain the 1 : 1 competitor/target ratios, which are optimal for quantitative analysis. In our experience, we needed less competitors (about 0.04 to 0.08 amol) to get the 1 : 1 ratio in DNA from breast cancer tissue in comparison to the DNA from leukocytes where we needed about 0.32 amol. The 1 : 1 ratio was even different for DNA from oral carcinomas and from premalignant lesions of the oral cavity. This might be because of an enhanced DNA degradation in certain tumor tissues which results in a smaller intact gene copy number in comparison to the gene copy number in the same amount of DNA from leukocytes or benign tissues. Thus, it is reasonable to perform a titration experiment with different amounts of competitors (e.g., from 0.04 to 0.64 amol) whenever changing the source of DNA.

20. To exclude quantification errors due to contamination, every cdPCR assay should be accompanied by several controls: 1) one PCR without any template; 2) one PCR without competitors, but with DNA; 3) one PCR without DNA, but with competitors.

21. Staining of agarose gels with ethidium bromide and densitometric analysis of the photograph has to be optimized in every laboratory to avoid differences in staining intensity and nonlinearity of the photographs.

22. The evaluation of the method of double-differential PCR was established on silver stained polyacrylamide gels first. Electrophoresis and silver stain was performed on the automatic system Phast™ (Pharmacia, Freiburg, Germany) using precast 20% polyacrylamide gels (PhastGel™, homogeneous 20, Pharmacia). For details refer to (*4*).

23. The competitive-differential PCR method can be evaluated on a automatic genetic analyzer system (ABI Prism 310, Applied Biosystems, Weiterstadt, Germany) using primers labeled with a fluorescent dye.

## References

1. Wikstrand, C. J., Hale, L. P., Batra, S. K., Hill, M. L., Humphrey, P. A., Kurpad, S. N., et al. (1995) Monoclonal antibodies against EGFRvIII are tumor specific and react with breast and lung carcinomas and malignant gliomas. *Cancer Res.* **55**, 3140–3148.
2. Moscatello, D. K., Holgado-Madruga, M., Godwin, A. K., Ramirez, G., Gunn, G., Zoltick, P. W., et al. (1995) Frequent expression of a mutant epidermal growth factor receptor in multiple human tumors. *Cancer Res.* **55**, 5536–5539.
3. Lin, J. T., Wu, M. S., Shun, C. T., Lee, W. J., Sheu, J. C., and Wang, T. H. (1995) Occurrence of microsatellite instability in gastric carcinoma is associated with enhanced expression of c-erbB-2 oncoprotein. *Cancer Res.* **55**, 1428–1430.
4. Brandt, B., Vogt, U., Schlotter, C. M., Jackisch, C., Werkmeister, R., Thomas, M., et al. (1995) Prognostic relevance of aberrations of the erbB oncogenes in breast, ovarian, oral and lung cancer: double-differential PCR for clinical diagnosis. *Gene* **159**, 35–42.
5. Brandt, B., Beckmann, A., Gebhardt, F., Rötger, A., Jackisch, C., Assmann, G., and Zänker, K. S. (1997) Translational research studies of erbB oncogenes: selection strategies for breast cancer treatment. *Cancer Lett.* **118**, 143–151.

6. Slamon, D. J., Godolphin, W., Jones, L. A., Holt, J. A., Wong, S. G., Keith, D. E., et al. (1989) Studies of the HER-2/*neu* proto-oncogene in human breast and ovarian cancer. *Science* **244,** 707–712.

7. Bast, R. C., Boyer, C. M., Jacobs, I., Xu, F. J., Wu, S., Wiener, J., et al. (1993) Cell growth regulation in epithelial ovarian cancer. *Cancer* **71,** 597–601.

8. Bauknecht, T., Angel, P., Kohler, M., Kommoss, F., Birmelin, G., Pfleiderer, A., and Wagner, E. (1993) Gene structure and expression analysis of the epidermal growth factor receptor, transforming growth factor-alpha, myc, jun, and metallothionein in human ovarian carcinomas. *Cancer* **71,** 419–429.

9. Brandt, B., Vogt, U., Harms, F., Bosse, U., Zänker, K. S., Assmann, G. (1995) Double-differential PCR for gene dosage estimation of erbB oncogenes in benign and cancer tissue, and comparison to cellular DNA content. *Gene* **159,** 29–34.

10. Rötger, A., Brandt, B., and Barnekow, A. (1997) Competitive-differential PCR for gene dosage estimation of *erbB-1* (*egfr*), *erbB-2,* and *erbB-3* oncogenes. *DNA Cell Biol.* **16,** 443–448.

11. (1989) *Molecular Cloning,* 2nd ed. (Sambrock, J., Fritsch, E. F., and Maniatis, T., eds.), Cold Spring Harbor Laboratory Press, Cold Spring Harbor, pp. 1.25–1.31.

12. (1990) *PCR Protocols: A guide to methods and applications* (Inis, M. A., Gelfand, D. H., Sninsky, J. I., and White, T. J., eds.), Academic, New York.

13. Celi, F. S., Zenilman, M. E., Shuldiner, A. R. (1993). A rapid and versatile method to synthesize internal standards for competitive PCR. *Nucleic Acids Res.* **21,** 1047.

14. Warburg, O. and Christian, W. (1941) *Biochem. Z.* **310,** 384.

# 39

## One-Dimensional Genome Scanning—Detection of Genomic Changes in Ovarian Carcinoma

**Anthony Magliocco and Murray Brilliant**

## 1. Introduction

Genomic changes are a frequent underlying event in many malignancies, including ovarian cancers, and are intrinsic to the process of oncogenesis and tumor progression. Identification of recurrent nonrandom changes that affect specific genomic regions may provide prognostic information or lead to the discovery of new cancer related genes in somatic tissues.

One of the more convenient, but powerful, approaches that can be applied to evaluate DNA extracted from cells, blood, or tissue specimens is "one-dimensional genome scanning" (ODGS) method first described by Brilliant et al. *(1)*. This approach utilizes the existence of naturally occurring widespread repetitive genetic elements as markers for comparative analysis of nearly identical genomes (such as a normal tissue and its cancerous counterpart) to detect changes such as amplifications, deletions, and rearrangements in homologous segments of DNA. Evaluation of genomically dispersed, widely distributed repetitive elements as a marker enables rapid evaluation of a significant fraction of the genome for mutations in a single step. The approach is complementary to karyotype and ploidy analysis because it enables genomic assessment at a "finer" genetic scale and the evaluation of hundreds of separate genetic loci in one "snapshot" analysis. One additional, and highly exploitable, feature of this method of analysis is that genomic regions with detected alterations can be directly cloned and evaluated. ODGS was initially used to identify and characterize the pink-eye dilution gene locus in the mouse *(2)*. Later, the assay was successfully adapted to enable the evaluation of the genomes of human ovarian carcinoma specimens *(3)*.

ODGS is a modified Southern blot analysis using a probe to medium copynumber (i.e., 500–2000) repetitive elements. For ODGS, the conventional Southern blot is modified in two important ways. First, the length of the horizontal agarose gel slab should be as long as possible. Second, the quality of the DNA should be high to avoid potential artifacts from mechanical strand breaks. ODGS can successfully be applied to evaluate DNA extracted from tissue culture, organ preparations obtained from experimental animals, and blood and surgical specimens obtained from humans. The key to the success of ODGS is selecting and obtaining an appropriate probe to a suit-

From: *Methods in Molecular Medicine, Vol. 39: Ovarian Cancer: Methods and Protocols*
Edited by: J. M. S. Bartlett © Humana Press, Inc., Totowa, NJ

**Table 1**
**Copy Number of Selected Repetitive Elements Within the Human Genome**

| Element | Copy number per haploid genome | Homology |
|---|---|---|
| ERV-1 | 1 | Mammalian Type C retrovirus |
| HERV-R (ERV3) | 1 | Mammalian Type C retrovirus |
| S71 | 1 | Mammalian Type C retrovirus |
| HERV-E | 50–100 | |
| HERV-H (RTVL-H) | 800–1000 | |
| HERV-K | 50 | Mosaic |
| LINE | 10,000–50,000 | |
| alu | 500,000–900,000 | |

The HERV-H are the most suitable for One Dimensional Genome Scanning due to their intermediate copy number (800–1000 copies per haploid genome), but other elements such as HERV-K may produce acceptable results, but provide a lower resolution evaluation.

able repetitive element. There are several potential candidate repetitive elements occurring within the human genome (**Table 1**). In our studies using ODGS for evaluation of human DNA, we have utilized probes complementary to the endogenous retrovirus like element RTVL-H *(3)*.

Many characteristics of RTVL-H elements increase their value as potential genomic markers. The regulatory sequences in the RTVL-H LTRs may function as promoters for some adjacent human host genes or provide 3' processing signals for others *(4)*. Furthermore, RTVL-H elements may be sites for homologous recombination, a process that could lead to LOH, translocations, or deletions in somatic cancer cells *(5)*. Finally, RTVL-H and other similar elements are potentially transposable, a feature that likely explains their gradual expansion in copy number over evolutionary time, and could be a novel potential mechanism of genomic instability in cancers *(6–9)*.

## 2. Materials

### 2.1. Extraction of DNA

#### 2.1.1. Extraction of DNA from Frozen Tissue

1. Iso-High-pH buffer (0.14$M$ NaCl, 0.01$M$ Tris-HCl (pH 8.4), 1.5 m$M$ MgCl$_2$) with 0.1% NP40.
2. Digestion buffer: Iso-Hi-pH buffer, 2% SDS, and proteinase K (1 mg/mL).
3. 25:24:1 v:v:v phenol:chloroform:isoamyl alcohol.
4. 24:1 v:v chloroform:isoamyl alcohol.
5. Predialysis solution: 5 m$M$ EDTA 2% sodium bicarbonate.
6. Dialysis solution: 20 m$M$ Tris-HCl (pH 7.5), 10 m$M$ EDTA.

#### 2.1.2. Extraction of DNA from Frozen Blood

1. 1X phosphate-buffered saline (PBS) pH 7.4.
2. Extraction buffer (10 m$M$ Tris-HCl (pH 8.0); 0.1$M$ EDTA (pH 8.0); 20 μg/mL pancreatic RNaase; 0.5% SDS).
3. Protienase K solution 20 mg/ml.

4. 7.5*M* ammonium acetate.
5. Tris-EDTA (10 m*M* Tris-HCl, 0.1*M* EDTA pH 8.0).

## 2.2. DNA Digestion and Electrophoresis

1. Restriction endonucleases (we found SstI, StuI, EcoRI, EcoRV, and NdeI to give good results) and appropriate buffers (Life Technologies, Bethesda, MD, or Pharmacia, Uppsala, Sweden).
2. Running buffer 1X TBE buffer (90 m*M* Tris-borate, 1 m*M* EDTA, pH 8.3).
3. Bx Combo DNA running buffer: (0.1*M* EDTA, 60% sucrose, 2% ficoll, 0.04% xylene cyanol (w/v), 0.04% bromphenol blue (w/v).
4. Denaturation treatment 0.6*M* NaCl, 0.4*M* NaOH.
5. Neutralization solution (1.5*M* NaCl and 1.5*M* sodium citrate pH 7.0).
6. Transfer solution 10X SSC (1.5*M* NaCl and 0.15*M* sodium citrate pH 7.0).
7. Wash solution 2X SSC (dilute 10X SSC 1:5 for membrane wetting prior to prehybridization).
8. Prehybridization solution 0.5*M* NaPO$_4$ pH 7.1, 2 m*M* EDTA, 7% SDS, and 0.1% sodium pyrophosphate.
9. Agarose gel electrophoresis with 60 cm gel bed (special order DANKAR, Wilmington, MA).
10. 1X SSC, 0.1% SDS.
11. 0.5X SSC, 0.1% SDS.

## 3. Methods

### 3.1. DNA Extraction

#### 3.1.1. DNA Extraction from Frozen Tissue

Specimens of human cancer tissue and corresponding normal should be flash frozen as close to time of surgery as possible (*see* **Note 2**). Try to trim noncancerous tissues from around the cancer specimen. It is good practice to include a sample of "normal," if available, from adjacent, noninvolved tissue (fallopian tube or uterine wall are sometimes useful). Store the tissue wrapped in foil in a –80°C mechanical freezer until time of DNA extraction. Blood can be frozen in plain 10-cm$^3$ tubes until time of extraction.

1. Thaw, mince with a clean razor blade, and homogenize about 500 mg of frozen tumor tissue in a tight-fitting glass-Teflon homogenizer with 5 mL of ice-cold Iso-High buffer. (Keep this solution cold by immersing the bottom of the tube in a container filled with crushed ice while homogenizing, *see* **Note 3** for instructions regarding preparation of this solution.)
2. Centrifuge at 3000*g* at 4°C for 5 min.
3. Aspirate the supernatant and loose material above the pellet and discard. Homogenize the remaining pellet in 0.8 mL of ice-cold Iso-High at 0°C.
4. Vortex mix the resuspended nuclear pellet, and while still mixing, add an equal volume of ice-cold digestion buffer. The latter solution is a suspension when chilled incubate at 37°C for 2 to 3 h in a water bath.
5. Extract the nucleic acids gently by mixing with phenol: chloroform:isoamyl alcohol followed by extraction with chloroform: isoamyl alcohol. Spin at a low speed (400*g*) for 10 min at room temperature to separate phases and retain the aqueous (top) phase (*see* **Note 4**).
6. Place the aqueous phase *in* a prepared dialysis membrane Spectrapore 2, Spectrum Medical Industries. The membranes are prepared in advance by cutting the tubing into

approximately 20-cm lengths. Boil them for 10 min in 2 L of 5 m$M$ EDTA 2% sodium bicarbonate followed by boiling in 2 L of distilled water for three exchanges at 10 min for each exchange.

7. Dialyze against 3 L of dialysis solution (with three changes, about 1/h of the latter dialyzing solution) at room temperature for several hours.
8. Determine the concentration of the DNA spectrophotometrically using OD 260/280 ratios.
9. Store DNA at 4°C. The samples will remain stable for several months in this condition.

### 3.1.2. Extraction of DNA from Peripheral Blood

1. Thaw a frozen whole blood sample (10–20 mL) in a water bath at room temperature.
2. Transfer a 5-mL blood sample to a 15-mL centrifuge tube and dilute with an equal volume (5 mL) of 1X PBS.
3. Centrifuge the diluted blood at 3500$g$ for 15 min at room temperature and then discard the supernatant.
4. Resuspend the remaining pellet in 15 mL of extraction buffer.
5. Incubate at 37°C for 1 h.
6. Add proteinase K to make a final concentration of 100 µg/mL (75 µL of 20 mg/mL stock solution) and place in a water bath for 3 h at 50°C.
7. Extract DNA two times with phenol: chloroform: isoamyl alcohol followed by one time with chloroform: isoamyl alcohol, centrifuge at low speed (400$g$ for 10 min) each time to separate phases and always collect the aqueous phase.
8. Transfer the pooled aqueous phase to a fresh centrifuge tube and add 0.2 volume of 7.5$M$ ammonium acetate and two volumes of room temperature absolute ethanol.
9. Centrifuge to pellet the DNA at a low speed (1000$g$) for 10 min at room temperature.
10. Wash the DNA precipitate with 70% ethanol and recentrifuge to collect the pellet.
11. Let dry for several minutes.
12. Suspend in Tris-EDTA (pH 8.0) buffer.

### 3.2. Performing ODGS Assay

To perform ODGS, genomic DNA should be completely digested with a restriction endonuclease selected to cut within the unit length repetitive element. In the case of RTVL-H, we have found that several enzymes give acceptable patterns. These include *Stu*I, *Eco*RI, *Sst*I, and *Eco*RV *(3)*. Ideally, the digestion should theoretically cut the DNA at each RTVL-H element containing the site, producing fragments of DNA containing a portion of the RTVL-H element and a portion of flanking unique genomic DNA (of course there will also be a mix of a majority of fragments devoid of the RTVL-H element). *See* **Note 5** for additional details.

In our studies, we have used a selection of probes (a generous gift of Dr. D. Mager, B. C. Cancer Research Center, UBC, Vancouver, B. C., Canada V5Z 1L3) complementary to a variety of subtypes of RTVL-H including: 1) PRVHAII (1000 copies/ haploid genome) complementary to truncated RTVL-H. It contains 800 bp of the RTVL-H element from the 3′ end, adjacent to, but not including the 3′LTR cloned into pUC18; 2) probes to more "intact" RTVL-H elements (100 copies/haploid genome) which include p600 Env and pUC18 ΔC. p600 Env contains a 600 bp *Eco*RI/*Sst*I fragment of the env region cloned into pUC18. pUC18 ΔC contains a 403 bp fragment specific for the "C" pol region cloned into pUC18; 3) sequences complementary to the RTVL-H LTR (pAC160 and p70-1a). pAC160 (500–700 copies/haploid genome) is a 160 bp fragment specific for the type II subpopulation of LTRs, which is cloned into

Fig. 1. Principle of one dimensional genome scanning (ODGS). The top line represents a hypothetical portion of genomic DNA containing multiple repetitive elements indicated by solid boxes. Arrows indicate restriction enzyme locations. Roman numerals indicate result fragments containing portions of the repetitive element. The site of an amplification or deletion mutation is indicated by an open box. The predicted genome scan results are illustrated directly above. Amplification will result in an increased signal intensity of fragment II, whereas deletion will result in its loss. Cloning the wild type fragment or the amplified fragment fragment will enable isolation of non-repetitive unique flanking DNA (gray stretch). A transposition event will result in a new band (not shown). This approach enables direct detection and cloning of large scale deletions. Adapted from Gondo and Brilliant, *Electrophoresis* (1995) Feb; **16(2)**:174–178

the *Hinc*II site of pT7T3 18u. P70-1a (100 copies/haploid genome) is a 70 bp fragment specific for the type 1a subpopulation of LTRs. It is cloned into the *Hinc*II site of pUC. *See* **Fig. 1** for details regarding origin of probes.

1. Digest 5 μg of the genomic DNA from each sample overnight (to assure complete digestion) with 10 U of restriction endonuclease (try using either *Sst*I, *Stu*I, *Eco*RI, or *Nde*I from Life Tech or Pharmacia. *See* **Notes 5** and **6**).
2. Pour a 0.8% agarose gel (Seakem GTG) in 1X TBE buffer (for the custom gel bed, we used this required 700 mL total volume).
3. Mix samples with Bx Combo DNA running buffer and load gel with 5 μg of DNA.
4. Run gel for 4000 V h. If ethidium bromide is used in the running solution the gel can be examined under UV light to determine evenness of loading. This will be useful when assessing the hybridization results. Ethidium bromide staining can be performed after the run. Ethidium bromide is a potent carcinogen, so ensure safe handing and disposal (*see* **Notes 6** and **7**).
5. Following the run wash the gel twice with 3 L of wash buffer for 20 min with gentle agitation.
6. Neutralize gel by washing twice with 3 L 1.5*M* NaCl and 1.5*M* Na Citrate (pH 7.0).
7. The DNA was transferred to a nylon membrane (Hybond Plus, Amersham, Arlington Hts., IL) via capillary transfer with 10X SSC.

8. Following transfer, wash the membrane in 2X SSC solution for about 2 min to remove the gel adhered to the membrane and then bake in a vacuum oven at 80°C about 2 h.

9. Place the membrane in a plastic "seal-a-meal bag."

10. Prehybridize the dried membrane at 65°C with prehybridization solution for 4 to 8 h with gentle agitation **Do not allow the bag to cool** or the NaPO4 will crystalize and ruin the membrane at this point (*see* **Note 9**).

11. The cDNA used as a template for probe synthesis was purified by using DEAE-81 chromatography paper and labeled with $^{32}$PdCTP by using T7 polymerase and random primers (Oligolabelling Kits from Stratagene or Pharmacia).

12. $^{32}$PdCTP incorporated probes were isolated using a Chroma Spin 10 column (Clontech, Palo Alto, CA).

13. Determine the specific activity of the probe by counting activity of 1 µL of probe in a 1-µL capillary glass tube in a scintillation vial, without buffer (remember to boil probe prior to adding to hybridization solution).

14. Hybridize the membrane overnight at 65°C with agitation with $2–4 \times 10^6$ cpm per mL of the probe in prehybridization buffer.

15. Wash the membrane was in 1200 mL of 2X SSC for 20 min at 65°C, 3 washes of 1X SSC, 0.1% SDS for 20 min each, and 3 washes of 1200 mL 0.5X SSC, 0.1% SDS for 20 min each at 65°C, you can monitor the membrane with a hand-held geiger counter to avoid overwashing and loosing signal (*see* **Note 10**).

16. Place the membrane on a stiff card and wrap in cellophane wrap (to avoid drying).

17. Incubate at –70°C with Kodak XR film and an intensifying screen for 1–3 d.

## 4. Notes

1. The most demanding aspect of performing ODGS is the large physical size of the gels to be manipulated and processed without breaking them. The gel apparatus was custom built to our specification by DANKAR, Wilmington, MA. We also had to build the tanks for processing we used glued Lucite plastic plates to build "aquariums" that could easily accommodate the gel and the 3 L of fluid required for treatment. In our laboratory, it was necessary to custom build some equipment to enable appropriate processing. We also had a mechanical rotating platform built on a mobile cabinet to enable gentle agitation of the gels.

2. When selecting specimens for analysis care should be taken to harvest the material as quickly as possible from the time of surgery and to trim it to maximize the sampling of the malignant tissue. A sample of normal germline DNA should also be collected to enable the comparison of the complex banding patterns to identify differences. Samples such as uterine wall or fallopian tube (if uninvolved by cancer) function well. Peripheral blood also serves as an excellent sample. Fatty tissues tend to give lower yields of DNA and should be avoided if possible.

3. Make the proteinase K fresh on the day of the extraction. The iso-High Buffer is stable for extended periods in the refrigerator wrapped in aluminum foil to avoid light exposure.

4. During chloroform-phenol extractions, the DNA tends to be highly viscous and stringy, making isolation from the organic phase and interphase proteins difficult. We have found that use of a 5-mL disposable glass pipet (to avoid risk of dissolving in solvents use glass instead of plastic) with a wide mouth attached vertically to a ring stand with clamps and fitted with vacuum tubing and finally attached to a hand-operated bulb can provide the gentle suction necessary to remove the viscous aqueous layer without pulling up the interphase proteins. Care must be taken to appropriately dispose of the organic phase.

5. We do the overnight restriction enzyme digests in an incubator rather than a water bath to avoid evaporation and condensation of liquid on the inner surface of the lid of the microcentrifuge tubes.

Fig. 2. Example of ODGS. Example of conventional one dimensional genome scan on DNA from 4 breast cancers $T_{1-4}$ compared to DNA isolated from peripheral leukocytes in the same patients $N_{1-4}$ using a probe complementary to a portion of the RTVL-H element. The second panel on the right shows more detail from the 1.4–2.5 Kb region. Clear evidence of genomic DNA amplification (+) affecting a 1.9 Kb fragment containing part of the RTVL-H sequence is observed in two different breast cancers from unrelated individuals (efforts are underway to clone and characterize any unique host (non-repetitive) DNA on these amplified segments. Deletions are also observed. (–).

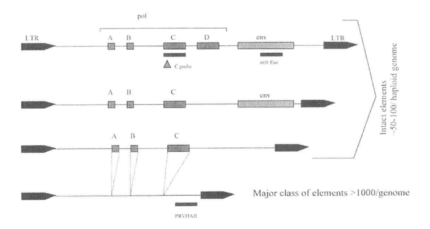

Fig. 3. Schematic representation of subclasses of RTVL-H elements and available probes (C-probe, 600 env, PRVHAII) from work of Mager et al. (personal communication). For details *see* **Subheading 3.2.**

6. Load the gel with the lanes to be directly compared adjacent to each other.
7. We usually try to photograph an ethidium bromide stained gel following electrophoresis to ensure that loading is even. This is important when interpreting the final ODGS results as unevenly loaded comparison lanes complicate analysis.
8. To obtain sufficient counts two separate standard labeling reactions are prepared and pooled. We find that best results are obtained by using as fresh radiolabel as possible and typically plan the hybridization reaction around the expected delivery of the isotope.
9. The hybridization solution has a tendency to crystallize at room temperature. The crystals can be forced back into solution be heating the bottle in a water bath. Do not allow the membrane when in hybridization solution to cool or it will ruin the membrane. This means that the step of adding probe to the bag must be accomplished relatively rapidly. We make a small cut in one corner of the seal a meal bag and inject the probe rapidly resealing the corner, agitating, and placing the bag back into the shaking water bath.
10. We wash the membrane in Pyrex cooking dishes and prepare all of the wash solutions in advance in 1200-mL containers, and place them in a water bath at the appropriate temperature to ensure equilibration by the time they are needed.
11. For a sample genome scan autoradiogram, *see* **Fig. 2**. The general concept of ODGS is illustrated in **Fig. 3**.

## References

1. Brilliant, M. H., Gondo, Y., and Eicher, E. M. (1991) Direct molecular identification of the mouse pink eyed unstable mutation by genome scanning. *Science* **252**, 566–569.
2. Brilliant, M. H., Gondo, Y., and Magliocco, A. (1995) One-dimensional genome scanning: identification of the basis of a mouse mutation and identification of genomic changes in ovarian carcinoma. *Electrophoresis* **16**, 163–167.
3. Magliocco, A. M. and Brilliant, M. H. (1994) Genome scanning detects genetic alterations in human ovarian carcinoma. *Hum. Mutat* **4**, 141–149.
4. Mager, D. L. (1989) Polyadenylation function and sequence variability of the long terminal repeats of the human endogenous retrovirus-like family RTVL-H. *Virology* **173**, 591–599.
5. Mager, D. L. and Goodchild, N. L. (1989) Homologous recombination between the LTRs of a human retrovirus-like element causes a 5-kb deletion in two siblings. *Am. J. Hum. Genet.* **45**, 848–854.
6. Kazmierczak, B., Pohnke, Y., and Bullerdiek, J. (1996) Fusion transcripts between the HMGIC gene and RTVL-H-related sequences in mesenchymal tumors without cytogenetic aberrations. *Genomics* **38**, 223–226.
7. Dahlberg, J. E. (1988) An overview of retrovirus replication and classification. *Adv. Vet. Sci. Comp. Med.* **32**, 1–35.
8. Asch, B. B., Asch, H. L., Stoler, D. L., and Anderson, G. R. (1993) De-regulation of endogenous retrotransposons in mouse mammary carcinomas of diverse etiologies. *Int. J. Cancer* **54**, 813–819.
9. Bratthauer, G. L., Cardiff, R. D., and Fanning, T. G. (1994) Expression of LINE-1 retrotransposons in human breast cancer. *Cancer* **73**, 2333–2336.

# 40

# Mapping of Tumor Suppressor Genes in Ovarian Cancers

## Ian G. Campbell and Emma J. Bryan

## 1. Introduction
### 1.1. Positional Cloning of Tumor Suppressor Genes (TSGs)
#### 1.1.1. Linkage Analysis

Although cancer is fundamentally a genetic disease, in the majority of cancers the mutations occur somatically (i.e., only in the tissue from which the cancer is derived). However, for many types of cancer, for example, breast, ovarian, and colorectal cancer there are a small number of cases that arise because of an inherited germline mutation. Genetic linkage analysis of such families enables the likely location of the TSG to be determined and has proven very successful in cloning some important TSGs. However, the genes responsible for inherited predisposition to cancer represent only a fraction of the total number of genetic defects that underlie the disease process.

#### 1.1.2. Loss of Heterozygosity Analysis

A more general approach to the mapping of TSGs is based on the fact that inhibition of tumor development will only be abolished if both copies of a TSG are inactivated (1). Frequently, one copy of a TSG will be inactivated by deletion of all or part of the chromosome, which is easily detectable by loss of heterozygosity (LOH) analysis using PCR amplifiable polymorphic markers (microsatellites), as illustrated in **Fig. 1**. In tumors, deletion of all or part of a chromosome will be evidenced by the absence of one of the alleles or LOH. By analyzing a large number of matched tumor and normal DNA pairs with a large number of DNA markers, the location of candidate TSGs may be determined. Once a candidate region has been refined to less than about 1000 kb, the actual TSG still needs to be identified from among the 10–30 genes which may reside in the interval.

The purpose of this chapter is to describe the use of LOH analysis for the mapping of TSGs. The technical requirements for LOH analysis are relatively straight forward and therefore this chapter will concentrate on the broader tactical considerations that will assist in assessing the feasibility and the execution of an LOH mapping program.

From: *Methods in Molecular Medicine, Vol. 39: Ovarian Cancer: Methods and Protocols*
Edited by: J. M. S. Bartlett © Humana Press, Inc., Totowa, NJ

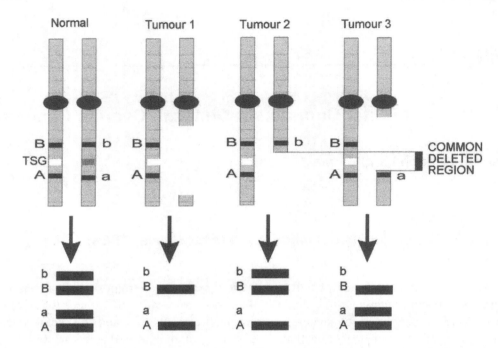

Fig. 1. The use of PCR amplifiable microsatellite markers for the identification of regions of deletions in tumors. A TSG is shown located between the markers A and B. The upper- and lower-case letters for A and B indicate different-sized alleles. PCR amplification of these alleles produces products of different sizes as indicated at the bottom of the figure. In the normal case, both alleles are present for each marker. In the tumor samples, one allele is missing in the tumor DNA indicating a DNA deletion event. Combining the data from the three tumors allows a common region of deletion to be defined.

## 2. Materials

### 2.1. DNA Extraction Buffers and Reagents

1. Sucrose/Triton lysis buffer: $0.319M$ sucrose, 5 m$M$ MgCl$_2$, 1% Triton X100 b (v/v), pH 7.5.
2. SDS lysis buffer: 75 m$M$ NaCl, 25 m$M$ EDTA, 1% SDS (v/v), pH 8.0.
3. Tween lysis buffer: 50 m$M$ Tris, 1 m$M$ EDTA, 0.5% Tween-20 (v/v), pH 8.3.
4. TE buffer: 10 m$M$ Tris-base, 1 m$M$ EDTA, pH 8.0.

### 2.2. Electrophoresis Buffers

1. TAE buffer (x50): $0.4M$ Tris-base, 5.71% glacial acetic acid (v/v), $0.06M$ EDTA, pH 7.6.
2. TBE buffer (x5): $0.44M$ Tris-base, $0.44M$ boric acid, 20 m$M$ EDTA, pH 8.0.
3. Electrophoresis loading buffer: 30% glycerol (v/v), 0.25% Xylene cyanol (w/v).

### 2.3. Microsatellite Analysis

Accurately mapped, PCR amplifiable, highly polymorphic microsatellite markers (*see* **Note 1**).

## 3. Methods

### *3.1. Preparation of Normal DNA from Blood (see Note 2)*

#### 3.1.1. Preparation of a Nuclear Pellet

1. The blood (10–20 mL) is stored in EDTA to prevent clotting. This can stored at 4°C for several days before proceeding with the extraction as follows.
2. The blood is centrifuged in a 30-mL Oak Ridge tube at 5000*g* for 10 min at 4°C (Hermle centrifuge Z382K, Germany). The serum is removed with a disposable Pasteur pipet and to the remaining volume is added an equal volume of ice-cold 2X sucrose/triton lysis buffer. The contents are mixed by inverting the tube several times and incubating for 10 min on ice to lyse the cell membranes of the RBC and WBC.
3. Centrifuge at 5000*g* at 4°C for 10 min to pellet the intact nuclei and remove the supernatant using a Pasteur pipet leaving a tight pellet at the bottom of the tube.
4. The pellet is resuspended in 5 mL of 1X sucrose/triton lysis buffer and centrifuged again at 5000*g* for 5 min.
5. Remove as much of the supernatant as possible. At this point, the pellet can be frozen at –20°C or processed immediately as described in **Subheading 3.1.2.**

#### 3.1.2. SDS/Proteinase-K DNA Extraction

1. The nuclear pellet is resuspended in 5 mL of SDS lysis buffer by drawing the pellet up and down several times into a 10-mL pipet.
2. Fifty µL of a 40 mg/mL solution of proteinase K is added and the mixture incubated overnight at 55°C.
3. 1.65 mL of prewarmed saturated NaCl solution is then added, followed by 7 mL of chloroform and mixed on a blood rotator for 1 h.
4. The phases are separated by centrifugation for 10 min at 5000*g* and the aqueous phase transferred to a new 30-mL Oak Ridge tube using a disposable Pasteur pipet.
5. The removal of the aqueous layer is done slowly to prevent the debris at the interface being drawn up as well.
6. DNA is precipitated by the addition of an equal volume of 2-propanol and recovered by centrifugation at 5000*g* for 20 min.
7. The supernatant is removed and the pellet washed in 5 mL of 75% ethanol. Following a final 5-min centrifugation at 5000*g*, the ethanol is removed and the pellet resuspended in 500 µL of TE buffer.
8. The DNA solution is then transferred to a 1.5-mL Eppendorf tube. An aliquot of the stock is then quantitated by measuring the absorbance at 260 nm. For PCR, a working solution at 50 ng/µL is prepared in 1X TE buffer and both the stock and working solution are stored at 4°C (*see* **Note 3**).

### *3.2. Preparation of Tumor DNA (see Note 4)*

#### 3.2.1. Preparation of DNA from Fresh Frozen Biopsies

1. About 200–1000 mg of fresh frozen tumor tissue (*see* **Note 5**) is finely mashed into powder using a Mikro-dismembrator (B.Braun Biotech International, Germany).
2. DNA is extracted using the SDS/proteinase-K DNA extraction protocol described above except that the tissue is lysed in 10 mL of lysis buffer and all subsequent volumes doubled.

### 3.2.2. Preparation of Normal and Tumor DNA
### from Microdissected Fresh and Archival Tissue

Microdissection is essential for cases where the tumor represents less than 50% of the tumor biopsy and can be performed on fresh or archival tissue. The choice of protocol will depend on local circumstances but many protocols are based on the method described by Pan et al. *(2)* (*see* **Note 6**).

## 3.3. Polymerase Chain Reaction (PCR)

1. The following reagents are added to a 0.5-mL microcentrifuge tube with a mineral oil overlay (*see* **Note 7**): 1 μL of template DNA; 0.5 μL of a nucleotide mix containing dGTP, dATP, and dTTP each at a concentration of 4 m$M$ and dCTP at a concentration of 0.4 m$M$ (*see* **Note 8**), 1 μL of a 10X reaction buffer with 1.5 m$M$ $MgCl_2$ (use the *Taq* DNA polymerase manufacturers recommended buffers), 1 μL of a primer mix containing 50 ng of each primer, 0.05 U of *Taq* DNA polymerase (any supplier), 0.5 μCi [α-$^{32}$P] dCTP at 3000 Ci/mmol (Amersham Life Sciences Ltd., UK, *see* **Note 9**), ultrapure water to give a final volume of 10 μL.
2. PCR is performed on a thermocycler with at least a 50 tube capacity (MJ Research Inc., USA or equivalent). The thermocycling conditions will depend on the properties of the particular microsatellite primer. In general, 30–35 cycles are sufficient when using DNA from fresh tissue but this may need to be increased to up to 40 cycles when using DNA from paraffin-embedded archival tissue.
3. After PCR cycling, add 2.5 μL of 5X loading dye and check the products on a 1.5% agarose gel. If the appropriate-sized product is visible (even if it is only just discernable) then proceed with polyacrylamide gel electrophoresis.

## 3.4. Contamination Control

Because of the sensitivity of PCR, extreme caution has to be taken to prevent contamination of reagents with extraneous DNA. This is not usually a problem when the DNA is from blood or from large portions of fresh tissue, but is problematical when using DNA from archival tissue which is present at very low concentrations and can easily be overwhelmed by minute levels of DNA contamination. To enable the PCR to be executed in a manner in which the risk of contamination is minimized, the following rules should be strictly applied;

1. Wear gloves during all stages of the PCR setup.
2. Dispense all reagents into small volumes using micropipets, which contain filters (e.g., Aerosol Resistant Tips, Promega, UK).
3. Include negative control tubes in every experiment to monitor the integrity of the PCR.

The generation of any products in these controls would be an indication of the presence of contaminants. In the event of contamination, all relevant batches of reagents should be discarded and the amplification repeated.

## 3.5. Polyacrylamide Gel Electrophoresis (PAGE)

Nondenaturing PAGE (*see* **Note 10**) is performed in 0.4 mm 20 × 45 cm or 40 × 43-cm sequencing rigs (S2 sequencing gel system, BRL Life Technologies, UK or equivalent) using shark tooth combs. Most microsatellite markers generate products in the range of 100–200 basepairs and resolution of these sizes are adequate in 8% polyacrylamide gels prepared from a 30% polyacrylamide-*bis*-acrylamide (29:1) stock solution (Anachem, UK or any equivalent supplier) and run in 1X TBE. If the DNA products are larger than 250 basepairs, then 6% polyacrylamide gels should be used.

### 3.5.1. Electrophoresis Running Conditions

Load 2 µL of the PCR products containing tracking dye onto the gel. Load the matching normal DNA adjacent to the tumor DNA. Electrophoresis is carried out at 300 V for approximately 18 h. The exact length of the run will depend on the size of the PCR products and can be monitored by observing the migration of the xylene cyanol marker dye, which will comigrate with double stranded DNA fragments of 160 bp in an 8% PAG.

### 3.5.2. Gel Drying and Autoradiography

1. After electrophoresis, the plates are dismantled and the gel transferred onto Whatman 3MM filter paper, then covered with plastic wrap (Saran Film, UK), and dried on a gel dryer (AE-3750, Genetic Research Instrumentation Ltd., England) at 80°C for about 30 min.
2. The gels are loaded into autoradiography cassettes with intensifying screens (Amersham Life Sciences) and exposed to X-ray film (Kodak X-AR or equivalent) at room temperature or at −80°C from a few hours to a few days. Film exposed at −80°C is about four times faster than room temperature, but the images will have a poorer resolution.

### 3.6. Interpretation of Autoradiographs

LOH is indicated by the loss of one of the alleles in the tumor bands compared with the matching normal track. **Figure 2** shows a typical autoradiograph and demonstrates the three possible results. First, the normal may be homozygous (as in the case of tumors 1 and 4) in which there will only be one band (plus a heteroduplex above) (*see* **Note 11**) in which case LOH cannot be assessed in the tumor and is usually described as not informative (NI). Second, the normal may be heterozygous (case 2, 3, and 5) in which case 2 bands will be discernable (plus 2 heteroduplex bands). If the matching tumor track also shows 2 bands (case 3), then this is referred to as informative with no loss of heterozygosity, or simply heterozygous (Het). If the tumor track has lost one of the alleles (cases 2 and 5) then this is referred to as informative with loss of heterozygosity or simply LOH. It should be noted that in virtually all cases, the smaller allele will appear darker than the larger allele which is presumably owing to amplification bias toward the smaller product. This is not a problem if the tumor DNA is essentially free of normal DNA contamination as LOH will be clearly identifiable as complete loss of one allele. However, with increasing levels of normal DNA contamination, the interpretation becomes more difficult. In these circumstances, it is important to remember that it is the relative intensities of the alleles and not the absolute intensities that are important. In case 5 for example, allele b is still visible in the tumor track, but is greatly diminished compared to allele b in the matching normal track. Similarly, allele c in the tumor track is greatly enhanced compared with allele c in the matching normal track. This pattern is indicative of LOH albeit with approximately 20% normal contamination (*see* **Note 12**). Clearly, as the level of contamination increases the reliability of LOH detection will be decreased.

Fig. 2. Representative autoradiograph of an LOH analysis using microsatellite marker run on a nondenaturing polyacrylamide gel. Matched normal (N) and tumor (T) DNA analyzed with a chromosome 22q microsatellite marker. 2 μL of $^{32}$P-dCTP-labeled PCR product was loaded onto an 8% polyacrylamide gel with 1X TBE running buffer and electrophoresis carried out at 300 V for 18 h. The gel was dried and exposed to X-ray film for 24 h at room temperature. Three different-sized alleles **a**, **b**, and **c** (bold) are indicated by the bold arrows. The matching "shadow" band for alleles a, b, and c (outline pen) are indicated by the outline pen arrows. The interpretation of autoradiograph for each tumor is indicated at the bottom of the figure. Cases 1 and 5 are homozygous for alleles b and c, respectively. Cases 2 and 4 are informative as in the normal track two alleles (b and c) are detected. In both cases, LOH is observed in the tumor tracks. Case 2 shows loss of allele c and case 5 shows loss of allele b. Note that in case 5, allele b is still visible, but is greatly diminished in intensity compared to allele b in the matching normal track. Correspondingly, allele c in the tumor track is darker than allele c in the matching normal track. Case 3 is heterozygous for alleles a and b and the tumor remains heterozygous.

### 3.7. Strategic Considerations

#### 3.7.1. The Number and Histological Subtype of the Tumors

A critical requirement for an LOH study is the availability of sufficient numbers of tumors because the mapping of a TSG loci is dependent on the finding of rare tumors, which have lost only part of the chromosome under investigation. Although it is difficult to assign a value to the number of tumors required, anything less than about 50 is unlikely to identify a candidate TSG loci with any accuracy. Because advanced ovarian cancers generally harbor large chromosomal alterations, some attempt should be made to maximize the number of early stage and/or low grade tumors.

It is likely that the different histological subtypes of ovarian cancer may arise by different mechanisms and therefore involve the inactivation of distinct TSGs. Analysis of all ovarian cancers as a single disease may result in an underestimation of the relevance of LOH at a particular loci. In addition, if 2 TSGs with different histological subtype involvement reside on the same chromosome arm combining the LOH data may result in a completely spurious assignment of a TSG locus.

#### 3.7.2. Polymorphic PCR Amplifiable Microsatellite Markers

With the advent of PCR and the discovery of highly polymorphic di-, tri- and tetranucleotide repeat sequences at frequent intervals in the genome, the assessment of

LOH has been revolutionized. The number of accurately mapped microsatellite markers is increasing steadily and hundreds are available for each chromosome arm. The primer sequences for amplification of these polymorphisms, as well as information on the product size and estimated heterozygosity, are available from a number of genome databases accessible on the world wide web. A good starting point is the National Human Genome Research Institute at the National Institutes of Health, USA (http://www.nhgri.nih.gov/) which provides links to genome and genetic data worldwide.

Several factors need to be considered when selecting the microsatellite markers that depend on the scale of the analysis to be undertaken. If a pan genomic "allelotype" is to be undertaken, then initially a few evenly spaced markers per chromosome should be selected. Choose markers that are informative (i.e., heterozygous) in at least 75% of cases as this will provide the most data for the least effort. If a limited analysis is to be undertaken on a chromosome arm or a smaller chromosomal segment, then a layered analysis is probably the most efficient approach as illustrated in **Fig. 3**. The first step is to analyze the region with a few highly informative widely spaced markers in order to identify the few tumors showing LOH on only part of the region. In most cases, the ovarian cancers will either show no LOH (tumor 1 in **Fig. 3**) with any marker or show LOH with all informative markers across the region (tumor 2 in **Fig. 3**). Initially, these cases can be set aside and further analysis restricted to the relatively few cases showing LOH with only some markers (tumor 3 in **Fig. 3**). In **Fig. 3**, an interstitial deletion is present in the interval flanked by markers A and B. On the second screen, the region is refined between microsatellite markers F and G, and on the third screen between markers J and G. The only limitation to this process is the availability of suitable markers in the breakpoint regions. Initially, the choice of markers will be based both on the location of the marker and on a high-estimated heterozygosity, but as the candidate region is refined, the choice of markers will be limited and may require the use of markers with a low chance of being informative.

Once the data for the tumors showing LOH in only part of the region has been completed and a candidate region(s) has been identified, this information can be used to reassess the tumors which were heterozygous or showed LOH across the region in the first screen. The reasoning behind this is that the tumors that appeared heterozygous may harbor very small deletions which can now be detected as the candidate region has been partially defined. The tumors with apparent LOH across the entire region may harbor homozygous deletions (i.e., they may have lost both copies of the gene) which would be detected by apparent retention of heterozygosity in the candidate region *(14)*.

## 4. Notes

1. Links for information on available microsatellite markers are listed on the National Human Genome Research Institute World Wide Web site (http://nhgri.nih.gov/).
2. The source of the normal DNA is not critical and may be taken from normal ovarian tissue, but it is usually convenient to obtain this from blood lymphocytes. In general, 10 mL of blood will provide sufficient DNA for thousands of PCR assays.
3. The DNA can be safely stored at 4°C for years. Freezing of a part of the stock may be useful for very long-term storage, but repeated freeze thawing will cause shearing of the DNA which may reduce the usefulness of the DNA for procedures such as Southern blotting.

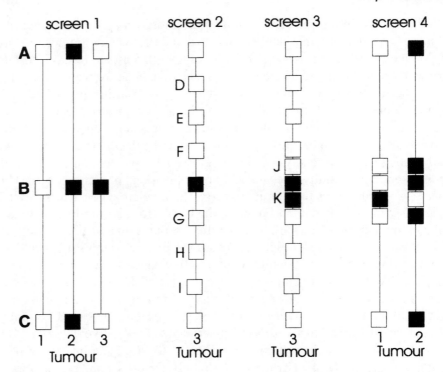

Fig. 3. LOH analysis screening strategy. **Screen 1:** LOH analysis is performed with only a small number of evenly spaced microsatellite markers (A, B, and C) in order to identify the few tumors with partial LOH. Tumor 1 shows no LOH with any marker indicating that it either harbors no areas of LOH or they are small. Tumor 2 shows LOH with all markers suggesting that it has lost the entire chromosome. In rare cases, these tumors may harbor a second deletion in the retained chromosome (termed a homozygous deletion). Tumor 3 shows LOH only with marker B indicating the presence of an interstitial deletion between markers A and C. **Screen 2:** Only tumor 3 is analyzed with additional markers within the breakpoint region which refines the deletion to the interval between markers F and G. **Screen 3:** Additional markers refine the candidate TSG locus to between markers G and J. **Screen 4:** Tumors 1 and 2 are now screened using only the markers within the candidate TSG locus. Tumor 1 shows LOH with marker K only refining the candidate region to the interval between markers B and G. Tumor 2 shows "apparent LOH" *(6)* with marker K suggestive of a homozygous deletion, which is consistent with the presence of a TSG between markers B and K.

4. Fresh snap-frozen tumors are the best source of good quality DNA and priority should be given to obtaining as many of these as possible. However, DNA can be extracted from archival paraffin-embedded tumors, which has the advantage of providing access to a larger cohort of tumors from which specific histological subtype and grade and stage tumors can be selected. The major disadvantage is that the quantity of DNA is small and the quality of DNA is poor and in a proportion of the cases the data obtained may be difficult or impossible to interpret.

5. The detection of LOH is highly dependent on the exclusion of contaminating normal DNA that is derived from the normal stroma that is invariably present within the tumor biopsy. Ideally, the DNA should have less than 5% contamination with normal DNA, but provided the extent of normal DNA contamination can be estimated, interpretation of LOH analysis may still be possible with 50% contamination. To minimize stromal contamina-

tion, frozen sections are taken from representative parts of each tumor and stained with haematoxylin and eosin. Only those sections containing the highest percentage of tumor should be used for DNA extraction. The amount of tumor tissue required depends entirely on the number of analyses to be undertaken. As a guide, a pea-sized portion of tumor will provide sufficient DNA for several thousand PCR reactions.

6. Microdissection is essential for cases where the tumor represents less than 50% of the tumor biopsy. Microdissection from fresh tissue produces DNA of high quality, but it is important to extract DNA from as many cells as possible to reduce the possibility of introducing amplification bias of the microsatellite alleles which can simulate LOH. Many microdissection protocols *(3–5)* are based on that described by Pan et al. *(2)*.

7. Only 2–3 µL of the PCR product is used for electrophoresis, therefore a 10-µL volume PCR is more than adequate and reduces the expense, as well as the radiation hazard as less reagents are required. Depending on circumstances, a microtiter plate format may be used.

8. Using a low concentration of dCTP dramatically increases the activity of the PCR product as this reduces the competition with $[\alpha\text{-}^{32}P]$ dCTP. The low dCTP concentration may reduce slightly the product yield, but this will be overwhelmingly compensated by the increase in specific activity.

9. It is possible to perform the LOH analysis without radio labeling by running the PCR products on 1-mm thick 20 cm × 20 cm polyacrylamide gels and staining with ethidium bromide or equivalent. However, in our experience the sensitivity of other detection methods do not match that of radioisotope labeling. To reduce the radiation hazard $^{33}$phospate labeled dCTP can be substituted.

10. Analysis can be performed on denaturing or nondenaturing polyacrylamide gels and there are advantages and disadvantages with each system. When run on a nondenaturing gel, a heterozygous pattern will appear as four bands rather than two bands. The homoduplex products will always run faster than the heteroduplexes, but the separation will vary from marker to marker. Denaturing polyacrylamide gels should eliminate heteroduplexes, but because the products all run as single strands the total number of bands will be double, which may complicate the analysis. In some circumstances, denaturing polyacrylamide gels may be advantageous and this can only be assessed by comparing the two methods with each marker.

11. It is advisable to load all the samples analyzed with the same marker together rather than loading a single normal and tumor pair analyzed with a number of markers. Running all cases analyzed with the same marker together will assist in interpreting which are the homoduplexes bands and which are heteroduplex bands.

12. The relative intensities of the allele can be quantitated using any of the densitometry systems available commercially. However, our rule of thumb has been that if LOH is not discernable by eye then it is either not LOH or there is overwhelming normal DNA contamination so that it is better to be conservative and record the result as heterozygous. One of the advantages of using radioactively labeled PCR products is that different exposures can be made of the gel which can assist in determining the relative allele intensities.

## References

1. Knudson, A. G. (1993) Anti-oncogenes and human cancer. *Proc. Natl. Acad. Sci. USA* **90,** 10,914–10,921.
2. Pan, L. X., Diss, T. C., Peng, H. Z., and Isaacson, P. G. (1994) Clonality analysis of defined B-cell populations in archival tissue sections using microdissection and the polymerase chain reaction. *Histopathology* **24,** 323–327.
3. Jiang, X., Hitchcock, A., Bryan, E. J., Watson, R. H., Englefield, P., Thomas, E. J., and Campbell, I. G. (1996) Microsatellite analysis of endometriosis reveals loss of heterozygosity at candidate ovarian TSG loci. *Cancer Res.* **56,** 3534–3539.

4. Watson, R. H., Roy, W. J., Jr., Davis, M., Hitchcock, A., and Campbell, I. G. (1997) Loss of heterozygosity at the -inhibin locus on chromosome 2q is not a feature of human granulosa cell tumors. *Gynecol. Oncol.* **65,** 387–390.
5. Roy, W. J., Jr., Watson, R. H., Hitchcock, A., and Campbell, I. G. (1997) Frequent loss of heterozygosity on chromosomes 7 and 9 in benign epithelial ovarian tumors. *Oncogene* **15,** 2031–2035.
6. Larson, A. A., Kern, S., Curtiss, S., Gordon, R., Cavenee, W. K., and Hampton, G. M. (1997) High resolution analysis of chromosome 3p alterations in cervical carcinoma. *Cancer Res.* **57,** 4082–4090.

# 41

## Detection of the Replication Error Phenotype in Ovarian Cancer—PCR Analysis of Microsatellite Instability

**Gillian L. Hirst and Robert Brown**

## 1. Introduction

Microsatellites are simple, tandemly repeated DNA sequences that are abundantly distributed throughout the human genome, and because of their polymorphic nature have been widely utilized as genetic markers *(1)*. They consist of a repeating unit of 1 to 5 basepairs, averaging 25 to 60 bases in length, and are commonly found in the form $d(CA)n : d(GT)n$ *(2)*. It has been estimated that there are approximately 100,000 CA/GT repeat sequences in the human genome *(3)*. Studies in patients with HNPCC (hereditary nonpolyposis colorectal cancer) first reported the appearance of instability at microsatellites sequences involving either an expansion or contraction of the repeat sequence *(4,5)*. The suggestion that this might reflect a defect in DNA repair was vindicated when subsequent work demonstrated defects in one of four mismatch repair genes [reviewed in *(6)*]. Such microsatellite instability (MI) has now been reported in a variety of different tumor types including lung, breast, ovary, stomach, endometrium, and bladder [reviewed in *(7)*].

Work from several groups has also shown that a number of tumor cell lines tolerant to methylating agents are also mismatch repair defective and show MI. Moreover, loss of mismatch repair has also been implicated in the tolerance of tumor cells to a number of other classes of cytotoxic drugs including cisplatin and doxorubicin, and it is becoming apparent that mismatch repair may play an important role in the cytotoxic nature of certain drugs [reviewed in *(8)*].

Acquisition of an RER+ (replication error) phenotype as demonstrated by MI is now widely used as a measure of mismatch repair deficiency *(9,10)*. MI has been shown to correlate with reduced survival and poor disease prognosis in breast cancer *(11)*. Conversely, MI correlates with good prognosis in colon cancer *(12)*. These differences may reflect the different impact of a mutator phenotype on tumor progression vs lack of mismatch repair on drug sensitivity. MI has been suggested to occur in 15–20% of sporadic ovarian tumors and two separate studies have raised the possibility that this may have prognostic significance *(13,14)*. A possible correlation with response to chemotherapy has been suggested *(15)* but further larger studies are needed.

From: *Methods in Molecular Medicine, Vol. 39: Ovarian Cancer: Methods and Protocols*
Edited by: J. M. S. Bartlett © Humana Press, Inc., Totowa, NJ

The acquisition of an RER+ phenotype will lead to greater levels of genomic instability and higher mutation rates at genes throughout the genome. This has the possibility of increasing the mutation rate at genes involved in drug resistance or in tumor progression *(16)*. Thus, if a tumor does recur with resistant disease owing to defects in mismatch repair, it may be more likely to progress to a more advanced, aggressive neoplasm.

No consensus exists as to how many or which type of microsatellites should be studied. However, a panel of microsatellites has been recommended to be used for MI analysis in HNPCC *(17)*, as well as correlating MI with loss of expression of mismatch repair proteins *(18)*. This proposes a panel of five microsatellite loci consisting of repeats with different lengths to be analyzed in the initial analysis. When less than two marker loci display shifts in the microsatellites, the panel should be enlarged to include an additional set of five marker loci. The number of marker loci analyzed, as well as the number of unstable loci found, should always be identified. A typical panel of microsatellite markers fulfilling the above criteria is given in **Table 1**.

A protocol for PCR amplification of microsatellite sequences using internal radiolabeling and a touchdown protocol which has been successfully used to analyze microsatellite instability in human, mouse, and canine DNA is given.

## 2. Materials

### 2.1. Polymerase Chain Reaction (PCR)

1. *Taq* DNA polymerase, 5 U/μL supplied with 10X PCR buffer: 100 m$M$ Tris-HCl, 15 m$M$ MgCl$_2$, 500 m$M$ KCl, pH 8.3 (20°C) (Boehringer Mannheim, Mannheim, Germany).
2. PCR dNTP mixture containing premixed dATP, dCTP, dGTP, and dTTP, 10 m$M$ each, (Boehringer Mannheim).
3. Microsatellite primers (e.g., MapPairs™ from Research Genetics, Huntsville, AL).

### 2.2. Detection of PCR Products by Agarose and Polyacrylamide Gel Electrophoresis

#### 2.2.1. Agarose Gel Electrophoresis

1. Running buffer: 1X TBE buffer diluted from 10X stock : 0.89$M$ Tris, 0.89$M$ boric acid, 2 m$M$ EDTA pH 8.0.
2. 5X sample loading buffer: 30% v/v glycerol, 0.25% w/v bromophenol blue, 0.25% w/v xylene cyanol FF.

#### 2.2.2. Polyacrylamide Gel Electrophoresis

1. Polyacrylamide gel mixture: 6% w/v acrylamide, 0.3% w/v bisacrylamide, 7$M$ urea, 1X TBE, ratio 19.1 (e.g., EASIGEL, Scotlab, Coatbridge, Scotland).
2. 10% Ammonium persulphate—make fresh as required.
3. Formamide sample loading buffer: 10 mL formamide, 10 mg xylene cyanol FF, 10 mg bromophenol blue, 200 μL 0.5$M$ EDTA.
4. M13 DNA sequencing ladder, made up according to kit instructions and stored ready to use; e.g., Sequenase 2.0 kit (Amersham International, Amersham, UK).

## Table 1
## A Proposed Panel of Microsatellite Markers

| Marker | CL[a] | Repeat Motif | Primer sequence (5' to 3')[b] | Size (bp)[c] |
|---|---|---|---|---|
| **1st Set** | | | | |
| Bat-26 | 2p | $(T)_5\ldots(A)_{26}$ | (a) TGACTACTTTGACTTCAGCC<br>(b) AACCATTCAACATTTTAACCC | 80–100 |
| BAT-40 | 1p13.1 | $TTTT.TT..(T)_7\ldots TTTT.(T)_{40}$ | (a) ATTAACTTCCTACACCACAAC<br>(b) GTAGAGCAAGACCACCTTG | 80–100 |
| APC | 5q21/22 | $(CA)_{26}$ | (a) ACTCACTCTAGTGATAAATCG<br>(b) AGCAGATAAGACAGTATTACTAGTT | 96–122 |
| Mfd15CA | 17q11.2-q12 | $(TA)_7\ldots(CA)_{24}$ | (a) GGAAGAATCAAATAGACAT<br>(b) GCTGGCCATATATATTTAAACC | 150 |
| D2S123 | 2p16 | $(CA)_{13}TA(CA)_{15}(T/G\ A)_7$ | (a) AAACAGGATGCCTGCCTTTA<br>(b) GGACTT TCCACCTATGGGAC | 197–227 |
| **2nd set** | | | | |
| BAT-25 | 4q12 | $TTTT.T.TTTT.(T)_7.A(T)_{25}$ | (a) TCGCCTCCAAGAATGTAAGT<br>(b) TCTGCATTTTAACTATGGCTC | 90 |
| D18S58 | 18q22.3 | $(GC)_5GA(CA)_{17}$ | (a) GCTCCCGGCTGGTTT<br>(b) GCAGGAAATCGCAGGAACTT | 144–160 |
| D18S69 | 18q21 | $(CA)_4AA(CA)_{14}(T)_6$ | (a) CTCTTTCTCTGACTCTGACC<br>(b) GACTTCTAAGTTCTTGCCAG | 110 |
| D10S197 | 10qter | $CACCAGA(CA)_7.A.A(CA)_{12}(AGAAA)_2$ | (a) ACCACTCGACTTCAGGTGAC<br>(b) GTGATACTGTCCTCAGGTCTCC | 161–173 |
| MYCL1 | 1p32 | $GAAAA(GAAAA)_2TAAAA(A/G)_{10}$<br>$GAAAGA(GAAA)_{14}$<br>$GAAA(GAAAAA)_8GAAAAAA(GAAAAA)_2$ | (a) TGGCGAGACTCCATCAAAG<br>(b) CTTTTTAAGCTGCAACAATTTC | 140–209 |
| F710/711[d] | 17 centromere | | (a) AATTCGTTGGAAACGGGATAATTTCAGCTG<br>(b) CTTCTGAGGATGCTTCTGTCTCTAGATGGC | 227 |

The first set contains five markers for microsatellites of differing repeat lengths. If less than two marker loci display microsatellite instability, the panel should be enlarged to incorporate an additional five markers as given in the second set.
[a] Chromosomal location of marker.
[b] Forward and reverse primers.
[c] Expected size of product.
[d] Positive control primers.

## 3. Methods

### 3.1. PCR

1. Thaw DNA samples (50–100 ng/μL) and PCR reagents, except the DNA polymerase on wet ice (*see* **Note 1**).

2. Determine the quantity of PCR master mix required for the number of samples + 1 using the following PCR set up for a reaction of 25 μL total volume: 2.5 μL 10X PCR buffer including $MgCl_2$ at 15 m$M$, 0.8 μL dNTP mix, 0.1 μL $\alpha^{32}$P CTP (Redivue, stock at 110 TBq/mL) (*see* **Note 2**), 0.1 μL *Taq* polymerase, 18.5 μL autoclaved $dH_2O$. Remember to include a negative control consisting of all the PCR reagents minus the template DNA, for each different set of primers. Another useful control is a reaction containing all the reagents minus primers (*see* **Note 3**).

3. Add 1 μL (50–100 ng) of DNA and 1 μL of each primer (4 μ$M$) to autoclaved thin-walled microcentrifuge tubes and keep on ice. Make up the PCR master mix and add the *Taq* DNA polymerase last, straight from –20°C. Vortex and briefly pulse the master mix in a benchtop minifuge (*see* **Note 4**). Add 22 μL to each reaction, vortex, and pulse briefly again. Overlay reactions with 30 μL of mineral oil if PCR thermal cycler does not have a heated lid.

4. Having calculated the theoretical annealing temperature (*Tm*) of the primers (*see* **Note 5**), perform a suitable PCR touchdown protocol following the parameters given in **Table 1**, which uses an example where the theoretical *Tm* of the primers is 56°C, and the touchdown goes from 60°C–56°C.

5. To check for a successful PCR, visualise products on a 1.8% TBE agarose minigel. For a 100ml gel, 1.8g agarose in 100ml 1X TBE. Ethidium bromide can be added to the gel (5 μl of 10mg/ml stock solution in 100ml gel). Load approximately 8 μl of sample mixed with 2 μL 5X sample loading buffer into each lane, and also reserve a lane for 100–250 ng of an appropriate DNA molecular weight marker, e.g., 123 bp ladder. Run at 180 V for approximately 30 min in 1X TBE buffer (*see* **Note 6**). Detect bands using an UV transilluminator. Products may be stored at 4°C or –20°C until use, however it is expedient to run them within a few days if they are radiolabeled with $^{32}$P.

### 3.2. Polyacrylamide Gel Electrophoresis

1. Following successful PCR, samples are visualized on a 6% denaturing polyacrylamide gel to separate alleles and determine size (*see* **Note 7**). Clean sequencing gel plates, combs (0.4 mm), and spacers (0.4 mm) with hot water and detergent, and rinse with $dH_2O$. If necessary, plates can be cleaned with a solution of KOH/methanol, made by adding approximately 5 g KOH in 100 mL methanol. Spray clean plates with alcohol and allow to dry. One plate can be coated with silicone treatment, such as Repelcote (BDH, Poole Dorset) to ensure that the gel remains attached to only one of the glass plates when they are separated after electrophoresis (*see* **Note 8**).

2. Insert spacers and seal the sides and bottom of the two glass plates together tightly with electrical tape (3M). First prepare a sealing gel (*see* **Note 9**): 2 mL acrylamide solution, 2 μL Temed (N,N,N'-tetramethylethylene-diamine), 30 μL 10% ammonium persulphate. Mix by swirling. Immediately pour in between glass plates using a 10-mL glass pipet, or a plastic syringe and allow to coat the bottom of the plates. As this is setting, prepare the main gel: 70 mL acrylamide gel mixture, 27.6 μL Temed, 554 μL 10% ammonium persulphate. Mix by swirling and draw up into a pipet or 50-mL plastic syringe barrel. Immediately pour, in a continuous stream, between the glass plates, holding the plates at a 45° angle on one bottom corner so that the gel flows evenly along the lower part of the side spacer. Make sure that no air bubbles are trapped (*see* **Note 10**). Lie plates horizon-

tally, but raise the loading end slightly, at an angle of approximately 10° to the bench to ensure polyacrylamide does not leak out. Insert a 0.4-mm shark tooth comb between the two gel plates (straight edge first) in order to create a trough the width of the comb in the top of the gel, and clamp in place with a large bulldog clip. Clamp further bulldog clips on the sides of the gel plates to prevent leakage. Do not clamp clips on the bottom edge without a spacer as this will distort the gel. Then allow the gel to set at room temperature for approximately 1 h.

3. Remove the bulldog clips and electrical tape from the bottom edge of the plates with a scalpel, and fit into sequencing gel apparatus. Fill tanks with 1X TBE and prerun the gel, for 30–60 min at approximately 35–40 mA/1500–1900 V, 60 W for a 0.4-mm gel. Meanwhile, set up a water bath or a PCR or heating block at 94°C.

4. Mix 4 μL of labeled PCR product with 4 μL of formamide sample loading buffer. Denature samples and premade molecular weight markers at 94°C for 5 min. Remove and place on ice for 2–5 min.

5. Meanwhile, switch off gel apparatus and remove shark tooth comb. Clean the comb, and the trough formed in the gel to remove unpolymerized acrylamide, by syringing with 1X TBE buffer. Reinsert the comb, teeth in first, into the preformed trough, allowing teeth to touch the top surface of the gel causing a slight indentation. Do not allow teeth to pierce the gel.

6. Load approximately 7 μL of sample into each well using flat-edged pipet tips. Add 4 μL of molecular weight markers to each well (*see* **Note 11**).

7. Run the gel at 35–40 mA/1500–1900 V for about 2 h until the xylene cyanol FF marker dye (light blue) reaches the bottom of the gel.

8. Switch off electrical supply and remove glass plates. Remove the electrical tape from the two sides of the gel with a scalpel and place the plates flat onto the laboratory bench. Also remove the comb. Gently separate the glass plates with a palette knife or large flat spatula, taking care not to wrinkle or rip the gel. Start by inserting the knife into one corner and pry the plates apart slowly. Make sure the gel sticks to the bottom plate, otherwise turn the plates around so the other plate is on bottom. Once separated, the gel should be totally stuck to one of the glass plates. Remove the spacers. Place 3MM Whatman paper (cut to size) on top of the gel and gently smooth out any air bubbles. Slowly remove the paper with the gel attached and cover with Saran wrap.

9. Dry the gel under vacuum for 30–60 min at 80°C.

10. Place gel in an autoradiograph cassette with intensifying screens and expose to X-ray film at –70°C for 24–72 h.

## 4. Notes

1. To prevent cross contamination when performing PCR, it is important to separate your PCR reactions from previous DNA preparations. Conduct PCR reactions in a bench area apart from other laboratory work, or use a tray to keep work isolated. It is also good practice to keep a separate set of pipets for pre-PCR work. Keep your own stock of PCR reagents in small aliquots frozen at –20°C. Use sterile techniques and autoclaved equipment. Exposure to UV irradiation in a UV DNA crosslinker (e.g., Stratagene) can sterilize pipets and other equipment from contaminating DNA.

2. PCR primers can be end labeled with $^{32}$P or $^{35}$S γATP, or as described here, an internal radiolabel is added with {α-$^{32}$P}dCTP in the PCR reaction. Dye-labeled primers have also become available, which may be detected on fluorescent detection apparatus, e.g., 373A DNA fragment analyser (Applied Biosystems, Foster City, CA).

3. It is useful and less costly to optimize the PCR conditions for each primer conditions without radiolabel first. In the event of PCR not working, there are a number of trouble-

shooting approaches that can be taken and there are several excellent review chapters, e.g., *(19)*. One of the most critical factors influencing PCR is the magnesium ($Mg^{2+}$) concentration, which may vary from 0.5 m$M$–5 m$M$, depending on the influence of components in the reaction mixture including dNTP's, free pyrophosphate (PPi), and EDTA. The sequence of the primers will influence the success of a PCR greatly. However, commercially available and published primers should already be optimally designed. Sequences and/or information relating to microsatellite primers for a variety of species can be obtained from the GenBank database. Primer concentration may also affect a PCR reaction, as high primer concentration may promote mispriming, and low primer concentrations affect yield, but generally a concentration of between 0.1 and 0.5 µ$M$ is optimal. Other factors that may be altered are the cycling conditions, template concentration, and the *Taq* polymerase concentration, which is usually optimal between 0.5 and 2.5 U. There are now a number of commercially available PCR trouble-shooting kits, e.g., Boehringer Mannheim, which includes buffers of different pH and magnesium content, and may be of use in determining the PCR correct conditions.

4. Remember to vortex all solutions before pipeting, and briefly pulse in a microcentrifuge to bring reagents down from the sides and underneath the lid.

5. The theoretical annealing temperature of the primers may be calculated from the following simplified formula: $2°C \times (A+T) + 4°C \times (G+C)$ *(29)*. It is probably the most crucial factor in the design of a highly specific PCR, as too high an annealing temperature will result in no product and too low an annealing temperature may result in nonspecific products. A standard PCR protocol, each cycle or round of PCR consists of three steps: a DNA denaturation step at 94°C, a primer annealing step, and a primer extension step at 72°C. Use of a "touchdown" protocol *(20)*, which utilizes the exponential nature of PCR can greatly improve the quality of microsatellite profiles by decreasing the chance for mispriming. The early rounds of the PCR reaction use annealing temperatures several degrees above the theoretical annealing temperature of the primers, and each subsequent round drops the annealing temperature by one or two degrees until the touchdown temperature is reached. For example, *see* **Table 2**. In optimising a PCR protocol, it may be necessary to try several "theoretical" *Tm*.

6. An alternative option is to add ethidium bromide solution to the running buffer at 0.5 mg/mL). Alternatively, the gel can be stained afterwards in a solution of ethidium bromide (0.5 mg/mL in 1X TBE).

7. The PCR products are usually run on denaturing polyacrylamide gels so that single-stranded DNA can be separated and the two alleles resolved. The sizes of the alleles on the autoradiograph are determined by referring to an M13 sequencing ladder run alongside samples as a molecular-weight marker. Theoretically, one allele should produce one band on a gel, but in practice several bands are seen, which is thought to be owing to events such as mispriming, strand slippage, and the terminal transferase activity of *Taq* DNA polymerase *(20)*. This can make interpretation of gels difficult. In addition, extra bands may arise if PCR products are internally radiolabeled using {α-$^{32}$P}dCTP because of separation of the CA and TG strands on the gel. If these products differ sufficiently in their nucleotide content, then one strand will be preferentially labeled compared to the other and will cause little interference in scoring gels. This is usually the case when primers are located close to the repeat sequence, but problems may arise if primers are located farther upstream and downstream, producing much flanking sequence in the PCR product.

8. Denaturing polyacrylamide gels can be made in advance, e.g., the day before kept at 4°C, ensuring the exposed edges are kept covered in Saran wrap and moist paper towels. The M13 sequencing ladder used as a molecular-weight marker can also be made in advance and stored at 4°C. To silicone-treat the sequencing plates, pour a small amount of silicone

**Table 2**
**Example of a Typical Touchdown PCR Protocol**
**for Primers Whose Optimal Annealing Temperature (*Tm*) is 56°C[a]**

| PCR Stage | Cycling Temperature | Number of Cycles |
|---|---|---|
| Stage 1 | Denature DNA for 5 min at 94°C | 1 cycle |
| Stage 2 | 94°C, 1 min | |
| | 60°C, 1 min | 2 cycles |
| | 72°C, 1 min | |
| Stage 3 | 94°C, 1 min | |
| | 59°C, 1 min | 2 cycles |
| | 72°C, 1 min | Reduce annealing temperature by 1°C every two cycles until *Tm* achieved |
| Stage 6 | 94°C 1 min | |
| | 56°C 1 min | 25 cycles |
| | 72°C 1 min | |
| Stage 7 | 72°C, 5 min | 1 cycle |
| Stage 8 | 4°C | Hold |

[a]The initial annealing temperature starts several degrees above the optimal annealing temperature of the primers and drops by one degree every two cycles of PCR until the desired "touchdown" annealing temperature is achieved, at which point 10–25 rounds of cycling are performed.

solution onto one of the glass plates, wipe over with a paper towel pad ensuring the entire surface is covered with the silicone, and rinse with dH$_2$O. Allow the plate to dry.

9. Remember to use acrylamide solution immediately after adding Temed and ammonium persulphate.

10. If air bubbles do appear while pouring the gel, they can sometimes be eliminated by gently squeezing the plates together just below the bubble. If the bubble persists, the gel can be poured out, and repoured, or failing that, the plates recleaned and a new gel solution made. Additionally, bubble-getters are now available commercially, which are the width of a spacer and can be inserted inbetween the plates to remove the bubble.

11. To conserve time, it may be possible to load several samples in one lane on a polyacrylamide gel, providing there is sufficient separation between the expected sizes of the products. It is useful to load molecular-weight markers in the first and/or last lanes of the gel and note position. This will help to orientate the gel once processed.

## References

1. Hearne, C. M., Ghosh, S., and Todd, J. A. (1992) Microsatellites for linkage analysis of genetic traits. *Trends Genet.* **8**, 288–294.
2. Beckmann, J. S. and Weber, J. L. (1992) Survey of human and rat microsatellites. *Genomics* **12**, 627–631.
3. Loeb, L. A. (1994) Microsatellite instability: marker of a mutator phenotype in cancer. *Cancer Res.* **54**, 5059–5063.
4. Aaltonen, L. A., Peltomaki, P., Leach, P. S., Sistonen, P., Pylkkanen, L., Maklin, J., et al. (1993) Clues to the pathogenesis of Familial Colorectal Cancer. *Science* **260**, 812–815.
5. Thibodeau, S. N., Bren, G., and Schaid, D. (1993) Microsatellite instability of the proximal colon. *Science* **260**, 816–819.
6. Karran, P. (1996) Microsatellite instability and DNA mismatch repair in human cancer. *Seminars Cancer Biol.* **7**, 15–24.
7. Eshleman, J. R. and Markowitz, S. D. (1995) Microsatellite instability in inherited and sporadic neoplasms. *Current Opin. Oncol.* **7**, 83–89.

8. Modrich, P. (1997) Strand specific mismatch repair in mammalian cells. *J. Biol. Chem.* **272,** 24,727–24,730.

9. Parsons, R., Li, G. M., Longley, M. J., Fang, W. H., Papadopoulos, N., Jen, J., et al. (1993) Hypermutability and mismatch repair deficiency in RER⁺ tumor cells. *Cell* **75,** 1227–1236.

10. Karran, P. and Bignami, M. (1994) DNA damage tolerance, mismatch repair and genome instability. *BioEssays* **16,** 833–839.

11. Paulson, T. G., Wright, F. A., Parker, B. A., Russack, V., and Wahl, G. M. (1996) Microsatellite instability correlates with reduced survival and poor disease prognosis in breast cancer. *Cancer Res.* **56,** 4021–4026.

12. Bubb, V. J., Curtis, L. J., Cunningham, C., Dunlop, M. G., Carothers, A. D., Morris, R. G., et al. (1996) Microsatellite instability and the role of hmsh2 in sporadic colorectal-cancer. *Oncogene* **12,** 2641–2649.

13. King, B. L., Carcangiu, M. L., Carter, D., Kiechle, M., Pfisterer, J., Pfleiderer, A., and Kacinski, B. M. (1995) Microsatellite instability in ovarian neoplasms. *Brit. J. Cancer* **72,** 376–382.

14. Fujita, M., Enomoto, T., Yoshino, K., Nomura, T., Buzard, G. S., and Inoue, M. (1995) Microsatellite instability and alterations in the hMSH2 gene in human ovarian cancer. *Int. J. Cancer* **64,** 361–366.

15. Brown, R., Hirst, G. L., Gallagher, W. M., McIlwrath, A. J., Margison, G. P., van der Zee, A. G., and Anthoney, D. A. (1997) hMLH1 expression and cellular responses of ovarian tumor cells to treatment with cytotoxic anticancer agents. *Oncogene* **15,** 45–52.

16. Markowitz, S., Wang, J., Myeroff, L., Parsons, R., Sun, L., Lutterbaugh, J., et al. (1995) Inactivation of the type ii tgf-beta receptor in colon cancer cells with microsatellite instability. *Science* **268,** 1336–1338.

17. Bocker, T., Diermann, J., Friedl, W., Gebert, J., Holinski-Feder, E., Karner-Hanusch, J., et al. (1997) Microsatellite instability analysis: a multicenter study for reliability and quality control. *Cancer Res.* **57,** 4739–4743.

18. Dietmaier, W., Wallinger, S., Bocker, T., Kullmann, F., Fishel, R., and Ruschoff, J. (1997) Diagnostic microsatellite instability: definition and correlation with mismatch repair protein expression. *Cancer Res.* **57,** 4749–4756.

19. Kidd, K. K. and Ruano, G. (1995) Optimizing PCR, in *PCR2: A Practical Approach* (McPherson, M. J., Hames, B. D., and Taylor, G. R., eds.), IRL, Oxford, pp. 1–22.

20. Don, R. H., Cox, P. T., Wainwright, B. J., Baker, K., and Mattick, J. S. (1991) "Touchdown" PCR to circumvent spurious priming during gene amplification. *Nucleic Acids Res.* **19,** 4008–4009.

# 42

## Immunostaining Human Paraffin-Embedded Sections for Mismatch Repair Proteins

**Melanie Mackean and Robert Brown**

## 1. Introduction

The loss of the function in any one of four human DNA mismatch repair genes, *hMSH2*, *hMLH1*, *hPMS1*, and *hPMS2*, is thought to lead to deficient mismatch repair (MMR) of DNA in the somatic cells leading to increased mutations and thereby cancer development. Microsatellite instability (MI) detected by PCR analysis has, to date, been the hallmark of loss of the function of these genes. Western and Northern blotting has confirmed the loss of MMR protein expression with MI. However, this technique relies on fresh samples for DNA extraction and requires a normal tissue sample (*see* Chapter 41). Expression of MMR proteins can now be examined in both fresh and archival paraffin-embedded tissue samples by immunohistochemistry. This was first described for polyclonal *hMSH2* antibody, in paraffin-embedded tissue, by Wilson et al. *(1)* and confirmed by Leach et al. *(2)*, who showed that *hMSH2* is highly expressed in the nuclei cells of the gastrointestinal epithelium that undergo rapid renewal in both the ileum, colon, and esophagus. Thibodeau et al. *(3)* examined paraffin-embedded tissue from colorectal tumors for both *hMLH1* and *hMSH2* genes and function by DNA sequence analysis, MI analysis by PCR, and immunohistochemistry. They showed that loss of immunohistochemical staining for these MMR proteins corresponded very closely with loss of function of these genes detected by microsatellite analysis. Of 19 tumors showing MI, 14 had loss of either or both *hMLH1* and *hMSH2* immunostaining. Of eight tumors showing a germline mutation in either *hMLH1* or *hMSH2*, seven had a corresponding loss of immunostaining for the protein. Of 14 tumors showing a negative immunostain for one or both of *hMLH1* and *hMSH2*, all had MI on PCR analysis and seven had a germline mutation in the DNA sequence of at least one of the MMR genes. Fink et al. *(4)* have performed immunohistochemistry for *hMLH1* and hPMS2 on fresh frozen tissue sections. They confirmed a high nuclear expression in the epithelium of the digestive tract and in the testis and ovary. We describe here a method for immunohistochemistry for *hMSH2*, *hMLH1*, and *hPMS2* in both fresh and paraffin-embedded material.

Immunohistochemistry has undergone numerous refinements over the past 20 years and is now routinely performed for both diagnostic and prognostic information on

From: *Methods in Molecular Medicine, Vol. 39: Ovarian Cancer: Methods and Protocols*
Edited by: J. M. S. Bartlett © Humana Press, Inc., Totowa, NJ

patient tissue samples in pathology laboratories. Numerous kits are commercially available and choice is normally based on local experience and the cost of the monoclonal antibodies used. Microwaving as a technique for exposing antigens to the antibodies has been developed over the last 14 years *(5)*. The technique used below employs the streptavidin-biotin technique coupled to peroxidase activity for use as a label. A small amount of primary antibody when bound to the antigen of interest in the tissue will be detected by a cascade of two further antibody–antibody reactions and finally activation of the peroxidase activity bound to the third antibody. Diaminobenzidine (DAB) is then used as a substrate for the bound antibody complex, which produces a brown color after undergoing oxidation. If no primary antibody is bound to the tissue there will be no peroxidase activity and the tissue will not stain brown with DAB. In order to visualize negative tissue samples, they are counterstained with a routine haematoxylin stain (blue). The method below is divided into several steps for clarity. The whole procedure should take approximately 6 h for 20 slides.

## 2. Materials

Using Vectastain® Elite ABC Kit (*see* **Note 4**).

### 2.1. Stable Solutions for Immunostaining

All stable at 20°C.

1. Phosphate-buffered saline (PBS).
2. 0.1% hydrogen peroxide (per 1 L): 1 mL 100 vol hydrogen peroxide + 1 L distilled water.
3. Sodium tricitrate buffer (per 1 L): 2.94 g sodium tricitrate + 1 L distilled water. Adjust to pH 6.0 with HCl.
4. Antidote to DAB (per 100 mL): 3 g potassium permanganate ($KMnO_4$) + 2 g sodium carbonate ($Na_2CO_3$) + 100 mL distilled water.

### 2.2. Unstable Solutions for Immunostaining

Keep on ice and make up fresh. Solutions stain approx 20 slides (*see* **Note 5**).

1. Blocking Serum (Vectastain® Yellow—10 mL): 10 mL PBS + 150 µL normal horse serum (i.e., 3 drops yellow block).
2. Biotinylated Antibody (Vectastain Blue—10 mL): 10 mL PBS + 150 µL normal horse serum (i.e., 3 drops yellow block) + 50 µL biotinylated antimouse IgG (i.e. 1 drop blue block).
3. ABC reagent (Vectastain Grey). **Make up 30 min before use.** 5 mL PBS + drops solution A + 2 drops solution B.
4. DAB diaminobenzidine tetrahydrochloride (per 5 mL): 5 mL distilled water + 2 drops Vectastain buffer + 2 drops hydrogen peroxide + 4 drops Vectastain® DAB reagent. *Note*—possible carcinogen. Use gloves.

### 2.3. Primary Antibodies

(Per 2 mL = approx 20 slides, *see* **Notes 6** and **7**).

1. Anti-*hMLH1*: 20 mL *MLH1* antibody (500 µg/mL purified antihuman mouse monoclonal IgG, clone G168-15, PharMingen®, stock solution kept at 4°C) + 1980 µL PBS, i.e., 5 µg/mL solution.
2. Anti-*hMSH2*: 20 µL *MSH2* antibody (100 µg/mL purified antihuman mouse monoclonal IgG, Ab-2 clone FE11, Calbiochem® stock solution kept at 4°C) + 1980 µL PBS, i.e., 1 µg/mL solution.

3. Anti-hPMS2: 40 µL *PMS2* antibody (100 µg/mL purified antihuman mouse monoclonal IgG, Ab-1 clone 9, Calbiochem stock solution kept at 4°C) + 1960 µL PBS, i.e., 2 µg/mL solution.

### 2.4. Solutions for Counterstaining

1. Haematoxylin: Harris formula filtered before use, Surgipath®.
2. Graded ethanols (100%, 70% ethanol).
3. Histo-clear®, Fischer Scientific Ltd. (Pittsburgh, PA).
4. Scott's Tap Water: 1 in 10 dilution in distilled water of Surgipath Scott's tap water substitute. **Warning:** can cause skin irritation. Use gloves.
5. Acid Alcohol: 10 mL concentrated hydrogen chloride (specific gravity 1.16 g/mL—approx 33%) in 990 mL 70% ethanol.
6. Hystomount®, Hughes and Hughes Ltd.

## 3. Methods

### 3.1. Dewaxing of Slides in a Laminar Flow Hood (see Note 8)

1. Place slides in metal rack (maximum 20). Wash in bath of Histo-clear for 20 min.
2. Rinse in bath of 100% ethanol for 1 min (*see* **Note 9**).
3. Rinse in bath of 70% ethanol for 1 min.
4. Rinse in tap water for 1 min.
5. Wash in bath of PBS for 5 min (*see* **Note 10**).

### 3.2. Removal of Endogenous Peroxidase Activity (see Note 11)

1. Wash in bath of 0.1% hydrogen peroxide for 20 min.
2. Wash in bath of PBS for 5 min.

### 3.3. Antigen Retrieval (see Note 12)

1. Fill microwave box with 750 mL of sodium tricitrate buffer (*see* **Note 13**).
2. Place slides in plastic rack and place rack into box, cover with cling film, pierce three times.
3. Microwave on full power (650 W microwave) for 15 min (*see* **Note 14**).
4. Leave to cool for 20 min.

### 3.4. Isolate the Tissue Section (see Note 15)

1. Wipe each slide in turn around tissue section with tissue paper to dry.
2. Circle tissue section with 5 mm margin with PAP-pen.

### 3.5. Vectastain ABC Technique

1. Fill bottom of immunostaining box with damp tissue paper (*see* **Note 16**). Place slides, one at a time, into immunostaining box. Cover tissue section with 3–5 drops (approx 100–200 µL) of yellow block and leave for 20 min.
2. Tap off yellow block, one slide at a time, and cover tissue section with 100 µL (2–3 drops) of primary antibody of interest (i.e., *hMLH1*, *hMSH2*, or *hPMS2*). Leave for 30 min.
3. Place slides in metal rack and wash in PBS for 5 min.
4. Place slides into immunostaining box and cover tissue section with 3–5 drops (100–200 µL) of blue block. Make up ABC solution at this point and leave for 30 min.
5. Place slides in metal rack and wash in PBS for 5 minutes.
6. Place slides in immunobox and cover tissue section with 3–5 drops (100–200 µL) of gray block. Leave for 30 min.
7. Place slides in metal rack and wash in fresh PBS for 5 min.

8. Place slides in immunobox and cover tissue section with 3–5 (100–200 μL) drops of DAB (*see* **Note 17**). Leave for 10 min.
9. Place slides in metal rack and wash in PBS for 5 min.
10. Use 5 mL of antidote to DAB over the immunobox.

### *3.6. Counterstain with Haematoxylin in a Laminar Flow Hood (see Note 8)*

1. Rinse in tap water.
2. Wash in haematoxylin for 60 s (*see* **Note 18**) and then rinse in tap water.
3. Rinse in acid alcohol for 2–10 s (*see* **Note 18**) and then rinse in tap water.
4. Wash in Scott's tap water for 60 s and then rinse in tap water.
5. Wash in 70% alcohol for 60 s.
6. Wash in 100% alcohol for 60 s.
7. Place in Histo-clear for at least 5 min.

### *3.7. Mount Slides*

Perform in laminar air flow hood.

1. Place 20 cover slips on filter paper and place a drop of Hystomount on each cover slip (*see* **Note 19**).
2. Take each slide in turn and wipe off excess Histo-clear around tissue section. Place tissue section face down onto cover slip and leave for 10 s.
3. Invert slide and cover slip so that the cover slip is face up and leave to set for at least 1 h.

## 4. Notes

1. Tissue sections will be brown if positive for the MMR protein and blue if negative. It is essential for each run to include a known positive and negative slide control. We use a sectioned paraffin-embedded samples of cell line with known MMR protein status. i.e., Ovarian A2780 as a positive control, Ovarian A2780/CP70 for *hMLH1* and *hPMS2* negative, and Colon LOVO 1 as negative for *hMSH2 (7,8)*.
2. To immunostain fresh fixed samples, omit **step 1** and place directly into PBS. Start with removal of endogenous peroxidase activity (**Subheading 3.2., step 2**).
3. Be gentle with the slides. The tissue sections can wash off if moved in solutions too vigorously. Using APES (Sigma, St. Louis, MO) coated slides to mount the tissue sections. This will help them to stick.
4. The use of the Vectastain *Elite* ABC kit is a personal choice. It does allow a small amount of expensive antibody to be used for a positive result.
5. Vortex all solutions before using to ensure even mixing.
6. Different batches of primary antibody give variable staining. With a new batch it is a good idea to run positive and negative controls with dilutions suggested, but also 50% and 200% of these. We have found *hPMS2* in particular to vary and require different dilutions depending on the batch.
7. To prevent variability of staining try to keep the stock solutions of primary antibody on ice at all times and return to storage as promptly as possible.
8. Histo-clear and Hystomount emit noxious fumes. Perform all steps involving these in a laminar flow hood.
9. Check the slides when in 100% ethanol (**Subheading 3.1.**) for dewaxing. If they are adequately dewaxed, the section will be the shape of the tissue section. If they are not adequately dewaxed, the section will still be the square shape of the original paraffin block. If this is the case, place back into the Histo-clear for another 10 min and check again. Better to check at this stage than to perform the whole immunostain and find out at the end it has not worked because of persistent wax!

10. When washing in PBS, place the metal rack with the slides into a glass bath containing enough PBS to cover the tops of the slides (usually 350 mL). Place the bath on a rocker table for 5 min to ensure even washing. Change the PBS after each wash ideally, but certainly after the peroxide step and the gray block to prevent false positive staining.

11. All tissue sections of interest must be checked for endogenous peroxidase activity (which will give a false positive result). Normally, the 0.1% hydrogen peroxidase step should solve this problem, but it is worthwhile to check each block by running a slide through the whole immunostain leaving out the primary antibody step. This slide should be negative (blue) if there is no endogenous activity.

12. We have tried different forms of antigen retrieval with saponin, trypsin, and different times of microwaving and found 15 min in a microwave to give the most consistent results.

13. Make sure there is enough buffer in the microwave box so that the top of the slides are covered after 15 min of boiling. If this is a problem, perform the microwaving in three separate 5-min steps and top up with buffer after each 5 min. If the slides do dry out, there will be brown "hot spots" as artifact on the final slides. Use a microwave with a turntable to prevent "hot spots" and place the box eccentrically on the table, not in the middle.

14. Watch yourself with the microwave step. The buffer is boiling hot after 15 min in the microwave. Use protected ovengloves to remove the box from the microwave and leave the cling film on until it is cooled.

15. The PAP-pen step allows you to use smaller amounts of primary antibody and prevents the tissue sections from drying out. After each step in the immunobox, doublecheck each slide to make sure the solution is up to the edge of the circle drawn with the PAP-pen.

16. It is critical to consistent immunostaining not to let the tissue section on the slide dry out at any stage. This means covering each slide with the next solution on a one-by-one basis. Do not be tempted to take all 20 slides out of the bath, place into the immunobox, and then cover with solutions. They will dry out giving artifact staining on the final slide. Ensure the immunobox is kept humid by lining the bottom with tissue paper soaked in warm water and cover the box with a plastic lid during the incubation times for the slides.

17. DAB is a potential carcinogen. Always use gloves when handling and soak all equipment that touches DAB in an equal amount of antidote afterward for at least 30 min.

18. The depth of counterstain is of personal choice. The slides will be more blue by leaving in haematoxylin for longer (**Subheading 3.6., step 2**) or leaving in acid alcohol, which leaches out the color (**Subheading 3.6., step 3**), for a shorter time.

19. Using too much Hystomount will make the final slides messy to handle. Using too little might allow the tissue section to dry out with time. The ideal amount spreads from a central drop to cover the square of the cover slip in about 10 s. The amount to use will vary with the size of the cover slip. Always choose a cover slip size that adequately covers the tissue section.

20. When the slides are prepared from the paraffin-embedded material, they loose antigenicity and will stain false negative (blue) over a period of months if stored at room temperature (*6*). Store prepared slides at 4°C prior to immunostaining.

21. Scoring the immunostain is a matter of personal preference. It is usual for each slide to be scored for both the intensity of the stain and the percentage of cells stained. Automated systems, e.g., CAS system, exist for automated counting of the percentage of cells stained. It is good practice for the slides to be independently scored by at least two observers, blind of any clinical information. Interobserver and intraobserver variation should be calculated with kappa scores ideally above 0.5.

## References

1. Wilson, T. M., Ewel, A., Duguid, J. R., et al. (1995) Differential cellular expression of the human MSH2 repair enzyme in small and large intestine. *Cancer Res.* **55,** 5146–5150.

2. Leach, F. S., Polyak, K., Burrell, M., et al. (1996) Expression of the human mismatch repair gene hMSH2 in normal and neoplastic tissues. *Cancer Res.* **56,** 235–240.

3. Thibodeau, S. N., French, A. J., Roche, P. C., et al. (1996) Altered expression of hMSH2 and hMLH1 in tumor with microsatellite instability and genetic alterations in mismatch repair genes. *Cancer Res.* **56,** 4836–4840.

4. Fink, D., Nebel, S., Aebi, S., et al. (1997) Expression of the DNA mismatch repair proteins hMLH1 and hPMS2 in normal human tissues. *Brit. J. Cancer* **76,** 890–893.

5. Leong, A. S. Y. (1996) Microwave technology in immunohistochemistry. *J. Cellular Path.* **1,** 99–108.

6. Jacobs, T. W., Prioleau, J. E., Stillman, I. E., and Schnitt, S. J. (1996) Loss of tumor marker immunostaining intensity on stored paraffin slides of breast cancer. *J. Natl. Cancer Inst.* **88,** 1054–1059.

7. Brown, R., Hust, G. L., Gallagher, W. M., et al. (1997) LMLH1 expression and cellular responses of ovarian cancer tumor cells to treatment with cytotoxic anticancer agents. *Oncogene* **15,** 45–52.

8. Mackay, H. J., Cameron, D., Rahilly, M., et al. (2000) Reduced MLH1 expression in breast tumors after primary chemotherapy predicts disease free survival. *J. Clin. Oncol.*, in press.

# 43

## Quantitative PCR Detection of c-*erbB-2* Gene Amplification

### Karl Dobianer, Michael Medl, and Jürgen Spona

### 1. Introduction

The association of c-*erbB-2* oncogene amplification and prognostic factors was intensively studied in human gynecological carcinomas, especially in mammary carcinoma *(1)*. Positive lymph nodes, estrogen and progesterone receptor negative tumors, and short survival time correlate with c-*erbB-2* amplification.

The need for short and reliable tests for the determination of c-*erbB-2* amplification led to the development of quantitative PCR systems, which have several advantages compared to quantitative Southern blotting: no extensive purification of the samples, even in the presence of highly degraded DNA (e.g., in paraffin-embedded tissue); 100 times smaller sample volumes and PCR techniques are fast, nontoxic and nonradioactive. Therefore, these methods are useful for prospective, as well as retrospective studies *(2–5)* in which the problem of degraded DNA and small sample volumes arises.

The idea of a quantitative PCR system for the detection of gene amplification is to design PCR primers including the amplified region of the c-*erbB-2* gene and primers for a reference gene, which is not amplified with high probability. The two primer pairs are used in the same reaction and therefore produce concurrently two PCR products in a ratio reflecting the copy numbers of oncogene and reference gene in the original DNA. The signal strengths of both genes are compared and the amplification is calculated as the ratio of c-*erbB-2* signal vs reference gene signal. This technique can be easily adapted to other genes and is extremely useful for measuring large sample numbers at low cost in short time. A technically skilled person can measure about 100 to 200 samples a day, depending on the laboratory equipment.

The method outlined in this chapter consists of the following steps: DNA extraction and purification of various tissues; PCR reaction; gel electrophoresis; detection and densitometry; calculation of results.

### 2. Materials

#### 2.1. DNA Extraction and Purification

##### 2.1.1. Paraffin-Embedded Tissue

1. Heatable vacuum centrifuge (minimum 40°C) (e.g., SpeedVac™), explosion-proof, if available.

From: *Methods in Molecular Medicine, Vol. 39: Ovarian Cancer: Methods and Protocols*
Edited by: J. M. S. Bartlett © Humana Press, Inc., Totowa, NJ

2. Isooctane analytical grade: store at room temperature. *Caution*: highly flammable, vapors toxic, perform all manipulation under a hood.

3. Proteinase K lysis buffer 1: 1 m$M$ CaCl$_2$, 0.5% v/v Tween-20, 10 m$M$ Tris-HCl pH 8.0, 267 µg proteinase K per mL buffer in bidistilled sterile water (all reagents analytical grade), stable at 4°C for 2 wk, adjust pH before adding proteinase K.

### 2.1.2. Frozen Tissue Sections, Fresh Tissue, and Cultured Cells

1. Proteinase K lysis buffer 2: 1 m$M$ CaCl$_2$, 0.5% v/v Tween-20, 10 m$M$ Tris-HCl pH 8.0, 300 µg proteinase K per mL buffer in bidistilled sterile water (all reagents analytical grade), stable at 4°C for 2 wk, adjust pH before adding proteinase K.

## 2.2. Quantitative PCR Reaction

1. 10X PCR reaction buffer: 1$M$ KCl, 30 m$M$ MgCl$_2$, 100 m$M$ Tris-HCl, pH 8.4, 0.01% w/v gelatin G2500 (Sigma, St. Louis, MO) in bidistilled sterile water (all reagents analytical grade), stable at 4°C for 2 wk (*see* **Note 1**).

2. dNTP mix: 10 m$M$ dNTP (i.e., 10 m$M$ each of dATP, dTTP, dGTP, dCTP) in bidistilled sterile water stable at 4°C for 2 wk (*see* **Notes 1–4**).

3. Primers:
   PC03 (5′ACACAACTGTGTTCACTAGC3′) (*see* **ref. 7**).
   KM38 (5′TGGTCTCCTTAAACCTGTCTT3′) (*see* **ref. 7**).
   HER2a (5′CCTCTGACGTCCATCATCTC3′) (*2–5*).
   HER2b (5′ATCTTCTGCTGCCGTCGCTT3′) (*2–5*) (*see* **Notes 3** and **5**).

4. *Taq* polymerase (USB or Promega, Madison, WI) stable at –20°C for 3 mo.

## 2.3. Gel Electrophoresis

1. 1X TAE: 4.84 g Tris-HCl, 1.14 mL concentrated acetic acid, 2 mL EDTA (0.5 mol/L) pH 8.0 make up to 1000 mL with distilled or deionized water, stable at 4°C for 6 mo, if sterile-filtered.

2. 3% low-melting-point agarose gel: 2% Nusieve GTG, 1% low-melting agarose Bio-Rad, 0.01% SybrGreen I™ in 1X TAE. Stable liquid at 60°C for 2 wk in a closed vessel, stable solid at 4°C for 1 wk, if kept in 1X TAE.

3. 10X loading buffer: 0.01% bromophenol blue, 40% saccharose in 1X TAE or sterile bidistilled water. Stable at –20°C for several years.

4. Any low-molecular-weight length standard: e.g., Lambda/*BstE* II or pBR322/*Hae*III.

## 2.4. Detection and Densitometry

1. Photographic camera or video imaging equipment.
2. Densitometer or densitometry software.

# 3. Methods

## 3.1. DNA Extraction and Purification (see Notes 6, 8, and 9)

### 3.1.1. Paraffin-Embedded Tissue

**Caution:** isooctane and its vapors are highly flammable and potentially toxic, so **steps 1–7** must be performed under explosion-proof conditions with explosion-proof apparatuses in a explosion-proof hood.

1. Add 1.5 mL isooctane to 2 10-µm stroma-free paraffin-embedded tissue sections (each about 1 cm$^2$). In the same way, prepare 2 10-µm paraffin-embedded tissue sections (each about 1 cm$^2$) from normal human placenta.

2. Vortex thoroughly.

3. Incubate at 70°C for 5 min (*see* **Note 10**).
4. Spin down in a centrifuge at about 5000*g*.
5. Discard the supernatant (*see* **Note 11**).
6. Repeat **steps 1–5** four times.
7. Dry the pellet in a vacuum centrifuge at 40°C for 10 min (*see* **Note 12**).
8. Suspend the dried pellet in 75 mL proteinase K lysis buffer 1 and vortex thoroughly.
9. Incubate at 56°C for 4 h, vortex every 30 min (*see* **Note 13**).
10. Deactivate proteinase K by boiling the sample for 20 min (*see* **Note 14**).
11. Centrifuge the sample at 12,000*g* for 5 min at room temperature.
12. The supernatant is ready for use in the PCR reaction (*see* **Note 15**).

### 3.1.2. Frozen Tissue Sections, Fresh Tissue, and Cultured Cells (see **Note 7**)

1. Suspend two 10-μm stroma-free frozen tissue sections (each about 1 cm²) or 1 to 5 mg fresh tissue or 1 to 5 μL cultured cell pellet in 100 μL proteinase K lysis buffer 2, and vortex thoroughly. In the same way prepare two 10 μm frozen tissue sections (each about 1 cm²) or 1 to 5 mg fresh tissue from normal human placenta.
2. Incubate at 56°C for 6 h, vortex every 30 min (*see* **Note 13**).
3. Deactivate proteinase K by boiling the sample for 20 min (*see* **Note 14**).
4. Centrifuge the sample at 12,000*g* for 5 min at room temperature.
5. The supernatant is ready for use in the PCR reaction (*see* **Note 15**).

### 3.2. Quantitative PCR Reaction (see also Subheading 4.)

1. Program the thermocycler:

   | 1 | cycle | 94°C | 2 min |
   |---|---|---|---|
   | | | 55°C | 2 min |
   | | | 72°C | 2 min |
   | 30 | cycles | 94°C | 30 s |
   | | | 55°C | 30 s |
   | | | 72°C | 90 s extension +1-s/cycle |
   | 1 | cycle | 72°C | 5 min |

   Preheat the thermocycler to 94°C (*see* **Note 16**).
2. On a tray with crushed ice, pipet 1 μL of DNA preparation into the reaction tubes (*see* **Notes 17** and **18**).
3. Add an additional tube with 1 μL placenta DNA preparation in bidistilled sterile water as single copy control.
4. Add an additional tube with 1 μL bidistilled sterile water as contamination control (*see* **Note 19**).
5. On a tray with crushed ice prepare the master mix (*see* **Note 20**):
6. Determine the multiplication factor (*MF*) using the following formula: $MF$ = (number of samples+2)*1.1 (e.g., 30 samples => MF=(30+2)*1.1 = 35.2) (*see* **Note 21**).
7. On crushed ice, in a plastic reaction tube with a volume greater than MF*99 μL pipet in the following order:
   79*$MF$ μL bidistilled sterile water
   10*$MF$ μL 10X PCR reaction buffer
   2*$MF$ μL dNTP mix
   2*$MF$ μL Primer PC03
   2*$MF$ μL Primer KM38
   2*$MF$ μL Primer HER2a
   2*$MF$ μL Primer HER2b
   2*$MF$ U *Taq* polymerase

8. Immediately after adding the *Taq* polymerase vortex gently and add 99 µL of the master mix to each sample, without taking them out of the ice (*see* **Note 22**).
9. Close the caps of the reaction tubes, take them out of the ice, and put them directly in the preheated (94°C) thermocycler (*see* **Note 23**).
10. Start the program.

### 3.3. Gel Electrophoresis (see Note 24)

Standard agarose gel electrophoresis is performed with the PCR products.

1. Prepare a 3% low-melting agarose gel in 1X TAE (*see* **Note 25**).
2. Pipet 2 µL 10x loading buffer into 18 µL PCR products (*see* **Note 26**).
3. Load the gel with this mix.
4. Load one slot with the molecular-weight standard (*see* **Note 27**).
5. Run the gel in 1X TAE with an electric field strength of 5–10 V/cm for about 1 h at room temperature (*see* **Note 28**).

### 3.4. Detection and Densitometry (see Note 29)

1. Visualize the gel with a 302 UV transilluminator.
2. Take a picture of the gel with video or photo equipment.
3. Perform densitometry of the bands.

### 3.5. Calculation of the Results (see Note 30)

1. Determine the signal strength ratio of the 98 bp product (c-*erbB-2*) and the 168 bp product (reference gene: β-globin) for each sample.
2. In the same way, determine the signal-strength ratio for placenta DNA.
3. Divide the sample ratios from **step 1** by the placenta ratio from **step 2**.
4. The result is the amplification of the c-*erbB-2* gene in relation to β-globin.

## 4. Notes

1. It is advisable to produce the PCR reagents (except *Taq* polymerase) in greater amounts in higher concentrations (e.g., fivefold) and to store aliquots of these stock solutions at –20°C. In this form, they are stable up to 2 yr. When a new aliquot is needed, simply add the amount of bidistilled sterile water needed for the ready-to-use concentration to the aliquot. Vortex thoroughly to homogenize the solution.
2. Although the system was adjusted to the specified reaction buffer and *Taq* polymerase, it may also work with commercially available PCR reaction buffers and *Taq* polymerase from other companies.
3. Primers were synthesized by several companies; they all worked equally well.
4. The specified concentrations serve for most tissue preparations. However, sometimes in unusual tissues, adaptation of parameters may be necessary. If no or unspecific PCR products are obtained with these conditions, $MgCl_2$ concentration may be varied from 10 m$M$ to 50 m$M$, KCl can be decreased to 0.05$M$, gelatine can be omitted in the 10X PCR reaction buffer.
5. For the quantification of c-*erbB-2* amplification the β-globin gene serves as reference gene. The primers PC03 (5′ACACAACTGTGTTCACTAGC3′) and KM38 (5′TGG TCTCCTTAAACCTGTCTT3′) yield a 168 bp product as published previously (*7*). c-*erbB-2* primers *HER2a* (5′CCTCTGACGTCCATCATCTC3′) and *HER2b* (5′ATCTT CTGCTGCCGTCGCTT3′) are computer designed and derive from sequences flanking the transmembrane region. They result in a 98 bp product.

6. Because PCR is a molecular technique that does not need highly purified sample material, the purification techniques for different types of tissue are similar and uncomplicated. Cell break-up is followed by proteolytic digestion of nucleic acid-bound proteins such as histones to make the DNA accessible to *Taq* polymerase, the DNA synthesis enzyme of PCR. Sometimes it is even possible to omit the cell lysis step and to use the tissue directly for digestion.

7. If tissue or cultured cells are not used immediately for histologic fixation or PCR analysis, they should be frozen in liquid nitrogen immediately after biopsy or harvest, because DNases released by cell autolysis may degrade cell DNA.

8. In general, it is possible to use paraffin-embedded tissue sections with any histologic tissue fixation. However, best results are obtained with unbuffered formalin.

9. Sometimes it is possible to use the paraffin-embedded tissue sections directly in the PCR reaction without further purification. Although this technique is very simple and rapid, the yields are poor and the resulting electrophoresis bands may be smeared by side products and cell proteins.

10. Caution, this is the most dangerous step in the purification: vapor pressure of isooctane at 70°C can pop the cap of the reaction tube. Although the evaporation of some isooctane does not interfere with the purification, isooctane and its vapors are highly flammable.

11. Be careful not to discard the pellet. Sometimes the pellet is very small and tends to float on the surface of isooctane. In this case, use a pipet to discard the isooctane.

12. The dried pellet is easily whirled up if the centrifuge is ventilated, therefore first ventilate, then stop the centrifuge. Alternatively, the pellets can be dried for 1 h upside down at room temperature on a sheet of paper, but be careful not to loose the pellet.

13. Although vortexing is not essential, it enhances the digestion. The incubation time can be extended up to 12 h without damage to the DNA.

14. An incomplete deactivation of proteinase K interferes with the PCR reaction by digestion of *Taq* polymerase by proteinase K, so never shorten this step. However, extension of this step up to 1 h is possible.

15. The sample is stable at 4°C for about 2 wk, at –20°C for 1 yr, in liquid nitrogen for several years. Aliquot the sample before freezing because repeated thawing-freezing cycles degrade DNA, so do not use a refrozen sample. With 13.3 pg DNA per human cell (*6*), this extraction yields about 40 ng DNA/μL.

16. The specified times and temperatures refer to the sample, not to the heater, therefore actual parameters can be adjusted for different thermocyclers by measuring the temperatures inside the reaction tubes.

17. Avoid any warming of the sample, especially if primers and or *Taq* polymerase are already present in the reaction mix. Warming may result in the formation of unspecific products, such as primer dimers.

18. Although DNA from one cell is theoretically sufficient for quantitative PCR analysis, it is advisable to use at least DNA from about 3000 cells per PCR reaction.

19. If PCR products are detected in the contamination control, at least one reagent was contaminated with DNA or PCR products from previous experiments, leading to false results. If possible, always set up PCR reactions in a room separated from sample purification and gel electrophoresis. A good idea to avoid contamination is to use filter tips for the PCR reaction and a different set of pipets for DNA extraction, PCR, and gel electrophoresis.

20. A master mix is prepared to avoid fluctuations in reagent concentrations because of inexact pipeting.

21. Ten percent more than needed is prepared because especially with large sample numbers one may run out of master mix if the pipets and tips are not 100% exact.

22. After addition of *Taq* polymerase, work as fast as possible. Even at 0°C *Taq* polymerase has a certain activity. Because DNA duplex formation at 0°C is very nonspecific, this may lead to nonspecific products.

23. This technique is called "hot-start." Any nonspecific DNA duplexes formed during preparation are destroyed before the *Taq* polymerase achieves high activity.

24. The conditions specified in this section are not crucial. Wide variations are possible.

25. The use of other low-melting agaroses is possible. However, the concentration of the gel should be kept at 3%.

26. The amount of reaction products loaded on the gel depends on the yield of the reaction and the linearity of detection. A good volume to start with is 18 µL. Any loading buffer can be used.

27. Any length standard can be used, as long as it covers the length of the PCR products (98 and 168 bp).

28. With cooling, it is possible to rise the field up to 15 V/cm for half an hour. However, the bands are less sharp.

29. It is important to determine the linearity range of gel detection, imaging, and densitometry. First, determine the linearity of densitometry. Frequently, you can find the linear range in the technical specifications of the densitometer. Usual values are up to 2 OD or 4 OD. Any scanned image must be under this upper limit. Peaks with higher maxima than the linearity range have a plateau. The next step is to determine the linearity of the imaging unit, i.e., a photo or an digitalized video image. The signal strength of the highest peak must be always lower than upper linearity limit of densitometry. Capture images of a bright band on the same gel with different exposure times or apertures. Draw the density of the band vs the amount of light emitted (calculated form apertures or exposure times) and determine the upper linear density limit. Gel detection linearity is measured by loading different amounts of DNA (e.g., from the length standard) on the same gel and to determine the signal strengths of corresponding bands. Adjust the exposure time and/or the aperture so that the signal of the brightest band is lower than the upper linear density limit. DNA amount vs signal strength leads to the upper linear gel detection limit. For the evaluation, only use signal strengths that are lower than all three upper linear limits. If a signal is too strong, first try to reduce aperture or exposure time. If it is then lower than the upper linear density limit, but still higher than the upper linear gel detection limit, you have to repeat the electrophoresis with less PCR product. Because densitometers have usually a wider linearity range than imaging units, this procedures are sufficient to give linear densitometry signals.

30. Placenta ratio should theoretically be 1.0, but ranges from about 0.7–1.4 because of different reactivity of PCR primers.

## References

1. Slamon, D. J., Clark, G. M., Wong, S. G., Levin, W. J., Ullrich, A., and McGuire, W. L. (1987) Human breast cancer: correlation of relapse and survival with amplification of the HER-2/neu oncogene. *Science* **235,** 177–181.

2. Dobianer, K., Zhao, M., Kury, F., Schemper, M., Jakesz, R., Reiner, G., et al. (1992) Prognostic implication of growth factors and oncogenes in mammary carcinoma, in *Senology* Elsevier Science, New York, pp. 235–240.

3. Dobianer, K., Hruza, Ch., Ehrlich, G., Sevelda, P., Czerwenka, K., Soreq, H., et al. (1995) HER-2 amplification but not butyrylcholinesterase (BCHE) mutability reflects aggressiveness of European-originated ovarian tumors. *Gynecol. Oncol.* **56,** 200–206.

4. Stühlinger, M., Rosen, A., Dobianer, K., Hruza, Ch., Helmer, H., Kein, M., et al. (1995) HER-2 oncogene is not amplified in primary carcinoma of the fallopian tube. *Oncology* **52,** 397–399.

5. Medl, M., Sevelda, P., Czerwenka, K., Dobianer, K., Hanak, H., Hruza, Ch., et al. (1995) DNA Amplification of HER-2/neu and INT-2 oncogenes in epithelial ovarian cancer. *Gynecol. Oncol.* **59,** 321–326.

6. Innis, M. A., Gelfand, D. H., Sninsky, J. J., and White, T. J. (1989) *PCR protocols—A guide to methods and applications.* Academic, New York.
7. Saiki, R. K., Gelfand, D. H., Stoffel, S., Scharf, S. J., Higuchi, R., Horn, G. T., et al. (1987) Primer-directed enzymatic amplification of DNA with a thermostable DNA polymerase. *Science* **239,** 487–491.

# VI

## mRNA Analysis

# mRNA Analyses

*A Technical Overview*

## John M. S. Bartlett

## 1. Introduction

This section deals with techniques of mRNA analysis, both qualitative and quantitative. The technical details for the techniques described in this section are included in the chapters themselves. In this overview, some of the fundamentals that researchers need to understand in approaching this area are highlighted. This is by no means exhaustive, but the aim is to provide an overview of some basic techniques that can be applied to analysis of gene expression, both in cell lines and in tumor biopsies. Detailed descriptions of the practical background of a wide range of molecular techniques can be found in most molecular biology texts. Further protocols can be found in other volumes from this series, which cover specifically the areas of differential display *(1)*, oligonucleotide primed *in situ* synthesis (PRINS) and polymerase chain reaction (PCR) *in situ (2)*, and basic PCR protocols *(3,4)*. Further protocols are also available on the World Wide Web (e.g., **ref. 5**).

As with any such research approach, it is imperative that the researcher have a clear goal in mind at the outset of the experimental procedure and that the techniques selected to achieve that goal are appropriate. There are, therefore, a few basic principles that bear stating at this stage prior to the examination of the techniques available in this area.

The most significant principle, commonly overlooked by those researching RNA expression, is that although proteins are effectors, RNA is a blueprint. In examining the expression of RNA molecules, one gains insight into the regulation of expression and stability of the RNA species under examination and extrapolates this into an understanding of the regulation of the protein derived from this RNA blueprint. It is important that this extrapolation is made with care. As with any blueprint, the existence of the blueprint does not prove the material for which its codes has been produced and conversely, failure to detect the template does not mean the protein is not present. It is therefore essential to link RNA analyses with analyses of protein expression and function.

In addition, owing to the extreme sensitivity of modern analytical techniques, especially PCR, it is possible to detect extremely low copy numbers of mRNA species

From: *Methods in Molecular Medicine, Vol. 39: Ovarian Cancer: Methods and Protocols*
Edited by: J. M. S. Bartlett © Humana Press, Inc., Totowa, NJ

within cell populations and the relative importance of these molecules must be related to the copy numbers detected. Indeed, with such sensitive methods available, the possibility of stromal or other contamination sources must be borne in mind. In common with all analytical techniques, it is imperative that the composition of the tumor tissue under examination be understood before correct interpretation can be carried out. This is particularly important in solution phase studies where mRNA is extracted from entire tissues and the possibility of incorrectly assigning expression to tumor, rather than stromal, components exist.

So why use mRNA analyses at all? There are a number of significant advantages to mRNA analyses over conventional protein analyses, affecting sensitivity, ease of execution, sample throughput, and evaluation of expression levels.

The advent of the reverse transcriptase polymerase chain reaction (RT-PCR) increased sensitivity of mRNA detection fold significantly when compared with Northern blots or RNase protection assays (RPA). The ability to detect copies of mRNA in the low hundreds [attomolar ($10^{-21}$M) range (6)] meant that the amounts of tissue required could be reduced significantly, or conversely the number of products screened could be increased. Using modern PCR systems it is now feasible to PCR up to 384 reactions in a 2–3 hour incubation, providing sufficient throughput for most screening applications. Furthermore, the use of reverse transcription of mRNA to stabilize material for long term storage is an additional advantage of this approach (7,8).

Because detecting the expression of mRNA transcripts is an important first step in any investigation, questions relating to level of expression, regulation, and location (tumor or stroma, proliferative or nonproliferative cells) are immediately raised. mRNA studies are extremely powerful for the detection of dynamic changes in expression within and between cell populations. Quantification of expression (either with respect to an internal control or with full molar quantification) can be performed using Northern blotting, RNase protection assays, or increasingly with RT-PCR (7–10). These methods can be applied to the study of differential expression between tissues and induction or clearance of mRNA species. Although care is required in the individual experimental design, mRNA studies give an immediate and sensitive method for the investigation of dynamics of gene expression.

Increasingly, conventional targeted strategies for comparing expression between tissues are being expanded to provide global comparisons of gene expression between, for example, neoplastic and nonneoplastic tissues. Formally, the domain of those able to perform complex RNA subtraction library analyses with the recent development of techniques relating to differential display (displaying the RNA profiles from separate sources and noting differences) has been widely applied to the study of tumor-specific gene regulation. Such techniques are reliant on careful validation of the approach taken by repeat experiments using targeted sequences (e.g., PCR or RPA). However, these techniques can be immensely powerful in the detection of novel or known genes that are up- or downregulated in transformed tissues (11,12).

All the aforementioned techniques can be compromised by the fact that all tissues are not homogeneous in their cellular composition. The presence of blood vessels, inflammatory cells, stromal components, and a mixture of tumor and normal tissue cells can complicate analyses. It is imperative, at some stage of the investigation to determine the tissue source of the mRNA detected in order to avoid ascribing a tumor origin to a stromal protein or mRNA. The ability to use both archival (paraffin embedded) and fresh (frozen) material has been the major advantage to the development of *in situ* hybridization techniques involving mRNA detection. Whereas sensitivity can be compromised, the ability to localize gene products and also to make use of archival material with significant patient follow-data, makes this an extremely attractive approach. Recent developments in the technique of *in situ* RT-PCR, have overcome many of the sensitivity issues, meaning that cellular localization of gene products is now achievable with the sensitivity and specificity of the PCR technique.

Each individual approach will present specific problems, which must be sufficiently addressed to allow accurate and reliable data to be gathered if the effort expended is to be worthwhile. The sections below cover, in broad outline, the technical challenges relating to the approaches described hereafter.

## 2. RT-PCR

The reverse transcriptase polymerase chain reaction (RT-PCR) is now arguably the method most commonly used for detection of mRNA species. It is essentially a two-stage technique, the first of which, reverse transcription, is required in order to exploit the sensitivity and specificity of the second (PCR).

Reverse transcription comprises the transcription of the mRNA of choice into DNA (more accurately termed copy DNA or cDNA). This stage of the reaction is performed using RNA virus enzymes whose role in vivo is to transcribe viral RNA genome into a template for host transcription systems. The earliest RT enzymes used were derived from the Molony murine leukaemia virus (Mo-MLV reverse transcriptase) and the avian myeloblastosis virus (AMV reverse transcriptase). More recently, genetically modified forms of these enzymes with enhanced activity have become the agents of choice. The enzymes are relatively heat labile (particularly in comparison to *Taq* polymerase and reactions are performed at 42°C with mRNA and nucleotides). The reaction must be "primed," as the enzymes are dependent upon double-stranded nucleic acid template. The primer is usually allowed to anneal to the RNA following a short incubation (in the absence of enzyme) at 85°C to denature RNA tertiary structure. Primer selection is very important. Either a primer specific for the target sequence may be used or, more commonly, primers targeted at copying the entire mRNA population can be employed. The use of poly (dT) primers will target mRNA poly A tails and transcribe from this point. In this case, between 2–4 kilobases of cDNA can be routinely copied, which may place a constraint on PCR primer design. RNA can be transcribed with random hexanucleotide primers (more efficient than poly dT and produce cDNAs from the entire RNA pool), however, in this case separation of mRNA from ribosomal and transfer RNAs is recommended as these will also be copied diluting the target sequences *(13,14)*. The cDNA produced is then utilized for multiple PCRs using specific sequence primers.

A further novel development has been the use of rTth DNA polymerase (from the bacterium *Thermus thermophilus*), which allows reverse transcription and PCR to be performed in a single reaction tube using this thermostable DNA polymerase with reverse transcriptase activity. Use of higher temperatures for the RT step with this system allows more efficient transcription, particularly from mRNAs with high GC content *(3,4)*.

PCR involves the geometric amplification of specific regions of DNA (or cDNA) using a thermocycling chain reaction. Using this system, it is possible to produce millions of copies from a single cDNA template. The reaction is therefore extremely sensitive and can be highly robust and allows high throughput. However, there are a number of steps of the PCR reaction, which must be carefully optimized (even when working from published primer sequences) before successful PCR can be achieved.

The aspects of the PCR reaction that are most likely to influence the efficiency and specificity are (in order or importance) PCR primers, *Tm* (annealing temperature), magnesium chloride concentration, buffer system, and enzyme concentration. Of these, PCR primers are by far the most critical component of any PCR. As with the RT step of the reaction priming, it is essential to allow DNA synthesis to occur. With the PCR, amplification is achieved using a pair of PCR primers targeted on complementary DNA strands. The PCR "product" is then delimited by these two primers and becomes both the target for, and product of, further cycles of amplification *(3–5)*. Primers are generally between 16–30 bases long. The two primers should both have a G/C content of approximately 50% and similar (or identical) melting temperatures (*Tm* is the temperature at which 50% of the primer is bound to DNA). The *Tm* is usually calculated by a complex formula, which takes into account both the base composition (% G/C) and the sequence and is usually quoted with the synthesis report supplied with commercially supplied primers. However, a rough guide can be given from the formula: $Tm = 81.5°C + 16.6(\log_{10}[Na^+]) + 0.41(\%G + C) - 675/n$, $[Na^+]$ = molar salt concentration ($Na^+ = K^+$ in PCR buffer) and $n$ = oligonucleotide length (bases) *(14)*. Care should be taken to avoid stretches of any nucleotide of more than 2–3 bases (especially at the 3' end). Secondary structures such as loops or primer dimerization sites should be avoided. Primer design can also be optimized to reduce artefacts arising from contamination. In the case of RT-PCR, genomic DNA can often be carried over in the purification of RNA. To avoid false positive signals resulting from the amplification of such DNA, it is possible to perform a digest with RNase free DNase preparations. However, this involves further enzyme steps while RNA is in a highly labile form. Designing PCR primers to span introns will both reduce the amplification of genomic DNA and provide a means of distinguishing such contamination from the RNA/cDNA product of interest. It cannot be overstressed at this point that the single most common reason for poor PCR results is poor primer design.

The quoted melting temperature of PCR primers is rarely, if ever, the optimal annealing temperature for use in PCR reactions. A general principle is to set the annealing temperature approximately 5°C below the *Tm* of the primers in use. Where this results in false priming (demonstrated by the production of multiple bands in the PCR reaction) the reaction can be optimized by raising the annealing temperature, reducing the magnesium chloride concentration, modifying the buffer conditions, or modifying the enzyme concentration.

The magnesium chloride concentration is critical to the PCR reaction. The thermostable DNA polymerases are members of the family of magnesium dependent ATPases. At low magnesium concentrations, enzyme activity is virtually absent. However, at high magnesium concentrations, magnesium ions can bind to the negatively charged backbone of DNA and produce sites that prevent primer binding or lead to mismatches in primer binding. Therefore, it is necessary for each individual PCR reaction to optimize the magnesium ion concentration. This optimization is essentially a playoff between efficiency of enzyme action and specificity of primer annealing, for most reactions magnesium chloride concentrations between 0.5–4.0 *mM* will be optimal.

Buffer compositions vary both in salt concentration and in pH. There are implications for variations on enzyme activity, but more particularly, on annealing temperature (*see* formula above). It is unlikely that a "homemade" mix will improve a PCR that cannot be optimized using proprietary buffers. Varying the enzyme concentration will have a similar overall effect to variation of magnesium concentration. High concentrations of enzyme will allow production of false priming products, whereas low concentrations will reduce the amount of specific product produces. Overall, however, the effect of varying enzyme concentrations is relatively minor.

Various modifications of the PCR, such as "touch down" and "hot-start" PCR can be employed to improve specificity of the primer annealing. However, often the most effective means of improving PCR selectivity and specificity is to redesign the primers used (*3,4,14*).

As it can be surmised, the value of RT-PCR for the identification will be as much a direct consequence of the amount of care given to the validation of the reaction itself as it is of the care taken in tissue and patient selection.

## 3. Quantitative RT-PCR

All the caveats applied to the PCR reaction itself (*see* **Subheading 2.**) and to the quantification of PCR products (*see* Chapter 48) are valid when approaching the quantification of RT-PCR reactions with the additional problem of the reverse transcription step. Critical to the determination of RNA concentrations for a specific mRNA species are the cellularity of the tissue, the purity of the mRNA, and use of internal and external standards (*3,4,6,15,16*).

The first of these issues is one over which the researcher has little control, unless established cell-culture models are being used, but one that must be addressed. Take for example, two tissue samples: one expressing 100 copies of mRNA "X" and the other expressing 300 copies of the same mRNA. Superficially, we might conclude that the second sample expresses higher levels of the tumor specific mRNA than the first. Now assume that sample 1 is comprised of 10% tumor, whereas sample 2 is 95% tumor material. In this case, it would be clear that tumor levels of mRNA "X" were, in fact, greater in sample 1 than in sample 2. However, accurate and valid the method of quantification is, failure to determine the tumor/stroma ratio in the sample can result in erroneous conclusions being drawn. This principle applies equally to analyses performed by RNase protection assays, Northerns, or indeed differential display techniques (*see* Chapters 47 and 50).

The quality of mRNA extracted is an issue that might have been addressed earlier, however, the supreme sensitivity of the PCR technique makes this less of a problem than in the case of enzymic amplification prior to quantification. Even with conventional and proprietary mRNA extraction techniques some carry over of polymerase or transcriptase inhibitors can be observed. In extreme cases, this may reduce the efficiency of the RT-PCR to an extent which causes errors in quantification. Every effort should therefore be made to ensure that mRNA preparations for quantification are as pure as possible.

*Quantification* of mRNA by the RT-PCR method can apparently be achieved relatively easily by simply comparing the intensity of products following RT-PCR of, for example, c-*erbB-2* and GAPDH. However, whereas this approach may be acceptable for semiquantitative analysis of gene copy number there are more problems associated with quantification of RT-PCR products in this way. First, the differences in expression levels may be much more divergent (50–100-fold vs 2–4-fold). Second, such an approach takes no account of the considerable potential variation in reverse transcription rates for different gene products. The recommended approach to quantification using RT-PCR is to either separate the RT and PCR or assess efficiency of each separately *(15)* or to combine these assessments by using mRNA control templates *(17,18)*. Both these techniques require extensive molecular modification of both the control and target gene sequence and are therefore omitted from this section.

## 4. RNase Protection Assays (RPA) and Northern Blots

Northern blotting techniques are a derivative of the DNA blotting procedures originally developed by Southern. RNA fragments are denatured and size separated on agarose gels by electrophoresis. The RNA "ladder" is then transferred, usually onto "nitrocellulose" by the process of Northern blotting. Probes specific for the species of mRNA of interest are labeled and hybridized to the membrane to detect full-length mRNAs that can be sized by reference to 28S, 18S, and 5S ribosomal RNA bands (which can also be used for assessment of mRNA quality). By assessing the amount of RNA signal-bound relative concentrations between differing RNA species can be assessed. By comparison with many more "modern" methods this approach is now time consuming and cumbersome. Nonetheless, it has the value that it detects and sizes mRNA species (not normally a function of either PCR or RPA) and can therefore be used to isolate complete novel transcripts from mRNA pools.

RNase protection assays provide a level of sensitivity some 20–50-fold greater than Northern blots, and can be used to accurately identify and quantify different mRNA species within gene families even when a high degree of sequence homology exists. Sequence homology between, for example, FGFs, TGFβs, and c-*erbB1-4* mRNAs is extremely high. Identification of gene superfamily members by Northern is often complicated by crosshybridization of probes. In the RNase protection assay, detection of mRNA relies on the formation of a RNA:RNA hybrid of absolute specificity. Single-stranded RNA is digested with a single strand-specific RNase mixture and even single basepair mismatches will lead to loss of hybridization signal. Therefore, this technique provides a readily quantifiable means of detecting multiple RNA species, either individually or simultaneously.

Northern blots require relatively little equipment to perform, although electroblotting is now the method of choice for RNA transfer, capillary transfer remains highly efficient for most applications. Therefore, this technique can be readily carried out using a flat-bed electrophoresis system and a reasonable radioactive facility. With the advent of biotin-labeled probes, even the latter is now less common.

Most problems encountered with Northern blotting approaches relate to the specific hybridization of the probe and subsequent detection. The stringency (i.e., an arbitrary measure of specificity) of probe hybridization to the membrane and of post hybridization washes is governed by salt and formamide concentrations and by temperature *(13,14)*. Increasing temperature and formamide concentration will decrease hybridization (i.e., increase stringency), whereas decreasing salt concentration will have the same effect. The use of formamide can enable high stringency washes to be performed at relatively low temperatures. The optimum DNA:DNA hybridization temperature can be defined by the following formula: $T = 81.5°C + 16.6(\log 10[Na^+]) + 0.41(\%G + C) - 820/l - 0.6(\%F) - 1.4(\%mismatch)$. In this formula $[Na^+]$ = molar salt concentration, $l$ = probe length (bases), $\%F$ = % formamide, % mismatch = % noncomplementary basepairs between hybridizing strands (13,14). For applications such as use of riboprobes and the RNase protection assay systems, it should be remembered that DNA:RNA heteroduplexes and RNA:RNA duplexes are more stable and require a moderately higher *Tm*. It is common, in both Northern and Southern blotting, to use a relatively low stringency during probe hybridization to ensure that some labeling of the blot occurs and then to increase in a stepwise manner the degree of stringency in a series of posthybridization washes. In RNase protection assays, this stringency is applied by use of single-strand-specific RNases, which will digest any nonspecifically bound probe and result in the digestion of false positive signals. These assays are therefore highly specific and sensitive.

Northern blots and RNase protection assays can be readily quantified in a number of ways, the simplest of which is to use preflashed X-ray film (which sensitizes the photographic emulsion and produces a linear relationship between band intensity and counts) followed by scanning and image analysis. A cheaper, albeit more labor-intensive method for quantification involves using the film as a template to excise and count the bands of interest. In either case, unless a range of standards of known mRNA concentration (produced from plasmids, and so on.) are included as a control, these results are at best semiquantitative (13,14).

Northern blots are relatively labor intensive and require significant effort in the validation of posthybridization washes to ensure a reproducible and clear signal. However, the membranes, once produced, can be reprobed a number of times and stored for long periods. RNase protection assays lend themselves more readily to high throughput screening of multiple transcripts simultaneously. However, when used in conjunction with radioactively labeled probes, these assays used large amounts of radioactivity. Furthermore, because nonspecifically bound mRNA is digested, these techniques require relatively high levels of mRNA to be purified (1–3 (μg mRNA or 10–20 (μg total RNA per assay). They also require the synthesis of probes in specific vectors, which allow enzyme priming of RNA synthesis. Nonetheless, this method is more readily executed, quantified, and adapted to large numbers of samples than Northern blotting.

## 5. Differential Display

One of the most intriguing questions facing any researcher in the study of tissues is which genes are over/under expressed in this tissue or which are specifically expressed only within this tissue. Particularly in the field of cancer research, the ability to perform a global screen of expressed genes is of great significance in detected genes associated with tumor initiation, invasion, and metastases. Prior to 1991, these approaches were limited to those with extensive molecular biology expertise and with access to facilities which allowed the cloning and screening of large numbers of expressed genes from different tissues. Following the development of differential display techniques, *these approaches have been greatly simplified* by the application of PCR techniques to differential gene expression studies. Differential display techniques are as varied as the questions they are used to answer, however, in general they combine three separate techniques to address this single question.

1. Production of cDNA from mRNA by reverse transcription.
2. Design of arbitrary primers to allow parts of the cDNA (tags) to be amplified by PCR.
3. Use of sequencing quality resolution by acrylamide electrophoresis.

This approach builds up a "fingerprint" of the RNA species expressed in different tissue or cell samples. Comparison of these fingerprints identifies those genes that are up- or downregulated in different tissues. The technique is quite elegant in both its simplicity and power. However, as with many such techniques, the secret lies in the careful design and interpretation of the results.

The model is best suited to the study of gene regulation in tissue culture where conditions can be varied under careful control to avoid artefacts. Even then, extreme care must be taken to ensure that results are reproducible between experiments, the control of tissue-culture conditions is in fact the most critical phase of the experiment in the production of accurate differential display results. Use of tissue samples makes the approach all the more complex. Although there is obvious value in investigations seeking to identify metastasis-related gene expression, care must be taken to ensure that differences between pre- and postmetastatic tissues are related to metastasis and not a consequence of altered tumor–stroma interactions, differences between primary tumors, and so on. In addition, extreme care must be taken to ensure samples to be compared are treated exactly the same to avoid artefacts being introduced during storage, extraction, or subsequent amplification.

Once novel regulatory changes are identified using differential display techniques it remains common to doublecheck these changes using a second system, such as RPA, PCR, or Northerns, to confirm the result. This is an important confirmatory step prior to investing significant effort into the study of novel genes or gene transcripts identified by differential display (1).

Even with these caveats, differential display has already proven itself as a highly valuable system for the study of gene expression changes during neoplastic progression.

## 6. In Situ Hybridization and In Situ RT-PCR

*In situ* hybridization of mRNA has long been established as an invaluable complement to immunocytochemistry for the localization of mRNA expressing cells within tissues. As discussed above, defining changes in mRNA expression, quantifying alterations in gene expression or identification of novel genes expressed within tumor tissues is only the first half of the overall picture. Determining the site at which such gene expression occurs is equally important to an understanding of the complex interactions which are known to occur within tissue samples. In addition, use of *in situ* hybridization has meant that many mRNA studies could be extended from fresh or frozen samples to include archival material from routine pathological evaluation of tumor stage and grade. In essence, the principles of *in situ* hybridization techniques, and even of RT-PCR *in situ* are similar to those of liquid phase analysis by PCR and Northern blotting. However, there is added the further complication of seeking to identify gene expression within tissues in which the 3-dimensional architecture is intact and in which many of the contaminants (e.g., DNA and protein) normally excluded from the reaction are still present. The technical problems of both *in situ* hybridization and *in situ* RT-PCR are those of Northerns and of RT-PCR in general with these additional factors included.

*In situ* hybridization (ISH) involves production of a labeled DNA or RNA probe, introduction of the probe onto a tissue section, and access of the probe to the mRNA within cells where it hybridizes as in a Northern blot. All the discussions above relating to stringency apply equally to the technique as applied to tissue sections.

*In situ* reverse transcriptase polymerase chain reaction (*in situ* RT-PCR) represents a fairly recent application of RT-PCR to tissue sections. Essentially the RT-PCR is performed *in situ* within the cells of the tissue section. The advantage over ISH is that a markedly greater level of sensitivity can be achieved. ISH can detect between 20–200 copies of mRNA per cell whereas *in situ* RT-PCR is often able to detect single copies of mRNA per cell *(2)*. In both ISH and *in situ* RT-PCR, signal can be detected either directly by radiolabeling or fluorescently labeling the probe itself, or by use of secondary signal amplification by means of antibodies following the incorporation of biotin or some other antigen into the probe. In the case of *in situ* RT-PCR, the amplification products can also be unlabeled and detected by a secondary ISH method.

As with some immunocytochemical techniques, ISH and *in situ* RT-PCR techniques are relatively vigorous when compared with conventional histochemical stains, in order to prevent loss because of sections and cells detaching during staining coated slides are used. Either silane or TESPA (3-aminopropyltriethoxysilane) precoated microscope slides coated can be used followed by baking *(2,19)*. Once such coated slides are prepared, the crucial choice between fixed or frozen tissue sections must be addressed. Frozen tissue sections will provide a greater opportunity for detection of mRNA levels, particularly in the context of *in situ* RT-PCR, however, morphology is significantly better with fixed materials. Even with *in situ* RT-PCR the use of extremely short-length PCR products can allow the use of this technique with archival material. If fixed material is to be used, then the method of fixation must be appropriate to the technique used. Crosslinking fixatives, such as those used in most conventional pathology are preferred (e.g., formaldehyde or paraformaldehyde) *(2,19–22)*. Glutaraldehyde can be readily used for ISH, however, for *in situ* RT-PCR this fixative reduces tissue permeability. All tissues, either frozen or fixed, will require a degree of permeabilization to enable reagents to penetrate tissues to where the RNA is housed *(19–22)*.

A variety of steps are performed to enable tissue permeabilization to be optimized. Each parameter must be validated for the tissues under study. Acid exposure is thought to denature basic proteins and to reduce nonspecific binding. Detergents are used to solubilize membranes. However, by far the most significant stage in this process is the use of proteinases to remove endogenous proteins from the sections and allow reagent access. In our experience, proteinase K offers the optimal method for exposure of intracellular components. Other pretreatments may be used to reduce nonspecific binding of probes.

The use of positive and negative controls can be enhanced by incubation with DNA- or RNA-specific nucleases. In all RNA detection methods, the use of a control in which the RNA is digested as a confirmation that signal is specific to RNA hybridization is invaluable. This is naturally even more important in techniques such as *in situ* RT-PCR where the potential for signal amplification is so great.

Conventionally both ISH and PCR use isotopic methods of detection, however, these can be time consuming and delay collection of results and extend the period required for technical validation. Use of nonisotopic methods (enzymes/fluorescence) can reduce the time required for experiments to be completed and evaluated, however, such methods have their own problems. In this approach, once the DNA probe is hybridized, the problem of detection becomes an immunohistochemical one. In this case, (as described in Chapter 51) endogenous enzymes with similar activity to reporter enzymes must be inactivated and endogenous biotin must be blocked. In some cases, efforts to reduce tissue autofluorescence may also be required.

*In situ* RT-PCR conditions differ from those used for conventional RT-PCR in several ways (*see* Chapter 46). These differences must be addressed if this is technique is to be adequately validated.

## 7. Conclusions

Evaluation of mRNA expression provides much valuable information which can aid in the study of transformed and nontransformed tissues and in the direct comparison of disease and regulatory systems. Care must be taken to ensure adequate controls. Precautions are in place to prevent artefacts from compromising data. Nonetheless, RNA analysis represents an invaluable approach to the study of ovarian cancer as evidenced by significant numbers of ground breaking studies using the techniques described below.

## References

1. Liang, P. and Pardee, A. B., eds. (1998) *Differential Display Methods and Protocols*, vol. 85 (Methods in Molecular Biology) Humana, Totowa, NJ.
2. Gosden, J. R., ed. (1984) *PRINS and In Situ PCR Protocols*, vol. 71 (Methods in Molecular Biology) Humana, Totowa, NJ.
3. White B. A., ed. (1984) *PCR Protocols, Current Methods and Applications,* vol. 15 (Methods in Molecular Biology) Humana, Totowa, NJ.
4. Bartlett, J. M. S. and Stirling, D., eds. *PCR Protocols, Current Methods and Applications,* 2nd ed. (Methods in Molecular Biology) Humana, Totowa, NJ, in press.
5. US Dept. Commerce Molecular Biology Techniques Forum http://research nwfsc.noaa.gov/protocols/methods/
6. Miller, W. R., Hulme, M. J., Bartlett, J. M. S., MacCallum, J., and Dixon, J. M. (1997) Changes in messenger RNA expression of protein kinase a regulatory subunit Ialpha in breast cancer patients treated with tamoxifen. *Clinic. Cancer Res.* **3,** 2399–2404.
7. Bartlett, J. M., Langdon, S. P., Scott, W. N., Love, S. B., Miller, E. P., Katsaros, D., et al. (1997) Transforming growth factor-beta isoform expression in human ovarian tumors. *Euro. J. Cancer* **33,** 2397–2403.
8. Crickard, K., Gross, J. L., Crickard, U., Yoonessi, M., Lele, S., Herblin, W. F., and Eidsvoog, K. (1994) Basic fibroblast growth factor and receptor expression in human ovarian cancer. *Gynecol. Oncol.* **55,** 277–284.
9. Ji, H. J., Zhang, Q. Q., and Leung, B. S. (1990) Survey of oncogene and growth factor/receptor gene expression in cancer cells by intron-differential RNA/PCR. *Biochem. Biophys. Res. Commun.* **170,** 569–575
10. Jindal, S. K., Ishii, E., Letarte, M., Vera, S., Teerds, K. J., and Dorrington, J. H. (1995) Regulation of transforming growth factor alpha gene expression in an ovarian surface epithelial cell line derived from a human carcinoma. *Biol. Reprod.* **52,** 1027–1037.
11. Diachenko, L. B., Ledesma, J., Chenchik, A. A., and Siebert, P. D. (1996) Combining the technique of rna fingerprinting and differential display to obtain differentially expressed messenger-rna [full text delivery]. *Biochem. Biophys. Res. Commun.* **219,** 824–828.
12. Schneeberger, C., Eder, S., Speiser, P., and Zeillinger, R. (1996) Competitive reverse transcriptase-PCR: an improved method for determination of c-erbB-2 gene expression. *Anticancer Res.* **16,** 849–852.

13. Sambrook, J., Fritsch, E. F., and Maniatis, T. (1989) *Molecular Cloning: A Laboratory Manual.* Cold Spring Harbor Laboratory Press, Cold Spring Harbor, New York, NY.
14. Doyle, K., ed. (1996) Protocols and applications guide. Promega Corp., Madison, WI (available free of charge).
15. Bartlett, J. M. S., Hulme, M. J., and Miller, W. R. (1996) Analysis of cAMP RI-alpha messenger-RNA expression in breast-cancer—evaluation of quantitative polymerase chain-reaction for routine use. *Brit. J. Cancer* **73,** 1538–1544.
16. Underwood, M. A., Bartlett, J. M. S., and Cooke, T. G. (1994) An improved method for semiquantification of gene amplification from archival material. *PCR Meth. Applicat.* **4,** 178–184.
17. Peck, K., Sher, Y-P., Shih, J-Y., Roffler, S. R., Wu, C. W., and Yang, P-C. (1998) Detection and quantitation of circulating cancer cells in the peripheral blood of lung cancer patients. *Cancer Res.* **58,** 2761–2765.
18. Ozawa, K., Seo, M., and Imamura, T. (1997) A quantitative method for evaluation of FGF family and FGF receptor family gene expression by RT-PCR. *Brain Res. Protocols* **1,** 211–216.
19. Waller, H. A. and Savage, A. K. (1994) Analysis of gene transcription *in situ*: methodological considerations and applications in pathology. *J. Histotechnol.* **17,** 203–218
20. Lewis, F. (1996) *An Approach to in situ PCR.* PE Applied Biosystems, CA.
21. Nuovo, G. J., Gallery, F., Hom, R., MacConnell, P., and Bloch, W. (1993) Importance of different variables for enhancing *in situ* detection of PCR-amplified DNA. *PCR Meth. Applicat.* **2,** 305–312.
22. O'Leary, J. J., Browne, G., Landers, R. J., Crowley, M., Healy, I. B., Street, J. T., et al. (1994) The importance of fixation procedures on DNA template and its suitability for solution-phase polymerase chain reaction and PCR *in situ* hybridization. *Histochem. J.* **26,** 337–346.

# 45

## *In Situ* Hybridization Detection of TGF-β mRNA

### Anders Gobl and Rudi Henriksen

### 1. Introduction

Immunohistochemical techniques and molecular hybridization enable demonstration of specific proteins and DNA or RNA sequences, respectively. *In situ* hybridization is a variant of molecular hybridization that allows detection of specific DNA or RNA sequences in tissue sections or cell preparations, as well as in chromosome preparations and was first described by Pardue and Gall *(1)*. Basically, a single-stranded probe of mRNA or DNA containing complementary sequences are hybridized to RNA or DNA in the sample. The probe is radioactively or nonisotopically labeled for localization and eventually quantification of the product.

Single-stranded antisense RNA probes (riboprobes) harbor several advantages compared to DNA probes. Being single stranded, riboprobes do not reanneal in solution, cRNA–mRNA hybrids have been reported to be more stable than cDNA–mRNA hybrids *(2)*, competitive hybridization to the complementary strand is not possible, and RNase treatment can digest unhybridized probe. These advantages contribute to a very high sensitivity and low background. Finally, being an expression of gene function, detection of transcripts in several occasions will be preferable to DNA hybridization.

In this chapter, we shall focus on detection of TGF-β mRNA by *in situ* hybridization. TGF-β is a growth factor family playing several roles in physiology and pathology (for some recent reviews *see* **refs.** *3* and *4*). *In situ* hybridization allows cellular localization for the production of the single members of the family and have thereby contributed to understanding their role in biology. Recent examples illustrating the significance of *in situ* hybridization detection of TGF-β mRNA in various aspects of nonmalignant *(5–7)* as well as malignant *(8–10)* biological conditions have been included in the reference list.

### 2. Materials
#### 2.1. Preparation of Slides

1. Paraformaldehyde/PBS (Sigma, St. Louis, MO P-6148). Add 4 g of paraformaldehyde to 100 mL PBS (pH 7.4) in an Erlenmeyer flask and cover it with aluminum foil. In a fume hood, heat the mixture until the paraformaldehyde dissolves (just before boiling). Cool

From: *Methods in Molecular Medicine, Vol. 39: Ovarian Cancer: Methods and Protocols*
Edited by: J. M. S. Bartlett © Humana Press, Inc., Totowa, NJ

down to room temperature and filter the solution through a 0.45-μm filter. Store at +4°C for not more than 1 mo.

2. Silanized Glass-slides. Rinse the slides with water and let them dry. Treat the slides for 5 min with 2% silane (Sigma, A-3648) solution (dilute with acetone). Then wash the slides twice with acetone and twice with water, air-dry, and store at room temperature.

## 2.2. cDNA Probes

1. A 1050-bp *Eco*RI fragment of TGF-β1 cloned in pBluescript (Stratagene, La Jolla, CA) *(11)* (*see* **Note 1**).
2. A 2.3-kb *Eco*RI fragment of TGF-β2 cloned in pBluescript *(12)*.
3. A 463-bp *Kpn*I-*Eco*RI of TGF-β3 cloned in pBluescript *(13)*.
4. A 499-bp *Bam*HI-*Hin*dIII fragment of latent TGF-β1 binding protein cloned in pGEM3 (Promega, Madison, WI) *(14)*.
5. To check the integrity of cellular RNA, tissue sections were hybridized with β-actin probe made from a 1.7-kb *Bam*HI cDNA fragment cloned in pSP65 (Promega) *(15)*.

## 2.3. cRNA Probes

1. 5X *in vitro* transcription buffer for T7 RNA polymerase: 0.2$M$ Tris-HCl (pH 8.0), 40 m$M$ MgCl$_2$, 10 m$M$ spermidine-(HCl), 125 m$M$ NaCl. Store at –20°C.
2. 5X *in vitro* transcription buffer for SP6 RNA polymerase: 0.2$M$ Tris-HCl (pH 7.9), 30 m$M$ MgCl$_2$, 10 m$M$ spermidine-(HCl). Store at –20°C.
3. r(AGC)TP, 5 m$M$ solution is made from 100-m$M$ stock solutions of ATP, GTP, and CTP (Amersham-Pharmacia Biotech, Uppsala, Sweden) using water. Store at –20°C.
4. [$^{35}$S]-UTPαS, 20 mCi/mL, >1000 Ci/mmol (Amersham-Pharmacia Biotech, SJ 603). Store at –80°C. Handle in a fume hood because [$^{35}$S] isotopes can give off radioactive SO$_2$ gas.
5. T7 or SP6 RNA polymerase, 50 U/mL, and 15 U/mL, respectively. Use 0.5–1 μL per reaction.
6. 10X DNase I buffer. 0.1$M$ Tris-HCl (pH 7.5), 50 m$M$ MgSO$_4$. Store at –20°C.
7. *Escherichia coli* tRNA (Boehringer Mannheim, Mannheim, Germany). Make 10 mg/mL stock solution in water. Store at –20°C.
8. Ammonium acetate, 4$M$. Dissolve 154.2 g ammonium acetate in 500 mL water. Store at room temperature.
9. RNase free DNase I, (10 U/μL; Boehringer Mannheim). Store at –20°C.
10. RNasin, RNase inhibitor (40 U/μL; Promega). Store at –20°C.

## 2.4. In Situ Hybridization

1. Diethyl pyrocarbonate (DEPC)-treated 20X SSC stock solution. Per liter: Dissolve 175.3 g NaCl and 88.2 g Na-citrate and adjust the pH to 7.0. Add 1 mL DEPC (Sigma, D-5758) and shake well. Incubate overnight at room temperature or 37°C. Autoclave and store at room temperature.
2. 10X Triethanolamine (TEA) solution (Sigma, T 1377). Measure 133 mL TEA and add H$_2$O up to 800 mL. Mix and adjust pH to 8.0 with HCl. Add water to 1 L. Autoclave and store at room temperature.
3. 10X Tris-Glycine solution. 1$M$ Tris-HCl (pH 7.0) containing 1$M$ glycine. Autoclave and store at room temperature.
4. Acetylation mixture. Just before use, add acetic anhydride (Sigma, A-6404) to 0.25% in 1X TEA. Mix well.
5. Sheared salmon testes DNA (Sigma, D-1626). Dissolve DNA in water at a concentration of 10 mg/mL. This usually takes about 12 h. Shear the DNA by passing it 10–15 times rapidly through a 18-gage needle. Extract the DNA twice with phenol-chloroform and

then precipitate with 2 vol of ethanol. Recover the DNA by centrifugation and redissolve in water. Determine the exact concentration by measuring the optical density at 260 nm. Then boil the solution for 10 min and store at –20°C in aliquots.

6. Formamide buffer. 50% formamide, 2X SSC, and 10 m*M* dithiothreitol (DTT; Sigma, D-9779. Make 1*M* stock solution in water). Can be made in advance. Store at room temperature. Add DTT just before use.

7. Hybridization mixture. Per 1 mL: 500 µL formamide containing 20% dextran sulfate (Amersham-Pharmacia Biotech), 100 µL 20X SSC, 100 µL 10-mg/mL *E. coli* tRNA (Boehringer Mannheim), 100 µL 10-mg/mL sheared salmon sperm DNA, 100 µL 20-mg/mL RNase free BSA (Sigma, B-8894), 100 µL 1*M* DTT. Can be made in advance (50–100 mL) and stored at –20°C.

8. RNase A solution. Stock solution of RNase A (Boehringer). Dissolve RNase A at a concentration of 10 mg/mL in 10 m*M* Tris-HCl (pH 7.5), 1 m*M* EDTA. Store at –20°C. RNase A is diluted with 2X SSC to a final concentration of 20 µg/mL just before use.

## 2.5. Autoradiography

1. NTB-2 nuclear track emulsion (Eastman Kodak, Rochester, NY).

# 3. Methods

## 3.1. Preparation of Slides

1. Make 4-µm tissue sections using a cryostat and washed, silane-treated glass-slides.
2. Fix tissue sections for 5 min at room temperature in 4% paraformaldehyde/PBS.
3. Transfer slides to cuvettes containing 70% ethanol. Store at +4°C for up to 3 mo.

## 3.2. Labeling of RNA Probes

1. Assemble the following components in a 1.5-mL or 0.5-mL microfuge tube at room temperature: 1.2 µL 5X transcription buffer (SP6 or T7), 2.5 µL (50 µCi) [$^{35}$S-UTP, 0.5 µL r(AGC)TP, 1 µL (100 ng-1 µg) linearized DNA template, and 0.8 µL RNA polymerase (SP6 or T7). Final reaction volume is 6 µL (*see* **Note 2**).
2. Incubate in an air incubator at 37°C for 60-120 minutes (*see* **Note 3**).
3. To the reaction, add 50 µL solution containing 1X DNase buffer, 1 µL DNase I (10 U/µL), and 0.5 µL RNasin (40 U/µL). Incubate at 37°C for 10 min. This will eliminate the DNA template.
4. To the reaction, add 50 µL 4*M* ammonium acetate (dissolve 154.2 g ammonium acetate in 500 mL water, store at room temperature) containing 5 µL tRNA (10 mg/mL stock solution in water; store at –20°C), and 2–3 vol of ethanol. Mix and precipitate for 5 min at room temperature. Centrifuge for 5 min in a microfuge at maximum speed (about 15,000*g*). Carefully remove and safely discard the supernatant.
5. Dissolve the pellet in 50 µL H$_2$O. Add 50 µL 4*M* ammonium acetate and 2–3 vol ethanol. Precipitate for 5 min at room temperature, centrifuge for 5 min in a microfuge (15,000*g*). Remove and discard the supernatant (*see* **Note 4**).
6. Dry the pellet in a Speed Vac for approximately 2 min, or air-dry in a heat block set at +50°C for 10 min. Dissolve the pellet in 50 µL 10 m*M* Tris-HCl (pH 7.0) containing 20 m*M* DTT (*see* **Note 5**). Remove 1 µL of the probe and determine the cpm in a β-scintillation counter. After successful labeling, 1 µL probe will contain between 0.5– × 10$^6$ cpm. Store probes at –80°C. Use 1 µL probe per slide.

## 3.3. In Situ *Hybridization*

1. Rinse slides in two changes of 2X SSC about 1 min each time at room temperature. Agitate frequently.

2. Acetylate by immersion of slides in freshly prepared acetylation mixture for 10 min with gentle agitation at room temperature.
3. Rinse slides as in **step 1**.
4. Immerse in 1X Tris-glycine solution for 30 min with gentle agitation at room temperature.
5. Prepare hybridization mixture. For each slide use 20 μL hybridization mixture containing 1 μL (about $10^6$ cpm) cRNA probe. Heat probes at 95°C for 5 min and then transfer to a heatblock set at 55°C.
6. Rinse slides twice in 2X SSC for 1 min. Let slides set in second 2X SSC until hybridized (up to several hours). Approximately 5 min before loading probe transfer slides to formamide buffer at 55°C.
7. Apply probe to slides individually as follows: remove slide from formamide buffer, wipe back, blot excess liquid around tissue or cell spot by means of Kleenex tissue. Add probe, mount cover slip, and transfer to a humidified chamber.
8. Hybridize overnight at 50°C.
9. Transfer slides to formamide buffer at 55°C until cover slips slide off. Transfer to a second change of formamide buffer at 55°C and rinse with constant agitation for 5 min.
10. Transfer to a third change of formamide buffer and rinse for 20 min with frequent agitation at 55°C.
11. Rinse slides well in 4 changes of 2X SSC at room temperature, 1 min each (*see* **Note 6**).
12. Transfer slides to prewarmed RNase A solution. Incubate at 37°C for 30 min (*see* **Note 7**).
13. Rinse in two changes 2X SSC, 1 min each.
14. Transfer slides to formamide buffer at 55°C with constant agitation for 5 min.
15. Rinse in two changes 2X SSC, 1 min each.
16. Sequentially dehydrate in 70%, 80%, and 95% ethanol, 1 min each.
17. Dry at room temperature for at least 30 min.

### 3.4. Autoradiography

1. In the darkroom, liquefy the NTB-2 emulsion by incubating in a water bath at +45°C for 20 min. Be sure to cover any light coming from the water bath with aluminum foil. Aliquot the emulsion in 25-mL aliquots in 50-mL Falcon tubes. Wrap the tubes with aluminum foil and store in a light-proof box at +4°C. Each tube will suffice for autoradiography of 100–200 slides. Before use, liquefy the emulsion and add 25 mL water containing 2% glycerol prewarmed at +45°C. Mix gently several times, remove the cap, and put back in the water bath. Dip the slides in the emulsion and then blot away excess emulsion on a tissue of Kleenex.
2. Put the slides in horizontal position in a light-proof box and let dry for 1 h at room temperature.
3. Transfer slides (vertical position) to light-proof box containing drying substance (Blue gel; Kebo, Stockholm, Sweden). Expose at 4°C for 1–3 wk (*see* **Note 8**).
4. Let the box equilibrate at room temperature for 1 h.
5. Develop slides at room temperature for 5 min with Dental X-Ray or D-19 developer (Eastman Kodak) diluted five times with water. After a brief wash in water, fix the slides at room temperature for 5 min with Unifix (Eastman Kodak) diluted five times in water.
6. Counterstain 5–10 min with hematoxylin (Sigma, HHS 1-16). Rinse with tap water several times to remove excess hematoxylin.
7. Let the slides dry at room temperature.

## 4. Notes

1. The plasmids containing the probes are linearized with suitable restriction endonucleases to generate templates for antisense or sense (as a negative control) cRNA probes. Only antisense cRNA probe is made for β-actin.

2. It is important to assemble the components at room temperature because spermidine can precipitate DNA at low temperatures $(0 - +4°C)$. The reaction described will normally yield about $50 \times 10^6$ cpm, which is enough for approximately 50 slides. It is possible to scale up or down the reaction. Store [$^{35}$]S isotopes at $-80°C$. [$^{35}$]S isotopes can give off radioactive $SO_2$ gas and should therefore be handled in a fume hood.

3. Using a water bath or heat block for the incubation may reduce the volume of the reaction caused by evaporation and, therefore, reduce the efficiency of the RNA synthesis.

4. Precipitation two times in the presence of ammonium ions will remove about 99% of the unincorporated ribonucleotides. Carefully transfer the supernatant to a new microfuge tube and cap it tightly. The tube is then discarded in a box assigned for radioactive waste. After performing labeling, always check yourself and your work area for radioactive contamination using a Geiger–Müller monitor. A microfuge specially assigned for work with radioactive samples is recommended.

5. It is important to include DTT to stabilize the probe.

6. This rinsing will remove all traces of formamide which could inhibit RNase A.

7. The RNase A will degrade single-stranded RNA, but not hybridized (double-stranded) RNA. Unspecific bound probe to the tissue will be eliminated and markedly increase signal-to-noise ratio.

8. Exposure time will, of course, depend on the level of gene expression. Sometimes, 3 d of exposure is enough. If possible, hybridize sets of slides that can be developed after different exposure times.

## Acknowledgment

This work was supported by the Swedish Cancer Foundation and Lion's Cancer Fund.

## References

1. Pardue, M. L. and Gall, I. G. (1969) Molecular hybridization of radioactive DNA to the DNA of cytological preparations. *Proc. Natl. Acad. Sci. USA* **64,** 600–604.
2. Wetmur, J. G., Ruyechan, W. T., and Douthart, R. I. (1981) Denaturation and renaturation of Penicillum chrysogenum mycophage double-stranded ribonucleic acid in tetraalkylammonium salt solutions. *Biochemistry* **20,** 2999–3002.
3. Lawrence, D. A. (1996) Transforming growth factor-beta: a general review. *Eur. Cytokine Netw.* **7,** 363–374.
4. Pepper, M. S. (1997) Transforming growth factor-beta: vasculogenesis, angiogenesis, and vessel wall integrity. *Cytokine Growth Factor Rev.* **8,** 21–43.
5. Newcom, S. R. and Gu, L. (1995) Transforming growth factor beta 1 messenger RNA in Reed-Sternberg cells in nodular sclerosing Hodgkin's disease. *J. Clin. Pathol.* **48,** 160–163.
6. Minshall, E. M., Leung, D. Y., Martin, R. J., Song, Y. L., Cameron, L., Ernst, P., et al. (1997) Eosinophil-associated TGF-beta1 mRNA expression and airways fibrosis in bronchial asthma. *Am. J. Respir. Cell Mol. Biol.* **17,** 326–333.
7. Coker, R. K., Laurent, G. J., Shahzeidi, S., Hernandez-Rodriguez, N. A., Pantelidis, P., du Bois, R. M., et al. (1996) Diverse cellular TGF-beta 1 and TGF-beta 3 gene expression in normal human and murine lung. *Eur. Respir. J.* **9,** 2501–2507.
8. Henriksen, R., Gobl, A., Wilander, E., Öberg, K., and Funa, K. (1995) Expression and prognostic significance of TGF-β-isotypes, latent TGF-β1-binding protein, TGF-β type I and type II receptors and endoglin in normal ovary and ovarian neoplasms. *Lab. Invest.* **73,** 213–220.
9. Walker, R. A. and Gallacher, B. (1995) Determination of transforming growth factor beta 1 mRNA expression in breast carcinomas by in situ hybridization. *J. Pathol.* **177,** 123–127.
10. Schmid, P., Itin, P., and Rufli, T. (1995) In situ analysis of transforming growth factor-beta s (TGF-beta 1, TGF-beta 2, TGF-beta 3), and TGF-beta type II receptor expression in malignant melanoma. *Carcinogenesis* **16,** 1499–1503.
11. Derynck, R., Jarrett, J. A., Chen, E. Y., Eaton, D. H., Bell, J. R., Assoian, R. K., et al. (1985) Human transforming growth factor-beta complementary DNA sequence and expression in normal and transformed cells. *Nature* **316,** 701–705.
12. Madisen, L., Webb, N. R., Rose, T. M., Marquardt, H., Ikeda, T., Twardzik, D., et al. (1988) Transforming growth factor-beta 2: cDNA cloning and sequence analysis. *DNA* **7,** 1–8.

13. Derynck, R., Lindquist, P. B., Lee, A., Wen, D., Tamm, J., Graycar, J. L., et al. (1988) A new type of transforming growth factor-beta, TGF-beta 3. *EMBO J.* **7,** 3737–3743.
14. Kanzaki, T., Olofsson, A., Moren, A., Wernstedt, C., Hellman, U., Miyazono, K., et al. (1990) TGF-beta 1 binding protein: a component of the large latent complex of TGF-beta 1 with multiple repeat sequences. *Cell* **61,** 1051–1061.
15. Ponte, P., Ng, S. Y., Engel, J., Gunning, P., and Kedes, L. (1984) Evolutionary conservation in the untranslated regions of actin mRNAs: DNA sequence of a human beta-actin cDNA. *Nucl. Acids Res.* **12,** 1687–1696.

# mRNA Detection by *In Situ* RT-PCR

## H. Anne Waller and A. Kay Savage

## 1. Introduction

*In situ* polymerase chain reaction (PCR) is a recently developed technique whereby DNA (or cDNA) is enzymically amplified within cells or tissue sections, enabling the localization of specific low copy number sequences within a heterogeneous cell population. *In situ* reverse transcriptase PCR (RT-PCR) is an adaptation of the technique in which mRNA sequences are reverse transcribed to give a DNA copy (i.e., cDNA), which is subsequently amplified by PCR. The technique provides significantly enhanced sensitivity of detection over conventional mRNA *in situ* hybridization (ISH) as successful amplification can be achieved from a single mRNA target sequence. Amplification products are detected directly by incorporation of label during thermal cycling, or indirectly using a labeled probe and ISH *(1–9)*. **Figure 1** shows the basic principal of the technique.

The technique is not easy to perform and is very expensive. Dedicated reagents and equipment are required for both RNA handling (to avoid RNase contamination leading to false negative results) and for PCR amplification (to avoid contamination with amplification product leading to false positive results). The method has become technically less demanding with the emergence of thermocycling systems, which are specifically adapted for *in situ* PCR (e.g., Hybaid Omnislide™ thermocycler system and Perkin-Elmer GeneAmp *in situ* PCR System 1000) as they provide reliable sealing of the specimen enabling reproducible reaction conditions to be achieved. These systems also allow more samples to be processed per batch test, which is particularly important when establishing optimal parameters.

In conventional RT-PCR, provided that the template is of adequate purity and does not contain inhibitors, optimization is relatively simple *(10,11)*. However, optimization of *in situ* RT-PCR is extremely complex *(1–8)*. Factors that need to be considered include tissue fixation (to preserve morphology and prevent loss or diffusion of target and/or amplified sequences), tissue permeabilization (to allow access of amplification and detection reagents), choice of primers (to achieve specific amplification and adequate length of product to avoid diffusion), PCR reagents (e.g., increased enzyme levels and optimization of buffers), thermal cycling parameters (to achieve specific amplification and avoid over amplification and diffusion of product), and post-PCR detection strategies (including ISH for indirect methods) *(1–9)*.

From: *Methods in Molecular Medicine, Vol. 39: Ovarian Cancer: Methods and Protocols*
Edited by: J. M. S. Bartlett © Humana Press, Inc., Totowa, NJ

Fig. 1. Basic Principal of *in situ* RT-PCR. Oligonucleotide primers, i.e. oligo (dT), random hexamer or specific primers, are hybridized to intracellular mRNA within whole cells or tissue sections. First strand cDNA synthesis is then performed in the presence of RT and dNTPs. Specimens are then subjected to repeated cycles of denaturation, specific primer annealing and extension in the presence of thermostable DNA polymerase resulting in amplification of the target sequence, enabling detection of rare mRNA sequences *in situ*.

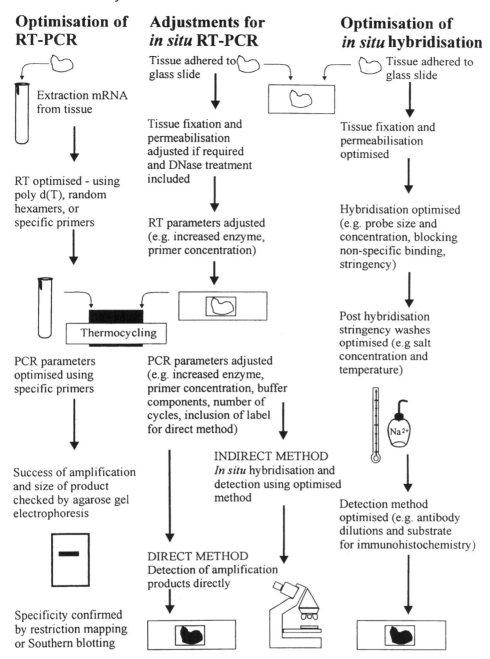

**Optimisation of RT-PCR**

Extraction mRNA from tissue

RT optimised - using poly d(T), random hexamers, or specific primers

Thermocycling

PCR parameters optimised using specific primers

Success of amplification and size of product checked by agarose gel electrophoresis

Specificity confirmed by restriction mapping or Southern blotting

**Adjustments for *in situ* RT-PCR**

Tissue adhered to glass slide

Tissue fixation and permeabilisation adjusted if required and DNase treatment included

RT parameters adjusted (e.g. increased enzyme, primer concentration)

PCR parameters adjusted (e.g. increased enzyme, primer concentration, buffer components, number of cycles, inclusion of label for direct method)

INDIRECT METHOD
*In situ* hybridisation and detection using optimised method

DIRECT METHOD
Detection of amplification products directly

**Optimisation of *in situ* hybridisation**

Tissue adhered to glass slide

Tissue fixation and permeabilisation optimised

Hybridisation optimised (e.g. probe size and concentration, blocking non-specific binding, stringency)

Post hybridisation stringency washes optimised (e.g salt concentration and temperature)

Na²⁺

Detection method optimised (e.g. antibody dilutions and substrate for immunohistochemistry)

Fig. 2. Optimization of *in situ* RT-PCR. Initially RT-PCR and ISH methods are optimized separately using known positive and negative control specimens. Adjustments are then made for *in situ* RT-PCR.

While establishing *in situ* RT-PCR methods, we recommend the use of cell smears or cytospins before commencing with tissue sections. Optimal fixation and permeabilization steps can easily be determined and standardized, thereby simplifying the optimization of other steps in the procedure. Cells are also less prone to false positive results. Indirect methods of detection employing ISH give more reliable results with fewer background problems. Although indirect methods are technically more demanding, they have the major advantage of adding another level of specificity, which is determined by the ISH probe sequence and stringency conditions used.

It is important to establish the optimal parameters for conventional RT-PCR and ISH separately, using known positive and negative control samples, before commencing with *in situ* RT-PCR *(9–12)*. Once this is achieved many of the parameters for the combined technique will have been established (*see* **Fig. 2**). A variety of positive and negative controls must be included when performing *in situ* RT-PCR, and we have indicated these in the appropriate steps of our method. Known positive and negative control tissues must also be included in every batch test, and repeated experiments must be carried out to ensure reproducibility and reliability of the results.

## 2. Materials

### 2.1. Tissue Fixation and Permeabilization

#### 2.1.1. Tissue Section Preparation and Permeabilization

1. 1.2 mm *in situ* PCR-silane coated glass slides, preprinted to aid localization of up to three samples per slide (Perkin-Elmer Applied Biosystems, Cheshire, U.K.) (*see* **Note 2**).
2. PBS (phosphate-buffered saline; 10 m$M$ sodium dihydrogen orthophosphate, 20 m$M$ disodium hydrogen orthophosphate, 0.14$M$ NaCl, pH7.4), stored at 4°C.
3. 10mg/mL proteinase K (Sigma molecular biology grade, 15–20 U/mg) prepared in nuclease-free water, stored in aliquots at –20°C (unused stock being discarded after thawing). Proteinase K dilution buffer (0.1$M$ Tris pH 8.0, 50 m$M$ EDTA pH 8.0), stored at 4°C.

#### 2.1.2. Reduction of Nonspecific Interactions

1. "DNAse master mix" freshly prepared as multiples of the following (to give 50 μL per test sample): 1 μL RNasin ribonuclease inhibitor (40 U/μL), 5 μL RQ1 RNase-free DNase (1 U/μL), 5 μL 10X DNase buffer (500 m$M$ Tris pH 7.5, 10 m$M$ MgCl$_2$, 1 mg/mL BSA) plus 39 μL nuclease-free water (components from Promega Ltd, Southampton, U.K.) (*see* **Note 5**).
2. 10 mg/mL RNase A (Sigma, 100 U/mg solid) prepared in sterile water, stored in aliquots at –20°C. Working solution freshly prepared as 500 μg/mL RNase in prewarmed (37°C) RNase dilution buffer (0.5 $M$ NaCl, 10 m$M$ Tris pH 8.0, 1 m$M$ EDTA pH 8.0).
3. Freshly prepared 4% w/v paraformaldehyde in PBS and dissolved by warming to 60–65°C with stirring and addition of NaOH pellets (a couple) until dissolved. The solution is cooled to room temperature before use. Fixatives are toxic and must be used in a fume hood.
4. Freshly prepared 0.1$M$ triethanolamine pH 8.0 containing acetic anhydride (250 μL per 100 mL). The acetic anhydride must be added just prior to use, with vigorous stirring. **Care:** Use in a fume hood.

### 2.2. In Situ RT-PCR

#### 2.2.1. Reverse Transcription of mRNA In Situ

1. 100 m$M$ ultrapure dATP, dCTP, dGTP, and dTTP (Pharmacia Ltd., Milton Keynes, U.K.). Equal volumes mixed to give 25 m$M$ for each dNTP, stored at –20°C in aliquots (*see* **Note 5**).

2. "RT master mix" freshly prepared as multiples of the following (to give 25 µL per sample): 10 µL 5X RT buffer (250 m$M$ Tris pH 8.3, 375 m$M$ KCl, 15 m$M$ MgCl$_2$, 50 m$M$ DTT), 5 µL 40 m$M$ sodium pyrophosphate, 1 µL RNasin, 0.25 µL M-MLV reverse transcriptase (200 U/µL), 2 µL dNTP mix, 6.75 µL nuclease-free water (components from Promega) (*see* **Note 5**).

3. "Primer master mix" freshly prepared as multiples of the following (to give 25 µL per sample): 5 µL random hexamer primers (0.5 µg/µL, Promega) and 20 µL nuclease-free water, heat denatured in a boiling water bath for 5 min, and rapidly cooled (*see* **Note 5**).

4. "RT reaction mix" freshly prepared as multiples of 25 µL "RT master mix" and 25 µL "primer master mix" (making a sample volume of 50 µL). The final RT reaction mix being 1X RT buffer (with 10 m$M$ DTT), 4 m$M$ sodium pyrophosphate, 1 m$M$ each dNTP (with 40 U RNasin, 50 U RT, and 2.5 µg primers).

### 2.2.2. Amplification of cDNA In Situ

1. GeneAmp *in situ* PCR system 1000 (PE Applied Biosystems). Includes an assembly tool to enable sealing of reaction components with AmpliCover™ disks and AmpliCover™ Clips (giving 35–50 µL reaction volume over the sample). The thermocycler has vertical slots for up to ten slides.

2. Oligonucleotide PCR primers (R&D Systems Europe Ltd., Oxon, U.K.) diluted to 10 pmol/ µL in nuclease-free water, stored in aliquots at –20°C (*see* **Note 5**). The specific primer sequence is user defined and dependent on the particular application (*see* **Notes 7** and **8**).

3. A "PCR primer master mix" is freshly prepared as multiples of the following (allowing 25 µL per sample); 1–5 µL each primer made up to 25 µL with nuclease-free water (optimal concentration being determined empirically), heat denatured in a boiling water bath for 5 min, then rapidly cooled (*see* **Note 7**).

4. 100 m$M$ ultrapure dATP, dCTP, dGTP, and dTTP (Pharmacia, Uppsala, Sweden). Stock prepared as a 10 m$M$ mix of each dNTP in nuclease-free water, stored at –20°C in aliquots (*see* **Note 5**).

5. A "PCR buffer master mix" is freshly prepared as multiples of the following (allowing 25 µL per sample): 5 µL 10X PCR buffer (100 m$M$ Tris pH 9.0, 500 m$M$ KCl, 1% Triton X-100), 1 µL dNTP mix, 3–5 µL 25 m$M$ MgCl$_2$ (optimum determined empirically), 2 µL *Taq* DNA polymerase (5 U/µL) and 1 µL 2.5% BSA made up to 25 µL with nuclease-free water (components from Promega, Madison, WI).

6. "PCR master mix" freshly prepared as multiples of 25 µL "PCR buffer master mix" and 25 µL "PCR primer master mix" (making a sample volume of 50 µL). The final PCR reaction mix being 1× PCR buffer, 0.2 m$M$ each dNTP, 10–50 pmol of each primer (i.e., 0.2–1 µ$M$), 10 U *Taq* polymerase, 1.5–2.5 m$M$ MgCl$_2$, 0.05% BSA.

### 2.3. Probe Labeling for Post-RT-PCR In Situ Hybridization

1. Linearized recombinant transcription vectors (1-2 µg/µL) containing appropriate cDNA sequence (for hybridization) and viral polymerase sites (i.e., SP6, T7, or T3); e.g., pSP65, pSP73, and pGEM-3Zf+ (Promega), pBluescript II KS+ (Stratagene Ltd., Cambridge, U.K.), stored at –20°C (*see* **Notes 10–13**).

2. DNA-dependent RNA polymerases SP6, T7, and T3 (10–20 U/µL), 5X transcription buffer (200 m$M$ Tris pH 7.9, 30 m$M$ MgCl$_2$, 10 m$M$ spermidine, 50 m$M$ NaCl) (Promega) and Digoxigenin (DIG) NTP labeling mix (10 m$M$ each ATP, CTP, and GTP, 6.5 m$M$ UTP, 3.5 m$M$ DIG-11-UTP) (Boehringer Mannheim, East Sussex, U.K.), all stored at –20°C (*see* **Note 5**).

3. 7$M$ ammonium acetate and TE pH 8.0 (10 m$M$ Tris pH 8.0, 1 m$M$ EDTA) prepared in nuclease-free water.

4.  DIG quantification test strips (coated with positively charged nylon) and DIG-labeled control RNA (100 µg/mL) (Boehringer Mannheim). **Care:** do not handle the membrane.
5.  RNA dilution buffer prepared as 5:3:2 nuclease-free water: 20X SSC (3*M* NaCl, 0.3*M* Tri-sodium citrate): formalin (i.e., 40% formaldehyde), stored at 4°C.
6.  Maleic acid buffer (0.1*M* maleic acid, 0.15*M* NaCl, pH 7.5 with NaOH pellets), stored at 4°C.
7.  10X blocking solution prepared as 10% w/v DIG blocking agent (Boehringer Mannheim) in maleic acid buffer, dissolved by heating to 65°C) autoclaved (11 min at 15 psi) and stored in aliquots at –20°C. **Note:** the solution remains cloudy.
8.  TBS developer buffer (100 m*M* Tris, 100 m*M* NaCl, 5 m*M* MgCl$_2$, pH 9.5), stored at 4°C.
9.  Alkaline phosphatase-conjugated anti-DIG antibody (Fab fragments), stored at 4°C (Boehringer Mannheim).
10. Sigma Fast™ NBT/BCIP buffered substrate tablets, stored at –20°C (Sigma, St. Louis, MO). Substrate freshly prepared as 1 tablet in 10 mL water (making 0.3 mg/mL nitro blue tetrazolium, 0.15 mg/mL 5-bromo-4-chloro-3-indolyl phosphate, 100 m*M* Tris pH 9.5, 5 m*M* MgCl$_2$). **Note:** the substrate is light sensitive.

### 2.4. Post-RT-PCR In Situ *Hybridization*

#### 2.4.1. In Situ *Hybridization*

1.  Hybridization buffer prepared as 50% formamide, 2X SSC, 10% dextran sulphate (from freshly prepared stock), 0.25% BSA, 0.25% Ficoll (MWt 400,000), 0.25% polyvinylpyrolidone (PVP-40, MWt 40,000), 10 m*M* Tris pH 7.5, 0.5% sodium dodecyl sulphate (SDS), 250 µg/mL denatured salmon sperm DNA (molecular biology grade components from Sigma). Buffer aliquots are stored at –20°C until required, and once thawed unused buffer is discarded (*see* **Note 5**).

#### 2.4.2. Posthybridization Washes and Detection of Signal

1.  TBS diluent buffer (0.1*M* Tris, 0.1*M* NaCl, pH 7.5).
2.  Blocking solution prepared as 10% BSA in TBS containing 0.3% w/v Triton X-100, and antibody diluent prepared as 2% Normal Sheep Serum (Sigma) in TBS with 0.3% w/v Triton X-100, both stored at –20°C in aliquots.
3.  Methyl green nuclear counterstain (Vector Labs., Peterborough, U.K.) and Loctite 358 UV curing adhesive (BSL, Essex, U.K.).

## 3. Methods

Precautions must be adopted to avoid contamination with nucleases (particularly RNases) and cross-contamination of pre-PCR amplification reagents with amplification products (*see* **Note 1**).

### 3.1. Tissue Fixation and Permeabilization

#### 3.1.1. Tissue Section Preparation and Permeabilization

1.  4–6 µm formalin-fixed paraffin-embedded sections are mounted onto coated slides (up to three per slide) and dried overnight at 37°C prior to baking 60°C for 48 h. The slides are baked lying flat to avoid loss of melted paraffin. Blocks and sections are stored at room temperature in a dust-free container until use (*see* **Notes 2** and **3**).
2.  Sections are dewaxed in xylene (2 × 15 min) and rehydrated by successive immersion in graded ethanol (100% × 2, 75 and 50% for 5 min each) then distilled water.
3.  Slides are then washed in PBS (2 × 5 min) and are permeabilized with 0.3% w/v Triton X-100 in PBS for 15 min, followed by washing in PBS (2 × 5 min).

4. Slides are equilibrated in prewarmed proteinase K dilution buffer for 10–15 min prior to digestion with proteinase K (freshly diluted from stock) for 30 min at 37°C. The optimal proteinase K digestion will need to be determined empirically for each tissue tested (*see* **Note 4**). Digestion is carried out in a Coplin jar for low enzyme levels. Where higher levels are needed, 30-50 μL of enzyme is pipeted onto individual slides (after carefully wiping around the samples with a clean tissue) and sealed using parafilm "cover slips." Incubation is then carried out in an oven (in a moist chamber). Care must be taken to avoid drying out of the samples.

5. Proteinase K is inhibited by incubation in 0.1*M* glycine in PBS for 5 min. Slides are then washed in PBS (2 × 5 minutes) and rinsed in distilled water.

### 3.1.2. Reduction of Nonspecific Interactions

1. After carefully wiping around samples with a clean tissue, all tissues are predigested with 50 μL "DNase master mix" to prevent amplification of genomic sequences. Incubation is carried out overnight at room temperature under parafilm "cover slips" (in a moist chamber). Slides are then washed in PBS (2 × 5 min).

2. To confirm signals are from an RNA target RNase predigestion is carried out for every sample tested (negative control). Slides are incubated with 50 μL RNase at 37°C for 1 h under parafilm "cover slips" (in a moist chamber). The remaining test slides are kept in PBS (*see* **Note 6**).

3. All slides are then washed in PBS (2 × 5 min), postfixed in 4% paraformaldehyde for 3 min and washed in PBS (2 × 5 min). Care must be taken to avoid cross-contamination of test slides with RNase.

4. To reduce nonspecific interactions specimens are acetylated for 10 min in Triethanolamine/acetic anhydride with constant stirring.

5. To inhibit endogenous alkaline phosphatases slides are dipped in prechilled 20% glacial acetic acid for 15 s (at 4°C).

6. Slides are rinsed well with PBS, dehydrated through graded ethanols (50, 75, then 100% for 5 min each) and air-dried.

## 3.2. In Situ *RT-PCR*

### 3.2.1. Reverse Transcription of mRNA In Situ

For each tissue tested a negative control is included, with omission of RT from the reaction. This is an additional control to confirm amplification is from an mRNA target (*see* **Note 6**).

1. First-strand cDNA synthesis is carried out by adding 50 μL RT reaction mix per sample and incubating for 2 h at 37°C under parafilm "cover slips."

2. The slides are then rinsed well with water, dehydrated in graded ethanols (*see* **Subheading 3.1.2., step 6**), and air-dried ready for PCR.

### 3.2.2. Amplification of cDNA In Situ

For each tissue tested, a negative control is included, omitting *Taq* polymerase from the reaction. PCR conditions will need to be adjusted for each application, particularly the primer concentration and cycling parameters (including annealing temperature, and annealing and extension times). We generally use the same $MgCl_2$ concentration as optimized for conventional RT-PCR, and three sets of cycling parameters (5, 10, and 20 cycles) per test (*see* **Notes 7–9**).

1. The Assembly Tool and GeneAmp thermocycler are preheated to 70°C. Slides are placed on the Assembly Tool (with the writing area to the right) and 50 µL of "PCR master mix" is pipeted onto the sample. The reaction is enclosed with the Amplicover™ Disc and Amplicover™ clip, and the slide pushed to the left (i.e., onto the next sample). Sealed slides are transferred to the thermocycler while further slides are set up.

2. Reactions are cycled at 95°C for 1.5 min (1 cycle); 95°C for 1 min (denaturation), 50–60°C for 1–2 min (primer annealing usually 5°C below primer Tm), 72°C for 2–3 min (extension) for 5, 10, and 20 cycles; 72°C for 10 min (1 cycle) (*see* **Note 8**).

3. Slides are disassembled using the Disassembly Tool and washed in PBS (2 × 5 min), postfixed in 0.4% paraformaldehyde/PBS for 15 min, rinsed in water and dehydrated through graded ethanols (*see* **subheading 3.1.2., step 6**) and air-dried. Slides from 5, 10, and 20 cycle batches are pooled for the ISH detection steps.

### 3.3. Probe Labeling for Post-RT-PCR In Situ Hybridization

Sense or antisense RNA probes (complementary to the amplified target) may be used for ISH detection as the target is double stranded (*see* **Notes 10–13**). Probes which span intron boundaries will prevent detection of amplified genomic sequences. Templates are generally prepared to give RNA probe sizes in the range of 100–300 b (*see* **Note 12**).

1. Transcription reactions are set up at room temperature in a 20 µL volume (made up with nuclease-free water): 4 µL 5X transcription buffer, 2 µL 100 m*M* DTT, 1 µL RNasin, 0.5 µL template DNA, 2 µL DIG NTP mix and 1 µL appropriate polymerase (i.e., SP6, T7, or T3). Reactions are carried out for 1.5 h at 37°C with a further addition of enzyme after 45 min (*see* **Note 12**).

2. Reactions are terminated by the addition of 1 µL DNase and 1 µL RNasin, and digesting for 10 min at 37°C.

3. 1 µL of tRNA (10 µg/µL), 75 µL nuclease-free water and 5 µL 4M NaCl are then added, and RNA is then precipitated with 100 µL ammonium acetate and 750 µL chilled (–20°C) ethanol and pelleted by centrifugation for 15 min (12,000*g*).

4. The pellet is air-dried and resuspended in 10 µL TE pH 8.0. Labeled probes are stored at –20°C until required (stable for at least 1 y).

5. An aliquot of probe is assessed for DIG incorporation using DIG quantification test strips (according to manufacturers direction). Control DIG-labeled RNA and labeled probe are diluted in RNA dilution buffer to give a range of between 0.01–10 pg/µL, and 1 µL (of 5 dilutions in the range) is spotted onto the DIG test strips and air-dried, then baked at 80°C for 30 min under vacuum.

6. Membranes are then developed back to back (control and test). Strips are blocked for 2 min in 1X blocking solution (in maleic acid buffer), incubated with 1:2000 labeled antibody (in 1X blocking solution) for 3 min, blocked again for 1 min, washed in maleic acid buffer for 1 min, equilibrated in TBS developer buffer for 1 min, and developed in substrate.

7. After 30 min to 1 h substrate development is stopped by rinsing the strips in water. Strips are blotted onto clean filter paper and air-dried. Probe concentration is then estimated by comparison of signal intensities given on the control strip (taking dilution factors into account).

### 3.4. Post-RT-PCR In Situ Hybridization

The optimal conditions for ISH detection will need to be determined empirically (*see* **Notes 13–16**).

### 3.4.1. In Situ *Hybridization*

1. Probes are diluted in prewarmed hybridization buffer (70–80°C, to aid dispensing). Optimal probe concentrations will need to be determined empirically for each probe. We usually use concentrations of around 0.1–0.5 ng/μL (*see* **Note 14**).
2. 35 μL diluted probe is pipeted onto the samples on the Assembly Tool and sealed using Amplicover™ discs and clips. Sample cDNA and RNA probe (secondary structure) are then denatured at 95°C for 5 min, prior to hybridization overnight at 42°C (*see* **Note 15**).

### 3.4.2. Posthybridization Washes and Signal Detection

Posthybridization stringency washes will need to be determined empirically and are dependant on the probe length and sequence (*see* **Note 15**). Prior to dispensing antibody and substrate onto the sections, slides are carefully wiped dry (using clean tissues) while leaving the individual samples wet. Great care must be exercised to avoid samples from drying out at any stage during the immunohistochemical detection procedure (*see* **Notes 16** and **17**).

1. Slides are washed in 4X SSC containing 0.1% SDS at room temperature (2 × 10 min), followed by 4X SSC at 37°C (3 × 20 min).
2. Unhybridized RNA probe is then removed by incubation with 500 μg/mL DNase-free RNase A (in 2X SSC) at 37°C for 30 min.
3. Sections are washed in 2X SSC, followed by 0.1X SSC at 37°C for 30 min each.
4. Slides are then washed in TBS diluent (2 × 10 min) prior to blocking with BSA for 30 min under parafilm cover slips.
5. Excess blocking agent is removed and samples are then incubated with 1:300 antibody (in antibody diluent) for 2 h at room temperature under parafilm cover slips (*see* **Note 16**).
6. Slides are then washed in TBS diluent containing 0.3% w/v Triton X-100 (2 × 10 min), followed by TBS diluent (3 × 10 min).
7. Slides are equilibrated in TBS developer buffer for 5 min prior to incubation with substrate under parafilm cover slips, in the dark. Development is carried out for 2–5 h in a humid chamber (further development giving unacceptable background).
8. Slides are then washed in distilled water and counterstained with methyl green (2 min), rinsed with water, blotted, and air-dried. Glass cover slips are mounted using Loctite 358 adhesive (cured for 2 min on a UV transilluminator) (*see* **Note 18**).

## 4. Notes

1. Gloves must be worn at all stages during the preparation of materials and solutions, and during all manipulations up to and including hybridisation. We have found that some powdered gloves can lead to spurious results, and we therefore recommend that powder-free gloves are used.

   All solutions should be prepared using nuclease-free chemicals, glassware, and plasticware that have been reserved for RNA work. DEPC (diethylpyrocarbonate, Sigma) treatment of solutions to inhibit RNases is not essential if you have a good supply of deionised water (such as Milli Q), autoclaving is sufficient (11 min at 126°C under 15 psi pressure). Otherwise, all solutions (used up to and including hybridization) should be pretreated with 0.1% v/v DEPC for at least 12 h at 37°C and double autoclaved to remove all residual DEPC. Solutions containing Tris (hydroxymethyl methylamine) or DTT (DL-dithiothreitol) must not be treated directly with DEPC (reacts with amines and sulphydryl groups), but are made up in sterile DEPC treated water. DEPC is a suspected carcinogen and corrosive, handle with care. Concentrated stocks should be handled in a fume hood.

Sterile disposable plasticware is essentially nuclease-free and can be used without special pretreatment. Glassware must be thoroughly cleaned (with detergent, and well rinsed with distilled water, then rinsed with ethanol and air-dried) and sterilized by baking at 180°C for 4 h. Nonbakeable/autoclaveable equipment and plasticware (such as slide incubation trays and electrophoresis equipment) should be thoroughly cleaned immediately after use, rinsed with sterile water, and air-dried. Separate solutions, glassware and plasticware are also used for RT and PCR, and we recommend that RT-PCR reagent mixtures are made up in a class II tissue culture cabinet (to avoid cross-contamination with amplification products).

2. If you wish to prepare your own RNase-free coated slides they must be cleaned and baked, then treated with 2% TESPA (3-aminopropyltriethoxysilane) in acetone for 5 min, followed by rinsing in sterile water. Coated slides are dried at 50–60°C and stored in a dust-free container until required.

3. Routine histology laboratories and theatres generally use 10% neutral buffered formalin as a standard fixative, and this is fine for *in situ* RT-PCR (the use of nuclease-free/DEPC treated PBS for making up the fixative is not essential). It is important that specimens are fixed quickly (within 15 min of excision) to avoid degradation of target mRNA. The length of fixation is often determined by laboratory rotas for processing and embedding. If possible, limit the length of fixation to 3–6 h for small tissue blocks (<2 mm thick), and 12–24 h for larger blocks (up to 1 cm thick). We have used tissues that have undergone extensive fixation and usually overcome permeabilisation problems by increasing proteinase K digestion. We have also used decalcified specimens (5–10% formic acid or preferably 20% EDTA pH 8.0). Formic acid can reduce the detectable mRNA, so may give false negative results for very rare mRNA species.

The protocol may be adapted for application to snap frozen tissues or cell smears/cytospins. Unfixed tissues are snap frozen in cryo-embedding medium (Bright Instruments Co Ltd., Cambridge, U.K.) and are stored at –80°C until required. 4–6 μm sections are mounted onto coated slides and air dried for 5 min prior to washing in PBS (2 × 5 min) to remove all traces of mounting medium. Slides are then fixed for 30 min in 4% paraformaldehyde/PBS and washed in PBS (2 × 5 min). Fixed-frozen sections may be dehydrated though graded ethanol, air-dried, and stored at 4°C for up to 1 w (in air-tight boxes with desiccant) prior to further pretreatment (this is useful when preparing several different blocks for analysis).

Cell-culture suspensions must be washed in PBS (X2) to remove culture medium (particularly important if biotin is used as a reporter as the medium contains high levels of endogenous biotin). Washed cell pellets are then resuspended in 4% paraformaldehyde and fixed for 30 min prior to the preparation of cytospins onto coated slides. Alternatively, slides can be prepared by allowing fixed cells to settle onto the coated slides, or by preparing smears with a device such as Cytoshuttle (*6*). Slides are then washed in PBS (2 × 5 min) followed by rinsing in distilled water and drying overnight at 37°C. Slides are stored in sealed boxes with silica gel at –80°C (in usable batches to avoid repeated thawing) until required. Slide boxes are brought to room temperature before opening to avoid ice crystal artefacts. Cells are rehydrated in water and washed in PBS prior to use.

4. Optimal proteinase K digestion is critical. Under fixation or over digestion with protease will result in a weak or absent cytoplasmic signal and inadequate tissue morphology. Extracellular signal may be evident due to diffusion and/or solution phase amplification. Weak or absent signal will also result from delayed fixation, contamination of pre-amplification reagents with RNase, or over fixation (with inadequate permeabilization). Short-fixed paraffin-embedded specimens (3–24 h) will generally require 0.5–5 μg/mL proteinase K, and extensively fixed specimens up to 50 μg/mL proteinase K. Cytospins/smears or fixed-frozen sections will generally require 0-0.5 μg/mL proteinase K.

5. Care must be exercised when using molecular biology enzymes, to ensure that stocks do not lose activity as a result of repeated warming. Remember to ensure adequate mixing of the components. Any droplets on the inner surface of the tube or lid should be spun down by brief centrifugation. Care should also be exercised to avoid repeat freeze-thawing of stock DNA, RNA, and nucleotide solutions. They should be stored in usable aliquots and discarded after a few thawing cycles. Some reaction buffers contain components that may precipitate from solution on freezing (e.g., spermidine, SDS, DTT, sodium pyrophosphate). If this occurs, they should be warmed to 37°C to aid dissolution.

6. Signals present on the RNase or No RT controls will indicate incomplete DNase digestion and amplification of genomic sequences, or nonspecific background occurring during ISH detection. Positive signals on the No *Taq* control will indicate nonspecific background occurring during ISH detection. Mispriming and amplification of nonspecific sequences (or primer-dimers), or unsuccessful amplification, will result in weak or absent signal. Contamination of PCR reagents with amplification product will lead to solution phase amplification and background over the sample (including RNase and No RT controls).

7. We use a single primer pair (primers 18–25 bp) and generally ensure that amplification products are around 200–400 bp. We also try and use primers that span intron boundaries to reduce amplification of any residual genomic DNA that may be present. Primer concentrations need to be determined empirically, but optimal concentrations are generally around 0.2–1 μ*M*.

8. Specificity of amplification is critical for successful *in situ* RT-PCR. As with conventional PCR, primers should have close to 50% GC content and have the same melting temperature (*Tm*, being the temperature at which 50% hybrids are dissociated). Primers with multiple repeats of G or C nucleotides (particularly at the 3′ end), or hairpin loops should be avoided. The 3′ ends of the primers should not be complementary, otherwise primer dimers will be amplified *(10,11)*.

$$Tm = 81.5°C + 16.6(\log_{10}[Na^+]) + 0.41(\%G+C) - 675/n$$

Where $[Na^+]$ = molar salt concentration ($Na^+ = K^+$ in PCR reaction buffer) and $n$ = oligonucleotide length (bases) *(10)*.

While optimizing and establishing the method, amplified cDNA should be extracted from tissues and checked by agarose gel electrophoresis to confirm correct size of amplification product. Restriction digestion or Southern blotting may be used to confirm the sequence. Different primers to the same mRNA target should be used to confirm consistency of results.

9. The use of several cycling parameters is not only important when establishing the *in situ* RT-PCR method, but also when using tissue sections. The efficiency of amplification will be variable in different tissues, and levels of expression of target mRNA will differ between samples. Overamplification of target sequences will result in background because of diffusion of product.

10. We have routinely used single-stranded RNA probes for our mRNA ISH studies, and therefore use RNA probes for *in situ* RT-PCR detection. However, as sensitivity of detection is not limiting, you may prefer to use cDNA or oligonucleotide probes, which are easier to handle and labeling can be performed using one of the many commercially available kits.

11. When preparing plasmids, we use a method adapted from Sambrook *et al. (11)* and the Promega protocols and applications guide *(10)*, allowing rapid isolation of plasmid DNA (1–5 μg/mL of culture) of suitable quality for *in vitro* transcription without the need for purification by column chromatography or CsCl density gradient centrifugation.

We have also synthesized *in vitro* transcription templates by PCR. The technique is based on the allowance of mismatch basepairing of sequences (for T7, T3, or SP6) at the

5′ end of the PCR primer during initial cycles (with low annealing temperature), with the 3′ end (18 bases) being specific to the desired cDNA (allowing amplification). This method allows direct generation of templates possessing RNA polymerase sites without the need for laborious subcloning of cDNA into riboprobe vectors.

12. To enable the production of specific "run-off" transcripts (without vector sequences) plasmid templates must be fully linearized using appropriate restriction sites downstream of the RNA polymerase promoter. Restriction enzymes are used according to manufacturers direction and linearised templates are purified by phenol:chloroform extraction and ethanol precipitation *(10,11)*. Success of linearization is established by agarose gel electrophoresis *(11)*.

When preparing linearized transcription templates, restriction enzymes that yield 3′ overhangs should be avoided where possible to prevent aberrant initiation of transcription. However, where this cannot be avoided, 3′ overhangs are removed using the Klenow fragment of DNA polymerase I prior to transcription. Standard transcription reactions are set up without nucleotides or RNA polymerase, and 1 U of Klenow added. Templates are incubated for 15 min at 22°C, then transcription proceeded by the addition of nucleotides and polymerase.

Where necessary, limited alkaline hydrolysis of RNA transcripts is used to achieve optimal probe size (100–300 b) for ISH. RNA probes may be checked by denaturing agarose gel electrophoresis *(11)* to ensure success of labeling incorporation into transcripts of the correct size (and to ensure the success of hydrolysis when performed). Labeled transcripts from PGEMEX-1 and riboprobe Gemini control vectors (Promega) can be used as molecular-weight markers to verify transcript sizes. This step is important for unestablished probes, but otherwise need only be included if problems are evident with the ISH detection.

13. The ISH probe must be checked by Southern blotting to establish specificity, and aid optimization of hybridization stringency when establishing the ISH method. When establishing the *in situ* RT-PCR detection, we compare signals achieved with both the sense and antisense RNA probes to confirm consistency of results (both strands should give the same signal, provided that levels of original target mRNA are outside of the detection limit for standard ISH). During establishment of the ISH method omission of probe is used to assess levels of nonspecific background signal (i.e., because of the detection method). An unrelated probe of similar size and GC content is also used to establish any background due to nonspecific binding of labeled probe.

14. Nonspecific binding of ISH probe will result in false positive signal (uniform background, or background over connective tissue). If this occurs, tissue pretreatments may need to be adjusted (e.g., increased protease, or acid treatment). Try increasing the unlabeled nucleic acids (salmon sperm or tRNA) during hybridization or include a prehybridization step to block nonspecific binding sites. Increase the number and length of posthybridization washes and include a detergent (such as SDS, Tween-20, or Triton X-100). If excessive probe levels are used, nonspecific background will result. Insufficient probe will give a weak or absent signal. Degradation of RNA probe used for detection will result in a weak or an absent signal, or may give unacceptable background all over the sample.

15. Mismatch hybridization is avoided by controling the stringency of hybridization and posthybridization washes. Stringency may be increased (i.e., mismatched hybrids reduced) by increasing temperature, decreasing salt concentration, or increasing formamide concentration *(9,12)*. The inclusion of formamide allows hybridization and stringency washes to be performed at lower temperatures, preserving cellular morphology. Optimal hybridization is generally around 15–35°C below the melt temperature *(Tm)*.

$$Tm = 81.5°C + 16.6(\log 10[Na^+]) + 0.41(\%G+C) - 820/l - 0.6(\%F) - 1.4(\%mismatch)$$

Where [Na$^+$] = molar salt concentration, $l$ = probe length (bases), %F = % formamide, % mismatch = % noncomplementary basepairs between hybridizing strands *(12)*. Note that RNA:DNA (and RNA:RNA) duplexes form more stable hybrids with slightly increased *Tm*. *Tm* is also slightly lower (by around 5°C) *in situ* than in solution *(12)*.

We usually perform the hybridization step at fairly low stringency, and perform higher posthybridization stringency washes (increasing temperature and/or decreasing salt) as required to achieve a specific signal. Mismatched hybrids on ISH detection will yield false positive cytoplasmic signals (which are not removed on posthybridization treatment with RNase). If the stringency of hybridization or post washes is too high, ISH signals will be weak or absent.

16. It is important to include negative controls with omission of primary antibody to confirm background because of endogenous enzyme (which usually gives a localized signal, variable between different tissues). Lysosomal phosphatases can be further inhibited by inclusion of levamisole in the substrate (0.24 mg/mL) if required. Excessive antibody levels (or incubation times), or over development in substrate, will result in nonspecific background (particularly over the connective tissue). If the primary antibody is too dilute, or substrate not active, signals will be weak or absent.

17. Patchy signal indicates poor mixing of reagents, air bubbles present during incubations, or drying out of sections during immunohistochemical detection. It should also be noted that patchy signal may also result on tissue sections as whole cells are not always present (target mRNA may have been present in the part of the cell cut away during sectioning).

18. Alternatively, nuclei may be weakly counterstained with haematoxylin (or other water insoluble counterstain) and sections mounted using aqueous mount (e.g., glycerol mount from Dako Ltd, High Wycombe, UK).

## References

1. Chen, R. H. and Fuggle, S. V. (1997) *In situ* PCR amplification of intracellular mRNA. *Methods Molec. Biol.* **71,** 123–132.
2. Long, A. A. and Komminoth, P. (1997) *In situ* PCR. An overview. *Methods Molec. Biol.* **71,** 141–161.
3. Nuovo, G. J. (1994) *In situ* detection of PCR-amplified DNA and cDNA: a review. *J. Histotechnol.* **17,** 235–246.
4. Teo, I. A. and Shaunak, S (1995). Polymerase chain reaction *in situ*: an appraisal of an emerging technique. *Histochem. J.* **27,** 647–659.
5. Nuovo, G. J. (1992) *PCR in situ Hybridization: Protocols and Applications.* Raven, New York.
6. Lewis, F. (1996) *An Approach to in situ PCR.* PE Applied Biosystems, CA.
7. Martínez, A., Miller, M. J., Quinn, K., Unsworth, E. J., Ebina, M., and Cuttitta, F. (1995) Non-radioactive localisation of nucleic acids by direct *in situ* PCR and *in situ* RT-PCR in paraffin-embedded sections. *J. Histochem. Cytochem.* **43,** 739–747.
8. Embelton, M. J., Gorochov, G., Jones, P. T., and Winter, G. (1992) In-cell PCR from mRNA: amplifying and linking the rearranged immunoglobulin heavy and light chain V-genes with single cells. *Nucleic Acids Res.* **20,** 3831–3837.
9. Waller, H. A. and Savage, A. K. (1994) Analysis of gene transcription *in situ*: methodological considerations and applications in pathology. *J. Histotechnol.* **17,** 203–218.
10. Doyle, K., ed., (1996) *Protocols and Applications Guide.* Promega Corporation, Madison, WI.
11. Sambrook, J., Fritsch, E. F., and Maniatis, T. (1989) *Molecular Cloning: A Laboratory Manual.* Cold Spring Harbor Laboratory Press, Cold Spring Harbor, New York.
12. Valentino, K. L., Eberwine, J. H., and Barchas, J. D., eds. (1987) *In situ Hybridisation: Applications to Neurobiology.* Oxford University Press, Oxford, England.

# 47

# RNase Protection Assay Analysis of mRNA for TGFβ$_{1-3}$ in Ovarian Tumors

## John M. S. Bartlett

## 1. Introduction

RNase protection assays provide a level of sensitivity some 20–50-fold greater than Northern blots, and can be used to accurately identify and quantify different mRNA species within gene families even when a high degree of sequence homology exists. Sequence homology between TGFβ$_1$, TGFβ$_2$, and TGFβ$_3$ mRNAs is approximately 70%. Identification of these subspecies by Northern is often complicated by cross-hybridization of probes. In the RNase protection assay, detection of mRNA relies on the formation of a RNA:RNA hybrid of absolute specificity. Single-stranded RNA is digested with a single-strand specific RNase mixture and even single basepair mismatches will lead to loss of hybridization signal. Therefore, this technique provides a readily quantifiable means of detecting multiple RNA species, either individually or simultaneously. This technique has been applied to the study of both ovarian carcinoma cell lines *(1)* and tumors *(2)* yielding valuable insights into the role of TGFβs in ovarian carcinomas.

## 2. Materials

All chemicals, unless otherwise noted, are molecular biology grade and obtained from Sigma U.K. (Poole, Dorset). All glassware was pretreated with di-ethylpyrocarbonate (DEPC). All deionized distilled water was pretreated with DEPC and autoclaved (DEPC water). DEPC is a potent anti-RNase agent.

### 2.1. DEPC Treatment of Glassware/Distilled Water

1. 0.1% DEPC is added to distilled deionized water and glassware filled and left to stand overnight. The water was decanted and autoclaved (DEPC treated water) and glassware sterilised at 220°C for 2 h (DEPC treated glassware). DEPC is driven off by both procedures.

### 2.2. RNA Extraction

1. 3 *M* lithium chloride 6*M* urea: Dissolve in 800 mL DEPC water and make up to 1 L. Store at 4°C for 3–6 mo.

From: *Methods in Molecular Medicine, Vol. 39: Ovarian Cancer: Methods and Protocols*
Edited by: J. M. S. Bartlett © Humana Press, Inc., Totowa, NJ

2. 10 m*M* Tris-HCl, 0.5% sodium dodecyl sulphate (SDS) pH 7.5. Prepare stock solutions of 10% SDS, 0.5*M* Tris-HCl (pH 7.5) in DEPC water. Stocks are stable at room temperature for up to 12 mo.
3. Proteinase K: Prepare 1 mg/mL w/v DEPC water stock, store at –20°C for up to 12 mo. Dilute in 10 m*M* Tris-Cl/0.5% SDS as required, discard unused diluted enzyme.
4. Phenol:Chloroform:Isoamyl alcohol: Phenol is presaturated with 10 m*M* Tris-HCl pH 7.5. Prepare a mixture of 25:24:1 Phenol:Chloroform:Isoamyl alcohol (v/v/v). Store at room temperature for up to 6 mo, shield from light.

## 2.3. Electrophoresis and Purification of Riboprobes

1. Gel Loading Buffer: 8 mL deionized formamide, 40 µL 250 m*M* EDTA, 10 mg bromophenol blue, 10 mg xylene cyanol, 2 mL distilled water. Store at 4°C for 6 mo.
2. 40% Acrylamide (stock solution): Dissolve 38 gm acrylamide (Bio-Rad, Richmond, CA, Cat. 161-0101), 2 gm *bis*-acrylamide (Bio-Rad Cat. 161-0201) in 100 mL distilled water. Check that pH is <7.0. Store in dark at 4°C for 3 mo (*see* **Note 3**).
3. 5X TBE Buffer: 54.0 gm Tris Base, 27.5 gm boric acid, 20 mL 0.5*M* EDTA (pH 8.0). Dissolve and make up to 1 L with distilled water. Store at room temperature. Dilute 1:5 before use.
4. Gel solution (for an 8% denaturing gel): 42 gm Urea, 20 mL 40% acrylamide stock solution, 20 mL 5X TBE, 25 mL distilled water. Stir at room temperature until urea dissolves, use fresh.
5. Potassium hydroxide/methanol (for plate washing): Dissolve 50 gm KOH pellets in 1 L methanol.
6. Maxim & Gilbert's Elution Buffer: 0.5*M* ammonium acetate, 0.1% SDS, 1 m*M* EDTA in DEPC water.
7. Hybridization buffer: 8 mL deionized formamide, 2 mL 200 m*M* PIPES (pH 6.7), 2*M* NaCl, 5 m*M* EDTA. Final concentration 80% formamide, 40 m*M* PIPES, 400 m*M* NaCl, 1 m*M* EDTA. Store at 4°C for 6 mo.

## 2.4. RNA:RNA Hybridization

1. 3*M* sodium acetate pH 5.2 Dissolve in DEPC water, adjust pH.
2. RNA hybridization buffer: For 6 mL (20 tubes): Mix 60 µL 1*M* Tris pH 7.5, 1.8 mL 1*M* NaCl, 120 µL 0.25*M* EDTA, 4 mL DEPC water, 24 µL T1 RNase, 6 µL RNase A (both 100,000 U/mL, Boehringer Mannheim, Mannheim, Germany) (*see* **Note 4**).

# 3. Methods

## 3.1. RNA Extraction

1. Tumors should ideally be collected fresh and stored in liquid nitrogen. Routinely samples are collected on ice and transported for freezing within 30–60 min.
2. Tumors are disaggregated using a Braun-micro dismembranator. Teflon vessels and steel ball bearings are cooled in liquid nitrogen prior to use. Frozen tissue (50–500 mg) is placed in the vessel with a single ball bearing and agitated at 1000 cycles/second for 60 s. The vessel is then recooled in liquid nitrogen. This process is repeated until tumor tissue is powdered, usually 2 times (*see* **Note 5**).
3. Immediately after disaggregation of tissue tumor material is resuspended from frozen in 1.5 mL LiCl/Urea and transferred to a separate tube. The vessel is washed a further 2 times with 1.5 mL LiCl/Urea and the washing combined with the original sample. The resuspended medium is made up to 6 mL in LiCl/Urea and sonicated for 2 × 30 s at maximum power using a probe sonicator. The sonicated samples are stored overnight at 4°C (*see* **Note 6**).

4. Centrifuge at 15,000$g$, 4°C for 30 min. The supernatant is discarded and the pellet washed with a further 6 mL of lithium chloride/urea, recentrifuged (15,000$g$, 4°C for 30 min) and the supernatant again discarded.

5. The pellet is resuspended in 6 mL Tris-HCl/SDS with 50 µg/mL proteinase K (Boehringer Mannheim, UK), and incubated at 37°C for 20 min.

6. Samples are extracted with 100% phenol, followed by phenol:chloroform:isoamyl-alcohol. Following each extraction the sample is centrifuged at 2000$g$ at room temperature for 10 min and the aqueous phase recovered.

7. Following the final extraction, 300 µL 8$M$ LiCl and 2.5 vol absolute alcohol are added and samples stored at –20°C for 30 min- overnight. RNA is pelleted by centrifugation at 4000$g$, 4°C for 45 min. The supernatant is discarded and the RNA pelleted dried and resuspended in DEPC treated distilled water. Concentrations are estimated by optical density at 260 nm/280 nm.

## 3.2. Preparation of Riboprobes

1. Labeled RNA (both sense and antisense) is prepared from 1.0 µg/µL linearized template DNA (*see* **Note 1**) using a Gemini II/Riboprobe system (Promega Ltd., Southampton UK). The reaction mixture contained:

    4.0 µL 5X Transcription Buffer
    2.0 µL 100 m$M$ Dithiothreotol
    0.8 µL RNasin (Human placental RNase inhibitor; Amersham, UK, Cat. N120Y)
    4.0 µL 2.5 m$M$ rATP, rGTP, rUTP
    2.4 µL 100 µ$M$ rCTP
    1.0 µL Linearized template DNA (1 µg)
    5.0 µL α-32P-CTP (Amersham, UK, PB10162)
    1.0 µL RNA polymerase (SP6, T3, or T7 as appropriate)

    Incubate at 37°C for 60 min.

2. Add 1.0 µL RQ1 DNase to each mixture and incubated at 37°C for 15 min. (RQ1 is an RNase free preparation of DNase I added to digest the DNA template and prevent formation of DNA/RNA hybrids).

3. Add 78 µL distilled water, 20 µg tRNA carrier (20 µL of 1 mg/mL tRNA in distilled water, Sigma, UK) and 20 µL 10$M$ ammonium acetate together with 300 µL absolute ethanol. Mix and place on dry ice for at least 10 min.

4. Centrifuge at 12,000–15,000$g$ for 10 min and decant ethanol (**caution:** this mixture is very radioactive). Wash pellet in 500 µL cold (–20°C) 70% ethanol, recentrifuge and decant supernatant. Dry pellet.

## 3.3. Purification of Labeled RNA ("Riboprobe")

1. Resuspend labeled riboprobe in 30 µL gel loading buffer and place on ice prior to loading on an acrylamide gel. Prior to loading denature at 85°C for 5 min and place immediately on ice.

2. Electrophorese in a 8% denaturing acrylamide gel in TBE buffer (*see* **Note 7**). Load 30 µL of gel loading buffer to each well (without sample) and prerun gel for 15-20 min at a constant current of 25 mA to equilibrate the gel. Load samples and run for a further 2.5 h at 25 mA. (Shorter/longer riboprobes will require modification of running times.) Care should be taken when dismantling gel rig after run as all solutions will be highly radioactive, wear goggles and work behind shields. Remove upper gel plate. Position gel using

radioactive ink-marked Whatman filter paper wrap in Saran Wrap/clingfilm. Place in perspex box for transport to dark room. Expose gel to film for 5–30 s (Kodak X-Omat, UK) and develop autoradiograph.

3. Using a scalpel cut the bands from the autoradiograph to form a template. Place the template over the gel and excise bands containing riboprobe, (use a fresh blade for each probe), and place gel slices in 1.5-mL Eppendorf tubes. Add 400 µL Maxim & Gilbert's elution buffer, vortex strongly, and incubate overnight at 37°C.

4. Vortex gel/elution buffer and centrifuge for 30 s at 12,000*g*. Pipet off the supernatant (containing riboprobe) to a separate Eppendorf. Add 1 µL 10 µg/mL tRNA per sample followed by 2.5 vol of cold (–20°C) absolute ethanol. Vortex and place on dry ice for 10 min.

5. Pellet RNA by centrifugation at 15,000*g* for 10 min at room temperature. Discard supernatant and pellet with 500 µL 70% ethanol. Recentrifuge and discard supernatant. Dry pellet under vacuum for 10 min.

6. Resuspend pellet in 50 µL hybridization buffer. Count 1 µL aliquot (*see* **Note 8**). Store on ice until required (riboprobe may be stored up to 7 d before use, for best results use as soon as possible).

## 3.4. RNA:RNA Hybridization

1. Prepare 20 µg of total tumor RNA for hybridization in a 1.5-mL Eppendorf as follows: Add 1:10th vol of 3*M* sodium acetate (pH 5.2) and 2.5 vol absolute ethanol. Vortex and place on dry ice for 10 min. Centrifuge at 15,000*g* for 10 min and discard supernatant. Wash once with 250 µL 70% ethanol (–20°C) and recentrifuge and discard supernatant. Air-dry pellet and resuspend in 30 µL hybridization buffer.

2. Add $10^6$ counts for each probe to be analysed (usually minimum of β-actin and one other) to the hybridization mix, vortex, and spin down. Denature to 85°C for 20 min and incubate at 51°C overnight.

3. Prepare RNA digestion buffer. Add 300 µL digestion buffer to each sample and incubate for 30 min at 37°C.

4. Spin samples briefly and add 20 µL 10% SDS and 2 µL proteinase K (10 mg/mL). Vortex, spin, and incubate for 15 min at 37°C.

5. Add 350 µL of phenol:chloroform:isoamylalcohol. Vortex vigorously and centrifuge at 12,000*g* for 10 min.

6. Remove 300 µL of upper aqueous layer (avoiding phenol) to a new tube.

7. Add 5 µg tRNA and 750 µL absolute ethanol (–20°C), vortex, and place on dry ice for 10–30 min.

8. Centrifuge at 15,000*g* for 10 min and decant ethanol.

9. Wash in 500 µL 70% ethanol (–20°C), vortex, and centrifuge at 15,000*g* for 10 min and decant ethanol. Repeat once.

10. Dry pellet under vacuum and resuspend in 3 µL gel loading buffer, place on ice.

## 3.5. Electrophoresis and Detection of RNA:RNA Hybrids

1. Prepare a 6% denaturing acrylamide gel. Wash wells with TBE, load 3 µL of gel loading buffer into all wells, and prerun gel at 25 mA for 10–20 min.

2. Prepare the following controls: $10^3$ cpm of each riboprobe in 3 µL loading buffer. 35S labeled molecular weight markers (*see* **Note 9**).

3. Heat all samples to 85°C for 2–3 min and cool on ice immediately. Load samples on gel, and run at 25 mA for 2 h.

4. Remove gel from rig and separate glass plates, immerse gel in gel fixing solution (10% acetic acid, 10% methanol in distilled water) for 15 min at room temperature.

5. Carefully remove gel from fixing solution and place a piece of 3 MM Whatman filter paper on the gel. Either invert the gel and lift the glass plate away or lift the paper from the plate, the gel should stick to the filter. Cover the exposed surface of the gel with cling film and place on a gel dryer for 1 h.

6. Preflash X-Omat autoradiography film and place directly on the gel. Expose overnight at –70°C and develop film. Identify positive/negatives by presence of bands corresponding to the size of the cloned cDNA fragment. For quantification, gel documentation and scanning systems can be used (*see* **Note 10**).

## 4. Discussion

The RNase protection assay was developed originally to allow rapid, simultaneous quantitation of relatively low copy mRNAs and quantitation of gene expression. This technique is robust and an experienced operator can process around 100 samples in a single assay. However, as described here, the method requires significant levels of radio-isotope representing a high level of risk to the operator. The synthesis of biotinylated nucleotides may circumvent the need for using isotopes, but will extend the complexity of the assay, requiring blotting and detection steps to be added. The major advantage of this technique is the ability to simultaneously detect and quantify multiple mRNA species without the need for enzymatic modification (as in reverse-transcriptase PCR) and the ability to detect splice variants without the need for ARMS PCR technology *(3)*. It is readily applicable to tumor samples and results in ovarian cancers using this model have been used to demonstrate the expression of FGFs, TGFα, and the TGFβ supergene family. Whereas quantitative PCR methods are rapidly superseding this technology, there remain significant question marks over the accuracy of such quantitative methods particularly at the level of the reverse transcription step which can be modified markedly by variation in RNA quality and protein carryover from RNA purification. To this extent, both the reverse transcription and PCR steps of quantitative PCR remain highly susceptible to contaminants from tumor tissue and the laboratory environment. Further quantitation using PCR requires the mutagenesis of control templates and extensive validation. The RNase protection assay has proven a reliable and robust method for rapid and accurate quantitation of mRNAs direct from tissue RNA samples and is widely used for studies of subjects as diverse as growth factor expression *(1,2)*, drug resistance *(4)*, gene transcription activation *(5)*, and differentiation of expression patterns *(6,7)*.

## 5. Notes

1. To synthesize mRNA probes from cloned DNA fragments, plasmids incorporating RNA polymerase promotors (T3, T7, or SP6) are required. Ideally, two promotors should be present either side of the multiple cloning site to allow synthesis of mRNA in both the sense and antisense direction, to allow production of control sense RNA strands for quantitation. Bluescript™ is an ideal choice for cloning fragments, as it is a high copy number plasmid which can be readily linearized in either direction. Linearized DNA reduces wastage in the RNA synthesis caused by copying plasmid sequence.

2. The high levels of radioactive P-32 used in this assay system present a considerable hazard to the operator. To generate multiple riboprobes (4 in this instance), over 5 MBq of isotope are used. Appropriate shielding (perspex boxes, face shields, and so on) and monitoring (finger badges, film badges) must be in place. Although replacement of P32-CTP

with biotinylated CTP is feasible detection of biotinylated CTP requires blotting and antibody detection that extends greatly the time required for this protocol.

3. Acrylamide is a potent neurotoxin. In view of this hazard, predissolved acrylamide solutions are recommended.

4. These RNases are very concentrated and stable; contamination of any other part of the method with these enzymes will degrade RNA. When pipeting RNases, wear two pairs of gloves. Uncap tubes, discard outer gloves **before** picking up pipets. Aliquot RNases, cap tubes, and discard gloves again.

5. Disaggregation is critically dependent on tissue structure. Most tumors of serous, endometriod, or mucinous subtypes are readily disaggregated in $2 \times 60$ s bursts. Other tumor types (Brenner, thecoma) may require longer periods to disrupt tissue.

6. Extraction of RNA from solid tumors can be problematic, many of the commercial systems available for RNA extraction are validated for extraction of RNA from cell-culture material or blood lymphocytes. These kits have often been less successful with tumor derived material.

7. Unless glass plates are used exclusively for RNA work, scrub with 5% potassium hydroxide in methanol (w/v) prior to use. In all cases, scrub with concentrated detergent (Fairy liquid), rinse with tap water, and copiously with deionized water, followed by detergent and methanol. Dry and set aside for use. For riboprobes with sufficient separation (30+ basepairs) it is not necessary to use 0.4-mm gels and sequence length reads (40 cm). Routinely these assays can be performed on 16–20-cm reads using 1-mm gels (such as those used for protein separation prior to Western blots).

8. Yield is routinely $50–100 \times 10^6$ counts. Yields below $0.75 \times 10^6$ counts/µL are not viable if large numbers of samples are required.

9. Synthesis of 35-S labeled markers. 35-S labeled markers are prepared using a Hinf1 restriction enzyme digest of pBR322: 2 µg of plasmid was incubated with 10 U Hinf1 overnight at 37°C. Digestion was check on an agarose minigel. Hinf1 restricts the sequence 5'GANTC3' leaving 5' protruding ends, which are labeled with Klenow fragment (Promega). 1 µg (1 µL) Hinf1 digest is incubated with 2 µL 10X Klenow Buffer, 1 µL 2 m$M$ dGTP/dCTP/dTTP, 2 µL 35-S dATP (Amersham), 1 µL Klenow, 9 µL distilled water for 30 min at room temperature. The reaction is halted by adding 2 µL 0.25$M$ EDTA. Markers are stored at –20°C and 0.1–0.5 µL run on each gel as a size markers.

10. Use of antisense control RNA. Whereas gel scanning of preflashed autoradiographs gives accurate **relative** quantitation, that is quantitation of samples related to control values, it is not possible to calculate absolute mRNA concentrations in this way. In order to provide such quantitation the synthesis of unlabelled antisense RNA from the plasmid containing the cDNA under investigation is required. In vectors such as Bluescript where two RNA polymerase promotors are present, this is achieved by digesting the vector such that use of the Riboprobe kit generates antisense RNA. This control RNA is synthesized unlabeled and can be quantified and diluted in the assay system to provide a "standard curve" of known RNA concentrations against which unknowns can be quantified.

## References

1. Bartlett, J. M. S., Langdon, S. P., Scott, W. N., Love. S. B., Miller, E. P., Katsaros, D., et al. (1997) Transforming growth factor-β Isoform expression in human ovarian tumors. *Eur. J. Cancer* **33,** 2397–2403.

2. Bartlett, J. M. S., Rabiasz, G. J., Scott, W. N., Langdon, S. P., Smyth, J. F., and Miller, W. R. (1992) Transforming growth factor-β mRNA expression in growth control of human ovarian carcinoma cells. *Brit. J. Cancer* **65,** 655–660.

3. Brooks, D. J., Woodward, S., Thompson, F. H., Dossantos, B., Russell, M., Yang, J. M., et al. (1996) Expression of the zinc finger gene EVI-1 in ovarian and other cancers. *Brit. J. Cancer* **74,** 1518–1525

4. Nooter, K., Westerman, A. M., Flens, M. J., Zaman, G. J. R., Scheper, R. J., Vanwingerden, K. E., et al. (1995) Expression of the multidrug resistance-associated protein (mrp) gene in human cancers(1). *Clinic. Cancer Res.* **1,** 1301–1310.

5. Spinner, D. M., Brandstetter, T., Kiechleschwarz, M., Dubois, A., Angel, P., and Bauknecht, T. (1995) C-jun expression and growth-stimulation in human ovarian-carcinoma cell-lines following exposure to cytokines. *Int. J. Cancer* **63,** 423–427.

6. Li, J., Ding, S. F., Habib, N. A., Fermor, B. F., Wood, C. B., and Gilmour, R. S. (1994) Partial characterization of a cdna for human stearoyl-coa desaturase and changes in its messenger-rna expression in some normal and malignant-tissues. *Int. J. Cancer* **57,** 348–352.

7. Siyanova, E. Y., Serfas, M. S., Mazo, I. A., and Tyner, A. L. (1994) Tyrosine kinase gene-expression in the mouse small-intestine. *Oncogene* **9,** 2053–2057.

# 48

# RT-PCR Quantitation of HSP60 mRNA Expression

**Raymond P. Perez, Lakshmi Pendyala, Zeyad Elakawi, and Mahmoud Abu-hadid**

## 1. Introduction

Heat shock protein 60 (HSP60, HSPD1) is a "chaperonin" that facilitates folding of nascent proteins into proper conformations (*1*). It is thought to play a critical role in the assembly, folding, and transport of proteins in the mitochondria. HSP60 also interacts with nascent cellular proteins to prevent their denaturation under heat stress (*2*). The HSP60 gene sequence is known and is highly conserved (*3*). Expression of the HSP60 gene has been associated with cisplatin resistance in several preclinical model systems and in ovarian carcinoma patients (*4–6*); we quantitated HSP60 mRNA expression in preclinical human ovarian and bladder carcinoma models.

In general terms, quantitation of RT-PCR products can be accomplished by either: 1) determination of the amount of products formed after a given number of amplification cycles following titration of the amount of cDNA template (titration analysis), or 2) determination of the amount of products formed at several consecutive cycles for given amounts of template (kinetic analysis). Depending on the amount of template in reactions, PCR product quantities typically increase exponentially for a finite number of cycles, followed by a plateau. For either type of analysis, quantitation is performed in the log-linear portion of the reaction (*7*). Within the linear range, the amount of PCR product formed is directly proportional to the number of copies of the target mRNA. The relationship between the initial cDNA concentration and amount of product is described by the slope of the linear portion of the curve.

The method we used for quantitation is conceptually straightforward. HSP60 mRNA levels were quantitated by a titration RT-PCR relative to expression of an endogenous standard ("housekeeping") gene, β-actin, within the linear range of amplification for each reaction. Standardization relative to a housekeeping gene allows for differences in RNA quantity, RNA purity, and efficiency of cDNA synthesis to be controlled. PCR products were separated by ion-exchange HPLC and detected by UV absorbance at 260 nm. Thus separation, detection, and quantitation of the product depends mainly on physical properties of the dsDNA product formed during the PCR.

Previous studies of HSP60 mRNA· expression used Northern blotting for quantitation. The PCR method we used is similar to Northern blotting in that expression of HSP60 was quantitated relative to levels of an endogenous standard. Like North-

From: *Methods in Molecular Medicine, Vol. 39: Ovarian Cancer: Methods and Protocols*
Edited by: J. M. S. Bartlett © Humana Press, Inc., Totowa, NJ

ern blotting, our PCR method is probably most correctly described as "semiquantitative," because expression is quantitated in relative terms instead of in absolute copy numbers. However, RT-PCR offers potentially significant advantages over Northern blotting, including the ability to assay much smaller amounts of RNA and greater speed.

## 2. Materials

### 2.1. Cell Lines and Growth Media

1. Platinum-resistant ovarian carcinoma cell lines: The A2780 human ovarian carcinoma cell line and a subline selected for cisplatin resistance (2780/CP) by chronic in vitro treatment were originally provided by Drs. R. Ozols and T. Hamilton (Fox Chase Cancer Center, Philadelphia, PA) *(8)*. Oxaliplatin-resistant sublines were developed by chronic in vitro exposure to the drug in Dr. Pendyala's laboratory *(9)*. Cells were grown at 37°C in a humidified atmosphere of 5% $CO_2$ in air. Cisplatin-resistant bladder carcinoma cell line: The UCRU-BL13 human bladder carcinoma cell line *(10)* was provided by Dr. D. Raghavan and D. Glaves-Rapp, Roswell Park Cancer Institute. A clonal, cisplatin-resistant subline (BL13/CR24D) was derived by chronic in vitro selection, in the laboratory of Dr. Glaves-Rapp.
2. Growth medium for ovarian carcinoma cell lines: RPMI-1640 medium supplemented with 10% FBS (Gibco, Grand Island, NY), 0.28 U/mL insulin, 100 g/mL streptomycin, 100 U/mL penicillin, and 0.3 mg/mL glutamine. All media components were filter (0.2 µ) sterilized and complete media was stored at 4°C.
3. Growth medium for bladder carcinoma cell lines: RPMI-1640 medium supplemented with 10% FBS (Gibco), 100 g/mL streptomycin, 100 U/mL penicillin, 0.56 mg/mL $NaHCO_3$, and 0.3 mg/mL glutamine. All media components were filter (0.2 µ) sterilized and complete media was stored at 4°C. Cells were grown at 37°C in a humidified atmosphere of 5% $CO_2$ in air.
4. Primers were synthesized in the RPCI biopolymer facility on an ABI prism synthesizer, based on previously published sequences for β-actin and HSP60 (GenBank accession numbers 10278 and M34664, respectively). Primer sequences are as follows:
   HSP60 5′: AGACGTTCAGCCTCATGACTTAGGA
   HSP60 3′: GGAGGGCACAACCCCCTCCCAA
   Actin 5′: GCGCTCGTCGTCGACAACGG
   Actin 3′: GCCACACGCAGCTCATTGTAGA
5. Reaction buffer: 1X = 60 m$M$ Tris (pH 9.0), 15 m$M$ $(NH_4)_2SO_4$; buffer is prepared and stored at room temperature as a 5X stock solution (i.e., 300 m$M$ Tris, 75 m$M$ $(NH_4)_2SO_4$; all buffer components purchased from Sigma, St. Louis, MO).

### 2.2. HPLC

1. Buffer A: 25 m$M$ Tris-HCl with 1 m$M$ EDTA (pH 8.0); all buffer components were purchased from Sigma.
2. Buffer B: Buffer A + 1.0$M$ NaCl. Buffers were stored at either room temperature or at 4°C. Buffers were generally consumed very rapidly, so stability studies were not performed.
3. The HPLC system consisted of Waters Associates M6000A pump and an automatic sample injector WISP, with an Autochrome-one pump gradient maker and a Waters Associates model 470 UV detector. Column: Gen-Pak Fax (4.6 × 100 mm; Waters Associates). The HPLC system is interfaced with a Hewlett-Packard computer with chromatography data acquisition by Nelson Analytical Chromatography software.

## 3. Methods

### 3.1. Cell Culture/Harvest

1. Each cell line was plated into 25-cm$^2$ disposable tissue-culture flasks (Falcon, Los Angeles, CA; purchased from VWR Scientific) at a sufficient initial density to yield approximately 60% confluence by 48 h postplating, depending on the known growth rates of the individual cell lines. Cells were routinely harvested at that time-point.
2. Media was aspirated and cells were washed three times with 1X PBS (purchased from Gibco/BRL.
3. Cells were lysed directly in flasks in 1 mL Trizol® reagent (Gibco/BRL) with gentle swirling.

### 3.2. RNA Isolation

RNA isolation was performed essentially according to the manufacturer's protocol for Trizol reagent, without modification *(11)*.

1. Cultured cells were lysed for 5 min at room temperature in Trizol reagent (2.5 mL) added directly to tissue culture flasks.
2. Lysates were mixed with chloroform (0.5 mL), followed by centrifugation at 12,000$g$ for 15 min at 4°C.
3. The aqueous phase (containing RNA) was transferred to fresh microcentrifuge tubes, RNA was precipitated with isopropanol (1.25 mL) and pelleted by centrifugation at 12,000$g$ for 10 min.
4. The RNA pellet was washed with 75% ethanol, air-dried, and resuspended in nuclease-free (i.e., DEPC-treated) water.
5. RNA quantity ($A_{260}$) and purity ($A_{260/280}$) were determined by UV spectrometry. Aliquots of resuspended RNA were diluted into water to a final volume of 1 mL, and $A_{260}$ and $A_{280}$ were read on a UV spectrophotometer (Perkin-Elmer #552), relative diluent blanks in matched quartz cuvetes. RNA quantity was calculated assuming that 40 µg/mL yields an $A_{260}$ = 1.0. RNA purity was checked against expected values for $A_{260/280}$ ratio = 1.8–2.0.
6. Reconstituted RNA was stored at –70°C. Our samples have been stable > 2 yr under these conditions. However, given the susceptibility of RNA to nuclease digestion and chemical degradation, some variability in stability should be anticipated.

### 3.3. cDNA Synthesis

1. Each reaction contained 20 µg total RNA, 2.5 µL of 100 pmol/µL oligo-dT primer (Gibco/BRL), 10 µL of 5X Superscript II® reaction buffer, 5 µL 0.1$M$ DTT, 5 µL of 10 m$M$ working solution of DTPs, 500 U Superscript II reverse-transcriptase (2.5 µL), and 5 µL sterile DEPC-treated water in a final volume of 50 µL. Oligo-dT primers (dT12-18) and Superscript II reverse transcriptase (including 0.1$M$ DTT and reaction buffer) were purchased from Gibco/BRL.
2. 20 µL of 1 µg/µL total RNA plus 2.5 µL oligo-dT primer were incubated at 90°C for 10 min in a heat block.
3. The reaction was rapidly cooled in an ice-water bath for 2 min.
4. The remaining reaction components (10 µL buffer, 5 µL DTT, 5 µL water, 2.5 µL reverse transcriptase) were added and the reaction incubated at 43°C for 1 h.
5. The reaction was rapidly cooled on an ice-water bath, then stored at –20°C. cDNA prepared in this manner has been stable for > 2 yrs.

### 3.4. Polymerase Chain Reaction (PCR)

1. Each reaction contained: cDNA, 100 $\mu M$ each dNTP, reaction buffer, $Mg^{++}$ 1.5 m$M$, 50 pmol of each primer, 2.5 U *Taq* polymerase, and sterile DEPC-treated water in a final volume of 50 $\mu$L. Deoxynucleotide triphosphates (100 m$M$ stock solutions, pH 7.0) and $MgCl_2$ (25 m$M$ solution; PCR grade) were purchased from Sigma; native *Taq* polymerase was purchased from Perkin-Elmer. All PCR reagents were stored at –20°C; stability studies were not performed.
2. A master mix containing all components, except cDNA and *Taq* polymerase, was prepared on the benchtop at room temperature, in quantity sufficient for ($n$+1) reactions (i.e., if 10 reactions were to be performed, sufficient master mix was prepared for 11 reactions, to account for potential losses during repeated pipeting). Master mix (18 $\mu$L) was distributed to each reaction tube. Thin-walled PCR tubes (0.2 mL) were purchased from Laboratory Products Supply (Rochester, NY). Comparable thin-walled reaction tubes from other sources could reasonably be substituted.
3. cDNA (1 $\mu$L of appropriate dilution; *see* **Subheading 3.6., step 1**) was added to each reaction tube.
4. Reactions were overlaid with 20 $\mu$L mineral oil (molecular biology grade, Sigma).
5. Reaction tubes were transferred to the thermal cycler block, which was preheated to 94°C, and incubated at this temperature for 2 min.
6. *Taq* polymerase was added to each reaction (i.e., manual "hot start"; *see* **Note 6**).
7. Thirty cycles of amplification were performed, with denaturation at 94°C for 1 min, followed by annealing/extension at 72°C for 2 min, on an Ericomp Powerblock® thermal cycler.

### 3.5. HPLC (see Notes 1–4)

1. PCRs were diluted by addition of 50 $\mu$L water; 80 $\mu$L of the resulting solution was pipeted into HPLC autosampler inserts and loaded onto the autosampler carousel.
2. Quantitation of the PCR product was performed by anion exchange chromatography with gradient elution *(12)*.
3. The HPLC gradient was from 30:70 of buffer A: buffer B to 100% buffer B in a 30 min linear gradient. Detection was with UV at 260 nm.

### 3.6. Quantitative PCR

1. The linear range of amplification is established prior to quantitation. Serial dilutions of cDNA are prepared in water and used as template for PCRs. Products are separated by HPLC and detected/quantitated by A260. Integrated peak areas for the absorbance vs time chromatograms are plotted relative to the amount of cDNA in each reaction (expressed in ng of total RNA; **Fig. 1**). Inspection of such a plot allows determination of the linear range for HSP60 and β-actin.
2. Quantitation is performed for one (or more) cDNA quantities within the linear range. The amount of PCR product (integrated peak area) formed for HSP60 can then be expressed relative to the amount of product formed for β-actin at a given initial quantity of template cDNA. Quantitation can alternatively be done using several different concentrations of cDNA, provided all are within the linear range. In this case, slopes of the line for HSP60 can be divided by the slope of the line for β-actin to quantitate relative HSP60 mRNA levels.

## 4. Notes

1. In general, the sensitivity of our HPLC system was comparable or exceeded that of ethidium bromide staining. For example, the detection limit for PCR products by HPLC

Fig. 1. Quantities of PCR products formed for HSP60 and β-actin, following titration of cDNA concentration. The cDNA concentration is expressed in terms of the amount of total RNA present in an equivalent volume of cDNA reaction mixture. Data shown are means (± standard deviation) of at least two independent experiments. Arrows indicate that the quantity of cDNA per PCR (10 ng) used for relative quantitation of HSP60 and β-actin was within the log-linear portion of the curves.

was 1 ng, whereas quantities of DNA ≥ 10 ng could be seen on ethidium bromide stained gels. We did not compare the sensitivity of this HPLC system to alternative DNA intercalating fluorescent dyes that are purported to have greater sensitivity than ethidium bromide (such as Sybr green I®, Molecular Probes, Inc., Eugene, OR).

2. The HPLC conditions used produced excellent separation of DNA fragments ranging in size from 100 to 800 bp (**Fig. 2**). A linear correlation was observed between integrated peak areas and the amount of injected DNA ($r = 0.998$). Gradient conditions for optimal separation of PCR products of other sizes would need to be empirically determined. Investigators may wish to routinely inject known DNA size/quantity standards as a quality control check for detection sensitivity and product size discrimination. The DNA mass ladder (Gibco/BRL) allows monitoring of both separation and sensitivity with a single sample injection.

3. Conditions for PCR and HPLC were optimized for our specific instrumentation. Alternative instruments can be used, but additional optimization may be required.

4. Alternative HPLC columns for quantitation of PCR products are available from Perkin-Elmer (TSK DEAE-NPR column) and DuPont (Zorbax GF-250 sizing column); we have no direct experience with these products.

5. The HSP60 and β-actin primers yield products of 328 and 271 bp from cDNA, respectively. Reaction products can be checked relative to known size standards (such as 100 bp ladder, Gibco/BRL) on ethidium bromide stained agarose gels (1–2% agarose, in TAE or TBE) following electrophoresis.

6. A manual "hot start" (i.e., addition of *Taq* polymerase while reactions were held at the denaturing temperature) was included in our protocol because this method reportedly improves the specificity and yield of PCRs by minimizing false-priming *(13)*. Manual addition of enzyme can be difficult, especially if oil/wax overlays are used. Investigators must be certain that the pipete tip is below the hydrophobic overlay, to insure delivery of the polymerase into the reaction mixture. Pipeting for manual hot start must be done

Fig. 2. HPLC separation of DNA fragments from 100 to 2000 bp size (DNA mass ladder, Gibco/BRL). Reproduced from **ref. 16** with permission from Elsevier Science.

quickly, as pipete tips may warp or seal within seconds at high temperatures, potentially compromising delivery of the intended volume. Alternatively, manual polymerase addition can be replaced by a 2-step wax-mediated hot start *(14)*. Numerous commercial products have recently become available to "automate" hot starts, including precast paraffin beads (± one or more reaction components; multiple vendors), a version of *Taq* polymerase that is inactive until heated to denaturation temperature (AmpliTaq Gold®, Perkin-Elmer), and an anti-*Taq* monoclonal antibody that is added to the master mix and which dissociates from the polymerase upon heating (TaqStart®, Clontech).

7. If desired, product identity can be confirmed by sequencing. Following HPLC separation, eluted fractions containing PCR can be collected, then desalted and concentrated on a Centrex UF-0.5 3K molecular weight cutoff filter (Schleicher & Scheuell, Dassel, Germany). Alternatively, PCR products can be subjected to agarose gel electrophoresis (as in **Note 8**), followed by recovery of DNA from bands excised from the gel. Numerous methods and commercial reagents are available for this purpose. We generally recover excised DNA fragments by centrifugation (15,000$g$) over 0.45 μ cellulose acetate filters (Lida), followed by desalting over 3 K mw cutoff filters (Schleicher & Scheull) as above. Recovered DNA purified by either method can then be subjected to automated sequencing using the same primers as for PCR or cloned into a suitable plasmid vector prior to sequencing.

8. PCR product identity can alternatively be verified by restriction mapping. PCR products can be recovered from gels as above and digested with endonucleases that cut each product once. For example, the following fragment sizes are expected following restriction of the HSP60 product with various endonucleases: *Alu*I (292 + 36 bp), *Mae*I (149 + 179), and *Spe*I (148 + 180). For β-actin, expected fragment sizes for some commonly used endonucleases are: *Bgl*I (64 + 207), *Hae*II (92 + 179), and *Sma*I (64 + 207). These endonucleases were selected from a larger list of restriction enzymes expected to cut each PCR product once, using the "map" program from the Wisconsin Package (version 8.1, Genetics Computer Group, Madison, WI). Complete maps of potential restriction sites could be generated with this software, or with a variety of similar software packages available

commercially (such as Gene Construction Kit, Textco, Inc.) or as freeware (such as DNAid+, available from the Indiana University Molecular Biology software archives at FTP://iubio.bio.indiana.edu/molbio/).

9. PCR products (and primers, primer-dimers, secondary products, etc.) can be recovered from agarose gels as in **Note 10** for injection onto the HPLC column. This allows retention times for reaction products to be determined and, if necessary, for optimization of HPLC conditions for quantitation of products of interest.

10. RNA preparations may occasionally contain contaminating genomic DNA. Genomic DNA will yield a PCR product of 404 bp for the β-actin primer pair when amplification is performed with denaturation at $96° \times 30s$ followed by annealing/extension at $68° \times 60s$. Thus, β-actin products from genomic DNA and cDNA can be distinguished by size on agarose gels (and, usually, by different HPLC retention times) under these conditions. Genomic DNA contamination could directly interfere with quantitation of HSP60 because this gene lacks introns (hence, genomic and cDNA yield products of identical size and sequence). Contaminating genomic DNA can be eliminated by 1) treatment of RNA with RNase-free DNase; 2) isolation of mRNA from total RNA; or 3) direct isolation of mRNA. Reagents for each of these approaches are available from a variety of commercial vendors.

11. It is generally prudent to include positive and negative controls in each set of reactions. Negative controls are identical to quantitative reactions except that no template is added. The presence of bands at the expected product size in no-template controls usually indicates carryover contamination from setup of a concurrent reaction or contamination of one or more reagents with cDNA, genomic DNA, or product from a prior PCR. Nonspecific bands (especially primer-dimers) can be seen in no-template controls in the absence of contamination. Positive controls are useful for verifying the integrity of the reaction mix. Any sample known to yield a strong reaction for the gene of interest can be used as a positive control. For example, RNA isolated from either of the ovarian carcinoma cell lines used in our investigations could serve as a positive control. Alternatively, one could isolate PCR product following agarose gel electrophoresis of a known positive reaction (as in **Note 10**) and reamplify this as a positive control.

To avoid overcycling during reamplification (overcycling can generate smears, increased nonspecific background, and unintended products larger than expected size) *(15)*, isolated PCR product should be diluted substantially (dilution in the range of $10^{-3}–10^{-6}$ is usually necessary). Also, particular care should be taken to avoid contamination of pipetors and reagents when handling concentrated purified PCR products. Aerosol-resistant pipete tips should be used and dilutions should be prepared in a location remote from where PCRs are usually set up.

12. It is important to establish that expression of the endogenous standard remains stable under the experimental conditions used. We previously published data showing comparable expression of β-actin (relative to μg of total RNA) in the A2780, 2780/C10, and 2780/C25 cell lines *(16)*; similar data were obtained for the A2780-2780/CP and UCRU-BL13-BL13/CR24D cell line pairs in preliminary experiments (data not shown). Other frequently expressed genes could alternatively be used as endogenous standards (for example, Glucose-6-phosphate dehydrogenase(G6PD), aldolase, 18s or 28s ribosomal RNA, and so on) if their expression is relatively stable under the experimental conditions used.

13. Quantitative PCR offers potentially powerful approaches to further characterize mechanisms responsible for observed differences in HSP60 mRNA expression. For example, quantitative conditions for amplification of genomic DNA can be determined, allowing quantitation of relative HSP60 gene copy number. Increased HSP60 mRNA levels that correlated with cisplatin resistance were observed in our model systems. Quantitation of HSP60 gene copy number in the various cell lines showed the same relative gene copy

number in each cell line, which suggests that increased mRNA levels in platinum-resistant cell lines was not becuase of gene amplification *(17)*. Alternatively, mRNA stability can be compared by harvesting cell lines at various times during incubation with an RNA synthesis inhibitor (such as Actinomycin-D ($\geq 50$ µg/mL final concentration); note that actinomycin-D is a teratogen and carcinogen—it should be handled in a chemical fume hood and gloves/mask should be worn). These examples illustrate how the same general PCR approach can be adapted to several interrelated quantitative endpoints.

14. The use of HPLC for quantitation was convenient in light of our group's considerable experience with this methodology. In addition, the use of an HPLC setup that incorporated an autosampler and on-line quantitation allowed high throughput at relatively low labor intensity. However, HPLC instrumentation and operation are fairly expensive and our approach may not be cost-effective for investigators who are not already performing HPLC. Moreover, some PCRs might reach plateau before enough product is formed to allow quantitation by HPLC. Although space does not permit detailed consideration of all possible approaches to PCR product quantitation, several potential alternative approaches could be used for product quantitation. For example, very sensitive dsDNA fluorescent dyes, such as Sybr green I (Molecular Probes, Inc.) could allow photodetection of PCR products within the linear range of amplification on agarose gels and their subsequent quantitation by densitometry. Similarly, methods for quantitation of PCR products in solution by a different dsDNA intercalating dye, Picogreen® (Molecular Probes, Inc.), has been reported *(18)*. Numerous laboratories have included labeled nucleotides in PCRs for quantitation of radioactivity or chemiluminescence incorporated into products by Southern / dot blotting, scintillation counting, and so on. Regardless of the ultimate means of product detection / quantitation, extreme care must be taken to insure that quantitation is being performed in the linear range of amplification.

15. The method we have described is relatively straightforward. However, we are available to answer any questions that may arise. Please feel free to contact Dr. Perez by e-mail at Raymond.P.Perez@Hitchcock.org, by telephone at (603) 650-6633, by FAX at (603) 650-7791, or by mail at Dartmouth-Hithcock Medical Center, One Medical Center Drive, Lebanon, NH 03756.

## References

1. Craig, E. A., Gambill, B. D., and Nelson, R. J. (1993) Heat shock proteins: molecular chaperones of protein biogenesis. *Microbiol. Rev.* **57,** 402–414.
2. Martin, J., Horwich, A. L., and Hartl, F. U. (1992) Prevention of protein denaturation under heat stress by the chaperonin Hsp60. *Science* **258,** 995–998.
3. Venner, T. J., Singh, B., and Gupta, R. S. (1990) Nucleotide sequences and novel structural features of human and Chinese hamster hsp60 (chaperonin) gene families. *DNA Cell Biol.* **9,** 545–552.
4. Enns, R. E., Hom, D. K., Thiebaut, F., and Howell, S. B. (1991) An amplified mitochondrial chaperonin gene causes resistance to cisplatin in human ovarian tumor cells. *Proc. Amer. Assoc. Cancer Res.* **32,** 2088–2090 (abstract).
5. Kimura, E., Enns, R. E., Alcaraz, J. E., Arboleda, J., Slamon, D. J., and Howell, S. B. (1993) Correlation of the survival of ovarian cancer patients with mRNA expression of the 60-kD heat shock protein HSP-60. *J. Clin. Oncol.* **11,** 891–898.
6. Shen, D-W., Pastan, I., and Gottesman, M. (1994) A 52 kD protein is overexpressed in cisplatin-resistant human liver carcinoma cells and in cisplatin-resistant mouse cells after DNA-mediated transformation. *Proc. Amer. Assoc. Cancer Res.* **35,** 2630 (abstract).
7. Gause, W. and Adamovicz, J. (1994) The use of PCR to quantitate gene expression. *PCR Meth. Applicat.* **3,** s123–s135.
8. Behrens, B. C., Hamilton, T. C., and Masuda, H. (1987) Characterization of a cis-diamminedichloroplatinim (II)-resistant human ovarian cancer cell line and its use in evaluation of platinum analogues. *Cancer Res.* **47,** 414–418.
9. Glavy, J., Pendyala, L., Creaven, P. J., Perez, R., Zdanowicz, J., and Elakawi, Z. (1994) Isolation and preliminary characterization of oxaliplatin resistant A2780 ovarian carcinoma sublines. *Proc. Amer. Assoc. Cancer Res.* **35,** 2590 (abstract).

10. Russell, P. J., Raghavan, D., Gregory, P., Phillips, J., Wills, E. J., Jelbart, M., et al. (1986) Bladder cancer xenografts: a model of tumor cell heterogeneity. *Cancer Res.* **46,** 2035–2040.
11. Chomczynski, P. (1993) A reagent for the single-step simultaneous isolation of RNA, DNA, and proteins from cell and tissue samples. *Biotechniques* **15,** 532–536.
12. Warren, W., Wheat, T., and Knudsen, P. (1991) Rapid analysis and quantitation of PCR products by high-performance liquid chromatography. *Biotechniques* **11,** 250–255.
13. D'Aquila, R. T., Bechtel, L. J., Videler, J. A., Eron, J. J., Gorczyza, P., and Kaplan, J. C. (1991) Maximizing sensitivity and specificity of PCR by pre-amplification heating. *Nucl. Acids Res.* **19,** 3749.
14. Sparkman, D. R. (1992) Paraffin wax as a vapor barrier for the PCR. *PCR Meth. Appl.* **2,** 180,181.
15. Bell, D. A. and DeMarini, D. (1991) Excessive cycling converts PCR products to random-length higher molecular weight fragments. *Nucl. Acids Res.* **19,** 5079.
16. El-akawi, Z., Abu-hadid, M., Perez, R., Glavy, J., Zdanowicz, J., Creaven, P. J., et al. (1996) Altered glutathione metabolism in oxaliplatin resistant ovarian carcinoma cells. *Cancer Lett.* **105,** 5–14.
17. Abu-hadid, M., Wilkes, J. D., Elakawi, Z., Pendyala, L., and Perez, R. P. (1997) Relationship between heat shock protein 60 (HSP60) mRNA expression and resistance to platinum analogues in human ovarian and bladder carcinoma cell lines. *Cancer Lett.* **119,** 63–70.
18. Enger, O. (1996) Use of the fluorescent dye PicoGreen for quantitation of PCR products after agarose gel electrophoresis. *Biotechniques* **21,** 372–374.

# 49

## The Effects of Butyrate and the Role of *c-myc* in N.1 Ovarian Carcinoma Cells Determined by Northern Blotting

### Georg Krupitza

## 1. Introduction

Two hypothetical concepts are discussed as means to cure cancer: 1) extinction of the neoplastic cell pool which forms the tumor and 2) induction of terminal differentiation to park tumor cells in growth arrest *(1)*. Sodium butyrate (NaB) has been shown to promote differentiation of HL-60 cells to mature monocytes *(2)* or an eosinophil-commited HL-60 subline to eosinophils *(3)*. NaB also triggers terminal differentiation of keratinocytes *(4)*. However, application of NaB to colon carcinoma cells (but not to normal colon cells) induces apoptosis *(5)*. Therefore, a pharmacological agent that elicits differentiation in one cell type can trigger an entirely different response, apoptosis, in another.

The human ovarian adenocarcinoma cell line HOC-7 was shown to exhibit a phenotype of advanced differentiation when treated with well-known differentiation inducing agents such as DMF (N,N-dimethylformamide), DMSO (dimethylsulfoxide), and TGFβ (transforming growth factor beta; *(6–8)*. Because HOC-7 is polyclonal, monoclonal sublines have been selected *(9)*. One subclone, N.1, has been chosen for further studies because it most closely resembles the parental HOC-7 cell line *(10)*. N.1 cells, such as HOC-7, arrest growth upon NaB treatment *(11)*. This is accompanied by morphological changes, which are typical for a differentiated cell phenotype such as cell flattening and cell enlargement. During NaB treatment, biochemical markers of differentiation include efficient downregulation of the protooncogenes c-*myc*, cyclin D1, and of the invasiveness-related protease plasminogen activator/urokinase [upa; *(11,12)*] and N.1 cells are growth arrested as long as c-*myc* is repressed.

However, c-*myc*, cyclin D1, and upa expression levels recover and N.1 cells resume proliferation as soon as NaB is withdrawn from the growth medium. Thus, the morphological phenotype of cell differentiation and the regulation of gene expression is only owing to the permanent presence of NaB, but it is not terminal.

Recent experiments evidence that N.1 cells undergo c-*myc*-dependent apoptosis *(13,14)*. Therefore, NaB does not allow for eradication of N.1 carcinoma cells because it is a potent downregulator of c-*myc*, which inhibits apoptosis.

From: *Methods in Molecular Medicine, Vol. 39: Ovarian Cancer: Methods and Protocols*
Edited by: J. M. S. Bartlett © Humana Press, Inc., Totowa, NJ

The fact that NaB, nevertheless, induces apoptosis of colon carcinoma cells might be because of swift interruption of transduction of survival signals. Alternatively, apoptosis of colon carcinoma cells which was shown to be *p53*-independent *(5)*, might also be independent of c-*myc*. Upa induces detachment of N.1 cells from extracellular matrix *(13)*, which renders cells even more susceptible to apoptosis *(15)*. Down-regulation of upa by NaB, therefore, further supports the apoptosis-protected state of N.1 ovarian carcinoma cells, which are shifted into dormancy by c-*myc* inhibition.

It is concluded that studying c-*myc* and upa expression is relevant to estimate if pharmacological treatment might support apoptotic cell destruction or if it rescues transformed cells by allowing the escape into cell cycle arrest *(16)*.

In order to study gene expression on a routinely basis, a nonradioactive (cheap and ready to hand) Northern blot method was established. The detailed method is outlined below (*see* **Note 1**).

## 2. Materials

### 2.1. Cell Culture and Experiments

1. α-Minimal essential medium (αMEM); store at 4°C + fetal calf serum (FCS); store at –20°C.
2. 350 m*M* sodium butyrate (100X stock; store at –20°C, protect from light).
3. PBS (phosphate-buffered saline pH 7.2).

### 2.2. Separation of Total RNA, Capillary Transfer, and Immobilization

1. 37% formaldehyde (filter sterilize to remove particulate matter which reduces background; store at room temperature [RT], protect from light).
2. 10X MOPS buffer, pH 7.0 (200 m*M* 3-[N-morpholino]propanesulfonic acid- hemisodium salt, 50 m*M* sodium acetate, 10 m*M* EDTA (ethylenediaminetetraacetic acid); filter steril-ize; store at RT, protect from light).

### 2.3. cDNA-Probe Labeling

1. NEBlot Phototope Kit (New England Biolabs, Beverly, MA, Cat. No. 7550). Components include: 5X labeling mix (biotinylated random primer octamers), dNTP mix (1 m*M* dCTP, 1 m*M* dGTP, 1 m*M* dTTP, 1 m*M* dATP/biotin dATP), Klenow polymerase (3′–5′ exonu-clease, 5 U/μL); all components are stored at –20°C.

### 2.4. RNA Blot Hybridization

1. 1*M* phosphate buffer pH 7.2 (autoclaved stock; store at RT).
2. Hybridization buffer (500 m*M* phosphate buffer pH 7.2, 7% SDS, 1% BSA, 1 m*M* EDTA; store at RT. Compose from filter sterilized stock solutions. The hybridization buffer suggested by the NEB kit-protocol produces unacceptable background for northern blot analysis).
3. Saline sodium citrate (SSC) pH 7.0; 150 m*M* NaCl, 15 m*M* sodium citrate; 20X SSC stock, filter sterilized, store at RT.

### 2.5. Signal Development

1. NEK Phototope 6K Detection Kit (New England Biolabs Cat. No. 7006). Components: biotinylated alkaline phosphatase 380 ng/μL (= 0.4 U/μL; store at 4°C), streptavidin (reconstitute with buffer S to 1 μg/μL = 0.015 U/μL; store at 4°C), Lumigen-PPD (store at 4°C), Lumigen PPD-diluent (2-amino-2-methyl-1-propanol buffer; store at RT).

2. Streptavidin reconstitution buffer (buffer S: 10 m$M$ phosphate buffer pH 7.2, 150 m$M$ NaCl, 0.05% sodium azide, filter sterilized; store at 4°C).

3. Blocking solution (5% SDS [sodium dodecyl sulfate], 25 m$M$ phosphate buffer pH 7.2, filter sterilized, store at RT).

4. Streptavidin washing buffer (0.5% SDS, 2.5 m$M$ phosphate buffer pH 7.2, which is 1/10 of the concentration of blocking solution; store at RT).

5. 10X alkaline phosphatase washing buffer (100 m$M$ Tris pH 9.5, 100 m$M$ NaCl, 10 m$M$ MgCl$_2$, filter sterilized; store at RT).

## 3. Methods

### 3.1. Cell Culture and Experiments

Typically, N.1 cells are grown in 25 cm$^2$ cell-culture flasks (7 mL αMEM, 10% FCS) in a humidified 5% CO$_2$ atmosphere to 80–90% confluence. Experiments are started by addition of 70 µL of, e.g., 350 m$M$ NaB solution containing 25% ethanol (100x stock). Controls are treated with 70 µL 25% ethanol only. For dose response experiments appropriate 100x stocks containing 25% ethanol are prepared. After considerable time (between 6–24 h) the mRNA of c-*myc* and upa is repressed in N.1 cells.

### 3.2. RNA Isolation

1. Experiments are terminated by discarding the cell-culture medium and by washing the cell layer twice with 5 mL ice cold, sterile PBS (1–2 min each; *see* **Note 2**).

2. 1 mL RNAzol™B is added into each cell-culture flask taking care to distribute the liquid equally across the surface on which the cells are grown.

3. Leave the flask standing on the benchtop (in a horizontal position just as cells grow in the incubator) for 5–8 min and gently agitate every 2 min to allow mixing of RNAzolB with the cells.

4. When cells are completely dissolved, collect the lysate in one corner of the flask and pump the lysate through a blue tip mounted to a 1000 µL Gilson pipetman to shear genomic DNA. Thereby the lysate loses viscosity (*see* **Note 3**).

5. Collect the lysate in a sterile Eppendorf tube (1.5 mL). At this point, lysates can be stored at –80°C for several months without losing RNA integrity (thaw before use).

6. Add 200 µL chloroform to the RNAzolB-cell lysate (which is approx 1 mL), vigorously vortex the samples for 15–20 s and put back on ice for 5 min.

7. Quickly vortex the samples again and spin at 11,500$g$ for 15 min at 0–4°C.

8. The organic (lower) phase which contains protein and DNA is separated from the aqueous (upper) phase which contains total RNA. The aqueous phase (approx 550 µL) is carefully aspirated and collected in a new Eppendorf tube (*see* **Note 4**).

9. An equal volume of isopropanol (550 µL) is added to the rescued aqueous phase, vortexed, and left on ice for 15 min.

10. Pellet the precipitated RNA by centrifugation (11,500$g$, 15 min, 0–4°C) and drain off supernatant (the pellet will appear drop-shaped near the tip of the tube; *see* **Note 5**).

11. Add 700 µL of ice-cold 80% ethanol and vortex for some 2 s only until the pellet swirls off the tube wall.

12. Quickly centrifuge the pellet to the tube tip and aspirate ethanol with Pasteur pipet.

13. Quickly spin the sample again and completely aspirate residual ethanol with a Pasteur *pipet with a very fine capillary* (*see* **Note 5**).

14. Allow the pellet to dry for a few minutes to redissolve in 7–12 µL sterile H$_2$O 30 min on ice.

15. Carefully vortex the tube so that the droplet goes into a rotating motion (avoid the droplet splashing and jumping during vortexing). RNA samples can be stored at –80°C for several months.

16. Before storing the samples, it is advised to determine the amount of isolated total RNA by reading the absorbance of 1 μL in 999 μL distilled $H_2O$ at 260 nm by spectrophotometry using 1 mL quartz cuvets.

17. Multiply the $A_{260}$ by 40. This gives the RNA concentration in μg/mL. Because 1 μL of the RNA sample was measured the calculated value gives the sample concentration in μg/μL. Typically, an average RNA pellet dissolved in 12 μL $H_2O$ contains approx 6–9 μg total RNA /μL sample.

## 3.3. Separation of Total RNA, Capillary Transfer, and Immobilization

### 3.3.1. Gel Preparation

1. Melt 400 mg agarose by boiling in 30 mL double distilled $H_2O$.
2. Add 4 mL 10X MOPS and 6.7 mL 37% formaldehyde, mix gently (avoid air bubbles), and pour into the gel form.
3. After the gel has solidified let it rest at 4°C for 30 min.
4. Prerun the gel with 1X MOPS buffer, pH 7.0, at 50 V (constant) in the cold room for 20 min.

### 3.3.2. Sample Preparation

1. Pipet the volume of sample that contains 20 μg RNA into a sterile 1.5-mL reaction vial and add sterile $H_2O$ (if necessary) to make up to a total of 5 μL.
2. Add 1 μL 10X MOPS pH 7.0, 3.5 μL 37% formaldehyde, 10 μL formamide, and mix (sample buffer; always prepare fresh).
3. Denature secondary RNA-structures by heating the sample-mix to 70°C for 20 min.
4. Thereafter, add 6 μL gel loading solution (Sigma No. G-2526; contains glycerol and bromophenol blue) and mix.
5. Apply sample-mix onto the prerun agarose-formaldehyde gel. Additives that stain RNA such as Radiant Red fluorescent RNA stain (BioRad) are not recommended because it inhibits sensitivity by 60–80%

### 3.3.3. Gel Electrophoresis

1. Denatured RNA-preparations are immediately loaded into the sample wells and the gel is run at 50 V (const.) in the cold room for 60 min.
2. Then the electrophoresis buffer (MOPS buffer pH 7.0; *see* **Subheading 2.2., item 2**) has to be remixed (*see* **Note 6**).
3. Continue the RNA separation at 80 V (const.) in the cold room for another 60–90 min (*see* **Note 7**).

### 3.3.4. Gel Treatment for Capillary Transfer

1. The gel is removed from the electrophoresis apparatus and gently agitated in 250 mL of 50 m*M* NaOH, 100 m*M* NaCl (add 2.5 mL of 5*M* NaOH stock, 5 mL of 5*M* NaCl stock [autoclaved] into 250 mL sterile aqua dest.) on a rocker platform at RT for 20 min.
2. Equilibrate the gel in 250 mL of 100 m*M* Tris pH 7.5 (1*M* Tris-HCl stock; autoclaved) for 20 min (RT, gently rocking).
3. Finally treat the gel in 250 mL 2X SSC for 20 min (RT, gently rocking).
4. Transfer RNA from the gel to Immobilon S membrane (Millipore No. MBBU IMS 02), which was prewetted in 2X SSC for a few min, by the capillary method using 10X SSC as transfer buffer, overnight (*see* **Fig. 1** for transfer setup).

Fig. 1. Capillary transfer set up. A glass plate is put across a plastic tray which contains 500 mL 10X SSC. 3 layers of Whatman 3MM filter paper are folded around the glass plate and immersed into 10X SSC transfer buffer and moistened all over. Rolling a 10 mL pipet across the moistened filter paper squeezes out trapped air. The agarose gel with the sample slots facing the filter paper is placed on top and trapped air is squeezed out. Saran wrap is put around all four sides of the gel to avoid capillary bypass (only one side is shown). Immobilon S (cut to size and prewetted) is placed on top and trapped air squeezed out. Three layers of Whatman 3MM filter paper (cut to size, dry) are put on top of the membrane. A pile of paper towels (some 5–6 cm high) is positioned and positive pressure applied.

5. Remove the membrane (do not forget to mark one corner to identify the orientation of sample application) and clip it to Whatman 3MM chromatography paper (RNA-side up; clips prevent the membrane from curling).

6. Allow the membrane, clipped to Whatman 3MM, to dry completely either at RT or in a dry-oven (do not exceed 70°C).

7. Expose the membrane to 50 mJ in a UV crosslinker (the RNA-side of the membrane has to face the UV lamps).

8. At this stage, the membrane can be stored at –20°C for several weeks (both sides of the membrane physically protected with Whatman 3MM paper and wrapped in aluminium foil).

### 3.4. cDNA-Probe Labeling

1. cDNA probes are labeled with NEBlot Phototope Kit (New England Biolabs Cat. No. 7550; *see* **Note 8**). 1–2 µg of double-stranded cDNA probe (which does not include extended vector sequences), 10 µL 5X labeling mix (kit component), and $H_2O$ to a final volume of 44 µL are immersed in a boiling water bath for 3 min to separate double strands.
2. Immediately chill the probe-mix on ice for 3 min to prevent strand rejoining.
3. Keep the probe on ice, add 5 µL dNTPs (kit component), 1 µL Klenow polymerase (3′-5′ exo⁻; kit component), and incubate at 15°C overnight (*see* **Note 9**).
4. The reaction is terminated by the addition of 6 µL 200 m$M$ EDTA pH 8.0 (autoclaved; store at RT), 1 µL salmon sperm DNA (10 µg/µL; store at –20°C), 6 µL sodium acetate pH 5.5 and 150 µL 98% ethanol.
5. Mix and put the reaction mixture at –20°C for several hours or overnight to precipitate the probe (*see* **Note 10**).
6. Pellet DNA by centrifugation (11,500$g$, 0–4°C, 15 min).
7. Redissolve the pellet in TE (10 m$M$ Tris-HCl pH 8.0, 1 m$M$ EDTA; autoclaved, store at RT) to an estimated final concentration of 10 ng/µL and store at –20°C.

### 3.5. RNA Blot Hybridization

1. Prewet the membrane with 6X SSC (*see* **Subheading 2.4., item 3**).
2. Put the filter into a plastic bag, fill with 6 mL hybridization buffer (which has to be pre-heated to 68°C to reduce viscosity), seal the plastic bag using a sealer, and incubate the membrane at 68°C for 1–2 h to block nonspecific binding sites.
3. Dilute 12 µL (120 ng) of labeled probe in distilled water (human c-*myc* exon 3 probe; human upa probe ATCC No. 57329; rat GAPDH [glyceraldehyde 3-phosphate dehydro-genase] probe, entire coding region; also hybridizes with human GAPDH mRNA) to a final volume of 200 µL, immerse into a boiling water bath for 3 min to separate labeled from nonlabeled cDNA strands. (Store biotinylated probes at –20°C.)
4. Immediately chill the probe on ice for 3 min to prevent strand rejoining.
5. Incubate the membrane with the denatured probe (20 ng/mL hybridization buffer, final concentration). Remove the plastic bag containing the membrane from the 68°C water bath. Open the bag on one side, add the denatured biotinylated probe directly into the hybridization buffer, mix to distribute the probe, remove air bubbles, reseal the bag. To prevent cooling down of the hybridization buffer which would increase viscosity, this procedure has to be done swiftly.
6. Put the membrane back to 68°C water bath, leave it overnight, and make sure that the membrane is in a flat, horizontal position by putting weight on the corners of the plastic bag.

### 3.6. Signal Development

1. After overnight incubation the membrane is removed from the plastic bag (*see* **Note 11**).
2. Wash the membrane in 2X SSC, 0.1% SDS (2 × 5 min each at RT).
3. Thereafter, the membrane is subjected to stringent washing conditions in 0.1X SSC, 0.1% SDS (2 × 10 min each, at 68°C; *see* **Note 12**).
4. Put the membrane back into a plastic bag which is cut considerably larger than the membrane size (*see* **Note 13**).
5. Fill the plastic bag with 40 mL of blocking solution and wash the membrane at RT for 1 h using a rocker platform (*see* **Note 13**).
6. Incubate the membrane in 3 mL blocking solution which contains 3 µL of streptavidin (add directly before use) and gently agitate at RT for 5 min.
7. Wash the membrane in 40 mL streptavidin washing buffer at RT using a rocker platform (3 × 20 min each, *see* **Note 13**).

8. Gently agitate the membrane with 3 mL blocking solution which contains 4–5 µL alkaline phosphatase (biotinylated) at RT, for 5 min (*see* **Note 14**).
9. Wash the membrane in 40 mL alkaline phosphatase washing buffer at RT using a rocker platform (3 × 10 min each; *see* **Note 13**).
10. Incubate the membrane in 1.5 mL Lumigen-PDD-diluent, 15 µL Lumigen-PDD for 5 min.
11. Drain off solution thoroughly, reseal the plastic bag to prevent moistening of the X-ray film, and leave in the dark for 90 min to allow for the development of light emission (without film).
12. Expose the membrane to Kodak X-OMAT DS films for 40–60 min and develop. If the signal is too strong the membrane has to be reexposed for considerably shorter time.
13. For further use, the membrane can be stored sealed in a plastic bag in 6 mL streptavidin washing buffer at 4°C for several month (*see* **Note 15**).

### 3.7. Membrane Stripping

1. The membrane is washed in sterile, double-distilled water (3 × 2 min each; RT) and immersed in 500 mL 2 m*M* EDTA, 0.1% SDS at 80°C (which is already preheated to 80°C) for 10–15 min.
2. Equilibrate the membrane in 6X SSC for 2 min.
3. Pre-saturate the membrane with hybridization buffer.
4. Add upa and/or GAPDH cDNA-probe, which serves as internal control to examine equivalent sample loading.

Typically, a membrane can be stripped and rehybridized 3–5 times. It is advised to start with those DNA probes which gives the weakest signal (GAPDH and upa give a stronger signal than c-*myc*. For other genes find out empirically).

## 4. Notes

1. All buffers have to be autoclaved or filter sterilized. Pipet tips and reaction tubes may be touched with gloves only. They have to be autoclaved and protected from dust. Fingertips and dust are a prominent source of RNase activity. Use powder-free gloves, because powdered gloves produce background on the blot. The gel apparatus has to be dedicated for Northern analysis only and pipetman and so on have to be cleaned frequently. Before use trays, glass plates and electrophoresis equipment have to be washed with liquid household soap (a cleaning sponge has to be used for this purpose only). Soap is washed off with tap water and equipment finally rinsed with double-distilled water.
2. After washing the cell layer twice, PBS has to be removed thoroughly to avoid dilution of RNAzolB in which cells will be subsequently dissolved. This is achieved when PBS is aspirated with a Pasteur pipet connected to a suction pump.
3. Do not pipet RNAzolB lysate too vigorously. Because of its viscosity the liquid might "jump" into the suction cylinder of the pipetman. This will destroy the RNA preparation. When the lysate is getting less and less viscous pipet the lysate across the growth surface of the T-25 flask for another 5–6 times to collect residual cell material which might still stick there.
4. Take care to avoid collection of the white and fluffy interphase. It is better to take less aqueous phase instead of contaminating the sample preparation with interphase; "less is more!" On average, some 550 µL of aqueous phase can be collected.
5. The supernatant will be aspirated with a Pasteur pipet which was melted and drawn out to create a very fine capillary (the narrow capillary allows for the quantitative removal of tiny droplets. This is necessary to completely redissolve total RNA in not more than 7–12 µL H$_2$O).

6. Electrophoresis buffer has to be re-mixed because it exhausts rapidly resulting in a pH- gradient between the buffer tanks which would destroy RNA and gel. To regenerate the electrophoresis buffer, aspirate electrophoresis buffer with a sterile 25-mL pipet from the tank with the [+]- pole and reapply it to the buffer tank with the [-]-pole (repeat 10X).

7. If the gel runs longer, degradation of RNA has been observed due to buffer exhaustion. For most purposes, separation across half of the possible running length of the minigel proved to be sufficient for a Northern analysis.

8. cDNA probes should preferably have a minimum length of 800 bp. Smaller probe size will result in gradually decreasing labeling efficiency because the random octamer primers provided with the kit hybridize only on an average basis.

9. Execute the probe labeling reaction in the sequence and at the temperatures described. This results in labeled probe, which has approximately the same size as unlabeled probe, hybridizes with utmost specificity, and will produce the least background. If the labeling procedure is performed as it is described by the NEB-protocol, the size of labeled probes will increase tremendously. Klenow polymerase (3'-5' exo⁻) is a major improvement over normal Klenow polymerase for DNA labeling because it does not degrade the probe when dNTPs are gradually consumed. When a cryostat is not available adjust a water bath to 15°C and put it to the cold room.

10. Do not store at −80°C because this destroys the biotin label. The labeled probe can be stored at least for 1 yr at −20°C, which is a major advantage over radioactively labeled probes.

11. Collect the probe, which is diluted in hybridization solution (20 ng/mL) and store at −20°C. It can be reused up to four times. Usually, a reused probe gives less background. Before a membrane is incubated with used probe, the hybridization solution (containing probe) has to be immersed into a boiling water bath for 5 min. Nonspecific binding sites of the membrane have to be presaturated with probe-free hybridization buffer.

12. Do not exceed washing times because this may disrupt specific RNA–DNA hybrids.

13. The membrane size is determined by the size of the Bio-Rrad electrophoresis chamber which measures 10 × 6.5 cm. The plastic bag should measure approximately 15 × 15 cm, which provides optimal physical washing conditions because it allows the membrane to float freely in, e.g., 40 mL of blocking solution (or washing buffers) which will rinse both membrane surfaces. This is a relevant step to minimize background! For the same reason, blocking and washing steps have to be extended severalfold over the washing times given in the original NEB kit-protocol.

14. When transferred to blocking solution alkaline phosphatase precipitates but rapidly redissolves when mixed gently—do not vortex. Biotinylated alkaline phosphatase and streptavidin have to be diluted in blocking solution directly before use, because protein and enzyme activity is not stable in 5% SDS.

15. The light signal develops at pH 9.0–9.5. However, high pH degrades RNA. Therefore, the membrane is stored in streptavidin wash buffer pH 7.2. c-*myc* mRNA typically migrates at 2.4 kb, upa mRNA at 2.4 kb, and GAPDH mRNA at 1.4 kb. 18S and 28S control rRNA migrate at 1.8 kb and 4.7 kb, respectively.

## References

1. Bloch, A. (1984) Induced cell differentiation in cancer therapy. *Cancer Treat. Rep.* **68,** 199–205.
2. Yen, A. and Chandler, S. (1992) Inducers of leukemic cell differentiation cause down-regulation of RB gene expression. *Proc. Soc. Exp. Biol. Med.* **199,** 291–297.
3. Gomolin, H., Yamaguchi, Y., Paulpillai, A., Dvorak, L., Ackerman, S., and Tenen, D. (1993) Human eosinophil Charcot-Leyden crystal protein: cloning and characterisation of a lysophospholipase gene promotor. *Blood* **82,** 1868–1874.

4. Staiano-Coico, L. and Higgins, P. (1992) Cell shape changes during transition of basal keratinocytes to mature enucleate-cornified envelopes: Modulation of terminal differentiation by fibronectin. *Exp. Cell Res.* **201,** 126–136.

5. Hague, A., Manning, A., Hanlow, K., Huschtscha, L., Hart, D., and Paraskeva, C. (1993) Sodium butyrate induces apoptosis in human colonic tumor cell lines in a p53-independent pathway: implications for the possible role of dietary fibre in the prevention of large bowl cancer. *Int. J. Cancer* **55,** 498–505.

6. Grunt, T., Oeller, H., Somay, C., Dittrich, E., Fazeny, B., Mannhalter, C., and Dittrich, C. (1993) Modulation of the immunophenotype of ovarian cancer cells by DMF and TGFβ-1. *J. Cell Physiol.* **156,** 358–366.

7. Grunt, T., Somay, C., Oeller, H., Dittrich, E., and Dittrich, C. (1992) Comparative analysis of the effects of DMSO and retinoic acid on the antigenic pattern of human ovarian carcinoma cells. *J. Cell Sci.* **103,** 501–509.

8. Somay, C., Grunt, T., Mannhalter, C., and Dittrich, C. (1992) Relationship of Myc protein expression to the phenotype and to the growth potential of HOC-7 ovarian cancer cells. *Br. J. Cancer* **66,** 93–98.

9. Grunt, T., Dittrich, E., Somay, C., Wagner, T., and Dittrich, C. (1991) Separation of clonogenic and differentiated cell phenotypes of ovarian cancer cells HOC-7 by discontinuous density gradient centrifugation. *Cancer Lett.* **58,** 7–16.

10. Grunt, T., Oeller, H., Somay, C., and Dittrich, C. (1993) Different propensity for spontaneous differentiation in cell clones isolated from the human ovarian surface epithelial cell line HOC-7. *Differentiation* **53,** 45–50.

11. Krupitza, G., Harant, H., Dittrich, E., Szekeres, T., Huber, H., et al. (1995) Sodium butyrate inhibits c-myc splicing and interferes with signal transduction in ovarian carcinoma cells. *Carcinogenesis* **16,** 1199–1205.

12. Krupitza, G., Grill, S., Harant, H., Hulla, W., Szekeres, T., Huber, H., et al. (1996) Genes related to growth and invasiveness are repressed by sodium butyrate in ovarian cancer cells. *Br. J. Cancer* **73,** 433–438.

13. Simonitsch, I. and Krupitza, G. (1998) Autocrine self elimination of cultured ovarian cancer cells by TNFα. *Br. J. Cancer* **78,** 862–870.

14. Krupitza, G., Grusch, M., Braun, K., Fuhrmann, G., Steinbrugger, R., Hulla W., et al. (1998) TNFα-mediated cell death is independent of *Cdc25A. Cell Death Diff.* **5,** 758–764.

15. Frisch, S. and Francis, H. (1994) Disruption of epithelial cell-matrix interactions induces apoptosis. *J. Cell Biol.* **124,** 619–626.

16. Wawra, E., Poeckl, E., Muellner, E., and Wintersberger, E. (1981) Effect of sodium butyrate on induction of cellular and viral DNA synthesis in polyoma infected mouse kidney cells. *J. Virol.* **38,** 973–981.

# 50

# Differential Display

## Grant C. Sellar, Genevieve J. Rabiasz, Barbara Smith, and Jennifer Southgate

## 1. Introduction

Differential display reverse transcriptase polymerase chain reaction (DDRT-PCR) is an extremely powerful method for analyzing differences in gene expression between matched tissue/cell samples. Liang and Pardee originally described the technique in 1992 in their seminal paper (1). DDRT-PCR is now firmly established as a widespread powerful and commonly used method for identifying differentially expressed genes.

The method couples the power of PCR with the high resolution afforded by poly-acrylamide gel electrophoresis (PAGE). DDRT-PCR provides a direct visual representation or profile of gene expression between samples under test. It is not limited to pairwise comparisons as is the case with subtractive hybridization-based techniques. DDRT-PCR also allows the identification of the more subtle changes in gene expression and not merely large differences or "on–off" situations. Reagents for DDRT-PCR are now commercially available in kit form; for example, the RNAimage kit marketed by GenHunter Corporation. We, however, assemble all our reagents individually, and these are outlined in this method.

This chapter will provide a background to the method, a protocol routinely used in our laboratories, and finally a discussion describing variations on DDRT-PCR, and also comparisons with other difference analysis methodologies.

### 1.1. Differential Display RT-PCR

#### 1.1.1. Overview

Total RNA is isolated from tissues or from cell lines grown in culture. In order for truly differentially expressed genes to be isolated, it is important that the samples are matched as closely as possible. In addition, the samples should be processed simultaneously and cells should be at the same growth stage when harvested. If they are not, it is likely that differences owing to individual variation will be identified, complicating downstream analyses. Isolated RNA is treated with DNaseI (RNase-free) in order to remove contaminating DNA, which may interfere with subsequent analysis. For DDRT-PCR from whole tissues the total RNA must be polyA-selected and DNaseI-treated to remove contaminants that may inhibit subsequent stages.

From: *Methods in Molecular Medicine, Vol. 39: Ovarian Cancer: Methods and Protocols*
Edited by: J. M. S. Bartlett © Humana Press, Inc., Totowa, NJ

Reverse transcription (RT) reactions are performed, including controls without reverse transcriptase (-RT), on the DNaseI-treated total RNA using one of three single-base anchored oligo dT primers. PCR is then performed under conditions of low-dNTP concentration and low-annealing temperature using the same anchored primer as was used in the RT reaction, in combination with one of a series of arbitrary 13′mer primers. The anchored and arbitrary primers incorporate an *Hind*III restriction site on the 5′ end that allows for easy release of inserts from plasmid vectors following subcloning.

Our standard procedure is to perform PCR reactions in triplicate on a set of first-strand cDNA samples. Only differences that are reproducible across three separate PCR reactions are considered to be real and isolated for further analysis. This increases the fidelity of the procedure thereby reducing the incidence of false positive isolation.

DDRT-PCR products are identified following separation by polyacrylamide gel electrophoresis and overnight exposure to X-ray film. Differentially expressed bands are excised from the gel and eluted from the polyacrylamide. To confirm that the correct band has been isolated, the product is reamplified under the original conditions using the eluate as template. The products of the reamplification reaction are separated on polyacrylamide co-run with the original DDRT-PCR reaction for comparison. A flow-diagram outlining the DDRT-PCR method is shown in **Fig. 1**.

Following confirmation, products are reamplified "cold," i.e., without the incorporation of a radioactive nucleotide. The products are sized on agarose gels where they tend to be between 100 basepairs (bp) and 500 bp in length. Products are then excised from low-melting point agarose, purified, and subcloned into plasmid vectors. Subsequently, products can be used as probes for Northern blots, ribonuclease protection assays, and cDNA library screening, targets for Reverse Northern blots, and templates for sequencing.

## 2. Reagents

### 2.1. General Reagents

1. Acrylamide: Acrylamide/Bis Acrylamide Sequencing Solution [19:1] with $7M$ Urea/ 1XTBE (Severn Biotech. Ltd. Cat. No. 20-2700-05).
2. DEPC-treated $H_2O$: Add 1 mL DEPC (Diethyl Pyrocarbonate; Sigma, St. Louis, MO, Cat. No. D-5758) per 1000 mL $H_2O$ (0.1% v/v). Mix well by shaking bottle. Allow to stand overnight in a fume hood. Autoclave to destroy DEPC.
3. DNaseI: MessageClean Kit (GenHunter Corp. Cat. No. M601). Alternative sources of DNaseI (RNase-free) may be used, e.g., Pharmacia Biotech, Uppsala, Sweden, Cat. No. 27-0514-02.
4. DNA Size marker: 100 bp DNA ladder (GibcoBRL, Gaitherersburg, MD, Cat. No. 15628-019).
5. dNTPs: Ultrapure dNTP set, 100 m$M$ solutions, $4 \times 25$ pmol (Pharmacia Biotech. Cat. No. 27-2035-01). Make a stock containing 10 m$M$ of each dNTP in DEPC-treated $H_2O$ and store at −20°C. This is then diluted to 1 m$M$ in DEPC $H_2O$ for use in the DD RT-PCR reaction.
6. Filter Paper: Whatman 3MM Chromatography Paper (Cat. No. 3030 917).
7. Isotope: [α-$^{32}$P] dATP Redivue Ambient 3000 Ci/mol (Amersham, Arlington Heights, IL, Cat. No. AA0004).
8. Low-melting point agarose: Sea Plaque (FMC BioProducts, Rockland, ME, Cat. No. 50100).

Fig. 1. Flow diagram outlining the Differential Display method. Differentially expressed bands identified between the three RNA samples, A, B, and C, under comparison are boxed.

9. Mineral oil (Sigma Cat. No. M-5904).
10. Orientation Marker for X-ray film: Tracker tape (Amersham, Arlington Heights, IL, Cat. No. RPN2050).
11. PAGE Loading Dye: 95% Formamide (deionized), 20 m*M* EDTA, pH 7.6, 0.05% bromphenol blue, 0.05% xylene cyanol FF. Prepare in DEPC $H_2O$ and store in aliquots at −20°C.

### 2.2. Plasmid DNA Isolation

1. QIAprep Spin Miniprep Kit (Qiagen, Chatsworth, CA, Cat. No. 27106).

### 2.3. PCR Product Purification

1. WIZARD PCR Preps DNA Purification System (Promega, Madison, WI, Cat. No. A7170).
2. PCR Tubes: 0.6-mL RNase-free microcentrifuge tubes, sterilized by autoclaving. (Robbins Scientific Europe Ltd., Sunnyvale, CA, Cat. No. 1048-00-0).

### 2.4. Primers

Primer sequences were taken from Bauer et al. 1993 *(2)*. For the subsequent easy release of *DDRT-PCR* products from plasmid vectors following subcloning, an *Hind*III restriction site (H: 5′-AAGCTT-3′) has been incorporated onto the 5′-end of the primers.

1. Anchored Primers (20 µ*M* stock in DEPC-treated H₂O):
   HT₁₁A:      5′-AAGCTTTTTTTTTTTA-3′
   HT11G:      5′-AAGCTTTTTTTTTTTG-3′
   HT₁₁C:      5′-AAGCTTTTTTTTTTTC-3′
2. Arbitrary Primers (20 µ*M* stock in DEPC-treated H₂O):
   H03:        5′-AAGCTTCTACCC-3′
   H04:        5′-AAGCTTTGGCTCC-3′
   H07:        5′-AAGCTTATACAGG-3′
   H09:        5′-AAGCTTGTCATAG-3′
   H14:        5′-AAGCTTCAAGTCC-3′
   H17:        5′-AAGCTTCTGACAC-3′
   H21:        5′-AAGCTTCTAACCG-3′

## 2.5. Reverse Northern Blotting

1. ReversePrime RNA labeling kit (GenHunter Corp.; R701).

## 2.6. Reverse Transcription

1. Moloney Murine leukemia Virus (MMLV) Reverse Transcriptase, FPLC pure, 1000 U. (Pharmacia Biotech. Cat. No. 27-0925-02.). Store at –20°C.

## 2.7. Sequence Analysis

1. BLAST2.0 search program and sequence databases are available at the National Center for Biotechnology Information (NCBI) Blast server: http://www.ncbi.nlm.nih.gov/BLAST

## 2.8. TA Cloning

1. pGEM-T Easy Vector System II (Promega Cat. No. A1380).
2. AmpliTaq DNA Polymerase (5 U/µL) with 10X PCR Buffer II and 25 m*M* MgCl₂) (PE Applied Biosystems, Foster City, CA, Cat No. N8080161). Aliquot the 10X buffer and 25 m*M* MgCl₂ out in PCR tubes and store at –20°C.
3. TBE Electrophoresis Buffer: 10X Stock: 0.9*M* Tris-borate/0.02*M* EDTA.
4. Tris-Cl/EDTA buffer: TE pH 7.4: 10 m*M* Tris-Cl/1 m*M* EDTA.

## 2.9. Total RNA Isolation

1. Tri Reagent (Sigma Cat. No. T9424) or alternatively Ultraspec (Biogenesis Ltd., Poole, U.K.).

# 3. Methods

## 3.1. Isolation of Total RNA

1. Isolate total RNA from tissue samples or from cells growing in culture using either Tri Reagent or Ultraspec according to manufacturer's instructions.
2. The presence of contaminating DNA in the RNA samples will hinder the DDRT-PCR analysis. DNA is therefore removed by DNaseI treatment using the MessageClean Kit or Ultraspec, according to the manufacturers' protocols. Either of these methods yield consistently satisfactory results.
3. DNaseI-treated RNA should be stored at –70°C in small aliquots of at least 1 µg/µL ready for use in RT-PCR reaction.
4. Prior to carrying out DDRT-PCR, verify:
   a. that the RNA is intact by running out a 3–5 µg aliquot on a formaldehyde/agarose mini gel in 1XTBE, using DEPC- H₂O at all stages and

b. that it is free from contaminating DNA by performing an RT-PCR reaction with a PCR primer pair which amplifies different size products on cDNA and genomic DNA.

## 3.2. Reverse Transcription (RT) Reaction

The conditions given are per sample and can therefore be scaled up as appropriate.

1. 200 ng of RNA is required per RT reaction. Dilute the 1 µg/µL stock of DNaseI-treated total RNA to 0.1 µg/µL with DEPC $H_2O$ and keep on ice.
2. Thaw the 10X PCR Buffer II and 25 m$M$ $MgCl_2$, primers, and dNTPs and keep on ice.
3. Combine the RNA, DEPC $H_2O$, and anchored primer in a 0.6 mL PCR tube. For each RNA under test set up two tubes.

| Reagent | Stock Concentration | Volume |
|---|---|---|
| RNA (200 ng) | 0.1 µg/µL | 2.0 µL |
| $HT_{11}N$ (N=A/C/G) | 20 µ$M$ | 2.5 µL |
| DEPC $H_2O$ | | 4.7 µl |
| Total Volume | | 9.2 µL |

4. Incubate in a PCR block at 65°C for 10 min.
5. Immediately place samples on ice for 5 min.
6. Add the following reagents. Prepare appropriate master mixes, one with and one without reverse transcriptase (+RT and –RT, respectively), sufficient for all samples.

| Reagent | Stock Concentration | Volumes | |
|---|---|---|---|
| | | +RT | –RT |
| RNA/Primer | | 9.2 µL | 9.2 µL |
| PCR Buffer II | 10X | 2.0 µL | 2.0 µL |
| $MgCl_2$ | 25 m$M$ | 6.4 µL | 6.4 µL |
| dNTPs | 1 m$M$ | 0.4 µL | 0.4 µL |
| MMLV RT | 15.6 U/µL | 2.0 µL | 0.0 µL |
| DEPC $H_2O$ | | 0.0 µL | 2.0 µL |
| Total Volume | | 20.0 µL | 20.0 µL |

7. Briefly whirlimix and then spin samples.
8. Incubate reactions at 37°C for 60 min in a PCR block.
9. Incubate reactions at 95°C for 10 min in a PCR block.
10. Immediately place samples onto ice. Samples can then be used for PCR, or alternatively, may be stored at –70°C for future use.

## 3.3. Polymerase Chain Reaction (PCR)

PCR is performed using the same anchored primer as used in the RT reaction in combination with an arbitrary primer.

1. In a 0.6-mL PCR tube, add the following per reaction. Make a PCR master mix sufficient for all samples, omitting the [α-$^{32}$P]dATP from the mix.

| Reagent | Stock Concentration | Volume |
|---|---|---|
| PCR buffer II | 10X | 1.8 µL |
| $HT_{11}N$ | 20 µ$M$ | 2.25 µL |
| Arbitrary primer | 20 µ$M$ | 2.5 µL |
| $MgCl_2$ | 25 m$M$ | 0.56 µL |
| dNTPs | 1 m$M$ | 0.4 µL |
| *Taq* polymerase | 5 U/µL | 0.2 µL |
| ([α-$^{32}$P]dATP | 10 µCi/µL | 0.1 µL) |
| DEPC $H_2O$ | | 10.2 µL |
| Total | | 18.01 µL |

2. Place 2 μL of cDNA reaction in a fresh 0.6-mL PCR tube on ice, in triplicate, for each cDNA under test.
3. Add 0.1 μL [α-$^{32}$P]dATP per PCR to the master mix. Whirlimix and spin briefly.
4. Add 18.01 μL of "hot" PCR mix to the tube containing 2 μL of cDNA. Pipet up and down to mix samples.
5. Overlay the PCR mix with light mineral oil and close the tubes.
6. PCR samples using the following conditions. Store samples at +4°C until ready to separate on a polyacrylamide sequencing gel, or alternatively for longer periods, at –20°C.

PCR Conditions: 95°C for 2 mins, 1 cycle followed by 40 cycles of (94°C for 30 s, 32°C for 2 min and 72°C for 30 s) with a final extension time of 5 min at 72°C.

### 3.4. Polyacrylamide Gel Electrophoresis (PAGE)

1. Pour a 6% acrylamide/1X TBE sequencing gel. Allow sufficient time (approximately 2 h) for complete polymerization of the acrylamide to occur. Gels can be poured the previous day and then stored overnight at +4°C. In this case, equilibrate to room temperature prior to using. Prerun the gel in 1X TBE electrophoresis buffer for approximately 30 min to 1 h at constant 80 W to bring the gel running temperature to 50°C.
2. Add 5 μL of PAGE loading dye to 5 μL of PCR sample in a 0.6-mL tube, heat denature for 2 min at 72°C, and then load 5 μL onto the gel. Prior to loading the gel, flush the wells with 1X TBE buffer using a fine-tip pasteur pipet to remove urea.
3. Run for approximately 2 h at 80 W, allowing the first blue dye to run off the bottom of the gel. The buffer in the bottom chamber of the electrophoresis apparatus will be radioactive at the end of the run.
4. After the run, carefully separate the gel plates, transfer the gel on to a sheet of Whatman 3MM paper, cover with cling film, and dry in a vacuum gel drier for 2 h at 80°C. It is unnecessary to fix the gel in acetic acid/methanol prior to drying as this renders the DNA inhibitory to subsequent reamplification.
5. Expose the dried down gel overnight to X-ray film at –70°C. Accurate alignment of the developed autoradiograph with the dried down gel is vital for recovery of the correct bands from the gel. Therefore, use a marker to allow correct positioning of the autoradiograph, e.g, radioactive marker spots or Tracker Tape. We usually put two pieces of film into the cassette. One is used as a template for excising the bands of interest; the other can be retained for both record and publication purposes.

### 3.5. Isolation of Differentially Expressed Bands

1. Up- and downregulated bands between RNAs of interest are identified from the auto-radiograph. Only recover bands that are reproducibly differentially expressed in each of the three independent PCR reactions (*see* **Note 1**). Using one piece of film, cut out the area surrounding the identified band using a scalpel blade making a window in the autoradiograph.
2. Overlay the autoradiograph on top of the dried down gel and position as accurately as possible. This is crucial in recovering the correct bands of interest. This is where the use of either radioactive marker spots or Tracker Tape when exposing the dried down gel to X-ray film is important. The windows in the film define the DDRT-PCR products. Excise products from the gel using a scalpel blade.
3. Place the excised band into a 1.5-mL screw cap Eppendorf tube containing 100 μL TE buffer.
4. Elute the products into TE by overnight incubation of the tubes at 65°C.
5. Remove the piece of gel slice and discard.

6. Eluted products can be stored at –20°C until required.
7. Reamplify the differentially expressed product.

## 3.6. Reamplification of Differentially Expressed Products (see Note 3)

1. Set up a PCR with the same combination of primers and amplification conditions as used previously. Use 2 µL of the eluted DNA in a 20 µL reaction, incorporating [α-$^{32}$P] dATP as for the initial DDRT-PCR reaction.
2. Prepare a 6% (w/v) acrylamide/1X TBE sequencing gel.
3. Add 5 µL of loading dye to 5 µL of PCR sample, heat denature for 2 min at 72°C and then load 5 µL onto the gel. Co-run the original PCR reaction alongside the reamplified products for comparison.
4. Run the PAGE gel as before, transfer onto Whatman 3MM filter paper, dry and expose to X-ray film overnight at –70°C.
5. Overnight autoradiography will confirm that the DDRT-PCR product has been reamplified, and is the same as that originally identified.
6. To obtain sufficient DDRT-PCR products for subsequent downstream analyses, a "cold" PCR, i.e., without incorporation of radioactive label, is performed. Set up a 20 µL PCR with the same combination of anchored and arbitrary primers and use 2 µL of the eluted DNA as template. Increase the concentration of dNTPs in the reaction to standard levels for PCR (200 µ$M$).

| Reagent | Stock Concentration | Volume |
|---|---|---|
| Eluted DNA | | 2 µL |
| PCR buffer II | 10X | 2 µL |
| HT$_{11}$N | 20 µ$M$ | 0.5 µL |
| Arbitrary primer | 20 µ$M$ | 0.5 µL |
| MgCl$_2$ | 25 m$M$ | 1.6 µL |
| dNTPs | 1 m$M$ | 4 µL |
| *Taq* polymerase | 5 U/µL | 0.5 µL |
| DEPC H$_2$O | | 8.9 µL |
| Total | | 20 µL |

7. Run 5 µL of PCR product on a 2% (w/v) agarose minigel in 1X TBE co-run with 100 bp ladder as a size marker. This will confirm that the product has been recovered, and also establish the size of the product. Should the product fail to reamplify at this stage, then successful recovery may be achieved by repeating the "cold" PCR using 2.5 µL of the failed reaction mix as template and/or repeating the PCR using a range of magnesium concentrations.

## 3.7. Downstream Analyses

Having identified and successfully reamplified DDRT-PCR products the question arises as to "what happens next."

1. Separate products on a 2% (w/v) low melting point gel and excise DNA bands from the gel, trimming off as much surrounding agarose as possible.
2. Purify the band from agarose using the WIZARD PCR DNA Purification System following the manufacturer's protocol.
3. Confirm that products have been recovered by running a small aliquot (5–10 µL) on a 2% (w/v) agarose mini-gel.
4. Clone the recovered products into pGEM-T Easy cloning vector. Follow the protocol supplied by Promega for the ligation and transformation steps, and use blue/white colour selection to aid identification of insert-containing plasmids.

5. Select up to six independent white colonies for each DDRT-PCR product and isolate plasmid DNA using a QIAprep Spin Miniprep kit (QIAGEN).

If automated sequencing is available (*see* **Notes 2** and **3**), it is useful at this stage to select and sequence up to six clones from each cloned DDRT-PCR product before any further analysis. This will confirm that the bands each represent single products (which is often not the case) and, in addition, give initial information about the nature of differentially expressed genes. Using the BLAST2.0 program at the NCBI search the gene and mRNA sequence databases to identify DDRT-PCR products. Not all the products will be readily identifiable as known genes. It is also worth searching the databases of Expressed Sequence Tags (ESTs) as EST clones are readily obtainable and can facilitate the isolation and analysis of unknown differentially expressed gene products.

## 3.8. Conclusion

DDRT-PCR is a powerful technique for the identification of differentially expressed genes. It is firmly established and its successful implementation is well documented in the literature. It has advantages over other difference analysis methods, but also has drawbacks. The method of choice is dependent upon both the system under investigation and also the setup in individual laboratories. The equipment required is probably available in most laboratories and is therefore relatively straightforward to set up and successfully identify differentially expressed genes (*see* **Notes 4–6**). The high rate of false positives are a problem, but with the implementation of a good screening method these can be eliminated and remove a potential bottleneck in the analysis procedure.

## 4. Notes

1. Confirmation of Differential Expression: DDRT-PCR tends to have quite a high rate of false positives that come through the initial PCR amplifications. False positive rates can easily be greater than 50%. Confirming that isolated bands are differentially expressed can become a bottleneck area in the analysis, especially if large numbers of products have been identified. It is necessary, therefore, that a screening method be undertaken to identify the true differentially expressed products and eliminate the false positives that have come through the system. This streamlines the subsequent analyses to be performed. If DDRT-PCR has been carried out on a small scale and the number of products to be analyzed is limited, it may be beneficial to proceed directly with hybridizations of Northern blots using probes generated from DD products. If possible, it is recommended that the Northern blots be generated with RNA from the same samples as those used in the DDRT-PCR experiment. However, this approach is expensive both on time and reagents. In addition, products less than 150 bp may not yield good hybridization probes owing to inefficient incorporation of radioactive label, and therefore, products of this size may have to be removed from the analysis. If the products have already been sequenced, EST clones corresponding to smaller products can be obtained and used as hybridization probes. Also, Northern blots may not be sensitive enough to detect mRNA species expressed at low levels, which may be identified by DDRT-PCR. Alternative approaches are to use Ribonuclease Protection Assays or Reverse Northern blotting.

   Reverse Northerns (RN) provide a rapid and sensitive method for screening all DDRT-PCR products using a small number of hybridizations. Equal amounts of plasmid DNA (1 µg) from cloned DD products are dotted onto duplicate blotting membranes using either a slot blot or 96-well dot blot vacuum manifold. Alternatively, performing PCR across the insert using primers that flank the cloning site, e.g., SP6/T7 can readily generate target

DNAs. In this case, 200 ng of PCR product are sufficient. In RNs, the probe is generated from the RNA population and is radioactively labeled using the ReversePrime kit. The number of blots and probes used is dependent upon the conditions of the experiment. Blots are hybridized and washed according to standard protocols and blots exposed for various lengths of time to obtain interpretable results.

2. Identification of DDRT-PCR Products: Products that are confirmed as being differentially expressed form a streamlined subset from the original population. These products now require to be sequenced, if this was not performed after the cloning step. The method used for sequencing, whether radioactive or fluorescent, is dependent upon the available methodology in individual laboratories. The sequence generated is used to search the available public databases. We routinely use the BLAST2.0 search program at the NCBI to search the nonredundant nucleotide databases containing gene information and also the Expressed Sequence Tag and Sequence Tag Site (STS) databases to identify the products. DDRT-PCR gives information from the 3'-end of genes and little in the way of coding information. Consequently, some products will be identified as known genes, some will be identified as ESTs or STSs, and some will be novel. The amount of genome mapping information for each gene/EST/STS will depend upon the detail available in the databases. With the current explosion in sequencing information and genome mapping data, the databases are being continually updated. It is worth periodically researching the databases to establish over time the identity of all the isolated DDRT-PCR products.

3. The initial identification of DDRT-PCR products is a relatively rapid process and can easily be carried out by one individual. For optimum results, the radioactive label should be used prior to decaying through half-lives. Therefore, the DDRT-PCR experiments should be completed in as short a period of time as possible. The analysis of subsequent primer pair combinations can be combined with the reamplification of previously identified products, and samples can be separated on the same polyacrylamide gel. It is practically quite difficult, however, for one person to simultaneously be performing DDRT-PCR reactions, elution, reamplifications, product purification, cloning and sequencing. It is recommended that following the "cold" reamplification reaction, subsequent steps be carried out by a second individual, thereby preventing delays in the process.

4. Adaptation of DDRT-PCR: Reciprocal subtraction DDRT-PCR (RSDD) has recently been described as an adaptation of DD, which allows the identification of both abundant and rare differentially expressed genes *(3)*. RSDD couples subtractive hybridization with DDRT-PCR, thereby reducing the complexity of products generated by DD alone. The subtraction step requires the construction of good cDNA libraries prior to performing DDRT-PCR, thereby increasing the time required for the technique. RSDD products are again generated from the 3'-end of genes. These can be used to screen the cDNA libraries for longer clones that will aid in their identification. In addition, following sequencing of products, corresponding ESTs can be obtained which may yield further information.

5. Comparison of DDRT-PCR with Other Difference Analysis Technologies: DDRT-PCR provides a direct visual representation or profile of gene expression between samples. Unlike subtractive hybridization techniques such as PCR Select from Clontech or cDNA-representational difference analysis [cDNA-RDA; *(4)*], it is not limited to pairwise comparisons. It also allows for the direct identification of both up- and downregulated differentially expressed genes. DDRT-PCR also enables the identification of more subtle changes in gene expression and not merely large changes or on-off differences. However, it is probably not very good for identifying low-level differences in gene expression. cDNA-RDA is the most stringent of the techniques and has the benefit that a limited number of products are identified, and these almost certainly represent true differences. cDNA-RDA allows the identification of changes in low-level gene expression. Conse-

quently, Northern blotting may not be sufficiently sensitive, and RT-PCR analysis may therefore be required to detect such low-level transcripts *(5)*. PCR Select is not as stringent as cDNA-RDA, and consequently libraries of difference products are constructed. Screenings of the difference libraries using the Reverse Northern technique is then required to identify true differences and eliminate "noise." In addition, products that are represented multiple times in the library also require identification by screening prior to sequencing. Alternatively, of course, large-scale sequencing could be performed relatively rapidly if the libraries are gridded in a 96-well format. It may also be possible to couple DDRT-PCR with microarrays as has recently been reported for cDNA-RDA *(6)*.

6. The major drawback of DDRT-PCR is that it requires incorporation of a radioactive nucleotide, which necessitates experiments being carried out taking appropriate safety precautions. In addition, it relies on reverse transcription using an anchored oligo dT primer, and consequently, products that are isolated originate from the 3′-untranslated region (3′-UTR) of genes, and yield very little protein coding information. In the PCR Select and cDNA-RDA subtraction techniques, amplicons are generated from each RNA population by restriction enzyme digestion of synthesized second strand cDNAs. Therefore, the products from these methods are not limited to the 3′-end of the gene, and may yield more protein coding information, thus making product identification more readily achievable.

## Acknowledgments

We would like to thank Dr. Hani Gabra (ICRF Medical Oncology Unit, Edinburgh) for his stimulating discussions and critical reading of this manuscript.

## References

1. Liang, P. and Pardee, A. B. (1992) Differential display of eukaryotic messenger RNA by means of the polymerase chain reaction. *Science* **257,** 967–971.
2. Bauer, D., Muller, H., Reich, J., Riedel, H., Ahrenkiel, V., Warthoe, P., et al. (1993) Identification of differentially expressed mRNA species by an improved display technique (DDRT-PCR). *Nucleic Acids Res.* **21,** 4272–4280.
3. Kang, D.-C., LaFrance, R., Su, Z.-Z., and Fisher, P. B. (1998) Reciprocal subtraction differential RNA: an efficient and rapid procedure for isolating differentially expressed gene sequences. *Proc. Natl. Acad. Sci. USA* **95,** 13,788–13,793.
4. Hubank, M. and Schatz, D. G. (1994) Identifying differences in mRNA expression by representational difference analysis of cDNA. *Nucleic Acids Res.* **25,** 5640–5648.
5. Gress, T. M., Wallrapp, C., Frohme, M., Muller-Pillasch, F., Lacher, U., Friess, H., et al. (1997) Identification of genes with specific expression in pancreatic cancer by cDNA representational difference analysis. *Genes Chromosomes Cancer* **19,** 97–103.
6. Welford, S. M., Gregg, J., Chen, E., Garrison, D., Sorensen, P. H., Denny, C. T., et al. (1998) Detection of differentially expressed genes in primary tumor tissues using representational differences analysis coupled to microarray hybridization. *Nucleic Acids Res.* **26,** 3059–3065.

# VII

## PROTEIN EXPRESSION

# 51

## Measurement of Protein Expression

*A Technical Overview*

### Jonathan R. Reeves and John M. S. Bartlett

### 1. Introduction

In common with other tumor types, ovarian cancer is a genetic disease and work at the DNA or RNA level is crucial to gain an understanding of the genetic changes leading to tumor formation. Phenotypic change, however, is the result of loss or aberrant expression of normal protein or expression of a mutated form. Proteins are the front end of biology and for this reason, analysis of protein expression is of paramount importance. Any researcher detecting changes in DNA or RNA without corresponding changes in protein levels or turnover should question whether the changes are artefactual or coincidental. Often researchers are put off measuring proteins because of the relative complexity and perceived lack of sensitivity that protein detection systems exhibit. When it is possible to design reverse transcription polymerase chain reaction (RT-PCR) and PCR reactions capable of detecting and quantifying single mRNA/DNA copies, then it is often easier to demonstrate mRNA expression rather than investigating proteins.

Measurements of protein in tissues is often more demanding technically than analysis of DNA or RNA. Oligonucleotides recognizing any nucleic acid sequence can be obtained relatively quickly and inexpensively and the tissue preparation and methods of analysis are, to some extent, common for different genes. Detection of proteins, however, requires the molecule to retain some biological activity or antigenicity so an appropriate method of tissue preparation is of paramount importance for such studies.

For immunological methods of protein analysis, the specificity of each antibody is crucial for each method of tissue preparation. All too frequently, antibodies that have been shown to recognize a molecule of approximately the correct molecular weight in Western blots or immunoprecipitations of cell lines, vastly overexpressing that molecule, perform poorly or not at all in fixed or frozen tissue sections containing lesser amounts of protein. In these cases, the risk of misinterpreting nonspecific for specific labeling is very real. If the antibody is well characterized and the levels of expression in control tissues is known, then with appropriate controls the researcher can be confident in immunolabeling. However, with a less well-characterized antibody, more stringent controls will need to be performed in the experimental setting.

This review will predominantly address methods for measuring protein in tissues in two broad categories:

From: *Methods in Molecular Medicine, Vol. 39: Ovarian Cancer: Methods and Protocols*
Edited by: J. M. S. Bartlett © Humana Press, Inc., Totowa, NJ

1.  tissue homogenate methods such as ELISA, Western blotting, or ligand binding assays;
2.  *in situ* techniques or immunohistochemistry.

Each type of assay has advantages and disadvantages and it is important to select the most appropriate method for the questions being posed and for the resources available. In particular, the decision to choose *in situ* vs homogenate methods may have a considerable impact on the data to be gathered.

## 2. Homogenate Methods

### 2.1. General Issues

Included under this heading are protein blots, ELISAs, radioimmunoassays, and various ligand binding assays that require a homogenized and partially purified form of the cellular material prior to analysis. These methods are particularly suited to the analysis of *in vitro* tumor models such as immortalized "monoclonal" cell lines in which setting they can be used to provide highly accurate analyses of expression and cellular content of various protein substrates. Such results can similarly be extended to homogeneous tissues, such as tumor xenografts and indeed body tissues of relatively uniform composition (e.g., liver).

The attraction of such methods is that they are readily quality-controlled and yield accurate and consistent quantitative estimates of protein expression. They can also be more readily adapted to allow assessment of protein characteristics such as enzyme activities, kinetic measurements of receptor occupation and also give some measures of protein interactions by immunoprecipitation and other investigations. These methods are, therefore, well suited to some aspects of the investigation of protein function (*see* PART VIII on cell signaling and apoptosis). Additionally, Western blots can give information on protein modification (glycosylation/phosphorylation, and so on) and degradation products. In cell systems and in functional investigations, these methods are often more powerful than *in situ* analyses.

Tumor samples recovered at surgery at composed of a variety of cell types (including tumor cells, blood vessels, stromal cells, normal epithelial cells, and infiltrating lymphocytes) in some cases with only a small proportion being carcinoma cells. Even then the carcinoma cell population may be heterogeneous. Homogenization results in equal treatment of noncancer cells and cancer cells so any measurement of protein expression or function represents an average garnered from all cell types present and not a true quantitative measurement of the molecule within the tumor. The researcher should be aware of this and the likely effect on data prior to embarking on a large study. Without cell fractionation, either by flow cytometry or by isopycnic centrifugation, prior to analysis, it is difficult to determine whether the measured molecule is predominantly expressed in the tumor or nontumor cells.

Therefore, as a first principle, analysis of uncharacterized tumor samples should be avoided or approached only with caution. This must of course be counterbalanced by the caveat that many model systems are just that, models, which function in isolation and may display mechanisms that differ distinctly from the complex interactions of tumor cells in the true host. How far any analysis can be interpolated from model systems into tumor biology will necessarily remain in tension with the purist approach of analysing all tissues *in situ*. Wherever possible, biological systems must be evaluated in clonal models and then measured against dual culture or in vivo models. When a full and practicable understanding has been developed, measurement of carefully characterized and evaluated tumor samples may be reasonably approached.

Another feature of homogenate methods is that they generally require large amounts of fresh frozen tissue. Tissue samples of 500 mg may be sufficient for a modest number of protein blots or points on a Scatchard plot, but will provide up to 1000 5 μm 1 cm² histological sections. Although large amounts of tissue may seem to be a disadvantage, this reduces the level of heterogeneity in expression levels. Nonetheless, researchers are increasingly seeking to gain the most value from often small tumor banks that are difficult to resource and the pressure to avoid approaches that utilize significant amounts of tissue for relatively little gain is high. In this context, methods that allow simultaneous analysis of DNA/RNA and protein from the same tissue sample are recommended, providing the quality of the protein product is not sacrificed. This will depend upon the application in question.

## 2.2. Controling the Homogenization Process

Homogenization is performed to disrupt the tissue and cellular structures in place in order to isolate the protein(s) of interest, however, in so doing a number of undesirable side effects may occur including the release of lysozymes and proteases from intracellular compartments. Similarly, disruption of the normal cellular structure may adversely affect the stability of protein modifications such as phosphorylation and destabilize protein protein interactions. High salt, oxidative stress, extremes of pH freeze/thawing, and heavy metals are all contributors to protein instability. Thus, perhaps the most frequent problem encountered with any isolation process is loss of protein activity. To circumvent this, lysis buffers should be designed with a view to the end point in mind. In almost all cases, the inclusion of protease inhibitors is essential and often inhibitors of phosphatases, kinases, and other enzyme systems may be desirable. The use of low temperatures and speed in processing the samples can also be essential in maintaining the integrity of the proteins to be analyzed.

### 2.2.1. Buffer Selection

The use of buffered solutions in cell lysis and protein purification steps seeks to avoid exposure of proteins to high salt and pH extremes. The intracellular environment is *generally* one in which high protein concentrations, moderate ionic strength, and near neutral pH are present. In certain intracellular microenvironments, these conditions may vary and extraction procedures may require modification to suit this context. In general, however, the following additives to a basic buffering agent (Tris/HEPES) are beneficial.

1. Addition of chelating agents to remove heavy metal ions (EDTA).
2. Addition of reducing agents such as dithiothreitol or more commonly 2-mercaptoethanol to prevent oxidative damage to which cysteine residues and disulphide bridges may be particularly vunerable.
3. Inclusion of additives such as glycerol and detergent can aid stability and detergents are valuable aids to disruption of membranes to release bound proteins or lyse organelles *(1,2)*.

### 2.2.2. Protease Inhibitors

Many molecules, including cell surface receptors, are extremely sensitive to protease digestion. Inclusion of broad-spectrum protease inhibitors will often reduce the

**Table 1**
**Frequently Used Protease Inhibitors**

| Name | Class | Recommended Concentration |
|------|-------|---------------------------|
| Phenylmethylsulfonyl fluoride | Serine proteases | 0.1–1.0 m$M$ |
| Benazamidine | Serine proteases | approx 1 m$M$ |
| Aprotinin | Serine proteases | approx 5 µg/mL |
| Chelating agents: EDTA/EGTA | Metalloproteases | 0.1–1.0 m$M$ |
| Pepstatin A | Acid proteases | approx 1 µg/mL |
| Leupeptin | Thiol proteases | approx 5 µg/mL |
| Antipain | Thiol proteases | approx 1 µg/mL |

rate of such protease digestion (*see* **Table 1**) and for the majority of proteins careful combination of protease inhibitors with low temperature will maintain protein stability *(1)*. These can either remove required cofactors (such as metal ions in the case of EDTA) or act as surrogate substrates in either a competitive or noncompetitive fashion. In general, a spectrum of protease inhibitors is added to most tissue homogenization protocols where recovery of labile proteins is the objective *(1)*.

### 2.2.3. Preservation of Enzyme Activities

This is a complex area as the proteins under investigation may be highly varied and have varied activities. However, it is of particular relevance when extrapolations from experimental findings to physiological functions are to be made. A few examples drawn from the authors' experience, may indicate the problems to be faced. Activation/inactivation of enzymes within cell systems is often a complex balance under tight control. In the context of growth factor receptors, a complex balance between ligand binding, receptor phosphorylation and dephosphorylation exists that can be dramatically disturbed during cellular lysis. Release of ligand can inappropriately activate receptors and mask the true in vivo/in vitro picture along an entire signaling pathway or compete with receptors in ligand binding assays for receptor concentration determination. Alternatively, release/activation of phosphatases can reduce or eliminate cellular responses. Consideration of these points should be made and tailored to individual proteins under investigation.

### 2.2.4. Protein Compartmentalization

Once again, this is a highly complex area, however, in its simplest form, it is essential that consideration is given to the intracellular localization of proteins under investigation. Most studies described here and in Parts VIII and IX (signal transduction/apoptosis) deal with cell membrane or cytosolic proteins that can be readily isolated in a one step protocol. Alternative approaches will apply to nuclear or mitochondrial proteins *(2)*.

Often all the above points can be covered by either a careful consideration of the question under investigation coupled with a literature review. However, particular in the isolation of novel proteins, a degree of empiricism will exist and a process of iteration toward the desired goal may be required.

## 2.3. Choice of Screening Methods

Once a protein is successfully isolated, the method of detection and assay becomes of paramount interest. This choice will depend largely on the end point that the researcher has in view. Is a simple quantitation of the protein required, or some functional information also useful. Is information on the binding affinity, activation status of the protein *in situ* paramount or is further information on the interaction of proteins likely to be informative. This latter area is adequately covered in Part VIII (signal transduction), where kinase assays and other dynamic evaluations are described.

### 2.3.1. Immunoassay

In Chapter 52, Beck et al. describes immunoassay approaches for the analysis of IGFI receptor in tissue homogenates. The advantages of this system over receptor binding assays for IGFI receptor are clearly described, and where an appropriate antibody is available, immunoassays are clearly of significant value. However, they also have potential drawbacks. First, if the antibody is inappropriately selected, it may either cross-react with other species with high-protein sequence homology (e.g., TGFβ1 and TGFβ2 81%), or may not recognize altered conformation states (e.g., following ligand binding). Second, particularly in the case of IGFI, the ligand for IGFI receptor, binding proteins may sequester the protein in question and mask the true concentration present. Third, many growth factor systems are highly permissive with respect to ligands (e.g., FGF receptor, TGFβ receptor, EGF receptor, IGF receptor) and measurement of a single ligand may not reflect the true biological situation. Finally, detection of an immune-reactive protein gives no information about its biological activity.

Conversely, immunoassays are generally more accurate, reproducible, and more readily applied to large numbers of samples than binding assays.

### 2.3.2. Binding Assays ("Scatchards")

The principle of ligand binding assays is clearly set out in Chapter 53 (Scambia et al.), with a clear review of the kinetics involved. This immediately provides an insight into the possible applications of this technology, it provides information on the dynamic interaction between receptor and ligand(s). It can also be adapted as described by Scambia et al. to the measurement of total receptor levels and in other situations to the analysis of total ligand present within the tissue sample (4). No antibody is required and if a tissue is particularly rich in receptors, it can be used as a pool for receptor-based ligand quantitiation.

The drawbacks of such assays have to be set against these potential gains. First, such assays require relatively large amounts of sample (for receptor measurements) or tissue (for ligand measurements). Second, the sensitivity and accuracy of such assays is considerably lower than for immunoassays and can be confused by background nonspecific binding sites. No discrimination between ligands is made and although subclasses of receptors can be distinguished based on affinity differences (e.g., IGFI receptor and insulin receptor) this complicates analysis.

### 2.3.3. Western Blotting

The use of Western blotting, as described by Scambia et al. in Chapter 54, provides additional information regarding protein size and structural integrity and can also be used to provide additional functional information on posttranslational modifications (phosphorylation, and so on). This technique can, therefore, be used to quantitate and analyze proteins from complex mixtures, as well as to track structural integrity through a purification schedule. It requires, however, a multistep analysis of the protein and subsequent antibody detection. A simple protocol will involve electrophoresis of proteins (usually in one dimension, but two-dimensional analysis is also possible), transfer of proteins onto a support membrane, blocking binding sites, and detection with antibody systems.

### 2.3.3.1. GEL ELECTROPHORESIS

By and large, this is the most flexible aspect of the western blotting procedure, the use of denaturing or nondenaturing conditions, immunoprecipitation and two-dimensional procedures (*see* **ref. 5**) can greatly increase the information gathered about the protein. Each of these procedures is, however, highly complex and should be researched carefully before use. The most frequent aspect of Western blotting applied to the understanding of protein expression in tumor biology is the simple detection and quantitation of proteins separated on denaturing acrylamide gels. Denaturing gels are used as the method of choice because nondenatured protein electrophoresis is complicated by variable charge and shape as well as size; in SDS gels under denaturing conditions, the components of charge and shape are largely excluded leading to separations based almost exclusively on molecular size *(6)*. This method thus provides information both on expression and size of proteins and can also be used to detect significant protein modifications such as phosphorylation, and so on. The conditions used for electrophoresis are governed by the size and mobility of the protein under investigation. In general, the larger the protein, the lower the acrylamide concentration used for adequate separation *(6)*. If proteins are only present at low concentrations, the use of a "stacker" gel allows further sample concentration at the interface of the stacking and resolving gels. Once proteins are resolved by electrophoresis, the gel is removed and proteins transferred onto a stable membrane support.

### 2.3.3.2. PROTEIN BLOTTING

The blotting aspect of this procedure allows the transfer of proteins from the matrix of the resolving gel onto a stable and permanent support. A variety of membranes can be used for this procedure, each of which has benefits and drawbacks. Traditionally, nitrocellulose membranes were the agents of choice because of a high-binding capacity (approx 250 µg protein/cm$^2$) and relatively short blocking times required, however, these membranes tend to be brittle and this can affect long-term storage and handling. Nylon membranes are more flexible, but have a much lower (approx 150 µg protein/cm$^2$) capacity and require extensive blocking that can still leave high backgrounds. As a result, polyvinylidene fluoride (PVDF) membranes have become widely accepted as a "standard" for most routine blotting. PVDF represents a compromise with an intermediate affinity for protein (approx 175 µg protein/cm$^2$) with good flexibility and shorter blocking times than required for nylon membranes *(7)*. Nonetheless, choice of membranes may still influence greatly the success of this procedure.

Once the membrane has been chosen, transfer conditions should be optimized *(8)*. Blotting can be carried out by capillary action or by electrophoresis in either submersed tanks or semidry blotters. Capillary blotting has become less popular with the advent of rapid semidry electroblotting procedures that can be completed within 30–60 min. Most proteins will transfer under standard conditions, but for high-molecular weight proteins (>100 kDa) addition of 0.1% SDS can improve transfer, whereas the addition of 20% methanol can improve binding of small molecular weight proteins to membranes *(8)*. The choice of semidry (rapid) vs wet (slow) electroblotting is predominantly one determined by access and preference.

### 2.3.3.3. BLOCKING OF MEMBRANES

The very property of membranes that makes them ideal for blotting can preempt clear immunodetection of nonspecific binding of antibodies (which are proteins too). Blocking of membranes following transfer saturates these binding sites and allows for specific antibody–protein interactions thereafter. Again a variety of blockers are available from the widely used milk fat proteins (dried milk) to ovalbumin and bovine serum albumin. These are all commonly available, and cheap sources of protein without any apparent merits/demerits, nonetheless empirical experience will demonstrate that some work better than others with individual systems. In addition, inclusion of a low concentration of detergents reduces background, although high concentrations (>0.05% Tween-20) can elute proteins from PVDF *(9)*.

### 2.3.3.4. SELECTION OF PRIMARY ANTIBODY

Antibodies which work on Western blots may or may not work in other systems and vice versa. There does not appear to be any clear means of selecting antibodies that have a high degree of efficiency in difference conditions. Polyclonal antibodies give a higher chance of detection of the protein in question, but this is coupled with a greater risk of cross reactivity. Monoclonals, when validated provide a highly specific screen which, in theory at least, is available in limitless supply. However, in practice, the high cost of commercial monoclonals can limit their usefulness. If an antibody has a low affinity for the protein in question, high concentrations and long incubation times may improve sensitivity *(6,9)*.

### 2.3.3.5. DETECTION SYSTEMS/SECONDARY ANTIBODIES

Again, a wide range of systems are now available, iodination of antibodies is by and large out of fashion. Biotinylated or more commonly enzyme-linked secondary antibodies provide highly sensitive, and in most cases, semiquantitative screening systems. In this context, the choice between permanent records on the blot using colored substrates and luminescence autoradiography depends on the desire to reprobe the blot for other proteins thereafter *(9,10)*.

### 2.3.3.6. REPROBING BLOTS

A further advantage of Western blots is that the membrane can be stored for prolonged periods and then stripped of the primary assay system and reprobed with other antibodies. Each stripping protocol can reduce the sensitivity of the blot, but blots can be reprobed 3–4 times *(9)*.

## 2.4. Summary: Analysis of Proteins in Cellular Homogenates

Once tissues are homogenized, intracellular proteins become accessible for a wide range of biochemical evaluations, including functional and physical assays. Each system has merits and demerits, which should be considered, with the overall experimental aim in view, prior to work starting. Included in this evaluation should be the amount of tissue required, the availability of material for other assays, and the information required from the experimental approach.

## 3. *In Situ* Methods (Immunohistochemistry)

### 3.1. General Issues

The major advantage of *in situ* techniques over methods based on tissue disruption is that the molecule is demonstrated within histological sections and it is thus possible to identify which cells within the tissue express the molecule of interest. Pathology departments frequently have extensive archives of tissue, usually fixed in formalin and embedded in paraffin wax, and this forms an attractive resource for researchers, with hundreds of sections available from a single block. Information regarding tumor pathology and patient follow-up is generally attainable for such material giving a disease endpoint. Such archival tissue would seem to be the material of choice for immunohistochemical studies, but this is not necessarily the case and the researcher should be aware of certain limitations. Formalin fixation and paraffin-embedding methods have changed little over the last century and they certainly were not designed with the immunohistochemist in mind. The solvents and heat used during tissue processing denature proteins and the fixatives create crosslinks affecting, to a lesser or greater degree, the antigenicity of the molecule of interest. A number of methods have been developed to "retrieve" antigens including proteolytic digestion and heat treatments *(11)* and these are effective in many systems, but it would seem prudent to start with material that does not require retrieval of antigens concealed or lost at an earlier stage of tissue preparation. The researcher might legitimately ask a number of questions when assessing a series of immunohistochemically labeled paraffin sections.

- How much signal would there have been if the tissue was fresh frozen instead of fixed?
- Is the fading towards the center of the section because of a lower degree of formalin penetration or does the centre actually express less of the molecule?
- I see that specimen A was fixed on Friday and processed on Monday, does this give the same degree of labeling as specimen B fixed on Tuesday and processed on Wednesday?

For the immunohistochemist to be fully aware of the limitations of studying archival material a pilot study comparing labeling in fresh frozen material with the same cases fixed and embedded in paraffin should be considered. Then it will be possible to determine the extent of information loss due to fixation and paraffin embedding and to establish whether either method yields data of sufficient quality to answer the questions posed. Working on frozen material avoids many of the problems likely to be experienced with paraffin-embedded tissues. Although the histological quality of frozen sections is frequently criticized, with careful tissue storage and competent cryostat work, sections of high quality can be obtained (*see* Note 2 on radioimmunohistochemistry, Chapter 59 by Reeves). Brief fixation of the sections (for example in 1% buffered formaldehyde) prior to immunohistochemistry often leaves antigens intact resulting in significantly improved histology. Although frozen section immunohistochemistry avoids many of the problems associated with working on formalin fixed and paraffin-embedded material, the data produced is at best semiquantitative. If it is thought that quantitation of protein expression will enable a more complete analysis, then the time and effort employing quantitative immunohistochemistry should be considered (*see* Chapter 59 on radioimmunohistochemistry). The different quality and types of information that can be produced from paraffin section immunohistochemsitry, frozen section immunohistochemistry and quantitative methods are illustrated by the frequency distribution histograms in **Fig. 1**.

### 3.2. Analysis of Labeled Sections

After generating a series of immunohistochemical sections, the researcher is presented with the task of interpretation with the aim of turning the images under the microscope into meaningful data for analysis. There are many published scoring protocols for immunohistochemical sections ranging from simple positive negative categorization, through estimations of percentage of positive cells or nuclei, to combinations of intensity and labeled proportion (histoscore) *(12,13)*. Whichever method is selected, an evaluation of interobserver variability is encouraged to enable an assessment of the accuracy of the scoring method and the data generated. The most appropriate method of analysis is dependent on the nature of the relationship between the molecule being studied and the biological endpoint. If this is a clear cut relationship with zero or very low expression resulting in one outcome and high expression resulting in another, then division of cases into positive and negative categories may be all that is needed. However, rarely does the immunohistochemist have the luxury of such a clearly defined relationship. There may be a subtle critical threshold of protein expression and a more thorough evaluation of the sections is warranted. At best, conventional frozen or paraffin section immunohistochemistry is semiquantitative and even the most careful evaluation may not be able to divide cases accurately either side of a critical threshold. If there are multiple thresholds or a continuum between expression and biological parameter, then the chances of meaningful interpretation of immunohistochemical sections becomes slim.

Unfortunately, the researcher is often faced initially with the very task of attempting to define the relationship between protein expression and tumor biology. With unlimited resources and time, the nature of the relationship should be defined first with the most accurate and quantitative method available and those data can then be used to establish how the more simple methods are robust. However, time and resources are generally limited so the researcher should be aware of the limitations of the technique being employed and open to the suggestion that quantitative analysis may yield a more accurate and thorough interpretation (as illustrated in **Fig. 1**).

### 3.3. Controls

#### 3.3.1. General Issues

This section is written with the immunohistochemist in mind, but it is equally relevant for researchers using other antibody-based methods of protein analysis. It is of paramount importance for the specificity of each antibody to be established in each test system. All too frequently, antibodies that have been shown to recognize a molecule of approximately the correct molecular weight in Western blots or immunoprecipitates of cell lines vastly overexpressing that molecule perform poorly or not at all in fixed or frozen tissue sections that may contain lesser amounts of protein. For the uninitiated,

Fig. 1. Frequency distribution histograms illustrating c-*erb*B-2 expression in 60 breast carcinomas by three different immunohistochemical methods. (**A**) Paraffin section immunohistochemistry, with results expressed as a histoscore, where the observer estimates the labeling
intensity and the proportion of labeled tumor cells for each case and calculates the sum of
(1 × % weakly positive) + (2 × % moderately positive) + (3 × % strongly positive) to give a
maximum score of 300. Note that in paraffin sections, no information is available from two
thirds of the cases with a score of zero. (**B**) In frozen sections, there is no loss of antigenicity
owing to formalin fixation and paraffin embedding, consequently, at least some specific labeling was demonstrable in all but two cases. (**C**) Radioimmunohistochemistry (expressed as log *x* the
expression within normal breast paranchyma) gives a quantitative assessment of c-*erb*B-2 in all
but one case. Note that c-*erb*B-2 expression ranges from a little below normal to about 500

the risk of misinterpreting nonspecific for specific labeling can be very real, especially if the researcher is expecting to see expression in the test system. Always beware of the immunohistochemical study that requires nonstandard methods to produce labeling. For example, the methods section of such a publication may state that optimal labeling was only achieved by using a nonstandard blocker of nonspecific binding. It is clear that in these cases labeling was not readily attainable by standard means and a considerable amount of method "optimization" was required. The critic should look carefully at the experimental controls to be convinced of specificity. Generally, if an antibody works, it will work with standard immunohistochemical procedures.

If an antibody is well characterized in the experimental system being exploited, and the levels of expression in control tissues have been well established by complementary means, then with simple controls (using a known positive control, and an isotype-matched control antibody in the place of the primary antibody as a negative control) the researcher can be relatively confident in his or her immunolabeling. Being presented with a less well-characterized antibody, the researcher should find as much information as possible about the reagent and the molecule that is recognizes and should perform more stringent controls to be confident about labeling in the selected test system. Beware of manufacturers' own data as they have a vested interest in selling the product. The following section details some of the controls that may be considered when the specificity of an antibody is under question. It is important to understand the strengths and weaknesses of each type of control.

### 3.3.2. Isotype-Matched Control Antibody/No Primary Antibody

In many immunohistochemical studies, the methods section will state that negative controls were performed by running a parallel set of sections with no primary antibody *(14)*. This simply indicates whether the secondary reagents are specific or whether there is a problem with endogenous proteins (e.g., biotin, peroxidase, alkaline, and phosphatase). It gives no indication as to the specificity of the primary reagent. If a monoclonal antibody is being used, an isotype-matched control antibody recognizing a protein not present in the tissue should be used in the place of the primary antibody. For example, if the primary antibody is a mouse monoclonal IgG2a used at 2 µg/mL, then the control antibody should also be mouse IgG2a at 2 µg/mL. If the primary antibody is, for example, a purified rabbit polyclonal used at 5 µg/mL, then preimmune rabbit immunoglobulins should be used as the control at 5 µg/mL. Isotype-matched controls will not indicate whether the primary antibody crossreacts with other proteins within the section, but will indicate whether the blockers of nonspecific binding being used are sufficiently effective to prevent nonspecific protein–protein interactions between the labeling reagents and molecules within the sections.

---

Fig. 1. *(continued)* times the normal level and there are two distinct populations. The population with the highest expression corresponds to those with maximal or near maximal frozen section immunohistochemical histoscores (275 to 300), but actual level of expression within these ranges by a factor of 20. Most of these, but not all, show a degree of labeling in the paraffin sections. In subsequent studies, the quantitative c-*erb*B-2 expression data were shown to be significantly better at predicting patient survival than the conventional methods (data not shown). Reproduced with permission from **ref. *12***.

### 3.3.3. Antigen Blocking Controls

If the antigen to which the antibody was raised is available in reasonable quantities, then antigen blocking controls can be performed. Although these do provide information about specificity, it is important to be clear on exactly what they do tell us. Generally, the primary antibody is incubated with an excess of the antigen and the antigen-antibody complex is applied to the sections. Continued presence of labeling in such controls would indicate nonspecific binding of the primary antibody probably through protein–protein interactions. Although an absence of labeling confirms specificity of the antibody (and we would hope it recognizes the antigen to which it was raised), it does not confirm that the labeling in the absence of blocking antigen is specific. Incubation of the primary antibody with free antigen will prevent binding to specific and crossreacting molecules. Antigen-blocking controls are generally overrated and inappropriate conclusions are often drawn from them.

### 3.3.4. Controls Specific for an Individual Antibody

The researcher should have his eyes open for antibody-specific control opportunities and these should not be missed. For example, one antibody that recognizes the c-*erb*B-3 protein is specific for the ligand binding site. By preincubation of the sections with ligand (heregulin β1), it is possible to show that antibody labeling is reduced thus confirming that the labelling is indeed due to the c-*erb*B-3 protein.

### 3.3.5. Established Positive/Negative Control Tissues

There is no substitute for good positive and negative controls in immunohistochemical studies. If there are data on control tissues with known levels of protein expression, tissue distribution and subcellular localization, such as normal tissues, cell lines, or transfected cell lines, then, if possible, these should be obtained for positive controls. Ideally, a panel of cell lines with expression levels quantified by complementary means, such as ligand binding assay, ELISA, or protein blot assay can be used to confirm that the immunohistochemical labeling is indeed present in the proportions expected *(12)*.

### 3.3.6. Panel of Other Antibodies

If there are other antibodies available recognizing the same molecule, then these can be used to support the specificity of the test antibody in a pilot study. It is often possible to obtain test amounts of antibody from suppliers at a nominal charge. If other researchers have generally opted for another reagent to detect the molecule then there may be very good reasons why this is the case.

### 3.3.7. Independent Data

Depending on the system being examined, it may be possible to confirm protein expression by an independent nonantibody-based method. For example, in an immunohistochemical study looking at epidermal growth factor receptors using the EGFR1 monoclonal antibody, it was possible to demonstrate identical labeling in a panel of normal tissues and tumors using labeled ligand (epidermal growth factor) as the primary reagent *(15)*.

### 3.4. Power Analysis

Many readers of this section will want to study a series of ovarian tumors with the intention of relating their measured parameter with some biological measure of the disease process, such as existing pathological variables or patient survival. Such a study requires statistical analysis and, at the end of the study, the researcher is frequently left with results of marginal significance and wondering whether analysis of just a few more cases would have given statistics with a greater degree of confidence. Before embarking on this sort of study, the researcher should ask questions to estimate whether the resources and methods available are likely to yield data with sufficient statistical power. What is the likely extent of the measured difference between cases and is this change subtle or clear cut? What proportion of cases fall into each of the measured categories? How many cases will it be necessary to analyze before detecting a statistically significant difference between the categories? If the answers are not in existing literature, then a pilot study should be considered to address these problems before embarking on a more ambitious project. Frequently, through poor experimental design, the project intending to answer all the questions itself becomes the pilot study. Further suggested reading on the importance of statistical power is given in the reference list *(16–18)*.

### References

1. Deutscher, M. P. (1990) Maintaining protein stability, in *Methods in Enzymology* Vol. 182 (Deutscher, M. P., ed.), Academic, London, U.K. ch. 8, pp. 83–93.
2. *Protein Purification Protocols* (1996) (Doonan, S., ed.), Humana, Totowa, NJ.
3. *Cell Biology: A Laboratory Handbook* (Celis, J. E., ed.) (1994) Academic, London, U.K. (See volume 1 for various isolation protocols.)
4. Scatchard, G. (1949) The attraction of protein for small molecules and ions. *Ann. N.Y. Acad. Sci.* **51,** 660–672.
5. Sambrook, J., Fritsch, E. F., and Maniatis, T. (1989) Molecular cloning. A laboratory manual, in *Detection and Analysis of Proteins Expressed from Cloned Genes. Second Edition*, Cold Spring Harbor Laboratory, Cold Spring Harbor, NY, ch. 18.
6. Garfin, D. E. (1990) One-dimensional gel electrophoresis, in *Methods in Enzymology* (Deutscher, M. P., ed.), vol. 182, Academic, London, U.K., ch. 33, pp. 425–441.
7. Burnette, W. N. (1981) "Western blotting": electrophoretic transfer of proteins from sodium dodecyl sulfate-polyacrylamine gels to unmodified nitrocellulose and radiographic detection with antibody and radioiodinated protein A. *Anal. Biochem.* **112,** 195–203.
8. Towbin, H., Staehelin, T., and Gordon, J. (1979) Electrophoretic transfer of proteins from polyacrylamide gels to nitrocellulose sheets: procedure and some applications. *Proc. Natl. Acad. Sci. USA* **76,** 4350–4534.
9. Promega Protein Guide: Tips and Techniques (1993) Promega Corp., Madison, WI.
10. Knecht, D. A. and Randall, L. D. (1984) Visualization of antigenic proteins on Western blots. *Anal. Biochem.* **136,** 180–184.
11. Shi, S. R., Cote, P. J., and Taylor, C. R. (1997) Antigen retrieval immunohistochemistry: past, present and future. *J. Histochem. Cytochem.* **45,** 327–343.
12. Reeves, J. R., Going, J. J., Smith, G., Cooke, T. G., Ozanne, B. W., and Stanton, P. D. (1996) Quantitative radioimmunohistochemical measurements of p185(erbB-2) in frozen tissue sections. *J. Histochem. Cytochem.* **44,** 1251–1259.
13. Detre, S., Saccani Jotti, G., and Dowsett, M. (1995) A quickscore method of immunohistochemical semiquantitation: validation for oestrogen receptors in breast carcinomas. *J. Clin. Path.* **48,** 876–878.
14. Simpson, B. J. B., Weatherill, J., Miller, E. P., Lessells, A. M., Langdon, S. P., and Miller, W. R. (1995) C-erbB-2 protein expression in ovarian tumors. *Br. J. Cancer* **71,** 758–762.
15. Reeves, J. R., Cooke, T. G., Fenton Lee, D., McNicol, A. M., Ozanne, B. W., Richards, R. C., and Walsh, A. (1994) Localization of EGF receptors in frozen tissue sections by antibody and biotinylated EGF-based techniques. *J. Histochem Cytochem.* **42,** 307–314.
16. A'Hern, R. P. (1995) Statistical power: a measure of the quality of a study. *Br. J. Urol.* **75,** 5–8.
17. Simon, R. and Altman, D. G. (1994) Statistical aspects of prognostic factor studies in oncology. *Br. J. Cancer* **69,** 979–985.
18. Fayers, P. M. and Machin, D. (1995) Sample size: how many patients are necessary? *Br. J. Cancer* **72,** 1–9.

# 52

# Measurement of IGF-1 Receptor Content in Tissues and Cell Lines by Radioimmunoassay (RIA) and ELISA Techniques

**Eberhard P. Beck, Laura Sciacca, Giuseppe Pandini, Wolfram Jaeger, and Vincenzo Pezzino**

## 1. Introduction

The IGF-1 receptor (IGF-1-R) belongs to the tyrosine kinase growth factor receptor family. It is structurally similar to, but distinct from, the insulin receptor, with which it shares a 70% homology. As expected, it crossreacts with insulin and, vice versa, insulin receptor crossreacts with IGF-1. Numerous studies suggest that IGF-1-R is very important for mitogenesis and is essential for phenotype transformation, at least in rodents (*1*). In particular, the IGF-1-R has been described in human breast cancer (*2–4*) and ovarian cancer (*5*) tissues and in cultured human breast cancer cell lines (*6,7*).

The possibility of measuring IGF-1 receptors in human tissues and cultured cell lines would certainly be of interest in several neoplastic disorders both for clinical investigators in oncology and for basic science researchers.

To quantitate IGF-1-R levels, specific $^{125}$I-labeled IGF-1 binding to the receptor is generally used (*8*). Although the binding assay is sensitive and easy, there are several drawbacks. The binding assay can only detect active and unoccupied receptors. Scatchard plots are sometimes linear, but often curvilinear (*8,9*), which makes the determination of the receptor number difficult. Most important is that significant amounts of IGF binding proteins could interfere with an accurate quantitation of the IGF-1-R, because they can also bind $^{125}$I-labeled IGF-1.

In the past years, we have set up two different methods that are readily applicable to the measurement of IGF-1 receptors in tissues and cell lines. The first is a sensitive and specific radioimmunoassay (RIA) (*10*), and the second is a recently developed ELISA method for the IGF-1 receptor. The potential utility of such techniques has already been described in studies of breast cancer (*11*) and ovarian cancer (*5*).

## 2. Materials

1. Culture medium: modified Eagle's medium (MEM) containing 10% fetal calf serum (FCS), 2 mmol/L glutamine, 1X nonessential amino acids, and 40 µg/mL gentamycin.
2. Serum-free medium: culture medium without FCS, containing 0.1% bovine serum albumin (BSA) RIA grade, and 10 µg/mL transferrin.

From: *Methods in Molecular Medicine, Vol. 39: Ovarian Cancer: Methods and Protocols*
Edited by: J. M. S. Bartlett © Humana Press, Inc., Totowa, NJ

3. Solubilization buffer: 50 m*M* HEPES buffer, pH 7.4, containing 2 mg/mL bacitracin, 1 m*M* phenylmethylsulfonylfluoride (PMSF), and 1% Triton X-100.
4. RIA buffer: 50 m*M* HEPES, pH 7.6, 150 m*M* NaCl, 0.1% Triton X-100, 0.2% BSA, and 0.2 m*M* PMSF.
5. ELISA buffer A (TBST): 20 m*M* Tris-HCl, pH 7.4, 150 m*M* NaCl, 0.05% Tween-20.
6. ELISA buffer B: 50 m*M* HEPES, pH 7.6, 150 m*M* NaCl, 0.05% Tween-20, 1% BSA, 2 m*M* sodium orthovanadate, 1 mg/mL bacitracin, and 1 m*M* PMSF.
7. TMB buffer: 3,3',5,5'-tetramethylbenzidine 0.4 mg/mL in 0.1*M* citrate-phosphate buffer, pH 5.0 with 0.4 µL/mL of 30% $H_2O_2$ (Kirkegaard and Perry Laboratories, Gaithersburg, MD).

## 3. Methods

### 3.1. Tissue Sample Preparation

1. Tissue specimens of human breast and ovary were collected during surgery, dissected free from adjacent tissue, and then frozen in liquid nitrogen immediately. Informed consent was obtained from each patient.
2. 0.1–2.0 g of tissues were minced using scissors.
3. The material was suspended at 0.1–0.2 g/mL in solubilization buffer without Triton X-100, and homogenized with a polytron homogenizer at 4°C.
4. The homogenized material was then incubated with Triton X-100 (1% final concentration) for 60 min at 4°C under continuous shaking.
5. The solubilized material was centrifuged at 10,000*g* for 5 min at 4°C in a microfuge, and the supernatant was frozen at –80°C until assayed.
6. The protein content in tissue specimens was determined by the Bradford method *(12)*.

### 3.2. Cell Sample Preparation

1. Human breast cancer cell lines (MCF-7, ZR-75-1, MDA-MB231, T47-D) were grown in culture medium at 37°C in 5% $CO_2$.
2. The medium was changed every 2 d.
3. Cell monolayers were preincubated for 24 h in serum-free medium.
4. Cells were harvested with phosphate-buffered saline (PBS) and 0.2 % EDTA (5–10 min at 37°C).
5. Cells were counted in a Neubauer chamber.
6. Cells ($2–3 \times 10^6$) were solubilized in 1 mL of solubilization buffer for 60 min at 4°C under continuous shaking.
7. The solubilized material was then centrifuged at 10,000*g* for 5 min at 4°C in a microfuge, and the supernatant was frozen at –80°C until assayed.
8. The protein content in cells was determined by the Bradford method *(12)*.

### 3.3. RIA Technique

#### 3.3.1. Purification of IGF-1 Receptor (IGF-1-R)

The IGF-1-R was purified by sequential affinity chromatography, as described in **ref. 9**. Human placenta membranes were solubilized with Triton X-100. A glycoprotein fraction was first purified on a Sepharose column. WGA-Sepharose eluate fractions containing IGF-1 binding activity were pooled and applied to a second Sepharose column coupled with the monoclonal antibody αIR-3, that is specific to the human IGF-1-R (Oncogene Research Cambridge, MA). Purified receptor concentration in this latter eluate was measured by amino acid analysis *(9)*. The same preparation was used for the ELISA technique. Occasionally, IGF-1-R purified from CHO cells transfected with IGF-1-R cDNA and calibrated with purified IGF-1-R from human placenta was used.

### 3.3.2. Preparation of $^{125}$I-labeled IGF-1 Receptor

1. Purified human placental IGF-1 receptor (3.2 µg) was incubated for 90 min with 500 µCi $^{125}$I-Bolton-Hunter reagent (New England Nuclear, Boston, MA) in 45 µL of 50 m$M$ borate buffer, pH 8.5.
2. The reaction was performed at 22°C under continuous shaking and stopped by the addition of 250 µL of ice cold borate buffer containing 0.5$M$ glycine and 0.1% Triton X-100.
3. The subsequent procedure of $^{125}$I-IGF-1-R separation was run at 4°C. The entire mixture was applied to a 4-mL WGA-agarose column (Miles Scientific, Naperville, IL), which had been equilibrated with 50 m$M$ HEPES buffer, pH 7.4, containing 150 m$M$ NaCl, 0.1% Triton-X 100, 0.2% BSA, and 0.2 m$M$ PMSF.
4. After 10 min, the column was washed with 20 mL of the same buffer.
5. $^{125}$I-labeled IGF-1 receptors were eluted with the same buffer containing 0.4$M$ N-acetylglucosamine without BSA. Fractions of 500 µL were collected and counted.

### 3.3.3. Preparation of Polyclonal Antibody to the Human IGF-1 Receptor

The polyclonal antibody to the human IGF-1 receptor was prepared as described in **ref. 9**. Rabbits were immunized by injecting 10 to 20 µg of purified human placental IGF-1-R mixed with complete Freund adjuvant into the popliteal lymph node. Three weeks later, 5 to 10 µg of the purified receptor mixed with incomplete adjuvant were subcutaneously injected at multiple sites on the back. Sera from the rabbits were obtained 1 wk after the second injection. IgG fractions were prepared by ammonium sulfate precipitation followed by DEAE-cellulose chromatography. Polyclonal antibody N-20 (Santa Cruz Biotechnology Inc., Santa Cruz, CA) might be used.

### 3.3.4. RIA Procedure

1. To 9 × 70-mm plastic tubes were added, in a total volume of 200 µL of RIA buffer, 0 to 60 ng of unlabeled IGF-1-R or multiple dilutions of unknown sample.
2. After the addition of 100 µL of the anti-IGF-1-R antibody (final dilution 1:10,000 in RIA buffer) plus nonimmune rabbit serum (final dilution 1:400) as carrier for protein precipitation, the tubes were incubated for 24 h at 4°C.
3. 100 µL of RIA buffer containing 12,000 to 18,000 cpm of $^{125}$I-labeled IGF-1-R was added.
4. After 24 h at 4°C, 100 µL of goat antirabbit γ-globulin serum (Antibodies Inc., Davis, CA) (final dilution 1:150 in RIA buffer) was added.
5. After an additional 24 h incubation at 4°C, the tubes were centrifuged at 3000$g$ for 20 min, the supernatants aspirated with a pump, and the radioactivity counted. IGF-1 receptor content was expressed as ng per 0.1 mg protein.

### 3.4. ELISA Technique

The standard IGF-1-R used for the ELISA technique was the same preparation used for RIA. The following antibodies were used: monoclonal antibodies αIR-3 and 17-69, that reacts with the α-subunit at residues 440-586 (kindly supplied by Dr. K. Siddle, Cambridge, UK).

### 3.4.1. Preparation of Biotinylated anti-IGF-1 Receptor Antibody

1. Purified monoclonal antibody 17–69 (2 mg/mL) was diluted 1:2 with 0.1$M$ NaHCO$_3$.
2. It was dialyzed 3 times for 2 h at 4°C against 0.1$M$ NaHCO$_3$.

3. After dialysis, proteins were measured using mouse IgG as a standard, and the sample protein adjusted to 800 μg/mL.
4. 0.2 μg Biotin (Calbiochem, La Jolla, CA) (2 mg/mL in Dimethylformamide)/μg antibody was added to the sample, shaken vigorously, and rotated end over end at 22°C for 2 h.
5. The solution was then dialyzed three times for 16–18 h at 4°C against 50 m$M$ HEPES, 150 m$M$ NaCl pH 7.6.

### 3.4.2. ELISA Procedure

1. IGF-1 receptors were captured by incubating 100 μL of standard receptor or multiple dilution of cellular and tissue extract, in Maxisorp immunoplates (Nunc, Roskilde, Denmark) precoated overnight at 4° C with 2 μg/mL αIR-3.
2. After 16 h at 4° C the plates were washed with 300 μL of ELISA buffer A.
3. The immunocaptured receptors were incubated for 2 h at 22° C, with 0.3 μg/mL of the biotinylated anti-IGF-1-R 17-69 antibody in 100 μL of ELISA buffer B.
4. Unbound biotinylated antibody was washed with 300 μL of ELISA buffer A.
5. 100 μL of peroxidase-conjugated streptavidin (0.1 μg/mL in ELISA buffer B) was added and incubated for 30 min at 22° C.
6. The reaction was enhanced by an ELAST ELISA Amplification Sistem (New England Nuclear, Boston, MA).
7. The peroxidase activity was determined colorimetrically by adding 100 μL of TMB buffer.
8. The reaction was stopped within 30 min by the addition of 100 μL of 1$M$ $H_3PO_4$.
9. The absorbance was measured at 450 nm.

For quantitative calculations a standard curve drawn with known concentrations of IGF-1-R was used. By comparing the absorbance obtained from a sample containing an unknown amount of IGF-1-R with those obtained from the standards, the concentration of IGF-1-R in the sample was determined. IGF-1 receptor content was expressed as ng per 0.1 mg protein.

## 4. Technical Notes

### 4.1. Standardization and Validation of RIA Procedure

Unlabeled purified IGF-1 receptor competed with the radioactive receptor binding to the antibody (**Fig. 1**). Detectable binding inhibition was seen with 2.0 ng of the unlabeled IGF-1 receptor and over 80% of the binding was inhibited in the presence of 60 ng of the receptor. In 10 experiments, half maximal displacement was at 19 ± 5 ng (mean ± SE). In contrast to the IGF-1 receptor, unlabeled insulin receptor (from NIH/3T3 cells transfected with human insulin receptor cDNA) did not readily compete for the binding, because 60 ng of insulin receptor inhibited only 10%. The ligand, IGF-1, did not compete at all.

The interassay coefficient of variation was 10% and the intraassay coefficient of variation was 5%. In addition, the competition-inhibition curve obtained from Triton X-100 extracts of MCF-7 breast cancer cells was similar to that seen with the purified IGF-1 receptor.

Multiple dilutions of cellular extracts prepared from placenta and breast cancer tissues also produced competition-inhibition curves that were parallel to that of the pure IGF-1 receptor standard.

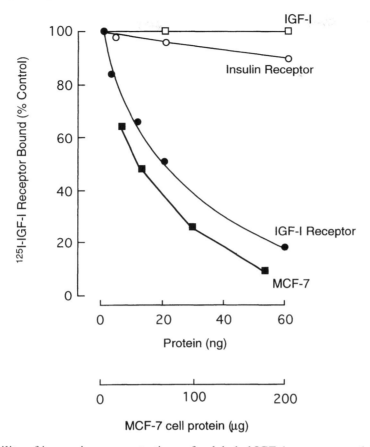

Fig. 1. Ability of increasing concentrations of unlabeled IGF-1 receptors, unlabeled insulin receptors, unlabeled IGF-1, and MCF-7 cell extracts to compete with labeled IGF-1 receptor for the antireceptor antibody.

## 4.2. Standardization and Validation of ELISA Technique

The assay was linear from 0.125 to 1.0 ng IGF-1-R/well. The minimal detectable amount of IGF-1-R was between 0.1–0.2 ng. Purified insulin receptor did not react in the assay (**Fig. 2**). In addition, the dose-response curve obtained with increasing concentrations of MDA-MB231 cell extracts was similar to that seen with IGF-1 receptor. Increasing concentrations of extracts from placenta and breast cancer produced dose-response curves parallel to that obtained with the purified IGF-1-R standard. The intraassay coefficient of variation was 7% at 0.3 ng and 5% at 0.6 ng. The interassay coefficient of variation was 10 and 8%, respectively.

## 4.3. IGF-1 Receptor Content in Cell Lines

The content of IGF-1-R was measured in four cultured human epithelial breast cancer cells. In these cell lines the IGF-1-R content ranged from 5.9 to 56.2 ng/0.1 mg protein measured by RIA, and from 2.6 to 34.0 ng/0.1 mg protein by ELISA. $^{125}$I-IGF-1 ligand binding studies performed in the same breast cancer cell lines showed a good

Fig. 2. Dose-response curves of increasing concentrations of IGF-1 receptors (IGF-1-R), insulin receptors (IR), and MDA-MB231 cell extracts in the ELISA assay.

agreement between IGF-1 binding and IGF-1 receptor content measured by both RIA and ELISA (**Table 1**).

## 5. Discussion

The present study demonstrates the feasibility of carrying out routine determinations of the IGF-1 receptor. Employing a labeled-purified IGF-1 receptor and a polyclonal antireceptor antibody, we developed a sensitive and specific RIA, which can be used to measure IGF-1 receptors in tissues and cells. An alternative method, developed as an ELISA technique, which utilizes two monoclonal antibodies to the human IGF-1 receptor, yielded similar results. These assays could be useful to study the IGF-1 receptor both in vivo and in vitro.

The RIA technique is sensitive to concentrations of unlabeled IGF-1 receptors as low as 2.0 ng. This sensitivity allows the measurement of IGF-1 receptors in very small quantities of biological materials. In addition, this assay is highly specific for the IGF-1 receptor, because the closely related receptor of insulin, which has major sequence homology to the IGF-1 receptor *(13)*, reacted only weakly. Unlabeled IGF-1 at a concentration as high as 60 ng/mL did not interfere with the assay, indicating that occupancy of the IGF-1 receptor by the ligand did not influence its immunoreactivity in the radioimmunoassay.

**Table 1**
**IGF-1 receptor (IGF-1-R) Content in Cultured Breast Cancer Cell Lines**
**Measured by Radioimmunoassay (RIA), ELISA, and Ligand Binding Methods**

| Cell Line | IGF-1-R RIA (ng/0.1 mg protein) | IGF-1-R ELISA (ng/0.1 mg protein) | % B/T per 0.1 mg protein |
|---|---|---|---|
| MCF-7 | 56.2 | 34.0 | 15.6 |
| MDA-MB231 | 5.9 | 2.6 | 1.6 |
| T-47D | 14.7 | 10.0 | 7.0 |
| ZR-75-1 | 11.0 | 10.0 | 8.3 |

Moreover, increasing concentrations of extracts of both cell lines and tissues produced dose-response curves that were parallel to the standard curve, thus indicating that no interference was present in the tested material in our conditions.

The same characteristics of sensitivity, specificity, and good parallelism of unknown cell or tissue samples were also true for the ELISA technique. In particular, the ELISA assay was approximately 10-fold more sensitive than the radioimmunoassay (lowest detectable level 0.2 ng vs 2.0 ng). On the other hand, amounts of receptor greater than 1 ng could not be accurately measured with ELISA. With this latter technique, therefore, a narrower range of receptor concentration can be utilized, thus making IGF-1-receptor determination somewhat more difficult, unless appropriate and multiple dilutions of the sample are tested.

Both techniques have certain advantages over ligand-binding assays. First, smaller biological specimens are needed. Second, multiple samples can be stored and thereafter their receptor content measured in the same assay. In addition, a precise quantitation of receptor number does not require Scatchard analysis, which is more difficult to carry out than these immunoassays. It should be also pointed out that the two methods described in the present study provide data that are potentially different from data obtained by ligand-binding assays. In fact, our techniques quantitate the total number of receptor molecules present in the sample, independent of their binding ability, whereas the binding assay quantitates only the number of receptors whose binding sites are accessible to the hormone.

Combined with functional studies of IGF-1 binding, RIA and ELISA methods provide, therefore, an additional approach to understanding conditions of altered IGF-1 action. When we examined IGF-1 receptor content in breast cancer tissues and cell lines, significant amounts of IGF-1 receptors were detected in tissue samples and cultured cells. In addition, measurement of IGF-1 receptor content was similar with both techniques and also correlated with IGF-1 ligand binding.

IGF-1-receptor content in ovarian cancer tissues was highly variable. This may well reflect a great heterogeneity of IGF-1 receptor expression in this type of malignancy. It has been reported that breast cancer cells express more IGF-1 receptors than normal breast cells, as measured by ligand binding studies *(14)*. By using the RIA, IGF-1 receptors were also found to be elevated in human breast cancer *(15)*. In addition, this latter study suggested that a high IGF-1-receptor content was a favorable prognostic indicator. The present techniques, therefore, confirm and extend previous data obtained with ligand binding studies.

We believe that the radioimmunoassay and the ELISA techniques for the measurement of IGF-1 receptors can be useful for many types of investigations, including screening large number of samples in studies of breast, ovarian, and other cancer tissues.

## References

1. Baserga, R. (1995) The insulin-like growth factor-I receptor: a key to tumor growth? *Cancer Res.* **55,** 249–252.
2. Yee, D., Paik, S., Lebovic, G. S., Marcus, R., Favoni, R., Cullen, K., et al. (1989) Analysis of insulin-like growth factor-I gene expression in malignancy: evidence for a paracrine role in human breast cancer. *Mol. Endocrinol.* **3,** 509–517.
3. Peyrat, J. P., Bonneterre, J., Beuscart, R., Djiane, J., and Demaille, A. (1988) Insulin-like growth factor-I receptors in human breast cancer and their relation to estradiol and progesterone receptors. *Cancer Res.* **48,** 6429–6433.
4. Foekens, J. A., Portengen, H., Jansen, M., and Klijn, G. (1989) Insulin-like growth factor-I receptors and insulin-like growth factor-I-like activity in human primary breast cancer. *Cancer (Phila.)* **63,** 2139–2147.
5. Beck, E. P., Russo, P., Gliozzo, B. M., Jaeger, W., Papa, V., Wildt, L., et al. (1994) Identification of insulin and insulin-like growth factor I (IGF-I) receptors in ovarian cancer tissue. *Gynecol. Oncol.* **53,** 196–201.
6. Furlanetto, R. and Di Carlo, J. N. (1984) Somatomedin-C receptors and growth effects in human breast cells maintained in long-term tissue culture. *Cancer Res.* **44,** 2122–2128.
7. Pollak, M. N., Polychronakos, C., Yousefi, S., and Richard, M. (1988) Characterization of insulin-like growth factor-I (IGF-I) receptors of human breast cancer cells. *Biochem. Biophys. Res. Commun.* **154,** 326–331.
8. Tollefsen, S.E. and Thompson, K. (1988) The structural basis for insulin-like growth factor I receptor high affinity binding. *J. Biol. Chem.* **263,** 16,267–16,273.
9. LeBon, T. R., Jacobs, S., Cuatrecasas, P., Kathuria, S., and Fujita-Yamaguchi, Y. (1986) Purification of insulin-like growth factor I receptor human placental membranes. *J. Biol. Chem.* **261,** 7685–7689.
10. Pezzino, V., Milazzo, G., Frittitta, L., Vigneri, R., Ezaki, O., Kasahara, M., et al. (1991) Radioimmunoassay for human insulin-like growth factor-I receptor: applicability to breast carcinoma specimens and cells lines. *Metabolism* **40,** 861–865.
11. Milazzo, G., Giorgino, F., Damante, G., Sung, C., Stampfer, M. R., Vigneri, R., et al. (1992) Insulin receptor expression and function in human breast cancer cell lines. *Cancer Res.* **52,** 3924–3930.
12. Bradford, M. M. (1978) A rapid and sensitive method for the quantitation of microgram quantities of protein utilizing the principle of protein-dye binding. *Anal Biochem.* **72,** 248–254.
13. Goldfine, I. D. (1987) The insulin receptor: molecular biology and transmembrane signalling. *Endocr. Rev.* **8,** 235–255.
14. Peyrat, J. P., Bonneterre, J., Beuscart, R., Djiane, J., and Demaille, A. (1988) Insulin-like growth factor receptors in human breast cancer and their relation to estradiol and progesterone receptors. *Cancer Res.* **48,** 6429–6433.
15. Papa, V., Gliozzo, B. M., Clark, G. M., McGuire, W. L., Moore, D., Fujita-Yamaguchi, Y., et al. (1993) Insulin-like growth factor-I receptors are overexpressed and predict a low risk in human breast cancer. *Cancer Res.* **53,** 3736–3740.

# 53

# Radioreceptor Measurement of ER/PR

## Giovanni Scambia, Gabriella Ferrandina, G. D'Agostino, A. De Dilectis, and Salvatore Mancuso

## 1. Introduction

Evidence that steroid hormones can play an important role in gynecological malignancies has been provided since 1896, when Sir George Beatson reported remissions in two patients with breast cancer after bilateral oophorectomy. All steroid hormones act on their target cells by binding to cellular receptors. Thus, the presence of the appropriate receptor in a tissue can be taken as a good indication that that tissue is hormone-sensitive. Following these observations, many studies in this century have demonstrated that the knowledge of the steroid-receptor status of gynecological tumors, especially breast and endometrial cancer, can offer important information about the differentiation, response to endocrine therapy, and prognosis of the disease.

In this chapter, the most common radioreceptor methods used for the steroid-hormone receptor determination in neoplastic tissues are reviewed. In order to introduce the principles of the radioreceptor binding measurement, the theory of ligand–receptor interaction is briefly summarized here.

### 1.1. Equations Describing Ligand–Receptor Interaction

Interaction of the ligand with its receptor is described by the equation:

$$(H) + (R) \overset{K1 \rightarrow}{\underset{\leftarrow K2}{}} (HR)$$

where $K1$ and $K2$ express the association and dissociation speed constants of the $HR$ complex. In conditions of equilibrium, the speed of association reaction $K1 (H) (R)$ is equal to the speed of dissociation reaction $K2 (HR)$:

$$K1 (H) (R) = K2 (HR), \text{ that is}$$

$$K1/K2 = (HR) / (H) (R)$$

The ratio $K1/K2$ represents the dissociation constant $(Kd) = (H) (R) / (HR)$.

By using the symbols $B$ for $HR$, $RT$ to express the total number of sites, and $F$, $H$ (free-ligand concentration), we obtain, by simple mathematic passages, the classic formulation

From: *Methods in Molecular Medicine, Vol. 39: Ovarian Cancer: Methods and Protocols*
Edited by: J. M. S. Bartlett © Humana Press, Inc., Totowa, NJ

Fig. 1. Free-ligand concentration and bound-ligand concentration where the total number of sites (RT) is represented by the plateau, which is the saturation curve, and Kd corresponds to ligand concentration.

$$B = RT\,(F)\,/\,Kd + F$$

derived from the Michaelis-Menten equation.

In **Fig. 1**, the total number of sites (*RT*) is represented by the plateau of the hyperbole that constitutes the saturation curve, whereas *Kd* corresponds to the ligand concentration at which 50% of receptors is bound to the ligand.

In fact, from

$$(Kd) = (H)\,(R)\,/\,(HR)$$

derives that, if half the receptors present in the system is bound to the hormone, the number of free receptors *(R)* will be equal to *(HR)*, that is the number of complexes formed. Then the previous equation becomes $Kd = (H)$, where the dissociation constant at equilibrium represents the concentration of free hormone at which there is 50% of saturation of binding sites.

Therefore, from the saturation curve it is possible to know the number and affinity of receptors. A better valuation of these parameters can be made by the conversion of the saturation curve data according to the Scatchard *(1)* analysis (**Fig. 2**). It consists of expressing the ratio of bound/free ligand in function of the slope of bound ligand. It is like a linearization of the saturation curve where the *Kd* may be determined from the slope of the plot according to the equation:

$$\text{Slope} = 1/Kd \text{ where } Kd = 1/Ka = K\text{-}1/K1.$$

The binding capacity is (*n o Rt*) estimated from the intercept on the abscissa. By definition, the higher the affinity of the binding site, the lower the dissociation constant, which is a measure of the tendency of the steroid-receptor complex to dissociate. It is worth mentioning that some factors could produce artefacts in the saturation curve:

1. When the concentration of labeled ligand in the system is too high, the bound ligand could be overestimated.

Fig. 2. The Scatchard analysis: a linear depiction of the saturation curve.

2. In the absence of saturation conditions, bound ligands could be underestimated and free ligands overestimated, with possible alterations of Scatchard plot.
3. Presence of high levels of endogenous ligands, can alter the equilibrium of receptor-ligand interactions in a experimental system.
4. Interactions of receptor–ligand are not well described by the equation at the equilibrium.

$$(H) + (R) \; K1 \leftrightarrow K2 \; (HR)$$

5. Instability of either ligand or receptor could also alter the saturation curve.

## 2. Materials

1. TENMG Buffer: consisting of 25 m$M$ Tris-Cl, 1.5 m$M$ EDTA, 5 m$M$ NaN$_3$, 0.1% Monothioglycerol, 20% glycerol (TENMG) pH 7.4.
2. 2,4,6,7-[$^3$H]estradiol-17β at 250 n$M$, or [$^3$H]Organon 2058 at 250 μ$M$ in ethanol.
3. 2,4,6,7-estradiol-17β at 75 μ$M$, or [$^3$H]Organon 2058 at 75 μ$M$ in ethanol as unlabeled competitor at 300 fold higher concentrations. Ethanol concentration should never exceed 1% in each tube.
4. DCC suspension: prepared monthly and stored at 4°C is composed of: Charcoal Norit A, 500 mg, Dextran T 70, 50 mg, phosphate-buffer solution, 100 mL. Shake overnight at 4°C. to dissolve dextran, store at 4°C.

## 3. Methods
### 3.1. Dextran-Coated Charcoal Method

This method is based on the ability of charcoal to adsorb free steroids and of Dextran to protect the steroid-receptor complex *(2)*. The DCC suspension must remove the whole free steroid, so that background radioactivity has to be, after separation, not *higher than* 1% of total cpm in the control samples. The incubation is stopped by ice-cold DCC, which is then removed by a 20 min centrifugation at 7000*g* and the radioactivity of the supernatant determined by liquid scintillation counting (*see* **Note 1**).

### 3.2. Assay Protocol

The details of the protocol that have been set up in our laboratories are the following *(3,4)*:

1. Homogenize tissue sample in ice-cold TENMG buffer (1:5 weight/volume) by using 3–4 bursts an Ultra-Turrax homogenizer at intervals of 15 s (*see* **Note 2**).
2. Centrifuge at 7000*g* for 20'– at 4°C.
3. Take the supernatant and ultracentrifuge it at 105,000*g* for 75'– at 4°C.
4. Incubate 100-µL aliquots of the resulting cytosol fraction [1–2 mg protein/mL, determined according to the Bradford's method *(5)*] overnight at 4°C in presence of labeled steroids: 40 µL 2,4,6,7-[$^3$H]estradiol-17β at increasing concentrations from 0.5 to 5 n*M*, or 40 µL [$^3$H]Organon 2058 at increasing concentrations from 0.5 to 40 n*M*, to measure, respectively, ER and PR, with or without 50 µL of the specific unlabeled competitor at 300-fold-higher concentrations. Ethanol concentration should never exceed 1% in each tube (*see* **Note 3**).
5. Stop reaction in the tubes by adding 400 µL of ice-cold DCC suspension and mix.
6. Centrifuge at 7000*g* for 20' at 4°C.
7. Gently transfer with Gilson dispensors 400 µL of the supernatant into minivials.
8. Add 4 mL scintillation liquid.
9. Determine radioactivity by β-counter.
10. Convert the measured radioactivity (cpm deriving from the arithmetical difference between total bound steroid and nonspecific bound) to concentration of steroid bound and express it in femtomoles/mg protein.

## 4. Notes

1. Any satisfactory assay must:
   - measure only cellular receptor, not steroid, metabolizing enzymes, plasma-binding proteins, or other lower affinity binding proteins;
   - reflect biological specificity of the ligand;
   - be quantitatively reproducible.

   The utilization of biochemical methods offers the advantage of a quantitative evaluation and allows a characterization of the binding parameters (dissociation constant, *Kd*) of the receptor. On the other hand, drawbacks of this methods are the interference of normal, stromal, and inflammatory components of the tissue; the specimen size, that is, often a limiting condition; and finally, the biochemical method allows only the determination of the free receptor, i.e., the receptor that is not occupied by the endogenous ligand.
2. Tissue procurement, specimen handling, and preparation. Tissue specimens should be excised expeditiously and without trauma from the surgical technique. The specimens, well trimmed of normal and necrotic tissue, must be transported as soon as possible to the laboratory in the frozen state. If the assay cannot be performed on fresh tissue, it is preferable to freeze them in liquid nitrogen immediately after surgery and then store at –80°C until assay which, however, should be carried out within few weeks.

   Specimens must be maintained on ice to retard steroid hormone receptor degradation. Recent studies, in fact, indicate the half-lives of oestrogen and progestin receptors are highly variable in intact tumor biopsy specimens, ranging from 30 min to 6 h at room temperature. If the laboratory is far away from the surgery room, the snap cap vials used for grid storage by electron microscopists can be utilized for freezing in liquid nitrogen or dry ice.

   The biopsy sent for receptor analyses must be representative of the tissue procured, and the specimen must be of sufficient volume (at least 200 mg) for receptor determination.

Intratumoral regional differences in steroid receptor status have been observed, suggesting a clonal heterogeneity relative to receptor status, that is, why the submission of a representative sample is preferable. In general, the quantity of receptors in each sample can vary from undetectable to several hundred femtomoles/mg cytosol protein, independently from the proportion of tumor epithelium, but, in order to check that the specimens really contain tumor tissue, fixation and staining of a small sample of the biopsy is necessary.

The time interval between cytosol preparation and introduction of ligand should be as short as possible, because it has been reported that the rapid, temperature-dependent degradation of receptors can be avoided by the association of ligand *(6)*.

3. Choice of labeled ligand, competitor, and concentration range. Although various synthetic ligands have been utilized, labeled oestradiol is still the ligand of choice for ER determination. It is preferable to use 2,4,6,7-[$^3$H]oestradiol-17β because it has a longer half-life than iodine-labeled oestradiol, and a higher specific activity with respect to 6,7-[$^3$H]oestradiol-17β. The competitor used to eliminate nonspecific binding is diethylstilbestrol (DES), which is chosen because of its very poor affinity for plasma transport proteins and so no competitive binding can be ascribed to such contaminants. The concentration range selected should span the known *Kd* of ER. For human ovarian tissue, an appropriate range is $2$–$30 \times 10^{-10} M$. As far as the PR assay is concerned, the radiolabeled progesterone was used in early assays, but binding to glucocorticoid receptor had to be eliminated with excess cortisol. Among the synthetic analogs readily available, [$^3$H]Organon 2058 has proved, in our experience, to be the best ligand. Moreover, it is available in the unlabeled form and can be used as competitor. The appropriate concentration range for human tissue is $5$–$50 \times 10^{-10} M$ [$^3$H]ORG 2058.

## References

1. Scatchard, G. (1949) The attraction of protein for small molecules and ions. *Ann. N.Y. Acad. Sci.* **51,** 660–672.
2. EORTC (1980) Breast Cancer Cooperative Group Revision of the standards for the assessment of hormone receptors in human breast cancer. *Eur. J. Cancer* **16,** 1513–1515.
3. Scambia, G., Benedetti-Panici, P., Baiocchi, G., Battaglia, F., Ferrandina, G., Greggi, S., and Mancuso, S. (1990) Steroid hormone receptors in carcinoma of the cervix: lack of response to an antiestrogen. *Gynecol. Oncol.* **37,** 323–326.
4. Scambia, G., Benedetti-Panici, P., Ferrandina, G., Distefano, M., Salerno, G., Romanini, M. E., et al. (1995) Epidermal growth factor, oestrogen and progesterone receptor expression in primary ovarian cancer: correlation with clinical outcome and response to chemotherapy. *Br. J. Cancer* **72,** 361–366.
5. Bradford, M. M. (1976) A rapid and sensitive method for the quantitation of microgram quantities of proteins utilizing the principle of protein-dye binding. *Anal. Biochem.* **72,** 248–254.
6. Wittliff, J. L., Pasic, R., and Bland, K. I. (1991) Steroid and peptide hormone receptors identified in breast tissue, in *The Breast* (Bland and Copeland, eds.), pp. 900–936.

# 54

## nm23 Protein Expression by Western Blotting in Patients with Epithelial Ovarian Carcinoma

**Giovanni Scambia, Maria Marone, Gabriella Ferrandina, Gabriella Macchia, and Salvatore Mancuso**

## 1. Introduction

Western blotting is utilized to detect and quantify the amount of a specific protein in a complex mixture of proteins and at the same time to determine its molecular weight. In particular, by Western blotting it is also possible to detect and discriminate the two isoforms of nm23, H1, and H2 (1, 2). nm23-H1 is about 18.5 kD (3) and nm23-H2 is 17 kD (4), hence, they migrate as two distinct bands on a standard SDS polyacrylamide gel. Because the two isoforms are very highly conserved (4), they retain most of the same epitopes; thus any polyclonal antibody raised against one of the two isoforms or a monoclonal antibody against a conserved epitope will recognize both nm23-H1 and -H2 at the same time. Analysis by immunohistochemistry, on the other hand would require two distinct reactions with two specific antibodies for H1 and H2 raised against the least conserved epitopes to avoid crossreaction.

Western blotting (5,6) requires five main steps:

1. preparation of a total protein lysate from the tissue sample;
2. separation of the proteins by SDS polyacrylamide gel electrophoresis according to their molecular weight;
3. transfer of the separated proteins from the gel to a suitable membrane;
4. binding of the antibody to the specific proteins; and
5. visualization of the bound antibody.

The total protein lysate is prepared by homogenizing the tissue sample in a buffer containing detergents which dissociate the membranes and solubilize the proteins. The total protein content is then measured by binding to a dye (Coomassie blue) and comparing the intensity of binding to that of a known standard. Electrophoresis of a known amount of proteins is carried out in SDS-polyacrylamide gels in a discontinuous buffer system (7). The strongly anionic detergent SDS is used in combination with a reducing agent (β-mercaptoethanol) and heat to dissociate the proteins before they are loaded on the gel (7). The denatured proteins bind SDS and become negatively charged to an extent that is dependent on their size, hence, SDS-bound proteins migrate through polyacrylamide gels according to their molecular weight. The effective range of separation

From: *Methods in Molecular Medicine, Vol. 39: Ovarian Cancer: Methods and Protocols*
Edited by: J. M. S. Bartlett © Humana Press, Inc., Totowa, NJ

of SDS-polyacrylamide gels depends mostly on the concentration of polyacrylamide used *(8)*. nm23-H1 and -H2 are most effectively separated on a 12 % gel.

After separation by SDS-PAGE, the proteins are electrophoretically transferred and bound to a solid support, a microporous filter made of polyvinylidene fluoride (PVDF). The filter is subsequently exposed to an antibody specific for the target protein. Prior to the addition of the antibody, the membrane is coated with a blocking agent, such as nonfat dry milk, so that antibodies do not bind nonspecifically to the membrane and to other proteins. The filter is then incubated with a secondary antibody which recognizes the Fc portion of the first antibody. The secondary antibody is conjugated with an enzyme, for example alkaline phosphatase *(9)*, which will develop a colored reaction corresponding to the protein of interest when the filter is exposed to the specific substrates.

## 2. Materials

### 2.1. Preparation of a Total Protein Lysate from The Tissue Sample

1. Lysis buffer: 20 m$M$ Tris-HCl pH 7.4, 0.1$M$ NaCl, 5 m$M$ MgCl$_2$, 1% Nonidet P-40 (can be substituted with Sigma IGEPAL CA 630), 0.5 % sodium deoxycholate, 2 U/mL aprotinin (kallikrein inhibitor U) and sterile double-distilled H$_2$O (ddH$_2$O) to the final volume. N.B. Sodium Deoxycholate tends to precipitate out. Dissolve it into Tris-HCl, by stirring and lightly heating. When it has dissolved, slowly add NaCl and MgCl$_2$ while stirring. You can make a stock of lysis buffer without aprotinin and store it for months at 4°C. Aprotinin can be diluted into water to 200 U/μL and stored in aliquots at –20°C. When diluted in lysis buffer, aprotinin is stable for 1 wk at 4°C.

### 2.2. Separation of the Proteins by SDS Polyacrylamide Gel Electrophoresis

1. 30% Acrylamide/bisacrylamide 29:1. Acrylamide: bisacrylamide stock solution can be stored at 4°C in the dark. Powder can be used to make a stock that can be stored for a few months. Because acrylamide (in form of powder and unpolymerized solution) is neurotoxic, both the powder and solution should be handled carefully and with gloves. We prefer to buy a 30% ready stock solution, which is stable for 12 mo at 4°C.
2. Resolving gel: 12% (from stock - acrylamide/bisacrylamide 29:1), 0.26% 1$M$ Tris-HCl (pH 8.8) 0.1% SDS, ddH$_2$O to the final volume of the gel. Ammonium persulfate 0.1%, TEMED (6.6$M$) 2.64 m$M$.
3. Stacking gel: 4.95% (from stock - acrylamide/bisacrylamide 29:1), 0.125% 1$M$ Tris-HCl pH 6.8, 0.1% SDS, ddH$_2$O to the final volume of the gel. Ammonium persulfate 0.1%, TEMED (6.6 M) 2.64 m$M$. To facilitate visualization of the gel wells, add bromophenol blue to a final concentration of 1 mg/mL in the stacking gel.
4. Ammonium Persulfate should be stored as a 10% solution in ddH$_2$O at 4°C for a few months. TEMED (N,N,N′,N′-Tetramethylethylendiamine) should be stored at 4°C.
5. Tris-glycine electrophoresis buffer (running buffer): 25 m$M$ Tris, 250 m$M$ glycine, 0.1% (w/v) SDS, pH 8.3. It can be made as a 5X stock and stored indefinitely at room temperature. 6. 5X SDS sample buffer: 60 m$M$ Tris-HCl pH 6.8, 25% glycerol, 2% SDS, 0.715$M$ β-mercaptoethanol, 0.1 % bromophenol blue. Store at –20°C.

### 2.3. Transfer

1. 10X Transfer Buffer: 390 m$M$ glycine, 480 m$M$ Tris base. To prepare 1X transfer buffer, dilute 1 part of 10X stock with seven of ddH$_2$O then add two of methanol to make it 20%.

Do not add methanol directly to the 10X stock as the glycine would precipitate out. Transfer buffer (1X) will be: 39 m$M$ glycine, 48 m$M$ Tris base, 20% methanol, pH 8.3.
2  Ponceau-S-red: 0.2 % Ponceau-S in 3 % trichloroacetic acid.

### 2.4. Binding of the Antibody to the Specific Proteins

1. 10X TBS: 1$M$ Tris base, 1.5$M$ NaCl, adjust the pH to 7.4 with concentrated HCl.
2. 1X TBST: Dilute TBS 1 : 10 in water and add 0.5 mL Tween-20 per liter to make 1X TBST, which will be: 0.1 M Tris, 0.15 M NaCl, 0.05 % Tween-20. Inclusion of Tween-20 in the 10x stock may cause formation of a precipitate. Formation of a light foggy precipitate in the 1X solution will not affect the experiments. If the precipitate becomes heavier and/or cloudy, prepare a fresh dilution.

### 2.5. Other Reagents

1. Bio-Rad (Richmond, CA) protein assay reagent.
2. PVDF transfer membrane, 0.45-µ$M$ pore size.
3. Carnation™ nonfat dry milk (other brands do not work as well and should be tested). Dissolve in 1X TBST just before use; then store at 4°C for 1 wk.
4. Antihuman NDP kinase/nm23 rabbit polyclonal antibody (Neomarkers). Store at 4°C.
5. Alkaline phosphatase conjugated goat antirabbit IgG (Bio-Rad). Store at 4°C.
6. BCIP/NBT phosphatase substrate system (Kirkegaard & Perry). The kit consists of the following: 2.5 g/L BCIP (5-bromo-4-chloro-3-indolil-phosphate); 5.0 g/L NBT (Nitroblue tetrazolium); Tris buffer solution (0.1$M$ Tris-HCl pH 9.0); it is stable for several months at 4°C. Stocks can be made from powder or tablets (Sigma,) but sensitivity is more variable from batch to batch.

## 3. Methods

### 3.1. Preparation of a Total Protein Lysate

### 3.1.1. Lysis

1. Immediately after surgical resection, trim out necrotic, haemorragic, or fat tissue portions out. Then place the biopsy in a cryovial, freeze it in liquid nitrogen and stored at –80 °C.
2. Add four to five volumes of cold lysis buffer (generally 300–800 µL for our usual bioptic samples) to the frozen sample and homogenized with 4–5 strokes of an Ultra-Turrax or Polytron homogenizer. The solution should be kept ice cold (*see* **Note 1**).
3. Spin at 9000$g$ for 10 min at 4°C. When dealing with small tissue samples, transfer them to microfuge tubes and spin in a microfuge for 5 min at 4°C. Store the supernatant at –20°C.

In our experiments, we use the A2780 ovarian cancer cell line as a positive control. A pellet containing 5–10 × 10$^6$ cells is resuspended in 500 µL buffer, kept for 20 min on ice, spun for 3–5 min at 4°C in the microfuge. The supernatant is stored at –20°C.

### 3.1.2 Determination of Protein Concentration by the Bio-Rad Protein Assay (Microassay Procedure)

This method is based essentially on the procedure described by Bradford *(10)*. Any similar procedure can be used.

A standard curve has to be prepared each time the assay is performed.

1. Prepare serial dilutions of BSA from 25 to about 1 µg/mL (for example 25, 12.5, 6.25, 3.125, 1.56 µg/ml) in H$_2$O. Place 0.8 mL of each dilution in microfuge tubes.

2. Place the appropriately diluted samples in microfuge tubes. For our ovarian cancer samples the working dilution is in the range of 1:200–800. Commonly a 1:500 dilution works well. Place 0.8 mL diluted sample buffer in "blank" tube.

3. Add 0.2 mL Dye Reagent Concentrate to the samples to be tested and to the BSA dilitions.

4. Mix well to avoid excess foaming and, after 5 min to 1 h, measure $OD_{595}$ (absorbance set at 595 nm) vs blank in disposable 1.5-mL cuvets. Plot $OD_{595}$ vs concentration of standards on graph paper and read unknown concentration of samples from the curve.

5. Multiply the figures obtained by the dilution factor (for example, 500) to obtain the concentration in µg per mL (*see* **Note 2**).

## *3.2. SDS-PAGE*

### *3.2.1. Pouring SDS Polyacrylamide Gels*

1. Assemble the glass plates according to the manufacturer's instructions. We generally use 1-mm thick minigels (8 by 7–8 cm) which give good resolution, an efficient separation between the two nm23 bands and run much faster than large size gels.

2. For a minigel, prepare 5 ml of 12% acrylamide mix for the resolving gel. Mix the components in the order listed in **Subheading 2**. Polymerization will begin as soon as the TEMED is added. Pour the acrylamide solution into the gap between the glass plates. Leave sufficient space for the stacking gel (the length of the teeth of the comb plus 1–1.5 cm). Overlay the acrylamide solution with 70% ethanol by dropping the ethanol with a Pasteur pipet (the overlay prevents oxygen from diffusing into the gel and inhibiting polymerization and allows the formation of a straight line between the two gels—*see* **Notes 3** and **4**).

3. After polymerization is complete (10–30 min), pour off the overlay. You can check if polymerization is complete by gently tilting the gel: The gel will not move, moreover, the line between the two phases (gel and ethanol) becomes sharper after polymerization.

4. Prepare the stacking gel. solution and pour it onto the surface of the polymerized resolving gel. Insert a clean Teflon comb into the stacking gel solution, being careful to avoid trapping air bubbles at the bottom of the teeth. If necessary add more stacking gel solution to fill the spaces completely. Keep the gel in a vertical position at room temperature till it has polymerized.

5. After polymerization is complete (about 30 min), remove the Teflon comb carefully. Mount the gel in the electrophoresis apparatus. Add 1X running buffer to the top and bottom reservoirs. With some apparatus it is necessary to seal the chambers with agarose or with grease (the latter is messier). Gels can be stored at 4°C for a few days. In this case keep the comb in the gel, cover the gel with a few layers of Kimwipes soaked in water and the whole system with Saran Wrap™.

### *3.2.2. Preparing the Samples and Loading the Gel*

1. Thaw the samples, including the control on ice. Take an aliquot containing 40 µg of total proteins. Add 5X SDS sample buffer to make it 1X final. Add 1X SDS sample buffer to take all the samples to the same volume. Up to 40 µL can be easily loaded in standard size wells (10-well comb).

2. Boil for 10 min, spin briefly. Prepare the control sample and the molecular weight standards in the same way. If the samples have been previously diluted in SDS sample buffer, boiled, and stored at –20°C, heat them briefly.

3. Load the samples into the bottom of the wells. Long tips (for sequencing gels) are very convenient. Attach the apparatus to a power supply and apply a constant current of 20–25 mA per gel (2 gels can run at 40–50 mA) until the migration front (bromophenol

blue) reaches the bottom of the gel (1.5–2 h). Some sources claim that constant voltage is required. If you opt for constant voltage (100 V), do not double voltage when running two gels (*see* **Notes 5–13**).

4. Turn off the power supply. Remove the glass plates from the electrophoresis apparatus and by gently twisting one of the spacers, pry the plates apart. Keep the gel on one of the plates.

## 3.3. Transfer

### 3.3.1. Electroblotting

1. Prepare 1X transfer buffer with methanol and cool to 4°C.
2. Equilibrate the gel in transfer buffer for 5–15 min (30 min for thick gels). This reduces bubble formation between gel and filter during the transfer. Keep the gel on the glass plate.
3. Cut the transfer membrane to the dimensions of the gel. If using PVDF, which is hydrophobic, soak it in 100% methanol for a few seconds, then into transfer buffer for 10–15 min. Never let it dry at any time during the procedure. If this happens, soak it in methanol again before transferring it to any aqueous solution. If using nitrocellulose, wet in transfer buffer directly.
4. Cut two pieces of 3MM paper per gel to the size of the membrane and soak them in transfer buffer. Soak the fiber pads in transfer buffer.
5. Assemble the unit as follows: Place a prewetted fiber pad on the gray panel of the holder. Place the transfer membrane on top of the gel, then place a piece of saturated 3MM paper on top of the transfer membrane. Turn the gel over, remove the glass plate and place a piece of wet 3MM paper on top of the gel. Roll a pipet over the sandwich to remove bubbles. Place the sandwich on top of the pad and cover it with the other pad. Close and insert into the transfer unit. Make sure that the filter is facing the anode and the gel the cathode. The sandwich should be assembled as follows:

- (cathode = black)
black side of the holder
fiber pad
3MM paper
gel
transfer membrane
MM paper
fiber pad
clear side of the holder
+ (anode = red)

6. Place in the tank filled with transfer buffer. Use enough buffer to cover the gel. Place a stir bar in the unit. Set up the cooling system or run in the cold room. This is optional for low-power transfers (70 mA), otherwise, it is essential. Place the unit on top of a stirrer and turn it on. Stirring will help to maintain uniform conductivity and temperature during transfer (*see* **Note 14**).
7. Transfer overnight at 70 mA. Alternatively, transfer can be done at 400 mA for 1 h 30 min. It works well, especially with minigels, but there is an increased chance of getting small bubbles between the gel and the filter, which can affect transfer. The total amperage dispensed (mA × h) should be at least 600. Thicker gels will require a longer time (mA × h = 800—*see* **Notes 15–18**).
8. Take off the sandwich. Do not let the membrane dry.

### 3.3.2. Staining in Ponceau-S-Red

The filter is stained with Ponceau-S-red to provide visual evidence that electrophoretic transfer of proteins has taken place. Staining with Ponceau is completely compatible with all further steps of immunological probing because the staining washes away during processing of the blot (*see* **Note 19**).

1. Transfer the PVDF filter to a tray containing a working solution of Ponceau-S-Red. Incubate the filter for 2 min at room temperature with gentle agitation.
2. Wash the PVDF filter in several changes of deionized water. If necessary, mark the positions of the proteins used as molecular-weight standards with pencil or waterproof ink. If required, this is the time to trim the filter to a thin strip containing the protein of interest and remove the rest, so as to minimize the volume of the solutions required for the following steps.

## 3.4. Binding of the Antibody to the Specific Proteins

For the following incubations, use as small a glass container as possible to reduce volumes to a minimum. Some kinds of plastic may bind antibodies and should not be used.

### 3.4.1. Blocking

1. Incubate in 6% (up to 10%) Carnation nonfat dry milk in 1X TBST for 30 min—2–3 h (or overnight) while shaking. Protocols vary: some say that you should incubate at 37°C, some at room temperature, some at 4°C. Thirty min at room temperature are sufficient to obtain efficient blocking. If the incubation has to be extended to more than 4 h, it is advisable to do it at 4°C. 5–10 mL of solution are sufficient to cover a filter the size of a minigel. 2 mL will be sufficient for a thin strip.
2. Wash in 1X TBST for 10 min to remove excess milk.

### 3.4.2. Incubation With the Primary Antibody

1. Use 2–4 mL of 3% (maximum 5%) milk in 1X TBST. The amount of antibody depends on the antibody itself. Usually a dilution of 1:100–1:500 works well for most monoclonal and polyclonal antibodies. For nm23, we currently use a 1:200 dilution.
2. Incubate overnight to 20 h at 4°C with gentle shaking. Incubation for 4–5 h at room temperature will work equally well. Shorter incubation times may yield a fainter signal.
3. Wash in 1X TBST for 10 min, then twice for 5 min.

### 3.4.3. Incubation With the Secondary Antibody

1. Use the appropriate secondary antibody, which this specific case will be an alkaline phosphatase conjugated goat antirabbit antibody diluted 1:2000. A dilution of 1:1000–1:5000 in 3% (maximum 5%) milk in 1X TBST. Make up 2–2.5 mL solution for a small blot.
2. Incubate for 30 min to 3 h (usually 1–2 h) at room temperature. Longer incubation time may increase nonspecific binding. Wash in 1X TBST.

## 3.5. Detection of Proteins by Alkaline Phosphatase

We use the BCIP/NBT phosphatase substrate system, which is very easy to use and whose color is stable on the filter for a long time.

1. Wash three times in 1X TBST over 10–15 min at room temperature.
2. Just before use, prepare the substrate as follows:

Fig. 1. Representative example of Western blotting for nm23-H1 and H2. Lanes 1 to 5 are ovarian cancer samples. Lane 6 is the A2780 ovarian cancer cell line used as a positive control. 40 µg of total proteins were loaded in each lane. Size of molecular-weight markers is indicated.

Mix 10 parts of Tris buffer solution with 1 part of BCIP concentrate and 1 of NBT concentrate. Use at room temperature. For a minigel, mix 5 mL Tris, 0.5 mL BCIP, 0.5 mL NBT. Reduce the volumes for smaller blots.

3. Pour over the blot, after removing the TBST, and keep on the shaker till the signal develops. It may take 30 s to 30 min. The reaction should be stopped before background color becomes too intense or before the liquid becomes a darken purple and forms a black precipitate. If this happens before the signal is satisfactory, remove the used solution and prepare a fresh one.
4. Stop the reaction by rinsing the blot with water to remove excess substrate. Rinse several times. Dry the membrane and keep. If using PVDF filters, most background disappears after drying (*see* **Notes 19–24**).

A typical Western blot for nm23-H1 and H2 in a series of ovarian cancer patients is shown in **Fig. 1**.

## 4. Notes

1. During sample preparation, the sample buffer turns yellow. The SDS sample buffer has become too acidic and the protein sample may migrate anomalously; add 0.1 *N* NaOH until the solution turns blue.
2. Impossible to quantify the amount of proteins in a sample. The amount of proteins loaded does not correspond to the intensity of Ponceau-S staining. Various chemicals can interfere with the adsorbance reading, because of chemical/proteins or chemical/dye interactions. A standard tissue sample in lysis buffer can be read at a dilution as low as 1:50 without interference. If particles can be seen in the sample, tissue debris could still be present. Centrifuge for 5 min, transfer the supernatant to a new microfuge tube and repeat the reading.
3. The gel does not polymerize. Make sure you have included both APS and TEMED in the mix. Old APS, or APS kept at room temperature for too long (several hours or more), may become ineffective. In this case, prepare a fresh APS stock, a new gel mix and pour the gel again.
4. The gel polymerizes too fast. Polymerization is accelerated by high temperature, which usually occurs in the summer in poorly air-conditioned labs. If the amount of APS and TEMED are correct, cool the mix on ice before adding APS and TEMED and pouring.

5. Edge effect, i.e., distortion at the edges of the lanes. This can be caused by uneven electrical flow. Adding 1X sample buffer to unused wells may help.

6. Tracking dye is diffuse. Either the buffer is not made correctly, or acrylamide solution was improperly stored. Prepare fresh buffers and acrylamide: bisacrylamide stock. Acrylamide and bisacrylamide slowly convert to acrylic acid and bisacrylic acid.

7. The protein bands are diffuse. Migration is too slow or gel pore size is too large. Increase the operating current by 25 to 50% or use a higher percentage of acrylamide. "Smiling" or reduced mobility of samples at the edge of the gel may happen if the center of the gel is hotter than the sides. Decreasing the power setting may help. If using a chamber as the Bio-Rad mini Protean, it is also possible to fill up the lower buffer reservoir to distribute heat more evenly over the surface of the gel.

8. Protein bands are vertically streaked. This may be because of a variety of reasons, such as overloading, high current, high protein concentration, DNA in the sample. Decrease the amount of proteins loaded on the gel or reduce the operating current by 50%. Another cause can be precipitation of proteins, which can sometimes be overcome by centrifuging the sample before loading. Streaking may also result from precipitation of very high protein concentrations in the stacking gel. The aggregated proteins dissolve during the course of electrophoresis. If the samples have been properly heated up and centrifuged, dilution may help. High DNA content in the sample is also said to cause streaking. This can be avoided by sonicating the sample. This can be a problem mostly for lysates which were not processed with a homogenizer.

9. Protein bands spread laterally from the gel lanes. The sample is absorbed on the sides of the well. The time between applying the sample and running the gel should be reduced to decrease the diffusion out of the wells. Alternatively, percentage of acrylamide in the stacking gel can be increased up to 5%.

10. Uneven protein bands. Stacking gel may not have been adequately polymerized; the electrical current flow may be uneven; wells may be overloaded; salt content in the sample may be too high. Wait a longer time before removing the gel comb. Make sure that electrophoresis buffer in both upper and lower chambers is making good contact with the gel. Reduce the amount of sample loaded per well or dilute it.

11. Bands are skewed. This can be because of an uneven interface between stacking and resolving gel. Do not move the gel until the resolving gel has completely polymerized or pay extra care in layering the ethanol over the gel.

12. The run takes too long. The buffer may be too concentrated or operating current too low. Prepare a new stock of buffer or increase current (it should never be higher than 28–30 mA per gel).

13. The run is too short. The buffer may be too diluted or operating current too high. Prepare a new stock of buffer or decrease current (18–20 mA per gel). A very low current setting (below 12–15 mA) will cause diffusion of bands.

14. Transfer. Note that transfer is not the same on both sides of the membrane. Be sure to look at the right side of the membrane. PVDF can be seen through only when wet. Nitrocellulose is more fragile, has a lower binding capacity, gives a fainter signal than PVDF, and background remains after drying the membrane. For all these reasons, PVDF is our choice. For proteins expressed at high levels and with high affinity antibodies, nitrocellulose can be used as well. It can be successfully used for nm23.

15. No transfer, clear filter after Ponceau-S staining. No current flow, gel and filter placed in the wrong orientation. Check the power supply and blotting apparatus. Also, check the orientation of the gel and filter relative to the anode and cathode.

16. Protein bands are diffuse. Gel and filter were not in tight contact. Check the plastic holders and pads.

17. Clear white bubbles on the filter after blotting and staining. Bubbles block the current flow in specific spots. Take extra care to remove all bubbles which can be trapped between the gel and the filter.

18. Unusually high current reading. It is most likely because of improper preparation of the transfer buffer and will create problems owing to excess heat generation during the transfer period. Prepare a new transfer buffer. During transfer electrolytes elute from the gel, increasing buffer conductivity and decreasing the resistance. It may help to incubate the gel in transfer buffer for 15–30 min prior to transfer to equilibrate the gel. This is useful mostly for fast transfers. Alternatively, reduce power setting and increase time accordingly.

19. Appearance of low molecular weight bands as seen by Ponceau-S staining. Protein degradation. One of the main problems in this step is the handling of the samples before they are actually frozen. If the time which spans between the actual surgery, i.e., when the biopsy is taken, and stocking is too long, degradation of the most sensitive proteins may occur. Degradation can be detected at two steps in the procedure: on the Ponceau-stained membranes by an unusual increase in low molecular-weight bands at the bottom of the gel and a corresponding decrease in the intensity of staining of high molecular-weight proteins or, after detection, by the appearance of extra bands below the specific ones on the filter. In both cases, quantification of the specific bands is difficult and unprecise and it may not be possible to discriminated the specific low molecular-weight degradation products from nonspecific background. Great care should then be taken at the time of bioptic resection. Ideally, a small tank containing liquid nitrogen should be taken in the surgery room so that the biopsy can be transferred to a cryotube and frozen immediately. Later, the samples can be recovered from the tank and transferred to the appropriate container for long time storage at –80°C. Repeated freezing and thawing can also cause degradation. If a sample has to be used several times, store it in small aliquots which can be stored at –20°C for years.

20. Diffuse background on the filter. Blocking was insufficient. Increase time of blocking or the amount of milk in TBST (up to 10%).

21. Lanes are streaked. Antibody/antibodies bound nonspecifically. Try reducing the concentration of the primary or secondary antibody and/or the time of incubation to reduce the level of nonspecific binding.

22. Presence of extra bands of various molecular weight. Concentration of the primary or secondary antibody was too high. Washing between incubations was insufficient. Reduce the amount of antibody or the time of incubation. Increase washing time.

23. Absence of signal. First or second antibody is inactive or nonsaturating because of improper storage or excess dilution of the antibodies. A control for first antibody activity may involve spotting the antigen directly on a piece of membrane and performing the immunoassay. The secondary antibody can be tested for binding to a different first antibody produced in the same species. Alternatively, antigen on the membrane is limiting. Include a known amount of control antigen on the gel. Load a higher amount of total proteins. Moreover, NBT and/or BCIP may have become inactive owing to prolonged or improper storage. Use a fresh stock of NBT and BCIP. Note that BCIP may develop a blue color over time, which does not affect product performance.

24. Double bands. Proteins are oxidized. β-mercaptoethanol may have evaporated from the sample buffer or the sample itself. Prepare a fresh stock of SDS sample buffer.

## References

1. Scambia, G., Ferrandina, G., Marone, M., et al. (1996) Nm 23 in ovarian cancer: correlation with clinical outcome and other clinico-pathological and biochemical prognostic parameters. *J. Clin. Oncol.* **14,** 334–342.
2. Marone, M., Scambia, G., Ferrandina, G., et al. (1996) Expression of nm 23 in endometrial and cervical cancer. *Brit. J. Cancer* **74,** 1063–1068.

3. Steeg, P. S., Bevilacqua, G., Kopper, L., et al. (1988) Evidence for a novel gene associated with a low tumor metastatic potential. *Natl. Cancer Inst.* **80,** 200–204.

4. Stahl, J. A., Leone, A., Rosegard, A. M., et al. (1991) Identification of a second human nm 23 gene, nm 23-H2. *Cancer Res.* **51,** 445–449.

5. Towbin, H., Staehelin, T., and Gordon, J. (1979) Electrophoretic transfer of proteins from polyacrylamide gels to nitrocellulose sheets: procedure and some applications. *Proc. Natl. Acad. Sci. USA* **76,** 4350–4534.

6. Burnette, W. N. (1981) "Western blotting": Electrophoretic transfer of proteins from sodium dodecyl sulfate-polyacrylamine gels to unmodified nitrocellulose and radiographic detection with antibody and radioiodinated protein A. *Anal. Biochem.* **112,** 195–203.

7. Laemmli, U. K. (1970) Cleavage of structural proteins during the assembly of the head of bacteriophage T4. *Nature* **227,** 680–685.

8. Sambrook, J., Fritsch, E. F., and Maniatis, T. (1989) *Molecular cloning. A laboratory manual.* Second ed., Cold Spring Harbor Lab., Cold Spring Harbor, NY.

9. Knecht, D. A. and Randall, L. D. (1984) Visualization of antigenic proteins on Western blots. *Anal. Biochem.* **136,** 180–184.

10. Bradford, M. M. (1976) A rapid and sensitive method for the quantitation of microgram quantities of protein utilizing the principle of protein-dye bindinig. *Anal. Biochem.* **72,** 248–254.

## Further Reading

Hames, B. D. and Rickwood, D., eds. (1990) Gel *Electrophoresis of Proteins. A practical approach.* Second ed., Oxford University Press, Oxford, U.K.

Ausubel, F. M., Brent, R., et al. (1994) Current protocols in molecular biology. Mass. General Hospital, Harvard Medical School, Boston, MA.

Bollag, D. M., Rozycki, M. D., and Edelstein, S. J. (1996) *Protein Methods.* Wiley-Liss, New York.

Walker, J. (1996) *The Protein Protocols Handbook.* Humana, Totowa, NJ.

# 55

# Detection and Quantitation of Matrix Metalloproteases by Zymography

## Thomas M. Leber and Rupert P. M. Negus

## 1. Introduction

Matrix metalloproteases (MMPs) are a family of structurally and functionally related endopeptidases. They have in common a zinc ion at the active site and are released as an inactive proform (zymogen). Proteolytic activation enables MMPs to degrade components of the extracellular matrix such as collagens, fibronectin, and laminin [for review *see (1–4)*].

MMP activity is controled at several levels. Gene expression is regulated by cytokines such as tumor necrosis factor $\alpha$ and transforming growth factor $\beta$ [for review *see (2–5)*], activation of MMPs can be triggered in vitro by proteases and other MMPs *(2–4,6)* and finally, their proteolytic activity is counterbalanced by tissue inhibitors of metalloproteases (TIMPs) *(1–4)*.

MMPs play an important role in tissue remodeling during embryogenesis and wound healing *(2,7)*. In addition, these enzymes may contribute to the pathology of chronic diseases such as osteo- and rheumatoid arthritis *(8–10)*, and malignancy *(8,10–12)*. Events like angiogenesis, intra- and extravasation, and migration of tumor or host immune cells have been associated with MMP activity *(12,13)*. However, the exact role of MMPs/TIMPs in the pathology of cancer and other diseases is still being defined and further investigation into their mechanism of action in vivo is required *(14)*.

In this chapter, we present the method of quantitative gelatinolytic zymography for the detection and quantitation of MMPs. The protocol is based on a recently published and validated method that uses an improved single step staining/destaining procedure *(15)*.

## 2. Materials

1. 1.2% gelatin solution: Add 1.2 g gelatin (e.g., porcine skin, 300 bloom, Sigma, St. Louis, MO) to 100 mL deionized water, microwave slowly until fully dissolved, aliquot in samples of 5 mL and store at 4°C. Melt in microwave prior to use (10–15s).
2. Running gels (for 2 slab gels, $140 \times 100 \times 1$ mm): Mix 11 mL 40% acrylamide (29:1, National Diagnostics, Hull, UK), 10 mL running gel buffer (National Diagnostics), 15 mL deionized water and 4 mL 1.2% gelatin (*see* **Note 1**). Add 80 µL TEMED (N,N,N′,N′-tetramethylethylenediamine) and 160 µL of a 10% (w/v) ammonium persulfate (APS) solution prepared in deionized water and pour gels. Overlay gels with 1 mL butanol and

From: *Methods in Molecular Medicine, Vol. 39: Ovarian Cancer: Methods and Protocols*
Edited by: J. M. S. Bartlett © Humana Press, Inc., Totowa, NJ

leave to set for at least 20 min. Once gel has set thoroughly, drain off butanol by inverting the gels.

3. Stacking gels (for 2 gels): Mix 2.5 mL 40% acrylamide (29:1, National Diagnostics), 5 mL stacking gel buffer (National Diagnostics), and 12.5 mL deionized water. Add 40 μL TEMED and 80 μL of a 10% (w/v) APS solution, pour gels, insert combs, and leave gels to set for at least 20 min (*see* **Note 2**).

4. Running buffer (10X): Mix 30.28 g Tris base, 144.12 g glycine, and add water to 1 L (*see* **Note 3**). For a 1X working solution, mix 100 mL stock solution with 5 mL 20% (w/v) sodium dodecylsulphate (SDS) prepared in deionized water and 895 mL deionized water.

5. Sample buffer (5X): Mix 5 mL 0.5*M* Tris-HCl (pH 6.8), 5 mL glycerol, and 0.5 g SDS. Add a few crystals of bromophenol blue. Store at room temperature. If SDS precipitates, dissolve by microwaving briefly (2–4 s).

6. Low-salt collagenase buffer (10x): Mix 60.6 g Tris base, 117 g NaCl, 5.5 g $CaCl_2$, and make up to 900 mL with deionized water. Adjust to pH 7.6 with conc. HCl, top up to 1 L with deionized water and store at 4°C. For a 1x working solution mix 100 mL stock solution with 900 mL deionized water and add 670 μL Brij-35 (30%w/v, Sigma).

7. Destain solution: Mix 200 mL glacial acetic acid, 600 mL methanol, and 1200 mL tap water. Store at room temperature.

8. PhastGel-Blue-R Coomassie blue tablets (Pharmacia, Uppsala, Sweden). Prepare 0.2% stock solution according to manufacturers instructions. Filter through Whatman filter paper No. 1 (Whatman, Maidstone, UK) and store at 4°C (*see* **Note 4**). For a working dilution, mix 10 mL stock solution with 190 mL destain solution.

9. Step tablet No. 2 (Kodak, Rochester, NY).

10. Image analysis program (e.g., NIH Image 1.58 or later, National Institute of Health, USA, http://rsb.info.nih.gov/nih-image/download.html).

## 3. Methods

### 3.1. Collection and Preparation of Tissue Samples

1. Tumor samples are best collected directly from the operating theatre.

2. Cut tissue samples to approx 5 mm thick using sterile forceps and scalpels or scissors. Cool isopentane in a plastic container to near the freezing point on liquid nitrogen and snap freeze tissue in it. Isopentane penetrates tissues faster than liquid nitrogen and leads to more rapid freezing. This is particularly important if samples are also to be used for histology or *in situ* hybridization, when good preservation of morphology is important.

3. Tissue samples should be transported on carbon dioxide ice and stored at –70°C.

### 3.2. Zymography

### 3.2.1. Preparation and Processing of Gels

1. Prepare gels as described, carefully remove the combs, and rinse wells with 1x running buffer. Prepare samples in 1x sample buffer (*see* **Note 5**).

2. Run gel at 180 V until blue marker runs off the gel (approx 3.5 h).

3. Processing of gels: Lay plates flat on bench (on tissue paper) and gently lever apart glass plates using a spatula. Moisten gel with 2.5% (w/v) Triton X-100 prepared with deionized water. With a scalpel, cut off stacking gel, mark a corner for orientation, and cut along spacers to facilitate detachment of the gel. Carefully lift off gel and transfer it into a suitable plastic box with lid containing approx. 200 mL 2.5% Triton X-100. Incubate gel at room temperature for 1 h with gentle shaking. Prepare 1X collagenase buffer (500 mL per gel). Pour off Triton X-100 solution, rinse gel twice in 150 mL collagenase buffer and incubate gel in remaining 200 mL collagenase buffer overnight (16 h) at 37°C.

4. Staining of gel: Rinse gel briefly with water, add stain at working dilution (200 mL per gel) and incubate for 1–4 h with gentle shaking (*see* **Note 6**). Pour off staining solution and discard, rinse gel briefly with water, and wrap it in Saran wrap (Dow Chemicals) for analysis.

5. Analyzed gels can be dried for storage. Soak gel for 20 min in water containing 10% (v/v) glycerol and place between two prewetted sheets of cellophane (Bio-Rad, Hercules, CA). Dry gel either on a heated vacuum drier (approx 1 h, 80°C) or, for better results, fixed in a plastic frame permitting the liquid to evaporate (room temperature, 1–2 d).

### 3.2.2. Zymogram Analysis

1. Evaluation of zymogram: Scan gels using a flat bed scanner (e.g., UMAX Astra 1200 S) in transmissive mode using gray scale and the following parameters: gamma = 1, shadow = 0, range = 1–255. Do not use autoadjust functions. The density of each pixel is encoded on a scale ranging from 1 (clear) to 255 (opaque). A resolution of 150 dots per inch (dpi) leads to satisfactory results without excessively large files. The flat bed scanner has to be calibrated prior to evaluation of zymogram scans (*see* **Note 7**). Once the scanner has been calibrated, zymogram gels can be analyzed according to the instructions in the manual of the NIH image program (*see* **Notes 8** and **9**). Briefly, start NIH Image, reset to remove any previous measurements ("Reset" in the "Analyze" menu), load the "gel plotting macro" (in "Special" menu), and open the file containing the scanned gel. Next, open the calibration file (go to "Calibrate" in the "Analyze" menu, then "Open" the saved calibration file). Use the Rodbard function as the calibration function. (The procedure of resetting, opening the file to be analysed and calibrating the scan has to be done every time a new gel is analyzed.) Use the "rectangular tool" in the tool bar to select an area consisting of the band and approx 2 cm background above and below the band. Use the command "mark first lane," "mark next lane," and "plot lanes" offered by the "gel plotting macro" in the "Special" menu to plot the pixel intensity of each lane. After plotting the lanes use the "line tool" to close the area under the curve by joining the horizontal background line before and after the peak. To determine the integrated density of the band apply the "wand tool" on the enclosed area. Comparison of the integrated densities against a comigrated standard allows quantification of the proteolytic activity in a particular sample. This, however, is only possible in the linear range of the assay which needs to be determined for each protease using, for example, commercially available proteins or cell culture supernatants containing the protease of interest (*see* **Note 10**). A typical example for the quantitation of proMMP-9 by zymography is shown in **Fig. 1**. For limitations of the zymography method *see* **Note 11**.

## 4. Notes

1. Noncommercial buffers for the running and stacking buffers can also been used (**16**). Because these do not contain SDS, add 200 µL 20% (w/v) SDS to the running gel preparation and 100 µL 20% (w/v) SDS to the stacking gel preparations described in this protocol.

2. If wells do not set properly, increase the amount of TEMED and APS added to the stacking gel (e.g., to 45 µL TEMED and 90 µL APS). Make sure that the wells do not collapse while removing the comb. In our experience, Teflon combs are better than other plastic materials. Siliconizing of combs, e.g., with SigmaCote (Sigma) facilitates their removal and reduces the risk of wells collapsing.

3. In our experience, noncommercial 10X running buffer worked better than commercially available 10X running buffer.

4. We found that PhastGel-Blue-R tablets provided better batch to batch staining results than did powdered Coomassie blue from other sources. Filtration using Whatman filter paper No.1 is very slow and should be done overnight at 4°C.

Fig. 1. Linear range of proMMP-9 quantitation by zymography. ProMMP-9 (TCS Biologicals, Botolph Claydon, UK) was diluted to 1000 pg/mL in 60 m$M$ Tris-HCl (pH 7.2), 15 m$M$ CaCl$_2$, 80 m$M$ NaCl$_2$, 0.1% bovine serum albumin (BSA) and stored at –20°C. For zymograms doubling dilutions were prepared in the same buffer and 8 µL loaded onto a gel. **A** shows the same zymogram after staining for 1 h and 2 h of staining, respectively. Quantitation of the bands after 2 h of staining is shown in **B** and the linear range shown in **C**. Modified from **ref. *15***.

5. Sample preparation and storage. Tissue culture medium should be centrifuged (14,000$g$, 5 min) to remove cells and cell fragments prior to immediate use for zymography or storage at –20°C. Sample preparation from tissue biopsies requires mechanical disruption of the tissue with a tissue homogenizer in the presence of a detergent such as 1–2% SDS or Triton X-100 in 50 m$M$ Tris-HCl (pH 7.5). These extracts often contain large amounts of fat and DNA both of which can interfere with the migration and quantitation of proteolytic activity on zymograms. One way of reducing these contaminants is to extract tissue material with 1.5% Triton X-114 followed by separation of the hydrophobic and the aqueous phase *(17)*. For complete MMP extraction from the Triton X-114 phase, it might be necessary to repeat extraction several times. Note, that presence of Mg$^{2+}$ and Ca$^{2+}$ can influence the amount of MMP extracted from the hydrophilic phase *(17)*.

6. Strong bands of proteolysis are usually visible within 10–20 min. To achieve better background staining, the staining process should be extended to several hours. Length of staining does not affect the linearity of the assay, but may affect its sensitivity *(15)*.

7. Calibration of a scanner using a step tablet and the NIH Image program. Calibration of the scanner is crucial because the relationship between the densities scanned and the coding

from 1–255 is not linear. Calibration has to be done once for every scanner used. The results can be stored in the form of a file for later use. The procedure is described in detail in the NIH Image hand book. Briefly, place a step tablet on the scanner and scan in the same way as a gel. Reset the measurements ("Analyze" menu, "Reset"). Draw a box in the clearest area on the scan and measure the densities ("Measure" in "Analyze" menu). Repeat this with successively increasing density. Go into the "Analyze" menu and then "Calibrate." The values measured will be listed on the left side of the table. Fill in the right column with the known densities of the step tablet. Save the data as a file for later use. Activate the Rodbard-function and press "OK." A window containing the linearised densities will appear. Note that the curve itself is not a straight line, but the increase between each step is now uniform. Close this window.

8. This protocol refers to the NIH 1.58 program, but other image-analysis programs might also be used. Calibration of the scanner remains essential whatever software package is used.

9. Some useful changes in the NIH settings. To change the setting of the NIH program to obtain density scans in which the opaque represents the bottom of the y-axis and clear represents the top, go into "Options," "Preferences," and click on "invert Y co-ordinates." In the same window, set the "Undo & Clipboard" buffer size to 1000 K. Make sure that the program is working in "Greyscale" mode (see "Options" menu). Finally, go into "Options," "Profile Plot Options," and make sure the box "Invert" is activated. Save this setting by "Record Preferences" in the "File" menu.

10. In our experience, the use of $140 \times 100 \times 1$ mm gels resulted in a longer linear range for MMP-9 than mini gels ($90 \times 60 \times 1$ mm).

11. Limitations of zymography. Because of the presence of SDS during the run of a zymogram, the complex between an MMP and its natural inhibitor (e.g., TIMPs, tissue inhibitor of MMPs) dissociates. Zymography will therefore reveal the total gelatinolytic activity on the sample loaded, but not the net proteolytic activity in the sample. In addition, the proteolytic activity of the pro- and activated forms of MMPs cannot be compared on an absolute scale. The proform of MMPs shows proteolytic activity on zymograms because it becomes activated during the process of renaturation *(18)*. The extent of this activation has not been investigated in detail, but it is unlikely to be complete. Therefore, 1 ng proMMP-9, for example, might lead to different proteolytic activity on a zymogram than 1 ng active MMP-9. In addition, zymogram data always need to be backed up by other methods, e.g., Western blotting to actually prove the identity of the protease analyzed. Supplementing of collagenase buffer with inhibitors to proteases (e.g., 1 m*M* 1,10-phenanthroline (Sigma) for MMPs) can be used to classify the proteolytic activity analysed.

## References

1. Murphy, G. and Knauper, V. (1997) Relating matrix metalloproteinase structure to function: why the "hemopexin" domain? *Matrix Biol.* **15,** 511–518.
2. Matrisian, L. M. (1992) The matrix-degrading metalloproteinases. *Bioessays* **14,** 455–463.
3. Mauch, C., Krieg, T., and Bauer, E. A. (1994) Role of the extracellular matrix in the degradation of connective tissue. *Arch. Dermatol. Res.* **287,** 107–114.
4. Murphy, G. (1995) Matrix metalloproteinases and their inhibitors. *Acta. Orthop. Scand. Suppl.* **266,** 55–60.
5. Mauviel, A. (1993) Cytokine regulation of metalloproteinase gene expression. *J. Cell Biochem.* **53,** 288–295.
6. Sang, Q. X., Birkedal Hansen, H., and Van Wart, H. E. (1995) Proteolytic and non-proteolytic activation of human neutrophil progelatinase B. *Biochim. Biophys. Acta.* **1251,** 99–108.
7. Bullen, E. C., Longaker, M. T., Updike, D. L., Benton, R., Ladin, D., Hou, Z., et al. (1995) Tissue inhibitor of metalloproteinases-1 is decreased and activated gelatinases are increased in chronic wounds. *J. Invest. Dermatol.* **104,** 236–240.
8. Stetlerstevenson, W. G. (1996) Dynamics of matrix turnover during pathological remodeling of the extracellular-matrix. *Am. J. Pathol.* **148,** 1345–1350.

9. Woessner, J. F., Jr. and Gunja Smith, Z. (1991) Role of metalloproteinases in human osteoarthritis. *J. Rheumatol. Suppl.* **27,** 99–101.

10. Woessner, J. F., Jr. (1991) Matrix metalloproteinases and their inhibitors in connective tissue remodeling. *Faseb J.* **5,** 2145–2154.

11. Basset, P., Okada, A., Chenard, M. P., Kannan, R., Stoll, I., Anglard, P., et al. (1997) Matrix metalloproteinases as stromal effectors of human carcinoma progression: therapeutic implications. *Matrix Biol.* **15,** 535–541.

12. Liotta, L. A. and Stetler Stevenson, W. G. (1991) Tumor invasion and metastasis: an imbalance of positive and negative regulation. *Cancer Res.* **51,** 5054s–5059s.

13. Karelina, T. V., Goldberg, G. I., and Eisen, A. Z. (1995) Matrix metalloproteinases in blood vessel development in human fetal skin and in cutaneous tumors. *J. Invest. Dermatol.* **105,** 411–417.

14. Chambers, A. F. and Matrisian, L. M. (1997) Changing views on the role of matrix metalloproteinases in metastasis. *J. Nat. Cancer Inst.* **89,** 1260–1270.

15. Leber, T. M. and Balkwill, F. R. (1997) Zymography: a single step staining method for quantitation of proteolytic activity on substrate gels. *Analyt. Biochem.* **249,** 24–28.

16. Brown, P. D., Bloxidge, R. E., Anderson, E., and Howell, A. (1993) Expression of activated gelatinase in human invasive breast carcinoma. *Clin. Exp. Metastasis* **11,** 183–189.

17. Monsky, W. L., Kelly, T., Lin, C. Y., Yeh, Y., Stetler-Stevenson, W. G., Mueller, S. C., et al. (1993) Binding and localization of M(r) 72,000 matrix metalloproteinase at cell surface invadopodia. *Cancer Res.* **53,** 3159–3164.

18. Kleiner, D. E. and Stetler Stevenson, W. G. (1994) Quantitative zymography: detection of picogram quantities of gelatinases. *Anal. Biochem.* **218,** 325–329.

# 56

## Simultaneous Flow Cytometric Detection of DNA and Cellular Protein Molecules

### Willem E. Corver and Cees J. Cornelisse

## 1. Introduction

Flow cytometry (FCM) is a sophisticated technique for rapid simultaneous analysis of multiple cellular parameters. The technique is based on the interception of a hydrodynamically focused stream of single cells in suspension by an excitation light beam at high speed. As a result, each cell produces light scattering and fluorescence, proportional to the cell size, shape, structure, and fluorescently labeled cellular components, respectively.

Multiparameter FCM of cellular protein molecules (e.g., surface protein molecules) combined with DNA content measurement requires single cell suspensions from intact cells. Cell suspensions from cultured monolayer cells can easily be obtained by scraping, or treating the cells with EDTA or trypsin/EDTA, provided that chemical or enzymatic treatment of the cells does not have an adverse effect on the target protein (*1*). Cytology specimens, e.g., cervical smears, fine-needle aspirates as well as pleural and peritoneal effusions are suitable for flow cytometric analysis. Also ascites tumor cells growing in cell clumps can be dissociated using trypsin/EDTA (*2*). So far, there is still no generally accepted procedure for optimal dissociation of tumor tissue available. A dissociation method suitable for one type of tumor, might not work for a second one (*3*). In general, enzymatic dissociation results in higher cell yields and viability (*4*). The effect of mechanical or enzymatic dissociation on the yield of DNA-aneuploid cells from fresh ovarian tumors still needs to be investigated.

Although proteolytic enzymes might have an effect on membrane-associated molecules, several surface proteins of ovarian cancer ascites—and solid ovarian tumor cells can readily be detected in combination with DNA content measurements after enzymatic dissociation (*2*). Beside the dissociation method, other variables also affect the flow cytometric outcome. Next to sampling and DNA staining, prolonged fixation with protein crosslinkers like formalin, paraformaldehyde (PF), and glutaraldehyde have an adverse effect on the coefficient of variation (CV) of the DNA-histogram peaks and should therefore be omitted. Good results can be obtained with short fixations using 1.0% paraformaldehyde combined with lysolecithin (*5*) or followed by methanol denaturation. These fixation procedures allow the simultaneous detection of intracellular and intranuclear protein molecules (*see* **Note 1**).

From: *Methods in Molecular Medicine, Vol. 39: Ovarian Cancer: Methods and Protocols*
Edited by: J. M. S. Bartlett © Humana Press, Inc., Totowa, NJ

Fig. 1. Simultaneous measurement of Ep-CAM (FITC, green fluorescence), keratin 8/18 (RPE, orange fluorescence) and DNA (PI, red fluorescence) of a human ovarian cancer ascites using a FACScan flow cytometer. Cells were isolated by centrifugation and microscopically analyzed for aggregates. No trypsin treatment was necessary in this case (*see* **Subheading 3.2.**). Cells were indirectly stained for Ep-CAM, fixed, and permeabilized by the simultaneous action of PF and LL, and stained for keratin 8/18

The following methods describe protocols that have been used successfully on cultured tumor cells as well as on cells obtained from ovarian tumors to measure cellular protein molecules by single parameter or multiparameter FCM in combination with DNA content analysis. The first protocol is used for cell surface staining. Briefly, cells are isolated using proteolytic enzymes (**Subheading 3.1.–3.3.**) and indirectly stained for one or multiple cell surface proteins using fluorescein isothiocyanate (FITC) and/or R-phycoerythrin (RPE) as fluorescent reporter molecules (**Subheading 3.4.1.**). Dead cells can be discriminated from live cells using low concentrations of propidium iodide (PI) (*see* **Note 2**). The second series of protocols are used for staining of multiple cellular protein molecules, which differ in their cellular localization (membrane, cytoplasmic, and nuclear). Briefly, cells are stained for surface molecules (FITC fluorescence), washed, and fixed using PF, while simultaneously permeabilized using lysolecithin (**Subheading 3.4.2.**). Then, cells are stained for intermediate filaments (e.g., keratin or vimentin, RPE fluorescence). Cells can also be stained for DNA using a high concentration of PI to allow simultaneous measurement of cellular proteins and DNA content. It is recommended to use a different fixation protocol for the simultaneous staining of intermediate filaments and nuclear-associated protein molecules (**Subheading 3.4.3.**) (*see* **Note 1**).

Using a combination of monoclonal antibodies (MAbs) and subclass specific FITC or RPE conjugated secondary reagents in conjunction with DNA content measurements is a powerful technique in identifying tumor subpopulations by FCM *(2,6)*. It can be performed using a single-laser bench-top flow cytometer *(2,7)*. This technique is, therefore, within the reach of many clinical laboratories. An example of a human ovarian ascites stained for the epithelial cellular adhesion molecule (Ep-CAM) (FL1, FITC, green fluorescence), keratin 8/18 (FL2, RPE, orange fluorescence) and DNA (FL3-A, PI, red fluorescence) is shown by **Fig. 1**.

## 2. Materials

### 2.1. Harvesting Monolayer Tumor Cells From Culture

1. Roswell Park Memorial Institute (RPMI-1640) culture medium (GibcoBRL, Gaithersburg, MA) or Dulbecco's Modified Eagles medium (DMEM) culture medium (GibcoBRL) supplemented with 10% Fetal calf serum (FCS, e.g., GibcoBRL), Penicillin - Streptomycin (ICN Biomedicals, Inc., High Wycomb, U.K.) and L-Glutamine (ICN Biomedicals, Inc.).

---

Fig. 1. *(continued)* (*see* **Subheading 3.4.2.**). Then DNA was stained with PI (*see* **Subheading 3.5.**). Note the presence of a tumor population with a DNA Index of 3.04. The level of protein expression is slightly higher to that of the cell population with the DNA Index of 1.51. Furthermore, Ep-CAM and keratin 8/18 positive cells can be observed in the DNA-diploid fraction. These cells might represent tumor cells *(6)* (*see* also Chapter 56). Controls are shown in the upper row (**A–C**). Ep-CAM and keratin 8/18 positive cells are shown in the lower row (**E–G**). (**A**) GaMIgG2a-FITC (FL1) vs GaMIgG1-RPE (FL2), (**B**) GaMIgG2a-FITC (FL1) vs DNA PI (FL3-A), (**C**) GaMIgG1-RPE vs DNA PI (FL3-A), (**D**) corresponding DNA histogram of the control cells DNA PI (FL3-A). (**E**) Ep-CAM FITC (FL1) vs keratin 8/18 RPE (FL2), (**B**) Ep-CAM FITC (FL1) vs DNA PI (FL3-A), (**C**) Keratin 8/18 RPE vs DNA PI (FL3-A), (**D**) corresponding DNA histogram of the positive stained cells DNA PI (FL3-A).

2. Trypsin 0.25% (GibcoBRL)/EDTA 2 m*M* (disodium ethylenediaminetetra-acetic acid, Sigma, St. Louis, MD) made from 10X stock solution trypsin (2.5%) and from 50X stock solution of 100 m*M* disodium-EDTA, pH 7.6.
3. Trypan Blue 0.4%, prepared in phosphate buffered saline, pH 7.4.

## 2.2. Isolation of Cells from Ovarian Ascites Specimen

1. Standard ammonium chloride erythrocyte lysing buffer. 1.0 L contains: 167 m*M* NH$_4$Cl (Merck, Darmstadt, Germany), 10 m*M* KHCO$_3$ (Merck), 0.1 m*M* EDTA (ethylenediaminetetra-acetic acid, Sigma). Adjust pH to 7.4 and store at 4°C.

## 2.3. Isolation of Cells from Solid Ovarian Tumors

1. Collagenase Type IA and IV (Sigma), hyaluronidase type V (Sigma), trypsin (GibcoBRL), DNase I, Type II (Sigma). A mixture of enzymes can be prepared in DMEM, without FCS, and stored in the freezer. Aliquots of 10 mL are suitable. The mixture contains: 0.05% collagenase type IA, 0.1% collagenase type IV, hyaluronidase type V (0.05%) and 0.001% DNase I, type II. Avoid repeatedly freezing and thawing.
2. 2.5% trypsin stock solution (GibcoBRL), stored at –20°C.

## 2.4. Staining of Cellular Proteins

1. MAbs directed against surface antigens (e.g., antiepithelial cell adhesion molecule (Ep-CAM), clone Ber-Ep4 (DAKO, Glostrup, Denmark), directed against intermediate filaments (e.g., antikeratin or vimentin, DAKO) or directed against nuclear associated proteins [e.g., anti-Ki-67 (clone Ki-67, DAKO), antiproliferating cell nuclear antigen (PCNA, clone PC10, Dako)].
2. FITC or RPE conjugated goat antimouse IgG or IgG subclass specific secondary reagents (e.g., Southern Biotechnology Associates, Birmingham, AL).
3. Phosphate buffered (PBS, pH 7.4) paraformaldehyde (E.M. grade, methanol free, e.g., Merck), freshly prepared from 8X stock solution (8.0% PF), (*see* Note 3).
4. Lysolecithin from egg yolk (Sigma), stock solution 10 mg/mL, dissolved in 100% methanol and stored in the freezer.
5. Phosphate buffered paraformaldehyde/lysolecithin solution (80–160 µg/mL).
6. PBS containing 0.5% bovine serum albumin (PBA) (BSA fraction V, Sigma), pH 7.4. Store at 4°C.

## 2.5 DNA Staining

1. RNase (Sigma), 10X stock dissolved in PBS, stored at –20°C.
2. 100 m*M* Propidium Iodide (Molecular Probes), made from 1*M* 10X stock solution dissolved in PBS, stored at –20°C (*see* **Notes 4** and **5**, about DNA stains).

## 2.6. Special Equipment

1. A flow cytometer (e.g., Becton Dickinson/Pharmingen, San Jose, CA, Beckmann/Coulter or DAKO).
2. Sheath fluid (e.g., Becton Dickinson/Pharmingen or Beckmann/Coulter) or (home made) phosphate-buffered saline (PBS): 150 m*M* NaCl (e.g., Merck), 1.165 m*M* Na$_2$HPO$_4$.2H$_2$O (Merck) and 0.234 m*M* KH$_2$PO$_4$ (Merck). This solution must be prepared in highly purified H$_2$O, filtered over a 0.22-µm filter. A 10X stock solution of 10 L (100 L of sheath fluid) is easily prepared and can be stored at room temperature. pH 7.5 after dilution.

**Summary of Staining Procedures**

| 2 surface proteins and DNA | 1 surface and 1 cytoplasmic or nuclear protein and DNA | 1 cytoplasmic and 1 nuclear protein and DNA |
|---|---|---|
| wash cells 2 times with PBA ↓ | wash cells 2 times with PBA ↓ | wash cells 2 times with PBS ↓ |
| primary MAbs, 30 min, 4°C ↓ | primary MAb, 30 min, 4°C ↓ | 1% PF, 5 min, 4°C ↓ |
| wash 2 times with PBA ↓ | wash 2 times with PBA ↓ | wash once with PBA ↓ |
| secondary reagents GaMIgX FITC/RPE, 30 min, 4°C ↓ | secondary reagent GaMIgX RPE, 30 min, 4°C ↓ | 100% methanol, 10 min, -20°C ↓ |
| wash 2 times with PBS ↓ | wash 2 times with PBS ↓ | wash 2 times with PBA ↓ |
| 1% PF, 5 min, 4°C, 80-160 µg/mL Lysolecithin(1 mL) ↓ | 1% PF, 5 min, 4°C, 80-160 µg/mL Lysolecithin(1 mL) ↓ | primary MAbs, 30 min, 4°C ↓ |
| add 1 mL PBA ↓ | add 1 mL PBA ↓ | wash 2 times with PBA ↓ |
| wash 2 times with PBA ↓ | wash 2 times with PBA ↓ | secondary reagents GaMIgX FITC/RPE, 30 min, 4°C ↓ |
| PI/RNase, 30 min, 37°C ↓ | primary MAb, 30 min, 4°C ↓ | wash 2 times with PBA ↓ |
| Store at 4°C | wash 2 times with PBA ↓ | PI/RNase, 30 min, 37°C ↓ |
| | secondary reagent GaMIgX FITC, 30 min, 4°C ↓ | Store at 4°C |
| | wash 2 times with PBA ↓ | |
| | PI/RNase, 30 min, 37°C ↓ | |
| | Store at 4°C | |

Fig. 2. Schematic presentation of indirect staining and fixation procedures for multiparameter DNA flow cytometry of disaggregated human solid tumors. IgX = IgG1, or IgG2a, or IgG2b, or IgG3.

3. Analysis software (e.g., Becton Dickinson/Pharmingen, Beckmann/Coulter, DAKO, Verity Software House.

## 3. Methods

The tumor sample that is going to be processed for flow cytometric analysis can be weighed before dissociation to allow monitoring the yield and viability of the tumor cells obtained from the specimen using the Trypan blue method. The staining procedures are summarized by **Fig. 2**.

## 3.1. Harvesting Cultured Cells

### 3.1.1. Monolayer Tumor Cells

1. Culture monolayer cells in culture flasks till the cells reach confluence. Refresh the culture medium every 2 d (*see* **Note 6**).
2. Collect the culture medium in a 50-mL tube (e.g., Falcon, Los Angeles, CA) and spin cell debris down at 1000*g* for 5 min.
3. Meanwhile, wash cells in culture flask twice with 10 mL Hank's Balanced Salt Solution (HBSS) type I (Sigma) for 5–10 min, using an incubator at 37°C.
4. Add 2.5 mL HBSS containing 0.25% trypsin/0.2 m*M* EDTA (pH 7.6) and detach cells using an incubator at 37°C.
5. Examine the process using a microscope after a few minutes of incubation. (Duration of dissociation is cell line dependent).
6. Stop the process when cells are just releasing from the culture flask bottom by pouring the spun down culture medium (**step 2**) by one stroke in the culture flask and mix gently.
7. Spin harvested cells down (250*g*, 5 min) and wash once with HBSS.
8. Vortex cell pellet gently and add 10 mL of HBSS. Filter cells over a nylon sieve with a 50 mM pore size (e.g., DAKO).
9. Count the cells using the Trypan blue method applying a hemocytometer (Bürker) chamber. Adjust the cell concentration to $1 \times 10^6$/mL and store cells on ice (4°C) until further preparation.

### 3.1.2. Cells Growing in Suspension

1. Culture the cells in culture flasks till the culture reached a cell concentration of about $2 \times 10^6$. Refresh the culture medium every 2 d (*see* **Note 6**).
2. Collect the culture medium in a 50-mL tube and spin cells down at 250*g* for 5 min.
3. Repeat **step 8** and **9** (**Subheading 3.1.1.**). Filtering the cells can be omitted.

## 3.2. Isolation of Cells from Ovarian Ascites Specimen

1. Isolate ovarian ascites cells by centrifugation (250*g*, 5 min) and measure the volume of the cell pellet. Use 50-mL tubes (e.g., Falcon).
2. Resuspend pellet gently using a Vortex and add three times the volume of the cell pellet of the standard lysing buffer. Lyse the erythrocytes for 10 min at 37°C.
3. Fill the tube to a maximum of 50 mL with standard culture medium.
4. Spin cells down and wash three times with HBSS at room temperature. Finally, gently mix the cell pellet, add 10 mL of HBSS, and put on ice (4°C).
5. Take one drop of the cell suspension using a Pasteur's capillary pipet, put it on a microscope slide and cover it with a cover slip. Examine the specimen using a microscope. If tumor cells appear as single cells, go to **step 10**. However, if tumor cells appear as cell clusters dissociate the cell clusters as follows.
6. Spin cells down and incubate 1.0 mL of packed cells with 20-mL HBSS, containing 0.25% trypsin and 2 m*M* EDTA, pH 7.2, in a 75-cm$^2$ culture flask at 37°C.
7. Monitor the dissociation process microscopically.
8. Stop the process by adding 5.0-mL FCS, collect the cells and spin cells down (250*g*, 5 min).
9. Vortex the cell pellet gently and add HBSS dropwise. The volume can range from about 10–40 mL or more, depending on the size of the cell pellet.
10. Perform **step 9** (**Subheading 3.1.1.**).

### 3.3. Isolation of Cells from Solid Ovarian Tumors

1. Fill a flat polystyrene box with ice and put a Petri dish on top of it.
2. Weigh the tumor sample (Petri dish included) and weigh an empty Petri dish. Subtract the results (= sample weight). Put the sample with the Petri dish on ice.
3. Moisture the tissue with 1.0 mL of standard precooled (4°C) culture DMEM-medium, without FCS.
4. Cut the tumor sample into fragments of approximately 1–2 mm$^3$ using scalpel blades. Use a pair of tweezers to fix the tumor sample to Petri dish bottom.
5. Incubate fragments over night at 4°C with 10 mL of DMEM (GibcoBRL), without FCS, per 1.0 g tissue, containing the enzyme mix (*see* **Subheading 2.3.**)
6. Next day, dissociate tumor chunks at 37°C using an incubator.
7. After 2 h of incubation, add trypsin to a final concentration of 0.25%.
8. After 15 min of incubation at 37°C, gently pass the suspension several times through a 1.5-mm syringe needle and filter over a nylon sieve with a pore size of 100 mm.
9. Put the suspension on ice (4°C) and add FCS to a final concentration of 20% to block proteolytic activity.
10. Spin cells down at 250*g* for 5 min. A centrifuge with cooling facility (4°C) is preferred.
11. Vortex the cell pellet gently and add medium dropwise. The volume can range from about 1 to 10 or more milliliters, depending on the size of the cell pellet.
12. Perform **step 9** (**Subheading 3.1.1.**)

### 3.4. Staining of Cellular Proteins

#### 3.4.1. Staining of Surface Proteins (One Parameter, No Fixation)

1. Use 0.5–1*10$^6$ cells per test tube and spin cells down for 5 min at 250*g*. (A cooled centrifuge (4°C) is preferred.)
2. Discard the supernatant or other medium by turning the test tubes upside-down in one stroke. Keep the tubes upside-down and place the tubes in a tube rack containing a tissue, placed on the bottom of the tube rack. The last drop of supernatant will be taken up by the tissue.
3. Turn the tubes again, add 1.0 mL of cold PBA, vortex gently and spin cells down at 250*g*, for 5 min.
4. Discard the PBA in the same way as described by **step 2**.
5. Add 100 μL of diluted monoclonal antibody (MAb) (e.g., Ber-Ep4, DAKO) to the cells, vortex gently and incubate for 30 min on ice (4°C) (*see* **Note 7**).
6. Add 1.0 mL of cold PBA to the cells, vortex and spin cells down (250*g*, 5 min, 4°C).
7. Repeat **step 6** and add 100 μL of diluted secondary reagent, e.g., goat antimouse Ig-FITC (DAKO) (*see* **Note 8**).
8. Vortex gently and put the cells on ice for 30 min (4°C).
9. Repeat **step 6** twice.
10. Add 0.5 mL of ice cold PBA containing PI at a final concentration of 1.0 μ*M* to the cells, vortex gently, and store the cells on ice (4°C). Low concentrations of PI allow good discrimination between dead and viable cells (*see* **Note 2**).
11. Cells are ready for flow cytometric analysis after 30 min.

Note: **Steps 6–8** can be omitted when direct labeled antibodies are applied.

#### 3.4.2. Simultaneous Staining of Cell Surface Proteins and Cytoplasmic Proteins (Paraformaldehyde Fixation and Lysolecithin Permeabilization)

1. Perform **steps 1–8** of **Subheading 3.4.1.** to stain surface protein molecules (*see* **Note 9**).
2. Add 1.0 mL of cold PBS to the cells, vortex and spin cells down (250*g*, 5 min, 4°C) (*see* **Note 10**).

3.  Wash cells once with cold PBS
4.  Meanwhile, prepare an ice-cold 1.0% phosphate buffered PF solution containing 80–160 μg/mL of lysolecithin (LL) (*see* **Note 11**).
5.  Vortex the pelleted cells gently and add the PF/LL solution dropwise under constant swirling.
6.  Fix and permeabilize the cells for 5 min on ice (4°C), vortex gently, add 1.0 mL of PBA, and spin cells down (250*g*, 4°C).
7.  Wash the cells twice with cold PBA (250*g*, 5 min, 4°C).
8.  Perform **steps 5–9** of **Subheading 3.4.1.**
9.  Add 0.5 mL of ice-cold PBA. Cells are ready for flow cytometric analysis

Cells can now also be stained for DNA after **step 8** of **Subheading 3.4.2.** (*see* **Subheading 3.5.**)

### 3.4.3. Simultaneous Staining of Cytoplasmic and/or Nuclear Proteins (Paraformaldehyde Fixation and Methanol Denaturation)

1.  Perform **steps 1–3** (*see* **Subheading 3.4.1.**). Use cold PBS instead of cold PBA as washing buffer.
2.  Wash cells once again with cold PBS (250*g*, 5 min, 4°C ).
3.  Meanwhile, prepare an ice-cold 1.0% phosphate buffered PF solution.
4.  Vortex the pelleted cells gently and add the 1.0% PF solution dropwise under constant swirling.
5.  Fix the cells for 5 min on ice (4°C), vortex gently, add 1.0 mL of PBA, and spin cells down.
6.  Add 100 μL of cold PBS to the cells pellet, vortex gently, and add 900 μL of ice-cold (–20°C) 100% methanol dropwise under constant swirling.
7.  Put the cells in the freezer for 10 min.
8.  Spin cells down and add 100 μL of cold PBS to the cell pellet, vortex gently, and add 900 μL of PBA dropwise under constant swirling. This technique will prevent most cell clumping (*see* **Note 12**).
9.  Wash cells again with cold PBA (250*g*, 5 min, 4°C )
10. Perform **steps 5–9** of **Subheading 3.4.1.** (*see* **Note 9** for simultaneous staining of cytoplasmic and nuclear-associated protein molecules).
11. Add 0.5 mL of ice-cold PBA. Cells are ready for flow cytometric analysis.

The cells can also be stained for DNA (*see* **Subheading 3.5.**) directly after **step 10** of **Subheading 3.4.3.** This is recommended for proteins being studied, which expression is known to be cell cycle phase dependent (e.g., Ki-67).

### 3.5. DNA Staining

1.  Add 0.5 mL of 0.1% RNase (in PBA) containing 100 μ*M* of PI.
2.  Vortex gently and incubate the cells for 30 min at 37°C using a water heated incubator.
3.  Put the cells on ice (4°C). Cells are ready for flow cytometric analysis after 30 min (*see* **Note 13**).

## 4. Notes

1.  The PF/lysolecithin protocol is a mild fixation/permeabilization procedure not effecting cell surface staining (*see* **Figs. 3** and **4**). However, staining of nuclear antigens is less optimal using this procedure. Methanol or ethanol denaturation after PF fixation is therefore recommended for the staining of nuclear protein molecules. Unfortunately,

Fig. 3. Analysis of optimal lysolecithin concentration for simultaneous measurement of cell surface or cytoplasmic protein molecules. OVCAR-3 cells were treated as described by **Subheading 3.4.2.** and stained for keratin 8/18 using a GaMIgG-RPE (FL2, orange fluorescence). Permeabilized cells are monitored using 1.0 μ*M* PI (FL3, red fluorescence). (**A**) 0.63 μg LL/mL, (**B**) 1.25 μg LL/mL, (**C**) 5.0 μg LL/mL, (**D**) 80 μg LL/mL. Percentages in the quadrants indicate the nonpermeabilized (left corner) and permeabilized PI positive (upper left) and PI and keratin positive (upper right) cells. Note that all cells are stained for keratin only at high lysolecithin concentrations. This indicates that analysis of permeabilization by PI alone is not sufficient for monitoring the optimal permeabilization for labeling of intracellular proteins. This "delay" in permeability is probably caused by the relative large size of the immunoglobulin and the RPE molecule too which the cells are more resistant for penetration compared to a small molecule like PI.

postfixation with methanol after cell surface staining can negatively effect the fluorescence signals *(8)* (also authors observations). Therefore, it is advised to use the PF/lysolecithin protocol (**Subheading 3.4.2.**) for the simultaneous detection of surface and cytoplasmic protein molecules and PF/methanol protocol (**Subheading 3.4.3.**) for the simultaneous detection of cytoplasmic and nuclear-associated protein molecules.

2. The presence of dead cells might interfere with the analysis of viable cells, especially in cases with a relative low-specific fluorescence signal. Dead cells are permeable and can bind MAbs and secondary labeled antibodies nonspecifically. This can be avoided in cases of cell surface staining by adding low concentrations of DNA dyes, like PI, 7-AAD for

**A**

**B**

Fig. 4 (**A**). Analysis of optimal lysolecithin concentration for simultaneous measurement of two cell surface proteins and DNA content. NIH:OVCAR-3 cells were double stained for Ep-CAM (FITC, FL1 green fluorescence) and OV632 (RPE, FL2 orange fluorescence), fixed with 1.0% PF, while simultaneously exposed to different LL concentrations. Permeabilization was measured using 1.0 µ$M$ of PI (FL3, red fluorescence). Cell recovery was estimated by monitoring the event rate (●). Note the sharp increase of PI positive cells (■) over a relative small range of LL concentrations. (**B**) shows the effect of LL on retention of surface protein expression (+: Ep-CAM, Δ: OV632). Even at high LL concentrations the mean fluorescence intensity (MFI) is comparable to that of the untreated cells (black bar: Ep-CAM, dashed bar: OV632, no fixation and permeabilization).

single-laser excitation or TP3 for double-laser excitation. Dead cells are also permeable for these DNA dyes and stain strongly. The strong fluorescence signal from dead cells is easily separated from the autofluorescence of viable cells and they can be gated out during acquisition or during analysis *(9)* (*see* **Fig. 3**).

It is not possible to use DNA dyes for discrimination between viable and dead cells when the cells are also stained for intracellular proteins after fixation (all cells will be DNA stained). An elegant solution for this problem was introduced by O'Brien and Bolton, who used antitubulin antibodies as a probe for dead cells *(10)*.

3. Paraformaldehyde (PF) is a water soluble chemical protein crosslinker. An 8% stock can be prepared easily by dissolving 8 g. of PF in distilled water heated to 60°C, while stirring. Use a safety cabinet. Avoid evaporation. Add a few drops of 1 $M$ NaOH dropwise under constant swirling until the solution clears. Cool the solution down using running cold tab water. Filter the solution over a paper filter and store it at 4°C. A 1% PF working solution can be made by diluting the 8% PF stock in PBS. The pH should be between 7.2 and 7.4. The stock solution can be stored for several weeks at 4°C. A short fixation with PF (5 min on ice [4°C]) is sufficient for crosslinking membrane bound proteins and stabilizing the cells for permeabilization without significant loss of membrane antigen staining *(5)*. PF is unstable in solution and should be freshly prepared, because formic acid is gradually formed during storage. Discard the stock solution if pH drops below 7.2.

4. Propidium iodide (PI) is the most commonly used DNA stain for flow cytometric analysis of DNA content. This intercalating dye has a relative high affinity to both dsDNA and dsRNA, requiring RNase treatment of the cells before analysis. It has a broad excitation spectrum making it suitable for both ultraviolet (UV) excitation and visible blue light

excitation. The latter is one of the reasons why PI is a very popular DNA stain, because almost all modern bench-top flow cytometers are equipped with the blue 488-nm Argon-ion laser, allowing PI excitation. A disadvantage of the use of PI is the broad orange to red emission spectrum, requiring substantial compensation. This makes the combination of PI with other fluorochromes emitting in the orange range, e.g., RPE, of the spectrum less appropriate. However, proteins which are highly expressed, e.g., intermediate filaments like keratin and vimentin, and stained using RPE conjugated reagents can be easily detected in clinical samples, which were also stained for DNA-ploidy analysis using high concentrations of PI *(2,5)*. Also, spectral overlap of RPE/PI positive cells into the green fluorescence channel cannot entirely be corrected for using hardware compensation facilities.

7-Amino-actinomycin-D (7-AAD, Molecular Probes) is frequently used as an alternative for PI for measurements of multiple cellular proteins in combination with DNA-ploidy analysis using single laser excitation *(11,12)*. This G-C specific DNA dye has a larger "Stokes" shift (difference between excitation wavelength and maximum emission wavelength) than PI, allowing a better discrimination between RPE and 7-AAD fluorescent signals. However, Brockhoff et al. *(7)* clearly demonstrated that also 7-AAD shows considerable spectral overlap with RPE and that PI is still in favor owing to the low CV's of the DNA-histogram peaks and good stoichiometry of DNA binding. These findings were confirmed in our laboratory.

5. Flexibility in choice of DNA stain increases using flow cytometers with double (or more) excitation capability. Recently, DAKO and Becton Dickinson introduced bench-top flow cytometers capable of double excitation using a 488-nm Argon-ion laser line and a Mercury-Arc lamp (UV excitation) or a 488-nm Argon-ion laser line in combination with a red diode laser (approximate excitation: 635 nm), respectively. The Mercury Arc-lamp can be used for excitation of DAPI (2,4 diamidino-6-phenylindole, Molecular Probes, Eugene, OR), allowing analysis of multiple proteins and DNA with minimal spectral crossover problems *(13)*. DAPI is a DNA specific dye with excellent DNA binding characteristics. The red diode laser can be used for the excitation of TO-PRO-3 Iodide (TP3, Molecular Probes), a recently developed DNA dye *(14,15)*. Its usefulness as DNA dye has already been proven in clinical samples stained for two cellular proteins and DNA, analysed by a double-excitation flow cytometer *(16)*.

6. Culture conditions strongly effect levels of protein expression. It is, therefore, recommended to standardise intralaboratory culture conditions as much as possible, when levels of expression between different cell lines are going to be compared over a period of time *(1)*. Levels of protein expression are influenced by several factors like type of medium, percentage of fetal calf serum present in the medium, harvesting cells during log-growth phase or plateau phase, contact inhibition, temperature, and so on. Cultures must be initiated by the same quantity of cells and medium must be refreshed at given time intervals.

Levels of protein expression can be quantified using flow cytometry. Much effort has been put by the industry in developing highly uniform fluorescent beads containing defined amounts of fluorescent dyes like FITC, RPE (Flow Cytometry Standards) or broad spectrum dyes (Spherotec). (These beads are available from several companies.) In this way, levels of expression can be expressed in terms of molecules equivalent soluble fluorochrome (MESF or MEF). A second type of beads are coated with defined amounts of goat anti-mouse polyclonal antibodies or mouse monoclonal antibodies. These type of beads are treated the same way as the sample cells during the assay allowing quantification in terms of antibody binding capacity (ABC), giving an estimate of the amount of molecules present on the cells (available from Flow Cytometry Standards and DAKO).

7. One of the major drawbacks of flow cytometry is the lack of visual control of the stained cells being analyzed. MAbs that are going to be used for flow cytometric analysis must be

carefully selected, especially MAbs directed against intracellular antigens. Staining for intracellular antigens is sensitive to nonspecific binding of MAbs [e.g., p53 *(17)*]. Nonetheless, many antibodies suitable for immunohistochemistry can also be used for flow cytometry. However, the MAb must comply with certain criteria. The antibody must be titrated using cells expressing the target protein (positive control) and cells lacking the protein of interest (negative control) *(18)*. Cells must also be cultured on cover slips or spotted on glass sections allowing microscopic examination of protein localization using the same fixation, permeabilization, and staining procedure used for flow cytometry. Results should be compared to data from literature or the signals should at least be localized at the expected site of the cell. Standard immunohistochemistry on tissue section can contribute to verification of the antibody (e.g., antikeratin antibodies should not react with the stromal compartment of a tumor). Western blotting must confirm the expected size of the protein of interest.

8. Conjugated antimouse antibodies (secondary reagents) must be of high quality, especially in cases when intracellular proteins are stained. Poor quality secondary reagents can give severe background staining on fixed and permeabilized cells and thereby interfere with signal-to-noise ratios. Secondary reagents should be carefully titrated using labelled (positive signal) and unlabeled (background) cells. Signals must be compared to the autofluorescence signal from unstained cells. The optimal signal-to-noise ratio (titre) for the same secondary reagent can differ depending on its application. Higher concentration of the secondary reagent can be used when cells are stained for surface molecules (5–10 μg/mL). However, when cells are stained for intracellular proteins, the concentration of the secondary reagent is frequently lower (1–5 μg/mL), because of an increase of background staining on fixed and permeabilized cells and thereby interfering with the signal-to-noise ratio. FITC conjugated $F(ab_2)$ fragments are preferred for intracellular staining, because of their relative low background staining (authors observations). These secondary reagents are available from several companies specialized in antibodies.

9. The same protocol, utilized for staining of one surface antigen, can be used for simultaneous staining of multiple surface proteins or surface proteins and cytoplasmic associated proteins, provided that the MAbs applied are of a different IgG subclass, e.g., IgG1 and IgG2a. The antimouse subclass specific secondary reagents, goat antimouse IgG1 and goat antimouse IgG2a, conjugated to different fluorochromes (e.g., FITC, RPE, RPE/Cy5), can also be mixed. Thus, the preparation time is not increased. Secondary reagents conjugated to Cy5 can also be used in cases of a flow cytometer equipped with a red-diode laser or helium-neon laser.

Recent developments in our laboratory demonstrate the ability to measure three cellular proteins in combination with high-resolution DNA content measurements of cell suspensions prepared from human cervical carcinomas using a double-laser bench-top flow cytometer. Unfortunately, a limiting factor for these kind of studies is the lack of high-quality directly conjugated MAbs. At present, MAbs must be carefully selected according to IgG subtype and IgG subclass specific secondary reagents must be used. Widely available directly conjugated MAbs will certainly facilitate the analysis of solid tumors by multiparameter flow cytometry.

10. It is essential to wash the cells with PBS before fixing with 1.0% paraformaldehyde (PF). The action of PF can be neutralized in the presence of proteins from fetal calf serum (FCS) or BSA. Cell membranes will be partly fixed and the addition of an agent used for permeabilization can then disrupt the cell membranes leading to loss of fluorescent signals from membrane stained molecules and loss of cells.

11. Lysolecithin (L-α-lysophosphatidylcholine, Sigma, product # L-4129) is a naturally occurring phospholipid, which can be isolated from egg yolk. Lysolecithin replaces phos-

pholipids in the membrane bilayer, which results in the loss of membrane integrity *(19)*. Dent et al. *(20)* were the first to demonstrate that lysolecithin could be combined with the protein crosslinker paraformaldehyde, thereby stabilizing the membrane protein layer, while simultaneously the phospholipid bilayer is permeabilized. This allowed the simultaneous detection of surface proteins and DNA or intracellular proteins and DNA. Optimal titre's can be obtained by titration. Surface protein expression and/or intermediate filament expression can be used as parameters for cell membrane integrity and optimal permeabilization, respectively (*see* **Figs. 3** and **4**).

12. After centrifugation it is essential to swirl the cells gently before adding fixatives to the cells. Adding paraformaldehyde to the cell pellet without swirling allows rapid formation of cell aggregates caused by chemical crosslinking of cell surface proteins. Also, sudden changes in osmolarity, e.g., from washing in PBS to denaturation in 100% methanol, will cause cell aggregation and cell loss. It is, therefore, recommended to add 100 µL of PBS to the cell pellet, then vortex the cells gently before adding the methanol dropwise.

13. A prolonged storage of the cells at 4°C in the presence of PI will improve the CV's of the DNA histograms peaks *(21)*. Stained and PF-fixed, lysolecithin permeabilized cells can be stored for several days at 4°C without significant loss of cell surface fluorescence (authors' observations).

## References

1. Corver, W. E., Cornelisse, C. J., Hermans, J., and Fleuren, G. J. (1995) Limited loss of nine tumor-associated surface antigenic determinants after tryptic cell dissociation. *Cytometry* **19,** 267–272.
2. Corver, W. E., Bonsing, B. A., Abeln, E. C. A., Vlak-Theil, P. M., Cornelisse, C. J., and Fleuren, G. J. (1996) One tube triple staining method for the flow cytometric analysis of DNA ploidy and phenotypic heterogeneity of human solid tumors using single laser excitation. *Cytometry* **25,** 358–366.
3. Ensley, J. F., Maciorowski, Z., Hassan, M., Pietraszkiewicz, H., Sakr, W., and Heilbrun, L. K. (1993) Variations in DNA aneuploid cell content during tumor dissociation in human colon and head and neck cancers analyzed by flow cytometry. *Cytometry* **14,** 550–558.
4. Engelholm, S. A., Spang Thomsen, M., Brunner, N., Nohr, I., and Vindelov, L. L. (1985) Disaggregation of human solid tumors by combined mechanical and enzymatic methods. *Brit. J. Cancer* **51,** 93–98.
5. Corver, W. E., Cornelisse, C. J., and Fleuren, G. J. (1994) Simultaneous measurement of two cellular antigens and DNA using fluorescein-isothiocyanate, R-phycoerythrin, and propidium iodide on a standard FACScan. *Cytometry* **15,** 117–128.
6. Abeln, E. C. A., Corver, W. E., Kuipers-Dijkshoorn, N. J., Fleuren, G. J., and Cornelisse, C. J. (1994) Molecular genetic analysis of flow-sorted ovarian tumor cells: Improved detection of loss of heterozygosity. *Brit. J. Cancer* **70,** 255–262.
7. Brockhoff, G., Endl, E., Minuth, W., Hofstädter, F., and Knüchel, R. (1996) Options of flow cytometric three-colour DNA measurements to quantitate EGFR in subpopulations of human bladder cancer. *Anal. Cell. Pathol.* **11,** 55–70.
8. Toba, K., Winton, E. F., and Bray, R. A. (1992) Improved staining method for the simultaneous flow cytofluorometric analysis of DNA content, S-phase fraction, and surface phenotype using single laser instrumentation. *Cytometry* **13,** 60–67.
9. Sasaki, D. T., Dumas, S. E., and Engleman, E. G. (1987) Discrimination of viable and non-viable cells using propidium iodide in two color immunofluorescence. *Cytometry* **8,** 413–420.
10. O'Brien, M. C. and Bolton, W. E. (1995) Comparison of cell viability probes compatible with fixation and permeabilization for combined surface and intracellular staining in flow cytometry. *Cytometry* **19,** 243–255.
11. Rabinovitch, P. S., Torres, R. M., and Engel, D. (1986) Simultaneous cell cycle analysis and two-color surface immunofluorescence using 7-amino-actinomycin D and singel laser excitation. Applications to study of cell activation and the cell cycle of murine Ly-1 B cells. *J. Immunol.* **136,** 2769–2777.
12. Schmid, I., Uittenbogaart, C. H., and Giorgi, J. V. (1991) A gentle fixation and permeabilization method for combined cell surface and intracellular staining with improved precision in DNA quantification. *Cytometry* **12,** 279–285.
13. Li, B. D. L., Harlow, S. P., Budnick, R. M., Sheedy, D. L., and Stewart, C. C. (1994) Detection of HER-2/neu oncogene amplification in flow cytometry-sorted breast ductal cells by competitive polymerase chain reaction. *Cancer* **73,** 2771–2778.

14. Van Hooijdonk, C. A. E. M., Glade, C. P., and Van Erp, P. E. J. (1994) TO-PRO-3 iodide: A novel HeNe laser-excitable DNA stain as an alternative for propidium iodide in multiparameter flow cytometry. *Cytometry* **17,** 185–189.
15. Hirons, G. T., Fawcett, J. J., and Crissman, H. A. (1994) TOTO and YOYO: New very bright fluorochromes for DNA content analyses by flow cytometry. *Cytometry* **15,** 129–140.
16. Glade, C. P., Van Erp, P. E. J., and Van de Kerkhof, P. C. M. (1996) Epidermal cell DNA content and intermediate filaments keratin 10 and vimentin after treatment of psoriasis with calcipotriol cream once daily, twice daily and in combination with clobetasone 17-butyrate cream or betamethasone 17-valerate cream: A comparative flow cytometric study. *Brit. J. Dermatol.* **135,** 379–384.
17. Bonsing, B. A., Corver, W. E., Gorsira, M. C. B., van Vliet, M., Oud, P. S., Cornelisse, C. J., et al. (1997) Specificity of seven monoclonal antibodies against p53 evaluated with Western blotting, immunohistochemistry, confocal laser scanning microscopy and flow cytometry. *Cytometry* **28,** 11–24.
18. Stewart, C. C. (1992) Clinical applications of flow cytometry: Immunologic methods for measuring cell membrane and cytoplasmic antigens. *Cancer* **69 Suppl.,** 1543–1552.
19. Schroff, R. W., Bucana, C. D., Klein, R. A., Farrell, M. M., and Morgan, A. C. J. (1984) Detection of intracytoplasmic antigens by flow cytometry. *J. Immunol. Meth.* **70,** 167–177.
20. Dent, G. A., Leglise, M. C., Pryzwansky, K. B., and Ross, D. W. (1989) Simultaneous paired analysis by flow cytometry of surface markers, cytoplasmic antigens, or oncogene expression with DNA content. *Cytometry* **10,** 192–198.
21. Bauer, K. (1993) Quality control issues in DNA content flow cytometry. *Ann. NY Acad. Sci.* **677,** 59–77.

# c-*erb*B-2 Immunohistochemistry in Paraffin Tumors

## Gamal H. Eltabbakh

## 1. Introduction

Immunohistochemistry is the study of the intracellular distribution of antigens based on the formation of an immune complex. The concept is based on the application of a specific antibody to the antigen to be detected and visualization of the antigen–antibody reaction with a staining procedure. Immunohistochemical staining allows direct observation of antigenic expression at the cellular level.

c-*erb*B-2, a protooncogene located in humans on chromosome 17q, encodes a transmembrane cell surface glycoprotein of 185 kD. c-*erb*B-2 expression can be found in a number of normal human tissues, including the ovary (*1*). Evidence for a tumorigenic role is suggested by the finding that overexpression of c-*erb*B-2 in NIH/3T3 cells is transforming and that transgenic mice bearing the c-*erb*B-2 oncogene driven by a mouse mammary tumor virus promoter develop mammary carcinomas (*2*). Activation of c-*erb*B-2 protooncogene has been described in a wide range of adenocarcinomas (*3–6*). In human tumors, amplification and overexpression are the most common mechanisms of c-*erb*B-2 activation (*3*).

c-*erb*B-2, also known as *HER-2/neu*, is amplified or overexpressed in up to 35% of ovarian cancers (*1,4–7*). Several studies (*5,8,9*) have suggested that c-*erb*B-2 overexpression is associated with a poor prognosis among patients with metastatic breast cancer. Reports investigating the role of c-*erb*B-2 overexpression in ovarian cancer are controversial. Some authors (*1,5*) have associated a high expression with a poorer prognosis; others (*6,7*) have not found such an association. It has been reported that c-*erb*B-2 overexpression might be associated with resistance to chemotherapeutic agents (*9*), e.g., cisplatin. Hancock et al. (*10*) have demonstrated that downregulation of the cell surface levels of c-*erb*B-2 in breast and ovarian cancer cells that overexpress this protooncogene can increase sensitivity to cisplatinum.

The use of formalin-fixed paraffin-embedded sections has the practical advantage of permitting large retrospective studies of archival material, which is particularly important in uncommon types of cancers. However, concern has been raised about the sensitivity of immunohistochemical techniques in formalin-fixed tissues, especially those stored for a prolonged period of time (*5*).

When immunostaining in frozen tissue sections was compared with immunostaining in formalin-fixed paraffin-embedded tissue sections from the same breast cancers, the

From: *Methods in Molecular Medicine, Vol. 39: Ovarian Cancer: Methods and Protocols*
Edited by: J. M. S. Bartlett © Humana Press, Inc., Totowa, NJ

number of positive cases for both polyclonal and monoclonal antibodies was reduced. Press et al. *(11)* found that compared to immunostaining of frozen sections and DNA analysis, these antibodies demonstrated varying (6–100%) sensitivities, but high (92–100%) specificities. Singleton et al. *(12)* found a significant correlation between overexpression detected by immunohistochemical staining and gene amplification detected by Western blotting.

Tannapfel et al. *(13)* compared the levels of c-*erb*B-2 oncogene protein product obtained from Western blot analysis to overexpression by immunohistochemistry of formalin-fixed sections. These authors demonstrated that positive staining can only be considered specific for c-*erb*B-2 if: 1) there is definite staining along the tumor cell membrane, with no predominant immunoreactivity inside the tumor cell cytoplasm; 2) the intensity of immunoreactivity is comparable with a positive standard (e.g., breast carcinoma); and 3) the surrounding, normal, nonneoplastic tissue shows no immunoreactivity.

## 2. Materials

1. The c-*erb*B-2 Monoclonal Antibody (mAb1) [c-*erb*B-2, Triton, Alameda, CA] used in the method described here is a mouse antibody against the extracellular domain of the c-*erb*B-2 oncogene protein *(2)*. NIH/3T3 cells stably transfected with the c-*erb*B-2 oncogene are the source of immunogen. The antibody is supplied in a lyophilized form with 1% bovine serum albumin (BSA) and 0.1% sodium azide in a phosphate-buffered saline (PBS) buffer. The concentration of the antibody is 25 µg/mL per vial. The antibody is reconstituted with 1.0 mL deionized or distilled water. The reconstituted antibody stability is 2 mo at 2–8°C. For long-term storage, aliquots should be frozen at –20°C or below.
2. PBS at pH 7.4.
3. Rabbit antimouse IgG 1:100 dilution in PBS at pH of 7.4 (DAKO, Santa Barbara, CA).
4. Buffer: 0.06 m$M$ 3.3-diaminobenzidene and 2 m$M$ hydrogen peroxide in 0.05% Tris-HCl at pH 7.6.
5. 0.1% Trypsin in PBS at pH 7.4.
6. Ethanol series: 100%, 95%.
7. 0.3% Hydrogen peroxide in methanol. Make fresh daily.
8. 2% Normal rabbit serum in PBS at pH7.4.
9. Peroxidase-conjugated rabbit antimouse IgG (1:100 dilution in PBS, DAKO).

## 3. Methods

The following steps describe the technique using the standard avidin-biotin-peroxidase complex (ABC) detection system and c-*erb*B-2 monoclonal antibody (*see* **Notes 1** and **2**).

1. Prepare 5-µm-thick paraffin-embedded sections from tissue blocks containing the tumor fixed in formalin (*see* **Note 3**).
2. Examine one of the slides obtained from the same tissue block microscopically after staining with hematoxylin and eosin under low and high powers to confirm the presence of tumor tissue in the slides to be processed by immunohistochemistry.
3. Use negative and positive controls. The positive control can be obtained from a section of tumor known to stain positively for c-*erb*B-2. The negative control should be a section of the same area of tumor stained with nonimmune mouse immunoglobulin G, rather than specific monoclonal antibody. Sections obtained from normal ovaries should also be processed and stained in the same way as sections containing tumor.

4. Deparaffinize sections as follows:
   a. Slides are left in 100% xylene for 1 h at room temperature in a fume hood.
   b. Heat slides to 60°C for 15 min.
   c. Two changes in 100% ethanol, 3 min each.
   d. Two changes in 95% ethanol, 1 min each.
   e. Dip slides 10 times in distilled water and then keep them in microwave buffer.
5. Incubate sections for 10 min with 0.1% trypsin solution in a humidified chamber at 37°C (*see* **Note 4**).
6. Block endogenous peroxidase activity by incubating sections in a freshly prepared solution of 0.3% hydrogen peroxide in methanol for 30 min at room temperature (*see* **Note 5**).
7. Incubate sections with 2% normal rabbit serum in PBS for 30 min in a humidified chamber at room temperature.
8. Incubate sections with 5–10 µg/mL of monoclonal antibody for 90 min in a humidified chamber at room temperature (*see* **Notes 6–9**).
9. Incubate sections with peroxidase-conjugated rabbit antimouse IgG (1:100 dilution in PBS, DAKO) for 60 min in a humidified chamber; wash in PBS.
10. Immerse sections for 5–10 min in a solution of 0.06 m$M$ 3.3-diaminobenzidene and 2 m$M$ hydrogen peroxide in 0.05% Tris-HCl buffered at pH 7.6.
11. Wash sections, counterstain with hematoxylin, wash again, and mount.

In **Fig. 1**, positive staining is identified by a brownish color in the cell membrane. Cytoplasmic staining is considered nonspecific. The sample is considered positive for c-*erb*B-2 staining if the grade of staining is clearly higher than the faint staining obtained in the epithelial cells of the normal ovaries.

## 4. Notes

1. The use of an automated immunostainer, e.g., Ventana 320 (Ventana Medical Systems Inc., Tuscon, AZ) provides a standardized technique that avoids human errors.
2. The multitumor (Sausage) tissue block is a method of embedding 100 or more different tissue samples in a normal-sized paraffin block *(15)*. This method allows the simultaneous immunohistologic testing of numerous tissue samples on a single slide with one drop of antibody.
3. Sections obtained from formalin-fixed archival material may show a peripheral effect, a phenomenon in which the periphery of the section does not stain or, conversely, is the only part of the specimen that does stain, depending on which antigen is sought and by what method *(14)*. Sections showing the peripheral effect are those in which formalin fixation was too short (3–6 h). In these sections, the tissues are fixed partially in formalin and partially in alcohol.
4. Trypsinization was found to enhance antibody reactivity and reduce background staining.
5. If the background staining is high, a more prolonged or a higher concentration of hydrogen peroxide solution should be used.
6. Various antibodies have demonstrated activity in immunohistochemical staining for c-*erb*B-2, e.g., polyclonal antibody 21N and the monoclonal antibodies TA1, NCL-CB11, and mAb1. Monoclonal antibodies TA1 and mAb1 are specifically reactive with the extracellular domain of c-*erb*B-2 whereas NCL-CB11 recognizes the internal domain of c-*erb*B-2.
7. If staining is faint, a prolonged incubation with the primary antibody (e.g., overnight) might enhance reactivity.
8. By immunohistochemistry, the antibody shows strong staining of tumor cell membranes and some diffuse cytoplasmic staining. Crossreactivity with the epidermal growth factor receptor (EGFR) was not observed.

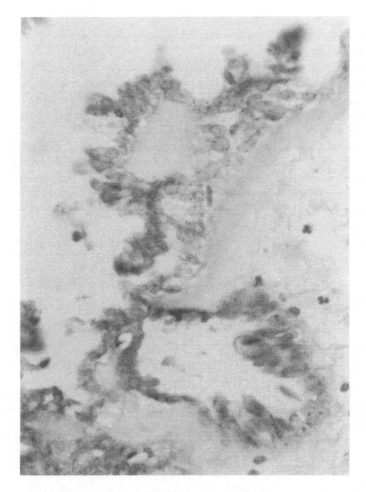

Fig. 1. A formalin-fixed section from an ovarian serous borderline tumor illustrating positive c-*erb*B-2 cytoplasmic membrane staining (original magnification × 486). Reproduced with
permission from Eltabbakh et al. *(7)*, W.B. Saunders, Inc.

9. An inherent disadvantage of immunohistochemical techniques, is the difficulty in quantitating expression levels precisely. Several semiquantitative methods have been described.
Sections could be graded for staining depending on the percentage of tumor cells
showing positive staining per 10 high-power fields, e.g., mild: 5–25%, moderate:
25–50%, strong: >50%. Microscope photometry and TV densitometry can be used for
more precise quantification.

## References

1. Berchuck, A., Kamel, A., Whitaker, R., Kerns, B., Olt, G., Kinney, R., et al. (1990) Overexpression
of *HER-2/neu* is associated with poor survival in advanced epithelial ovarian cancer. *Cancer Res.*
**50,** 4087–4091.
2. Di Fiore, P. P., Pierce, J. H., Kraus, M. H., King, C. R., Segatto, O., and Aaronson, S. A. (1987)
*erb*B-2 is a potent oncogene when overexpressed in NIH/3T3 cells. *Science* **237,** 178–182.
3. Slamon, D. J., Clark, G. M., Wong, S. G., Levin, W. J., Ullrich, A., and McGuire, W. L. (1987)
Human breast cancer: correlation of relapse and survival with amplification of the *HER-2/neu*
oncogene. *Science* **235,** 177–182.

4. Singleton, T. P. and Strickler, J. G. (1992) Clinical and pathologic significance of the c-erb-2 (HER-2/neu) oncogene. *Pathol. Annu.* **27,** 165–190.

5. Slamon, D. J., Godolphin, W., Jones, L. A., Holt, J. A., Wong, S. G., Keith, D. E., et al. (1989) Studies of the HER-2/neu proto-oncogene in human breast and ovarian cancer. *Science* **244,** 707–712.

6. Rubin, S. C., Finstad, C. L., Wong, G. Y., Almadrones, L., Plante, M., and Lloyd, K. O. (1993). Prognostic significance of HER-2/neu expression in advanced epithelial ovarian cancer: a multivariate analysis. *Am. J. Obstet. Gynecol.* **168,** 162–169.

7. Eltabbakh, G. H., Belinson, J. L., Kennedy, A. W., Biscotti, C. V., Casey, G., and Tubbs, R. R. (1997) P53 and HER-2/neu overexpression in ovarian borderline tumors. *Gynecol. Oncol.* **65,** 218–224.

8. Toikkanen, S., Helin, H., Isola, J., and Joensuu, H. (1992) Prognostic significance of HER-2 oncoprotein expression in breast cancer: a 30-year follow-up. *J. Clin. Oncol.* **10,** 1044–1048.

9. Gusterson, B. A., Goldhirsch, G. A., Price, K. N., Save-Soderborgh, J., Anbazhagan, R., Styles, J., et al. (1992) Prognostic importance of c-erbB-2 expression in breast cancer. *J. Clin. Oncol.* **10,** 1049–1056.

10. Hancock, M. C., Langton, B. C., Chan, T., Toy, P. Monahan, J. J., Mischak, R. P., and Shawver, L. K. (1991) A monoclonal antibody against the c-erbB-2 protein enhances the cytotoxicity of cis-diamminedichloroplatinum against human breast and ovarian tumor cell lines. *Cancer Res.* **51,** 4575–4580.

11. Press, M. F., Hung, G., Godolphin, W., and Slamon, D. J. (1994) Sensitivity of HER-2/neu antibodies in archival tissue samples: potential source of error in immunohistochemical studies of oncogene expression. *Cancer Res.* **54,** 2771–2777.

12. Singleton, T. P., Niehans, G. A., Gu, F., Litz, C. E., Hagen, K., Qiu, Q., et al. Detection of c-erbB-2 activation in paraffin-embedded tissue by immunohistochemistry. *Hum. Pathol.* **23,** 1141–1150.

13. Tannapfel, A., Kuhn, R., Kessler, H., and Wittekind, C. (1996) Expression of c-erbB-2 oncogene product in different tumors and its standardized evaluation. *Analy. Cell. Pathol.* **10,** 149–160.

14. Elias, J. M., Gown, A. M., Nakamura, R. M., Wilbur, D. C., Herman, G. E., Jaffe, E. S., et al. (1989) Special report: quality control in immunohistochemistry. Report of a workshop sponsored by the biological stain commission. *Am. J. Clin. Pathol.* **92,** 836–843.

15. Battifora, H. (1986) The multitumor (Sausage) tissue block: novel method for immunohistochemical antibody testing. *Lab Invest.* **55,** 244–248.

# 58

## Quantitative Immunohistochemistry of Estrogen and Progesterone Receptor Positivity in Ovarian Tumors

### A Rapid and Reliable Stereological Approach

**Gerrit A. Meijer, Paul J. van Diest, Jane Brugghe, and Jan P. A. Baak**

## 1. Introduction

Several assays exist to determine receptor status in ovarian cancers, like radio ligand binding assays, biochemical analysis, and even Northern blotting. However, pathologists generally prefer to judge the presence of biological markers in the context of tissue architecture, using immunohistochemistry (IHC). This allows for a better appreciation of exactly what in a tumor is positive for staining, and what is not.

However, the initial promising results of studies on the prognostic value of these markers could not always be confirmed *(1)*. This may be because of different methodological problems. First, there may have been selection of patients and differences in therapy. Second, there are often differences in tissue processing from study to study, especially with regard to the type of antibody and the application of antigen retrieval. Third, and possibly the most important, the interpretation of the staining and the presentation of the results are not standardized, with low intra- and interobserver reproducibility as a consequence. These problems are a very important obstruction for possible clinical applications. Therefore, a clear need exists for standardization of scoring of immunohistochemical staining, like ER/PR receptor in ovarian cancer.

For such a standardization, for the immunohistochemical scoring of ER/PR receptor, several items like staining patterns, tumor area to be assessed, sampling of fields of vision, scoring method, and decision thresholds need to be addressed (*see* Chapter 51).

### 1.1. Tissue Processing

There are several steps in tissue processing that may influence staining patterns and intensity. These include type and duration of fixation, section thickness, antigen retrieval procedures, type and concentrations of primary, second (and third) step antibodies, and way of staining development. For example, it has recently been reported that tumor marker-immunostaining intensity of several antigens including ER may be lost on stored paraffin slides of breast cancer *(2,3)*. For ER and PR, antibodies are available that work well on fresh frozen as well as formalin-fixed paraffin-embedded material. Staining of frozen material may be a little crisper and show less cytoplasmic

From: *Methods in Molecular Medicine, Vol. 39: Ovarian Cancer: Methods and Protocols*
Edited by: J. M. S. Bartlett © Humana Press, Inc., Totowa, NJ

staining, but using paraffin material is quite a good alternative. Obviously, proper positive and negative controls should be included in the staining batch.

## 1.2. Staining Patterns

In order to arrive at reproducible interpretation, there must be agreement on the significance of nuclear, diffuse cytoplasmic, or membrane staining for that specific antibody. Most antigens either localize (functionally) in the nucleus (such as *pRb*, *p53*, cyclin D1, steroid receptors), in the cytoplasm (*Bax*) or in the cellular membrane (*HER-2/neu*). Staining patterns other than the typical pattern for a given antibody (e.g., cytoplasmic instead of nuclear staining for steroid receptors or diffuse cytoplasmic instead of membrane staining for *HER-2/neu*) may have to be regarded as unfunctional and ignored. For ER and PR, only nuclear staining should be regarded as "real." Especially in paraffin sections, cytoplasmic staining is not uncommon, but this is rarely seen in fresh frozen material and should therefore be ignored.

## 1.3. Area to be Assessed

Although a purely random approach may sometimes be optimal, it will for most applications be necessary to define which part of the lesion contains the area of interest, in which the staining will be assessed. In general, several considerations can be made. For instance, invasive areas may be chosen over *in situ* parts, and for prognostic applications, as with ER/PR receptor status in ovarian cancers, the most poorly differentiated area of the tumor should be selected because this yields the best clinical correlations. However, for diagnostic applications the best differentiated tumor areas are usually most useful because typical antigen patterns are best preserved.

## 1.4. Sampling of Fields of Vision

Within the marked tumor area, it will usually be neither possible (considering the workload involved) nor necessary to assess all available fields of vision. Therefore, some form of sampling of fields of vision will have to be applied. It is a matter of experience *(4,5)* that this should not be left to the convenience of the observer because this will lead to interobserver variation and lack of reproducibility. Because some degree of clustering is usually present, the best way of sampling fields of vision is usually by systematically spreading them over the whole chosen tumor area. This assures that cells over the whole chosen area are assessed and will lead to the most representative sample and highest reproducibility *(4,5)*.

## 1.5. Assessment of Positivity of Immunohistochemical Staining

### 1.5.1. Qualitative Assessment

Qualitative assessment of immunohistochemical staining is widely used to visually judge whether any positivity of staining (as compared to the background) is present in the cells under study. This way of assessing positivity is in the daily practice often used for diagnostic reasons and is quite satisfactory for stains where the mere presence of antigens is informative irrespective of the degree of positivity or the fraction of positive cells, such as for keratins and CD31.

### 1.5.2. Quantitative Assessment

However, especially for antigens predictive of response to therapy or related to prognosis, as is the case with steroid receptors in ovarian cancers, one needs to be informed of the degree of positivity and the fraction of positive cells. A more sophisticated scoring procedure than qualitative assessment is then needed. Such staining has semiquantitatively been scored as – (negative), + (positive), ++ (strongly positive), or +++ (very strongly positive). Although this approach may be very intuitive, problems arise when there is heterogeneity in staining, e.g., it is usually not clear what to do with heavy staining in just a small number of cells. Some have advocated to report the staining intensity and the percentage of positive cells.

An even more refined method is the Histo-score *(6,7)*, where the fractions of negative (score 0), weakly positive (score 1), positive (score 2), strongly positive (score 3), and very strongly positive (score 4) cells are estimated, the fractions are multiplied with the scores and summed up, the total being the Histo-score. This method is widely applied to score steroid receptor positivity in breast cancer. However, in practice, the fractions are only roughly estimated without counting, and assigning a score to an individual nucleus is highly subjective. Studies have shown that the scoring of no staining (score 0) and 4 (very strong staining) is quite reproducible, but that there are many interobserver discrepancies in the scores 1–3 *(7)*. Therefore, this method is not optimal.

Alternatively, image analysis has been applied. Theoretically, image analysis allows the assessment of the amount of staining per cell by measuring absorption. However, in practice, IHC using di-aminobenzidine (DAB) as chromogen appeared to be only stoichiometric (meaning that there is a linear relationship between the amount of antigen and staining intensity as measured by degree of absorption) at low levels of intensity and not at the usual intensities used in daily immunohistochemistry *(8)*. This approach has therefore lost some of its initial popularity. Using the alkaline phosphatase antialkaline phosphatase (APAAP) approach or antibodies directly labeled with a fluorescent dye seems more promising to this end, but more experience has to be gained. Nevertheless, image analysis may well serve to objectively assess the number of positive cells *(9)*, although it remains a rather laborious and relatively expensive procedure.

Recently, an interactive approach for immunoscoring has been developed based on stereology *(10–12)* that is very quick, simple, and reproducible. In a defined area of the lesion, fields of vision systematically spread over the whole area of interest are chosen, as illustrated in **Fig. 1**. Because the first field is chosen at random, all fields are random, so this way of sampling is called systematic at random. This can be done manually, but is most efficiently done by means of a software-guided automatic scanning stage. In these fields of vision, cells are selected using a point grid, and the positivity of these cells is scored. The principle here is to sample relatively few cells from relatively many fields of vision, or the "do more less well" principle *(13,14)*. The number of fields of vision and cells to be assessed will vary from application to application and highly depends on the desired accuracy. In practice, for steroid receptor assessment in ovarian tumors, 200 cells sampled from 50–100 fields of vision will usually suffice to obtain a coefficient of variation < 5% *(11,13)*. However, on occasion (e.g., in case of values very close to the decision threshold) one may have to count more cells to reach an even higher accuracy. In general, it is not necessary to count 1000 cells as has been

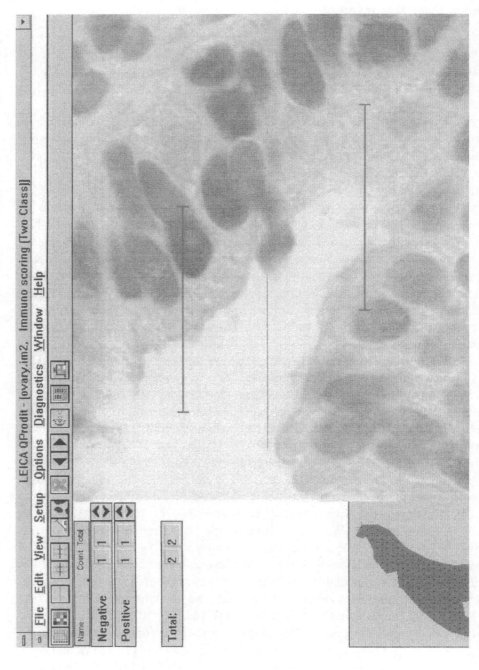

Fig. 1. Quantitative immunoscoring for estrogen receptor positivity in ovarian cancer with a video overlay system using systematic random sampling. The area of interest demarcated on the tissue section is represented by the dark field in the lower left corner. In each sampled field of vision, a line grid is projected over the image. Both ends of each line serve as probes for counting whether it hits a positive or a negative nucleus.

suggested *(15)*. Because fields spread over the whole area of interest are assessed (which copes best with clustering that is often observed) and selection of cells is done unbiased, this approach leads to highest reproducibility *(11)*. This approach is especially suitable for nuclear staining like steroid receptor staining in ovarian cancer, and allows to assess the percentage of positive cells, while as many categories for staining intensity (positive/ negative; positive/ weak/ negative; and so on) can be used if desired. However, it obviously does not overcome the problems involved in the subjective assessment of degree of positivity as pointed out above.

Nevertheless, the method proved to be robust in practice and good clinical correlations with this method already have been found for other nuclear immunohistochemical staining like *Ki76* and *p53* in Barrett's oesophagus *(12)*, *p53*, and cyclin D1 in breast cancer *(16)*, as well as the percentage of activated cytotoxic T-cells as a prognostic marker in Hodgkin's disease *(10)*. We have also applied this method to quantitation of ER in ovarian cancer. The results are described in detail below.

### 1.6. Choice of Cutoff Points

After having assessed the percentage of positive cells, the question is obviously how to choose the cutoff value for decision making on "positivity." To this end, different approaches may be followed. First, staining percentages may be compared with biochemical findings. Second, a cutoff point may be tuned to molecular biological results, e.g., presence of amplification on the DNA level or levels of mRNA. Third, one may derive a cutoff point from clinical studies taking clinical end points such as recurrence or survival, or response to a certain therapy. Preferably, such clinical cutoff points should be established in a learning set of patients and confirmed in an independent patient group. Also, cutoff points should be standardized from one study to another. This holds essentially, also, for semiquantitative scoring. For ER and PR in ovarian cancer, meaningful positivity thresholds have hardly been established.

### 1.7. Reporting

Results of immunoquantitation should preferably not just be reported as positive or negative, but the quantification method should be provided, as well as exact data from the quantitation and the decision threshold. This can be done by merely providing the data, but graphically presenting the data may be very illustrative and easy to understand. This also applies to the reporting of ER and PR quantitation in ovarian cancer.

## 2. Materials

### 2.1. Immunohistochemistry

1. Graded alcohols (95, 90, 80, 70, and 50%) in water.
2. 0.3% $H_2O_2$ in methanol.
3. Sodium citrate buffer (10 mmol, pH 6.0).
4. Phosphate-buffered saline (pH 7.4) (PBS).
5. Normal rabbit serum (NRS) (1:50 in PBS).
6. Normal swine serum (NSS) (1:10 in PBS).
7. Mouse antiestrogen receptor diluted 1:50 in PBS (DAKO, Glostrup, Denmark).
8. Biotinylated rabbit antimouse Ig diluted 1:100 in PBS (DAKO).

9. Rabbit antiprogesterone receptor 1:500 in PBS (DAKO).
10. Biotinylated swine antirabbit Ig 1:300 in PBS (DAKO).
11. StreptABComplex/HRP (DAKO).
12. Peroxidase substrate solution: 0.5 mg/mL 3,3'-diaminobenzidine tetrahydrochloride (DAB) (Sigma Chem. Co., St Louis, MO) and 0.02% (v/v) $H_2O_2$ in 100 mL PBS.
13. Storage medium: dissolve 17 g sucrose and 0.28 g $MgCl_2,6H_2O$ in 100 mL PBS, add 100 mL glycerol, mix well and store at $-20°C$.

## 2.2. Quantitative Analysis

1. A video-overlay measuring system consisting of a microscope equipped with: a CCD camera connected to a frame grabber card to display the microscope image on the computer screen (i.e., video overlay ), a motorized scanning stage that is software driven (optional).
2. Software: a computer program that: controls the scanning stage for the sampling of fields of vision (optional), handles video overlay, displays an adjustable point-grid over the microscopic image, provides counters and computes the area percentage of positive nuclei, and produces the required reports.

# 3. Methods

## 3.1. Immunohistochemistry

1. Cut 4-µm paraffin sections onto slides and dry at 37°C overnight.
2. Dewax in 100% acetone 2 × 5 min, rehydrate through graded alcohols 2 min each and (in case a mercury-containing fixative was used) depigment.
3. Rinse in tap water briefly.
4. Incubate in 0.3% $H_2O_2$ in methanol for 30 min at room temperature.
5. Rinse in tap water briefly.
6. Boil in citrate buffer (10 mmol, pH 6.0) in microwave oven for 3 × 5 min and allow to cool down to room temperature.
7. Rinse in tap water briefly.
8. Rinse in PBS 2 × 5 min.
9. Preincubate with: either normal rabbit serum (ER) or normal swine serum (PR) for 10 min.
10. Tap off serum and wipe away excess.
11. Incubate with primary antibody, either ER or PR, overnight at 4°C.
12. Rinse in PBS 3 × 10 min.
13. Incubate with secondary antibody for 30 min at room temperature (ER: rabbit anti-mouse Ig-biotin or PR: swine antirabbit Ig-biotin).
14. Incubate with streptABComplex/HRP kit according to the manufacturers instructions.
15. Rinse in PBS 3 × 10 min.
16. Incubate with peroxidase substrate solution for 3–5 min.
17. Rinse briefly in tap water and distilled water.
18. Counterstain and mount with cover slip.

## 3.2. Quantitative Analysis

In summary, for assessing steroid receptor status in ovarian cancer, we suggest an interactive stereological approach in a carefully defined part of the lesion. This approach consists of a systematic random sampling of fields of vision, preferentially guided by an automatic scanning stage, and assessment of positivity of cells in these fields selected with a point grid. Technically adequate slides are a prerequisite. An example of a protocol for such an approach is presented below:

1. Consider only the relevant staining pattern (i.e., nuclear staining for ER and PR receptor).
2. Define the area of the lesion to be assessed, which in the case of ovarian cancer should be epithelium rich with avoidance of necrosis, while only tumor cells should be judged.
3. In this area, apply a systematic random sampling approach for selection of a defined number of fields of vision.
4. In the fields of vision, assess positivity of cells selected with a point grid.
5. Define the number of cells to be assessed, using the principle that few cells should be sampled from many fields of vision (e.g., 2–4 cells from 50–100 fields of vision yielding a total of 200 counts).
6. Count the number of points falling either on positive nuclei ($P$) or on negative nuclei ($N$).
7. Calculate the area percentage of positive nuclei as $P/(P+N)*100$.
8. Define cutoff value and define how the results should be reported.

Such methods are fast, simple, and highly reproducible. Application of such protocols will yield to more objective data on the distribution of antigens in different lesions, which will be better comparable from study to study, and sooner lead to clinically applicable tests.

## 4. ER Assessment in Ovarian Cancer by Semiautomated Immunoquantitation: Clinical Correlations

Immunoquantitation as described above was carried out in a group of 21 patients with ovarian carcinomas of different stages, and results were correlated to a subjectively assessed Histo-score, and morphometrically assessed differentiation characteristics like nuclear area, mitotic activity, and volume percentage of epithelium. Immunohistochemical staining for ER was done on 4-µm paraffin sections with the Anti-ER monoclonal antibody (DAKO) in a 1:50 dilution, using a standard avidin-biotin-peroxidase complex (ABC) method by means of an automatic staining device (Ventana 320, Ventana Medical Systems Inc., Tucson, AZ), after antigen retrieval by boiling in citrate buffer for two times 10 min using a microwave oven. A modified Histo-score method was used for subjective scoring of positivity by estimating the percentages of negative (score 0), weakly positive (score 1), positive (score 2), and strongly positive (score 3), multiplying the percentages with the scores, and taking the total of these multiplications *(17)*. The percentage of ER positive nuclei was assessed with semiautomated immunoscoring as described above.

Mitoses were counted in 25 consecutive fields of vision at a magnification of x400 (field diameter 450 µm) in the most poorly differentiated area of the tumor, and the total was taken as the mitotic activity index (MAI). Volume percentage of epithelium (VPE), mean and standard deviation of nuclear area (MNA and SDNA, respectively) were measured using a video overlay system (QPRODIT, Leica, Cambridge, UK) as described before *(18)*. Correlations between these variables were assessed by linear regression analysis and the Mann-Whitney U test.

The Histo-score results correlated well with the percentage of ER positive nuclei ($r = 0.92$, $p = 0.000$, **Fig. 2**). Taking 10% positive nuclei (on quantitative immunohistochemistry) as cutoff, 13 cases were ER negative, and 8 were positive. Mean nuclear area and the standard deviation of nuclear area both were significantly higher ($p = 0.02$, $p = 0.02$, respectively) in ER negative ovarian cancers as compared to ER

Fig. 2. Correlation between histoscore and stereological assessment of the area percentage of ER positive nuclei in 21 ovarian cancers.

Fig. 3. Box plots for **(A)** mean nuclear area (MNA) and **(B)** standard deviation of nuclear area (SDNA) in 21 ovarian cancers. Cancers were grouped according to a stereologically assessed area percentage of ER positive nuclei < 10% (negative) or > 10% (positive).

542

Fig. 3B.

positive cancers (**Fig. 3**). For the mitotic activity index and the volume percentage of epithelium, trends were found in the same direction, but these differences did not reach statistical significance.

This shows that expression of the ER in ovarian cancer correlates with low mean and SD of nuclear area, which are correlated with a better prognosis *(18,19)*. Such correlations have also been described in breast cancer *(20)*, and indicate that ER expression parallels cytonuclear differentiation and low proliferation.

The results also indicate that in ovarian tumors, the assessment of the percentage positively stained by semiautomated immunoquantitation is as effective and possibly prognostically relevant as the much more subjective Histo-score, and that the staining intensity may be less relevant.

## Acknowledgments

We thank Mark Broeckaert and Brechje Harmsen for their help with the morphometric assessments, and Drs. Rik Mullink and Jaap Lagendijk for providing the immunohistochemically stained slides and Histo-score data.

## References

1. Brinkhuis, M., Meijer, G. A., and Baak, J. P. A. (1995) An evaluation of prognostic factors in advanced ovarian cancer. A review. *Eur. J. Obst. Gyn. Reprod. Biol.* **63,** 115–124.
2. Henson, D.E. (1996) Loss of p53-immunostaining intensity in breast cancer. *J. Natl. Cancer. Inst.* **88,** 1015,1016.
3. Jacobs, T. W., Prioleau, J. E., Stillman, I. E., and Schnitt, S. J. (1996) Loss of tumor marker-immunostaining intensity on stored paraffin slides of breast cancer. *J. Natl. Cancer Inst.* **88,** 1054–1059.

4. Fleege, J. C., van Diest, P. J., and Baak, J. P. A. (1990) Computer assisted efficiency-testing of different sampling methods for selective nuclear graphic tablet morphometry. *Lab. Invest.* **63**, 270–275.

5. Fleege, J. C., van Diest, P. J., and Baak J. P. A. (1993) Systematic random sampling for selective interactive nuclear morphometry in breast cancer sections. Refinement and multiobserver evaluation. *Anal. Quant. Cytol. Histol.* **15**, 281–289.

6. Bosman, F. T., Goeij, A. F. P. M., and de Rousch, M. (1992) Quality control in immunocytochemistry: experiences with the oestrogen receptor assay. *J. Clin. Pathol.* **45**, 120–124.

7. van Diest, P. J., Weger, A. R., and Lindholm, J. (1996) Reproducibility of subjective immunoscoring of steroid receptors in breast cancer. *Analyt. Quant. Cytol. Histol.* **18**, 351–354.

8. Fritz, P., Wu, X., Tuczek, H., Multhaupt, H., and Schwarzmann, P. (1995) Quantitation in immunohistochemistry. A research method or a diagnostic tool in surgical pathology? *Pathologica* **87**, 300–309.

9. Makkink-Nombrado, S. V., Baak, J. P. A., Schuurmans, L., Theeuwes, J. W., and vander Aa, T. (1995) Quantitative immunohistochemistry using the CAS 200/486 image analysis system in invasive breast carcinoma: a reproducibility study. *Anal. Cell. Pathol.* **8**, 227–245.

10. Oudejans, J. J., Jiwa, N. M., Kummer, J. A., Ossenkoppele, G. J., van Heerde, P., Baars, J. W., et al. (1997) Activated cytotoxic Tcells as prognostic marker in Hodgkin's disease. *Blood* **89**, 1376–1382.

11. Polkowski, W., Meijer, G. A., Baak, J. P. A, Kate, F. J. W., Obertop, H., Offerhaus, G. J. A., et al. (1997) Reproducibility of p53 and Ki67 immuno-quantitation in Barrett's oesophagus. *Analyt. Quant. Cytol. Histol.* **19**, 246–254.

12. Polkowski, W., Baak, J. P. A., van Lanschot, J. J. B., Meijer, G. A., Schuurmans, L. T., Kate, F. J. W., et al. (1998) Clinical decision making in Barrett's oesophagus can be supported by computerized immunoquantitation and morphometry of features associated with proliferation and differentiation. *J. Pathol.* **184**, 161–168.

13. Brugghe, J., Baak, J. P. A., Meijer, G. A., van Diest, P. J., and Brinkhuis, M. (1998) Rapid and reliable assessment of volume percentage of epithelium in borderline and invasive ovarian tumors. *Analyt. Quant. Cytol. Histol.* **20**, 14–20.

14. Gundersen, H. J. G. and Osterby, R. (1981) Optimizing sampling efficiency of stereological studies in biology: or "Do more less well!" *J. Microsc.* **121**, 65–73.

15. Hall, P. A., Richards, M. A., Gregory, W. M., d'Ardenne, A. J., Lister, T. A., and Stansfeld, A. G. (1988) The prognostic value of Ki67 immunostaining in non-Hodgkin's lymphoma. *J. Pathol.* **154**, 223–235.

16. van Diest, P. J., Michalides, R. J. A. M., Jannink, I., vander Valk, P., Peterse, J. L., de Jong, J. S., et al. (1997) Cyclin D1 expression in invasive breast cancer: correlations and prognostic value. *Am. J. Pathol.* **150**, 705–711.

17. Lagendijk, J. H., Mullink, H., van Diest, P. J., Meijer, G. A., and Meijer, C. J. L. M (1998) Tracing the origin of adenocarcinomas with unknown primary using immunohistochemistry. Differential diagnosis between colonic and ovarian carcinomas as primary sites. *Hum. Pathol.* **29**, 491–497.

18. Brinkhuis, M., Meijer, G. A., Lund, B., and Baak, J. P. A. (1996) Quantitative pathological variables as prognostic factors for overall survival in Danish patients with FIGO stage III ovarian cancer. *Int. J. Gynecol. Cancer* **6**, 168–174.

19. Brinkhuis, M., Baak, J. P. A., Meijer, G. A., van Diest, P. J., Mogensen, O., Bichel, P., and Neijt, J. P. (1996) Value of quantitative pathological variables as prognostic factors in advanced ovarian carcinoma. *J. Clin. Pathol.* **49**, 142–148.

20. Baak, J. P. A. and Persijn, J. P. (1984) In search for the best qualitative microscopical or morphometrical predictor of oestrogen receptor in breast cancer. *Path. Res. Pract.* **178**, 307–314.

# 59

# Radioimmunohistochemistry

*Quantitative Analysis of Cell Surface Receptors in Frozen Sections*

## Jonathan R. Reeves

## 1. Introduction

Radioimmunohistochemistry was developed for quantitation of epidermal growth factor receptors (EGFR) and the c-*erb*B-2 protein and applied in breast tumors. With appropriate preliminary development, the method can be extended to other antigens and tissues. Radioimmunohistochemistry has confirmed that relationships between EGFR and c-*erb*B-2 expression levels and disease endpoints exist that are not apparent when the receptors are measured with existing semiquantitative methods. The technique was pioneered in 1984 (*1*) for measurements of EGFR in squamous tumors and then modified (*2*) and applied to quantify the c-*erb*B-2 protein in breast carcinomas (*3*) using the ICR12 rat monoclonal antibody (*4*) (Dr. Chris Dean, Institute of Cancer Research, Sutton, London, U.K.). Although radioimmunohistochemistry is conceptually simple and reveals reliable quantitative data, considerable preliminary work is required for each new antigen and the technique itself is time consuming. For these reasons, careful consideration is necessary prior to being committed to a project based on the method. In this chapter, the application of radioimmunohistochemistry for the measurement of c-*erb*B-2 expression in frozen sections is described.

Radioimmunohistochemistry (summarized in **Fig. 1**) is a direct immunohistochemical method using [125]I labeled monoclonal antibodies. The method is truly quantitative because there is no risk of nonlinear amplification steps through secondary antibodies and tertiary reagents. Frozen sections are preferred because formalin fixation and paraffin embedding in archival tissues frequently results in inconsistent labeling requiring very careful controls for quantitation. After incubation with the radiolabeled antibody, the sections are washed, fixed, and dried before a rough idea of the amount of bound antibody on each section is obtained by film autoradiography. This allows an estimation of the appropriate duration of exposure for the final microautoradiography stage of the procedure where the sections are coated with autoradiographic emulsion. Correct exposure results in the development of a suitable density of single silver grains for counting. Too long and the grains merge and cannot be counted as single entities by image analysis, too short and insufficient grains develop. The density of silver grains is proportional to the amount of radioactivity, which in turn is proportional to the amount

From: *Methods in Molecular Medicine, Vol. 39: Ovarian Cancer: Methods and Protocols*
Edited by: J. M. S. Bartlett © Humana Press, Inc., Totowa, NJ

Fig. 1. Schematic of the steps involved in Radioimmunohistochemistry.

of bound antibody and so to the antigen concentration in the sections. Calibration standards of cell lines with known levels of the c-*erb*B-2 protein are processed in parallel to ensure quantitation and consistency between batches. These are, in ascending order of receptor density: MCF7 (almost negative), ZR-75-1 (low), MDAMB453 (low moderate), MDAMB361 (high moderate), SKBR3, SKOV3, and BT474 (high). Exceptionally high c-*erb*B-2 levels are found in the N87 gastric carcinoma cell line. (All available from the American-type cell-culture collection.)

## 2. Materials
### 2.1. Antibody Iodination

1. 15 µg antibody in about 150 µL PBS (10 m$M$ sodium phosphate, 140 m$M$ sodium chloride, pH 7.4) with no other protein.
2. 10 MBq $^{125}$I (iodination grade). Local rules for handling radioisotopes must be followed.
3. Iodogen coated silica glass tube (*see* **Note 1**).
4. Sephadex G25 gel filtration column equilibrated with four volumes of PBS (5 mL prepacked columns are convenient).
5. Xylene cyanole. 10 mg/mL in PBS.
6. Nonimmune rabbit serum.

### 2.2. Section Labeling

1. Silanized glass slides (*see* **Note 2**).
2. Frozen sections of control cell lines and tissues (*see* **Notes 3 and 4**).
3. Rabbit serum.
4. $^{125}$I labeled antibody (about 1 MBq or 3 µg per 100 cases) and unlabeled antibody (about 700 µg per 100 cases, *see* **Note 5**).
5. Acetone.
6. 2% formalin (50:50 mix of PBS and routine histological 4% formalin).

### 2.3. Film Autoradiography

1. Autoradiography cassettes.
2. Dupont Cronex film (other brands are probably as effective).

### 2.4. Microautoradiography

1. Autoradiographic emulsion. Kodak NTB2 emulsion (IBI Limited, 36 Clifton Road, Cambridge, U.K, *see* **Note 6**).
2. D19 developer. Commercially available or prepare by dissolving 2 g metol, 8 g hydroquinone, 90 g anhydrous sodium sulphite, 45 g anhydrous sodium carbonate, 5 g potassium bromide in 1 L distilled water. Store this stock solution at 4°C in the dark in an airtight bottle. If contents oxidize (go dark brown), discard and make fresh. Working solution is diluted 1:1 with distilled water and stored similarly.
3. Fixer. Use Kodak Unifix fixer, or an alternative suggested by the emulsion manufacturers. Some rapid-fix ammonium based fixers are not suitable for the emulsion.
4. Safranin (Basic Red). Dissolve 10 g of safranin in 1 L of distilled water. The stain is taken up by tissues under alkaline conditions, so before use, add a few drops of 2$M$ sodium hydroxide. If the solution loses effectiveness, add a few more drops of alkali or replace.

## 3. Methods
### 3.1. Antibody Iodination (Iodogen method)

1. Pipet the antibody into the base of the iodogen coated tube (*see* **Note 1**), and add the $^{125}$I.
2. Leave for 5 min and stop the reaction by making up to 1 mL with 50% rabbit serum. Add 50 µL of 10 mg/mL xylene cyanol (low molecular-weight marker).
3. Carefully load the labeled antibody mix onto the top of the equilibrated G25 gel filtration column and allow to flow into the column.
4. Elute with PBS and collect the high molecular weight fraction appearing before the xylene cyanole. (*see* **Note 7**.)

5. Determine the approximate specific activity by counting radioactivity associated with a fraction of the labeled antibody and by assuming that most of the antibody has been collected (*see* **Note 8**).

## 3.2. Section Labeling

1. Using properly frozen and stored tissues and cell lines (*see* **Note 3**) cut onto the bottom third of silanized slides *(2)* high-quality 5-μm frozen sections (*see* **Note 4**). For each specimen, cut two test sections and one control section. In addition, prepare sections for haematoxylin and eosin staining and conventional immunohistochemistry if required.
2. Ring sections with a water-impermeable pen (DAKO Ltd., High Wycombe, U.K.), fix in absolute acetone for 5 min and wash in PBS for 5 min.
3. Block nonspecific binding with 80 μL of 50% serum for 10 min (any species is acceptable, but we use rabbit serum). The control sections should have 5 μg of unlabelled antibody included in each 80 μL of blocking serum (*see* **Note 5**).
4. Prepare radiolabeled antibody stock by adjusting the specific activity with unlabeled antibody so that 1 mL contains 2.5 μg of antibody and 50 Kbq $^{125}$I.
5. Add 20 μL of radiolabeled antibody stock (each aliquot contains 50 ng of antibody and 1 Kbq $^{125}$I) directly to the blocking solution on each test and control section. Mix and allow the sections to incubate for 3 h in a humidified box. If the sections are large, double aliquots of blocking solution and antibody are acceptable.
6. Rinse off the unbound radiolabeled antibody with PBS and wash through three changes of PBS (2 min each).
7. Fix sections in 2% formalin for 10 min and wash through three changes of distilled water (2 min each) before air-drying the sections.

## 3.3. Film Autoradiography

1. Take one test section from each tissue specimen and tape down in an autoradiography cassette.
2. Lay film directly on sections (we use Dupont Cronex, but other brands are sufficient) and expose for approx 96 h.
3. Develop film and use to estimate the duration of exposure for the microautoradiography (*see* **Note 9**).

## 3.4. Microautoradiography

Dipping the sections in emulsion should be done in a suitably equipped clutter-free darkroom under a Wratten Number 2 safe lamp (very deep red).

1. Melt the working emulsion solution (1:1 emulsion:distilled water) by warming to 43°C in a water bath (*see* **Note 6**).
2. After about an hour, dip blank test slides to ensure that the emulsion is fully melted and bubble free. When satisfactory test slides have been obtained, start on the experimental ones.
3. Dip test slides into the emulsion vertically and withdraw slowly. Hold in a vertical position for a few seconds and wipe off excess emulsion from the back and base of the slide. Allow the slides to air-dry in a near vertical position for about 30 min. Check the slides under the safe lamp for even emulsion coating and no streaking over the section.
4. Once dry, load the sections up into microscope slide racks and place into lightproof boxes containing a desiccant such as silica gel and expose at 4°C.
5. After the appropriate exposure, place slides in a 1:1 dilution of D19 developer with distilled water at exactly 10°C for 4 min.

6. Rinse in distilled water for 1 min, and fix in Kodak Unifix fixer for 5 min.
7. After 20 min of washing in tap water, counterstain the sections lightly for 30 s with safranin, if necessary destain sections in 70% ethanol or 1% HCl in 70% ethanol in heavily overstained cases, dehydrate rapidly through alcohols (30 s in each) clear in two changes of xylene and mount in DPX. Dry for at least 1 wk before attempting counting.

## 3.5. Analysis

The precise make and model of image-analysis equipment is not crucial as long as it measures accurately the area of user-defined fields and number of silver grains within those areas. The equipment that we have the most experience with is a Joyce Loebl MiniMagiScan system connected to an Olympus OM-2 microscope via a monochrome video camera. Full or partial fields are selected by the operator and counted under a 40x objective and the grain counts from 10 such areas from different regions of the section are summed (10 full fields with this equipment is 0.1355 mm$^2$). During the counting procedure, the safranin counterstain is filtered out with a red filter to increase the contrast of the grains. The Joyce Loebl equipment was manufactured in the late 1980s and there are now more sophisticated and faster systems on the market. For each test and cell line control specimen, there should be three counts measured in grains per unit area, one for each test section and one for the negative control section. Determine the specific counts per unit area for each specimen and calculate the c-*erb*B-2 expression in the tissues (*see* **Notes 10–13**).

## 4. Notes

1. Preparation of iodogen coated glass tubes.
   a. Dissolve 0.5 mg of iodogen in 1 mL of chloroform.
   b. Pipet 50 μL aliquots of the dissolved iodogen solution in the base of 2 mL silica glass tubes.
   c. Allow the chloroform to evaporate and store the tubes in a dark and dry environment. Under these conditions the iodogen will remain stable for several years.
2. Silanized slides.
   a. Place clean slides in absolute acetone for 5 min.
   b. Transfer to acetone containing 20% 3-aminopropyl triethoxysilane for 5 min.
   c. Wash in running tap water for 30 min.
   c. Air-dry and store as for untreated slides.
3. Tissue freezing.
   a. Freeze fresh tissues (no more than 1 cm$^3$) directly in liquid nitrogen to minimize ice crystal formation and store short term at –70°C or in liquid nitrogen for the long term.
   b. For cell lines, scrape subconfluent cultures from the plastic (no trypsin), pellet at 300*g* for 5 min using a centrifuge tube with a conical base (a plastic 25-mL universal works well), aspirate the supernatant, and freeze pellets by holding the tube in liquid nitrogen. The frozen pellets can be detached by giving the base of the tube a sharp blow on the bench and stored as for the tissues.
4. Section cutting. With care, hundreds of quality 5-μm frozen sections can be obtained from a single piece of tissue or cell pellet. It is essential to have properly frozen and stored tissue, a cryostat that remains at cutting temperature (about –20°C for breast cancer tissues) and a sharp knife.
   a. Take stored tissue and transfer directly to the cryostat, when it attains cryostat temperature, place into a puddle of cooled cryostat mountant on a cork disk. It is essential

that the tissue does not approach thawing temperature at this point to prevent morphological damage, so the cork disk and tissue should be lowered gently into liquid nitrogen until the mountant is fully frozen.

b. Freeze the cork disk to the cryostat chuck using a small amount of water and cut sections.

c. Thaw sections onto silanized slides and allow to air-dry for about an hour. For dipping autoradiography, the sections should be placed on the lower third of the microscope slides.

d. After cutting sufficient sections, the cork disk can be detached by warming the chuck and the tissue block can be returned to cold storage.

e. Store sections by stacking with spacers between each slide (masking tape strips suffice) wrap in aluminium foil and place at –20°C for short-term or –70°C for longer term storage. It is essential to allow the foil packages to return fully to room temperature before unwrapping, otherwise condensation forms on the sections causing morphological damage.

5. Controls. If the antibody is not available in sufficiently large quantities, an iodinated isotype matched irrelevant control antibody can be used in place of the primary antibody.

6. NTB2 emulsion is supplied as a gel which melts on warming. A safe temperature for preparing the emulsion is 43°C; any warmer and background grains within the emulsion will increase. For radioimmunohistochemistry, slides should be dipped in a 1:1 mix of emulsion and distilled water. A dipping container with a diameter a little wider than a microscope slide will ensure minimal wastage of the emulsion. Both the concentrate and working emulsion can be stored at 4°C in lightproof containers. The shelf life is governed by the level of background grains in emulsion not exposed to radiation, and this can markedly exceed the expiry date suggested by the manufacturers.

7. The material eluting with the xylene cyanole will be the low molecular-weight fraction, or the unbound iodine. This can be left in the column and disposed of as solid waste or eluted as liquid waste depending on the local rules for radioactive disposal.

8. With EGF receptor and c-*erb*B-2 antibodies, we typically get about half of the radioactivity incorporated or 5 Mbq in 15 µg of antibody in a total volume of about 2.5 mL (volume dependent on the size of the gel filtration column). Using a gamma counter with 70% $^{125}$I counting efficiency, each microliter of the labeled antibody should give 84,000 counts per min (2 Kbq). The specific activity can be adjusted by varying the length of the iodogen reaction. If there is a very low specific activity, question the iodogen tubes or the gel filtration. The iodinated antibody can be used for up to 4 wk. Store in aliquots behind lead shielding at –20°C.

9. Film autoradiography. As a rough guide to estimate the exposure for microautoradiography, sections with less expression than ZR75 cells should have maximum exposure (100 or more hours). Those with similar levels to MDAMB453 cells about 48 h, MDAMB361 cells 24 h, and those with high expression about 4 h.

10. Analysis. For each cell line and test specimen, calculate the specific grain counts per mm$^2$ per h of emulsion exposure. For very long exposures, it may be necessary to correct for radioactive decay, but this should not be a significant source of error if all the sections from one batch are developed within 4 d. Using the counts from the calibration standards, calculate the conversion factor for the batch of sections using the following equation:

$$[(ZR75 \div 1100) + (MDAMB453 \div 4900) + (MDAMB361 \div 13000) \\ + (BT474 \div 58000) + (SKBR3 \div 60900] \div 5$$

Use this factor to multiply the grains/mm$^2$/h for each test specimen for an estimation of their c-*erb*B-2 densities in molecules per square micron *(2)*. If the conversion factor for each cell line is wildly different (more than a factor of two) then it may be necessary to reevaluate the controls for your own batches of cell lines.

11. Assay for epidermal growth factor receptors. This is essentially similar to the c-*erb*B-2 assay, except that we use 50 ng of the EGFR1 antibody (5) and 4 Kbq of $^{125}$I per section. This higher specific activity is used because EGFR expression is generally lower than that of c-*erb*B-2. Cell line standards are ZR75-1 and MCF7 (low), SKBR3 (moderate low), EJ bladder carcinoma line (moderate high), BT20 breast carcinoma cell line (high), and A431 vulval carcinoma line (very high).

12. Sensitivity. Radioimmunohistochemistry is quantitative over a wide range of expression levels primarily because the emulsion exposure is adjusted to suit the level of expression in each section. Using the procedure described here, radioimmunohistochemistry gives quantitative results in cases that label negatively with 3 step streptavidin biotin complex immunohistochemistry using the same primary antibody. Sensitivity can be further increased by extending the emulsion exposure (half-life of $^{125}$I is 60 d) or by increasing the specific activity of the antibody. This latter measure may result in elevated background counts though.

13. Time Scales. Generally we find it most economical to process batches of about 100 cases (about 400 sections in total) with each iodination. Section labeling is carried out over 3 d with about 130 slides being processed each day (test cases and cell line controls for each day). The film autoradiograph is exposed for 3 or 4 d (over the weekend) and the slides are organised into racks dependent on their planned emulsion exposure. Dipping and development of the emulsion requires organization but is a relatively efficient process. If the processing of these sections is completed within 3 wk of the iodination, it is possible to process a further batch of 100 cases. With our original Joyce Loebl image-analysis equipment, it was possible for one operator to obtain grain counts from 10 to 15 cases per day. However, there was considerable wastage of time waiting for the system. With the faster machines now available, results should be attainable from twice as many cases. Although radioimmunohistochemistry is time consuming relative to conventional immunohistochemistry, that time is often a small proportion of an entire study if the time taken to collect and store tissue, prepare sections, obtain follow-up data and generate manuscripts is taken into consideration. Radioimmunohistochemistry yields true quantitative data and can provide validation for or highlight limitations of simpler and less-precise methods.

## References

1. Hendler, F. J. and Ozanne, B. W. (1984) Human squamous cell lung cancers express increased epidermal growth factors. *J. Clin. Investigat.* **74**, 647–651.
2. Reeves, J. R., Going, J. J., Smith, G., Cooke, T. G., Ozanne, B. W., and Stanton, P. D. (1996) Quantitative radioimmunohistochemical measurements of p185(erbB-2) in frozen tissue sections. *J. Histochem. Cytochem.* **44**, 1251–1259.
3. Robertson, K. W., Reeves, J. R., Smith, G., Keith, W. N., Ozanne, B. W., Cooke, T. G., and Stanton, P. D. (1996) Quantitative estimation of epidermal growth factor receptor and c-erbb2 in human breast cancer. *Cancer Res.* **56**, 3823–3830.
4. Styles, J. M., Harrison, S., Gusterson, B. A., and Dean, C. J. (1990) Rat monoclonal antibodies to the external domain of the product of the C-erbB-2 proto-oncogene. *Int. J. Cancer* **45**, 320–324.
5. Waterfield, M. D., Mayes, E. L. V., Stroobant, P., Bennet, P. L. P., Young, S., Goodfellow, P. N., et al. (1982) A monoclonal antibody to the human epidermal growth factor receptor. *J. Cell. Biochem.* **20**, 149–161.

# VIII

# SIGNAL TRANSDUCTION

# 60

## Signal Transduction

*A Technical Overview*

### M. Jane Arboleda and Dennis J. Slamon

### 1. Introduction

Delineation of downstream signal transduction pathways is important for determining which intracellular signals contribute to the malignant phenotype of cancer cells. In this review, we discuss current methodologies used to study cell signaling. A number of factors that may influence the specificity of signaling will also be taken into consideration. Furthermore, because the *HER-2* receptor is amplified and overexpressed in ovarian cancers, we refer to this receptor and its downstream signaling pathways as model systems throughout this review.

Binding of growth factors to their cognate receptors results in receptor dimerization and transphosphorylation of specific tyrosine residue in the receptor carboxy terminal domain. These phosphorylated residues serve as docking sites for SH2-containing proteins and are necessary for further signal transmission. The *HER-2* receptor is activated by both receptor overexpression and by growth factor (heregulin) binding to *HER-2/HER-3* and *HER-2/HER-4* heterodimers. Activated receptor complex triggers the recruitment of *grb2/sos*, which in turn promotes *ras*-binding guanosine 5′-triphosphate (GTP) and the recruitment of *Raf* to the plasma membrane. Activated *Raf* phosphorylates and activates MEK, which in turn phosphorylates and activates MAP kinases. Activated MAP kinases then translocate to the nucleus and activate a variety of transcription factors, which ultimately govern the biological effects through induction of the requisite genes. A linear road map, such as the one described above, for the activation of the *ras* pathway can be elucidated for other growth-factor receptors or cytoplasmic-signaling molecules using several approaches.

### 2. Cell Signaling Turned "On" or "Off"

One approach to deciphering which signal pathways are important for a specific biological effect is to selectively turn signaling "on." Activation of a signal transduction pathway can be accomplished by expression of a constitutive active mutant where critical residues have been substituted *(1)* or deleted to mimic activation; by overexpression of critical genes in the pathways *(2)*; or by ligand binding to cognate receptors *(3,4)*.

From: *Methods in Molecular Medicine, Vol. 39: Ovarian Cancer: Methods and Protocols*
Edited by: J. M. S. Bartlett © Humana Press, Inc., Totowa, NJ

For example, N-terminal truncation of *Raf*, MEK, or ERK, which exerts a negative regulation on the catalytic domain, also results in an increase in kinase activity *(5)*. Furthermore, it is well established that cytoplasmic proteins such as *ras* and *Raf* require membrane localization for activity. Although it is not clear what occurs at the plasma membrane, artificial targeting of cytoplasmic signaling molecules to the plasma membrane by the CAAX or myristylation sequence can markedly increase their catalytic activity. "Raf-CAAX" is a fusion protein consisting of the Raf protein and the CAAX motif of *Ki-ras (6)*. Likewise, the "myr-AKT," which also has elevated activity, is a chimeric protein consisting of the myristylation sequence of the lck protein fused to the N-terminus of the AKT/PKB protein *(7)*. Another approach to directly activate signaling is by expression of chimeric proteins whose activity is tightly regulated by a conformational change induced by hormone binding (e.g., Raf-kinase domain fused to the estrogen binding domain) *(8,9)*.

Activation of signal cascades in response to receptor activation by ligand binding, receptor overexpression, or expression of a constitutively active mutant receptor can be detected using several methods. Using *HER-2* signaling as an example for growth-factor-initiated signaling, activation of the receptor by heregulin binding leads to the formation of heterodimeric complexes of *HER-2* with *HER-3* or *HER-4* receptors *(10,11)*. Tyrosine phosphorylation of both *HER-2* and *HER-3* or *HER-4* receptors can be detected by phosphate labeling followed by immunoprecipitation of the receptor or by Western blot analysis using an antiphosphotyrosine antibody.

Signaling proteins can also be identified by immunoprecipitating with antiphosphotyrosine antibody followed by immunoblotting with a specific antibody *(12)*. The immunoprecipitation/immunoblotting assay is also used frequently to detect proteins that physically associate with the receptor; or to identify components of a protein–protein complex *(13)*. Signaling activity of kinases can be measured by immune complex assays, which require first immunoprecipitating the kinase from whole cell lysates and then incubating the active kinase in the presence of radioactive adenosine triphosphate (ATP) and a specific or nonspecific substrate *(14)*. With a variety of commercially available antibodies, Western blot analyses and in vitro kinase assays are standard protocols used in signal transduction studies.

More recently, the availability of phospho-specific antibodies directed to many downstream signaling proteins allow for rapid determination of catalytic activity in whole-cell lysates *(15)*. However, because some antibodies are directed to only one phosphorylated site, data should be interpreted with caution. For example, the phospho-AKT antibody recognizes phosphorylation of serine residue 473, yet there is evidence that phosphorylation of threonine 308, which is phosphorylated by a different kinase, is involved in a 25-fold increase in AKT kinase activity *(16)*. Therefore, although in vitro kinase assays are still necessary in some instances to confirm any observations based on the use of activation specific antibodies, there are clear advantages to the use of these antibodies.

Immunohistochemical detection methods have been used successfully to stain cells with antiphosphotyrosine antibody *(17)*; and the same technique can be used with phospho-specific antibody to assay for activity directly in cells *(18)* or in clinical specimens *(19,20)*. Assaying for biochemical activity by either in vitro kinase assays or by Western blot analysis, as aforementioned, require an adequate supply of frozen tissue specimen *(21,22)*, but more importantly, all solid matrix blotting techniques, which require generation of crude tissue lysates, are subject to errors *(23)*. These potential errors are introduced by dilution of tumor cells with normal vascular, stromal, or inflammatory cells. With appropriate controls, the use of phospho-specific antibodies for immunohistochemical analysis of tissue sections can eliminate some errors in detection and the need to use large amounts of clinical material.

The second approach to decipher the biological significance of a signal transduction pathway is to selectively turn signaling "off." In the past, neutralizing antibodies to *ras (24,25)* or to *grb2/Ash (26)* have been used to successfully monitor biological effects, however, the need to microinject these antibodies into cells and the ability to only observe short term effects limit the use of this approach. Antisense to *grb2 (27)*, *ras (28,29)*, and *raf (30)* have also been used to inhibit signaling; yet, introduction of oligonucleotides into cells can produce cellular effects which are not limited to depletion of a particular mRNA *(31,32)*. "Dominant negative" proteins are mutant versions of signal transducers; and when they are expressed, they can interfere with the endogenous activities of the wild type protein. A mutation in a critical residuem, such as the lysine in the ATP binding site, results in elimination of enzymatic activity *(33,34)*. Dominant negative proteins comprised of just the regulatory or protein–protein interaction domain *(35–37)* can also interfere with signaling. The mechanism of interference by "dominant negative proteins," such as with N17*ras* or MEKS218/222A, is thought to be accomplished by binding to upstream activators thereby resulting in catalytically nonproductive complexes *(34,38,39)*. More recently, others have used proteins containing a point-mutated SH2 domain or simply expressed SH2/SH3 domains to successfully interfere with downstream signaling *(40)*.

Specific signals can also be turned "off" by using known chemical inhibitors of signal transduction pathways *(41–43)*; for example, wortmannin is a potent specific inhibitor of PI3 kinase *(44–47)*. Use of this inhibitor has identified several pathways that are dependent on PI3 kinase activity. Cellular exposure to wortmannin blocks PDGFR-mediated fibroblast motility and membrane ruffling *(48)*; prevents glucose uptake *(45)*; inhibits nerve growth factor (NGF)-dependent survival and differentiation of PC12 cells *(42,49)*; blocks vesicular sorting *(50)* and the endocytic pathway *(51)*; interferes with activities of glycogen synthase kinase 3 *(52)*, PKB/AKT kinase *(53,54)*, and Rac *(55)*. On the other hand, the PD098059 compound, which is a specific inhibitor of MEK activation *(56)*, inhibits growth factor stimulated microtubule-associated protein (MAP) kinase, anchorage independent growth of *ras* transformed cells *(43)*, and differentiation of PC12 cells *(57)*, but does not interfere with PI3 kinase activity *(58)*.

A particular signal pathway can be studied by using both genetic and chemical inhibitors in combination *(59)*. For example, overexpression of *HER-2/neu* constitutively activates Ras *(13)*. However, Ras itself has been shown to regulate several other pathways which can contribute to cellular transformation: Rac and Rho pathways *(60–62)* and the Raf/MEK pathway *(63)*. We have found that the ability of *HER-2* overexpressing cancer cell lines to grow in an anchorage-independent manner correlates with the level of MAP kinase activity (Arboleda, M. J. and Slamon, D. J., unpublished), suggesting that the Raf/MEK pathway may play a significant role in *HER-2* mediated transformation. Consistent with this observation, stable expression of dominant negative MEK is toxic to *HER-2* overexpressing (both natural and engineered) cell lines. In a panel of *ras*-mutated cell lines, where dominant negative MEK expression was tolerated, interference with MEK activity resulted in a consistent decrease in anchorage-independent growth (Arboleda, M. J. and Slamon, D. J., unpublished). Yet neither a block in the *rac* pathway nor the *rho* pathway, both of which have been placed downstream of PI3 kinase, led to a similar decrease in soft agar growth (Arboleda, M.J. and Slamon, D. J., unpublished). Like expression of dominant negative MEK, Ras-mutated cells treated with the MEK inhibitor PD098059 also resulted in inhibition of anchorage-independent growth *(43)* (Arboleda, M. J. and Slamon, D. J., unpublished). Inhibition of MEK activity, using either a genetic or chemical inhibitor, suggests that activities of Raf/MEK may dictate the anchorage-independent growth phenotype of human cancer cells.

The use of either genetic or chemical inhibitors should be interpreted with caution because of possible crosstalk between signal transduction pathways, and because the specificity of inhibition or the mechanism of inhibition is not clearly defined. For example, unlike expression of dominant negative MEK, the MEK inhibitor does not revert the malignant phenotype of cells transformed by oncogenic tyrosine kinases. One possibility for this discrepancy may be that high-level expression of dominant negative MEK may also interfere with other signaling pathways. For instance, integrin signaling also activates MAP kinase, but in a Ras and Raf-1-independent manner *(64)*. Therefore, the striking inhibitory effect on anchorage independent growth may, in part, be caused by nonspecific interference with other MEKK activity induced by integrin signaling. Similarly, concentrations of MEK inhibitor PD98059 required to inhibit growth of human *ras*-mutated cell lines in long-term soft agar assays (>100 μ*M*) were much higher than concentrations required to inhibit MEK in short term biochemical assays (5–10 μ*M*) *(43)* (Arboleda, M. J. and Slamon, D. J., unpublished). At high concentrations (>100 μ*M*), the compound may lose specificity *(65)*.

## 3. Specificity of Cell Signaling in Ovarian Cell Lines

As the field of signal transduction has matured, there are clear indications that many signaling pathways are repeatedly used to elicit a variety of cellular responses. Cells can receive a diverse set of extracellular signals, which appear to converge onto identical signaling pathways, and yet through some unknown mechanism, can process those signals to alter their behavior. As discussed in **Subheading 2.**, much work in signal transduction has been focused on simply turning signals "on" or "off." Yet, quantitative differences in signal intensity and duration, rather than qualitative differences of "on" or "off," have been shown to be critical factors in ultimately determining cell fate. A well-characterized example is the Raf/MEK/ERK signaling module in PC12 cells. For example, NGF, which induces differentiation of PC12 cells, activates both a transient and sustained phase of MAP kinase activity; whereas epidermal growth factor (EGF), which stimulates proliferation of PC12 cells, induces only a transient phase of MAP kinase activity *(66)*. However, when PC12 cells are engineered to overexpress epidermal growth factor-receptor (EGF-R,) EGF treatment of these cells, like NGF treatment, leads to sustained activation of MAP kinase and induces cellular differentiation *(67)*. Conversely, while MAP kinase signaling intensity is transiently stronger with heregulin-α and the duration of MAP kinase signaling is longer with heregulin-β *(68)*, both ligands stimulate cell proliferation *(69)*. The strength and duration of MAP kinase activity may be sufficient to determine the cellular responses in PC12 cells, but the activity does not appear to dictate responses to heregulin. Although extremely important, controling for quantitative differences in signaling, without fully understanding the internal cell circuitry involved, may be technically difficult. As we continue this discussion, we will focus on how to use the appropriate cell system as a way of further defining specificity of cell signaling.

Much work on growth factor receptor signaling has been performed in rodent fibroblast cell lines HEK 293 or COS-7, cell lines that abundantly express exogenous genes. But the use of these cell lines may be inappropriate for several reasons. First, the level of expression of transfected HER-2/*neu* into rodent fibroblast cell lines or in Cos7 cells are far in excess of those seen in human clinical specimens harboring the amplified gene. Such a high level of receptor expression can result in constitutive high-intensity signaling to downstream pathways which can potentially lead to conflicting biological effects. Several laboratories have reported that very-high-intensity Raf signaling can lead to growth inhibition instead of growth proliferation, which is ordinarily associated with increased Raf activity *(70,71)*. EGF treatment of A431 cells, which overexpress the EGF-R, causes growth inhibition by a similar mechanism *(72)*. These studies indicate that signal strength influences the cellular response. Therefore, if possible, the extent of activation in a particular cell system should be limited to levels that are physiologically relevant.

Second, even when expression levels can be controled, the biological effects of rodent fibroblast vs rodent epithelial cells are inconsistent, which suggests that variations in cell signaling are directly attributable to cell origin. For example, it has been shown that constitutive expression of active MEK is sufficient to transform normal rodent fibroblast cell lines *(63)*, whereas the same activity is not sufficient to transform rodent epithelial derived cell lines *(73)*. Therefore, because most human cancers are of epithelial origin, biological effects observed in rodent fibroblast cell lines, or even human fibroblast cell lines may not translate directly to human epithelial cell lines.

Third, the expression pattern of signaling molecules can vary in a tissue or organ-specific manner *(74,75)*; such that these differences in expression can lead to variations in cell signaling and cellular effect. For example, expression of heregulin homologs and heregulin receptors (*HER2–4*) are found in neuronal cells. In these cellular contexts, activation of heregulin receptors, which results in the activation of the same downstream signal transducers as in breast and ovarian cell lines *(76)*, control cell survival, maturation *(77)*, and regulate acetylcholine receptor levels in synapses of neuromuscular junctions *(78)* and in the brain *(79)*. In breast cells, the role of heregulin is controversial. The ligand has been reported to stimulate growth *(80)*, inhibit growth *(81)*, and induce cellular differentiation in breast cell lines *(82)*. These apparent conflicting reports may be caused by baseline Raf signaling *(71)* present in various cell lines before heregulin/NDF addition. In fact, growth inhibitory responses were observed when cells were treated with heregulin in 10% serum (a situation where Raf activity may be already at a maximum to signal mitogenesis) but not in 0.1% serum *(80)*. Using more than one representative cell line will eliminate observations that are unique to a specific cell line or tissue type. For example, because of the lack of effects on a few ovarian cell lines, one early study concluded that heregulin's activity may be restricted to breast cells *(83)*. Understandably, these earlier findings were complicated by the lack of knowledge about the Type 1 receptor tyrosine kinase (RTK)-receptor combinations present in a given cell. Nevertheless, the current literature indicates that heregulin's activity on a variety of cell types, including ovarian cells, is growth stimulatory and not growth inhibitory *(10,80,84–87)*. Collectively, these findings underscore the idea that differences in cell-signaling networks, which may be a function of cell origin or tissue type, can lead to differences in biological effects. Therefore, studies regarding ovarian cancer should be performed in ovarian cell lines.

The question arises whether it is technically feasible to generate panels of transfected human ovarian cell lines where signals have been turned "on" or "off." The retroviral-based gene-transfer technique has been successful for introducing genes into many different cell types *(88)*. However, because of toxicity to the helper virus cell line, inhibitory constructs do not package well in this system (Arboleda, M. J. and Slamon, D. J., unpublished). To avoid such problems, tetracycline-inducible promoters in retroviral constructs can be used instead *(89,90)*. There are now many commercially available lipid-based products that work well to transfect both human normal and malignant cell lines. We noted that transfection of normal cells was still technically more difficult; however, after testing a panel of commercially available reagents, we found pFx-7 (Invitrogen, San Diego, CA ) to be optimal in transfecting normal human ovarian surface epithelial cells (HOSE).

The significance of any signal-transduction pathway depends on the assay system used to evaluate the biological endpoint. Any conclusions derived from nonepithelial cell lines or cell lines that exhibit high-level gene expression should be used only as a foundation for further studies to be performed in the most appropriate, physiologically relevant system. Furthermore, in vitro assays can measure only one or a few aspects of malignant progression. For example, there is limited or no correlation with a cell's potential to invade through reconstituted basement membrane and its metastatic potential in vivo *(91)*. The important question depends on how activation or inhibition of a signal-transduction pathway ultimately influences the growth of cells in a physiological environment. Much confusion and controversy regarding the effects of heregulin has been resolved in this context. We have found that minor proliferative effects of heregulin in vitro can often translate to significant proliferative effects in vivo *(84)*. Moreover, the significant growth stimulatory effects of heregulin in vivo is confirmed by another report which states that heregulin/NDF expression targeted to mammary glands in transgenic mice model system results in mammary adenocarcinomas *(92)*. Therefore, whenever possible, confirmation of in vitro effects should be performed in vivo (*see* Stinson et al. for description of human xenograft models) *(93)*.

In this review, we have presented methods used in dissecting signal-transduction pathways and discussed various factors that may influence the specificity of cell signaling. We have chosen to focus on HER-2 signaling because amplification and overexpression of this gene has been detected in 20% of human ovarian cancer specimens, and because the *HER-2* gene has been shown to have the potential to play a direct role in the pathogenesis of those ovarian cancers in which it is altered. Much of the same techniques used in identifying proteins downstream of *HER-2* overexpression, and by heregulin activation of the receptor, can now be applied toward understanding the pharmacodynamic properties of signal-transduction inhibitors that are currently in clinical trials. For example, the 4D5 monoclonal antibody supposedly dampens signals from the *HER-2/neu* receptor by binding to the extracellular domain *(94,95)*. Despite the clinical effectiveness of the 4D5 monoclonal antibody on human breast and ovarian cancer, the mechanism of how this antibody inhibits growth of *HER-2* overexpressing cells remains unknown. Delineation of signal-transduction pathways downstream of *HER-2/neu* will help to elucidate the inhibitory mechanism of this antibody.

The following chapters offer new strategies to understand various components of signal transduction in ovarian cancer. This diverse set of new tools will undoubtedly lead to the identification of novel pathways and the validation of potential drug targets to aid in treatment of this disease.

## References

1. Mansour, S. J., Matten, W. T., Hermann, A. S., Candia, J. M., Rong, S., Fukasawa, K., et al. (1994) Transformation of mammalian cells by constitutively active MAP kinase kinase. *Science* **265,** 966–970.
2. Segatto, O., Lonardo, F., Helin, K., Wexler, D., Fazioli, F., Rhee, S. G., et al. (1992) erbB-2 autophosphorylation is required for mitogenic action and high- affinity substrate coupling. *Oncogene* **7,** 1339–1346.
3. Holmes, W. E., Sliwkowski, M. X., Akita, R. W., Henzel, W. J., Lee, J., Park, J. W., et al. (1992) Identification of heregulin, a specific activator of p185erbB2. *Science* **256,** 1205–1210.
4. Carraway, K. L. R. and Cantley, L. C. (1994) A neu acquaintance for erbB3 and erbB4: a role for receptor heterodimerization in growth signaling. *Cell* **78,** 5–8.
5. Mansour, S. J., Candia, J. M., Gloor, K. K., and Ahn, N. G. (1996) Constitutively active mitogen-activated protein kinase kinase 1 (MAPKK1) and MAPKK2 mediate similar transcriptional and morphological responses. *Cell Growth Differ.* **7,** 243–250.
6. Stokoe, D., Macdonald, S. G., Cadwallader, K., Symons, M., and Hancock, J. F. (1994) Activation of Raf as a result of recruitment to the plasma membrane [see comments] [published erratum appears in Science 1994 Dec 16;266(5192):1792-3]. *Science* **264,** 1463–1467.
7. Andjelkovic, M., Alessi, D. R., Meier, R., Fernandez, A., Lamb, N. J., Frech, M., et al. (1997) Role of translocation in the activation and function of protein kinase B. *J. Biol. Chem.* **272,** 31,515–31,524.
8. Samuels, M. L., Weber, M. J., Bishop, J. M., and McMahon, M. (1993) Conditional transformation of cells and rapid activation of the mitogen-activated protein kinase cascade by an estradiol-dependent human raf-1 protein kinase. *Mol. Cell Biol.* **13,** 6241–6252.
9. Greulich, H. and Erikson, R. L. (1998) An analysis of Mek1 signaling in cell proliferation and transformation. *J. Biol. Chem.* **273,** 13,280–13,288.
10. Carraway, K. L. R., Soltoff, S. P., Diamonti, A. J., and Cantley, L. C. (1995) Heregulin stimulates mitogenesis and phosphatidylinositol 3-kinase in mouse fibroblasts transfected with erbB2/neu and erbB3. *J. Biol. Chem.* **270,** 7111–7116.
11. Sliwkowski, M. X., Schaefer, G., Akita, R. W., Lofgren, J. A., Fitzpatrick, V. D., Nuijens, A., et al. (1994) Coexpression of erbB2 and erbB3 proteins reconstitutes a high affinity receptor for heregulin. *J. Biol. Chem.* **269,** 14,661–14,665.
12. Segatto, O., Pelicci, G., Giuli, S., Digiesi, G., Di Fiore, P. P., McGlade, J., et al. (1993) Shc products are substrates of erbB-2 kinase. *Oncogene* **8,** 2105–2112.
13. Janes, P. W., Daly, R. J., deFazio, A., and Sutherland, R. L. (1994) Activation of the Ras signalling pathway in human breast cancer cells overexpressing erbB-2. *Oncogene* **9,** 3601–3608.
14. Macdonald, S. G., Crews, C. M., Wu, L., Driller, J., Clark, R., Erikson, R. L., et al. (1993) Reconstitution of the Raf-1-MEK-ERK signal transduction pathway in vitro. *Mol. Cell. Biol.* **13,** 6615–6620.
15. Czernik, A. J., Girault, J. A., Nairn, A. C., Chen, J., Snyder, G., Kebabian, J., et al. (1991) Production of phosphorylation state-specific antibodies. *Meth. Enzymol.* **201,** 264–283.
16. Alessi, D. R., Andjelkovic, M., Caudwell, B., Cron, P., Morrice, N., Cohen, P., et al. (1996) Mechanism of activation of protein kinase B by insulin and IGF-1. *Embo J.* **15,** 6541–6551.
17. Landry, F., Chapdelaine, A., Begin, L. R., and Chevalier, S. (1996) Phosphotyrosine antibodies preferentially react with basal epithelial cells in the dog prostate. *J. Urol.* **155,** 386–390.
18. Philpott, K. L., McCarthy, M. J., Klippel, A., and Rubin, L. L. (1997) Activated phosphatidylinositol 3-kinase and Akt kinase promote survival of superior cervical neurons. *J. Cell Biol.* **139,** 809–815.
19. DiGiovanna, M. P., Carter, D., Flynn, S. D., and Stern, D. F. (1996) Functional assay for HER-2/neu demonstrates active signalling in a minority of HER-2/neu-overexpressing invasive human breast tumors. *Br. J. Cancer* **74,** 802–806.
20. Flick, M. B., Sapi, E., Perrotta, P. L., Maher, M. G., Halaban, R., Carter, D., et al. (1997) Recognition of activated CSF-1 receptor in breast carcinomas by a tyrosine 723 phosphospecific antibody. *Oncogene* **14,** 2553–2561.
21. Oka, H., Chatani, Y., Hoshino, R., Ogawa, O., Kakehi, Y., Terachi, T., et al. (1995) Constitutive activation of mitogen-activated protein (MAP) kinases in human renal cell carcinoma. *Cancer Res.* **55,** 4182–4187.
22. Sivaraman, V. S., Wang, H., Nuovo, G. J., and Malbon, C. C. (1997) Hyperexpression of mitogen-activated protein kinase in human breast cancer. *J. Clin. Invest.* **99,** 1478–1483.

23. Slamon, D. J., Godolphin, W., Jones, L. A., Holt, J. A., Wong, S. G., Keith, D. E., et al. (1989) Studies of the HER-2/neu proto-oncogene in human breast and ovarian cancer. *Science* **244,** 707–712.

24. Yamauchi, N., Kiessling, A. A., and Cooper, G. M. (1994) The Ras/Raf signaling pathway is required for progression of mouse embryos through the two-cell stage. *Mol. Cell Biol.* **14,** 6655–6662.

25. Kung, H. F., Smith, M. R., Bekesi, E., Manne, V., and Stacey, D. W. (1986) Reversal of transformed phenotype by monoclonal antibodies against Ha-ras p21 proteins. *Exp. Cell Res.* **162,** 363–371.

26. Matuoka, K., Shibasaki, F., Shibata, M., and Takenawa, T. (1993) Ash/Grb-2, a SH2/SH3-containing protein, couples to signaling for mitogenesis and cytoskeletal reorganization by EGF and PDGF. *Embo J.* **12,** 3467–3473.

27. Tari, A. M., Arlinghaus, R., and Lopez-Berestein, G. (1997) Inhibition of Grb2 and Crkl proteins results in growth inhibition of Philadelphia chromosome positive leukemic cells. *Biochem. Biophys. Res. Commun.* **235,** 383–388.

28. Chen, G., Oh, S., Monia, B. P., and Stacey, D. W. (1996) Antisense oligonucleotides demonstrate a dominant role of c-Ki-RAS proteins in regulating the proliferation of diploid human fibroblasts. *J. Biol. Chem.* **271,** 28,259–28,265.

29. Cowsert, L. M. (1997) In vitro and in vivo activity of antisense inhibitors of ras: potential for clinical development. *Anticancer Drug Des.* **12,** 359–371.

30. Monia, B. P., Johnston, J. F., Geiger, T., Muller, M., and Fabbro, D. (1996) Antitumor activity of a phosphorothioate antisense oligodeoxynucleotide targeted against C-raf kinase [see comments]. *Nat. Med.* **2,** 668–675.

31. Branch, A. D. (1998) A good antisense molecule is hard to find. *Trends Biochem. Sci.* **23,** 45–50.

32. Crooke, S. T. and Bennett, C. F. (1996) Progress in antisense oligonucleotide therapeutics. *Annu. Rev. Pharmacol. Toxicol.* **36,** 107–129.

33. Messerle, K., Schlegel, J., Hynes, N. E., and Groner, B. (1994) NIH/3T3 cells transformed with the activated erbB-2 oncogene can be phenotypically reverted by a kinase deficient, dominant negative erbB-2 variant. *Mol. Cell Endocrinol.* **105,** 1–10.

34. Stacey, D. W., Roudebush, M., Day, R., Mosser, S. D., Gibbs, J. B., and Feig, L. A. (1991) Dominant inhibitory Ras mutants demonstrate the requirement for Ras activity in the action of tyrosine kinase oncogenes. *Oncogene* **6,** 2297–2304.

35. Gishizky, M. L., Cortez, D., and Pendergast, A. M. (1995) Mutant forms of growth factor-binding protein-2 reverse BCR-ABL-induced transformation. *Proc. Natl. Acad. Sci. USA* **92,** 10,889–10,893.

36. Tanaka, M., Gupta, R., and Mayer, B. J. (1995) Differential inhibition of signaling pathways by dominant-negative SH2/SH3 adapter proteins. *Mol. Cell Biol.* **15,** 6829–6837.

37. Xie, Y., Pendergast, A. M., and Hung, M. C. (1995) Dominant-negative mutants of Grb2 induced reversal of the transformed phenotypes caused by the point mutation-activated rat HER-2/Neu. *J. Biol. Chem.* **270,** 30,717–30,724.

38. Wu, X., Noh, S. J., Zhou, G., Dixon, J. E., and Guan, K. L. (1996) Selective activation of MEK1 but not MEK2 by A-Raf from epidermal growth factor-stimulated Hela cells. *J. Biol. Chem.* **271,** 3265–3271.

39. Feig, L. A. and Cooper, G. M. (1988) Inhibition of NIH 3T3 cell proliferation by a mutant ras protein with preferential affinity for GDP. *Mol. Cell Biol.* **8,** 3235–3243.

40. O'Bryan, J. P., Lambert, Q. T., and Der, C. J. (1998) The src homology 2 and phosphotyrosine binding domains of the ShcC adaptor protein function as inhibitors of mitogenic signaling by the epidermal growth factor receptor. *J. Biol. Chem.* **273,** 20,431–20,437.

41. Clark, J. W., Santos-Moore, A., Stevenson, L. E., and Frackelton, A. R. Jr. (1996) Effects of tyrosine kinase inhibitors on the proliferation of human breast cancer cell lines and proteins important in the ras signaling pathway. *Int. J. Cancer* **65,** 186–191.

42. Kimura, K., Hattori, S., Kabuyama, Y., Shizawa, Y., Takayanagi, J., Nakamura, S., et al. (1994) Neurite outgrowth of PC12 cells is suppressed by wortmannin, a specific inhibitor of phosphatidylinositol 3-kinase. *J. Biol. Chem.* **269,** 18,961–18,967.

43. Dudley, D. T., Pang, L., Decker, S. J., Bridges, A. J., and Saltiel, A. R. (1995) A synthetic inhibitor of the mitogen-activated protein kinase cascade. *Proc. Natl. Acad. Sci. USA* **92,** 7686–7689.

44. Nakanishi, S., Kakita, S., Takahashi, I., Kawahara, K., Tsukuda, E., Sano, T., et al. (1992) Wortmannin, a microbial product inhibitor of myosin light chain kinase. *J. Biol. Chem.* **267,** 2157–2163.

45. Okada, T., Kawano, Y., Sakakibara, T., Hazeki, O., and Ui, M. (1994) Essential role of phosphatidylinositol 3-kinase in insulin-induced glucose transport and antilipolysis in rat adipocytes. Studies with a selective inhibitor wortmannin. *J. Biol. Chem.* **269,** 3568–3573.

46. Wymann, M. P., Bulgarelli-Leva, G., Zvelebil, M. J., Pirola, L., Vanhaesebroeck, B., Waterfield, M. D., et al. (1996) Wortmannin inactivates phosphoinositide 3-kinase by covalent modification of Lys-802, a residue involved in the phosphate transfer reaction. *Mol. Cell Biol.* **16,** 1722–1733.

47. Wymann, M. and Arcaro, A. (1994) Platelet-derived growth factor-induced phosphatidylinositol 3-kinase activation mediates actin rearrangements in fibroblasts. *Biochem. J.* **298,** 517–520.

48. Wennstrom, S., Hawkins, P., Cooke, F., Hara, K., Yonezawa, K., Kasuga, M., et al. (1994) Activation of phosphoinositide 3-kinase is required for PDGF-stimulated membrane ruffling. *Curr. Biol.* **4**, 385–393.

49. Yao, R. and Cooper, G. M. (1995) Requirement for phosphatidylinositol-3 kinase in the prevention of apoptosis by nerve growth factor. *Science* **267**, 2003–2006.

50. Brown, W. J., DeWald, D. B., Emr, S. D., Plutner, H., and Balch, W. E. (1995) Role for phosphatidylinositol 3-kinase in the sorting and transport of newly synthesized lysosomal enzymes in mammalian cells. *J. Cell Biol.* **130**, 781–796.

51. Shpetner, H., Joly, M., Hartley, D., and Corvera, S. (1996) Potential sites of PI-3 kinase function in the endocytic pathway revealed by the PI-3 kinase inhibitor, wortmannin. *J. Cell Biol.* **132**, 595–605.

52. Cross, D. A., Alessi, D. R., Vandenheede, J. R., McDowell, H. E., Hundal, H. S., and Cohen, P. (1994) The inhibition of glycogen synthase kinase-3 by insulin or insulin-like growth factor 1 in the rat skeletal muscle cell line L6 is blocked by wortmannin, but not by rapamycin: evidence that wortmannin blocks activation of the mitogen-activated protein kinase pathway in L6 cells between Ras and Raf. *Biochem. J.* **303**, 21–26.

53. Burgering, B. M. and Coffer, P. J. (1995) Protein kinase B (c-Akt) in phosphatidylinositol-3-OH kinase signal transduction [see comments]. *Nature* **376**, 599–602.

54. Franke, T. F., Yang, S. I., Chan, T. O., Datta, K., Kazlauskas, A., Morrison, D. K., et al. (1995) The protein kinase encoded by the Akt proto-oncogene is a target of the PDGF-activated phosphatidylinositol 3-kinase. *Cell* **81**, 727–736.

55. Hawkins, P. T., Eguinoa, A., Qiu, R. G., Stokoe, D., Cooke, F. T., Walters, R., et al. (1995) PDGF stimulates an increase in GTP-Rac via activation of phosphoinositide 3-kinase. *Curr. Biol.* **5**, 393–403.

56. Alessi, D. R., Cuenda, A., Cohen, P., Dudley, D. T., and Saltiel, A. R. (1995) PD 098059 is a specific inhibitor of the activation of mitogen- activated protein kinase kinase in vitro and in vivo. *J. Biol. Chem.* **270**, 27,489–27,494.

57. Pang, L., Sawada, T., Decker, S. J., and Saltiel, A. R. (1995) Inhibition of MAP kinase kinase blocks the differentiation of PC-12 cells induced by nerve growth factor. *J. Biol. Chem.* **270**, 13,585–13,588.

58. Lazar, D. F., Wiese, R. J., Brady, M. J., Mastick, C. C., Waters, S. B., Yamauchi, K., et al. (1995) Mitogen-activated protein kinase kinase inhibition does not block the stimulation of glucose utilization by insulin. *J. Biol. Chem.* **270**, 20,801–20,807.

59. Anand-Apte, B., Zetter, B. R., Viswanathan, A., Qiu, R. G., Chen, J., Ruggieri, R., et al. (1997) Platelet-derived growth factor and fibronectin-stimulated migration are differentially regulated by the Rac and extracellular signal-regulated kinase pathways. *J. Biol. Chem.* **272**, 30,688–30,692.

60. Khosravi-Far, R., Solski, P. A., Clark, G. J., Kinch, M. S., and Der, C. J. (1995) Activation of Rac1, RhoA and mitogen-activated protein kinases is required for Ras transformation. *Mol. Cell. Biol.* **15**, 6443–6453.

61. Prendergast, G., Khosravi-Far, R., Kurzawa, H., Solski, P., Lebowitz, P. F., and Der, C. (1995) Critical role of Rho in cell transformation by oncogenic Ras. *Oncogene,*

62. Qiu, R. G., Chen, J., Kirn, D., McCormick, F., and Symons, M. (1995) An essential role for Rac in Ras transformation. *Nature* **374**, 457–459.

63. Cowley, S., Paterson, H., Kemp, P., and Marshall, C. (1994) Activation of MAP kinase kinase is necessary and sufficient for PC12 differentiation and for transformation of NIH 3T3 cells. *Cell* **77**, 841–852.

64. Chen, Q., Lin, T. H., Der, C. J., and Juliano, R. L. (1996) Integrin-mediated activation of MEK and mitogen-activated protein kinase is independent of Ras [corrected] [published erratum appears in *J. Biol. Chem.* (1996) **271**, 22,280.] *J. Biol. Chem.* **271**, 18,122–18,127.

65. Levitzki, A., Gazit, A., Osherov, N., Posner, I., and Gilon, C. (1991) Inhibition of protein-tyrosine kinases by tyrphostins. *Meth. Enzymol.* **201**, 347–361.

66. Traverse, S., Gomez, N., Paterson, H., Marshall, C., and Cohen, P. (1992) Sustained activation of the mitogen-activated protein (MAP) kinase cascade may be required for differentiation of PC12 cells. Comparison of the effects of nerve growth factor and epidermal growth factor. *Biochem. J.* **288**, 351–355.

67. Traverse, S., Seedorf, K., Paterson, H., Marshall, C. J., Cohen, P., and Ullrich, A. (1994) EGF triggers neuronal differentiation of PC12 cells that overexpress the EGF receptor. *Curr. Biol.* **4**, 694–701.

68. Weiss, F. U., Wallasch, C., Campiglio, M., Issing, W., and Ullrich, A. (1997) Distinct characteristics of heregulin signals mediated by HER3 or HER4. *J. Cell Physiol.* **173**, 187–195.

69. Pinkas-Kramarski, R., Shelly, M., Glathe, S., Ratzkin, B. J., and Yarden, Y. (1996) Neu differentiation factor/neuregulin isoforms activate distinct receptor combinations. *J. Biol. Chem.* **271**, 19,029–19,032.

70. Woods, D., Parry, D., Cherwinski, H., Bosch, E., Lees, E., and McMahon, M. (1997) Raf-induced proliferation or cell cycle arrest is determined by the level of Raf activity with arrest mediated by p21Cip1. *Mol. Cell Biol.* **17**, 5598–5611.

71. Sewing, A., Wiseman, B., Lloyd, A. C., and Land, H. (1997) High-intensity Raf signal causes cell cycle arrest mediated by p21Cip1. *Mol. Cell Biol.* **17,** 5588–5597.

72. Fan, Z., Lu, Y., Wu, X., DeBlasio, A., Koff, A., and Mendelsohn, J. (1995) Prolonged induction of p21Cip1/WAF1/CDK2/PCNA complex by epidermal growth factor receptor activation mediates ligand-induced A431 cell growth inhibition. *J. Cell Biol.* **131,** 235–242.

73. Oldham, S. M., Clark, G. J., Gangarosa, L. M., Coffey, R. J. Jr., and Der, C. J. (1996) Activation of the Raf-1/MAP kinase cascade is not sufficient for Ras transformation of RIE-1 epithelial cells. *Proc. Natl. Acad. Sci. USA* **93,** 6924–6928.

74. Guerrero, C., Rojas, J. M., Chedid, M., Esteban, L. M., Zimonjic, D. B., Popescu, N. C., et al. (1996) Expression of alternative forms of Ras exchange factors GRF and SOS1 in different human tissues and cell lines. *Oncogene* **12,** 1097–1107.

75. Pinkas-Kramarski, R., Eilam, R., Alroy, I., Levkowitz, G., Lonai, P., and Yarden, Y. (1997) Differential expression of NDF/neuregulin receptors ErbB-3 and ErbB-4 and involvement in inhibition of neuronal differentiation. *Oncogene* **15,** 2803–2815.

76. Altiok, N., Altiok, S., and Changeux, J. P. (1997) Heregulin-stimulated acetylcholine receptor gene expression in muscle: requirement for MAP kinase and evidence for a parallel inhibitory pathway independent of electrical activity. *Embo J.* **16,** 717–725.

77. Pinkas-Kramarski, R., Eilam, R., Spiegler, O., Lavi, S., Liu, N., Chang, D., et al. (1994) Brain neurons and glial cells express Neu differentiation factor/heregulin: a survival factor for astrocytes. *Proc. Natl. Acad. Sci. USA* **91,** 9387–9391.

78. Jo, S. A., Zhu, X., Marchionni, M. A., and Burden, S. J. (1995) Neuregulins are concentrated at nerve-muscle synapses and activate ACh-receptor gene expression. *Nature* **373,** 158–161.

79. Ozaki, M., Sasner, M., Yano, R., Lu, H. S., and Buonanno, A. (1997) Neuregulin-beta induces expression of an NMDA-receptor subunit. *Nature* **390,** 691–694.

80. Lewis, G. D., Lofgren, J. A., McMurtrey, A. E., Nuijens, A., Fendly, B. M., Bauer, K. D., et al. (1996) Growth regulation of human breast and ovarian tumor cells by heregulin: Evidence for the requirement of ErbB2 as a critical component in mediating heregulin responsiveness. *Cancer Res.* **56,** 1457–1465.

81. Daly, J. M., Jannot, C. B., Beerli, R. R., Graus-Porta, D., Maurer, F. G., and Hynes, N. E. (1997) Neu differentiation factor induces ErbB2 down-regulation and apoptosis of ErbB2-overexpressing breast tumor cells. *Cancer Res.* **57,** 3804–3811.

82. Peles, E., Bacus, S. S., Koski, R. A., Lu, H. S., Wen, D., Ogden, S. G., et al. (1992) Isolation of the neu/HER-2 stimulatory ligand: a 44 kd glycoprotein that induces differentiation of mammary tumor cells. *Cell.* **69,** 205–216.

83. Peles, E., Ben-Levy, R., Tzahar, E., Liu, N., Wen, D., and Yarden, Y. (1993) Cell-type specific interaction of Neu differentiation factor (NDF/heregulin) with Neu/HER-2 suggests complex ligand-receptor relationships. *Embo J.* **12,** 961–971.

84. Aguilar, Z., Akita, R. W., Finn, R. S., Pietras, R. J., Ramos, B. L., Pegram, M. D., et al. Biological effects of heregulin on normal and malignant breast and ovarian epithelial cells, manuscript in preparation.

85. Ram, T. G., Kokeny, K. E., Dilts, C. A., and Ethier, S. P. (1995) Mitogenic activity of neu differentiation factor/heregulin mimics that of epidermal growth factor and insulin-like growth factor-I in human mammary epithelial cells. *J. Cell Physiol.* **163,** 589–596.

86. Marte, B. M., Jeschke, M., Graus-Porta, D., Taverna, D., Hofer, P., Groner, B., et al. (1995) Neu differentiation factor/heregulin modulates growth and differentiation of HC11 mammary epithelial cells. *Mol. Endocrinol.* **9,** 14–23.

87. Marikovsky, M., Lavi, S., Pinkas-Kramarski, R., Karunagaran, D., Liu, N., Wen, D., et al. (1995) ErbB-3 mediates differential mitogenic effects of NDF/heregulin isoforms on mouse keratinocytes. *Oncogene* **10,** 1403–1411.

88. Miller, A. D., Miller, D. G., Garcia, J. V., and Lynch, C. M. (1993) Use of retroviral vectors for gene transfer and expression. *Meth. Enzymol.* **217,** 581–599.

89. Hofmann, A., Nolan, G. P., and Blau, H. M. (1996) Rapid retroviral delivery of tetracycline-inducible genes in a single autoregulatory cassette. *Proc. Natl. Acad. Sci. USA* **93,** 5185–5190.

90. Shockett, P. E. and Schatz, D. G. (1996) Diverse strategies for tetracycline-regulated inducible gene expression. *Proc. Natl. Acad. Sci. USA* **93,** 5173–5176.

91. Noel, A. C., Calle, A., Emonard, H. P., Nusgens, B. V., Simar, L., Foidart, J., et al. (1991) Invasion of reconstituted basement membrane matrix is not correlated to the malignant metastatic cell phenotype. *Cancer Res.* **51,** 405–414.

92. Krane, I. M. and Leder, P. (1996) NDF/heregulin induces persistence of terminal end buds and adenocarcinomas in the mammary glands of transgenic mice. *Oncogene* **12,** 1781–1788.

93. Stinson, S. F., Alley, M. C., Kopp, W. C., Fiebig, H. H., Mullendore, L. A., Pittman, A. F., et al. (1992) Morphological and immunocytochemical characteristics of human tumor cell lines for use in a disease-oriented anticancer drug screen. *Anticancer Res.* **12,** 1035–1053.

94. Baselga, J., Tripathy, D., Mendelsohn, J., Baughman, S., Benz, C. C., Dantis, L., et al. (1996) Phase II study of weekly intravenous recombinant humanized anti-p185HER2 monoclonal antibody in patients with HER2/neu-overexpressing metastatic breast cancer. *J. Clin. Oncol.* **14,** 737–744.
95. Pegram, M., Lipton, A., Hayes, D., Weber, B., Baselga, J., Triphathy, D., et al. (1998) Phase II Study of receptor enhanced chemosensitivity using recombinant humanized anti p-185 monoclonal antibody plus cisplatin in patients with recurrent, with HER-2 overexpression, metastatic breast refractory to chemotherapeutic treatment. *J. Clin. Oncol.* **16,** 2659–2671.

# 61

## Immunoprecipitation to Determine JAK Kinase Activation in Response to Interleukins in Ovarian Cancer

### Takashi Murata

## 1. Introduction

In cytokine receptors, there is no consensus sequence motif for tyrosine and/or serine/threonine kinases in its intracellular domain (1). Cytokine receptors associate with and activate members of the Janus kinase family (JAK), which is phosphorylated following ligand binding (2). The JAK family consists of four kinase members, JAK1, JAK2, JAK3, and Tyk2. Recently, we have shown that in ovarian cancer cell lines, many IL-4 receptors were expressed and IL-4 inhibited the proliferation of ovarian carcinoma cell lines (3). Moreover, IL-4 induced the phosphorylation of JAK1, JAK2, Tyk2, STAT6, and IRS-1 proteins following ligand–receptor interaction (4).

After JAK stimulation, it is believed that the activation of signal transduction and activators of transcription (STAT) protein occurs (5). These proteins are phosphorylated in the cytosol on tyrosine residues and then translocated to the nucleus where they bind to DNA or DNA-binding protein and enhance the transcription of specific genes (6). IL-4 induces phosphorylation of IL-4 specific STAT termed IL4STAT or STAT6 (7,8) and then induces the binding of this protein to the consensus binding sequence, TTNCNNNAA or interferon-$\gamma$ activation sequence (GAS) (9).

In this section, the method of detection of JAK kinase tyrosine phosphorylation by using immunoprecipitation and Western blot technique is introduced.

## 2. Materials

1. Phosphatase inhibitor buffer (PI, 10X): 10 m$M$ sodium vanadate (Na$_3$VO$_4$), 250 m$M$ NaF, 100 m$M$ sodium pyrophosphate (Na$_4$P$_2$O$_7$), and 10 m$M$ EDTA. Make fresh in each experiment.
2. Binding buffer: 10 m$M$ HEPES (pH 7.4), 0.02% human serum albumin in 500 mL of RPMI-1640. Store at 4°C.
3. RIPA buffer (modified): 1% NP-40, 300 m$M$ NaCl, 50 m$M$ Tris-HCl (pH 7.4), leupeptin (10 µg/mL), aprotinin (10 µg/mL), pepstatin A (10 µg/mL), PMSF (2 m$M$). Make fresh each time.
4. Saline buffer (5X): 1.5$M$ NaCl, 250 m$M$ Tris-HCl (pH 7.4).
5. Tris-glycine-SDS running buffer for Western blot (10X): 250 m$M$ Tris-base, glycine 1.92$M$, SDS 1% (pH 8.3).

From: *Methods in Molecular Medicine, Vol. 39: Ovarian Cancer: Methods and Protocols*
Edited by: J. M. S. Bartlett © Humana Press, Inc., Totowa, NJ

6. Tris-glycine transfer buffer for Western blot (25X): 300 m$M$ Tris, 2.4$M$ glycine (pH 8.3).
7. Blocking buffer for Western blot: 1.25% BSA, 1.25% ovalbumin (Sigma, St. Louis, MO, A5378), 25 m$M$ Tris-HCl, 137 m$M$ NaCl, and 3.7 m$M$ KCl. Store at 4°C.
8. TBS-T buffer: 20 m$M$ Tris-HCl, 137 mm NaCl, 0.1% Tween-20.
9. Reprobing buffer: 100 m$M$ 2-mercaptoethanol, 2% SDS, 62.5 mm Tris-HCl pH 6.7.
10. Laemmli buffer (2X): 125 m$M$ Tris-HCl (pH 6.8), 20% glycerol, 4% SDS, 5% β-mercaptoethanol, 0.005% bromophenol blue.

## 3. Methods

### 3.1. Preparation of Ovarian Carcinoma Cell Lines

Because JAK and STAT proteins are expressed at low levels, it is difficult to visualize the protein without immunoprecipitation. To perform immunoprecipitation of target proteins, prepare at least $1–2 \times 10^7$ cells/sample. In the case of IGROV-1 cells, you can get $2 \times 10^7$ cells from one confluent 175-cm$^2$ flask.

1. Prepare $1–2 \times 10^7$ cells/sample. To analyze 10 samples, prepare $10 \times 175$ cm$^2$ confluent culture flasks.
2. Wash cells with 5 mL of PBS twice and incubate with 3 mL of 1X Trypsin EDTA (GIBCO-BRL, Gaithersburg, MD No.25300-054).
3. Remove cells with 7 mL of PBS into a 50-mL falcon tube and add 30 mL of PBS. Then, pellet cells by centrifuging at 400$g$, 5 min at 4 °C.
4. Discard supernatant and wash cells with 40 mL fresh PBS. Then, pellet cells by centrifuging at 400$g$, 5 min at 4°C.
5. Resuspend cells in 20 mL binding buffer (BB) and count the cell numbers (*see* **Note 1**).
6. Divide $2 \times 10^7$ cells into 15 mL of falcon tube and spin down the cells by centrifuging at 400$g$, 5 min at 4°C.
7. Discard BB and add 1 mL of fresh BB with or without appropriate cytokine.
8. Incubate samples at 37°C, 5–10 min (*see* **Note 2**). Then, quench the reaction with 10 mL of PBS plus 1X PI (PBS-PI). Pellet cells by centrifuging at 400$g$, 5 min at 4°C.
9. Discard supernatant and resuspend in 1 mL of fresh PBS. Transfer samples into 1.5-mL Eppendorf tubes. Then, pellet cells by microfuging at 12,000$g$, 2 min at 4°C.

### 3.2. Immunoprecipitation

In this step, all work should be performed below 4°C. Use crushed ice in an ice bucket and keep the samples cool at all times.

1. Discard supernatant and move all samples to an ice bucket.
2. Add 1 mL of modified RIPA buffer and incubate on ice for 30 min. After vortexing cells, spin down insoluble fraction by microcentrifuging at 12,000$g$, 15 min at 4°C.
3. Prepare two sets of screw-capped Eppendorf tubes and add either Protein A (Sigma, p9424) or Protein G (p3296) sepharose 4B fast flow beads 40 µL to both sets of tubes. Then, prewash tubes in saline buffer, three times (*see* **Notes 3** and **4**).
4. Transfer supernatant from **step 2** to one set of Eppendorf tubes prepared at **step 3**. (Mark this set A.)
5. Put 1 mL saline buffer with appropriate antibodies (1–5 µg) into the second set of Eppendorf tubes prepared at **step 3**. (Mark this set B.)
6. Both sets of tubes are incubated on a rotator for 1 h in a cold room.
7. B set: spin down beads and discard supernatant. Wash beads with saline buffer three times.
8. A set: spin down beads and transfer supernatant to B set of tubes. Then, B sets of tubes are incubated for 2 h or O/N in a cold room.

9. Spin down beads and discard supernatant. Then, wash beads with RIPA buffer five times (*see* **Note 5**).
10. Add 30 µL of 2X Laemmli buffer and store the samples at –20°C or go to Western blot.

## 3.3. Western Blotting

To visualize the phosphorylation of target proteins, separate proteins in SDS-PAGE gels and transfer to PVDF membrane. Then, biotinylated antiphosphotyrosine antibody, 4G10 is hybridized with phosphotyrosine in JAK kinase on the membrane and streptavidin-horseradish peroxidase attached with biotin. The phosphorylation reaction is visualized by chemiluminesant reaction using ECL reagent.

1. Boil the samples from **Subheading 3.2., step 10** in a water bath at 100°C for 5 min (pierce lids to prevent caps "popping").
2. Cool samples on ice for 1 min. Then, spin down the beads by microcentrifuging at 12,000$g$ for 1 min at 4°C. Load 30 µL of samples into the well of 8% SDS-PAGE minigel (ex. NOVEX, X cell II minicell, EI9002) and run at 125 V for 3 h (*see* **Note 6**).
3. Place gel in transfer apparatus (**Fig. 1**) and remove air carefully. Perform transfer to prewet PVDF membrane at 30 V for 1 h in ice bucket. (According to the manual of your transfer apparatus.)
4. Remove PVDF membrane and mark on the side facing gel.
5. Nonspecific binding sites are blocked by immersing the membrane in a plastic bag with 5 mL of blocking buffer for 1 h at room temperature (RT) on a rotator. Membranes may be left in the blocking buffer overnight in a refrigerator (2–8°C), if more convenient.
6. Wash the membrane in TBS-Tween buffer at RT once for 15 min and twice for 5 min with fresh changes of the washing buffer.
7. Incubate the membrane in diluted antiphosphotyrosine antibody (Biotinylated-4G10, Upstate Biotech. #16-103) in 5 mL TBS-T for 1 h at RT (*see* **Note 7**).
8. Wash the membrane as detailed in **step 6**.
9. Incubate the membrane in the diluted second antibody (streptavidin-HRP (Amersham, Arlington Heights, IL, RPN1231) 1:10000 ) for 0.5 h at RT (*see* **Note 8**).
10. Wash the membrane 1 × 15 min and 4 × 5 min in fresh changes of washing buffer.
11. Detection: It is necessary to work quickly once the blots have been exposed to the detection solution. All steps can be carried out in a dark room.
12. Take the detection reagents supplied and mix an equal volume of detection solution 1 and 2 to give sufficient to cover the membranes (0.125 mL/cm$^2$) and incubate membrane for 1 min at RT. Wrap the membrane in Saran Wrap and do not allow it to dry.
13. Expose on X-ray film for 1–30 min.

## 3.4. Reprobing Blots

The complete removal of primary and secondary antibodies from membranes is possible by following the method outlined below. The membranes may be stripped of bound antibodies and reprobed several times. Membranes should be stored wet, and wrapped in Saran Wrap in a refrigerator after each immunodetection.

1. Incubate the membrane with reprobing buffer at 65°C for 30 min.
2. Wash the membrane in TBS-T three times (15, 5, 5 min).
3. Block nonspecific binding in blocking buffer for 1 h at RT.
4. Wash the membrane in TBS-T three times (15, 5, 5 min).
5. Incubate the membrane with the antibody used for immunoprecipitation for 1 h at 4°C on the rotator.

6. Wash the membrane in TBS-T three times (15, 5, 5 min).

7. Incubate the membrane with antirabbit IgG HRP (1:20000) in 5 mL of TBS-T for 30 min at RT (*see* **Note 9**).

8. Wash the membrane in TBS-T three times (15, 5, 5 min).

9. Mix ECL reagents 1 and 2 immediately and incubate the membrane for 1 min. Wrap the membrane in Saran Wrap. Do not dry the membrane any time.

10. Expose the membrane to X-ray film for 1–30 min.

## 4. Notes

1. You can also use culture medium for this step. However, you should check whether JAK kinase is activated without interleukins or not.

2. JAK kinase phosphorylation is a very rapid reaction. First, perform a time-course (30 s–1 h) of JAK kinase phosphorylation to find the maximum point of phosphorylation of JAK.

3. You can also use Protein A/G agarose for immunoprecipitation. However, agarose is hard to visualize in the washing buffer.

4. You should use the appropriate Protein A or G beads for your antibody. In general, mouse monoclonal antibodies bind with Protein G, but rabbit polyclonal antibodies bind Protein A rather than Protein G.

5. This step is critical to get good results. Remove all wash buffer each time and do not leave wash buffer in the beads.

6. To get good results, using thick and narrow well-SDS-PAGE gel to concentrate a protein (i.e., 1.5-mm thick and 15-well precast gel from Novex).

7. You can reuse this antibody buffer one more time. Add 0.05% $NaN_3$ and store in 4°C.

8. It is recommended that the antibody dilution should be optimized to suit different blotting situations. This concentration of streptavidin HRP (Amersham, RPN1231) is optimized for Amersham's ECL kit (Amersham, RPN2106).

9. This concentration of antirabbit IgG HRP (Amersham, NA934) is optimized for Amersham's ECL kit.

## References

1. Kishimoto, T., Taga, T., and Akira, S. (1994) Cytokine signal transduction. *Cell* **76**, 253.
2. Ihle, J. N., Witthuhn, B. A., Quelle, F. W., Yamamoto, K., Thierfeider, W. E., Kreider, B., et al. (1994) Signaling by the cytokine receptor superfamily: JAKs and STATs. *TIBS* **19**, 222.
3. Obiri, N. I., Siegel, J., Varricchio, F., and Puri, R. K. (1994) Expression of high affinity IL-4 receptors on human melanoma, ovarian and breast carcinoma cells. *Clin. Exp. Immunol.* **95**, 148.
4. Murata, T., Obiri, N. I., and Puri, R. K. (1997) Human ovarian carcinoma cell lines express IL-4 and IL-13 receptors: Comparison between IL-4 and IL-13 induced signal transduction. *Int. J. Cancer* **70**, 230.
5. Ihle, J. N. and Kerr, I. M. (1995) Jaks and Stats in signaling by the cytokine receptor superfamily. *Trends Genet.* **11**, 69.
6. Darnell, J. E. Jr., Kerr, I. M., and Stark, G. R. (1994) Jak-STAT pathway and transcriptional activation in response to IFNs and other extracellular signaling proteins. *Science* **264**, 1415.
7. Hou, J., Schindler, U., Henkel, W. J., Ho, T. C., Brasseur, M., and McKnight, S. (1994) An interleukin-4-induced transcription factor. *IL-4 Stat. Science* **265**, 1701.
8. Quelle, F. W., Shimoda, K., Thierfelder, W., Fischer, C., Kim, A., Ruben, S. M., et al. (1995) Cloning of murine Stat6 and Human Stat6, Stat proteins that are tyrosine phosphorylated in responses to IL-4 and IL-3 but are not required for mitogenesis. *Mol. Cell. Biol.* **15**, 3336.
9. Ivashkiv, L. B. (1995) Cytokines and STATs: how can signals achieve specificity? *Immunity* **3**, 1.

# 62

## Detection of ErbB Receptor Family Tyrosyl Phosphorylation in Ovarian Carcinoma Cells

**Anne W. Hamburger**

## 1. Introduction

The epidermal growth factor receptor (EGFR) (ErbB) family of receptor tyrosine kinases is frequently overexpressed in ovarian cancer *(1)* . This receptor group is comprised of four members, EGFR (ErbB-1), HER2 (ErbB-2), HER3 (ErbB-3), and HER4 (ErbB-4). These receptors share a common molecular architecture, possessing a large glycosylated extracellular ligand-binding domain, a single hydrophobic transmembrane domain, and a cytoplasmic tyrosine kinase domain *(2)*. Amplification and over-expression of ErbB-2 have been reported in ovarian carcinoma, where high levels of ErbB-2 directly correlate with poor clinical prognosis *(3,4)*. Amplification of EGFR has also been reported, and may have prognostic significance *(5,6)*. Less is known about the clinical significance of ErbB-3 *(7)* and ErbB-4 *(8)*, which have been more recently identified.

Overexpression of ErbB receptors results in their enhanced tyrosine kinase activity and inappropriate activation of a variety of signal transduction pathways. A diversity of signaling molecules are preferentially activated by different ErbB receptors. The specificity of their binding is dictated by receptor sequences that flank a specific phosphotyrosine residue. For example, EGFR has been shown to associate with phospholipase C-γ, SHC, and Grb2 *(9)*. ErbB-2 can associate with PLCγ, SHC, RAS-GTPase, and Grb-2 activating proteins *(10)*. ErbB-3 has specific motifs allowing coupling to phosphatidylinositol 3-kinase (PI3K) and SHC, but not Grb-2 *(11)*. Inappropriate tyrosyl phosphorylation of these substrates has been postulated to be an important correlate of cellular transformation.

The results of these studies suggest that activation of specific ErbB signal transduction pathways may result in transformation of ovarian epithelial cells. We sought to understand the tyrosine phosphorylation profile of ovarian cancer cells. The ability of cytostatic proteins with potential therapeutic use, such as interferon and tumor necrosis factor, to affect tyrosine phosphorylation and ultimately cell growth was also explored *(12,13)*.

From: *Methods in Molecular Medicine, Vol. 39: Ovarian Cancer: Methods and Protocols*
Edited by: J. M. S. Bartlett © Humana Press, Inc., Totowa, NJ

## 2. Materials

### 2.1. Examination of Tyrosyl Phosphorylated Proteins

1. Phosphate-buffered saline (PBS): ($KH_2PO_4$(0.21 g/L), NaCl (9.9 g/L), $Na_2PO_4.7H_2O$ (0.726 g/L) pH 7.4.
2. SDS-polyacrylamide gel electrophoresis (PAGE) sample buffer (3X): 1.52 g Tris base, 2 g SDS, 2 mL β-mercaptoethanol, 20 mL glycerol, 1 mg bromophenol blue, 36 mg Na orthovanadate, 42 mg NaF. Adjust pH to 6.8 with 1 *N* HCl. Add $dH_2O$ to a final volume of 100 mL. Aliquot and freeze at –20°C.
3. 4X Tris-HCl/SDS gel buffer: 1.5 *M* Tris-HCl, pH 8.8, 0.4% SDS for separating gel; 1.5 *M* Tris-HCl, pH 6.8, 0.4% SDS for stacking gel. Store solutions at 4°C.
4. 30% acrylamide/0.8% bisacrylamide solution.
5. 5X SDS-PAGE running buffer: 15.1 g Tris base, 72.0 g glycine, 5.0 g SDS; add deionized water to 1 L. It is unnecessary to adjust pH of the stock solution. Final pH on dilution is 8.3.
6. Transfer buffer: 20 m*M* Tris/150 m*M* glycine, pH 8.0, 20% methanol. It is not necessary to adjust pH. Store at 4°C.
7. Blocking Solution. 5% bovine serum albumin in TBST (10 mM Tris-HCl, pH 8.0, 150 m*M* NaCl, 0.05% Tween-20).
8. Antibody dilution buffer: TBST with 2% BSA.
9. Stripping buffer (100 m*M* β-mercaptoethanol, 2% SDS, 62.5 m*M* Tris-HCl, pH 6.7).

### 2. 2. Kinase Activity of Immunoprecipitated ErbB-2

1. RIPA Buffer: 50 m*M* Tris HCl, pH 7.4, 150 m*M* NaCl, 1% Triton X-100, 1% Deoxycholic Acid, Na Salt, 0.1% SDS, aprotinin (1 µg/mL) PMSF (100 µg/mL) DTT (1 m*M*), Na-orthovanadate (1 m*M*).
2. Kinase Assay Buffer: 50 m*M* HEPES, pH 7.5, 0.1 m*M* EDTA, 0.015% Brij 35 (Sigma, St. Louis, MO) containing 0.1 mg/mL BSA and 0.2% β-mercaptoethanol.
3. ATP mixture [0.3 m*M* ATP, 30 m*M* $MgCl_2$, 200 mCi γ $^{32}$P-ATP (3000 Ci/mMol, Amersham, Arlington Heights, IL, AA0068)].

## 3. Methods

### 3.1. Examination of Tyrosyl Phosphorylated Proteins

1. Plate cells in monolayer in 60-mm dishes. Harvest cells when they have reached 80% confluence.
2. Rinse cells three times with cold PBS. Aspirate PBS.
3. Add SDS-PAGE sample buffer (400 µL/dish). Incubate rocking 10 min at 4°C. Collect cell lysates by scraping into microcentrifuge tubes.
4. Sonicate for 15 s. Store samples at –70°C prior to analysis.
5. Heat samples resuspended in SDS-PAGE sample buffer at 95°C in a heat block for 5 min.
6. Electrophorese samples (30 µL per lane) and prestained molecular weight markers (Bio-Rad, Richmond, CA, or equivalent) in Bio-Rad minigel apparatus 60 min 175 V (constant voltage).
7. Transfer proteins from gel to nitrocellulose at 35 V overnight at 4°C in Bio-Rad minigel blotting apparatus or equivalent (*see* **Note 1**).
8. Block membrane with 5% nonfat dried milk in TBST (1 mL per $cm^2$ of membrane) for 1 h at room temperature or overnight at 4°C.
9. Wash the membrane in two changes of TBST for 10 min at room temperature. All subsequent incubations and washes take place at room temperature.

Fig. 1. Inclusion of Na orthovanadate for detection of tyrosyl phosphorylation. SK-OV3 cells, grown in complete media, remained untreated (Lane 1) or received Na orthovanadate (100 µM) (lane 2) during the last hour of incubation.

10. Add primary antibody (antiphosphotyrosine, PY-20, Transduction Laboratories, Lexington, KY) in an appropriate volume of antibody dilution buffer to cover membrane at a dilution that has been predetermined to ensure maximum sensitivity and specificity. Incubate with shaking for 2 h (*see* **Note 2**).
11. Wash membrane in TBST for 15 min with three changes (*see* **Note 3**).
12. Add appropriate horseradish peroxidase-conjugated secondary antibody (Amersham Laboratories) at an appropriate predetermined dilution in antibody dilution buffer for 45 min.
13 Wash in TBST for 30 min with four changes of TBST.
14. Mix equal volumes of ECL detection reagents (A and B) (Amersham). Cover membrane and incubate for 1 min at room temperature.
15. Blot membrane on a paper towel. Place membrane on a piece of Whatman #1 filter paper placed in a stainless steel exposure cassette (8 × 10″) and cover the membrane with Saran Wrap.
16. Expose film (ECL Hyperfilm, Amersham) against membrane starting at 30 s and develop. After use, blot may be stored wet in TBST (*see* **Note 4**).
17. Strip the membrane by incubating at 50°C for 15 min in a large volume of stripping buffer with occasional agitation. Wash the membrane 2X in TBST using as large a volume of buffer as possible. Block the membrane in 7.5% nonfat dried milk in TBST for 1 h at room temperature. Perform immunodetection as previously described to ensure that the antibodies have been stripped off the blot. Proceed to immunoblot with the second antibody of choice. For example, blot first with antibody to phosphotyrosine. After developing the film, strip the blot and then reprobe with antibody to ErbB-2 to normalize phosphotyrosine levels to ErbB-2 protein levels.
18. Reprobe with the actin antibody (Boeringher Mannheim, Indianapolis, IN) as a loading control if quantitative changes are important.
19. Alternatively, ErbB antibodies or antibodies to signal transduction proteins may be used to immunoprecipitate specific proteins of interest (for immunoprecipitation protocol *see* **Subheading 3.2.**). Blots are probed first with antibody to phosphotyrosine, stripped, and then probed with antibody to the specific protein of interest (**Fig. 1**) (*see* **Notes 5** and **6**).

### 3.2. Assay of ErbB-2 Kinase Activity

1. Wash cells (plated as in **Subheading 3.1.**) in three changes of cold PBS.
2. Add RIPA buffer (0.4 mL/dish). Incubate with rocking for 10 min at 4°C.

3. Scrape cells and spin lysates at top speed in a microcentrifuge for 30 min at 4°C.

4. Preclear extracts by adding 20 µL of Protein G PLUS/Protein A Agarose (Calbiochem, La Jolla, CA) (referred to as beads) for 1 h at 4°C with rocking.

5. Centrifuge in microcentrifuge at 6500g for 5 min and transfer supernatant to a new tube for immunoprecipitation.

6. To a 1.5-mL microcentrifuge tube add:1 mL cell extract (protein concentration of approximately 1 mg), 1–2 µg of appropriate antibody [ErbB-2 antibody 5 (Calbiochem, *see* **Note 7**) for ErbB-2 kinase assays or a similar antibody that does not inhibit kinase activity].

7. Incubate for 4 h or overnight at 4°C.

8. Add 15 µL of beads and rock for 1 h at 4°C.

9. Collect the immunoprecipitates by centrifugation in a microcentrifuge at 6500g for 5 min at 4°C.

10. Carefully aspirate off media with a fine-tipped pipet or sequencing pipet tip.

11. Wash beads 4X with ice-cold RIPA buffer.

12. At this point, beads can be resuspended in sample buffer and used for immunoblot analysis. For the kinase assay proceed as follows:

13. Suspend pellet in 20 µL protein kinase assay buffer (*see* **Subheading 2.**).

14. Add 10 µL of Raytide™ (1 mg/mL) (Calbiochem) solution in kinase assay buffer to the beads (*see* **Notes 8** and **9**).

15. Start the reaction by adding 10 µL of ATP mix. Incubate at 30°C for 30 min.

16. Add 120 µL of 10% phosphoric acid to stop the reaction.

17. Vortex the reaction mixture and pipette 120 µL onto P81 papers ($2 \times 2$ cm).

18. Wash papers 3X with 0.5% phosphoric acid, and once with acetone. Dry under a heat lamp and quantitate phosphate incorporation by liquid scintillation counting.

## 4. Notes

1. The high-molecular weight proteins such as ErbB-2 are difficult to transfer. Overnight transfer at low voltage is recommended. The efficiency of transfer can be checked by following the transfer of the prestained standards and by staining the gel in 0.1% Commassie blue (45% methanol, 10% acetic acid).

2. The primary antibody can be left on overnight to increase the sensitivity of the assay.

3. Wash steps can be extended overnight if necessary.

4. Blots can be stored, completely wet, in TBST at 4°C for many months.

5. To quantitate changes in phosphotyrosine levels, a densitometer should be used to measure the amount of phosphotyrosylated protein as compared to the amount of the specific protein of interest.

6. Because of the constitutive activity of protein tyrosine phosphatases in many cell types, it may be necessary to incubate cells in 100 µ*M* Na orthovanadate for 1 h prior to harvesting cells *(14)*.

7. The activity of other receptors, such as EGFR, may be assayed this way using antibodies that preserve kinase activity.

8. We have successfully used Raytide but other synthetic substrates may be used.

9. The molecular weight of Raytide is 2116 Dalton.

## References

1. Simpson, B. J. B., Phillips, H. A., Lessells, A. M., Langdon, S. P., and Miller, W. R. (1995) C-erbB growth factor receptor proteins in ovarian tumors. *Int. J. Cancer* **64,** 202–206.
2. Hsuan, J. J. (1993) Oncogene regulation by growth factors. *Anticancer Res.* **13,** 2521–2532.
3. Cirisano, F. D. and Karlan, B. Y. (1996) The role of the HER-2/neu oncogene in gynecologic cancer. *J. Soc. Gynecol. Investig.* **3,** 99–105.

4. Meden, H. and Kuhn, W. (1997) Overexpression of the oncogene c-erbB-2 (HER/neu) in ovarian cancer: a new prognostic factor. *Euro. J. Obstet. Gynecol. Reprod. Biol.* **71,** 173–179.
5. Scambia, G., Benedetti-Panici, P., Ferrandina, G., Distefano, M., Salerno, G., Romanin, M. E., et al. (1995) Epidermal growth factor, oestrogen and progesterone receptor expression in primary ovarian cancer: correlation with clinical outcome and response to chemotherapy. *Brit. J. Cancer* **72,** 361–366.
6. Bartlett, J. M., Langdon, S. P., Simpson, B. J., Stewart, M., Katsaro, D., Sismond, P., et al. (1996) The prognostic value of epidermal growth factor receptor mRNA expression in primary ovarian cancer. *Br. J. Cancer* **73,** 301–306.
7. Simpson, B. J. B., Weatherill, J., Miller, E. P., Lessless, A. M., Langdon, S. P., and Miller, W. R. (1995) C-erbB-3 protein expression in ovarian tumors. *Br. J. Cancer* **71,** 758–762.
8. Plowman, G. D., Culouscou, J.-M., Whitney, G. S., Greene, J. M., Carlton, G. W., Foy, L., et al. (1993) Ligand-specific activation of HER4/p180$^{erbB4}$, a fourth member of the epidermal growth factor receptor family. *Proc. Natl. Acad. Sci. USA* **90,** 1746–1750.
9. Carpenter, G. (1992) Receptor tyrosine kinase substrates: *src* homology domains and signal transduction. *FASEB J.* **6,** 3283–3289.
10. Carraway, K. L. III and Cantley, L. C. (1994) A new acquaintance for erbB3 and erbB4: a role for receptor heterodimerization in growth signaling. *Cell* **78,** 5–8.
11. Kraus, M. H., Fedi, P., Starks, V., Muraro, R., and Aaronson, S. A. (1993) Demonstration of ligand-dependent signaling by the erbB-3 tyrosine kinase and its constitutive activation in human breast tumor cells. *Proc. Natl. Acad. Sci. USA* **90,** 2900–2904.
12. Mishra, S. and Hamburger, A. W. (1993) Exogenous phosphotyrosine modulates epidermal growth factor receptor tyrosine phosphorylation. *Carcinogenesis* **14,** 269–273.
13. Mishra, S. and Hamburger, A. W. (1994) Interferon Gamma-induced reduction in erbB-2 tyrosyl phosphorylation in human ovarian carcinoma cells. *Int. J. Cancer* **58,** 538–542.
14. Jallal, B., Schlessinger, J., and Ullrich, A. (1992) Tyrosine phosphatase inhibition permits analysis of signal transduction complexes in P185/her2 overexpressing human tumor cells. *J. Biol. Chem.* **267,** 4357–4363.

# 63

## Phosphotyrosine Kinase Assays as a Prescreen for Inhibitors of EGFr

**Joanne Edwards and John M. S. Bartlett**

## 1. Introduction

The epidermal growth factor receptor (EGFr) is a 170-kDa glycosylated transmembrane protein found in a wide variety of tissues *(1)*. It is the receptor for epidermal growth factor (EGF), transforming growth factor $\alpha$ (TGF$\alpha$), and other related growth factor peptides *(2,3)*. In 1980, EGF binding activity of receptor preparations was shown to be associated with a protein kinase activity. Subsequent studies demonstrated that the EGF binding activity and kinase activity were properties of the same protein *(4)*. In the absence of EGF, tyrosine kinase activity is low. Binding of EGF to the receptor domain results in receptor dimerisation and subsequent autophosphorylation of the cytoplasmic domain of EGFr at specific tyrosine residues. This autophosphorylation results in an activation of the tyrosine kinase activity of the EGFr. The phosphorylated tyrosine residues of the EGFr are involved in binding enzymes containing SH2 or SH3 domains *(5)*. Enzymes identified to date that bind tightly to EGFr phosphotyrosine residues include phosphatidyl inositol 3 kinase, phospholipase C$\gamma$ and ras GTPase activating protein *(6)*. Binding of these enzymes occurs at highly specific phosphotyrosine residues of the receptor and is believed to be a mechanism for signal transduction from the receptor to the final intracellular target.

EGF and TGF$\alpha$ are known to play important roles in regulation of growth in normal and malignant cell types, including ovarian cancer *(7,8)*. Approximately 50% of ovarian cancers have elevated levels of EGFr, this overexpression of EGFr correlates with a poor prognosis for patient survival *(9)*. Therefore, EGFr tyrosine kinase inhibitors (TKI) may, in the future, be used as treatment for ovarian cancer.

## 2. Materials

1. Cell lysis buffer (50 m$M$ HEPES pH 7.4, 1% Triton X-100, 150 m$M$ NaCl, 5 m$M$ ethyleneglycol tetra-acetic acid (EGTA), 100 μg /mL PMSF, 10 μg/mL aprotinin, 100 μg/mL benzamidine, 5 μg/mL leupeptin, and 100 μ$M$ sodium orthovanadate).
2. Substrate buffer (1.5 m$M$ peptide (RKGRAAENAEYLRV) (Genosys) in 135 m$M$ HEPES, 300 μ$M$ sodium orthovanadate, 3 m$M$ dithiothreitiol, 0.15% Triton X-100, 6% glycerol, and 0.05% sodium azide pH 7.4).
3. Epidermal growth factor (6 ng/μL) (Sigma, U.K.).

From: *Methods in Molecular Medicine, Vol. 39: Ovarian Cancer: Methods and Protocols*
Edited by: J. M. S. Bartlett © Humana Press, Inc., Totowa, NJ

4. Magnesium adenosine triphosphate (ATP) buffer. (6 μ*M* ATP, 30 m*M* HEPES and 72 m*M* MgCl$_2$ pH 7.4) (Sigma).
5. [γ$^{32}$P]ATP (40 μCi/mL) (Amersham plc, U.K.)
6. Stop reagent (300 m*M* orthophosphoric acid containing carmosine red).
7. Water bath at 30°C.
8. 1% acetic acid.
9. 20-mL scintillation counting vials.
10. Scintillation counter for phosphorus-32 counting.
11. Liquid scintillation cocktail and dispenser.
12. Peptide binding papers (P81 chromatography paper) (Whatman, U.K.).
13. Desk top centrifuge.
14. Dimethyl sulfoxide (DMSO).
15. Phosphate-buffered saline (PBS) (pH 7.4).
16. Rocking platform.
17. Wash tray.

## 3. Methods

### 3.1. Sample Preparation

1. Grow A431 cells in 80 cm$^3$ tissue culture flasks till 80% confluent (*see* **Note 1**).
2. Lyse cells in 0.7 mL lysis buffer.
3. Transfer cell lysate to a clean tube and incubated at 4°C for 20 min on a rocking platform.
4. Pellet by centrifugation, 400*g* max for 15 min at 4°C.
5. Decant supernatant into a fresh clean tube.
6. Store on ice, do not freeze.

Fresh samples must be used in the assay as a loss of EGFr activity often results following a freeze–thaw process (*see* **Note 2**).

### 3.2 Assay Methodology

This assay is designed to detect EGFr tyrosine kinase enzyme (EGFr TK) activity in solubilized cells. Enzyme present in the samples will catalyse the transfer of the γ-phosphate of adenosine 5' triphosphate to the tyrosine group on a peptide which is specific for EGFr TK. Specific detection of the enzyme is further guaranteed by using epidermal growth factor to activate the EGFr TK enzyme activity. Thus, EGF dependent tyrosine kinase activity may be determine from the difference in activity between the enzyme activity in the presence and absence of added EGF. The assay is performed at pH 7.4 in Hepes buffer with MgCl$_2$ as the essential metal ion. The assay will give linear incorporation of $^{32}$P into substrate peptide corresponding to a least 20% ATP incorporated, providing samples are suitable diluted (1–5 μg/mL). Phosphorylated peptide is separated on binding paper. After washing the paper the extent of phosphorylation may be detected by scintillation counting.

Dispense sufficient magnesium ATP buffer to perform the number of assays required. Add [$^{32}$P] ATP to a concentration of 200 μCi/mL. Each reaction requires 5 μL of magnesium [$^{32}$P] ATP buffer. Store on ice until required and do not refreeze for use at a later date. A summary of assay procedure is described in **Table 1**.

1. Label tubes for samples and place in a rack.
2. Pipet 8 μL of sample (10–50 μg) or lysis buffer into each appropriate tube (no enzyme control).

**Table 1**
**Summary of Assay Procedure**

|  | Samples | Zero Enzyme Blank | Zero EGF Blank | No Drug |
|---|---|---|---|---|
| Sample | 8 µL | 0 µL | 8 µL | 8 µL |
| Lysis Buffer | 0 µL | 8 µL | 0 µL | 0 µL |
| Drug | 2 µL | 2 µL | 2 µL | 0 µL |
| DMSO | 0 µL | 0 µL | 0 µL | 2 µL |
| EGF | 5 µL | 5 µL | 0 µL | 5 µL |
| Water | 0 µL | 0 µL | 5 µL | 0 µL |
| Substrate buffer | 10 µL | 10 µL | 10 µL | 10 µL |
| ATP | 5 µL | 5 µL | 5 µL | 5 µL |
| Mix, centrifuge for 15 s. Incubate at 30°C for 30 min. | | | | |
| Stop reagent | 10 µL | 10 µL | 10 µL | 10 µL |
| Centrifuge for 15 s. Aliquot 30 µL on to binding paper. Wash papers and count. | | | | |

3. Pipet 5 µL of EGF into each tube, or 5 µL of water (no EGF control).
4. Pipet 2 µL of drug ( dissolve in DMSO) into each tube or DMSO (no drug control).
5. Pipet 10 µL of substrate buffer into each tube or 10 µL of water ( no substrate control).
6. Start the reaction by adding 5 µL of magnesium [$^{32}$P]ATP buffer. Mix the contents of the tube. Microfuge for 15 s to wash all reagents into base of tube. Incubate for 30 min at 30°C.
7. Terminate the reaction with 10 µL stop reagent.
8. Mix the terminated reaction. Microfuge tubes for 15 s to wash all reagents into base of the tube.
9. Cut P81 Whatman paper into 2.5-cm$^2$ squares and number accordingly using pencil.
10. Pipet 30 µL of terminated reaction mixture onto the center of each paper square.
11. Place the squares into a wash tray and wash in 1% acetic acid. Incubate for 2 min on a rocking platform. Decant wash reagent and dispose of as phosphorus-32 liquid waste. Add a similar volume of wash reagent and repeat once.
12. Add 250 mL of distilled water to the wash tray. Rock for 2 min. Decant water and dispose of as phosphorus 32 liquid waste. Add a similar volume of water and repeat once.
13. Using forceps remove paper squares and place in a 20-mL scintillation vial. Dispose of water as phosphorus-32 waste.
14. Add 5 mL scintillant to each vial and count in an appropriate scintillation counter for phosphorus-32.
15. Count samples by scintillation counting for 1 min.
16. Expressed results in pmols/phosphate transferred/µg protein/minute.

### 3.3. Estimation of Protein Concentration in the Sample

Bradford's reagent (0.01% Commassie blue-G250, 4.5% ethanol, and 5.5% ortho-phosphoric acid) (200 µL) is added to 10 µL of cell homogenate, and 790 µL water; the color is allowed to develop for 5 min before the absorbance is read at 590 nm *(10)*. The amount of protein present is calculated from a standard curve constructed from samples containing 25, 20, 15, 10, 5, and 0 µg/mL bovine serum albumin.

### 3.4. Calculation of Results

The phosphorus-32 incorporated into the peptide is quantitatively measured by the binding papers. In the presence of enzyme sample and EGF the [$^{32}$P] counted on the

Fig. 1. Dose response curve of TKI inhibitor.

papers is the sum of nonspecific [$^{32}$P] ATP binding, specific binding of phosphorylated peptide, and binding of phosphorylated proteins in the cell extract (**A**).

In the absence of EGF and presence of enzyme, the [$^{32}$P] counted on the papers is the sum of nonspecific [$^{32}$P] ATP binding, and non-EGF-dependent tyrosine kinase phosphorylation of the peptide and cell extract proteins (**B**).

In the absence of enzyme and presence of EGF, the [$^{32}$P] counted on the papers is caused by nonspecific binding of [$^{32}$P] or its radiolytic decomposition products (**C**).

### 3.4.1. EGFr TK is Therefore Obtained from [A-B]

5 mL of 6 m$M$ Mg [$^{32}$P] ATP contains $3 \times 10^{-11}$ moles ATP
**R** = cpm per 5 mL Mg [$^{32}$P] ATP/ $3 \times 10^{-11}$

**R**= cpm per 5 mL Mg [$^{32}$P] ATP/3 cpm/pmol

Calculation of total phosphate (**T**) transferred to peptide and endogenous proteins
30 mL spotted on to binding paper
Total terminated volume 40 mL
$T$= [A-B] $\times$ [30/40]

$T$= [A-B] $\times$ 1.33

Calculation of pmoles phosphate (**P**) transferred per minute

**P**= **T/I** $\times$ **R** pmoles/min

Where **I** = incubation time (min)

p moles phosphate transferred/µg protein/minutes = **P**/µg of protein present in the assay

The data obtained by users will depend upon the type of experiment performed. **Figure 1** shows a typical dose response curve for a TKI with a IC 50 value of 30 μ*M*. A431 cells were used as a source of EGFr (*see* **Note 3**).

## 4. Notes

1. Samples must be prepared from cells of no greater than 80% confluence, as cells that have reached confluency have low expression of EGFr. If samples are prepared from confluent cells, almost no tyrosine kinase activity will be observed following EGF treatment.
2. Fresh samples must always be used as EGFr tyrosine kinase activity is lost following the freeze–thaw process.
3. It is advisable before starting a TKI dose response curve to conduct an assay with no drug present by repeatedly measuring the activity of solubilized A431 cells. This will test that the assay system is working and that you have a low interassay variation. This experiment should be repeated to measure intraassay variation.

## References

1. Gill, G. N., Santon, J. B., and Bertics, P. J. (1987) Regulatory features of the epidermal growth factor receptor. *J. Cell. Physiol.* **5,** 35–41.
2. Laurence, D. J. R. and Gusterson, B. A. (1990) The epidermal growth factor. A review of structural and functional relationships in the normal organism and in cancer cells. *Tumor Biol.* **11,** 229–261.
3. Johnson, G. R., Kannan, B., Shoyab, M., and Stomberg, K. (1993) Amphiregulin induces tyrosine phosphorylation of the epidermal growth factor receptor and p185erb B2. Evidence that amphiregulin acts exclusively through the epidermal growth factor receptor at the surface of human epithelial cells. *J. Biol. Chem.* **268,** 2924–2931.
4. Basu, A., Raghunath, M., Bishaylee, S., and Das, M. (1989) Inhibition of tyrosine kinase activity of the epidermal growth factor receptor by a truncated receptor form. *Mol. Cell. Biol.* **9,** 671–677.
5. Pronk, G., De Vries-Smits, A., Bunday, L., Downward, J., Maassen, J., Medema, R., and Bos, J. (1994) Involvement of Shc in insulin and epidermal growth factor induced activation of p21 ras. *Mol. Cell. Biol.* **14,** 1575–1580.
6. Downward, J., Yarden, Y., Mayes, E., Scrace, G., Torry, N., Stockwell, P., et al. (1984) Close similarity of epidermal growth factor receptor and v-erb B oncogene protein sequences. *Nature* **307,** 521–527.
7. Bartlett, J. M. S., Langdon, S. P., Simpson, B. J. B., Stewart, M., Katsaros, D., Sismondi, P., et al. (1996) The prognostic value of epidermal growth factor receptor mRNA expression in primary ovarian cancer. *Br. J. Cancer* **73,** 301–306.
8. Battaglia, F., Scambia, G., Benedetti Panici, P. I., Baiocchi, G., Peronne, I., Iacobelli, S., et al. (1989) Epidermal growth factor expression in gynaecological malignancies. *Gynecol. Obstet. Invest.* **37,** 855–862.
9. Berchuck, A., Rodriguex, G. C., Kamel, A., Dodge, R. K., Soper, J. T., Clarke-Pearson, D. L., et al. (1991) Epidermal growth factor receptor expression in normal ovarian epithelium and ovarian cancer. I. correlation of receptor expression with prognostic factors in patents with ovarian cancer. *Am. J. Obstet. Gynecol.* **164,** 669–674.
10. Bradford, M. (1976) A rapid and sensitive method for the quantitation of microgram quantities of proteins utilising the principle of protein-dye binding. *Anal. Biochem.* **72,** 248–254.

# 64

## Direct Kinase Assay Screening for Inhibitors of MAP Kinase

### Joanne Edwards and John M. S. Bartlett

## 1. Introduction

An important convergence point involved in the signal transduction pathways of many different growth factors, hormones, and cytokines are the p42 and p44 serine/threonine kinases called either MAP kinases (mitogen-activate protein kinases) or ERK 1 and ERK 2 (extracellular regulated kinases) *(2–4)*. MAP kinases are activated in cells upon stimulation with growth factors (e.g., insulin, platelet derived growth factor, epidermal growth factor) *(5–7)*, tumor promoters (e.g., phorbol 12-myristate 13-acetate) *(8)*, antigen binding to T-cell receptors, and infection of cells by *Salmonella sp*. MAP kinase is also involved in cell-cycle control and becomes activated during M-phase of the cell cycle *(9)*. As such, MAP kinase is of great interest in cancer studies including ovarian cancer. Studies on MAP kinase activation and regulation will lead to an improved understanding of intracellular signal transduction and involvement of this enzyme in key signaling process. It is therefore important to know how anticancer drugs if at all act on this kinase. MAP kinase is activated by sequential phosphorylation on both tyrosine and threonine residues by either the dual tyrosine/threonine kinase MEK (MAPK kinase) alone or by MEK in conjunction with an as yet undescribed kinase *(2)*. The serine/threonine kinases RAF and MEKK (MAPK kinase kinase) phosphorylate and activate MEK, in turn, during intracellular signaling *(6)*. Activation of MAPK is directly regulated by a specific MAPK phosphatase and indirectly regulated by protein kinase A activation, which results in inhibition of RAF activity in Mammalian cells *(11)*.

## 2. Materials

1. Cell lysis buffer (50 m$M$ HEPES pH 7.4, 1% Triton X-100, 150 m$M$ NaCl, 5 m$M$ ethyleneglycol tetra-acetic acid (EGTA), 100 µg/mL PMSF, 10 µg/mL aprotinin, 100 µg/mL benzamidine, 5 µg/mL leupeptin, and 100 µ$M$ sodium orthovanadate).
2. Substrate buffer (Amersham International plc U.K.).
3. Epidermal growth factor (10 ng/mL) (Sigma, U.K.).
4. Magnesium adenosine triphosphate (ATP) buffer (1.2 $M$ ATP, 30 m$M$ HEPES and 72 m$M$ MgCl$_2$ pH 7.4) (Sigma).
5. [$\gamma^{32}$P]ATP (40 µCi/ml) (Amersham International).

From: *Methods in Molecular Medicine, Vol. 39: Ovarian Cancer: Methods and Protocols*
Edited by: J. M. S. Bartlett © Humana Press, Inc., Totowa, NJ

6.  Stop reagent (300 m*M* orthophosphoric acid containing carmosine red).
7.  Activated Murine GST-p42 MAP kinase (Upstate biotechnology).
8.  Water bath at 30°C.
9.  1% acetic acid.
10. 20-mL scintillation counting vials.
11. Scintillation counter for phosphorus-32 counting.
12. Liquid scintillation cocktail and dispenser.
13. Peptide binding papers (P81 chromatography paper) (Whatman, U.K.).
14. Desk top centrifuge.
15. Dimethyl sulfoxide (DMSO).
16. Phosphate-buffered saline (PBS) (pH 7.4).
17. Rocking platform.
18. Wash tray.

## 3. Methods

### 3.1. Sample Preparation

1.  Grow cells of choice in 50-cm$^3$ tissue-culture flasks until 70% confluent.
2.  Cells are washed twice with PBS (pH 7.4) and cultured for 16 h in the presence of drug.
3.  Media are removed and the cells washed then incubated in serum-free media ± drug for 30 min prior to stimulation with EGF (10 ng/mL/5 min).
4.  Cells are washed twice and lysed (0.3 mL lysis buffer).
5.  Transfer cell lysate to a clean tube and incubated at 4°C for 20 min on a rocking platform.
6.  Pellet by centrifugation, 400$g_{max}$ for 15 min at 4°C.
7.  Decant supernatant into a fresh clean tube.
8.  Samples may be stored at –80°C or on ice for use in the assay protocol.

### 3.2. Assay Methodology

This assay is designed to detect MAP kinase activity in solubilized cells, however, slight modification allows direct screening for inhibitors of MAP kinase (refer to **Subheading 4.**). To assay for p42/p44 MAP kinase activity, the protein substrates myelin basic protein and microtubule associated protein 2 are commonly used. Amersham's MAP kinase substrate peptide is a synthetic peptide substrate based on the Thr$^{669}$ phosphorylation site of the EGFr and has been modified to contain only the phosphorylation sequence PLS/TP as a site for phosphorylation *(1)*. This peptide is although not totally specific for p42/p44 MAP kinase, is much more specific than the commonly used substrates myelin basic protein and microtubule associated protein 2 *(1)*. Enzyme present in the samples will catalyse the transfer of the γ-phosphate of adenosine 5′ triphosphate to the threonine group on the substrate peptide. The assay is performed at pH 7.4 in HEPES buffer with MgCl$_2$ as the essential metal ion. The assay will give linear incorporation of $^{32}$P into substrate peptide corresponding to a least 10% ATP incorporated, providing samples are suitable diluted (1–5 μg/mL). Phosphorylated peptide is separated from unincorporated label on binding paper. After washing the paper, the extent of phosphorylation may be detected by scintillation counting.

All assay components (substrate buffer, Magnesium/ATP buffer, and stop reagent) should be thawed at room temperature for around 20 min, before beginning the assay. The cell lysates should be thawed on ice. Once thawed, mix thoroughly be swirling and inversion and store on ice.

**Table 1**
**Summary of Assay Procedure**

|  | Samples | No Substrate Blank | Zero Enzyme Blank |
|---|---|---|---|
| Sample | 15 μL | 15 μL | 0 μL |
| Lysis Buffer | 0 μL | 0 μL | 15 μL |
| Water | 0 μL | 10 μL | 0 μL |
| Substrate buffer | 10 μL | 0 μL | 10 μL |
| ATP | 5 μL | 5 μL | 5 μL |
| Mix, centrifuge for 15 s. Incubate at 30°C for 30 min. |  |  |  |
| Stop reagent | 10 μL | 10 μL | 10 μL |
| Centrifuge for 15 s. Aliquot 30 μL on to binding paper. Wash papers and count. |  |  |  |

Dispense sufficient magnesium ATP buffer to perform the number of assays required. Add [$^{32}$P] ATP to a concentration of 200 μCi/mL. Each reaction requires 5 μL of magnesium [$^{32}$P] ATP buffer. Store on ice until required. Do not refreeze for use at a later date. A summary of assay procedure can be found in **Table 1**.

1. Label tubes for samples and place in a rack. For every sample you must have a substrate and a no-substrate tube.
2. Pipet 15 μL of sample (10–50 μg) or lysis buffer into each appropriate tube (no enzyme control).
3. Pipet 10 μL of substrate buffer into each tube or 10 μL of water (no substrate control).
4. Start the reaction by adding 5 μL of magnesium [$^{32}$P]ATP buffer. Mix the contents of the tube. Microfuge for 15 s to wash all reagents into base of tube. Incubate for 30 min at 30°C.
5. Terminate the reaction with 10 μL stop reagent.
6. Mix the terminated reaction. Microfuge tubes for 15 s to wash all reagents into base of the tube.
7. Cut P81 Whatman paper into 2.5-cm$^2$ squares and number accordingly using pencil.
8. Pipet 30 μL of terminated reaction mixture onto the center of each paper square.
9. Place the squares into a wash tray and wash in 1% acetic acid. Incubate for 2 min on a rocking platform. Decant wash reagent and dispose of as phosphorus-32 liquid waste. Add a similar volume of wash reagent and repeat once.
10. Add 250 mL of distilled water to the wash tray. Rock for 2 min. Decant water and dispose of as phosphorus-32 liquid waste. Add a similar volume of water and repeat once.
11. Using forceps remove paper squares and place in a 20-mL scintillation vial. Dispose of water as phosphorus-32 waste.
12. Add 5 mL scintillant to each vial and count in an appropriate scintillation counter for phosphorus-32.
13. Count samples by scintillation counting for 1 min.
14. Expressed results in pmols/phosphate transferred/μg protein/min.

### 3.3. Estimation of Protein Concentration in the Sample

Bradford's reagent (0.01% Commassie blue-G250, 4.5 % ethanol, and 5.5 % orthophosphoric acid) (200 μL) is added to 10 μL of cell homogenate, and 790 μL water; the color is allowed to develop for 5 min before the absorbance is read at 590 nm (**10**). The amount of protein present is calculated from a standard curve constructed from samples containing 25, 20, 15, 10, 5, and 0 μg/mL bovine serum albumin.

The no enzyme blank will correct for any nonspecific effects of [$^{32}$P] ATP or its radiolytic decomposition products binding to papers. The no-substrate control will assess the degree of endogenous protein phosphorylation.

### 3.4. Calculation of Results

The phosphorus-32 incorporated into the peptide is quantitatively measured by the binding papers. In the presence of enzyme sample, the [$^{32}$P] counted on the papers is the sum of nonspecific [$^{32}$P] ATP binding, specific binding of phosphorylated peptide, and binding of phosphorylated proteins in the cell extract (**A**).

In the absence of substrate, the [$^{32}$P] counted on the papers is caused by endogenous protein phosphorylation and nonspecific [$^{32}$P] ATP binding (**B**).

In the absence of the enzyme, the [$^{32}$P] counted on the papers is the nonspecific [$^{32}$P] ATP binding (**C**).

### 3.4.1. MAP Kinase Activity is Therefore Obtained from [A-B]

5 mL of 1.2 m*M* Mg [$^{32}$P] ATP contains $6 \times 10^{-9}$ moles ATP

**R** = cpm per 5 mL Mg [$^{32}$P] ATP/ $6 \times 10^{-9}$

**R**= cpm per 5 mL Mg [$^{32}$P] ATP/6 cpm/pmol

Calculation of total phosphate (**T**) transferred to peptide

30 mL spotted on to binding paper
Total terminated volume 40 mL
*T*= [**A-B**] × [30/40]

*T*= [**A-B**] × 1.33

Calculation of pmoles phosphate (**P**) transferred per minute

**P**= **T** × 1000/**I** × **R** pmoles/min

Where **I** = incubation time (min)

p moles phosphate transferred/μg protein/min = **P**/μg of protein present in the assay

The data obtained by users will depend upon the type of experiment performed. **Figure 1** shows MAP kinase activity in PEO1 cell lysates treated with EGF and MAP kinase inhibitors.

## 4. Notes

You may determine the direct effect of MAP kinase inhibitors in a cell-free system by following the assay system discussed above. However, to measure the direct effect of the drugs on MAP kinase activity, the assay is conducted in the presence of the drugs and the cell lysate (sample) is replaced with activated GST-MAP kinase (25–35 ng per tube). Stock-activated GST-MAP kinase (100 ng/ μL) is diluted to the appropriate concentration (approximately 2 ng/ μL) in assay dilution buffer (20 m*M* MOPS, pH 7.2,

Compound 1 concentration ($\mu$M)

Fig. 1. MAP kinase activity in cell lysates from PEO1 ovarian carcinoma cells without exogenous EGF (solid bars) or with exogenous EGF (hatched bars) in the presence of increasing concentrations of compound 1 a MAP kinase inhibitor. Compound 1 has an IC 50 value of 5 $\mu M$ in the presence of EGF.

**Table 2**
**Summary of Assay Procedure**

| | Samples | No Substrate Blank | Zero Enzyme Blank | No Drug |
|---|---|---|---|---|
| Activated MAP kinase | 13 μL | 13 μL | 0 μL | 13 μL |
| Assay dilution buffer | 0 μL | 0 μL | 13 μL | 0 μL |
| Drug | 2 μL | 2 μL | 2 μL | 0 μL |
| DMSO | 0 μL | 0 μL | 0 μL | 2 μL |
| Water | 0 μL | 10 μL | 0 μL | 10 μL |
| Substrate buffer | 10 μL | 0 μL | 10 μL | 0 μL |
| ATP | 5 μL | 5 μL | 5 μL | 5 μL |
| Mix, centrifuge for 15 s. Incubate at 30°C for 30 min. | | | | |
| Stop reagent | 10 μL | 10 μL | 10 μL | 10 μL |
| Centrifuge for 15 s. Aliquot 30 μL on to binding paper. Wash papers and count. | | | | |

25 m$M$ β-glycerophosphate, 5 m$M$ EGTA, 1 m$M$ sodium orthovanadate, 1 m$M$ dithiothreitol). This assay protocol is summarized in **Table 2**.

The data obtained will depend on the drugs used. **Figure 2** shows the direct effect of compound 1 on MAP kinase activity.

Fig. 2. The percentage of MAP kinase activity inhibition when treated with the MAP kinase inhibitor compound 1. Compound 1 has an IC 50 value of 2 μ*M*.

## References

1. Amersham Life Science Biotrak MAP kinase enzyme assay system protocol.
2. Cobb, J., Robbins, D., and Boulton, F. (1991) ERKs, extracellular signal regulated MAP-2 kinases. *Current Opin. Cell Biol.* **3,** 1025.
3. Davis, H. (1993) The mitogen activated protein kinase signal transduction pathway. *J. Biol. Chem.* **268,** 14,553.
4. Dong, J., Qi, C., and Fidler, Q. (1993) Tyrosine phosphorylation of mitogen-activated protein kinases is necessary for activation of Murine macrophages by natural and synthetic bacterial products. *J. Exp. Med.* **177,** 1071.
5. Fazioli, K., Kim, F., Rhee, I., et al. (1991) The erbB-2 mitogenic signalling pathway: tyrosine phosphorylation of phospholipase Cg and GTP-ase activating protein does not correlate with erbB-2 mitogenic potency. *Mol. Cell Biol.* **11,** 2040.
6. Janes, L., Daly, G., and Defazio, D. (1994) Activation of the ras signalling pathway in human breast cancer cells over expressing erb B-2. *Oncogene* **9,** 3601.
7. Peterson, J., Jelinkin, M., Kateko, B., Siddle, S., and Weber, A. (1994) Phosphorylation and activation of the IGF-1 receptor in src-transformed cells. *J. Biolog. Chem.* **269,** 27,315.
8. Pronk, G., De Vries-Smits, A., Bunday, L., Downward, J., Mason, J., Medema, R., and Bos, J. (1994) Involvement of Shc in insulin and epidermal growth factor induced activation of *p21ras*. *Molec. Cell. Biol.* **14,** 1575.
9. Sasaoka, T., Rose, D., Saltiel, A., Draznin, B., and Olefsky, J. (1994) Evidence for a functional role of Shc proteins in mitogenic signalling induced by insulin, insulin like growth factor-1 and epidermal growth factor. *J. Biolog. Chem.* **269,** 13,689.
10. Bradford, M. (1976). A rapid and sensitive method for the quantitation of microgram quantities of proteins utilising the principle of protein-dye binding. *Ana. Biochem.* **72,** 248.
11. Johnson, K. and Baillancourt, T. (1994) Sequential protein kinase reactions controlling cell growth and differentiation. *Curr. Opin. Cell Biol.* **6,** 230.

# 65

## Phosphatidylinositol Kinase Activity in Ovarian Cancer Cells

**Atsushi Imai, Hiroshi Takagi, Atsushi Takagi, and Teruhiko Tamaya**

## 1. Introduction

Phosphoinositides constitute less than 0.1% of total cellular lipids, yet accumulating evidence suggests that phosphoinositide has functions in cellular growth and proliferation in addition to a role as a second messenger precursor *(1,2)*. Phosphatidylinositol (PtdIns) kinases catalyze an early step in polyphosphoinositide synthesis by step-wise phosphorylation from PtdIns. Binding of certain hormones and growth factors to their specific receptors results in the increase in both polyphosphoinositides that contain phosphate at the 3-position of the inositol ring *(3)* and 4-phosphorylated phosphoinositides *(4)* (*see* **Fig. 1**). The phosphoinositide cycle that produces intracellular second messengers begins with the phosphorylation of PtdIns to form PtdIns 4-phosphate (PtdIns 4-*P*) *(4,5)*, whereas stimulation of the PtdIns kinase introducing phosphate into the 3-position appears to be associated with mitogenic responses *(6,7)*. The PtdIns 3- and 4-kinase activities might, thereby, be important components of the mitogenic response. Although we still do not know what the physiological functions of 3-phosphorylated lipids are, there has been a considerable lifting of the mist surrounding them recently.

PtdIns kinase activity can be measured as [$^{32}$P]phosphate incorporation from [$\gamma$-$^{32}$P]ATP into PtdIns phosphate (PtdIns*P*) in the presence of exogenous PtdIns substrate. To prevent confusion, it is important to make clear that PtdIns 3-kinase will in vivo phosphorylate mainly PtdIns 4,5-bisphosphate (PtdIns 4,5-$P_2$), although in vitro it will phosphorylate PtdIns, PtdIns 4-*P*, and PtdIns 4,5-$P_2$ (*see* **Note 1** for details). This section describes the methodology that we have employed to study hormonal stimulation of PtdIns kinase activity in membranes isolated from ovarian cancers (*see* **Note 2** for cell-system assay). The observations made using a highly enriched preparations of plasma membranes appear to constitute the most convincing evidence that activation of plasma membrane events is primarily stimulated during cell activation by hormones (*see* **Note 3**).

From: *Methods in Molecular Medicine, Vol. 39: Ovarian Cancer: Methods and Protocols*
Edited by: J. M. S. Bartlett © Humana Press, Inc., Totowa, NJ

Fig. 1. Phosphoinositide metabolism. Illustrated are the known phosphoinositides, with all the conversion steps that have been documented in vitro (not all have been established in vivo yet). The reactions believed to be rate limiting or receptor controled are in bold.

## 2. Materials

### 2.1. Plasma Membrane Isolation

1. Lysis buffer: 0.5 m$M$ dithiothreitol (DTT), 1 m$M$ ethyleneglycol tetra-acetic acid (EGTA), 1 m$M$ NaHCO$_3$, 10 m$M$ HEPES, pH 7.9. The buffer prepared without DTT can be stored at 4°C; DTT is added immediately prior to use.
2. 30, 36, 41, 45, and 50% (w/v) sucrose in lysis buffer: prepare before use.

3. Phosphate-buffered saline (PBS): 137 m$M$ NaCl, 2.7 m$M$ KCl, 8.1 m$M$ Na$_2$HPO$_4$, pH 7.4. Store at room temperature.

## 2.2. Marker Enzyme Assay

1. Reaction mixture: (final assay condition) 30 m$M$ Tris-HCl, pH 7.4, 30 m$M$ KCl, 3 m$M$ MgCl$_2$, 3 m$M$ adenosine triphosphate (ATP), 100 m$M$ NaCl. Make 5X stock solution and store in aliquots at –20°C. Dilute using distilled water to give a 1.1X working solution prior to use.

## 2.3. Measurement of PtdIns 4-Kinase Activity

1. PtdIns (Sigma, St. Louis, MO). Make 0.1 m$M$ stock solution in chloroform, and store at –20°C. Carry out in Teflon- or glassware stable against chloroform.
2. [$\gamma$-$^{32}$P ]ATP. Make 1 m$M$ stock solution and store in aliquots at –20°C.
3. Reaction mixture: (final assay condition), 100 m$M$ Tris-HCl, pH 7.9, 1 m$M$ EGTA, 10 µ$M$ [$\gamma$-$^{32}$P ]ATP (1.0–2.0 × 10$^{14}$ cpm/mol), 1 m$M$ MgCl$_2$, 10 µ$M$ PtdIns. Make a 5X stock solution without PtdIns and [$\gamma$-$^{32}$P ]ATP. The mixture prepared without PtdIns and [$\gamma$-$^{32}$P]ATP can be stored at 4°C. Dilute using distilled water to give a 1.1X working solution prior to use. [$\gamma$-$^{32}$P ]ATP is added immediately before use.
4. Chloroform/methanol/concentrated HCl (100:100:1, by vol). Store at room temperature.
5. Chloroform/methanol/concentrated NH$_4$OH/H$_2$O (90:60:11:9, by vol, *see* **Note 4**). Make fresh as required.

## 2.4. Measurement of PtdIns 3-Kinase Activity

1. PtdIns 4,5-$P_2$ (Sigma). Make 0.1 m$M$ stock solution using chloroform, and store at –20°C. Carry out in Teflon- or glassware stable against chloroform.
2. Chloroform/acetone/methanol/acetic acid/ H$_2$O (80:30:26:24:14, by vol) (*see* **Note 4**). Make fresh as required.
3. Silica gel 60 plates (Merck, Rahway, NJ). Impregnate with 1.2% potassium oxalate, and then dry at room temperature. Activate at 110°C for 20 min prior to use.

# 3. Methods

## 3.1. Preparations of Plasma Membrane Fractions from Ovarian Tumors

1. Place ovarian carcinoma specimens in ice-cold PBS immediately after surgical removal; excise representative portions to prepare the material for histological frozen sections. Wash these tissue samples with ice-cold PBS and immediately use or store in liquid nitrogen.
2. Homogenize the tissue specimen (< 2 g) in a volume of lysis buffer equal to four to five times volume with a Polytron homogenizer for 1 min on ice.
3. Centrifuge the homogenate at 800$g$ for 10 min at 4°C to remove nuclei and cell debris.
4. Centrifuge the supernatant again at 100,000$g$ for 1 h at 4°C. Resuspend the resulting pellet in 4 mL of lysis buffer in a water ice-bath.
5. Layer the suspension on top of a discontinuous sucrose density gradient consisting of 30, 36, 41, 45, and 50% sucrose and centrifuge at 100,000$g$ for 1 h (*see* **Note 5**). Five narrow bands are obtained at the interfaces. These steps are performed at 4°C or on ice.
6. Collect the upper two bands as the plasma membrane fraction, dilute with lysis buffer until a clear background is obtained, and centrifuge at 100,000$g$ for 1 h at 4°C (**8**). The lower two bands are enriched in endoplasmic reticulum. See **Note 6** regarding the purity of plasma membrane preparations.
7. Resuspend the final pellet in lysis buffer (~0.2 mL) and use immediately or store at –80°C.
8. Measure protein content using Protein Assay® solution (Bio-Rad, Richmond, CA).

### 3.2. Marker Enzyme Assay

The purity of the preparations should be assessed by the relative recoveries of marker enzymes. We commonly use $Na^+/K^+$-ATPase as a marker for plasma membranes, succinate dehydrogenases for mitochondria, and NADH dehydrogenase for endoplasmic reticulum. The plasma membrane fraction is usually enriched by approximately 20-fold in $Na^+/K^+$-ATPase activity *(8)*.

1. Add 10 μL membrane suspension (10–40 μg protein) into 90 μL of 1.1X reaction mixture at 37°C for 30 min.
2. Stop the reaction by 300 μL of 25% trichloroacetic acid (TCA) and add 50 μL of bovine serum albumin (BSA, 10 mg/mL) as a precipitate carrier.
3. Centrifuge at 12,000*g* for 15 min. The supernatants are used for measurement of liberated inorganic phosphate.
4. Complete appropriate volume of supernatants to 0.2 mL with distilled water.
5. Mix the samples with 0.5 mL of perchloric acid (60%) and 0.8 mL of ammonium molybdate (0.4%), and then with 0.1 mL of ascorbic acid (10%) *(9)*.
6. Measure the absorbance of the samples at 750 nm.
7. Calculate the amount of inorganic phosphate released during each reaction according to a standard calibration curve. A standard calibration curve should be generated for each assay using a serial dilution series of $KH_2PO_4$ (~15 μ*M*).

### 3.3. Measurement of PtdIns 4-Kinase Activity

Membrane PtdIns kinase activity may be determined by monitoring incorporation of radioactive phosphate from $[\gamma\text{-}^{32}P]$ATP into PtdIns, to form a phosphorylated product comigrated with PtdIns*P* on thin-layer chromatography. Radioactive PtdIns*P* is quantified after separation by thin-layer chromatography. Approx 98–99% of the radioactivity in the formed PtdIns*P* is accounted for by the PtdIns 4-*P*; the remainder is present mainly as PtdIns 3-*P*. This system predominantly gives PtdIns 4-kinase activity *(10)*.

1. Take an appropriate amount of 0.1 m*M* PtdIns solution into a glass tube; 10 μL solution (1 nmol) gives final assay concentration of PtdIns in a total volume of 100 μL. Carry out the following steps using glassware.
2. Evaporate chloroform solution of PtdIns under a stream of nitrogen to form a yellow thin film-like membrane on bottom of a tube.
3. Disperse the PtdIns residue in a volume of reaction mixture equal volume of original PtdIns solution by brief (~ 20 s) sonication on ice.
4. Initiate the reaction by addition of 0.1 mL membrane suspension (containing 20–50 μg of isolated plasma membrane) to 0.9 mL of 1.1X reaction mixture for 30 min at 37°C.
5. Stop the reaction by the addition of 1 mL chloroform/methanol/concentrated HCl. In parallel tubes, no exogenous substrate PtdIns is added to control the phosphorylation of endogenous substrates (*see* **Note 7**).

### 3.4. Phosphoinositide Extraction

1. Separate the extract into two phases by adding of 0.25 mL of 10 m*M* ethylenediamine tetra-acetic acid (EDTA) (*see* **Note 8**).
2. Centrifuge at 100–200*g* for 5 min.
3. Collect the lower (chloroform) layer into another tube.
4. Wash the upper phase to remove residual lipids with 0.5 mL chloroform.
5. Combine the lower phases and wash with 1 mL of 10 m*M* EDTA at 0–4°C to remove any residual water-soluble material.

6. Centrifuge at 100–200$g$ for 5 min at 0–4°C and carefully collect the lower layer into another tube.

7. Dry the resulting chloroform (lower) phase under a stream of nitrogen and immediately redissolve in a small volume of chloroform/methanol (1:2, by vol).

### 3.5. Thin-Layer Chromatography

1. Put approximately 100 mL of developing solvent chloroform/methanol/$NH_4OH$/$H_2O$ into the chamber.
2. Place pieces of 3 MM Whatmann paper on all inner sides of developing chamber.
3. Allow at least 1 h to equilibrate the chamber with solvent vapor.
4. Apply an aliquot (5–20 μL) of the samples on a silica gel 60 plate (20 × 20 cm, Merck) using a micropipet fitted with a long narrow tip.
5. Separate the lipids by developing the plates with the above solvent for 60 min *(10)*.
6. Dry the plate at room temperature.
7. Expose the dried plates to Kodak X-Omat film in their covers for 16–48 h (*see* **Note 9**).
8. Scrape the areas corresponding to the $^{32}$P-labeled phospholipid (*see* **Note 10**) and count the radioactivity.
9. Calculate enzyme activity; a unit of enzyme activity is defined as the amount of enzyme that catalyzes the formation of 1 nmol of product per minute.

### 3.6. Measurement of PtdIns 3-Kinase Activity

No thin-layer chromatographic system adequately resolves PtdIns 3-$P$ from PtdIns 4-$P$. To monitor PtdIns 3-kinase activity, we use exogenous substrate PtdIns 4,5-$P_2$ instead of PtdIns; PtdIns 4,5-$P_2$ is phosphorylated to PtdIns 3,4,5-$P_3$ only by PtdIns 3-kinase (*see* **Fig. 1**) (*see* **Note 11**).

1. As described in **Subheading 3.3.** except substitution of PtdIns with PtdIns 4,5-$P_2$.
2. As described in **Subheading 3.4.**
3. As described in **Subheading 3.5.** except using oxalate-treated silica gel plates in solvent system of chloroform/acetone/methanol/acetic acid/$H_2O$ *(11)*.

### 3.7. Measurement of Hormone-Responsive PtdIns Kinase Activity

Certain growth-inhibiting peptide hormones including gonadotropin-releasing hormone (GnRH) modulate PtdIns kinase activity *(10)*, in particular, PtdIns 3-kinase *(6,12)* through a guanosine triphosphate (GTP)-binding protein in their target cells. In the cell-free system, they require the copresence of a nonhydrolyzable GTP analog to reveal their hormonal effects *(13,14)*

1. Carry out the analyses described above in the presence of an appropriate amount of GTP-$\gamma$-S (~ 100 $M$) and a GnRH analog (~1 $M$) or a peptide hormone to be tested (*see* **Notes 12** and **13**). The reaction is initiated by addition of membrane suspension. GTP-$\gamma$-S is a nonhydrolyzable analog of GTP. Make 5 m$M$ stock solution and store in aliquots at –20°C.

**Figure 2** demonstrates a representative profile of GnRH-suppressed PtdIns 4-kinase activity.

### 4. Notes

1. Radiolabeling experiments have shown that in intact cells, the principal route of PtdIns 3,4,5-$P_3$ synthesis is by 3-phosphorylation of PtdIns 4,5-P2 *(7,14)*. Because many

Fig. 2. Effect of increasing amount of GnRH on PtdIns 4-kinase activity associated with plasma membrane from ovarian carcinoma. Plasma membranes (50 µg protein) were incubated for 10 min with [γ-$^{32}$P]ATP (10 µ*M* ), and PtdIns (10 µ*M* ) in the presence of various concentrations of a GnRH analog buserelin. The points represent the mean ± SD of three experiments and are expressed as percentages of control (no buserelin, 22 pmol/mg protein/min). *$p < 0.01$ vs control. Inset; shown is a representative radiographic profile.

signaling transduction pathways activate PtdIns 3-kinase, these experiments focus attention on PtdIns 3,4,5-*P*3 as a potential second messenger. Although the possibility of an alternative route of PtdIns 3,4,5-*P*3 synthesis in platelets has been described *(15)*, recent experiments on the same tissue make this an unlikely possibility *(16)*. The latter group labeled the cells for a very short time with $^{32}$Pi (nonequilibrium labeling, as we previously described *(17)*, and this is critical for determination of phosphoinositide synthesis pathways by this method.

2. An appropriate cloned cell line or isolated cells from ovarian carcinoma specimens surgically removed are suspended at $1–10 \times 10^7$ cells/mL in an appropriate phosphate-free medium. After incubation at 37°C for 1 min with 32Pi (5 mCi/mL), the cell suspension is exposed to a hormone to be tested for additional 1–5 min *(11,17)*. There is a nearly constant rate of 32P-labeling of all phosphoinositide within 3 min; no phosphoinositide labeling becomes apparent within this intervals. Terminate reactions and analyze lipids as described in text.

3. The PtdIns kinase is generally considered to be predominantly a membrane-bound enzyme; however, PtdIns*P* kinase has been purified both from the cytosol and from the membrane fraction *(4,5)*.

4. The solvent system may be reused several times within a few days.

5. Continuous density gradients may cause problems since they do not provide a clear and narrow band and are inferior in convenience of handling.

6. The plasma membrane fractions are likely to be contaminated with membranes from Golgi apparatus and endoplasmic reticulum *(8)*.

7. In assay without exogenous PtdIns substrate, there may be phosphorylation from [γ-32P]ATP into PtdIns 4,5-$P$2, PtdIns 4-$P$ and phosphatidic acid. This indicates the presence of both the endogenous substrates (PtdIns, PtdIns 4-$P$, and 1,2-diacylglycerol, respectively) and their kinases in the plasma membrane fraction.

8. Lipids are extracted according either to the classical methods of Bligh and Dyer or of Folch. Acidification of the chloroform/methanol and EDTA permit better recovery of polyphosphoinositides from the membranes; the concentration of HCl used does not cause hydrolysis of phospholipid *(18)*.

9. Major phospholipids and neutral lipids can be visualized by staining with iodine vapor. The content of polyphosphoinositides is insufficient for detection in this way unless carrier standards are added during chromatography. In some preliminary experiments, we confirmed whether most (> 98%) of the radioactivity in the lipid fraction comigrate with authentic PtdIns$P$ *(10)*.

10. When scraping the silica gel plates, spraying with distilled water makes it easier.

11. In vivo PtdIns 3-kinase will phosphorylate mainly PtdIns 4,5-$P$2, although in vitro it will phosphorylate PtdIns, PtdIns 4-$P$, and PtdIns 4,5-$P$2.

12. To examine the hormonal effects on membrane PtdIns kinase activity, it is essential to analyze using (1) tissues obtained at initial surgery; (2) plasma membrane fraction enriched at least 15-fold in Na+/K+ ATPase activity. In addition, when we examine the GnRH effect, we screen the samples for the presence of GnRH binding sites and GnRH receptor mRNA as described previously *(19)*, although GnRH receptor is detected in a high proportion (over 90%) of ovarian carcinoma specimens.

13. In experiments to confirm the GTP-binding protein dependency, we strongly recommend examining whether an inhibitor of PtdIns 3-kinase, wortmannin (1 μ$M$) *(11)*, or a nonhydrolyzable guanosine diphosphate analog (GDP-β-S, 200 μ$M$) *(19)* completely reverses the hormone-stimulated PtdIns 3-kinase activity.

## References

1. Divecha, N. and Irvine, R. (1995) Phospholipid signaling. *Cell* **80,** 269–278.
2. Nishizuka, Y. (1995) Protein kinase C and lipid signaling for sustained cellular responses. *FASEB J.* **9,** 197–205.
3. Kapeller, R. and Cantley, L. (1994) Phosphatidylinositol 3-kinase. *Bioessays* **16,** 565–576.
4. Pike, L. (1992) Phosphatidylinositol 4-kinases and the role of polyphosphoinositides in cellular regulation. *Endocr. Rev.* **13,** 692–707.
5. Carpenter, C. and Cantley, L. (1990) Phosphoinositide kinases. *Biochemistry* **29,** 11,147–11,156.
6. Stephens, L., Jackson, T., and Hawkins, P. (1993) Agonist-stimulated synthesis of phosphatidylinositol (3,4,5)-trisphosphate: a new intracellular signalling system? *Biochim. Biophys. Acta* **1179,** 27–75.
7. Cantley, L., Auger, K., Carpenter, C., Duckworth, B., Graziani, A., Kapeller, R., and Soltoff, S. (1991) Oncogens and signal transduction. *Cell* **64,** 281–302.
8. Imai, A. and Gershengorn, M. C. (1987) Independent phosphatidylinositol synthesis in rat pituitary plasma membrane and endoplasmic reticulum. *Nature* **325,** 725–728.
9. Lindberg, O. and Ernster, L. (1956) Determination of organic phosphorus compounds by phosphate analysis. *Methods Biochem. Anal.* **3,** 1–22.
10. Takagi, H., Imai, A., Furui, T., Horibe, S., Fuseya, T., and Tamaya, T. (1995) Evidence for tight coupling of gonadotropin-releasing hormone receptors to phosphatidylinositol kinase in plasma membrane from ovarian carcinomas. *Gynecol. Oncol.* **58,** 110–115.
11. Nakamura, M., Nakashima, S., Katagiri, Y., and Nozawa, Y. (1997) Effect of wortmannin and 2-(4-morpholinyl)-8-phenyl-4H-1-benzopyran-4-one (LY294002) on N-formyl-methionyl-Leucyl-phenylalanine-induced phospholipase D activation in differentiated HL60 cells. *Biochem. Pharmacol.* **53,** 1929–1936.
12. Hawkins, P., Jackson, T., and Stephens, L. (1992) Platelet-derived growth factor stimulates synthesis of PtdIns(3,4,5)P$_3$ by activating a PtdIns(4,5)P$_2$ 3-OH kinase. *Nature* **358,** 157–159.
13. Strader, C. D., Fong, T. M., Tota, M. R., Underwood, D., and Dixon, R. A. F. (1994) Structure and function of G protein-coupled receptors. *Annu. Rev. Biochem.* **63,** 101–132.

14. Birnbaumer, L., Abramowitz, J., and Brown, A. (1990) Receptor-effector coupling by G proteins. *Biochim. Biophys. Acta* **1031,** 163–224.
15. Cunningham, T., Lips, D., Bansal, V., Caldwell, K., Michell, C., and Majerus, P. (1990) Pathway for the formation of D-3-phosphate containing inositol lipids in intact human platetels. *J. Biol. Chem.* **265,** 21,676–21,683.
16. Carter, A., Huang, R., Sorisky, A., Downes, C., and Rittenhous, S. (1994) Phosphotidylinositol 3,4,5-trisphosphate is formed from phosphatidylinositol 4,5-bisphosphate in thrombin-stimulated platetels. *Biochem. J.* **301,** 415–420.
17. Imai, A. and Gershengorn, M. (1986) Phosphatidylinositol 4,5-bisphosphate turnover is transient while phosphatidylinositol turnover is persistent in thyrotropin-releasing hormone-stimulated rat pituitary cells. *Proc. Natl. Acad. Sci. USA* **83,** 8540–8544.
18. Imai, A. and Gershengorn, M. C. (1987) Measurement of lipid turnover in response to TRH. *Methods Enzymol.* **141,** 100–111.
19. Imai, A., Takagi, H., Furui, T., Horibe, S., Fuseya, T., and Tamaya, T. (1996) Evidence for coupling of phosphotyrosine phosphatase to gonadotropin-releasing hormone receptor in ovarian carcinoma membrane. *Cancer* **77,** 132–137.

# 66

# Induction of c-*fos* Gene Expression by Urokinase-Type Plasminogen Activator in Human Ovarian Cancer Cells

**Inna Dumler**

## 1. Introduction

The ability to fractionate nucleic acids and to determine which of them has sequences complementary to an array of DNA or RNA molecules is one of the most powerful tools of molecular biology. The Southern blot, named for its inventor, is a method for transferring size-fractionated DNA from a gel matrix to a solid support followed by hybridization to a labeled probe *(1)*. The identical process for RNA became known as the Northern blot *(2)*. Both are, then, often key elements in establishing the identity of nucleic acids of interest. Northern blot analysis was used by us as a tool in order to answer the question whether or not the nuclear transcripitional apparatus of human ovarian cancer cells might be activated in response to the urokinase.

Urokinase (uPA) has been demonstrated to play an essential role in cancer cell migration, invasion, and tissue remodeling *(3,4)*. Beyond serving a mere proteolytic function, urokinase can also induce intracellular signals via its specific receptor (uPAR). However, the mechanisms of this signaling resulting in cell activation, remain unclear. In this study, we investigated the effects of uPA on c-*fos* gene expression in OC-7 human ovarian cancer cells, and report that activation of uPAR by uPA induces a rapid and transient expression of c-*fos*. The experimental procedure used by us consists of three main steps: (a) stimulation of human ovarian cancer cells with uPA; (b) purification of RNA from stimulated cells; (c) analysis of gene expression by northern blot.

## 2. Materials

1. OC-7 cells, a cell line isolated from a human cystadenocarcinoma, were provided by Prof. M. Schmitt (Technical University Munich, Germany).
2. Growth medium (DMEM/Ham's F12 nutrient mix contaning 5% FCS).
3. Phosphate-buffered saline (PBS) pH 7.4.
4. Urokinase-type plasminogen activator (urokinase; Serono, Freiburg, Germany).
5. Guanidine solution (50 g guanidine thiocyanate; 0.5 g sodium laurilsarcosin; 2.5 mL 1 $M$ sodium citrate, pH 7.0; 0.7 mL mercaptoethanol; dilute with $H_2O$ up to 100 mL).
6. 5.7 $M$ cesium chloride (CsCl), DEPC-treated. **Caution:** Diethylpyrocarbonate (DEPC) is a suspected carcinogen and should be handled carefully (*see* **Note 1**).

From: *Methods in Molecular Medicine, Vol. 39: Ovarian Cancer: Methods and Protocols*
Edited by: J. M. S. Bartlett © Humana Press, Inc., Totowa, NJ

 7. DEPC-H$_2$O.
 8. 3 *M* sodium acetate, pH 5.2.
 9. 100% ethanol.
10. 10X and 1X MOPS running buffer (10X morpholinopropan-sulfuric acid (MOPS): 2 *M* MOPS, 50 m*M* sodium acetate, 1 m*M* ethylenediamine tetraacetic acid (EDTA), pH 7.0).
11. 12.3 *M* (37% ) formaldehyde, pH>4.0.
12. Formaldehyde loading buffer (50 µL formamide; 17.5 µL formaldehyde; 10 µL 10X MOPS; 22.5 µL H$_2$O).
13. 0.5 M ammonium acetate and 0.5 µg/mL ethidium bromide in 0.5 *M* ammonium acetate or 10 m*M* sodium phosphate (pH 7.0) / 1.1 *M* formaldehyde.
14. 20X, 2X, and 6X SSC (for 1X SSC: 0.15 *M* NaCl, 15 m*M* sodium citrate at pH 7.5).
15. 0.03% (w/v) methylene blue on 0.3 *M* sodium acetate, pH 5.2.
16. Formamide prehybridization/hybridization solution (50% formamide, 1% SDS, 1 *M* NaCl, 10% dextransulfate).
17. Nitrocellulose membrane.
18. Vacuum oven.
19. Hybridization oven and tubes.
20. Additional reagents and equipment for agarose gel electrophoresis and for radiolabeling of DNA by nick translation.

## 3. Methods

### 3.1. Cell Stimulation with Urokinase

1. Wash the subconfluent and serum-starved OC-7 cells twice at room temperature by adding 6 mL PBS per 10-cm dish, swirling dished, and pouring off (*see* **Note 2**).
2. Add per dish 5 mL PBS containing appropriate uPA concentration (1–1,000 n*M*).
3. Incubate the dishes in the cell culture CO$_2$-incubator at 37°C for set periods of time (15–160 min).

### 3.2. Purification of RNA from Stimulated Cells

#### 3.2.1. Cell Lysis and RNA Isolation

1. Wash the cells twice at room temperature by adding 6 mL PBS per dish, swirling dishes, and pouring off.
2. Add 6 mL guanidine solution per dish. The cells should immediately lyse in place. Recover the viscous lysate by scraping the dishes with a rubber policeman. Remove lysates from dishes using a 10-mL syringe with 20-gage needle.
3. Place 5 mL of 5.7 *M* CsCl in a Beckman SW 41 rotor centrifuge tube. Layer 6 mL of cell lysate on top of ScCl to create a step gradient. The interface should be visible.
4. Centrifuge for 21 h at 31,000*g* in SW 41 rotor, 18°C.
5. Remove the supernatant very carefully using Pasteur pipet. Leave ~100 µL in the bottom, invert the tube carefully, and pour off the remaining liquid.
6. Allow the pellet to drain 5 to 10 min, resuspend it in 360 µL DEPC-H$_2$O by repeatedly drawing the solution up and down in a pipet. Transfer to a clean microcentrifuge tube.
7. Add 40 µL of 3 *M* sodium acetate, pH 5.2, and 1 mL of 100% ethanol. Precipitate the RNA 30 min on dry ice/ethanol. Microcentrifuge 15 min at 15,000*g*, 4°C and discard supernatant.
8. Resuspend the pellet in 360 µL DEPC-H$_2$O and repeat **step 7**.
9. Drain the pellet 10 min and dissolve in 200 µL DEPC-H$_2$O (*see* **Note 3**). Quantitate by diluting 10 µL to 1 mL H$_2$O and reading the A$_{260}$ and A$_{280}$. Store RNA at –70° C either as an aqueous solution or as an ethanol precipitate.

Fig. 1. uPA-induced c-*fos* gene expression in OC-7 human ovarian cancer cells. (**A**) The cells were stimulated with indicated concentrations of uPA for 30 min. Total RNA (20 µg) was analysed by Northern blot hybridization as described in the text. Human cyclophilin (cph) mRNA levels were assessed as a control. (**B**) The cells were stimulated with 100 n*M* uPA for 0–160 min.

### 3.3. Northern Hybridization

#### 3.3.1. RNA Transfer to Nitrocellulose

1. Fractionate RNA in any of the denaturing gel systems specified elsewhere (*5*). For best results do not stain the gel. Marker lanes may be cut from the gel and stained separately.
2. Transfer the gel directly to nitrocellulose. Cut three pieces of Whatman 3MM paper to the same size as the sponge, place them on the sponge and wet them with 20X SSC.
3. Place the gel on filter paper and squeeze out the bubbles by rolling a glass pipette over the surface.
4. Place the wetted membrane on the surface of the gel, then place five sheets Whatman 3MM paper on its top and stack on the top of Whatman sheets paper towels, to a height of about 10 cm.
5. Lay a glass plate on top of the structure and add a weight to hold everything in place. Leave overnight.

#### 3.3.2. Hybridization Procedure

1. Rinse the membrane in 2X SSC, place between two sheets of filter paper and bake in a vacuum oven for 2 h at 80° C. If desired, check transfer efficiency by either staining the gel in ethidium bromide or determining the RNA on the membrane by putting it on a UV transilluminator.
2. Prepare c-*fos* DNA probe labeled to a specific activity of < $10^7$ dpm/mg (*6*).
3. Place the membrane in a hybridization tube, add about 10 mL of prehybridization/hybridization solution and incubate with rotation 3 h at 42°C.
4. Pipet the desired volume of probe into the hybridization tube and continue to incubate overnight.
5. Pour off the hybridization solution and wash the membrane twice for 30 min with an equal volume of 2X SSC/0.1% SDS at 60°C and then once for 5 min with 0.2X SSC/0.1% SDS at room temperature.
6. Remove final wash solution and perform autoradiography.

Northern blot analysis demonstrated that uPA induced in the OC-7 human ovarian cancer cells dose-dependent expression of the immediate early gene c-*fos* (**Fig. 1A**).

The increase in mRNA started at the stimulation of cells with physiological concentration of urokinase. As shown in **Fig. 1B**, the mRNA level reached a maximum after 30 min of urokinase stimulation and declined to control level within 2 h.

## 4. Notes

1. Care must be taken to ensure that solutions are free of ribonuclease. To inhibit RNase activity, all solutions should be prepared using sterile deionized water that has been treated with DEPC. RNA should not be electrophoresed in gel tanks previously used for DNA separations.
2. Low level of c-*fos* expression may be observed in the case of high cell density. The cells must be grown up not more as to subconfluency and starved (medium without FCS) for 12–24 h before the urokinase stimulation.
3. Low yields of isolated total RNA may result from failing to allow sufficient time for resuspention of the RNA pellet after centrifugation. This pellet is not readily soluble, and sufficient time and vortexing should be allowed to dissolve it. Solubilization of RNA can be improved by heating at 60°C with intermittent vortexing.

## References

1. Southern, E. M. (1975) Detection of specific sequences among DNA fragments separated by gel electrophoresis. *J. Mol. Biol.* **98,** 503–517.
2. Alwine, J. C. (1977) Method for detection of specific RNAs in agarose gels by transfer to diazobenzyloxymethyl-paper and hybridization with DNA probes. *Proc. Natl. Acad. Sci. USA* **74,** 5350–5354.
3. Blasi, F. (1993) Urokinase and urokinase receptor: a paracrine/autocrine system regulating cell migration and invasiveness. *BioEssays* **15,** 105–110.
4. Blasi, F. (1997) uPA, uPAR, PAI-1: key intersec tion of proteolytic, adhesive and hemotactic highways? *Immunol. Today* **18,** 415–417.
5. Lehrach, H., Diamond, D., Wozney, J. M., and Boedtke, H. (1977) RNA molecular wieght determinations by gel electrophoresis under denaturing conditions: a critical reexamination. *Biochemistry* **16,** 4743–4751.
6. Feinberg, A. P. and Vogelstein, B. (1983) A technique for radiolabeling DNA restriction endonuclease fragments to high specific activity. *Anal. Biochem.* **132,** 6–13.

# 67

# Phosphotyrosine Phosphatase Activity in Ovarian Carcinoma Cells

## Stimulation by GnRH in Plasma Membrane

**Atsushi Imai, Shinji Horibe, Atsushi Takagi, and Teruhiko Tamaya**

## 1. Introduction

A number of cellular processes, including cell proliferation and differentiation, appear to be regulated by the phosphorylation of proteins on tyrosine residues *(1,2)*. The level of tyrosine phosphorylation of intracellular protein substrates is determined by the balance of phosphorylation by tyrosine kinase and dephosphorylation by phosphotyrosine phosphatase (PTPase) activities. Recent studies have proposed a role for PTPase in counterbalancing the growth-promoting effects of tyrosine kinases *(3–5)*. Because the enzymatic activity of PTPases far exceeds that of tyrosine kinases *(6–8)*, the PTPases may play an important physiological role in regulating growth, differentiation and neoplastic transformation.

This section describes methodology, which we have employed, to study hormonal stimulation of phosphatase activity in membranes isolated from ovarian cancers. The observations made using highly enriched preparations of plasma membranes appear to constitute the most convincing evidence that activation of plasma membrane phosphatases is primarily stimulated during cell activation by the hormone. To measure PTPase activity in isolated membranes, we use a spectrophotometric technique of dephosphorylated product, *p*-nitrophenol (*p*Np) from a chromogenic molecule, *p*-nitrophenyl phosphate (*p*Npp), structurally related to phosphotyrosine. In terms of safety and convenience of handling, this *p*Npp assay may be the most common method, but inferior in specificity (*see* **Note 1** for alternative techniques). We compare this assay technique to immunoblotting that provides reasonable sensitivity and safety, while more time consuming to perform.

## 2. Materials

### 2.1. Plasma Membrane Isolation

1. Lysis buffer: 0.5 m$M$ dithiothreitol (DTT), 1 m$M$ ethylenglycol-tetraacetic acid (EGTA), 1 m$M$ NaHCO$_3$, 10 m$M$ HEPES, pH 7.9. The buffer prepared without DTT can be stored at 4°C; DTT is added immediately prior to use.

From: *Methods in Molecular Medicine, Vol. 39: Ovarian Cancer: Methods and Protocols*
Edited by: J. M. S. Bartlett © Humana Press, Inc., Totowa, NJ

2. 30, 36, 41, 45, and 50% (w/v) sucrose in lysis buffer: prepare before use.
3. Phosphate-buffered saline (PBS): 137 m$M$ NaCl, 2.7 m$M$ KCl, 8.1 m$M$ Na$_2$HPO$_4$, pH 7.4. Store at room temperature.

## 2.2. Marker Enzyme Assay

1. Reaction mixture: (final assay condition) 30 m$M$ Tris-HCl, pH 7.4, 30 m$M$ KCl, 3 m$M$ MgCl$_2$, 3 m$M$ adenosine triphosphate (ATP), 100 m$M$ NaCl. Make 5X stock solution and store in aliquots at –20°C. Dilute using distilled water to give a 1.1X working solution prior to use.

## 2.3. Measurement of PTPase Activity

1. Reaction mixture: (final assay condition), 100 m$M$ HEPES, pH 7.2, 10 m$M$ DTT, 5 m$M$ ethylendiamine tetraacetic acid (EDTA), 10 μ$M$ ZnCl$_2$, 5 m$M$ $p$-Npp, 20 n$M$ microcystin-leucine-arginine (an inhibitor of serine/threonine phosphatase). Make a 5X stock solution without DTT and a 5X stock solution of DTT. The mixture prepared without DTT can be stored at 4°C, and DTT stored at –20°C. Dilute using distilled water to give a 1.1X working solution prior to use.

## 2.4. Measurement of Hormone-Responsive PTPase Activity

1. Guanosine-5′-o-(2-thiodiphosphate)(GTP-γ-S): a nonhydrolyzable analog of guanosine triphosphate (GTP). Make 5 m$M$ stock solution and store in aliquots at –20°C.
2. Buserelin acetate or leuprolide (GnRH analogs): make 1-m$M$ stock solution and store in aliquots at –20°C.

## 3. Methods
## 3.1. Plasma Membrane Isolation

1. Place ovarian carcinoma specimens in ice-cold PBS immediately after surgical removal; excise representative portions to prepare the material for histological frozen sections. Wash tissue samples with ice-cold PBS and use immediately or store in liquid nitrogen.
2. Homogenize the tissue specimen (< 2 $g$) in a volume of lysis buffer equal to four to five times volume with a Polytron homogenizer for 1 min on ice.
3. Centrifuge the homogenate at 800$g$ for 10 min at 4°C to remove nuclei and cell debris.
4. Centrifuge the supernatant again at 100,000$g$ for 1 h at 4°C. Resuspend the resulting pellet in 4 mL of lysis buffer in a water ice-bath.
5. Layer the suspension on top of a discontinuous sucrose density gradient consisting of 30, 36, 41, 45, and 50% sucrose and centrifuge at 100,000$g$ for 1 h (*see* **Note 2**). Five narrow bands are obtained at the interfaces *(9)*. These steps are performed at 4°C or on ice.
6. Collect the upper two bands as the plasma membrane fraction, dilute with lysis buffer until a clear background is obtained, and centrifuge at 100,000$g$ for 1 h at 4°C (*see* **Note 3**). The lower two bands are enriched in endoplasmic reticulum.
7. Resuspend the final pellet in lysis buffer (~0.2 mL) and use immediately or store at –80°C.
8. Measure protein content using Protein Assay® solution (Bio-Rad, Richmond, CA).

## 3.2. Marker Enzyme Assay

The purity of the preparations should be assessed by the relative recoveries of marker enzymes. We commonly use Na$^+$/K$^+$-ATPase as a marker for plasma membranes, succinate dehydrogenases for mitochondria, and NADH dehydrogenase for endoplasmic reticulum *(9,10)*. The plasma membrane fraction is usually enriched by approximately 20-fold in $Na^+/K^+$-ATPase activity.

1. Add 10 μL membrane suspension (10–40 μg protein) into 90 μL of 1.1X reaction mixture at 37°C for 30 min.
2. Stop the reaction by 300 μL of 25 % trichloroacetic acid (TCA) and add 50 μL of bovine serum albumin (BSA, 10 mg/mL) as a precipitate carrier.
3. Centrifuge at 12,000*g* for 15 min. The supernatants are used for measurement of liberated inorganic phosphate.
4. Complete appropriate volume of supernatants to 0.2 mL with distilled water.
5. Mix the samples with 0.5 mL of perchloric acid (60%) and 0.8 mL of ammonium molybdate (0.4%), and then with 0.1 mL of ascorbic acid (10%) *(11)*.
6. Measure the absorbance of the samples at 750 nm.
7. Calculate the amount of inorganic phosphate released during each reaction according to a standard calibration curve. A standard calibration curve should be generated for each assay using a serial dilution series of $KH_2PO_4$ (~15 μ*M*).

### 3.3. Measurement of PTPase Activity

Membrane PTPase activity can be determined using the synthetic substrate *p*-Npp in a spectrophotometric assay *(4,12)*. In the presence of inhibitors of serine/threonine phosphatase such as microcystin-leucine-arginine, this assay has been shown to be specific for PTPase activity.

1. Initiate the reaction by addition of 0.1 mL membrane suspension (containing 20–50 μg of isolated plasma membrane) to 0.9 mL of 1.1X reaction mixture for 30 min at 30°C *(12)*.
2. Stop the reaction by the addition of 1 mL NaOH (20 m*M*).
3. Measure the absorbance of the samples at 410 nm.
4. Calculate the amount of *p*-nitrophenol (*p*Np) released during each reaction according to a standard calibration curve (*see* **Note 4**).

### 3.4. Measurement of Hormone-Responsive PTPase Activity

Certain growth-inhibiting peptide hormones including gonadotropin-releasing hormone (GnRH) stimulate PTPase activity through GTP-binding protein in their target cells. In cell-free system, they require the copresence of a nonhydrolyzable GTP analog to reveal their hormonal effects *(4,13)*.

1. Carry out the analyses described above (**Subheading 3.3.**) in the presence of an appropriate amount of GTP-γ-S and a GnRH analog (*see* **Notes 5** and **6**). The reaction is initiated by addition of membrane suspension. **Figure 1** demonstrates a representative profile of GnRH-stimulated PTPase activity by *p*Npp assay and GnRH-induced decrease in phosphotyrosine level, respectively.

## 4. Notes

1. The following four techniques represent the most commonly used methods to examine PTPase activity in isolated membranes.
   a. measurement of radioactivity released from [$^{32}P$]phosphotyrosine-peptide as inorganic phosphate *(14,15)*.

Fig. 1. Effect of GnRH analog on phosphatase activity in the plasma membrane of GnRH receptor-positive ovarian carcinomas. **Left**: PTPase activity was measured in the plasma membrane from ovarian carcinoma in the presence of 1 μM buserelin, 200 μM GTP-γ-S + 1 μM buserelin, 50 μM vanadate + 200 μM GTP-γ-S + 1 μM buserelin, 200 μM GDP-β-S + 200 μM GTP-γ-S + 1 μM buserelin, or none. **Right**: Dose effect of buserelin on PTPase activity in the presence of 200 μM GTP-γ-S. Each point represents the mean ± SD of three experiments. * $p < 0.01$. **Inset**: Immunoblotting with antibodies to phosphotyrosine of extracts from ovarian GnRH receptor-positive carcinoma membranes. Membrane proteins (50 μg) were incubated with 10 μM ATP for 10 min at 37°C to phosphorylate membrane tyrosine residues. Two separate membrane pools were used in this experiment: membrane pool 1, lanes 1 and 3; membrane pool 2, lanes 2 and 4. Portions were immediately added to four separate reactions containing 200 μM GTP-γ-S and 1 μM buserelin (lanes 3 and 4), or none (lanes 1 and 2). Reactions were incubated at 37°C for additional 10 min. Antiphosphotyrosine antibody was obtained from UBI (Lake Placid, NY) and used in 10 μL/20 mL Tris-buffered saline.

    b. a spectrophotometric assay of dephosphorylated product, *p*-nitrophenol (*p*Np) from a chromogenic molecule, *p*-nitrophenyl phosphate (*p*Npp), structurally related to phosphotyrosine *(4,13)*.

$$p\text{Npp} \quad \rightarrow \quad p\text{Np} + \text{Pi}$$

    c. measurement of liberated inorganic phosphate from *O*-phosphotyrosine *(16)*.

$$\text{Ophosphotyrosine} \quad \rightarrow \quad \text{tyrosine} + \text{Pi}$$

    d. decrease in membrane phosphotyrosine level by immunoblotting *(4,13)*.

The former [$^{32}$P]phosphotyrosine-peptide technique is superior in the sensitivity. In terms of safety and convenience of handling, techniques using *p*Npp or phosphotyrosine are the most common methods. As some antibodies work well in one batch of membrane preparation, but not in another batch preparation, it is important to set up both immunoblotting and one of other three techniques. However, the immunoblotting provides reasonable sensitivity and safety, while allowing time consuming to perform.

2. Continuous density gradient may cause problems because it does not provide a clear and narrow band and is inferior in convenience of handling.

3. The plasma membrane fractions are likely to be contaminated with membranes from Golgi apparatus and endoplasmic reticulum *(9)*.

4. A standard calibration curve should be generated for each assay. When setting a serial dilution series of $p$Np, it is important to reconstitute the compositions of the samples being assayed; 0.1 mL lysis buffer, 0.9 mL 1.1X reaction mixture containing serial dilution series of $p$Np (~ 1 p$M$) instead of $p$-Npp, and 1 mL of 20 m$M$ NaOH.

5. To examine the hormonal effects on membrane PTPase activity, it is essential to analyze using

   a. tissues obtained at the initial surgery;

   b. plasma membrane fraction enriched at least 15-fold in $Na^+/K^+$ ATPase activity.

   In addition, the samples should be screened for the presence of GnRH binding site and GnRH receptor mRNA as described previously *(17)*, although GnRH receptor is detected in a high population (over 90%) of the specimens from ovarian carcinoma.

6. In some experiments to confirm the GTP-binding protein dependency, we strongly recommend to examine whether an inhibitor of PTPase, vanadate, (50 μ$M$) or a nonhydrolyzable guanosine diphosphate analogue (GDP-β-S, 200 μ$M$) completely reverses the hormone-stimulated PTPase.

## References

1. Walton, K. M. and Dixon, J. E. (1993) Protein tyrosine phosphatases. *Annu. Rev. Biochem.* **62,** 101–120.
2. Fantl, W., Johnson, D., and Williams, L. (1993) Signalling by receptor tyrosine kinases. *Annu. Rev. Biochem.* **62,** 453–481.
3. Klarlund, J. (1985) Transformation of cells by an inhibitor of phosphatases acting on phosphotyrosine in proteins. *Cell* **41,** 707–717.
4. Pan, M. G., Florio, T., and Stork, P. J. S. (1992) G protein activation of a hormone-stimulated phosphatase in human tumor cells. *Science* **256,** 1215–1217.
5. Cicirelli, M., Tnks, N., Diltz, C., Weiel, J., Fischer, E., and Krebs, E. (1990) Microinjection of a protein-tyrosine-phosphatase inhibits insulin action in Xenopus oocytes. *Proc. Natl. Acad. Sci. USA* **87,** 5514–5518.
6. Maher, P. (1993) Activation of phosphotyrosine phosphatase activity by reduction of cell-substrate adhesion. *Proc. Natl. Acad. Sci. USA* **90,** 11,177–11,181.
7. Fischer, E., Charbonneau, H., and Tonks, N. (1991) Protein tyrosine phosphatases: a diverse family of intracellular and transmembrane enzymes. *Science* **253,** 401–406.
8. Ingebritsen, T. (1989) Phosphotyrosyl-protein phosphatases II; identification and characterization of two heat-stable protein inhibitors. *J. Biol. Chem.* **264,** 7754–7759.
9. Imai, A. and Gershengorn, M. C. (1987) Independent phosphatidylinositol synthesis in rat pituitary plasma membrane and endoplasmic reticulum. *Nature* **325,** 725–728.
10. Imai, A. and Gershengorn, M. C. (1987) Measurement of lipid turnover in response to TRH. *Meth. Enzymol.* **141,** 100–111.
11. Lindberg, O. and Ernster, L. (1956) Determination of organic phosphorus compounds by phosphate analysis. *Meth. Biochem. Analy.* **3,** 1–22.
12. Imai, A., Takagi, H., Furui, T., Horibe, S., Fuseya, T., and Tamaya, T. (1996) Evidence for coupling of phosphotyrosine phosphatase to gonadotropin-releasing hormone receptor in ovarian carcinoma membrane. *Cancer* **77,** 132–137.
13. Imai, A., Takagi, H., Horibe, S., Fuseya, T., and Tamaya, T. (1996) Coupling of gonadotropin-releasing hormone receptor to Gi protein in human reproductive tract tumors. *J. Clin. Endocrinol. Metab.* **81,** 3249–3253.
14. Streuli, M., Krueger, N., Tsai, A., and Saito, H. (1989) A family of receptor-linked protein tyrosine phosphatases in humans and Drosophila. *Proc. Natl. Acad. Sci. USA* **86,** 8698–8702.
15. Liebow, C., Lee, M., Kamer, A., and Schally, A. (1991) Regulation of luteinizing hormone-releasing hormone receptor binding by heterologous and autologous receptor-stimulated tyrosine phosphorylation. *Proc. Natl. Acad. Sci. USA* **88,** 2244–2248.
16. Mustelin, T., Coggeshall, K., and Altman, A. (1989) Rapid activation of the T-cell tyrosine protein kinase pp56lkc by the CD45 phosphotyrosine phosphatase. *Proc. Natl. Acad. Sci. USA* **86,** 6302–6306.
17. Imai, A., Ohno, T., Iida, K., Fuseya, T., Furui, T., and Tamaya, T. (1994) Gonadotropin-releasing hormone receptor in gynecologic tumors: frequent expression in adenocarcinoma histologic types. *Cancer* **74,** 2555–2561.

# 68

# Phosphatidylinositol 4-Kinase Assay in Ovarian Carcinoma Cells

**Seiji Isonishi, Aiko Okamoto, Kazunori Ochiai, Yoshio Saito, and Kazuo Umezawa**

## 1. Introduction

Membrane-constituting phospholipids include glycerol phospholipids such as phosphatidylcholine and phosphatidylinositol (PI) and sphingolipids. Recently, signal transduction starting from hydrolysis of these phospholipids have attracted attention as regulatory mechanisms for cell growth, differentiation, and apoptosis. During this process, phosphatidylcholine is hydrolyzed by phospholipase-D into phosphatidic acid and choline, and the former is dephosphophosphorylated into diacylglycerol (DAG). DAG stimulates protein kinase C and often promotes cell growth or differentiation. In case of PI, it is first phosphorylated by PI 3-kinase or PI 4-kinase. PI 3-kinase is often activated by phosphotyrosine of the activated growth factor receptors. Metabolic pathways including PI 4-kinase are now known as classical PI turnover pathways. PI-4-P formed with PI 4-kinase is then phosphorylated by PI-4-P kinase into PI-4,5-$P_2$. Phosphatidylinositol-specific phospholipase C(PI-PLC) is the rate-limiting enzyme of PI turnover (1), and catalyzes the hydrolysis of PI-4,5-$P_2$ to produce two second messengers, inositol 1,4,5-trisphosphate ($IP_3$) and DAG. The former mobilizes $Ca^{2+}$ from internal stores by binding to the receptor on endoplasmic reticulum. PI-PLC is activated in response to a wide variety of physiological stimuli such as growth factors and hormones and often shows enhanced activity in transformed cells.

PI 4-kinase has been reported to be a membrane-bound 55-kDa protein, and has been detected in many membrane structures, including lysosome (1), endoplasmic reticulum (2), nuclear envelope (3), and Golgi (4). The 2.6-kbp cDNA encodes a protein of 854 amino acids that is highly homologous to yeast PI 4-kinase, PIK1. Garcia-Bustos et al. (5) suggested that PIK1, a 125-kDa yeast PI 4-kinase, is nuclear-associated, and that PIK1 mutants arrest in G2 because of defects in cytokinesis. The PI 4-kinase activity was reported to be associated with cellular proliferation and malignancy (6) and also the inhibition of this enzyme would provide sensitive targets for designing new chemotherapy for patients with ovarian carcinomas (7).

We have screened for inhibitors of PI 4-kinase from microbial secondary metabolites and found that orobol isolated from *Streptomyces* strongly inhibits the enzyme

From: *Methods in Molecular Medicine, Vol. 39: Ovarian Cancer: Methods and Protocols*
Edited by: J. M. S. Bartlett © Humana Press, Inc., Totowa, NJ

*(8)*. Kinetic studies have indicated that orobol is competitive with ATP and uncompetitive with phosphatidylinositol *(8)*. It inhibited EGF-induced PI synthesis and inositol phosphate formation in A431 cells *(9)*. Although the successful introduction of cisplatin (DDP) and paclitaxel (PX) into the clinic of ovarian carcinoma, drug resistance represents the major limitation of these important anticancer drugs. DDP is one of the most clinically useful agents available in the management of malignant tumors arising in the ovary, testis, and bladder. Mechanisms proposed for the observed resistance include decreased DDP accumulation, increased cellular glutathione or metallothionein, and increased repair of platinum-induced DNA crosslinks, which have generally proved to be partly controlled by clinical approaches using high-dose or combination chemotherapy. Our biological effort toward identification of drugs for enhancing DDP and/or PX sensitivity should be a unique approach and we have focused on the signal transduction pathway that has proven to be involved in circumventing DDP resistance in selected tumor models.

The antimicrotubule agent PX has shown some efficacy in the treatment of ovarian and metastatic breast cancers, and particularly encouraging its utility in advanced ovarian cancers that are refractory to DNA damage-based chemotherapy. In contrast to tubulin depolymerizing toxins such as nocodazole or colcemid, PX stabilizes microtubule formation, and continuous treatment prevents completion of mitosis, resulting in cell-cycle blockage in mitosis and activation of apoptosis. At subnanomolar concentrations, PX suppresses microtubule dynamics by affecting shortening of microtubules. At higher concentrations, PX suppresses dynamics by inhibiting the growing and shortening of microtubules. Haber et al. *(10)* and other investigators *(11,12)* have reported altered expression of the β-tubulin isotype in a PX resistant cells.

Based on these data, we have examined the effect of orobol on cellular sensitivity to DDP and PX, and have suggested that PI 4-kinase is involved in the regulation of DDP and PX sensitivity in human ovarian carcinoma cells. Orobol treatment increased the sensitivity of 2008 cells to PX. The cellular PI 4-kinase was rather increased by orobol treatment.

## 2. Materials

1. Dissolve 1.0 mg of orobol in 0.1-mL dimethyl sulfoxide to give 10 mg/mL stock solution. The stock solution can be diluted in tissue-culture medium. Use orobol at 3–30 mg/mL for cell culture studies. Store the orobol in DMSO at –20°C. Orobol was isolated from *Streptomyces* as described previously *(8)*.
2. The human cell line 2008 was established from a patient with a serous cyst adenocarcinoma of the ovary *(13)*. A resistant subline, designated 2008/C13*5, was obtained by 13 monthly selections with 1 m$M$ DDP, followed by chronic exposure to DDP increased stepwise to 5 m$M$ *(14)*.
3. Culture medium: RPMI-1640 supplemented with 5% heat-inactivated fetal bovine serum, 2 m$M$ glutamine, 100 U/mL penicillin, and 100 μg/mL streptomycin (Irvine Scientific, Santa Ana, CA).
4. $Ca^{2+}$, $Mg^{2+}$-free Dulbecco's phosphate-buffered saline (PBS, pH 7.4).
5. Harvesting buffer: 0.05 $M$ $H_3BO_4$, 0.15 $M$ NaCl, 1 m$M$ $MgCl_2$,1 m$M$ $CaCl_2$ (pH 7.2).
6. Extraction buffer: 0.02 $M$ $H_3BO_4$, 0.2 m$M$ ethylenediaminetetraacetic acid (EDTA) at pH 2.0.
7. 0.5 $M$ boric acid, pH 10.2.
8. 20 m$M$ HEPES buffer pH 7.2.

9. 1 μg/μL PI in 20 mM HEPES pH 7.2. PI is supplied in an organic solvent. Transfer 60 μL to a new tube, evaporate solvent and add 60 μL 20 mM HEPES. Sonicate for 5 s to disperse PI in HEPES.
10. γ-$^{32}$P-adenosine triphosphate (ATP) (74-370GBq/mmol, NEN).
11. Chloroform/methanol/1 N HCl (4/1/2 v/v/v).
12. Packed silica gel column (1-mL packed column, Varian Associates).
13. Chloroform/methanol/4 N ammonium hydroxide (9/7/2, v/v/v/).
14. Chloroform/methanol (2/1 v/v).

# 3. Methods
## 3.1. Cell Culture

1. The cells are maintained in culture medium.
2. They are grown on tissue culture dishes in a humidified incubator at 37°C and 5% $CO_2$ atmosphere.

## 3.2. Membrane Preparation

1. The superconfluent 2008 cells are incubated with or without 20 μg/mL of orobol for 30 min in 60-mm plastic dishes at concentrations ranging from 3–30 mg/mL orobol.
2. The cells are washed twice by cold Ca, Mg-free PBS and scraped off by rubber policeman in 2.5 mL $Ca^{2+}$, $Mg^{2+}$-free PBS.
3. The cell suspension is centrifuged at 450$g$ for 10 min to collect the cells.
4. A volume equal to the packed cell volume of harvesting buffer is added. The mixture is vortexed and diluted by addition of 100 vol of extraction buffer.
5. The mixture is stirred on ice for 10 min. Then, 8 vol of 0.5 $M$ boric acid is added.
6. After 5 min, the cytoplasm is filtered by gravity through nylon mesh (*see* **Note 1**), and the filtrate is collected in a centrifuge tube.
7. The supernatant is centrifuged at 450$g$ for 10 min at 4°C and the supernatant transferred to a fresh centrifuge tube and recentrifuged at 12,000$g$ for 1 h at 4°C.
8. The supernatant is discarded and the precipitate is resuspended in 600 μL $Ca^{2+}$, $Mg^{2+}$-free PBS (adjust final volume to 1 mL with $Ca^{2+}$, $Mg^{2+}$-free PBS).

## 3.3. Phosphatidylinositol 4-Kinase Assay (see Note 2)

1. A mixture of 60 μg of phosphatidylinositol (Funakoshi) and membrane fraction (20 μL) of 2008 cells treated with or without orobol is incubated in 60 μL 20 mM HEPES buffer pH 7.2 for 10 min at 20°C. Then, 10 μL γ-$^{32}$P-ATP(74-370GBq/mmol, NEN) is added at a final concentration of 2 mM and the mixture is incubated at 20°C for 20 min.
2. The reaction is stopped by addition of 0.7 mL of chloroform/methanol/1 N HCl (4/1/2) and vortexed.
3. The mixture is centrifuged at 800$g$ for 10 min to separate phosphorylated lipid and unreacted radioactive ATP.
4. The lower layer (0.2 mL) is taken and applied to a packed silica gel column for removal of unreacted radioactive ATP.
5. Wash the column with 2 mL of chloroform.
6. The column is eluted with 1 mL of a mixture of chloroform/methanol/4 N ammonium hydroxide (9/7/2) and the eluted fraction is evaporated to dryness.
7. The residue is dissolved in 0.1 mL chloroform/methanol (2/1).
8. The solution is applied on a cellulose filter paper.
9. The paper is dried and counted for radioactivity in scintillation counter.

## 4. Notes

1. We use nylon stockings for this filtration.
2. This PI 4-kinase assay was modification of the method described in **ref. *15***. We have developed a rapid assay using a small packed silica gel column.

## References

1. Collins, C. A. and Wells, W. W. (1983) Identification of phosphatidylinositol kinase in rat liver lysosomal membranes. *J. Biol. Chem.* **258,** 2130–2134.
2. Cockcroft, S., Taylor, J. A., and Judah, J. D. (1985) Subcellular localization of inositol lipid kinases in rat liver. *Biochem. Biophys. Acta.* **845,** 163–170.
3. Smith, C. and Wells, W. (1983) Phosphorylation of rat liver nuclear envelopes. II. Characterization of in vitro lipid phosphorylation. *J. Biol. Chem.* **258,** 9368–9373.
4. Jergil, B. and Sundler, R. J. (1983) Phosphorylation of phosphatidylinositol in rat liver Golgi. *J. Biol. Chem.* **258,** 7968–7973.
5. Garcia-Bustos, J. F., Marini, F., Stevenson, I., Frei, C., and Hall, M. N. (1994) PIK1 an essential phosphatidylinositol 4-kinase assciated with the yeast nucleus. *EMBO J.* **13,** 2352–2361.
6. Rizzo, M. T. and Weber, G. (1994) 1-Phosphatidylinositol 4-kinase: an enzyme linked with proliferation and malignancy. *Cancer Res.* **54,** 2611–2614.
7. Look, K., Singhal, R., Moore, D. H., Sutton, G. P., and Weber, G. (1995) Increased phosphatidylinositol (PI) 4-kinase and PI 4-phosphate (PI) 5-kinase activities in extracts of malignant ovarian epithelium. *Proc. ASCO* **14,** 282.
8. Nishioka, H., Imoto, M., Sawa, T., Hamada, M., Naganawa, H., Takeuchi, T. and Umezawa, K. (1989) Screening of phosphatidylinositol 4-kinase inhibitors from *Streptomyces*. *J. Antibiotics* **42,** 823–825.
9. Nishioka, H., Sawa, T., Hamada, M., Shimura, N., Imoto, M., and Umezawa, K. (1990) Inhibition of phosphatidylinositol kinase by toyocamycin. *J. Antibiotics* **43,** 1586–1589.
10. Haber, M., Burkhart, C. A., Regl, D. L., Madafiglio, J., Norris, M. D., and Horwitz, S. B. (1995) Altered expression of Mb2, the class II β-tubulin isotype, in a murine J774.2 cell line with a high level of taxol resistance. *J. Biol. Chem.* **270,** 31,269–31,275.
11. Ranganathan, S., Dexter. D. W., Benetatos, C. A., Chapman, A. E., Tew, K. D., and Hudes, G. R. (1996) Increase of βIII- and βIVa-tubulin isotypes in human prostate carcinoma cells as a result of estramustine resistance. *Cancer Res.* **56,** 2584–2589.
12. Kavallaris, M., Kuo, D. Y.-S., Burhhart, C. A., Regl, D. L., Norris, M. D., Haber, M., and Horwitz, S. B. (1997) Taxol-resistant epithelial ovarian tumors are associated with altered expression of specific β-tubulin isotypes. *J. Clin. Invest.* **100,** 1282–1293.
13. Isonishi, S., Shiotsuka, S., Kimura, E., Ochiai, K., Yasuda, M., and Tanaka, T. (1997) Cell-cycle dependent enhancement of cisplatin sensitivity of a human ovarian carcinoma cell line by orobol. *Proc. Am. Assoc. Cancer Res.* **38,** 4137.
14. Andrews, P. A., Murphy, M. P., and Howell, S. B. (1985) Differential potentiation of alkylating and platinating agent cytotoxicity in human ovarian carcinoma cells by glutathione depletion. *Cancer Res.* **45,** 6250–6253.
15. Sugimoto, Y. and Erikson, R. L. (1985) Phosphatidylinositol kinase activities in normal and Rous sarcoma-transformed cells. *Mol. Cell. Biol.* **5,** 3194–3198.

# 69

## Calcium Mobilization in Ovarian Cancer Cells in Response to Lysophospholipids

**Yan Xu and Derek S. Damron**

## 1. Introduction

Intracellular free $Ca^{2+}$ concentration ($[Ca^{2+}]_i$) plays a critical role in regulating many diverse cellular functions including cell proliferation and programmed cell death (apoptosis) *(1)*. An elevation in $[Ca^{2+}]_i$ activates enzymes (phospholipase $A_2$, phospholipase D and some isoforms of protein kinase C) associated with the liberation of bioactive lipids such as arachidonic acid (AA) and lysophosphatidic acid (LPA) *(1,2)*. AA and its metabolites have been implicated in multiple steps of carcinogenesis *(3,4)*. LPA as well as several other bioactive lipids stimulate release of $Ca^{2+}$ from intracellular stores and regulate proliferation of ovarian cancer cells *(5–7)*.

Mobilization of cytosolic $Ca^{2+}$ can be induced by extracellular stimuli, such as growth factors, through $PLC\gamma$ activation. In addition, several other G protein-coupled receptor agonists (glycohormones, neurotransmitters, and peptides) mobilize intracellular $Ca^{2+}$ through activation of $PLC_\beta$ *(8)*. Both enzymes hydrolyze phosphatidyl inositol *bis*-phosphate ($PIP_2$) to produce inositol 1,4,5 *tris*-phosphate ($IP_3$) which activates receptors on the endoplasmic reticulum causing release of calcium into the cytosol. An elevation in $[Ca^{2+}]_i$ can also be achieved via influx of $Ca^{2+}$ through sarcolemmal calcium channels (voltage-operated, receptor-operated) located in the cell membrane. These channels are important for regulating $[Ca^{2+}]_i$ in excitable cells (muscle, neurons), but less important in ovarian cancer cells. This paper will focus on the measurement of calcium mobilization from intracellular stores.

## 2. Materials

### 2.1. Cell Culture

1. Serum containing medium: RPMI-1640 (Gibco, Gaithersburg, MD or Cellgro) with 10% fetal bovine serum (Gibco or Cellgro), 2 m$M$ glutamine (Gibco or Cellgro) and 10 µg/mL gentamycin (Gibco or Cellgro).
2. Serum free medium: RPMI-1640, 2 m$M$ glutamine and 10 µg/mL gentamycin.
3. 2 m$M$ ethylenediaminetetraacetic acid (EDTA) in PBS, pH 7.4.

From: *Methods in Molecular Medicine, Vol. 39: Ovarian Cancer: Methods and Protocols*
Edited by: J. M. S. Bartlett © Humana Press, Inc., Totowa, NJ

### 2.2. Buffers

1. Buffer A: 25 m$M$ HEPES, 140 m$M$ NaCl, 3 m$M$ KCl, 1 m$M$ MgCl$_2$, 1.8 m$M$, CaCl$_2$, and 10 m$M$ glucose, pH 7.4.
2. Buffer B: same as buffer A, but without CaCl$_2$.
3. Loading buffer: 125 m$M$ NaCl, 5m$M$ KCl, 1.2 m$M$ MgSO$_4$, 11 m$M$ glucose, 1.8 m$M$ CaCl$_2$, 25 m$M$ HEPES, and 0.2% BSA, pH 7.4.
4. Control Buffer A: 125 m$M$ NaCl, 5 m$M$ KCl, 1.2 m$M$ MgSO$_4$, 11 m$M$ glucose, 2.5 m$M$ CaCl$_2$, 25 m$M$ HEPES, pH 7.4.
5. Control Buffer B: same as control Buffer A, but without CaCl$_2$.
6. Prepare two pH 7.0 10 m$M$ ethyleneglycoltetraacetic acid (EGTA) buffers with 100 m$M$ KCl and 10 m$M$ K-MOPS, one containing 10 m$M$ CaCl$_2$, the other not containing CaCl$_2$. They will be referred to as CaEGTA and EGTA buffers, respectively.
7. Fura-2 stock solutions (1 m$M$ in dimetholsulfoxide) are kept frozen (in 50 µL quantities).

### 2.3. Lipids

1. LPA: dissolve oleyol-LPA in 10 m$M$ HEPES, pH 7.4 and 100 m$M$ NaCl to 3–5 m$M$; dissolve steroyl and palmitoyl LPA's in 50% methanol or 95% ethanol at concentrations of 1–2 m$M$ with sonication.
2. Lysophosphatidylserine (LPS): solubilize LPS in 50% ethanol to 3–5 m$M$ with sonication.
3. Sphingosinet-phosphate (SPP): make 1–2 m$M$ stock solution in Tris-saline, pH 10.0–11.0.
4. Sphingosylphosphoryl-choline (SPC): solubilize SPC in PBS or other physiological buffer (10 m$M$).

Aliquot lipids in single use vials and store at –80°C. Further dilutions of these lipids should be made using the assay buffer at the time of use (buffer A, B, or control buffer). Additional information on making lipid solutions is provided (*see* **Note 1**).

## 3. Methods
### 3.1. Cell Culture

1. Grow ovarian cancer cells in serum containing medium at 37°C, 5% carbon dioxide, 100% humidity.
2. Change the media to serum-free medium for 16–48 h before performing the calcium assays (*see* **Note 2**).

### 3.2. Dye Loading

Calcium assays may be performed on individual cells cultured on dishes under a microscope or on populations of cells suspended in a cuvet (*see* **Note 3** for the choice of selection). During and after dye loading, the cells should be kept in the dark (*see* **Note 4**).

### 3.2.1. Dye Loading Procedure for Cultured Cells on Dishes

1. Wash the cells (2 × 5 min) with loading buffer at pH 7.4.
2. Dilute fura-2/AM (1-m$M$ stock in DMSO, Molecular Probes) in loading buffer to final concentration of 1 µ$M$; add 1.5 mL to each dish.
3. Incubate at room temperature (30 min).
4. Wash cells (2 × 5 min) with loading buffer. Allow to stand in loading buffer for 20 min at room temperature.
5. Wash cells (2 × 5 min) with control buffer and allow to stand in control buffer A or B.

### 3.2.2. Dye Loading Procedure for Suspended Cells

1. Use 2 m$M$ EDTA/PBS (*see* **Note 5**) to detach cells from flasks.
2. Centrifuge cells at 800$g$ for 5 min.
3. Resuspend cells (1 × 10$^6$ cells/mL) and place in an incubator (37°C) for 2–3 h.
4. Centrifuge (800 × $g$/5 min) and resuspend cells in serum-free medium (5 × 10$^6$ cells/mL). Add fura-2/AM to a final concentration of 1 µ$M$.
5. Incubate cells at 37°C for 30 min.
6. Bring volume to 10–15 mL with serum-free medium and centrifuge (800$g$/5 min).
7. Wash twice with serum-free medium and harvest by centrifugation.
8. Resuspend cells in buffer A, or buffer B (1 × 10$^6$ cells/mL) and place in the incubator (37°C) for 30–60 min.

## 3.3. System Hardware (Spectrofluorometer and Fiber-Optic Cable)

1. The basic system consists of a patented RFK-6002 Delta-Scan high-speed dual-wavelength scanning illuminator and RF-0107D high-grade quartz fiber-optic bundle capable of adapting to either the epi-port of an inverted fluorescence microscope or alternatively to an MP1 sample compartment housing a temperature regulated cuvette holder (Photon Technology, Intl.). The Delta-Scan illuminator is high-speed alternating wavelength illumination system. Alternating wavelength exposure times can be varied from approximately one millisecond to hundreds of seconds, with no crosstalk between the two channels. Continuously variable micrometer-adjusted slits provide bandpass control for both monochromaters. The quartz fiber-optic bundle provides ease of optical alignment, freedom from vibration, and maximum flexibility in laboratory space utilization. The illumination produced by the arc lamp first encounters a rotating chopper disk, which alternately presents reflecting and transmitting segments to the lower monochromater or redirecting the beam to the upper monochromater via a focusing mirror (**Fig. 1**). The two separate monochromater outputs are collected by the ends of the bifurcated quartz fiber-optic bundle, brought to a common output end, and focused onto the sample. The output end of the fiber adapts to either a cuvette sample compartment for studies in suspensions of cells or to the epi-fluorescence port of a standard inverted fluorescence microscope.

### 3.3.1. Microscope-Based Photometry (Single Cells)

1. The microscope system hardware also includes a microscope and microscope adapter (Olympus America Inc., Lake Success, NY), a D-104B Single Channel Microscope Photometer (Photon Technology Intl.), one Model 710 photon-counting photomultiplier tube (PMT) housing with PMT (Photon Technology Intl.) connected to a Mirage 486 computer for data collection (**Fig. 1**). Data acquisition parameters and hardware settings are specified using software provided by Photon Technology Int'l (Felix™).
2. Illumination is delivered via the quartz fiber-optic bundle to the microscope via the epi-illumination port at the back of the microscope (**Fig. 1**). Fluorescence emission is collected through the microscope optics (containing a dichroic cube with a 400-nm dichroic mirror for fura-2) and directed to the photometer, which is attached directly to the side camera port of the microscope. In the photometer, the collected fluorescence first passes through a bilateral, continuously variable aperture. Four control knobs manually adjust the region of interest (ROI), which represents that portion of the field-of-view from which fluorescence emission will be measured. In this way, clusters of cells, single cells, or regions within cells as well as autofluorescence between cells (background) can be selected for study. After passing through the aperture, the light encounters a movable mirror. In the view position, this mirror redirects the emission beam up to a parfocal eyepiece for viewing by the user. In this mode, the user may directly observe the emission image to adjust

Fig. 1. Diagrammatic representation of the hardware used for microscope-based photometry.

the ROI. In the measure position, the mirror is removed from the optical path and the emission light then passes through a 1-in bandpass filter holder containing an emission barrier filter for fura-2 ($510 \pm 20$ nm) before finally striking the photon-counting PMT in the detector housing. Photon-counting PMT detection was chosen as the standard detection technique because its high sensitivity and fast time resolution make it ideal for rapid kinetics observation and low-level fluorescence measurements. Further, this system has a dynamic range of five orders of magnitude, and requires no high-voltage adjustments or zeroing associated with other detection technologies.

### 3.3.2. Sample Compartment-Based Photometry (Cell Suspension)

1. Illumination is delivered via the quartz fiber-optic bundle to an MP1 sample compartment (Photon Technology Intl.) via an access port in the back of a fully enclosed chamber. Quartz lenses are used for both incident and emission optical paths and can be easily aligned by the user. It also includes a variable temperature sample holder with a four-position cuvette turret and sample stirrer feature. An emission monochromater (101A) equipped with a PMT (Model 710) is directly attached to the chamber at a 90° angle to the incident beam for selection of emission wavelength (510 nm with band pass at 20 nm) and photon counting (Photon Technology Intl.). A lid-activated shutter protects the sensitive PMT detector from excessive light.

## 3.4. Microscope-Based Photometry (Individual Cells)

1. Culture dishes containing serum-starved (*see* **Note 2**) fura-2-loaded ovarian cancer cells (2000–20,000 cells/dish) are placed in a temperature regulated (37°C) chamber ($\Delta$TC3; Bioptechs, Inc.) mounted on the stage of an Olympus IX-70 inverted fluorescence microscope.
2. Fluorescence measurements are performed on individual cells at excitation wavelengths of 340 and 380 nm and an emission wavelength of 510 nm. The volume of the chamber is 1.5 mL.
3. Cells are washed and incubated in Control buffer A or B. The temperature of all solutions is maintained at 37°C in a water bath.
4. Just prior to data acquisition, background fluorescence between cells is measured and subtracted automatically from the subsequent experimental measurements.
5. Fura-2 fluorescence signals (340, 380, and 340/380 ratio) originating from single ovarian cancer cells are continuously monitored at a sampling frequency of 25-Hz, and are collected using Felix™ software.
6. For measuring intracellular calcium only, EGTA should be added to the buffer (1–2 m$M$ (*see* **Note 6**).
7. Reagents (lipids) may be added by superfusion of the cells. Alternatively, 1.5 mL control buffer with the appropriate amount of lipid (*see* **Note 7**) may be added directly to the dish after aspirating the control buffer.
8. To identify whether there is a densensitization of the response, a second addition of the same lipid or alternatively, a different lipid may be delivered to the cuvet (*see* **Note 8**).
9. To demonstrate intact, receptor-mediated $Ca^{2+}$ signaling, ATP (10–100 $\mu M$), thrombin (0.1–1 U/mL) or trypsin (2–25 $\mu$g/mL) may be added after the lipid-induced calcium signal returns to the baseline (**Fig. 2**).

## 3.5. Cuvet-Based Photometry (Suspensions of Cells)

1. Set the excitation at 340 and 380 nm and emission at 510 nm.
2. Data collection is acquired at 25 data points per second (25 Hz).
3. Set the bandwidth to 2 nm on the excitation monochromaters and 20 nm on the emission monochromater. Duration of the experiment is set at 15 min.

Fig. 2. LPA (1 $\mu M$) and ATP (100 $\mu M$) stimulated $Ca^{2+}$ release in ovarian cancer cells (HEY cells).

4. Aliquot dye-loaded cells (usually $2–5 \times 10^5$ cells) into a microcentrifuge tube.
5. Centrifuge ($1000g$) to gently pellet the cells.
6. Resuspend in 0.1 mL of buffer A or B and transfer to a cuvet containing 1.6 mL of prewarmed buffer A or B with a constant stirrer.
7. Begin to acquire baseline data by initiating data acquisition with Felix.
8. Wait for the baseline fluorescence to stabilize.
9. Add 1.7 µL of EGTA (1 $M$). Record baseline for ~1 min (*see* **Note 6**).
10. Add reagents (lipids) (≤17 µL) to the cuvet.
11. Perform **steps 8–9** from **Subheading 3.3.**

## 3.6. Calibration of Fura-2 and Determination of [Ca$^{2+}$]$_i$

Calibration of fura-2 can be performed either *in situ* or in cell-free conditions using fura-2 (free acid) in buffers with known $Ca^{2+}$ concentrations (*see* **Note 9** for choice of selection). We have included protocols for both types of calibration techniques.

### 3.6.1. In Situ *Calibration*

1. Prepare stock solutions of digitonin (10 m$M$ in ethanol) or ionomycin (10 m$M$ in ethanol) and EGTA (10 m$M$ in H$_2$O). At the end of each experimental protocol, wash away all interventions and lyse the cells to release intracellular fura-2 by adding digitonin or ionomycin (10 µ$M$, final concentration) to the cells on the dish or in the cuvet (1000-fold dilution of the stock).
2. If the experiment was performed in the absence of extracellular $Ca^{2+}$, add $Ca^{2+}$ back to the buffer to a final concentration of 1 m$M$. This will allow for the determination of the maximum fluorescence (Rmax) of fura-2 when bound to a saturating $Ca^{2+}$ concentration.

3. Once the fluorescence signal has stabilized following addition of digitonin or ionomycin, add 2 m$M$ EGTA (final concentration) to obtain the minimum fluorescence ratio (Rmin) for fura-2, i.e., when no $Ca^{2+}$ is bound to fura-2.

4. $[Ca^{2+}]_i$ is calculated as follows $[Ca^{2+}]_i$ = Kd × R-Rmin/Rmax-R × Sf2/Sb2 where Kd of fura-2 for $Ca^{2+}$ is taken as 224 nM, as described by Grynkiewicz et al. *(16)*. R is the fluorescence ratio of the cell. Rmin and Rmax are the fluorescence ratios of the calcium-free and $Ca^{2+}$-saturated fura-2 sample, respectively. Sf2 is the fluorescence intensity at 380 nm of the $Ca^{2+}$-free sample and Sb2 is the fluorescence intensity at 380 nm of the $Ca^{2+}$-bound sample.

### 3.6.2. Cell-Free Calibration

1 To a well-rinsed, cleaned test tube, add 8.991 mL of CaEGTA buffer and add 9 μL of fura-2 stock solution to obtain a final fura-2 concentration of 1 μ$M$. Seal tube with parafilm and mix by turning over several times.

2. In order to avoid $Ca^{2+}$ contamination of the $Ca^{2+}$-lacking EGTA buffer, place 2.997 mL of EGTA buffer into the dish or cuvet and introduce 3 μL of fura-2 *directly* using a 10 μL digital pipet. This results in a 1 μ$M$ final concentration of fura-2.

3. Measure the 340/380 fluorescence ratio of the EGTA buffer. It should be approximately 0.6–1.0.

4. Perform a titration of the dye in the following manner. Exchange 0.3 mL of the EGTA buffer with 0.3 mL of the CaEGTA buffer and again record the fluorescence ratio. The $Ca^{2+}$ concentration in the buffer is now 42 nM. Continue to exchange the following volumes (0.333, 0.375, 0.429, 0.5, 0.6, 0.75, 1.0, and 1.5 mL) and measure the fluorescence ratio. The $Ca^{2+}$ concentration in the buffer after the above exchanges should be 95, 162, 253, 380, 570, 880, 1520, and 3420 n$M$, respectively. A titration curve plotting the fluorescence ratio against the $[Ca^{2+}]_i$ can now been constructed.

## 4. Notes

1. The solubilities of different lysophospholipids are variable. One might consult the commercial vendor to obtain more information for the particular compound to be studied. Generally speaking, lipid stock solutions should be made at the highest concentrations in a buffer (for oleoyl-LPA, SIP or SPC) or a solvent that is soluble with $H_2O$, such as methanol, 50–95% ethanol, or DMSO. Dilutions should be made using the assay buffer. The volumes of the stock solution added to the cuvette or dish should not exceed 1%. The effect of the solvent used should be tested, particularly when greater than 1% volume of the stock solution is added. We noted that 1% methanol and 1% ethanol did not affect the calcium assay for ovarian cancer cells, such as HEY, OCC1, and SKOV3 cells. Distinct LPA species have different solubilities in aqueous solution. Oleyol-LPA can be solubilized in aqueous solution up to 5 m$M$. Routinely, we make this LPA in 10 m$M$ HEPES, pH 7.4 and 100 m$M$ NaCl to 2–4 m$M$ stock solution; aliquot and store at –80°C where it should remain stable for at least one year. At –20°C, it is stable for several months. Steroyl- and palmitoyl-LPAs are much less soluble in aqueous buffers (solubility less than 0.5 m$M$). Repetitive freezing and thawing does not affect LPA activity. However, prolonged exposure to room temperature should be minimized. Lipid solutions can be sterilized, if so desired, by passing through a sterile syringe filter (0.2 μ$M$). However, filtration usually results in loss of some lipid and is usually not necessary for calcium assays. Lipids, in particular, LPA, have been shown to bind to serum albumin. This association usually helps in solubilizing lipids, such as LPA. In addition, it has been shown that the presence of bovine serum albumin (BSA) does not affect the activity of LPA in calcium assays. Fatty acid free BSA (Sigma Chemical Co., St. Louis, MO) should be used.

2. Cell starvation before performing calcium assays is very important. Both LPA and SIP have been shown to be produced by activated platelets. Therefore, LPA and SIP are normal constituents of serum. The receptors for lysophospholipid on cells cultured in fetal bovine or fetal calf serum will be exposed to the agonists and will be desensitized. In addition, LPA and other lysophospholipids, not only desensitize themselves, but also possibly cross desensitize other lipids as we previously demonstrated *(1–3)*. The optimal time for cell starvation may vary depending on the cell line and needs to be determined empirically. Generally speaking, a minimum of 16 h and a maximum 48 h is required.

3. The advantage of the calcium assays performed in cell suspension is that this measures the average response of the entire population of cells, avoiding cell to cell variations. With this approach, a series of individual experiments can be performed using cells derived from the same batch allowing for direct comparisons between aliquots. However, assays in single cells, or clusters of cells on a cultured monolayer have recently become more popular. This allows us to study $Ca^{2+}$ mobilization at the single cell level where heterogeneity in the response between different cell types may be examined. In addition, the cells remain attached to the dish during the fura-2 loading procedure and therefore are not potentially damaged by enzymatic treatment with trypsin or EDTA, which is required to harvest cells for cell suspension studies. Although heterogeneity of the response between individual cells may impose limitations in some instances (primary cultures of cells) it is less of a problem in established cell lines.

4. Fura-2 AM is a membrane-permeant, $Ca^{2+}$-insensitive ester of the $Ca^{2+}$ fluorophore Fura-2, which becomes $Ca^{2+}$-sensitive and remains trapped intracellularly following hydrolysis by nonspecific intracellular esterases *(9)*. Dye loading at room temperature minimizes the sequestration of Fura-2 by intracellular organelles. If leakage of fura-2 is a problem, addition of the anion exchange blocker, probenecid (2.5 m$M$), helps to minimize fura-2 leakage from the cells.

5. To detach cells, trypsin should be avoided. We have found that ovarian cancer cell lines, including HEY OCC1 and SKOV3, react with thrombin and trypsin to release calcium, presumably through a thrombin and/or a protease receptor *(10)*. We have found that this activation partly cross desensitizes lysophospholipids, such LPA, LPS, and SPC-induced calcium mobilization. Therefore, cells should be detached using a PBS/EDTA solution.

6. EGTA pretreatment is used to chelate trace extracellular free calcium. Similar experiments can be performed in the same manner in calcium-containing buffers and omitting the EGTA-pretreatment. Some cell lines seem to be very sensitive to the absence of extracellular calcium and the EGTA pretreatment (they will not react to any agonist under these conditions, perhaps because they require extracellular $Ca^{2+}$ to fill intracellular stores). In these cases, calcium-containing buffer should be used. However, one should be aware that under these circumstances, the calcium changes observed could potentially represent both calcium release from intracellular stores and calcium influx.

7. The active concentrations of a lipid on calcium mobilization in ovarian cancer cells are likely in the range of 10 n$M$ to 10 μ$M$. At concentrations above 10 μ$M$, most lysophospholipids will have a detergent-like, nonspecific effect (lytic) on the plasma membrane, causing membrane leakage, and cell damage. Under these conditions, a prolonged (in contrast to a transient) calcium increase is often observed. Therefore, final concentrations of lipids should be kept below 10 μ$M$ and preferably in the n$M$ to low μ$M$ range.

8. The cross desensitizations between lipids may vary in different cell lines. We have found that LPA, LPS, and SPC completely crossdesensitize each other in HEY and OCC1 cell. In addition, we have observed that these homologous or heterogeneity desensitizations induced by lipid molecules may last for at least 8 h after stimulated cells recultured in lipid-free media.

9. Photobleaching and photochemical formation of fluorescent $Ca^{2+}$-insensitive forms is a general problem with both modes of calibration. Numerous difficulties in using the *in situ* method have been reviewed *(11)*, and include: (a) incomplete hydrolysis of fura-2 acetoxymethyl ester, resulting in $Ca^{2+}$ insensitive, but fluorescent compounds; (b) sequestration of fura-2 in noncytoplasmic compartments; (c) dye loss; (d) photobleaching and photochemical formation of fluorescent $Ca^{2+}$-insensitive forms; (e) shifts in excitation emission spectra and the dissociation constant (Kd) for $Ca^{2+}$ because of changes in ionic strength and viscosity. Similarly, estimation of $[Ca^{2+}]_i$ using a cell-free calibration protocol also has some limitations. Temperature, viscosity, ionic strength, and composition of the calibration buffer can all affect the Kd of the dye. Therefore, the dye may behave differently inside cells compared to a buffer designed to mimic the intracellular milieu. Because of confounding factors associated with both techniques, many authors prefer to use fura-2 as a qualitative indicator of $[Ca^{2+}]_i$ reported as the change in the 340/380 ratio.

# References

1. Clapham, D. E. (1995) Calcium signaling. *Cell* **80**, 259–268.
2. Fourcade, O., Simon, M. F., Viode, C., Rugani, N., Leballe, F., Ragab, A., et al. (1995) Secretory phospholipase A2 generates the novel lipid mediator lysophosphatidic acid in membrane microvesicles shed from activated cells. *Cell* **80**, 919–927.
3. elAttar, T. M. (1985) Cancer and the prostaglandins: a mini review on cancer research. *J. Oral Pathol.* **14**, 511–522.
4. Honn, K. V., Tang, D. G., Gao, X., Butovich, I. A., Liu, B., Timar, J., and Hagmann, W.(1994) 12-lipoxygenases and 12(S)-HETE: role in cancer metastasis. *Cancer Metastasis Rev.* **13**, 365–396.
5. Xu, Y. and Mills, G. B. (1995) Activation of human ovarian cancer cells: role of lipid factors in ascitic fluid, in *Ovarian Cancer* (Sharp, F., Mason, P., Blackett, T., and Berek, J., eds.), 3. Chapman and Hall Medical, London, New York, pp. 121–135.
6. Xu, Y., Gaudette, D. C., Boynton, J., Frankel, A., Fang, X-J., Sharma, A., et al. (1994) Characterization of an ovarian cancer activating factor (OCAF) in ascites from ovarian cancer patients. *Clin. Cancer Res.* **1**, 1223–1232.
7. Xu, Y., Fang, X. J., Casey, G., and Mills, G. B. (1995) Lysophospholipids activate ovarian and breast cancer cells. *Biochem. J.* **309**, 933–940.
8. Berridge, M. J. (1993) Inositol trisphosphate and calcium signalling. *Nature* **361**, 315–325.
9. Grynkiewicz, G., Poenie, M., and Tsien, R. Y. (1985) A new generation of $Ca^{2+}$ indicators with greatly imporved fluorescence properties. *J. Biol. Chem.* **260**, 3440–3450.
10. Ishihara, H., Connolly, A. J., Zeng, D., Kahn, M. L., Zheng, Y. W., Timmons, C., et al. (1997) Protease-activated receptor 3 is a second thrombin receptor in humans. *Nature* **386**, 502–506.
11. Roe, M. W., LeMasters, J. J., and Herman, B. (1990) Assessment of Fura-2 for measurements of cytosolic free calcium [Review]. *Cell Calcium* **11**, 63–73.

# Compartmentalized Protein Kinase C Activation in Ovarian Carcinoma Cells

## Alakananda Basu and Giridhar R. Akkaraju

## 1. Introduction

Protein kinase C (PKC), a family of phospholipid-dependent serine/threonine kinases, plays a cardinal role in malignancy (*1–5*). PKC isozymes can be categorized into three groups: Group A or conventional (c) PKC: $\alpha$, $\beta$I, $\beta$II, and $\gamma$; Group B or novel (n) PKC: $\delta$, $\varepsilon$, $\eta$, $\theta$, and $\mu$, and Group C or atypical (a) PKC: $\zeta$ and $\lambda$ ($\iota$) (*1,3,4*). Whereas cPKCs require $Ca^{2+}$ and diacylglycerol (DAG) phorbol esters for their activities, nPKCs and aPKCs are $Ca^{2+}$-independent. aPKCs are also insensitive to diacylglycerol and phorbol esters (*1,3,4*).

PKC usually resides in the cytoplasm or is loosely associated with the plasma membrane in an inactive form (*6*). Activators of PKC interact with the regulatory domain of PKC (**Fig. 1**), alter its conformation, and induce a redistribution of the cytosolic enzyme to the membrane compartments (*6,7*). This translocation is often used to monitor the activation state of the enzyme. Prolonged membrane association may lead to downregulation of PKC (*8*). Given the diversity of the PKC family, the subcellular distribution and proximity to specific substrates within the cell may be one mechanism by which the activity of different PKC isozymes is regulated (*9*).

As depicted in **Fig. 2**, compartmentalization of PKC can be monitored by biochemical assays, phorbol ester binding, Western blotting, and immunohistochemistry. Cells treated with or without PKC activator can be fractionated into cytosolic and particulate compartments and PKC assay or Western blot analysis can be performed with those fractions. Alternatively, cells may be analyzed by immunohistochemistry. To determine PKC activity, the cytosolic and particulate fractions are partially purified by anion exchange chromatography and $Ca^{2+}$-, phospholipid-dependent protein kinase activity is determined using histone as a substrate and by subtracting the activity determined in the absence of phosphatidylserine (PS) and DAG from that in the presence of PS and DAG. Novel and atypical PKCs are $Ca^{2+}$-independent and they do not utilize histone as the preferred substrate (*3*). Peptide substrates that correspond to the pseudosubstrate domain of PKCs can be used as substrates for these isozymes. These peptide substrates, however, have overlapping specificity and they lack isozyme selectivity (*10*). Therefore, although PKC assays can be used to monitor compartmentalization of cPKCs, it is

From: *Methods in Molecular Medicine, Vol. 39: Ovarian Cancer: Methods and Protocols*
Edited by: J. M. S. Bartlett © Humana Press, Inc., Totowa, NJ

Fig. 1. Model of protein kinase C activation by cofactors. Protein kinase C (Group A) contains 4 conserved (C1-C4) and 5 variable regions (V1-V5). The 80-kDa native enzyme consists of a 30-kDa regulatory domain and a 50-kDa catalytic domain connected through the V3 or hinge region. The regulatory domain of PKC contains a stretch of amino acids known as the pseudosubstrate sequence, which resembles a PKC substrate, but does not contain any serine or threonine residue that can be phosphorylated. In the unstimulated state, the regulatory domain interacts with the catalytic domain through the pseudosubstrate sequence and prevents access of substrate to the catalytic site. Allosteric activators or cofactors of PKC bind to the regulatory domain, induce a conformational change in the enzyme thereby exposing the substrate binding site, and catalysis takes place.

difficult to discriminate among PKC isozymes. Because PKC is the receptor for tumor-promoting phorbol esters, a radiolabeled phorbol ester [$^3$H]phorbol 12,13-dibutyrate is also used to monitor localization of PKC. This method does not require any purification step, but it also cannot discriminate among PKC isozymes. Western blot analysis and immunohistochemistry using PKC isozyme-specific antibodies are useful to detect individual PKC isozymes. Whereas Western blotting does not require any purification of PKC, it determines the abundance of PKC isozymes rather than their functional state. Immunohistochemistry also does not require any cell fractionation, but fixation of cells by some techniques may affect compartmentalization of PKC and it is difficult to quantify the abundance of PKC isozymes. Therefore, it is recommended to monitor subcellular distribution of PKC isozymes using more than one method. In this chapter,

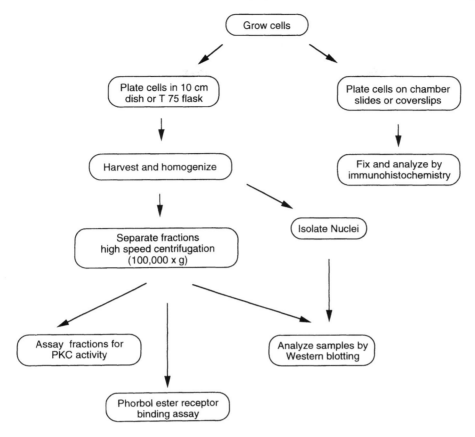

Fig. 2. Various appoaches to monitor compartmentalization of protein kinase C.

we have illustrated compartmentalization of PKC in ovarian carcinoma 2008 cells using a biochemical assay (**Fig. 3**) and Western blot analysis (**Fig. 4**), both of which are routinely used in our laboratory.

## 2. Materials
### 2.1. Subcellular Distribution
#### 2.1.1. Cell Culture

1. Complete medium [RPMI-1640 (Gibco, Gaithersburg, MD), 5% FBS (HyClone, Logan, UT), 2 mM glutamine (Gibco)].
2. Phosphate-buffered saline (PBS) [136 mM NaCl, 2.6 mM KCl, 10 mM $Na_2HPO_4$, 17 mM $KH_2PO_4$, pH 7.4].
3. Trypsin-ethylenediaminetetraacetic acid (EDTA) (0.05% trypsin, 0.53 mM EDTA-4Na) (Gibco).

#### 2.1.2. Cell Fractionation

1. 0.1 mM 12-O-tetradecanoylphorbol 13-acetate (TPA) in dimethyl sulfoxide (DMSO) (store in 50 µL aliquots at −20°C).
2. Buffer A: 20 mM Tris-HCl, pH 7.5, 0.5 mM EDTA, 0.5 mM ethyleneglycoltetraacetic acid (EGTA), 0.25 M sucrose, 10 mM β-mercaptoethanol (store at 4°C). To prepare 500 mL buffer A, mix the following: 10 mL 1.0 M Tris-HCl, pH 7.5, 2.5 mL 0.1 M EGTA,

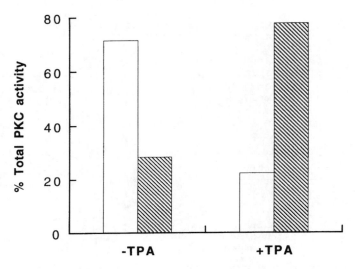

Fig. 3. Effect of TPA on PKC translocation. Ovarian carcinoma 2008 cells were treated with the vehicle DMSO or 100 n*M* TPA for 30 min. At the end of the incubation, cytosolic and membrane fractions were separated by high-speed centrifugation and subjected to DE-52 chromatography as described in **Subheading 3**. Ca$^{2+}$- and phospholipid-dependent PKC activity was determined by subtracting the activity determined in the absence of PS/DAG from that in the presence of PS/DAG. Open column, cytosolic PKC; hatched column, membrane PKC.

   0.5 mL 0.5 *M* EDTA, 43 g sucrose and H$_2$O to a final volume of 500 mL. Add 70 µL β-mercaptoethanol per 100 mL buffer A immediately before use.
3. Lysis buffer: 20 m*M* Tris-HCl, pH 7.5, 0.25 *M* sucrose, 2 m*M* EDTA, 5 m*M* EGTA, 10 m*M* β-mercaptoethanol, 1 m*M* PMSF, 25 µg/mL leupeptin, 25 µg/mL aprotinin, and 25 µg/mL soybean trypsin inhibitor. To prepare 10 mL lysis buffer mix the following: 30 µL 0.5 *M* EDTA, 0.45 mL 0.1 *M* EGTA, 25 µL 10 mg/mL leupeptin, aprotinin, and soybean trypsin inhibitor in H$_2$0, 10 µL 1 *M* PMSF in acetone and buffer A to 10 mL. Protease inhibitors are stored in aliquots at –20°C and added to the lysis buffer immediately before use.
4. Nuclei isolation buffer (buffer B): 10 m*M* HEPES, pH 7.9, 10 m*M* KCl, 0.1 m*M* EDTA, 0.1 m*M* EGTA, 1 m*M* dithiothreitol (DTT), 1 m*M* PMSF, 25 µg/mL leupeptin, 25 µg/mL aprotinin, 25 µg/mL soybean trypsin inhibitor, and H$_2$O to a final volume of 100 mL. Add DTT and protease inhibitors immediately before use.
5. Nuclei resuspension buffer (buffer C): 20 m*M* HEPES, pH 7.9, 0.4 *M* NaCl, 1 m*M* EDTA, 1 m*M* EGTA, 1 m*M* DTT, 25% glycerol, H$_2$O to a final volume of 10 mL. Add DTT immediately before use.

## 2.2. PKC Isolation

1. DE-52 (Whatman preswollen anion exchanger)-equilibrate in buffer A.
2. Elution buffer-0.15 *M* NaCl in buffer A.

## 2.3. PKC Assay

### 2.3.1. Reagents and Solutions

1. Lipid-Take 20 µL of 10 mg/mL phosphatidylserine (PS) in chloroform and 2.0 µL of 10 mg/mL diacylglycerol (DAG) in chloroform in a glass tube. Evaporate under nitrogen. Add 0.5 mL H$_2$O and vortex. Prepare fresh. Once the vial of PS and DAG are opened, they

should be stored in aliquots in glass vials under nitrogen at –20°C. Lipids should be reconstituted with the same volume of chloroform prior to use.

## 2.4. Western Blot Analysis

1. 4X sodium dodecyl sulfate (SDS) Sample buffer: 0.5 $M$ Tris-HCl, pH 6.8, 40% glycerol, 8% SDS, 0.05% bromophenol blue. Add 40 μL β-mercaptoethanol per 960 μL 4X sample buffer prior to use.
2. 4X Tris-HCl/SDS, pH 8.8 (1.5 $M$ Tris-HCl containing 0.4% SDS).
3. 4X Tris-HCl/SDS, pH 6.8 (0.5 $M$ Tris-HCl containing 0.4% SDS).
4. 30% acrylamide/0.8% *bis*-acrylamide, TEMED, 10% ammonium persulfate.
5. SDS electrophoresis buffer: 25 m$M$ Tris base, 192 m$M$ glycine, 0.1% SDS (15.1 g Tris base, 72.0 g glycine, 5.0 g SDS. Add $H_2O$ to 5000 mL).
6. Transfer buffer: 25 m$M$ Tris base, 192 m$M$ glycine, 15% methanol (15.1 g Tris base, 72 g glycine, 750 mL methanol. Water to 5000 mL).
7. TTBS: 20 m$M$ Tris-HCl, pH 7.5, 0.15 M NaCl, 0.05% Tween-20 (20 mL 1.0 $M$ Tris-HCl, pH 7.5, 8.7 g NaCl, 0.5 mL Tween-20. $H_2O$ to 1000 mL).
8. Blocking buffer and primary antibody dilution buffer (1% BSA, 0.02% azide): 1 g BSA and 0.02 g sodium azide per 100 mL TTBS.
9. Secondary antibody dilution buffer (5% nonfat dry milk in TTBS).
10. Stripping buffer: 100 mM β-mercaptoethanol, 2% SDS, 62.5 m$M$ Tris-HCl, pH 6.7.

## 3. Methods
### 3.1. Subcellular Distribution
#### 3.1.1. Separation of Cytosolic and Membrane Compartments

1. Ovarian cancer 2008 cells are maintained in complete medium and kept in a humidified incubator at 37°C with 95% air and 5% $CO_2$.
2. Cells are plated in T-75 flasks or 10-cm$^2$ tissue-culture dishes and incubated for at least 24 h. Cells in the logarithmic phase of the cell cycle are used in all experiments.
3. Cells are treated with vehicle or PKC activator. Usually, a 1000-fold stock solution is used (*see* **Note 1** and **Fig. 4**).
4. At the end of the incubation, aspirate off media, wash cells with PBS (*see* **Note 2**), and either harvest cells by trypsinization (tissue-culture flasks) or wash with cold PBS and collect cells by scraping (tissue culture dish) (*see* **Note 3**).
5. Count an aliquot of cells by hemocytometer or Coulter Counter.
6. Unless otherwise mentioned, all subsequent procedures described in **Subheading 3.1.1.** should be performed on ice or at 4°C.
7. Collect cells by centrifugation at 500$g$ for 3 min. Discard supernatant.
8. Wash cell pellet with PBS twice (500$g$, 3 min). Discard supernatant.
9. Add 1.0 mL lysis buffer per $10^7$ cells (*see* **Note 2**). Homogenize cells with Tissue-Tearor (setting 4, 30 s) (*see* **Note 4**).
10. Save an aliquot for protein determination and centrifuge 1.0 mL of the cell lysate at 100,000$g$ for 1 h. Keep track of the volume of the cell lysate.
11. Transfer the supernatant to an Eppendorf tube and measure the volume of the supernatant. This represents the cytosolic fraction.
12. Resuspend the pellet in 1 mL of lysis buffer by sonication or homogenization for 30 s. This can be used as particulate fraction for Western blot analysis.
13. Determine protein concentration in each fraction.

Fig. 4 Western blot analysis of PKC isozymes to monitor the effect of TPA on PKC compartmentalization. Ovarian carcinoma 2008 cells were treated with the DMSO or 100 n*M* TPA for 15 min or 30 min. Cells were fractionated to cytosolic and membrane compartments as described in **Subheading 3**. 25 µg of cytosolic fraction and an equivalent volume of membrane fractions were loaded onto an 8% SDS-PAGE. Proteins were transferred to PVDF membrane and incubated with antibodies to PKCα, -δ, -ε, or -ζ. The same blot was probed with different antibodies. This figure shows that the intracellular localization of PKC isozymes is distinct in 2008 cells. PKCα was present both in the cytosolic and membrane compartments. A 15 min exposure to TPA caused a significant translocation of cytosolic PKCα to the membrane compartment. nPKCδ and -ε were primarily membrane-bound. The abundance of PKCδ was much less compared to other PKC isozymes and could be detected only after prolonged exposure of the film to the immunoblot. aPKCζ was present both in the cytosolic and particulate fractions, but TPA had no effect on the translocation of aPKCζ.

### 3.1.2. Isolation of Nuclei

1. Treat cells with or without PKC activator (*see* **Notes 1** and **4**).
2. Wash cells with PBS and trypsinize or scrape and count.
3. Wash cell pellet with cold PBS and add 0.4 mL buffer B per $10^7$ cells.
4. Keep on ice for 15 min.
5. Add 10 µL of 25% NP-40 for 2 min.
6. Pellet nuclei by spinning for 1 min at 10,000*g* in a microcentrifuge.
7. Discard the postnuclear supernatant. Resuspend the pellet containing nuclei in 50 µL buffer C.
8. Vigorously rock for 15 min at 4°C.
9. Centrifuge at 16,000*g* for 20 min in a microcentrifuge.
10. Transfer the supernatant containing nuclei to a 0.5-mL microfuge tube.

### 3.2. PKC Isolation

1. Add 1% NP-40 (final concentration) to the particulate fractions obtained at **step 12** (**Subheading 3.1.1.**) and shake gently at 4°C for 30 min to release membrane-bound PKC (*see* **Note 5**).

2. Centrifuge the membrane lysate for 1 h at 100,000$g$. The supernatant represents membrane PKC.
3. Suspend 1.0 g DE-52 resin in 10 vol of 0.1 $M$ Tris-HCl, pH 7.5 containing 0.02% sodium azide in a beaker. Allow the resin to settle and decant the supernatant. Repeat this process five times. DE-52 can be stored at this stage at 4°C for at least 1 wk. Prior to use, replace 0.1 $M$ Tris-HCl with buffer A and repeat DE-52 wash until the supernatant has exactly the same pH and conductivity as buffer A.
4. Take approximately 500 µL of DE-52 slurry in 1.5-mL Eppendorf tubes and allow the resin to settle (*see* **Note 6**). Discard the supernatant.
5. Add high-speed supernatant from **step 12** (**Subheading 3.1.1.**) and **step 2** (**Subheading 3.2.**) that represent cytosolic and membrane fractions to DE-52 resin and shake at 4°C for 15 min.
6. Allow the resin to settle and discard the supernatant (*see* **Note 7**).
7. Wash DE-52 resin with 1.0 mL buffer A by repeating **step 6** four times.
8. Add 0.5 mL elution buffer (0.15 $M$ NaCl in buffer A) to DE-52 resin, shake for 10 min and allow the resin to settle (*see* **Note 8**). Save the supernatant, which represents partially purified PKC. Care should be taken so that the supernatant does not contain any cellulose particles.

## 3.3. PKC Assay

### 3.3.1. Assay Setup

1. Label Eppendorf tubes (duplicate or triplicate each condition) and keep them on ice. Mark Whatman P-81 phosphocellulose papers in the same manner with No. 2 pencil. Place them on a tray covered with aluminum foil.
2. Prepare master mix:

| Final concentration | Stock solution | µL/assay |
|---|---|---|
| 20 m$M$ Tris-HCl, pH 7.5 | 1.0 $M$ | 2.0 |
| 10 m$M$ MgCl$_2$ | 1.0 $M$ | 1.0 |
| Histone III-S | 5.0 mg/mL | 4.0 |
| 50 µ$M$ cold ATP | 20 m$M$ | 0.25 |
| [$\gamma$-$^{32}$P] ATP | 10 mCi/mL | 0.1 |
| H$_2$O to 60 µL | | |

If there are "$n$" number of tubes, then prepare master mix for "$n+1$" tubes to ensure that there is no pipeting problem while adding master mix to the last tube.
3. Take 5 to 20 µL of the cytosolic or particulate fraction in each tube (*see* **Note 9**) and adjust the volume to 20 µL with elution buffer. The volume will depend on the protein concentration. In a preliminary experiment, the linearity of the assay with time and protein has to be determined for each cell type.
4. Add 10 µL of 5 m$M$ CaCl$_2$ to each tube.
5. To one set add 10 µL H$_2$O and to the other set add 10 µL PS/DAG.
6. Add 60 µL master mix and vortex.
7. Incubate the reaction mixture at 30°C for 7 min. In our experience, the assay is linear for at least 10 min at 30°C.
8. At the end of the incubation, place the tubes on ice to stop the reaction. Add 30 µL of 325 m$M$ phosphoric acid and vortex.
9. Spot 25 µL of the reaction mixture onto a phosphocellulose paper. If the counts are low, 50 µL of the reaction mixture can be spotted.
10. Transfer the phosphocellulose papers to a beaker containing 0.5% phosphoric acid (10 mL/phosphocellulose paper) and shake gently for 10 min in a platform shaker. Discard the aluminum foil in the radioactive waste. Care must be taken to make sure that the

phosphocellulose papers are not stuck together during washing. Also, include one unspotted phosphocellulose paper to check for background counts.

11. Repeat wash three times (10 min each).
12. Air-dry the phosphocellulose filters on a tray. To expedite the drying process, the filter papers can be rinsed with a small volume of acetone or ethyl alcohol.
13. Label scintillation vials. Transfer phosphocellulose papers with forceps to scintillation vials. Add scintillation fluid to the vials and count $^{32}$P in a scintillation counter. Also, count 10 μL of the master mix to adjust for radioactive decay.

### 3.3.2. Calculations

$$\text{Specific Activity} = \text{pmol/min/mg}$$

If 50 μ*M* ATP is used per 0.1-mL assay, then each tube contains 5000 p*M* ATP.

$$\text{cpm/pmol phosphate} = \frac{\text{cpm per assay}}{5000 \text{ p}M}$$

$$\text{Specific Activity} = \frac{\text{cpm/pmol} \times (\text{dilution factor})}{\text{Vol (mL)} \times \text{Time of incubation (min)} \times (\text{protein in mg/mL})}$$

If 10 μL of 0.5 mg/mL PKC fraction is used, the reaction mixture is incubated for 7 min, and 50 μL of reaction mixture out of 130 μL (100 μL assay mixture+30 μL phosphoric acid) is spotted on phosphocellulose papers, then the specific activity is:

$$\text{Specific Activity} = \frac{\text{cpm (pmol)} \times 2.6 \text{ (dilution factor)}}{0.01 \text{ (mL)} \times 7 \text{ (min)} \times 0.5 \text{ (mg/mL)}}$$

Total PKC activity can be normalized to cell number or total protein used for the subcellular distribution study.

## 3.4. Western Blot Analysis

### 3.4.1. Electrophoresis and Transfer

1. For Western blot analysis, transfer an aliquot of cytosolic (**Subheading 3.1.1., step 11**) or particulate fractions (**Subheading 3.1.1., step 12**) or nuclear fractions (**Subheading 3.1.2., step 10**) to Eppendorf tubes. Add 1 vol 4X SDS sample buffer to three volume fractions, vortex, keep in the boiling water bath for 5 min and freeze samples at –20°C or –70°C. The samples can be stored at this stage for several months.
2. Pour an 8% SDS polyacrylamide separating gel (*see* **Note 11**). Cover the gel with a layer of isobutanol. Once the gel has polymerized (approximately 1 h), remove isobutanol and wash with dH$_2$O. Insert a comb, pour a 4% stacking gel and allow to polymerize.
3. Load approximately 25 μg of cytosolic fraction or equal volume of corresponding membrane fraction in each lane. In one lane, load 10 μL of prestained standard (*see* **Note 12**).
4. Run the gel at 20 mA per 0.75-mm thick gel (constant current) until the dye front is approximately 2 cm from the bottom.
5. Disassemble the gel and discard the stacking gel. Transfer the separating gel to a container containing 1X transfer buffer. Equilibrate the gel for 10 to 15 min in transfer buffer to remove any traces of SDS.
6. Cut out a piece of Immobilon-P (polyvinylidene difluoride) membrane to the size of the gel and wet in 100% methanol for 5 s. Place the membrane in water for 5 min to remove methanol and then equilibrate in transfer buffer for 15 min.

7. Presoak two pieces of Whatman filter paper and two fiber pads in transfer buffer. The transfer sandwich is assembled as follows: Open the gel holder and place one side on a flat, shallow tray containing transfer buffer. Place presoaked sponge, a piece of Whatman filter paper, gel, membrane, Whatman filter paper, and fiber pad (*see* **Note 10**). As each layer is added, remove air bubbles using a glass pipet. Close the gel holder firmly and insert into the transblot apparatus containing transfer buffer (half-filled). Make sure that the membrane side faces the anode so that negatively charged proteins are transferred from the gel to the membrane.
8. Fill the transblot apparatus with transfer buffer and transfer for 3 h at 60 V (constant voltage) (*see* **Note 11**).

### 3.4.2. Immunoblotting

1. After transfer, remove the membrane, rinse briefly with TTBS (*see* **Note 12**) and block nonspecific protein binding with 1% BSA in TTBS for 1 h.
2. Incubate the membrane with the primary antibody (anti-PKC) either overnight at 4°C or for 2 h at room temperature in a shaker. The antibody dilution will depend on the source of the antibody and should be determined in a preliminary experiment. The manufacturer's suggestion can be used as a guide (*see* **Note 13**).
3. Rinse the membrane with TTBS at least three times (10 min each).
4. Incubate the membrane in horseradish peroxidase-conjugated secondary antibody diluted in 5% nonfat dry milk in TTBS for 1.0 h.
5. Rinse the membrane with TTBS at least three times (10 min each). Thorough washing of the membrane is necessary because incomplete removal of unbound secondary antibody may give rise to higher background.
6. The proteins are visualized by incubation with ECL detection kit. Mix equal volumes of detection reagents 1 and 2, pour on the membrane (protein side up) and incubate for 1 min. The final volume of the detection reagent is approximately $0.125$ mL/cm$^2$ membrane. Drain off excess ECL reagent and wrap the membrane with plastic film. Place the membrane (protein-side up) in a film cassette and expose to autoradiography film in a dark room. The exposure time will vary depending on the intensity of the signal. Expose the first film for 1 min and then adjust the exposure time based on the signal.
7. The same blot can be stripped and reprobed with different antibodies. To strip the membrane, submerge the membrane in stripping buffer and incubate at 50°C for 30 min with shaking. Wash the membrane with large volume of TTBS ($3 \times 15$ min) and process for immunoblotting (*see* **Note 14**).

## 4. Notes

1. The translocation of PKC will depend on the agonists, cell type, and particular PKC isozyme. TPA is extremely hydrophobic and reasonably stable inside cells and it is easier to monitor translocation following treatment with TPA. Prolonged membrane association, however, may lead to downregulation of PKC. Some PKC agonists may induce transient or reversible translocation. Therefore, it is important to vary time and concentration for each agonist and with individual cell type to monitor translocation.
2. The composition of PKC isolation buffers and cellular fractionation procedures may affect subcellular distribution of PKC isozymes to some extent. For example, $Ca^{2+}$ will facilitate membrane association of PKC and EGTA will facilitate release of PKC. After treatment of cells with PKC activator, we wash cells with PBS containing no divalent cations and the lysis buffer contains 5 m*M* EGTA.
3. If cells are trypsinized for too long, cytosolic enzyme may be released. For the same reason, scraping should also be performed gently.

4. Dounce homogenization is the most commonly used method for homogenization. Cells can be homogenized with 50 strokes using a dounce homogenizer and centrifuged at 500*g* for 5 min to remove nuclei and cell debris. The postnuclear supernatant can be used to separate cytosol and nonnuclear membrane fractions and the nuclear fraction can be purified by sucrose gradient centrifugation. A large number of cells was required for efficient homogenization. In our experience, a large number of unbroken cells were sedimented when dounce homogenization was applied to ovarian carcinoma 2008 cells. It is also difficult to homogenize a large number of samples with 50 strokes using this method. Homogenization with a hand-held tissue homogenizer was most convenient and did not require processing of a large number of cells. To isolate nuclei, we run a parallel experiment and process cells from a different tissue culture flask or dish.

5. The extraction of particulate PKC may also be achieved with 0.3% to 0.5% Triton X-100. It is important to remember that high concentration of Triton X-100 may inhibit PKC activity.

6. We have performed anion exchange chromatography in a microfuge tube rather than using a column. This method is especially helpful when the amount of protein is low because elution of PKC from a column requires more elution buffer and PKC may be diluted.

7. It is important to make sure that PKC was bound to DE-52 cellulose. In an initial experiment, the eluate should be saved for PKC assay to check whether PKC remained bound to DE-52 resin or not.

8. The elution of PKC should be optimized for each cell type. Using a 0 to 0.4 $M$ NaCl gradient, we found that 0.15 $M$ NaCl contained most of the $Ca^{2+}$-, phospholipid-dependent PKC from 2008 cells. Therefore, we routinely use one-step bulk elution with 0.15 $M$ NaCl. Some novel PKCs may elute at higher salt concentration, but because they are $Ca^{2+}$-independent, it is difficult to monitor their activities.

9. DE-52 purified PKC should be used immediately for assay. It can be stored at 4°C for 2–3 d. Alternatively, it can also be stored in 50% glycerol at –70°C for several months.

10. It is important to have good contact between the gel and the membrane otherwise proteins may diffuse out. If necessary, use an extra blotting paper or fiber pad to make the gel sandwich.

11. The transfer time varies with the voltage, size of the protein, percentage of the gel, and type of the membrane. For PKC isozymes in the range of 70–90-kDa molecular mass, an 8% gel is recommended. Prolonged transfer time may result in leakage of protein out of the membrane, especially if pore size is big. This can be checked by adding an extra membrane.

12. During electrophoresis and transfer, prestained standards are useful to monitor the separation of proteins and efficiency of transfer. Sometimes lack of signal in the Western blot may be caused by inefficient transfer. The membrane can also be stained briefly with the dye Ponceau S (0.5% in acetic acid) after transfer. The dye is water soluble and can be removed by washing with water. This staining does not interfere with antibody binding.

13. If possible, it is better to check specificity of the PKC isozyme-specific antibodies using antibodies from different sources and/or that are raised against different epitopes. Often, blocking of signal by reincubation of primary antibody with the peptide that was used to generate the antibody is used to demonstrate specificity. In our experience, the peptide antigen often blocks most of the bands that are detected with the antibody. It, however, does not provide any information as to how specific the antibody is to a particular isozyme. We have recently found that monoclonal antibody to PKCγ often crossreacts strongly with PKCα. Antibody specificity can be determined with purified recombinant PKC isozymes that are commercially available from different sources.

13. Although we generally use PVDF membrane, nitrocellulose membrane can also be used. The stripping conditions may differ with different types of membrane. It is helpful to check manufacturer's recommendation.

## References

1. Nishizuka, Y. (1986) Studies and perspectives of protein kinase C. *Science* **233**, 305–312.
2. Blumberg, P. M. (1988) Protein kinase C as the receptor for the phorbol ester tumor promoters: Sixth Rhoads Memorial Award Lecture. *Cancer Res.* **48**, 1–8.
3. Basu, A. (1993) The potential of protein kinase C as a target for anticancer treatment. *Pharmacol. Ther.* **59**, 257–280.
4. Stabel, S. and Parker, P. J. (1991) Protein kinase C. *Pharmacol. Ther.* **51**, 71–95.
5. Goodnight, J., Mischak, H., and Mushinski, F. (1994) Selective involvement of protein kinase C isozymes in differentiation and neoplastic transformation. *Adv. Cancer Res.* **64**, 160–209.
6. Kraft, A. S. and Anderson, W. B. (1983) Phorbol esters increase the amount of Ca+2, phospholipid-dependent protein kinase associated with the plasma membrane. *Nature* **301**, 621–623.
7. Orr, J. W., Keranen, L. M., and Newton, A. C. (1992) Reversible exposure of the pseudo-substrate domain of protein kinase C by phosphatidylserine and diacylglycerol. *J. Biol. Chem.* **267**, 15,263–15,266.
8. Rodriguez-Pena, A. and Rozengurt, E. (1984) Disappearance of Ca+2-sensitive, phospholipid-dependent protein kinase activity in phorbol ester-treated 3T3 cells. *Biochem. Biophys. Res. Comm.* **120**, 1053–1059.
9. Kiley, S. C., Jaken, S., Whelan, R., and Parker, P. J. (1995) Intracellular targeting of protein kinase C isoenzymes: functional implications. *Biochem. Soc. Transac.* **23**, 601–605.
10. Basu, A. and Weixel, K. M. (1995) Comparison of protein kinase C activity and isoform expression in cisplatin-sensitive and -resistant ovarian carcinoma cells. *Int. J. Cancer* **62**, 457–460.

# 71

## A Novel and Simple Method to Assay the Activity of Individual Protein Kinases in a Crude Tissue Extract

**Basem S. Goueli, Kevin Hsiao, and Said A. Goueli**

## 1. Introduction

Protein kinases and phosphatases play an important role in a variety of cellular functions such as cell growth, development, and gene expression (1). It is estimated that one-third of the proteins in a typical mammalian cell are phosphorylated and about 200 protein kinases and 100 protein phosphatases have been identified. In addition, perhaps 2–3% of the genes in the entire genome of an eukaryotic cell may code for protein kinases and as many as 5% of the human genes may encode protein kinases and phosphatases (2). The fact that these protein kinases and phosphatases have multiple substrates in vivo may explain their diverse physiological functions (1–3). Thus, it is of considerable interest to develop an assay system that is specific for certain protein kinases and simple enough to be used by both the novice as well as the expert in the field.

The availability of peptides that serve as specific substrates for certain protein kinases made it possible to determine the activity of a specific protein kinase in a tissue or cellular extract with minimal interference from other enzymes (4). A widely used method to monitor the phosphopeptide product is the negatively charged phosphocellulose P-81 method, which requires the substrate to contain at least 2–3 basic amino acids because the binding is based on electrostatic interaction (5). The inclusion of basic amino acid residues, however, may alter the specificity of the substrate (6) and may give variable results depending on the sequence of the peptide, and in some instances, incomplete binding of phosphopeptides to the filters was observed (7). Because the binding of the phosphorylated proteins or peptides to the P-81 filter is electrostatic in nature, the washing protocol also may cause variability in the results and gentle washing is required to minimize the loss of the filter-bound peptide. In addition, any positively charged proteins (other than the phosphopeptide product) that are phosphorylated by protein kinase(s) including the autophosphorylated enzyme in the tissue extract will also bind to the P-81 filters. Thus, an assay method that can eliminate these pitfalls would offer important advantages over the existing methodologies. Here, we report on the development of an assay system that can be used to specifically determine the activity of an individual enzyme in crude tissue or cellular extract, circumvent the pitfalls associated with the phosphocellulose method, combine the

From: *Methods in Molecular Medicine, Vol. 39: Ovarian Cancer: Methods and Protocols*
Edited by: J. M. S. Bartlett © Humana Press, Inc., Totowa, NJ

attributes of simplicity and high sensitivity, and is amenable to both low and high through-put scales *(9,10)*.

## 1.1. Principle of the Assay System

The assay system is based on the high affinity and selective binding of biotin to streptavidin ($10^{-14}M$). Thus, when biotinylated derivative of a selective peptide substrate is phosphorylated by the cognate protein kinase, the phosphorylated/biotinylated product can be separated from both free adenosine triphosphate (ATP) and endogenously phosphorylated proteins that are nonbiotinylated using a streptavidin-linked matrix. The only phosphorylated product that binds to the matrix is the phosphoform of the biotinylated peptide. The excess free [γ-$^{32}$P] ATP can be readily removed by a simple washing procedure (i.e., 5–7 washes for 1–4 min each). The matrix bound phosphopeptide is dried and the $^{32}$P incorporated into the peptide substrate is quantified using a liquid scintillation counter *(9)*.

## 2. Materials
## 2.1. PKA Assays

1. Peptide Synthesis: The biotin-modified peptides were synthesized on a peptide synthesizer using established procedures of solid-phase peptide synthesis (Cambridge Res. Biochemicals, Wilmington, DE) and the C6-biotin moiety was added before cleavage of the peptide from the resin, and the peptide was purified by reverse-phase high-pressure liquid chromatography (HPLC). The identity and purity of the biotinylated peptides were confirmed by quantitative amino acid analysis, HPLC using two solvent systems and fast atom bombardment (FAB) mass spectrometry.

2. Peptide Substrates: Peptide substrates specific for various protein kinases were synthesized, i.e., cAMP-dependent protein kinase (PKA), $Ca^{2+}$ and phospholipid-dependent protein kinase (PKC), cyclin dependent (cdc2) protein kinase (cdc2), casein kinases (CK-1 and CK-2), DNA-dependent protein kinase (DNA-PK), and the tyrosine kinase of the epidermal growth factor receptor (EGFR). The amino acid sequence of each peptide is provided below under the description of the assay for the corresponding protein kinase.

3. Enzymes: The protein kinases PKA, PKC, cdc2, CK-1, CK-2, EGFR, and DNA-PK were obtained from Promega Corp., Madison, WI.

4. Extraction Buffer: 25 m*M* Tris-HCl, pH 7.4, 0.5 m*M* ethylenediaminetetraacetic acid (EDTA), 0.5 m*M* EGTA, 10 mM β-mercaptoethanol, 1 mg/mL leupeptin, 1 µg/mL aprotinin, and 0.5 m*M* phenylmethylsulfonylfluoride (PMSF). Store at 4°C or, for up to 6 mo, at –20°C. Just before use, add 0.5 mL of PMSF stock solution (100 m*M* PMSF in 100% ethanol) per 100 mL of extraction buffer.

5 Phosphate-buffered saline (PBS): 0.2 g/L KCl, 8.0 g/L NaCl, 0.2 g/L $KH_2PO_4$, and 1.15 g/L $Na_2HPO_4$.

6. PKA Assay Buffer (5X): 200 m*M* of Tris-HCl, pH 7.4, 100 m*M* $MgCl_2$, 0.5 mg/mL of bovine serum albumin (BSA).

7. Termination Buffer: 7.5 *M* guanidine hydrochloride in $H_2O$.

8. 2 *M* NaCl in 1% $H_3PO_4$: 116.9 g/L of NaCl, 11.8 mL/L of 85% $H_3PO_4$.

9. Other Reagents: The peptide inhibitor of PKA (PKI), the myristoylated peptide inhibitor of PKC, and streptavidin-linked membranes (SAM$^{2TM}$ Biotin Capture Membrane) (1.25 × 1.15 cm) were obtained from Promega Corp. All other reagents were of high research grade and obtained from Sigma Chemical Co. (St. Louis, MO).

## 2.2. Determination of PKC Enzymatic Activity

1. Extraction Buffer: PKA extraction buffer with 0.05% Triton® X-100.
2. Enzyme Dilution Buffer: 0.1 mg/mL BSA, 0.05% Triton® X-100.
3. PKC Coactivation 5X buffer, 1.25 m$M$ EGTA, 2 m$M$ CaCl$_2$, 0.5 mg/mL BSA.
4. Control Buffer 5X: 100 m$M$, Tris-HCl, pH 7.5, 50 m$M$ MgCl$_2$.
5. PKC Activation 5X buffer (*see* **Note 6** for preparation of this buffer): 1.6 mg/mL phosphatidylserine, 0.16 mg/mL diacylglycerol, 100 m$M$ Tris-HCl, pH 7.5, 50 m$M$ MgCl$_2$.

# 3. Methods

## 3.1. Determination of Protein Kinase Activity

The following are two fully detailed protocols used to assay the kinase activity of PKA and PKC to illustrate the utility and versatility of the assay system. Other enzymes can be assayed similarly using their selective biotinylated peptide substrates (*see* **Note 2**) and their optimal assay buffer and temperature conditions.

### 3.1.1. Preparation of Cellular or Tissue Extracts

1. Precool the appropriate homogenizer and extraction buffer to 0° to 4°C.
2. Tissue samples: Homogenize 1 g of tissue in 5 mL of cold extraction buffer with a cold homogenizer (e.g., a Polytron® homogenizer).
3. Cultured cells: Wash $5 \times 10^6$–$1 \times 10^7$ cells with PBS (5 mL per 100-mm dish) and remove the buffer completely. Suspend the cells in 0.5 mL of cold extraction buffer and homogenize using a cold homogenizer (e.g., a Dounce homogenizer).
4. Centrifuge the lysate for 5 min at 4°C at 14,000$g$ in a microcentrifuge and save the supernatant. Crude extracts should be assayed the same day they are prepared to retain maximal activity and obtain optimal results.

### 3.1.2. Determination of PKA Enzymatic Activity

1. Prepare the adenosine triphosphate (ATP) mix as follows:

| Component | Final per Reaction | 20 Reactions |
|---|---|---|
| 0.5 m$M$ ATP | 5.00 μL | 100 μL |
| [γ-$^{32}$P] ATP (3000 Ci/mmol) 10 μCi/μL | 0.05 μL | 1 μL |

2. Prepare the following reaction in 0.5–1.5 mL microcentrifuge tubes (a control reaction without substrate should also be performed to determine background counts):

| Component | Final per Reaction | |
|---|---|---|
| Number of Reactions | 5 | 20 |
| PKA Assay Buffer 5X | 5 μL | 100 μL |
| cAMP, 0.025 m$M$ (*see* **Note 1**) | 5 μL | 100 μL |
| PKA Biotinylated Peptide Substrate, 0.5 m$M$ (*see* **Note 2** and **3**) | 5 μL | 100 μL |
| [γ-$^{32}$P]ATP mix | 5 μL | 100 μL |

3. Prepare appropriate dilutions of the enzyme samples in 0.1 mg/mL BSA in H$_2$O. Place at 0°C. We recommend preparing and testing crude lysate samples undiluted and serially diluted 2- to 16-fold (a 1000-fold dilution is recommended for purified enzyme).
4. Mix gently and preincubate the reaction mix (**Subheading 3.1.2., step 2**) at 30°C for 1-5 minutes.

5. Initiate the reaction by adding 5 μL of the enzyme sample to the reactants. Total reaction volume will be 25 μL. Incubate the reaction at 30°C for 5 min. (Other time-points and temperatures may be tested, if desired).

6. Terminate the reaction by adding 12.5 μL of termination buffer to each reaction; mix well. This solution is stable at 4°C for at least 24 h, but can be kept at room temperature during processing.

7. Spot 10 μL from each terminated reaction onto a prenumbered SAM$^{2®}$ Membrane square. After all samples have been spotted follow the wash and rinse steps as described below. Save the reaction tubes to be used for standards as shown below (**Subheading 3.1.2., step 11**). For larger volumes, *see* **Note 4**.

8. Place the SAM$^{2®}$ Membrane squares (1.25 cm × 1.15 cm) containing samples from **Subheading 3.1.2., step 7** into a washing container. Wash using an orbital platform shaker set on low or by occasional manual shaking as follows:

   Wash 1 time for 30 s with 200 mL of 2 *M* NaCl
   ↓

   Wash 3 times for 2 min each with 200 mL of 2 *M* NaCl
   ↓

   Wash 4 times for 2 min each with 200 mL of 2 *M* NaCl in 1% $H_3PO_4$
   ↓

   Wash 2 times for 30 s each with 100 mL of deionized water
   *Total wash time <20 min.*

9. Dry the SAM$^{2®}$ Membrane squares on a piece of aluminum foil under a heat lamp for 5–10 min or air-dry at room temperature for 30–60 min. (If the SAM$^{2®}$ Membrane has been washed with ethanol, shorten the drying time to 2–5 min under a heat lamp or 10–15 min at room temperature).

10. Determine total counts for calculation of the specific activity of [γ-$^{32}$P] ATP as follows: Remove 5 μL aliquots from any 2 reaction tubes from **Subheading 3.1.2, step 7** and spot onto individual SAM$^{2®}$ Membrane squares or Whatman$^®$ 3mm filter disks. For this step, dry **without** washing. After analysis, use these results to calculate the specific activity of [γ-$^{32}$P] ATP as shown below. If 5 μL is not available from a single tube you may combine the contents of several tubes for this step.

11. Analysis by scintillation counting: If still connected, separate the SAM$^{2®}$ Membrane squares with samples (from **Subheading 3.1.2., steps 9** and **10**) using forceps, scissors, or a razor blade, and place the squares or 3 mm filter disks into individual scintillation vials. Add scintillation fluid to the vials and count.

12. PhosphorImager™ analysis: Alternatively, the SAM$^{2®}$ Membrane may remain intact and the intact SAM$^{2®}$ Membrane or 3 mm filter disks may be analyzed using a PhosphorImager.

### 3.1.3. Calculation of the Specific Activity of [γ-$^{32}$P] ATP

The specific activity of [γ-$^{32}$P]ATP in cpm/pmol of ATP $= \dfrac{(^{37.5}/_5)\,(X)}{2500}$

where 37.5 is the sum of the reaction volume (25 μL) + the termination buffer volume (12.5 μL), 5 is the volume in μL of the samples from **Subheading 3.1.2., step 10**, $X$ is the average cpm of the 5-μL samples from **Subheading 3.1.2., step 11**, and 2500 is the number of pmol of ATP in the reaction.

### 3.1.4. Calculation of Protein Kinase A Enzyme Activity

Enzyme specific activity in pmol ATP/min/μg of protein =

$$\frac{(cpm_{\text{reaction with substrate}} - cpm_{\text{reaction without substrate}}) \times (37.5)}{(10) \times (time_{\text{min}}) \times (\text{amount of protein in reaction}_{\mu g}) \times (\text{specific activity of } [\gamma\text{-}^{32}\text{P}]ATP)}$$

where 37.5 is the sum of the reaction volume (25 μL) + the termination buffer volume (12.5 μL) and10 is the volume in μL of the sample from **Subheading 3.1.2., step 7**.

### 3.1.5. Preparation of Tissue or Cell Samples for PKC Assay

Crude extracts should be assayed the same day they are prepared to retain maximal activity and obtain optimal results.

1. Precool the appropriate homogenizer and extraction buffer to 0° to 4°C.
2. *For tissue:* Homogenize 1 g of tissue in 5 mL of cold extraction buffer using a cold homogenizer (e.g., a Polytron® homogenizer). *For cultured cells:* Wash $5 \times 10^6$-$1 \times 10^7$ cells with PBS (5 mL per 100-mm dish) and remove the buffer completely. Suspend the cells in 0.5 mL of cold extraction buffer and homogenize using a cold homogenizer (e.g., a Dounce homogenizer).
3. Centrifuge the lysate for 5 min at 4°C, 14,000g in a microcentrifuge and save the supernatant.
4. Pass the supernatant over a 1-mL column of DEAE cellulose that has been preequilibrated in extraction buffer. Wash the column with 5 mL of extraction buffer, and then elute the PKC-containing fraction using 5 mL of extraction buffer containing 200 m*M* NaCl. Proceed to **Subheading 3.2.2.**

### 3.2.2. PKC Assay Protocol

1. Prepare the ATP mix as follows:

| Component | Final per Reaction | 20 Reactions |
|---|---|---|
| 0.5 m*M* ATP | 5.00 μL | 100 μL |
| [γ-$^{32}$P]ATP (3000 Ci/mmol) 10 μCi/μL | 0.05 μL | 1 μL |

2. Prepare the following reaction in 0.5–1.5 mL microcentrifuge tubes:
   a. Reactions in the presence of Phospholipids (Activated Reaction):

| Component | Final per Reaction | Final per 20 Reactions |
|---|---|---|
| PKC Coactivation 5X buffer | 5 μL | 100 μL |
| PKC Activation 5X buffer | 5 μL | 100 μL |
| PKC Biotinylated Peptide Substrate, 0.5 m*M* (*see* **Note 3**) | 5 μL | 100 μL |
| [γ-$^{32}$P]ATP mix | 5 μL | 100 μL |

   b. Reaction in the absence of phospholipids (control reaction):

| Component | Final per Reaction | Final per 20 Reactions |
|---|---|---|
| PKC Coactivation 5X buffer | 5 μL | 100 μL |
| PKC Control 5X buffer | 5 μL | 100 μL |
| PKC Biotinylated Peptide Substrate, 0.5 m*M* (*see* **Note 3**) | 5 μL | 100 μL |
| [γ-$^{32}$P]ATP mix | 5 μL | μL |

3. Prepare appropriate dilutions of the enzyme samples to be tested using enzyme dilution buffer. We recommend preparing and testing crude lysate samples undiluted and serially diluted 2- to 16- fold. Purified enzyme preparations may require greater dilution.
4. Mix gently and preincubate the reaction mix at 30°C for 1–5 min.

5. Initiate the reaction by adding 5 μL of the enzyme sample to the reactants. Total reaction volume will be 25 μL.

6. Incubate the reaction at 30°C for 5 min. (Other time-points and temperatures may be tested if desired.)

7. Terminate the reaction by adding 12.5 μL of termination buffer to each reaction; mix well. This solution is stable at 4°C for at least 24 h, but can be kept at room temperature during processing.

8. Repeat **Subheading 3.1.2., steps 7–12.**

### 3.2.3. Calculation of the Specific Activity of [γ-$^{32}$P] ATP:

The specific activity of [γ-$^{32}$P]ATP in cpm/pmol of ATP $= \dfrac{(^{37.5}/_5)\,(X)}{2500}$

where 37.5 is the sum of the reaction volume (25 μL) + the termination buffer volume (12.5 μL), 5 is the volume in microliters of the samples from **Subheading 3.2.2., step 10**. $X$ is the average counts/min of the 5 μL samples from **Subheading 3.2.2., step 11**, and 2500 is the number of pmol of ATP in the reaction.

### 3.2.4. Calculation of Protein Kinase C Enzyme Activity

The enzymatic activity of PKC can be determined by subtracting the activity of the enzyme in the absence of phospholipids (Control Buffer) from that of the enzyme in the presence of phospholipids (Activation Buffer).

Enzyme activity in pmol ATP/min/μg of protein =

$$\frac{(\text{cpm}_{\text{reaction with phospholipids}} - \text{cpm}_{\text{reaction without phospholipids}}) \times (37.5)}{(10) \times (\text{time}_{\text{min}}) \times (\text{amount of protein in reaction}_{\mu g}) \times (\text{specific activity of } [\gamma\text{-}^{32}\text{P}]\text{ATP})}$$

where 37.5 is the sum of the reaction volume (25 μL) + the termination buffer volume (12.5 μL) and 10 is the volume in μL of the sample.

### 3.3. Results and Discussions

As alluded to earlier, the basic principle of our assay system is to conjugate the selective peptide substrate of any protein kinase with biotin so that the biotinylated peptide can be used as a substrate to specifically assay for the activity of the enzyme of interest under its optimal condition using [γ-$^{32}$P] ATP. After completion of the reaction, the phosphorylated and unphosphorylated peptides are bound to streptavidin-linked matrix, and the free [γ-$^{32}$P] ATP can be removed by a simple washing procedure. The matrix can be membranes, streptavidin-linked magnetic particles, or membranes assembled into a 96-well plate format. The $^{32}$P incorporation into the filters, particles, or plates then can be counted in a liquid-scintillation spectrometer and used to calculate the activity of the enzyme under study. We have used this novel approach to characterize the enzymatic activity of several frequently used protein kinases including PKA, PKC, cdc2, DNA-PK, CK-1, CK-2, and the tyrosine kinase of EGFR, IR, pp60[src], and so on. In the current study, the results obtained with PKA and PKC using streptavidin-linked disks are presented to illustrate the utility of this method.

To begin to characterize the enzymatic activity of PKA and PKC using the streptavidin-linked disks, the effect of substrate concentration on the kinase activity was investigated. The results of **Fig. 1A** show an increase in the activity of PKA with increasing the concentration of the peptide substrate displaying a hyperbolic response curve that is typical of Michaelis-Menten saturation behavior. The substrate concentra-

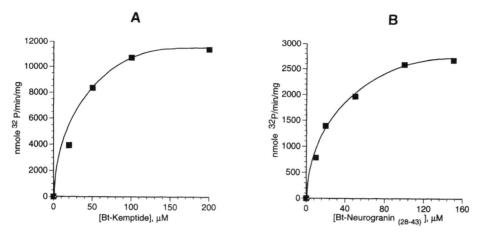

Fig. 1. Effect of peptide concentration on the protein kinase activity of PKA (**A**) and PKC (**B**). The protein kinase activity was determined as described in the methods section.

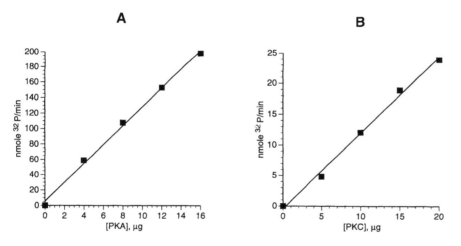

Fig. 2. Effect of enzyme concentration on the protein kinase activity of PKA (**A**) and PKC (**B**). The protein kinase activity was determined in the presence of 200 $\mu M$ of the corresponding biotinylated peptide substrates as described in the methods section.

tion required to achieve maximal activity was 150–200 $\mu M$. The transformation of the same data resulted in a Km Value for the substrate of 12 $\mu M$, and a $V_{max}$ value of 15 $\mu mol/min/mg$ of enzyme. Similar values have been reported for this enzyme using Kemptide as substrate (Km of 10 $\mu M$ and $V_{max}$ of 16 $\mu mol/min/mg$ of enzyme) (*5*). Similar enzyme substrate response curve was obtained with PKC using the peptide substrate neurogranin$_{(28-43)}$ (**Fig. 1B**). A maximum of PKC activity was reached at 100–150 $\mu M$ of peptide substrate. We have also observed that the basal activity of PKC (no phospholipids) was as low as the background (no enzyme added). This was an indication that all of the activity of PKC was absolutely dependent on the presence of activators.

Using saturating concentration of biotinylated peptide substrates for PKA and PKC (200 $\mu M$), we were able to demonstrate a linear response in the activity of PKA and PKC with increasing the amount of each enzyme in their corresponding reactions (**Fig. 2A,B**). We obtained a linear response in the activity of PKA up to about 16 ng of

Fig. 3. Effect of the specific peptide inhibitors of PKA and PKC on the kinase activity of the corresponding protein kinases. (**A**) shows the effect of PKA inhibitor on its kinase activity and (**B**) shows the effect of the myristoylated PKC inhibitor on its kinase activity. Both enzymes were tested using the corresponding peptide substrate at 200 $\mu M$ and under optimal enzyme conditions as described in the methods section.

pure PKA (**Fig. 2A**) and up to 20 ng of PKC (**Fig. 2B**). To confirm that the kinase activity of PKA we obtained is specifically catalyzed by the enzyme; we examined the effect of the specific inhibitor of PKA on the kinase activity. The results in **Fig. 3A** show that the addition of 10 $\mu M$ of the PKA inhibitor (PKI) drastically reduced the amount of $^{32}P$ incorporated into the peptide. Similarly, the addition of 100 M of the myristoylated peptide inhibitor of PKC resulted in complete inhibition of the $^{32}P$ incorporated into the peptide substrate (**Fig. 3B**).

To demonstrate the utility of this assay in determining the kinase activity of enzymes in tissue extract, the kinase activity of PKA and PKC was assayed in extracts of various rat tissues under optimal conditions for both enzymes. The basal activity of PKA (in the absence of cAMP) was significantly low in all tissues examined (**Fig. 4**, panel A). The addition of cAMP (5 M) increased the activity of the enzyme by 6-9 folds (Fig 4A, panel B). The addition of the PKI resulted in a remarkable inhibition of the basal, as well as the activatable kinase activity (more than 90%), thus confirming that the phosphate incorporation was catalyzed by PKA (**Fig. 4**, panels C and D). It is apparent that the remarkable low background observed in our assay attests to the fact that only the biotinylated phosphopeptide binds to the membranes. Thus the results obtained represent the true value for the $^{32}P$ that is incorporated into the peptide substrate and not in any additional proteins present in the extract. Similarly, PKC activity in extracts of various rat tissues was determined. The activity of the enzyme was stimulated by phospholipids (**Fig. 5**, panel A vs B) and inhibited by the addition of 100 $\mu M$ of the myristoylated PKC inhibitor (**Fig. 5**, panels C and D). It is noteworthy that the basal activities of PKC in various tissue extracts determined by our method (in the absence of activators) was as low as the background level (no enzyme added) and thus significantly high-fold stimulation was achieved.

An important consideration regarding this assay is that it can be easily scaled up to a high-throughput format by using high capacity streptavidin-linked sheets that are fitted into 96-well plate format. (These plates are available from Promega Corp.) They offer

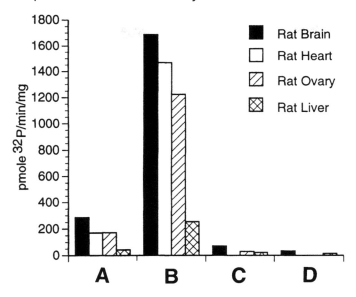

Fig. 4. The protein kinase activity of PKA in extracts of rat brain, heart, ovary, and liver as determined by the novel method as described in the methods section using 200 µM of the biotinylated peptide substrate under several conditions. Abbreviations: [a, none; b, plus 5 µM cAMP; c, plus 10 µM of PKA inhibitor; plus 5 µM cAMP, and 10 µM of PKA inhibitor].

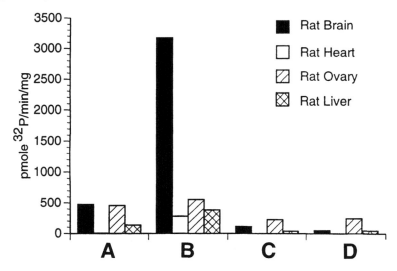

Fig. 5. The protein kinase activity of PKC in extracts of rat brain, heart, ovary, and liver as determined by the novel method as described in the methods section using 200 µM of the biotinylated peptide substrate. Abbreviations: [a, none; b, plus phospholipids; c, plus 100 µM of the myristoylated PKC inhibitor; and d, plus phospholipids and inhibitor].

several advantages that make them useful in pharmaceutical research for high-throughput drug screening assays of inhibitors/activators of protein kinases. The availability of equipment that facilitated complete automation of this assay such as automatic plate handling using robotics, automatic washers, and fully automated liquid-scintillation counters, provided the opportunity for efficient high-throughput analysis. We have demonstrated the feasibility of this system in a high-throughput format by using commercially available automatic washers and liquid-scintillation counters (Wallac's MicroBeta Trilux and Packard's TopCount MicroPlate liquid-scintillation counter) *(10)*.

## 4. Conclusion

We have developed a novel protein kinase assay system that uses an innovative approach to accurately measure the kinase activity of various protein kinases and circumvents the pitfalls of existing methodologies. The assay offers the following advantages that make it unique and the method of choice for determining the kinase activity of various enzymes in tissue or cellular extracts.

1. Versatility and Ease of Use: The kinase activity of individual protein kinases can be quantitated even in the presence of a mixture of other protein kinases as is the case when working with tissue or cellular extracts, and the assay can be completed in 10–15 min after reaction completion.
2. Low Background and High Sensitivity: Because only the phosphorylated peptide (and not other phosphorylated proteins present in cellular or tissue extracts) binds to the matrix, the background obtained is significantly lower than that observed with other methods and the results generated represent true estimates of enzymatic activity in the extract. This will also allow the investigator to detect enzyme activity of as little as few femtomoles to picomoles of an enzyme per reaction.
3. Correct Consensus Peptide Sequence: There is no need to alter the optimal substrate recognition sequence in order to be used as substrate for the corresponding enzyme in this assay as is the case with other assay systems such as the P-81 method. The only requirement is the addition of a biotin moiety to the N-terminus amino group of the peptide, which does not affect its specificity for the enzyme.
4. Reliability and Quantification of Results: Because the binding of biotin to streptavidin is the strongest known noncovalent biological interaction (Ka=$10^{15}$ $M^{-1}$), the phosphorylated biotinylated peptide strongly binds to the streptavidin-linked disk and is not affected by a wide range of conditions. These include extremes of pH (2.0–10.0), temperature, organic solvents, ionic, and nonionic detergents (SDS, CHAPS, Triton X-100, Tween-20, or Tween-80), and other denaturing agents (5-$M$ guanidine HCl and 2 $M$ urea) *(11)*. Therefore, the peptide is not likely to be washed off during the washing procedure, as is the case when the peptide substrate is bound to filters via weak electrostatic binding (e.g., phosphocellulose filter assay) *(7)*.
5. High-Binding Capacity: The binding capacity of the disk for the biotinylated peptide substrate is high (a minimum of 2.5 nmol/disk). This allows the use of high concentrations (up to 1 m$M$) of the peptide substrates under optimal enzyme assay conditions and maximizes the signal to noise ratio.
6. Adaptability to High-Throughput Assay Format: The assay has been successfully adapted to high-throughput 96-well plate format. The 96-well plates offer tremendous advantage *(10)* for scientists in pharmaceutical research or large- scale clinical studies to screen for activators and inhibitors of protein kinases.

## 5. Notes

1. This component is not required if the PKA catalytic subunit is the source of activity, replace with 5 µL of deionized water. Also replace with deionized water when measuring the basal activity of PKA.

| Protein Kinase | Peptide Sequence |
|---|---|
| PKA | Biotin-C6-Leu-Arg-Arg-Ala-Ser-Leu-Gly |
| PKC | Biotin-C6-Ala-Ala-Lys-Ile-Gln-Ala-Ser-Phe-Arg-Gly-His-Met-Ala-Arg-Lys-Lys |
| Cdc2 | Biot-C6-Pro-Lys-Thr-Pro-Lys-Lys-Ala-Lys-Lys-Leu |
| DNA-PK | Biot-C6-Glu-Pro-Pro-Leu-Ser-Gln-Glu-Ala-Phe-Ala-Asp-Leu-Trp-Lys-Lys |
| CK-1 | Biot-C6-Asp.Asp.Asp.Glu.Glu.Ser.Ile.Thr.Arg.Arg |
| CK-2 | Biot-C6-Arg.Arg.Arg.Glu.Glu.Glu.Thr.Glu.Glu.Glu |
| Tyrosine Kinases (EGFR, IR, src, and so on) | Two proprietary peptides (Promega Corp.) |

2. The appropriate peptide substrates for these kinases were obtained in the biotinylated form from Promega Corp. These are listed in the following table.

3. Final concentration is 100 $\mu M$, other concentrations may be used but should not exceed 200 $\mu M$.

4. Larger volumes may be spotted, however, if more than 15 $\mu$L is to be spotted, separate the squares first to prevent crosscontamination. Do NOT exceed 30 $\mu$L per square. (Minor seepage of liquid onto adjacent squares does not cause contamination as the biotinylated peptide is rapidly immobilized to the SAM$^{2®}$ Membrane before liquid migration is complete.) The linear capacity of the Membrane is 1.3 nmol/10 $\mu$L of terminated reaction volume.

5. More or less washing may be appropriate to achieve acceptably low background counts; this should be determined empirically.

6. Preparation of 5X PKC activation buffer. Reagents required:

   a. Prepare 200 mL of 5X PKC buffer:
      1. Add 10 mL of 2 $M$ Tris-HCl, pH 7.5 into 250-mL graduated cylinder.
      2. Add 10 mL of 1 $M$ MgCl$_2$ into the cylinder.
      3. Bring up the volume 200 mL by using nanopure water into the cylinder.

   b. Preparation of 1,2-dioleoyl-sn-glycerol (DAG):
      Add 6.4 mL of chloroform into one bottle of DAG (Sigma, 32 mg) to final concentration of 5 mg/mL.

      Protocol for making 5X activation buffer:
      i.   Prepare 20 (18 × 150-mm) test tubes.
      ii.  Prepare DAG to 5 mg/mL by using chloroform.
      iii. Pippet 0.16 mL of L-a-phosphatidyl-L-serine (PS) (10 mg/mL) and 0.032 mL of DAG (5 mg/mL) into 18X150-mm tube.
      iv.  Remove chloroform by using N$_2$ $_{(g)}$: It takes 5–10 min. **Steps i–iii** are performed in the ice bath.
      v.   Add 1 mL of 5X PKC buffer, then sonicate as described below:
           Use the sonicator VC500 (Sonics and Materials Inc., Danbury, CT), and use the Duty Cycle 20 on a scale of 1–100 and set the output control dial to 4 with the use of the microtip. Sonicate, *on ice*, 8 pulses (4 times), with a total of 32 pulses. After pulses each time, put the tube on wet ice for 15 s.
      vi.  This buffer should be prepared just an hour (on wet ice) before use. The final concentration of PS is 1.6 mg/mL, and DAG is 0.16 mg/mL.

## References

1. Hunter, T. (1995) Protein kinases and phosphatases: the yin and yang of protein phosphorylation and signaling. *Cell* **80,** 225–236.
2. Hubbard, M. J. and Cohen, P. (1993) On target with a new mechanism for the regulation of protein phosphorylation. *Trends Biochem. Sci.* **18,** 172–177.
3. Levitzki, A. and Gazit, A. (1995) Tyrosine kinase inhibition: an approach to drug development. *Science* **267,** 1782–1788.
4. Kemp, B. E. and Pearson, R. B. (1991) Design and use of peptide substrates for protein kinases. *Meth. Enzymol.* **200,** 121–134.
5. Casnellie, J. E. (1991) Assay of protein kinases using peptides with basic residues for phosphocellulose binding. *Meth. Enzymol.* **200,** 115–120.
6. Cisek, L. J. and Corden, J. L. (1991) Purification of protein kinases that phosphorylate the repetitive carboxyl-terminal domain of eukaryotic RNA polymerase II. *Meth. Enzymol.* **200,** 301–325.
7. Toomik, R., kman, P., and Engstrom, L. (1992) A potential pitfall in protein kinase assay: phosphocellulose paper as an unreliable adsorbent of produced phosphopeptides. *Anal. Biochem.* **204,** 311–314.
8. Hvalby, O., Hemmings, H. C. Jr., Paulsen, O., Czernik, A. J., Nairn, A. C., Godfraind, J.M., et al. (1994) Specificity of protein kinase inhibitor peptides and induction of long-term potentiation. *Proc. Natl. Acad. Sci. USA* **91,** 4761–4765.
9. Goueli, B.S., Hsiao, K., Tereba, A., and Goueli, S. A. (1995) A novel and simple method to assay the activity of individual protein kinases in a crude tissue extract. *Anal. Biochem.* **225,** 10–17.
10. Goueli, S. A., Hsiao, K., and Ruzicka, C. (1997) Advances in the SAM$^{2TM}$ membrane technology: high throughput biotin capture systems for use in rapid screening. *Promega Notes* **64,** 2–6.
11. Savage, D., et al. (1992) *Avidin-Biotin Chemistry: A Handbook*, Pierce Chemical Co., Rockland, IL.

# 72

# Photoaffinity Detection of cAMP Binding Proteins in Ovarian Cancer

**David J. Burns and Martin J. Hulme**

## 1. Introduction

Identification of individual cyclic AMP binding proteins in tumor cytosolic extracts is possibly owing to the ability of $^{32}$P-labeled 8-azido cyclic AMP to act as an effective analog of cAMP, to bind specifically to its protein effector sites, and on photoactivation to incorporate covalently to these sites by means of a highly reactive nitrene derivative. Resolution of labeled proteins can be achieved by SDS-PAGE and visualization by autoradiography *(1)*.

The principle cAMP binding proteins, which are the regulatory subunits of cAMP dependent protein kinase A, are represented by two main types, RI and RII. In breast cancer, these types migrate on SDS polyacrylamide gels that are run under reducing conditions at 48 and 52 kDa respectively, following photoaffinity typing *(2)*. More recently, photoaffinity detection of cAMP binding proteins has been used to analyze RI and RII components in ovarian tumor cytosols *(3)* and to relate expression to clinico-pathological features *(4)*.

With the aid of computer-assisted densitometry, resolved protein components can be semiquantified on the basis of relative expression of type, but not currently as an absolute measure of cytosolic protein expression. The method is easy to perform and has been a useful tool in the establishment of an association between cAMP binding proteins and serous histology, poor differentiation and poor patient survival in ovarian cancer.

## 2. Materials

### 2.1. Tumor Cytosol Preparation

1. Homogenization buffer: 20 m$M$ Tris, 0.25 m$M$ sucrose, 2 m$M$ magnesium chloride, 1 m$M$ calcium chloride, 10 m$M$ potassium chloride, 16.25 m$M$ hydrochloric acid. Adjust to pH 7.5, as necessary.

### 2.2. Protein Determination

1. BSA protein standard 1.3–1.5 mg/mL.
2. Bradford protein assay solution.

From: *Methods in Molecular Medicine, Vol. 39: Ovarian Cancer: Methods and Protocols*
Edited by: J. M. S. Bartlett © Humana Press, Inc., Totowa, NJ

### 2.3. Gel Preparation

1. A prepared acrylamide/*bis*-acrylamide solution should be used (e.g., 30% acrylamide/ 0.8% *bis*).
2. 1 *M* Tris buffer, pH 8.85 for the resolving gel (*see* **Note 1**).
3. 0.375 *M* Tris buffer, pH 6.8 for the stacking gel (*see* **Note 1**).
4. 10%(w/v) SDS solution made up in distilled water and filtered through Whatman No. 1 filter paper.
5. TEMED (N,N,N′,N′-Tetramethylethylenediamine).
6. 10%(w/v) ammonium persulphate in distilled water, make up fresh or a stock solution can be kept at 4°C for 2 wk.

### 2.4. Photoaffinity Labeling

1. $^{32}$P-8 Azido cAMP (ICN Radiochemicals catalog No. 37003).
2. MES/MgCl$_2$ buffer; dissolve 1.08 g of MgCl$_2$ and 5.2 g of MES (2-[N-Morpholino] ethanesulphonic acid) in 100 mL of distilled water, aliquot into 1 mL tubes and store at –20°C.
3. 3X sample buffer; 75mg Tris, 0.75g SDS, 3.75 mL Mercapto ethanol, 7.5 mL glycerol, 250 μL saturated solution of bromophenol blue, make volume up to 25 mL with distilled water (*see* **Note 2**).

### 2.5. Electrophoresis

1. $^{14}$C Methylated protein standard.
2. Electrophoresis buffer; 9.09 g Tris, 43.26 g glycine, 30 mL of a 10% SDS solution, dissolve and make up to 3 L with distilled water.
3. Gel fixative; 5% glacial acetic acid, 10% glycerol, 40% methanol. 500 mL per gel in a glass staining dish are adequate.

### 2.6. Autoradiography

1. Kodak X-ray developer diluted 1:5 with tap water.
2. Kodak X-ray fixative diluted 1:5 with tap water.

## 3. Methods

### 3.1. Tumor Cytosol Preparation

1. Weigh out 100–200 mg of tumor material into homogenization tubes.
2. Add 10X w/v of ice-cold homogenization buffer.
3. Using scissors, crudely mince the tumor.
4. Place the samples on ice.
5. Using a mechanical tissue homogenizer, homogenize on full power for 20 s, then return the samples to the ice tray.
6. Rinse homogenizer between samples using a beaker of water.
7. Homogenize samples for a further 15 s at full power.
8. Transfer samples to ultracentrifuge tubes.
9. Spin the homogenate in an ultracentrifuge at 100,000$g$ for 1 h at 4°C.
10. After spinning, collect the supernatant, keep an aliquot for a protein assay, and freeze the remaining cytosol in liquid nitrogen or in a –80°C freezer until needed.

### 3.2. Measurement of Cytosol Protein

1. Dilute the Bradford dye reagent as appropriate (e.g., Bio-Rad (Richmond, CA) premade reagent 1:5 with distilled water) and filter through Whatman No.1 filter paper.

2. Using a BSA protein standard of known concentration, prepare a standard curve (0.1~1.5 mg/mL).
3. Dilute an aliquot of the cytosol 1:5.
4. Mix 20 μL of the protein standards and dilute cytosols in duplicate with 1 mL of dilute dye reagent using 12 × 75-cm borosilicate glass tubes (e.g. Corning).
5. Add 200 μL of each sample to a 96-well flat-bottomed microtiter plate.
6. Measure the absorbance at 595 nm using a microtiter plate reader (e.g., Bio-Rad 2550 EIA reader, *see* **Note 3**).
7. Plot the standard curve and measure the absorbance for the cytosol. Most samples will be in the range 1–3 mg/mL (*see* **Note 4**).

## *3.3. Gel Preparation*

1. Assemble the gel system as per manufacturer's guidelines (e.g., Bio-Rad Protean II).
2. Put the gel comb into the plate assembly and mark a line on the plates 2 cm below the bottom of the comb then remove the comb.
3. Make up a 12% acrylamide gel solution (16 mL of 30% acrylamide, 15 mL. 1 $M$ Tris pH 8.85, 0.4 mL 10% SDS, 8.6 mL ddH$_2$O. 0.1 mL TEMED, 0.1 mL 10% ammonium persulphate per gel) and pour the gel to just above the line—this is the resolving gel.
4. Layer onto the top of the gel 2–3 mL of water saturated isobutanol and leave it for 20–30 min to allow the gel to polymerize.
5. When the gel has set, pour off the butanol and rinse with distilled water, then with a small volume of Tris buffer pH 6.8.
6. Replace the comb and pour the stacking gel (3.6 mL 30% acrylamide, 10 mL 0.375 $M$ Tris, 0.3 mL 10% SDS, 16 mL ddH$_2$O, 0.1 mL TEMED, 0.1 mL 10% ammonium persulphate) to the top. Allow the gel time to set.

## *3.4. Photoaffinity Labeling*

All radioactive procedures should, whenever possible, be carried out behind a perspex shield 1-cm thick, and with appropriate dosimetry.

1. Remove $^{32}$P-8 azido cAMP from the freezer and allow it to thaw.
2. Remove the cytosols from nitrogen and thaw rapidly.
3. Take 50 μL (1.85 MBq) of the isotope and dilute it with 285 μL of homogenization buffer. This is enough for 22 samples.
4. Add 50 μL of each cytosol (1–1.5 mg/mL) to separate wells of a round-bottom microtiter plate, add to each 15 μL MES/MgCl$_2$ buffer and 15 μL of dilute isotope.
5. Incubate the reaction mixture at room temperature in the dark for 1 h. (Wrap the plate in tin foil. Mark clearly and place behind a perspex shield.)
6. When sample incubation is complete, remove the tin foil and irradiate the plate for 30 s with 254-nm ultraviolet light.
7. Stop the reaction by adding 40 μL of 3X sample buffer to each well on the plate.
8. Carefully transfer the samples to screwcap Eppendorf tubes ensuring that the sample has been mixed.
9. Incubate the samples at 90°C for 3 min.

## *3.5. Electrophoresis*

1. Take out $^{14}$C methylated protein standard and let it thaw.
2. Add 10 μL of the $^{14}$C protein to the first well.
3. Add 20 μL of each prepared cytosol to each subsequent well.
4. Run the gel at 60 mA/gel through the stacking gel for 30 min or until into the resolving gel.

5. Run at 35 mA/gel through the resolving gel for 3–4 h (*see* **Note 5**).
6. The stacking gel can be easily detached from the resolving gel and discarded. Place the resolving gel in gel fixative in a sealable container for 1 h or overnight (*see* **Note 6**).
7. Place the gel on backing card (e.g., Whatman No.3 filter paper ) and cover it with "clingfilm," i.e., Saran Wrap.
8. Dry the gel down under vacuum for 2 h at 80°C (*see* **Note 7**).

### 3.6. Autoradiography

1. Place gel in an autoradiography cassette with film and store at –80°C overnight.
2. Process the autoradiograph with X-ray developer and fixer, each for 3 min, then rinse in tap water (*see* **Note 8**).
3. Band intensity will vary according to the exposure time. Optimize this time as required.

## 4. Notes

1. Use Tris base and pH with concentrated HCl, stirring the solution constantly.
2. In our experience, sample buffer can be stored indefinitely at 4°C.
3. If a plate reader is unavailable, a conventional spectrophotometer can be used, although larger volumes of reagents and protein cytosols may be required.
4. We have found that 1–1.5 mg/mL is optimal for photoaffinity labeling, and if direct comparisons between cytosols are required within each gel, then protein content for each cytosol must be equalized using homogenization buffer as the diluent.
5. Resolution of labeled bands is optimal if the gels are run slower for longer. As a rule, it is best to run the dye front off the end of the gel, as this contains unconjugated $^{32}$P, which can increase background after fixing and subsequent autoradiography.
6. Some shrinkage of the resolving gel will occur, but this does not significantly affect resolution of the protein bands.
7. Bio-Rad gel drying system, which incorporates a water pump with a model 583 gel dryer, has proved a good option, eliminating the need for a fume hood. If using a conventional oil-based pump, it must be solvent resistant (e.g., Genevac) and used in conjunction with a fume hood. There is no radioactive contamination of the pump.
8. If available, an automatic X-ray film processor is preferable.

## References

1. Pomerantz, A. H., Rudolph, S. A., Haley, B. E., and Greengard, P. (1975) Photoaffinity labeling of a protein kinase from bovine brain with 8-azidoadenosine 3′,5′-monophosphate. *Biochemistry* **14,** 3858–3862.
2. Miller, W. R., Hulme, M. J., Cho-Chung, Y. S., and Elton, R. A. (1993) Types of cyclic AMP binding proteins in human breast cancers. *Eur. J. Cancer* **29A,** 989–991.
3. Ramage, A. D. R., Burns, D. J., and Miller, W. R. (1994) Cyclic Adenosine 3′,5′-monophosphate-binding proteins in human ovarian cancers. *Br. J. Cancer* **69,** 186–190.
4. Simpson, B. J. B., Ramage, A. D. R., Hulme, M. J., Burns, D. J., Katsaros, D., Langdon, S. P., et al. (1996) Cyclic adenosine 3′,5′-monophosphate-binding proteins in human ovarian cancers: correlations with clinicopathological features. *Clin. Cancer Res.* **2,** 201–206.

# IX

## APOPTOSIS

# 73

## Apoptosis

*A Technical Overview*

### Susan M. Quirk

### 1. Introduction

Physiological or programmed cell death plays an important role during a variety of physiological and pathological processes *(1)*. It is an active form of cell death under tight regulation. Physiological cell death in mammals occurs during embryonic development of organs and tissues; for example, the loss of excess tissue between digits and the removal of excess neurons during development of the nervous system. Physiological cell death also maintains homeostasis of cell numbers during cyclic remodeling of many adult tissues including the intestinal epithelium, the uterine endometrium, and ovarian follicles, and is critical for the regulation of the immune response. Aberrant amplification of cell death occurs in AIDS and some neurodegenerative disorders. Conversely, cancers and autoimmune disease may arise when cells inappropriately fail to die or undergo mutations that inhibit normal cell death pathways *(2)*.

Apoptosis, the most common form of programmed cell death, is defined by distinct morphological features *(3)*. Apoptotic cells undergo shrinkage of the cytoplasm and nucleus. The chromatin becomes condensed and marginated beneath the nuclear envelope. An endogenous endonuclease becomes activated and preferentially cleaves internucleosomal (linker) regions of DNA. DNA is consequently fragmented into nucleosomal units. Mitochondria remain intact without swelling. The cell membrane remains intact during the beginning stages of apoptosis. However, membrane blebbing often occurs. The cell becomes broken up into fragments surrounded by intact membrane and containing intact organelles and fragments of nuclei. These apoptotic bodies are phagocytosed by macrophages or neighboring cells. Apoptosis is a relatively "clean" form of cell death in that it does not elicit an inflammatory immune response. These features are distinct from cells undergoing necrosis as a result of acute cell damage or "accidental" cell death. Necrotic cells immediately lose membrane integrity, cellular contents are released into the extracellular space and an inflammatory immune response is triggered. The distinct nuclear changes associated with apoptosis are absent in necrotic cells.

Apoptosis may be triggered by the removal of survival factors necessary for cell viability *(1,2)*. Examples are induction of apoptosis of cells in culture by removal of

From: *Methods in Molecular Medicine, Vol. 39: Ovarian Cancer: Methods and Protocols*
Edited by: J. M. S. Bartlett © Humana Press, Inc., Totowa, NJ

serum or growth factors, regression of the prostate epithelium and uterine epithelium following steroid hormone withdrawal, and the loss of neurons during development by insufficient stimulation by neurotrophic factors. Alternatively, depending on the cell type, apoptosis may be induced by a variety of cytotoxic stimuli such as radiation, oxidizing agents, cytokines [tumor necrosis factor (TNF), Fas ligand (FasL)], glucocorticoids, and chemotherapeutic drugs.

Extensive evidence indicates that there is a final common effector pathway for apoptosis regardless of the initiating stimulus. A class of proteases known as caspases (for cysteine-containing aspartate-specific proteases) are critical common intermediaries in the apoptotic pathway *(4)*. The first mammalian caspase gene identified was *ICE*, encoding the interleukin-1 (IL-1) converting enzyme *(5)*. *ICE* was cloned based on sequence homology with the nematode gene *CED*-3 which is essential for apoptosis during embryonic development. A family of caspases has since been identified and a numerical system of nomenclature has been developed (12 caspase family members to date) *(6)*. The caspases exist as inactive zymogens until activated by cleavage. Cleavage is generally initiated by another caspase, but may occur autocatalytically, at least in vitro. Apoptosis-inducing signals, such as TNF and FasL, activate a caspase cascade upon binding to their cell surface receptors *(4)*. Both receptors have cytoplasmic "death domain" regions that bind to accessory proteins that also contain death domains. By a series of protein–protein interactions caspase 8 (FLICE/MACH) is activated, and in turn, activates downstream caspases. Caspases are also activated by release of cytochrome-*c* from mitochondria. Cytochrome-*c* binds to and activates apoptotic protease activation factor-1 (APF-1). APF-1 then binds to and activates caspase-9. Bcl-2 and Bcl-$X_L$ proteins, members of the Bcl-2 family, have been shown to inhibit caspase activation and apoptosis by several different mechanisms *(7)*.

A relatively small number of cellular substrates for the caspases have been identified to date. These include procaspases, poly(ADP-ribose) polymerase, protein kinase C, nuclear lamins, and gelsolin. Importantly, one of the recently identified substrates is CAD, caspase-activated inhibitor of apoptosis-inducing deoxyribonuclease *(8)*. In healthy cells, CAD is bound to an apoptosis-inducing endonuclease that is responsible for fragmenting DNA and it maintains the endonuclease in an inactive state. When CAD is cleaved by a caspase, it releases the apoptosis-inducing endonuclease, which then moves into the nucleus and cleaves DNA.

Much current research focuses on the signaling pathways involved in induction and suppression of apoptosis. Numerous studies have analyzed changes in gene expression during apoptosis and have experimentally modified gene expression to induce or suppress apoptosis. Regardless of the stimulus for apoptosis, downstream events can be detected and used to characterize and to quantify apoptosis.

## 2. Methods for Detecting and Measuring Apoptosis

### 2.1. Electrophoretic Detection of Fragmented DNA

The fragmentation of DNA into nucleosomal units is recognized as the biochemical hallmark of apoptosis *(9)*. Nucleosomal units of approximately 180 bp can be detected by agarose gel electrophoresis of DNA isolated from cultured cells or tissue in which apoptosis is occurring. Staining of the gels with ethidium bromide reveals a ladder pattern of DNA fragments corresponding to single nucleosomes and progressive increments of multiple oligonucleosomal units. This method was first used to demonstrate the correlation between chromatin condensation, the first ultrastructurally visible sign of apoptosis, and DNA fragmentation in glucocorticoid-treated thymocytes *(9)*. The method indicates whether DNA fragmentation, typical of apoptosis, is occurring in a population of cells but does not indicate what is occurring in individual cells. Measuring the intensity of DNA ladders allows one to compare the relative amount of apoptosis occurring as a result of different treatments. However, the method does not indicate the proportion of cells in the population undergoing apoptosis. Fragmented DNA can be difficult to detect if the proportion of apoptotic cells in the population is small. To increase the sensitivity of the assay, DNA can be end-labeled with $^{32}$P-tagged nucleotides using the enzymes terminal deoxynucleotidyl transferase (TdT) *(10)* or Klenow polymerase *(11)* prior to separation by electrophoresis. In addition, DNA stains that are more sensitive than ethidium bromide such as SYBR Green I (Molecular Probes, Eugene, OR) are now available.

Examination of DNA in apoptotic cells using field inversion gel electrophoresis methods to detect large fragments of DNA, demonstrated that DNA is generally cleaved into large molecular weight fragments of 50 to 300-kb pairs and later broken down into nucleosomal units *(12,13)*. The formation of large DNA fragments was correlated with condensation of chromatin around the nuclear periphery *(14)*, one of the earliest ultrastructural features of apoptosis. However, in some cell types examined, fragmentation of DNA into 50-kbp units was not followed by internucleosomal cleavage *(12)*. These results indicate that although internucleosomal cleavage is a useful end point to identify apoptosis, it is not an essential step and other criteria must be considered. Furthermore, studies have shown that cleavage of DNA into kbp fragments occurs in some forms of necrosis, as well as apoptosis *(13)*. Another important point is that not all forms of programmed cell death are accompanied by fragmentation of DNA into oligonucleosomes *(15)*. Although it was once believed that fragmentation of DNA into nucleosomal units was one of the earliest events in apoptosis, it is now recognized that it occurs after nuclear condensation *(16)*.

The process of apoptosis does not absolutely require DNA fragmentation since it occurs in experimentally enucleated cells and cells in which DNA fragmentation is blocked *(14)*. These findings and others support the concept that apoptosis may be initiated by a cytoplasmic regulator(s) that has both cytoplasmic and nuclear targets. One experimental strategy that has been used to study cytoplasmic factors involved in apoptosis is to study effects of lysates prepared from treated cells on the integrity of isolated nuclei of test cells *(17)*. For example, this type of experiment provided an early clue that a CPP32-like caspase, together with a cytoplasmic component(s) causes apoptosis of nuclei *(18)*.

Other methods to examine DNA fragmentation during apoptosis include an enzyme-linked immunosorbent assay (ELISA) assay which quantifies nucleosomal units using antibodies directed against histones and DNA (commercially available from Oncogene Research Products, Cambridge, MA, and Boehringer Mannheim, Mannheim, Germany) and is reported to correlate well with DNA fragmentation *(19)*. The comet assay, originally proposed by Ostling and Johanson, measures the different patterns of DNA fragmentation occurring in individual cells *(20)*. A small number of cells are embedded in agarose on a microscope slide, lysed by incubation in a detergent solution, subjected to a weak electric field and stained with a fluorescent DNA-binding dye. Supercoiled

DNA from healthy cells does not migrate significantly whereas damaged DNA containing fragments and relaxed supercoils migrate varying distances to produce a comet pattern with the tail containing the damaged DNA. The comet assay has been applied to identification of cells within a population that are resistant to etoposide-induced DNA fragmentation *(21)*.

## 2.2. In Situ *Detection of DNA Fragmentation*

*In situ* techniques were developed to detect fragmentation of DNA in individual cells in cell cultures and tissue sections. DNA in fixed cells is labeled at free 3' ends with biotin- or digoxigenin-tagged nucleotides. In one version of the assay, the enzyme TdT is used for labeling and the assay is called TdT-mediated biotin-dUTP nick end labeling, or TUNEL *(22)*. In another version of the assay the enzyme DNA polymerase I is used and the assay is referred to as *in situ* nick translation *(23)*. There is some controversy over whether TdT or DNA polymerase I is more selective for detecting apoptotic versus necrotic cells *(24)*. However, there is general agreement that both assays suffer from the disadvantage that necrotic as well as apoptotic cells may be labeled, and that other methods must be used in conjunction to differentiate between apoptosis and necrosis *(24,25)*. For example, examination of cells for the nuclear morphology typical of apoptosis could be used to corroborate a positive TUNEL reaction. The major advantage of the *in situ* methods for studies of apoptosis is that they enable detection of DNA fragmentation in individual cells in a cultured population or tissue section and provide a means to monitor the temporal pattern of DNA fragmentation.

## 2.3. Nuclear Morphology

One of the most specific ways to determine whether apoptosis is occurring is to examine the ultrastructure of the cell. Using electron microscopy (EM) the characteristic early changes in the chromatin and other features of cell morphology associated with apoptosis can be detected. The obvious disadvantage of EM is that the number of cells in a population that can be viewed in a single field is small and can not be used to quantify the number of cells in a population undergoing apoptosis. However, a large variety of fluorescent stains for DNA are available that can be used in combination with fluorescence microscopy or flow cytometry to characterize and quantify apoptosis in a population of cells. Nuclei of apoptotic cells stained with fluorescent dyes are small (pycnotic) with condensed chromatin and are often fragmented. DNA dyes that are impermeant to intact cell membranes, such as propidium iodide (PI) and ethidium bromide, stain only dead cells or cells that have had membranes permeabilized by fixation or detergent. Nuclei of cells at early stages of apoptosis with intact cell membranes do not stain with these dyes. Other nuclear stains are permeant to cell membranes including Hoechst 33258, acridine orange and SYTO 13 (Molecular Probes) and therefore stain nuclei of both dead and live cells. In one technique to differentiate apoptosis and necrosis, cells are preloaded with SYTO-13 (green nuclear staining) followed by PI (red staining). Nuclei of necrotic cells stain progressively yellow (combination of green and red) and then red as staining by PI intensifies. Nuclei of viable cells remain green and are of normal size and appearance. Nuclei of apoptotic cells with intact membranes stain bright green and are pycnotic *(26)*.

Flow cytometric methods for detecting apoptosis use some of the same nuclear stains described for use in fluorescence microscopy *(27)*. By staining all cells in a population by permeabilizing membranes and using PI, the distribution of cells in various stages of the cell cycle can be determined. Alternatively, cells can be stained with membrane permeant dyes, such as Hoechst 33258, or SYTO-13 and SYTO-16 (Molecular Probes). Apoptotic cells form a distinct cell-cycle region in DNA histograms below the $G_0/G_1$ region (hypodiploid peak). Comparison of the flow cytometric pattern before and after treatment with a stimulus to induce apoptosis indicates whether cells in a particular phase of the cell cycle are susceptible to apoptosis. In addition, the flow cytometric pattern of cells can be followed at various times after an apoptotic stimulus to study progressive changes in cell size (measured by forward light scatter) and nuclear staining. Another major advantage of flow cytometry is that cells can be stained for chromatin simultaneously with antibodies to cell surface markers in order to identify and quantify the specific cells in a mixed population that are undergoing apoptosis. Changes in DNA content associated with apoptosis can be correlated with staining for proteins involved in regulation of apoptosis such as members of the bcl-2 and caspase families, p53 and others. The application of the TUNEL technique to label 3'-OH ends of fragmented DNA with fluorescently tagged nucleotide has been combined with flow cytometry *(28)*. The analysis can be used to test whether cells undergoing DNA fragmentation (TUNEL positive) have nuclear staining typical of condensed apoptotic nuclei. Flow cytometry is most easily used on nonadherent cells in single-cell suspensions (i.e., lymphocytes). Although possible, flow cytometry is more difficult to use on adherent cells that must be removed from the culture dish prior to analysis and for cells that tend to form extensive junctions and aggregate.

Nuclear matrix proteins comprise the structural framework of the nucleus and form complex interactions with the chromosomes. During apoptosis these proteins are released from the nucleus in a soluble form before DNA fragmentation occurs. The amount of nuclear matrix protein released is proportional to the number of dead cells. Immunocytochemistry of cells undergoing apoptosis reveals reduced staining for nuclear matrix proteins compared to healthy cells *(29)*. Immunoassays to detect the release of soluble nuclear matrix proteins *(29)* and antibodies directed against nuclear matrix proteins are commercially available (Oncogene Research Products, Cambridge, MA).

### 2.4. Plasma Membrane Asymmetry

Another feature of cells undergoing apoptosis is a change in the phospholipid character of the plasma membrane. In healthy cells, negatively charged phosphatidylserine residues are restricted to the inner side of the plasma membrane but in apoptotic cells these residues become exposed to the outer surface. Early cell surface changes in phosphatidylserine and other constituents are thought to signal engulfment by macrophages and to insure phagocytic removal of the cell before lysis. Studies have indicated that exposure of phosphatidylserine residues occurs very early in the apoptotic process, before nuclear condensation, cell shrinkage, and loss of membrane integrity *(30,31)*. Assays for early detection of apoptosis have been developed based on the selective binding of the calcium-dependent binding protein, annexin V (AV), to exposed phosphatidylserine residues on the outer cell surface *(30,31)*. Annexin V can be purchased commercially conjugated to fluorochromes such as FITC, or to biotin. Binding of annexin V to cells can be detected by fluorescence microscopy or flow cytometry. Annexin V binding is tested in combination with staining by a fluorescent DNA-binding dye impermeant to intact cell membranes, such as PI, to differentiate nonapoptotic live cells (PI–/AV–), cells in early stages of apoptosis (PI–/AV+), and cells in a late stage of apoptosis that have lost membrane integrity (PI+ and AV+). Annexin V will bind to phosphatidylserine on the inner cell membrane of necrotic cells as a consequence of membrane rupture and cells in late stages of apoptosis with disrupted membranes. Therefore, it is necessary to follow the time-course of staining of annexin V and PI in response to a given treatment in order to differentiate early staining by annexin V of the outer surface of membrane-intact apoptotic cells from staining of membrane-impaired necrotic or late apoptotic cells.

## 2.5. Caspase Activity

A goal of recent investigations has been to characterize the specific sequence of caspase activation required to elicit apoptosis in different cell types *(4)*. Primary reagents for these studies include a repertoire of peptide inhibitors specific for individual caspases *(32)*. For example, caspase-1 has a substrate specificity for the amino acid sequence YVAD and is inhibited by the tetrapeptide aldehyde, Ac-YVAD-CHO, whereas caspase-3 has substrate specificity for DEVD and is inhibited by Ac-DEVD-CHO. These inhibitors have been used to study caspase activity in cell-free systems and to inhibit apoptosis by cells in response to a variety of signals in vitro. Assays to measure caspase activity have been developed using small peptide substrates, encompassing the recognition site for the caspases, conjugated to a fluorophore. Cleavage of the peptide releases the fluorophore and signals are quantified by spectrofluorometry or flow cytometry. Many of these reagents are currently commercially available.

## 2.6. Biochemical Assays of Cell Death

A number of assays for the viability of cultured cells have been developed that are a useful first screen for cytotoxicity, but do not differentiate apoptotic from necrotic cell death. The LIVE/DEAD viability/cytotoxicity assay kit (Molecular Probes) stains cells using two probes: (1) Calcein AM, a fluorogenic esterase substrate that is hydrolyzed to a green fluorescent product in the cytoplasm of cells that have esterase activity. Only cells with intact membranes retain the esterase products; and (2) Ethidium homodimer-1, a red fluorescent nucleic acid stain that is membrane impermeable and stains only dead cells. This assay would result in similar staining for necrotic cells and cells in late stages of apoptosis with impaired membrane integrity. Another class of colorimetric assays uses tetrazolium salts to assess the redox potential of cells as a measure of cell viability, proliferation, and cytotoxicity *(33)*. In another type of assay, the activity of the cytosolic enzyme, lactate dehydrogenase, is measured in the supernatant of cultured cells that have lost membrane integrity *(34)*. Results obtained with this assay are comparable to results obtained with $^{51}$C-release assays. Use of these assays and a variety of other general cell-viability assays must be accompanied by additional tests to differentiate apoptosis and necrosis.

## References

1. Jacobson, M. D., Weil, M., and Raff, M. C. (1997) Programmed cell death in animal development. *Cell* **88,** 347–354.
2. Thompson, C. B. (1995) Apoptosis in the pathogenesis and treatment of disease. *Science* **267,** 1456–1462.
3. Kerr, J. F. R., Wyllie, A. H., and Currie, A. R. (1972) Apoptosis: A basic biological phenomenon with wide ranging implications in tissue kinetics. *Br. J. Cancer* **26,** 239–257.

4. Salvesen, G. S. and Dixit, V. M. (1997) Caspases: Intracellular signaling by proteolysis. *Cell* **91**, 443–446.

5. Yuan, J., Shaham, S., Ledoux, S., Ellis, H. M., and Horvitz, H. R. (1993) The C. elegans cell death gene *ced-3* encodes a protein similar to mammalian interleukin-1 beta-converting enzyme. *Cell* **75**, 641–652.

6. Alnemri, E. S., Livingston, D. J., Nicholson, D. W., Salvesen, G., Thornberry, N. A., Wong, W. W., and Yuan, J. (1996) Human ICE/CED-3 protease nomenclature. *Cell* **87**, 171.

7. Hengartner, M. O. (1998) Death cycle and Swiss army knives. *Nature* **391**, 441–442.

8. Enari, M., Sakahira, H., Yokoyama, H., Okawa, K., Iwamatsu, A., and Nagata, S. (1998) A caspase-activated DNase that degrades DNA during apoptosis, and its inhibitor ICAD. *Nature* **391**, 43–50.

9. Wyllie, A. H. (1980) Glucocorticoid-induced thymocyte apoptosis is associated with endogenous endonuclease activation. *Nature* **284**, 555,556.

10. Tilly, J. L. and Hsueh, A. J. W. (1993) Microscale autoradiographic method for the qualitative and quantitative analysis of apoptotic DNA fragmentation. *J. Cell Physiol.* **154**, 519–526.

11. Rosl, F. (1992) A simple and rapid method for detection of apoptosis in human cells. *Nucl. Acids Res.* **20**, 5243.

12. Oberhammer, F., Wilson, J. W., Dive, C., Morris, I. D., Hickman, J. A., Wakeling, A. E., et al. (1993) Apoptotic death in epithelial cells: cleavage of DNA to 300 and/or 50 kb fragments prior to or in the absence of internucleosomal fragmentation. *EMBO J.* **12**, 3679–3684.

13. Bicknell, G. R. and Cohen, G. M. (1995) Cleavage of DNA to large kilobase pair fragments occurs in some forms of necrosis as well as apoptosis. *Biochem. Biophys. Res. Comm.* **207**, 40–47.

14. Schulze-Osthoff, K., Walczak, H., Droge, W., and Krammer, P. H. (1994) Cell nucleus and DNA fragmentation are not required for apoptosis. *J. Cell Biol.* **127**, 15–20.

15. Zakeri, Z. F., Quaglino, D., Latham, T., and Lockshin, R. A. (1993) Delayed internucleosomal DNA fragmentation in programmed cell death. *FASEB J.* **7**, 470–478.

16. Cohen, G. M., Sun, X.-M., Snowden, R. T., Dinsdale, D., and Skilleter, D. N. (1992) Key morphological features of apoptosis may occur in the absence of internucleosomal DNA fragmentation. *Biochem. J.* **286**, 331–334.

17. Lazebnik, Y. A., Cole, S., Cooke, C. A., Nelson, W. G., and Earnshaw, W. C. (1993) Nuclear events of apoptosis in vitro in cell-free mitotic extracts: A model system for analysis of the active phase of apoptosis. *J. Cell Biol.* **123**, 7–22.

18. Enari, M., Talanian, R. V., Wong, W. W., and Nagata, S. (1996) Sequential activation of ICE-like and CPP32-like proteases during Fas-mediated apoptosis. *Nature* **380**, 723–726.

19. Bonfoco, E., Krainc, D., Ankarcrona, M., Nicotera, P., and Lipton, S. A. (1995) Apoptosis and necrosis: two distinct events induced, respectively, by mild and intense insults with *N*-methyl-D-aspartate or nitric oxide/superoxide in cortical cell cultures. *Proc. Natl. Acad. Sci. USA* **92**, 7162–7166.

20. Ostling, O. and Johanson, K. J. (1984) Microelectrophoretic study of radiation-induced DNA damages in individual mammalian cells. *Biochem. Biophys. Res. Comm.* **123**, 291–298.

21. Olive, P. L., Banáth, J. P., and Durand, R. E. (1990) Detection of etoposide resistance by measuring DNA damage in individual Chinese hamster cells. *J. Natl. Cancer Inst.* **82**, 779–782.

22. Gavrieli, Y., Sherman, Y., and Ben-Sasson, S. A. (1992) Identification of programmed cell death *in situ* via specific labeling of nuclear DNA fragmentation. *J. Cell Biol.* **119**, 493–501.

23. Wijsman, J. H., Jonker, R. R., Keijzer, R., Van de Velde, C. J. H., Cornelisse, C. J., and van Dierendonck, J. H. (1993) A new method to detect apoptosis in paraffin sections: *in situ* end-labeling of fragmented DNA. *J. Histochem. Cytochem.* **41**, 7–12.

24. Mundle, S. D. and Raza, A. (1996) The two *in situ* techniques do not differentiate between apoptosis and necrosis but rather reveal distinct patterns of DNA fragmentation in apoptosis. *Lab. Investigat.* **72**, 611,612.

25. Grasl-Kraupp, B., Ruttkay-Nedecky, B., Koudelka, H., Bukowska, K., Bursch, W., and Schulte-Hermann, R. (1995) *In situ* detection of fragmented DNA (TUNEL assay) fails to discriminate among apoptosis, necrosis, and autolytic cell death: A cautionary note. *Hepatology* **21**, 1465–1468.

26. Ankarcrona, M., Dypbukt, J. M., Bonfoco, E., Zhivotovsky, B., Orrenius, S., Lipton, S. A., and Nicotera, P. (1995) Glutamate-induced neuronal death: a succession of necrosis or apoptosis depending on mitochondrial function. *Neuron* **15**, 961–973.

27. Darzynkiewicz, Z., Juan, G., Li, X., Gorczyca, W., Murakami, T., and Traganos, F. (1997) Cytometry in cell necrobiology: Analysis of apoptosis and accidental cell death (necrosis). *Cytometry* **27**, 1–20.

28. Dolzhanskiy, A. and Basch, R. S. (1995) Flow cytometric determination of apoptosis in heterogeneous cell populations. *J. Immunol. Meth.* **180**, 131–140.

29. Miller, T. E., Beausang, L. A., Meneghini, M., and Lidgard, G. (1994) Cell death and nuclear matrix proteins, in *Apoptosis II: The Molecular Basis of Apoptosis in Disease* (Tomei, L. D. and Cope, F. O., eds.), Cold Spring Harbor Laboratory Press, Cold Spring Harbor, pp. 357–376.

30. Martin, S. J., Reutelingsperger, C. P. M., McGahon, A. J., Rader, J. A., van Schie, R. C. A. A., LaFace, D. M., et al. (1995) Early redistribution of plasma membrane phosphatidylserine is a general feature of apoptosis regardless of the initiating stimulus: Inhibition by overexpression of Bcl-2 and Abl. *J. Exp. Med.* **182,** 1545–1556.
31. Koopman, G., Reutelingsperger, C. P. M., Kuijten, G. A. M., Keehnen, R. M. J., Pals, S. T., and van Oers, M. H. J. (1994) Annexin V for flow cytometric detection of phosphatidylserine expression on B cells undergoing apoptosis. *Blood* **84,** 1415–1420.
32. Talanian, R. V., Quinlan, C., Trautz, S., Hackett, M. C., Mankovich, J. A., Banach, D., et al. (1997) Substrate specificities of caspase family proteases. *J. Biol. Chem.* **272,** 9677–9682.
33. Denizot, F. and Lang, R. (1986) Rapid colorimetric assay for cell growth and survival. *J. Immunol. Meth.* **89,** 271–277.
34. Decker, T. and Lohmann-Matthes, M. (1988) A quick and simple method for the quantitation of lactate dehydrogenase release in measurements of cellular cytotoxicity and tumor necrosis factor (TNF) activity. *J. Immunol. Meth.* **15,** 61–69.

# 74

## Detection of Low Levels of DNA Fragmentation in Ovarian Tumor Cell Lines

**Amanda J. McIlwrath**

## 1. Introduction

The techniques presented in this chapter describe the experimental procedure for the identification of the nonrandom DNA fragmentation associated with apoptosis. The major benefits of this method are its ability to detect a low level of DNA fragmentation and its ability to detect large DNA fragments (50 kb and 300–1000 kb) as opposed to the internucleosomal DNA ladder. It is a qualitative technique although it can be of limited quantitative value. It can be used to detect apoptosis in cell lines following exposure to a wide variety of agents.

In most cells that are undergoing apoptosis, the DNA is broken down into 180–200 bp internucleosomal fragments known as the DNA ladder (*1*). The DNA ladder can be visualized by ethidium bromide staining of DNA that has been subjected to agarose gel electrophoresis. The DNA ladder is not always observed and in some apoptosing cells only the large DNA fragments of 50 kb and/or 300–1000 kb are produced (*2*). The appearance of these large fragments are thought to be a precursor to DNA laddering. Apoptotic morphology may also be observed in the absence of DNA fragmentation (*3,4*). The absence of DNA fragmentation, therefore, is not necessarily diagnostic of lack of apoptosis although this appears to be in infrequent observation.

Because fragments of 50 kb and 300–1000 kb cannot be discriminated using normal agarose gel electrophoresis, field inversion gel electrophoresis must be employed. In order to sensitize the detection of DNA from potentially low numbers of apoptotic cells, I perform a Southern blot and detect the DNA with a radiolabeled probe. The Southern blot is hybridized with randomly sheared human DNA, which is [32]P-labeled by random priming. This allows visualization of the total human DNA that is present on the membrane caused by hybridization of the probe to repetitive DNA sequences. Before attempting to detect the large DNA fragments, it is worth trying to detect the DNA ladder, as this is a more rapid means for demonstrating the presence of apoptotic cells.

**Figure 1** shows an irradiation dose-dependent induction of DNA fragmentation in the A2780 ovarian adenocarcinoma cell line as measured by the appearance of 50 kb fragments. No evidence of internucleosomal, nonrandom DNA fragmentation was observed in the DNA from irradiated A2780 cells. Field inversion gel electrophoresis

From: *Methods in Molecular Medicine, Vol. 39: Ovarian Cancer: Methods and Protocols*
Edited by: J. M. S. Bartlett © Humana Press, Inc., Totowa, NJ

Fig. 1. An irradiation dose-dependent induction of DNA fragmentation in the A2780 ovarian adenocarcinoma cell line.

enabled discrimination between genomic DNA and 50 kb DNA fragments in irradiated A2780 cells. This method was also used to demonstrate reduced levels of cisplatin-induced apoptosis in cisplatin-resistant derivatives of A2780 cells (5). Instead of the lambda DNA marker, a lambda ladder marker (available from Promega Corp., Madison, WI) can be used. This covers the range of 50–1000 kb which allows for the confirmation of size for both the 50 kb band and the larger 300–1000 kb band.

## 2. Materials

All solutions are made using double-distilled water (ddH$_2$O).

1. L Buffer: 100 m$M$ ethylenediaminetetraacetic acid (EDTA) (pH 8.0), 10 m$M$ Tris-HCl (pH 7.6), 20 m$M$ NaCl.
2. Tris Acetate EDTA buffer (TAE): 40 m$M$ Tris-acetate, 1 m$M$ EDTA; for 1 L of 50X concentrated stock: 242 g Tris base, 57.1 mL glacial acetic acid, 100 mL 500 m$M$ EDTA (pH 8.0).
3. Denaturation buffer: 500 m$M$ NaOH (20 g/L), 1.5 $M$ NaCl (87.7 g/L).
4. Neutralization buffer: 1 $M$ Tris-HCl pH 7.4 (121.2 g/L), 1.5 $M$ NaCl (87.7 g/L).
5. Genescreen buffer: 500 m$M$ Na$_2$HPO$_4$ (345.9 g/5 L), 500 m$M$ NaH$_2$PO$_4$ (390.02 g/5 L).
6. Hybridization buffer: 50 m$M$ PIPES pH 6.8 (7.6 g/500 mL); 50 m$M$ NaH$_2$PO$_4$ (3.9 g/500 mL); 50 m$M$ Na$_2$HPO$_4$ (3.8 g/500 mL); 100 m$M$ NaCl (2.9 g/500 mL); 1 m$M$ EDTA (1 mL of 500 m$M$ EDTA/500 mL); SDS (25 g/500 mL).
7. 20X SSC: 3 $M$ NaCl (175.3 g/L), 300 m$M$ tri-sodium citrate (88.2 g/L) pH 7.0.

## 3. Methods

### 3.1. Preparation of DNA

The following protocol was used in the experiment described above. It therefore refers to monolayer tissue-culture cells that were irradiated and trypsinized 72 h after treatment.

**Steps 1–3** may vary according to the treatment required and the type of cells under investigation.

1. Seed cells into 10-cm$^2$ sterile tissue-culture plates at a density that will allow for exponential growth of control cells for the duration of the experiment.
2. Irradiate cells and harvest by trypsinization. The suspension cells are retained along with the monolayer cells (*see* **Note 1**).
3. Centrifuge at 200$g$, remove medium, and resuspend cells in ice-cold phosphate-buffered saline (PBS) at $4 \times 10^6$ cells/100 μL. Transfer cell suspension to Eppendorf tubes and keep on ice.
4. Melt 2% low gelling temperature (lgt) agarose in L buffer and keep at 42°C (*see* **Note 2**). Warm the cell suspensions to 42°C and add agarose to each tube to halve the cell concentration, i.e., to give a final concentration of $2 \times 10^6$ cells/100 μL 1% agarose.
5. Pipet cell suspension into a disposable plug mould (available from Bio-Rad, Richmond, CA) and allow to set at 4°C for 5–10 min (*see* **Note 3**). Transfer plugs into 500 m$M$ EDTA pH 8.0 in bijou bottles and store at 4°C until all plugs are ready for the lysis step (e.g., until the time-course is complete).
6. Lyse agarose-embedded cells in L buffer containing 1 mg/mL proteinase K and 1% SDS in bijou bottles at 50°C (*see* **Note 4**). Lyse a maximum of $10^7$ cells in 5 mL buffer. Lyse for 48 h replacing with fresh buffer after 24 h.

### 3.2. Field Inversion Gel Electrophoresis

1. Either lambda ladder (Promega, Ltd.) or denatured λ DNA (Life Technologies, Ltd., Bethesda, MD) can be run as a size marker (*see* **Note 5**). First linearize the λ DNA. Heat 5 μg of λ DNA at 56°C for 5 min and add 1% lgt agarose in L buffer to make up to 200 μL. Pipet into a plug mould, cool at 4°C, and store in 500 m$M$ EDTA pH 8.0, as for cell plugs. Run approximately 1 μg λ DNA per lane. The lambda ladder is supplied as an agarose plug (follow the manufacturers instructions).
2. Make a large (approx 450 mL volume, 24 cm wide × 20 cm long) horizontal 1% agarose gel in 1X TAE buffer. While the gel is setting, rinse agarose/cell plugs in 500 m$M$ EDTA and make up 5–10 mL of 1% lgt agarose (keep at 42°C until needed).
3. Load equal volumes of the plugs (i.e., approx equal cell numbers) into the wells (*see* **Note 6**). Load appropriate molecular weight markers and fill up all wells with 1% lgt agarose to prevent the plugs from floating out.
4. Place the gel in a large, horizontal gel electrophoresis tank and fill with 1X TAE. Run the gel at 4–15°C using a minipump to recirculate the buffer. Run the gel in a refrigerated room or, if this is unavailable, by using an electrophoresis tank with a cooling maze below the gel platform (*see* **Note 7**). Run the gel at 7–10 V/cm in 1X TAE for 48 h using a 500 V power supply and a Minipulse Polarity Switching System (IBI Technologies, Irvine, CA). Use the following parameters:

| | | |
|---|---|---|
| A | initial reverse time | 0.1 s |
| B | reverse increment | 0 |
| C | initial forward time | 0.3 s |
| D | forward increment | 0 |
| E | number of steps | 51 |
| F | reverse increment increment | 0.02 s |
| G | forward increment increment | 0.06 s |

These parameters allow for resolution to 1600 kb emphasizing the lower range (*see* **Note 8**).

Fig. 2. A diagram depicting the set up of a Southern blot.

## 3.3. Southern Blotting of DNA

1. Place the gel in a plastic container and denature gel for 15 min in denaturation buffer. Change denaturation buffer and denature for a further 15 min.
2. Discard the denaturation buffer and rinse the gel with a small volume of neutralization buffer. Neutralize for 30 min in neutralization buffer. Change buffer and neutralize for a further 30 min.
3. Southern blot onto Hybond-N membrane. Using Genescreen buffer rinse the gel and wet the nylon membrane. Set up the blot according to the diagram shown in **Fig. 2** (*see* **Note 9**). Transfer for at least 18 h (overnight).
4. Wrap the damp membrane in plastic wrap, crosslink the DNA using a UV crosslinker or UV box, and store at 4°C until ready to hybridize (*see* **Note 10**).

## 3.4. Random Priming

Human double-stranded DNA and λ DNA are randomly sheared using a hypodermic needle and end-labeled with $[\alpha^{32}P]dCTP$ using the Prime-It kit (Stratagene, Cambridge, UK; contains Klenow, primers, primer buffer without dCTP [also primer buffer without dATP], and Stop mix).

1. Shear some suitable DNA (e.g., human, mouse, λ) at a concentration of 10 ng/µL into random fragments with a disposable, 25-gage hypodermic needle (*see* **Note 11**).
2. Take 5 µL of sheared DNA (i.e., 50 ng) and add 19 µL ddH$_2$O and 10 µL primers (from Prime-It kit). Boil for 5 min to denature the DNA.
3. Add 10 µL primer buffer without dCTP, 8 µL $[\alpha^{32}P]dCTP$ (Amersham International plc, Little Chalfont, Bucks, UK) and 1 µL Klenow. Mix thoroughly with a pipet tip and incubate for a minimum of 1 h at 37°C (*see* **Note 12**).
4. Add 2 µL of Stop mix.
5. Separate unincorporated $[\alpha^{32}P]dCTP$ from labelled DNA using a disposable Sephadex G50 NICK column (Pharmacia Biotech). Wash column with 0.8 mL ddH$_2$O and dispose of eluent. Apply probe to centre of column and wash with 0.4 mL ddH$_2$O collecting eluent as waste. With a fresh Eppendorf under the column, add a further 0.4 mL ddH$_2$O and collect this fraction containing labeled DNA. Check the counts from 4 µL of the probe in a liquid-scintillation analyzer (should be about $1–2 \times 10^5$ cpm/µL).
6. Probes are denatured before hybridization by adding 0.1 volume of 3 $M$ NaOH for 5 min at room temperature, followed by 0.05 volumes of 1 $M$ Tris-HCl (pH 7.5) for 5 min on ice. Last, add 0.1 volume of 3 $M$ HCl for a further 5 min on ice.

### 3.5. Hybridization of Probes

All hybridization steps at 65°C are carried out in a hybridization oven containing a rotisserie.

1. Roll up the membrane and put in a hybridization bottle (*see* **Note 13**). Pour in 30 mL of hybridization buffer and prehybridize the membrane for 1 h at 65°C.
2. Add all of both probes to 10 mL of hybridization buffer and add to the bottle, having discarded the prehybridization buffer. Hybridize overnight at 65°C.
3. Wash with 1X SSC, 5% SDS three times: once for 15 min, once for 30 min, and once for 60 min (*see* **Note 14**).
4. Expose the side of the membrane which was next to the gel to X-ray film (usually for about 6 h minimum) and develop (*see* **Note 15**).

## 4. Notes

1. The number of apoptotic cells in a culture at any one time may be very low because the execution of apoptosis is rapid. The time over which one can detect any one particular apoptotic cell may be as little as 30 min (*6*). To produce as quantitative a result as possible, total cell cultures (suspension cells and trypsinized, monolayer cells) are resuspended and analyzed, thereby allowing the detection of apoptotic DNA fragments relative to the total amount of DNA obtained from the culture.
2. DNA extracted from cell cultures by phenol/chloroform is susceptible to random degradation and shearing during handling, resulting in a smear of DNA on the autoradiograph. To minimize random shearing, I embed cells in agarose plugs before lysing to liberate the DNA. Embed in molten agarose at a concentration of $2 \times 10^6$ cells/100 μL. An approximately equal volume of agarose is then loaded in each well (try to get about $10^6$ cells/ well). Lgt agarose melts at approximately 65°C and gels at approximately 30°C. The lgt agarose must be kept at 42°C to prevent gelling while the cell suspensions are being prepared. The most convenient way of achieving this is by using a dry block set to 42°C.
3. The 1% agarose blocks are quite delicate and it is therefore easiest to do all manipulations involving them in a 4°C room.
4. Proteinase K and SDS must be added fresh to the L buffer. Make sure that the proteinase K is DNase-free (store at −20°C). The very high concentration of proteinase K is required because the cells are embedded in agarose. This is 10 times the concentration that is used for cells in suspension. Agarose plugs should not be kept unlysed for more than 72 h.
5. Although λ DNA is used as a size marker for the 50-kb fragments it is actually 48.5 kb in length. The lambda ladder is a 20-step ladder ranging in size from approx 50–1000 kb. It is constructed from λ DNA concatamerized into oligomers. Again, each step actually differs by 48.5 kb. Store the markers at 4°C.
6. Cut equal volumes off each agarose plug using a scalpel on a glass plate in a 4°C room. Load into the wells of the gel with the aid of a small spatula.
7. Rubber tubing can be attached to adapters on the gel tank and to a cold water supply thereby allowing cold water to be pumped through the maze, cooling the gel above. One such electrophoresis unit incorporating a cooling maze is available from IBI. A minipump is required to recirculate the TAE in order to maintain the buffering capacity of the buffer. Place one end of the pump's tubing in one reservoir of the electrophoresis tank and the other end of the tubing in the second reservoir. Make sure that the valve between the two reservoirs is open.
8. Run on program 7 of IBI Minipulse Polarity Switching System. If you have a different switching system, the instruction manual may have a list of preprogrammed parameters

allowing resolution of 50–1000 kb. Alternatively, use the parameters listed in **Subheading 3.2., step 4**, to program your system.

9. Mark the side of the nylon membrane that is next to the gel and make sure that the gel, the membrane, the Whatman 3MM paper on top of the membrane, and paper towels are all the same size to ensure efficient capillary transfer. If, for example, the paper towels are over-hanging and in contact with the Whatman 3MM paper below the gel, the Genescreen buffer will bypass the gel and the DNA will not be transferred onto the nylon membrane. To ensure that this is avoided, cut strips off an unwanted autoradiograph and place around the gel on the lower layer of Whatman 3MM paper. This will prevent accidental "short-ing" of the system. The setup and volume of Genescreen buffer depends on the size of your gel. You may find that you need to balance a support on top of two reservoirs with one end of the Whatman paper hanging in each reservoir. Use about 2 L of Genescreen buffer for a 20 cm × 20 cm gel.

10. If a UV crosslinker is not available, expose the side of the membrane carrying the DNA to a total of 1.5 J/sq cm on a UV light box. Alternatively, membranes may be baked in an oven between two sheets of 3MM paper for 30 min to 2 h.

11. You will need a probe to hybridize to the DNA from your treated cells and also a probe to recognize the λ marker.

12. Appropriate safety guidelines for handling radioactivity should be followed. Use labora-tory space that is designated for work involving the use of radioactive substances. Use protective screening and wear two pairs of gloves. Monitor the work bench before and after use and decontaminate any spills. Dispose of radioactive waste (e.g., contaminated Sephadex column) according to safety guidelines.

13. Place the hybridization bottle on the rotisserie so the membrane sticks to the sides of the bottle when it rotates. If it is on the wrong way, the membrane will form a tight roll and hybridization will be uneven. If you are only hybridizing one blot, remember to put another bottle on the rotisserie for balance.

14. Wash the membrane until there is a low background activity. Take the membrane out of the bottle after the third wash and lay it on a piece of Whatman 3MM paper. Check the radioactive signal using a Geiger counter. If there is a high count coming from the bottom of the membrane (where there should be no DNA and therefore no hybridization of the probe) put the membrane back in the bottle and perform further washes until this is reduced.

15. I use Fuji photographic film and a Kodak automated X-ray developer. Other X-ray films of similar quality are suitable.

## References

1. Wyllie, A. H. (1980) Glucocorticoid-induced thymocyte apoptosis is associated with endogenous endonuclease activation. *Nature* **284,** 555,556.
2. Oberhammer, F., Wilson, J. W., Dive, C., Morris, I. D., Hickman, J. A., Wakeling, A. E., et al. (1993) Apoptotic death in epithelial cells: cleavage of DNA to 300 and/or 50 kb fragments prior to or in the absence of internucleosomal fragmentation. *EMBO J.* **12,** 3679–3684.
3. Sun, D. Y., Jiang, S., Zheng, L. M., Ojcius, D. M., and Young, J. D. (1994) Separate metabolic pathways leading to DNA fragmentation and apoptotic chromatin condensation. *J. Exp. Med.* **179,** 559–568.
4. Cohen, G. M., Sun, X. M., Snowden, R. T., Dinsdale, D., and Skilleter, D. N. (1992) Key morpho-logical features of apoptosis may occur in the absence of internucleosomal DNA fragmentation. *Biochem. J.* **286,** 331–334.
5. Anthoney, D. A., McIlwrath, A. J., Gallagher, W. M., Edlin, A. R. M., and Brown, R. (1996) Microsatellite instability, apoptosis and loss of p53 function in drug resistant tumor cells. *Cancer Res.* **56,** 1374–1381.
6. Evan, G. I., Wyllie, A. H., Gilbert, C. S., Littlewood, T. D., Land, H., Brooks, M., et al. (1992) Induction of apoptosis in fibroblasts by c-myc protein. *Cell* **69,** 119–128.

# Measurement of Apoptotic Cells by Flow Cytometry (Tunnel Assay)

## Michael G. Ormerod

## 1. Introduction

### 1.1. General Comments

Apoptotic cells were originally recognized by their characteristic morphology. Since then, a series of biochemical changes have been described. However, it has yet to be established whether any of these changes unequivocally identify an apoptotic cell. In any study of apoptosis, it is important that the presence, or absence, of apoptotic cells is confirmed by morphological examination.

Ovarian cell lines normally grow attached to the surface of a culture dish. During apoptosis, the cells may round up and detach from the surface of the culture dish *(1,2)*. The nuclei of the detached cells can be stained using acridine orange or a benzimidazole dye (for example, Hoechst 33342) and apoptotic cells recognized by the characteristic morphology of their nuclei and counted under a fluorescence microscope. Photomicrographs of conventionally stained apoptotic ovarian carcinoma cells can be found in **refs.** *(1–3)*. It may be found that at least 90% of the detached cells are apoptotic and over 90% of the attached cells have normal nuclear morphology. In this case, if quantification is all that is desired, apoptosis could be followed by counting the detached cells.

### 1.2. Measurement of Apoptosis in Ovarian Cells

The *in situ* end labeling (ISEL) method for detecting DNA strand breaks in cells is described in this chapter. The assay is also given the acronym, TUNEL (Tdt-mediated dUTP nick-end labeling). In most cells, at the end stage of apoptosis, the DNA is degraded by an endonuclease at the linker regions between the nucleosomes. This creates oligomers with a unit size of about 180 bp. If the DNA is extracted and analyzed by gel electrophoresis a series of bands consisting of 1, 2, 3, 4, .q.q. units are observed—the so-called DNA ladder. The degradation creates large numbers of DNA strand breaks in the apoptotic cells.

The method can only be applied if apoptosis proceeds to this final stage. In some human ovarian carcinoma cell lines, DNA degradation is incomplete and the method would not be appropriate *(1)*. However, DNA degradation has been observed in other

From: *Methods in Molecular Medicine, Vol. 39: Ovarian Cancer: Methods and Protocols*
Edited by: J. M. S. Bartlett © Humana Press, Inc., Totowa, NJ

Fig. 1. Cytograms from a flow cytometric ISEL assay of a murine haemopoetic cell line (BAF3) incubated for 16 h in the absence of the growth factor, interleukin-3. These cells are used by us as a positive control. **Panel A.** Red fluorescence (PI-DNA), peak signal vs integrated area. The region, R1, encloses single cells and excludes clumps of cells. **Panel B.** Log green fluorescence vs red (DNA/PI) fluorescence. The green positive, apoptotic (*A*) and the green negative, normal (*N*) cells are marked. *D* marks cells that had undergone "secondary necrosis" and whose DNA was heavily degraded.

human ovarian carcinoma cell lines [*see*, for example, **refs.** *(4,5)*] and in cells from biopsies of ovarian tumors *(6)*.

When working with cultured cells, both the cells remaining adherent to the culture dish and the detached cells in the culture supernatant should be collected. They can be examined separately or the two populations pooled, depending on the purpose of the experiment.

### *1.3. The ISEL Method*

The ends of the broken strands of DNA are labeled by incorporating either biotin-11-dUTP or digoxigenin-11-dUTP or 5'-deoxybromouridine triphosphate using terminal deoxynucleotidyl transferase. Cells are fixed in paraformaldehyde to crosslink the small fragments of DNA into the cell before further fixation in 70% ethanol. They are incubated with the enzyme and a labeled nucleotide, which is detected using FITC-avidin, FITC-anti-digoxigenin, or FITC-anti-BrdUdr. After the addition of propidium iodide (PI) to label the DNA, green (FITC) vs red (PI) fluorescence is recorded in the flow cytometer. The apoptotic cells fluoresce green, the DNA stain indicates the cell cycle compartment from which apoptosis was induced (**Fig. 1**). The additional information about the cell cycle is one of the major advantages of ISEL.

The method using biotin-dUTP is described below. Kits are available from several manufacturers containing the reagents for the three variants of the ISEL assay.

### 2. Materials

1. Phosphate-buffered saline (PBS). Dissolve 1.06 g $Na_2HPO_4$, 0.39 g $NaH_2PO_4$, 8.8 g NaCl in distilled water. Adjust pH to 7.2 and make up to 1 L.
2. Paraformaldehyde (Sigma, St. Louis, MO, cat. no. P6148). Make up a 1% solution in PBS by gentle warming. Adjust pH to 7.0. Either make up fresh or aliquot and store frozen.
3. Tris-buffered saline (TBS): 150 m*M* NaCl in 50 m*M* Tris-HCl buffer, pH 7.6. Dissolve 6.06 g Tris (base), 1.39 g Tris-HCl, and 8.8 g NaCl in distilled water and make up to 1 L.

4. Reaction buffer (x5): 1 *M* Na cacodylate, 125 m*M* Tris-HCl, pH 6.6, 1.25 mg/mL bovine serum albumen (BSA) (Cohn Fraction V, Sigma, cat. no. A2153). Dissolve 1.96 g Tris-HCl, 16 g Na cacodylate, and 0.125 g BSA in distilled water and make up to 100 mL. Store at 4°C (*see* **Note 1**).

5. Enzyme mixture: immediately before use, for each sample to be analyzed, mix 20 U terminal deoxynucleotidyl transferase (TdT) (Pharmacia, Uppsala, Sweden, cat. no. 27-0730-02), 0.5 nm biotin-dUTP (Sigma, cat. no. B6780), 5 µL 25 m*M* CoCl$_2$, 10 µL reaction buffer, and 35 µL distilled water.

6. Rinsing buffer: PBS, 0.1% Triton X-100, 5% nonfat dried milk. Add 100 µL Triton X-100 to 100 mL PBS; warm to 37° to dissolve Triton. Store at 4°C. On day of use, add 5 g nonfat dried milk. Coarse filter and then filter through a 2-µm filter.

7. Incubation buffer: 0.6 *M* NaCl, 60 m*M* Na citrate, 0.1% Triton X-100, 5% nonfat dried milk. Dissolve 3.5 g NaCl, 1.76 g Na citrate, and 100 µL Triton X-100 in 100 mL distilled water. Warm to 37°C. Store at 4°C. On day of use, add 5 g nonfat dried milk. Coarse filter and then filter through a 2-µm filter.

8. Incubation buffer containing avidin-FITC (Sigma, cat. no. A2050) at 2.5 mg/mL.

9. PI solution. Dissolve 40 mg PI (Sigma, cat. no. P-4170 or Molecular Probes, Eugene, OR, cat. no. P-1304) in 100 mL distilled water. Store at 4°C.

10. Ribonuclease (RNase) solution (Sigma, cat. no. R5503). Dissolve 1 mg in 1 mL distilled water. Make up fresh just before use.

## 3. Methods

1. Make a suspension of single cells at approximately $2 \times 10^6$ cells/mL (*see* **Notes 2** and **3**).

2. Centrifuge at 300*g* for 5 min at room temperature. Discard the supernatant and resuspend the pellet thoroughly in 100 µL PBS.

3. Add 1 mL ice-cold 1% paraformaldehyde solution and leave on ice for 15 min.

4. Centrifuge as in **step 2**. Resuspend the pellet in ice-cold PBS. Centrifuge again as in **step 2**. Resuspend cell pellet thoroughly in 200 µL PBS.

5. Add vigorously 2 mL ice-cold 70% ethanol. Leave at least 30 min on ice. The cells can be stored indefinitely at –20°C in this state.

6. Centrifuge cells at 400*g* for 5 min at room temperature, discard supernatant, resuspend pellet in TBS (*see* **Note 4**).

7. Centrifuge cells at 300*g* for 4 min, resuspend cell pellet in 50 µL enzyme mixture (*see* **Note 5**). Incubate at 37°C for 1 h.

8. Centrifuge cells at 300*g* for 4 min, resuspend cell pellet in rinsing buffer. Repeat this washing procedure and finally resuspend the cell pellet in 100 µL incubation buffer containing avidin-FITC. Incubate on ice for 30 min.

9. Wash and pellet cells twice in rinsing buffer (as in **step 8**) and resuspend final pellet in 400 µL PBS. Add 50 µL RNase solution, 50 µL PI solution. Incubate for 30 min at 37°C.

10. Analyze on the flow cytometer using blue light (argon-ion laser at 488 nm) and measuring forward and right angle light scatter (FALS and RALS), green fluorescence, and red fluorescence. If possible, use doublet discrimination by measuring area and either peak or width of the red fluorescent signal. Measure green fluorescence using a logarithmic amplifier, red using a linear amplifier. Set the discriminator (threshold) on the red fluorescent signal. Using pulse shape analysis of this signal (7), set a region on the single cells; use this region as a gate to display a cytogram of green fluorescence (fluorescein; strand breaks) vs red fluorescence (PI; DNA). The apoptotic cells are green positive. The display also shows the phase of the cycle from which apoptosis was triggered.

A typical result for some cells used as a positive control is shown in **Fig. 1** (*see* **Note 6**).

## 4. Notes

1. Protein in the incubation and rinsing buffers reduces the nonspecific binding of the reagents to the cells. Nonfat milk is effective but, without filtration, can give an artefactual peak in the flow cytometric data *(8)*.
2. For cell cultures, during sample preparation, ensure that the number of single cells is maximized and that there are as few clumps of cells as possible. For clinical samples, if the sample is bloody, the erythrocytes should be removed. If there is enough sample (for example, from a peritoneal exudate), remove the red blood cells by density gradient centrifugation; a suitable method is given in **ref. *9***.
3. It is helpful if a positive control is included consisting of cells that are known to be apoptotic. Many workers use the human promyelocytic cell line, HL-60, incubated with 0.15 µ*M* camptothecin for 4 h. We have used a murine haemopoetic cell line incubated overnight in the absence of an essential growth factor *(8)*.
4. The objective of this wash is to remove any remaining phosphate, which will inhibit the enzyme reaction.
5. It is helpful to include a negative control in which the enzyme has been omitted from reaction mixture.
6. Files of listed flow cytometric data from cells analyzed by this method can be found in **ref. *10***.

## Acknowledgments

The author would like to thank Dr. Francesca Di Stefano, Cancer Research Campaign Cancer Therapeutics Centre, Institute of Cancer Research, Sutton, England, who supplied the cells used to prepare the figures, and Simone Detre, Academic Department of Biochemistry, Royal Marsden NHS Trust, London, who labeled the cells used for **Fig. 1**.

## References

1. Ormerod, M. G., O'Neill, C. F., Robertson, D., and Harrap, K. R. (1994) Cisplatin induces apoptosis in a human ovarian carcinoma cell line without concomitant internucleosomal degradation of DNA. *Exp. Cell Res.* **206,** 231–237.
2. Ormerod, M. G., O'Neill, C. F., Robertson, D., Kelland, L., and Harrap, K. R. (1996) Cis-diamminedichloroplatinum(II) induced cell death through apoptosis in sensitive and resistant human ovarian carcinoma cell lines. *Cancer Chemother. Pharmacol.* **37,** 463–471.
3. O'Neill, C. F., Ormerod, M. G., Robertson, D., Titley, J. C., Cumber-Waalsweer, Y., and Kelland, L. R. (1996) Apoptotic and non-apoptotic cell death induced by cis and trans analogues of a novel ammine(cyclohexylamine)dihydrodichloroplatinum(IV) complex. *Brit. J. Cancer* **74,** 1037–1045.
4. Filipovich, I. V., Sorokina, N. I., Robillard, N., and Chatal, J. F. (1997) Radiation-induced apoptosis in human ovarian carcinoma cells growing as a monolayer and as multicell spheroids. *Int. J. Cancer* **72,** 851–859.
5. Henkels, K. M. and Turchi, J. J. (1997) Induction of apoptosis in cisplatin-sensitive and -resistant ovarian cancer cell lines. *Cancer Res.* **57,** 4488–4492.
6. Yamasaki, F., Tokunaga, O., and Sugimori, H. (1997) Apoptotic index in ovarian carcinoma: correlation with clinicopathological factors and prognosis. *Gynecol. Oncol.* **66,** 439–448.
7. Ormerod, M. G. (1994) Analysis of DNA—general methods, in *Flow Cytometry: A Practical Approach* (Ormerod, M. G., ed.), IRL Press at Oxford University Press, Oxford. 2nd Ed., pp. 119–135.
8. Detre S., Ormerod, M. G., Titley, J. C., and Dowsett, M. (1997) An unusual artefact in the terminal deoxynucleotidyl transferase assay for apoptotic cells. *Cytometry* **28,** 264–267.
9. Ormerod, M. G. (1994) Preparing suspensions of single cells, in *Flow Cytometry: A Practical Approach* (Ormerod, M. G., ed.), IRL Press at Oxford University Press, Oxford. 2nd Ed., pp. 45–54.
10. Ormerod, M. G. (1996) *Data Analysis in Flow Cytometry—A Practical Approach.* CD-ROM publ. by M. G. Ormerod.

# 76

# Detection of Apoptosis in Ovarian Cells In Vitro and In Vivo Using the Annexin V-Affinity Assay

Manon van Engeland, Stefan M. van den Eijnde,
Thijs van Aken, Christl Vermeij-Keers, Frans C.S. Ramaekers,
Bert Schutte, and Chris P. M. Reutelingsperger

## 1. Introduction

The ability of a cell to undergo apoptosis is crucial during development, tissue homeostasis, and in the pathogenesis and treatment of disease (1). To study apoptosis, it is important to be able to detect apoptotic cells reliably. Here we describe a method to detect apoptosis in vitro and in vivo on basis of the changes in phospholipid distribution in the plasma membrane that occur during this process. In healthy cells, phosphatidylserine (PS) is maintained predominantly in the inner plasma membrane surface by an aminophospholipid translocase (2). However, early during apoptosis, PS is translocated from the inner to the outer membrane surface and serves as a trigger for adjacent phagocytes to remove the dying cell (3–5). Exposure of PS can be detected in vitro and in vivo with fluorochrome- or biotin-labeled annexin V, a protein that binds to negatively charged phospholipids in the presence of calcium ions (6,7). In cells that are cultured in suspension, detection of apoptosis on the basis of PS exposure is relatively easy (8). However, sample handling of adherent cell lines, such as the ovarian cell line PA-1, might interfere with reliable detection of PS exposure. Therefore, we developed a method to detect PS exposure in adherent cell lines by labeling cells in a monolayer with annexin V and harvesting the cells afterwards by mechanical scraping (9) (**Figs. 1** and **2**). Fixation of annexin V-labeled cells also allows the study of the relationship between PS exposure and expression of intracellular antigens (10). We also present a method to detect apoptosis in vivo during follicular maturation in the mouse (**Fig. 3**). This method is based on in vivo studies of viable mouse embryos, which indicate that PS exposure is a pancellular phenomenon of apoptosis during mammalian development (11,12).

Other studies have shown that loss of PS plasma membrane asymmetry during apoptosis is not restricted to mammals, but also applies to avian, insect (13,14), and plant cells (15) and, hence, appears to be a phylogenetically conserved phenomenon. The annexin V-affinity assay thus appears widely applicable in vitro and in vivo to measure apoptosis regardless of species, cell type, and the apoptosis inducing trigger.

From: *Methods in Molecular Medicine, Vol. 39: Ovarian Cancer: Methods and Protocols*
Edited by: J. M. S. Bartlett © Humana Press, Inc., Totowa, NJ

Fig. 1. Confocal scanning laser microscopy analysis of PA-1 ovary teratocarcinoma cells. Apoptosis was induced by treating the cells for 6 h with 50 μ*M* roscovitine, a cyclin-dependent kinase inhibitor. Cells were labeled with annexin V-Oregon green to detect PS exposure, harvested by mechanical scraping, and labeled with propidium iodide (PI) to detect plasma membrane integrity. **A** and **B** show a linear projection of a stack of confocal images of early apoptotic cells after labeling with annexin V. At this stage, the plasma membrane integrity is preserved and, therefore, PI cannot enter the cell. **C** shows a secondary necrotic PA-1 cell, with clear annexin V staining at the plasma membrane (**C1**) and with PI staining of the condensed and fragmented chromatin (**C2**).

## 2. Materials

### 2.1. In Vitro Annexin V Labeling of Apoptotic Cells in Adherent Ovarian Cell Lines

#### 2.1.1. Viable Cell Analysis

1. Adherent cell line of interest, exponentially grown in a culture flask or grown on glass slides [for example PA-1 ovary teratocarcinoma cells (ATCC), cultured in Eagle's minimum essential medium (EMEM) (Gibco, Paisley, Scotland) supplemented with 10% fetal calf serum (FCS) (Integro b.v., Zaandam, The Netherlands), gentamycin (AUV, Cuyck, The Netherlands, 0.05 mg/mL final concentration), and 10% nonessential amino acids (Gibco)].
2. 50 μ*M* roscovitine (dissolved in dimethyl sulfoxide (DMSO), Calbiochem, La Jolla, CA) or apoptosis inducing agent of interest.
3. Annexin V binding buffer (25 m*M* HEPES, 125 m*M* NaCl, 2.5 m*M* CaCl$_2$, included in APOPTEST™-kit, Nexins Research B.V., Hoeven, The Netherlands).

4. Fluorochrome conjugated annexin V: APOPTEST-FITC, APOPTEST-OREGON GREEN, or APOPTEST-PHYCOERYTHRIN (Nexins Research B.V., store at 4°C).
5. Propidium iodide (PI) (included in APOPTEST-kit, stock solution of 250 µg/mL in PBS/RNase A (10 mg/mL), store at 4°C).

### 2.1.2. Combined Annexin V Labeling and Intracellular Antigen Staining

6. Biotin-conjugated annexin V (APOPTEST-BIOTIN, product B700, Nexins Research B.V., store at 4°C).
7. Phosphate-buffered saline (PBS: 137 m$M$ NaCl, 2.7 m$M$ KCl, 6.5 m$M$ Na$_2$HPO$_4$ .2 H$_2$O, 1.5 m$M$ KH$_2$PO$_4$).
8. PBS/BSA (1%, Sigma, St. Louis, MO).

## 2.2. In Vivo Annexin V Labeling of Apoptotic Cells During Follicular Maturation in Mice

1. HEPES buffer (20 m$M$ HEPES (pH 7.4), 132 m$M$ NaCl, 2.5 m$M$ CaCl$_2$, 6 m$M$ KCl, 1 m$M$ MgSO$_4$, 1.2 m$M$ K$_2$HPO$_4$, 5.5 m$M$ glucose, 0.5% BSA, store at –20°C, use at 4°C).
2. Biotin-conjugated annexin V (APOPTEST-BIOTIN, product B500, Nexins Research B.V.)
3. Avertine for anaesthesia of the mouse: to make a stock solution of avertine, dissolve 5 g of 2,2,2-tribromoethanol (T4, 840-2, Aldrich Chemie, Zwijndrecht, The Netherlands) in 10 mL 2-methyl-2-butanol (15,264-3, Aldrich Chemie) at 40°C (both compounds are toxic). For a working solution, dissolve 1 mL of the stock solution in 24 mL of saline at 50–55°C. Sterilize the solution using a Millipore filter. Store the stock and the working solution in the dark at 4°C.

## 3. Methods

## 3.1. In Vitro Annexin V Labeling of Apoptotic Cells in Adherent Ovarian Cell Lines

### 3.1.1. Viable Cell Analysis

1. Add direct-labeled annexin V (dilute according to the manufacturers instructions) to the apoptotic, adherent cells in the culture flask or the cells grown on slides without washing the cells (*see* **Note 1**).
2. Incubate for 3–5 min at room temperature. In case of cells grown on glass slides, cells labeled with annexin V-FITC or annexin V-Oregon green can be visualized immediately using fluorescence microscopy with or without the addition of PI (*see* **step 7**).
3. Collect the culture medium (this fraction contains detached apoptotic cells).
4. Wash the adherent cells in the culture flask three times with culture medium or annexin V-binding buffer to remove excess annexin V, collect the rinse solution and pool this rinse solution with the collected culture medium from **step 3**. Pellet these cells by centrifugation (400$g$, 5 min, 4°C), discard the supernatant, resuspend the cell pellet in culture medium or annexin V-binding buffer, pellet the cells by centrifugation (2000$g$, min), discard the rinse medium, and repeat this washing procedure.
5. Scrape the adherent cells in culture medium gently with a rubber policeman, pellet the cells by centrifugation, and discard the culture medium (*see* **Notes 2–4**).
6. Resuspend the pellet of scraped cells in medium or annexin V-binding buffer and pool these cells with the cells that detached from the culture flask (cells collected in **step 4**) to a final concentration of 10$^6$ cells/mL.
7. Add PI to the cell suspension (final concentration 10 µg/mL for flow cytometry and 1 µg/mL for microscopy) and incubate on ice for 15 min (*see* **Notes 5–7**).

**Membrane integrity**

Fig. 2. Dotplot of bivariate PI/annexin V flow cytometric analysis of adherent ovary cell line PA-1. Plasma membrane integrity is shown on the X-axis and annexin V immunofluorescence is shown on the Y-axis. Cells were treated with 50 $\mu M$ roscovitine to induce apoptosis. 6 h after roscovitine treatment, cells were labeled with annexin V-Oregon green, harvested by scraping, and labeled with PI. Four populations of cells can be identified: region R1: vital cells (annexin V negative/PI negative), region R2: apoptotic cells (annexin V positive/PI negative), region R3: dead cells (annexin V positive/ PI positive); and region R4: damaged cells (annexin V negative/PI positive). For technical details, *see* **ref. 9**.

8. Analyze the cells by flow cytometry, fluorescence microscopy, or confocal scanning laser microscopy *(9)*.

### 3.1.2. Combined Annexin V Labeling and Intracellular Antigen Staining

1. Repeat **steps 1–6** in **Subheading 3.1.1.**, but use annexin V-Oregon green or annexin V-biotin (*see* **Notes 8** and **9**).
2. Pellet the cells by centrifugation, resuspend the cells in PBS, pellet the cells by centrifugation, and discard the PBS.
3. Fix the cells in methanol for 5 min at –20°C.
4. Pellet the cells by centrifugation 2000*g*, min, 4°C, discard methanol, and resuspend the cells in PBS.
5. Pellet the cells by centrifugation 2000*g*, min, 4°C, discard PBS, and resuspend the cells in PBS/BSA (1%).
6. Incubate cells with the primary antibody directed against the antigen of interest (dilute according to the manufacturers instructions) for 60 min at room temperature.
7. Pellet the cells by centrifugation, discard PBS/BSA, and resuspend the cells in PBS/BSA, repeat once.

8. Incubate cells with the secondary antibody (dilute according to manufacturers instructions) and in case of annexin V-biotin labeling, incubate with FITC-conjugated avidin (Vector Laboratories, 1:100 dilution) for 60 min at room temperature.

9. Pellet the cells, discard PBS/BSA, and resuspend the cells in PBS/BSA, repeat once.

10. Prepare a cell suspension in PBS/BSA of $10^6$ cells/mL.

11. Add PI to the cell suspension (final concentration 10 µg/mL for flow cytometry and 1 µg/mL for microscopy) and incubate on ice for 15 minutes (*see* **Note 10**).

12. Fluorescence microscopy, flow cytometry, or confocal scanning laser microscopy (*10*).

## 3.2. In Vivo Annexin V Labeling of Apoptotic Cells During Follicular Maturation in Mice

1. Anaesthetize the mouse with ether.

2. Carefully inject in approximately 0.5–1.0 min biotin-conjugated annexin V (15 mg/kg body weight) at 37°C into the tail vein (*see* **Notes 12–14**). As negative control for endogenous peroxidase activity, i.e., nonspecific staining with 3,3′ di-amino-benzidine tetrahydrochloride (DAB; handle with care, carcinogenic), mice can be injected with HEPES buffer only (*see* **Note 15**).

3. Place the mouse back into the cage under a heating lamp, so that body temperature is preserved (*see* **Note 16**).

4. Make a 3.6% formaldehyde/HEPES solution by diluting the stock formaldehyde solution (36%) in ice-cold HEPES buffer (1:10 v/v).

5. Fill vessel (20-mL counter vessel, Coulter, Hialeah, FL) with 3.6% formaldehyde/HEPES solution and put the vessels on ice.

6. 30 min after injection with annexin V, anaesthetize the mouse with an intraperitoneal (ip) injection of 0.5 mL avertine (*see* **Note 17**).

7. With its ventral side upwards, fix the mouse with adhesive tape over the limbs on a cooled metal plate.

8. When the mouse does not show a pain reflex anymore, make a midline abdominal incision using a pair of scissors.

9. Locate and excise the ovaries and put these directly in the 3.6% formaldehyde/HEPES containing vessel (for in vivo detection of annexin V-biotin at electron microscopical level, *see* **Note 18**).

10. Take care to kill the mouse by decapitation of cervical dislocation after the tissue(s) of interest have been removed from the animal (*see* **Notes 19** and **20**).

11. Fix the tissue overnight at 4°C in 3.6% formaldehyde/HEPES.

12. Dehydrate the tissue in a graded series of ethanol at room temperature, followed by incubation with toluol, toluol/paraffin (1:1 v:v), and paraffin (Paraplast, Sigma) at 60°C; all steps in 1-d intervals.

13. Embed the paraffin-immersed tissue on the tissue-embedding station.

14. Cut 3-µm sections on the microtome and mount these on 3-amino-propyl-triethoxy-silane coated slides.

15. To dewax the slides, heat for 60 min at 60°C.
    All subsequent steps are at room temperature.

16. Rinse the slides with xylene (2 × 2 min) and 100% ethanol (2 × 1 min).

17. Inactivate endogenous peroxidase activity by incubating the slides with 2% $H_2O_2$/methanol.

18. Rinse the slides with distilled water (1 min) and 0.1 *M* PBS pH 7.3 (2 × 2 min).

19. Incubate the slides for 30 min with horseradish peroxidase conjugated avidin, prepared according to manufacturers protocol (ABC Elite kit, Vector Laboratories, Burlingame, CA).

Fig. 3. Micrographs of paraffin sections through mice ovaries that were perfused with biotinylated annexin V (**A–F**) or HEPES-buffer only (**G** and **H**). In A, annexin V labeled early apoptotic cells (arrowhead) and late apoptotic-pyknotic (arrow) granulosa cells are shown. During follicle maturation, initially apoptosis is absent (B). At later phases, annexin V labeled apoptotic granulosa cells (C, arrow) were observed in the primary (C) and secondary (D)

20. Wash the slides with 0.1 *M* PBS pH 7.3 (2 × 2 min).
21. Incubate slides for 7 min in the dark with a 0.75% DAB/PBS pH 7.3 (w/v) solution containing 0.075% $H_2O_2$.
22. Rinse the slides with tap water for 6 min.
23. Stain the sections for 10 s to 1 min with undiluted Gills Hematoxylin (Sigma Diagnostics, Deisenhofen, Germany).
24. Rinse the slides with tap water (10 s).
25. Differentiate staining by washing slides with 0.25% HCl/70% ethanol for 10 s.
26. Rinse the slides with tap water for 6 min.
27. Dehydrate slides with a graded series of ethanol followed by xylene (each step, 1 min).
28. Mount the slides (Permount, Fisher Scientific, Pittsburgh, PA).
29. Light microscopy.

## 4. Notes

1. Make sure that the culture medium contains 2.5 m*M* $Ca^{2+}$. Annexin V can only bind to PS in the presence of 2.5 m*M* $Ca^{2+}$.
2. Removal of annexin V before scraping the adherent cells prevents annexin V binding to internally located PS in cells that become damaged (permeable) caused by the scraping procedure.
3. Trypsin or ethylenedlaminetetraacetic acid (EDTA) harvesting of cells before annexin V labeling can induce changes in the plasma membrane, which leads to false positive results due to binding of annexin V to PS.
4. Trypsin or EDTA treatment after annexin V labeling interferes with the detection of bound annexin V, because trypsin and EDTA remove bound annexin V by proteolysis and chelation of $Ca^{2+}$ ions respectively. To avoid false positive results, use a rubber policeman for harvesting the cells.
5. Annexin V is able to detect PS at the outer surface of the plasma membrane, however, annexin V also binds internally located PS in necrotic cells in which the plasma membrane is permeable. Therefore, in in vitro assays, a membrane impermeable vital dye as propidium iodide (PI) must to be included in the assay to monitor plasma membrane integrity and to discriminate between apoptotic and necrotic cells (*12–15*).
6. In nonfixed cells, PI discriminates between viable and dead cells on the basis of membrane permeability of the dye.
7. Using the scraping method, four populations of cells can be detected after staining with annexin V and PI: (a) viable cells which are annexin V-negative/PI-negative; (b) apoptotic cells that are annexin V-positive/PI-negative; (c) (secondary) necrotic cells that are annexin V-positive/PI-positive; and (d) cells which are damaged during the scraping procedure and which are annexin V negative/PI positive.
8. The fluorescent properties of FITC are impaired by methanol fixation, therefore, the use of annexin V-Oregon green (low photo bleaching and pH insensitivity) or annexin V-biotin is recommended while fixing the cells.

---

Fig. 3. *(continued)* follicles. Unstained pyknotic cells were also observed (C, arrowhead), presumably these cells were already located in the phagosomes before perfusion with annexin V. Also in the Graafian follicle, apoptotic cells were present in large numbers (E). F shows an enlargement of the boxed area in E. Labeled apoptotic and postapoptotic necrotic cells that have been shed into the antrum are clearly visible (asterisk), as well as unlabeled late postapoptotic necrotic cells. Labeling of ingested (arrowhead) and noningested (arrow) apoptotic cells was absent in ovaries of specimen that were perfused with HEPES-buffer only (G: overview, H: detail of boxed area in G). Scale bars equal 10 μm (A), 25 μm (C, F, and H), 50 μm (B and D) and 100 μm (E and G).

9. APOPTEST-biotin, product B700 is recommended in in vitro experiments.

10. After fixation of cells, PI cannot be used to discriminate between apoptotic and necrotic cells by membrane permeability. In these cells, PI indicates DNA content of the cells.

11. Scraping of adherent cells introduces a population of annexin V-negative, PI- positive damaged cells. The proportion of this population of cells depends on the cell type and on the method of scraping.

12. APOPTEST-BIOTIN, product B500 is recommended in in vivo experiments.

13. Annexin V can be diluted in sterile HEPES buffer.

14. To avoid overload of the systemic volume of the mouse, do not inject more than 0.5 mL of annexin V solution.

15. As negative control, injection of mice with biotin-conjugated annexin V that has been heat inactivated at 56°C for 10 min can be used (16). In this manner, not only is tested for endogenous peroxidase activity, but also for nonspecific binding of biotinylated annexin V (11).

16. Annexin V inhibits blood coagulation: care should be taken to stop bleeding at the site of the puncture.

17. Keeping the mouse alive during removal of tissues limits the presence of postmortem artifacts. If only the ovaries are to be removed, this procedure may be done so quickly that excision can take place after killing the mouse by cervical dislocation directly after 30 min of perfusion with annexin V.

18. If necessary, tissues from specimens that have been perfused with biotin-conjugated annexin V can be tested for the presence of intracellular staining at the ultrastructural level (for technical details *see* **refs. 11,12**). This may help to asses whether the annexin V stained cells were indeed apoptotic (membrane labeling) or (postapoptotic) necrotic (intracellular staining). Under physiological conditions in vivo, the tissue-embedded apoptotic cells are cleared rapidly from the environment by phagocytes, before its plasma membrane has become disrupted, and the "so-called" postapoptotic necrotic cells elicit an inflammatory reaction. Hence, annexin V binding to tissue-embedded cells in vivo will normally be limited to staying at the outer layer of the plasma membrane. However, apoptotic cells that have been shed into a lumen are normally not cleared by phagocytosis, become postapoptotic necrotic, and also will stain with annexin V both intra- and extra-cellularly. Late necrotic cells will lose the ability to bind annexin V with the proceeding of the plasma membrane degradation. Apoptotic cells that were ingested by phagocytes before annexin V binding will not be labeled either, because annexin V does not pass the plasma membrane of viable phagocytes (11–14).

19. Annexin V is rapidly cleared from the blood, via the kidneys. This property can be used as a positive control for a correct systemic perfusion with biotinylated annexin V. For this control, in addition to ovaries, also dissect out the retroperitoneally located kidneys. Staining for annexin V labeling is similar to the procedures described for the ovaries. If the injection with biotinylated annexin V was successful, labeling should be present in the secondary tubes of the nephrons.

20. After systemic perfusion with annexin V, binding to apoptotic cells is not restricted to the ovaries, but present throughout the animal.

## References

1. Thompson, C. B. (1995) Apoptosis in the pathogenesis and treatment of disease. *Science* **267**, 1456–1462.

2. Diaz, C. and Schroit, A. J. (1996) Role of translocases in the generation of phosphatidylserine asymmetry. *J. Memb. Biol.* **151**, 1–9.

3. Fadok, V. A., Voelker, D. R., Campbell, P. A. S., Cohen, J. J., Bratton, D. L., and Henson, P. M. (1992a) Exposure of phosphatidylserine on the surface of apoptotic lymphocytes triggers specific recognition and removal by macrophages. *J. Immunol.* **148**, 2207–2216.

4. Fadok, V. A., Savill, J. S., Haslett, C., Bratton, D. L., Doherty, D. E., Campbell, P. A., et al. (1992b) Different populations of macrophages use either the vitronectin receptor or the phosphatidylserine receptor to recognize and remove apoptotic cells. *J. Immunol.* **149,** 4029–4035.

5. Savill, J. S. (1996) The innate immune system: recognition of apoptotic cells, in *Apoptosis and the Immune Response* (Gregory, C. D., ed.), Wiley Liss, New York, pp. 341–370.

6. van Heerde, W. L., de Groot, P. G., and Reutelingsperger, C. P. M. (1995) The complexity of the phospholipid binding protein annexin V. *Thromb. Haemost.* **73,** 172–179.

7. van Engeland, M., Nieland, L. J. W., Ramaekers, F. C. S., Schutte, B., and Reutelingsperger, C. P. M. (1998) Annexin V-affinity assay: a review on an apoptosis detection system based on phosphatidylserine exposure. *Cytometry* **31,** 1–9.

8. Koopman, G., Reutelingsperger, C. P. M., Kuijten, G. A. M., Keehnen, R. M. J., Pals, S. T., and van Oers, M. H. J. (1994) Annexin V for flow cytometric detection of phosphatidylserine expression on B cells undergoing apoptosis. *Blood* **84,** 1415–1420.

9. van Engeland, M., Ramaekers, F. C. S., Schutte, B., and Reutelingsperger, C. P. M. (1996) A novel assay to measure loss of plasma membrane asymmetry during apoptosis of adherent cells in culture. *Cytometry* **24,** 131–139.

10. van Engeland, M., Kuijpers, H. J. H., Ramaekers, F. C. S., Reutelingsperger, C. P. M., and Schutte, B. (1997) Plasma membrane alterations and cytoskeletal changes in apoptosis. *Exp. Cell Res.* **235,** 421–430.

11. van den Eijnde, S. M., Boshart, L., Reutelingsperger, C. P. M., de Zeeuw, C. I., and Vermeij-Keers, C. (1997) Phosphatidylserine plasma membrane asymmetry in vivo: a pancellular phenomenon which alters during apoptosis. *Cell Death Differ.* **4,** 311–317.

12. van den Eijnde, S. M., Luijsterburg, A. J. M., Boshart, L., de Zeeuw, C. I., van Dierendonck, J. H., Reutelingsperger, C. P. M., et al. (1997) In situ detection of apoptosis during embryogenesis with annexin V: from whole mount to ultrastructure. *Cytometry* **29,** 313–320.

13. van den Eijnde, S. M., Boshart, L., Baehrecke, E., de Zeeuw, C. I., Reutelingsperger, C. P. M., and Vermeij-Keers, C. (1998) Phosphatidylserine exposure by apoptotic cells is phylogenetically conserved. *Apoptosis* **3,** 9–16.

14. van den Eijnde, S. M., Boshart, L., Baehrecke, E., Reutelingsperger, C. P. M., and Vermeij-Keers, C. (1998) In: Pharmaceutical intervention in apoptotic pathways (Nagelkerke, J. F., van Dierendonck, J. M., and Noteborn, M. H. M., eds.), Amsterdam, Oxford, New York, Tokyo, pp. 63–74. Phosphatidylserine exposure by apoptotic cells; a phylogenetically conserved mechanism. *Proc. Royal Netherlands Acad. Sciences Colloquia,* in press.

15. O'Brien, I. E. W., Reutelingsperger, C. P. M., and Holdaway, K. M. (1997) Annexin V and TUNEL use in monitoring the progression of apoptosis in plants. *Cytometry* **29,** 28–33.

16. Reutelingsperger, C. P. M., Hornstra, G., and Hemker, H. C. (1985) Isolation and partial purification of a novel anticoagulant from arteries of human umbilical cord. *Eur. J. Biochem.* **151,** 625–629.

# 77

# Use of Diphenylamine in the Detection of Apoptosis

## Randall K. Gibb and Cicek Gercel-Taylor

## 1. Introduction

The diphenylamine assay is a very useful tool in measuring apoptosis by determining the percentage of fragmentation of known amounts of DNA into oligosomal-sized fragments. Another advantage of the diphenylamine assay is that apoptotic DNA fragmentation can be analyzed in both adherent and shed cells following treatment or experimentation. Data obtained from the experiment are expressed as a percentage relative to uninduced or untreated controls. This assay was first described by Dische (1,2) in the 1930s and later modified by Burton (3) in the mid-1950s. These modifications have resulted in an enhanced sensitivity of up to five times by adding sulfuric acid and acetaldehyde, and by allowing the colorimetric reaction to develop overnight at room temperature. These changes have also resulted in a reduction of the interference from other substances that were an initial drawback with the originally described method, further enhancing the sensitivity of the assay. The diphenylamine reaction takes advantage of the bonds between purines and deoxyribose, which are very labile. Once these bonds are broken, inorganic phosphates are liberated from the DNA and provide the substrate, which is measured by the reaction. The overall preparation time is approximately 3 h for 30 samples with incubation occurring overnight for 12 to 16 h. Reading of the results takes approximately 1 min per sample. This assay has been used to detect apoptotic fragmentation by others, and more recently by our group to evaluate cisplatin and Taxol induced fragmentation in ovarian carcinoma cell lines (4).

## 2. Materials

1. Phosphate-buffered saline (PBS): 10 m$M$ sodium phosphate, 150 m$M$ NaCl, pH 7.4.
2. Trichloroacetic acid: 10% and 5% solutions in double distilled water (ddH$_2$O).
3. Lysis buffer: 5 m$M$ Tris, 20 m$M$ ethylenediaminetetraacetic acid (EDTA), pH 8.0, 0.5% Triton X-100 (added immediately before use).
4. TE buffer: 10 m$M$ Tris, 1 m$M$ EDTA, pH 8.0.
5. Diphenylamine reagent: 1.5 g diphenylamine in 100 mL of acetic acid and 1.5 mL H$_2$SO$_4$, (store in the dark). Immediately before use, add acetaldehyde in the cold room to a final concentration of 16 μg/mL (see **Note 1**). This reagent is stable without acetaldehyde for at least 3 mo at 4°C (see **Note 2**).

From: *Methods in Molecular Medicine, Vol. 39: Ovarian Cancer: Methods and Protocols*
Edited by: J. M. S. Bartlett © Humana Press, Inc., Totowa, NJ

## 3. Methods

### 3.1. Quantitation of DNA Fragmentation

1. Harvest monolayer cultures with a rubber policeman (or directly into centrifuge tubes for suspension cultures) and centrifuge ($300g$) at 4°C for 10 min to pellet the cells (*see* **Note 3**).
2. Resuspend the cell pellet in 0.8 mL of 0.01 $M$ PBS, pH 7.4, and 0.7 mL of ice-cold lysis buffer. Transfer the cell lysate to microfuge tubes and incubate on ice for 15 min (*see* **Note 4**).
3. Centrifuge the lysates ($13,000g$) at 4°C for 15 min to separate fragmented DNA from high-molecular-weight DNA.
4. Transfer the entire supernatant (about 1.5 mL that contains fragmented DNA) to a 5-mL glass tube (*see* **Note 5**).
5. Resuspend the pellet that contains intact DNA in 1.5 mL TE, and again transfer to another 5-mL glass tube.
6. Add 1.5 mL of 10% TCA to each tube and incubate for 10 min at room temperature.
7. Centrifuge ($500g$) at 4°C for 15 min and discard the supernatant.
8. Resuspend the 10% TCA precipitates in 0.7 mL of 5% TCA, boil (100°C) for 15 min (*see* **Note 6**), cool to room temperature, and centrifuge ($300g$) at 4°C for 15 min.
9. Transfer 0.5 mL of the supernatant without disturbing the precipitate to a new glass tube, add 1 mL of the diphenylamine reagent, and incubate overnight at 30°C (*see* **Note 7**).
10. Measure the absorbance at 600 nm.
11. Percentage of DNA fragmentation = $OD_{600}$ of the supernatant / $OD_{600}$ of the supernatant + $OD_{600}$ of the pellet.

## 4. Notes

1. When mixing the acetic acid and sulfuric acid together, wear protective gloves as these substances are extremely caustic. Also note that a cold room is a designated place to add the diphenylamine so harmful vapors are kept to a minimum.
2. If the diphenylamine reagent has any trace of blue discoloration, we recommend that a new reagent be made because this can influence the $OD_{600}$ reading and affect your calculations in an uncontroled fashion.
3. We recommend a minimum of $2.5 \times 10^6$ cells for adequate DNA fragmentation determination, however, two times this amount ($5.0 \times 10^6$) is preferable.
4. Make sure that the suspension created after lysis is homogeneous prior to centrifugation to ensure adequate separation of the fragmented from intact DNA.
5. It is very important not to disturb the precipitate formed in **step 4** because this can interfere with subsequent readings between the fragmented and intact DNA. The use of a micropipet is highly recommended.
6. It is recommended that a water bath at 100°C is ready prior to processing the samples.
7. The time of incubation may be prolonged past 16 h if the colorimetric reaction is weak.

## References

1. Dische, Z. (1930) *Mikrochemise* **8,** 4.
2. Dische, Z. (1955) *The Nucleic Acids* (Chargraff, E. and Davidson, J. N., eds.), Academic, New York.
3. Burton, K. (1956) A study of the conditions and mechanisms of the diphenylamine reaction for the colorimetric estimation of deoxyribonucleic acid. *Biochem. J.* **62,** 315–323.
4. Gibb, R. K., Taylor, D. D., Wan, T., O'Connor, D. M., Doering, D. L., and GerHel-Taylor, Γ. (1997) Apoptosis as a measure of chemosensitivity to cisplatin and taxol therapy in ovarian cancer cell lines. *Gynecolog. Oncol.* **65,** 13–22.

# 78

## Activation of Caspase Protease
## During Apoptosis in Ovarian Cancer Cells

**Zhihong Chen, Mikihiko Naito, Tetsuo Mashima, Seimiya Hiroyuki, and Takashi Tsuruo**

## 1. Introduction

As a genetically controlled program, apoptosis has important roles in a variety of biological processes. The realization that chemotherapy can also induce apoptosis in some cancer cells both in vitro and in vivo indicates apoptosis may play a very important role in cancer and cancer therapy *(1,2)*. Many of the molecules that participate in the apoptotic cell suicide have been identified. At the heart of this pathway are a family of cysteine proteases, the "caspases" *(3)*.

Caspases are cysteine proteases and are specific for cleavage after Asp residues. Specific members of the caspase family have been identified as the enzymes responsible for the proteolysis of key proteins that are known to be selectively cleaved at the onset of apoptosis *(4)*, and potent inhibitors of these proteases such as Z-Asp-CH$_2$DCB, Z-EVD-CH$_2$DCB, Ac-YVAD-CHO, Ac-DEVD-CHO prevent apoptosis *(5–10)*. These observations indicate that the caspase family are involved in apoptosis.

Caspase-3 is a 32 kDa proenzyme. The active form is composed of two subunits, one of 17 kDa and one of 12 kDa, both of which are derived from the 32-kDa proenzyme by excision at Asp-x sites. The three-dimensional crystal structures of the mature forms of caspase-3 revealed that the consensus sequence for cleavage of macromolecular and peptide substrates by caspase-3 is DxxD, with the optimal peptide recognition motif DExD *(11)*. Therefore, fluorogenic substrate DEVD-MCA can be used to determine activation of caspase-3-like proteases.

Many proteins are believed to be cleaved by caspases during apoptosis. Actin is one of the substrates of caspase-3 *(12–14)*. In this chapter, we will describe caspase-3 (CPP32/Yama/Apopain), an actin-cleavable protease, activation during chemotherapy-induced apoptosis in ovarian cancer cells.

## 2. Materials

1. Lysis buffer. 10 m$M$ Tris-HCl, pH 8.1, 5 m$M$ dithiothreitol (DTT), 1 m$M$ phenylmethylsulfonylfluoride, 1 µg/mL leupeptin, 1 µg/mL pepstatin (*see* **Note 1**).

From: *Methods in Molecular Medicine, Vol. 39: Ovarian Cancer: Methods and Protocols*
Edited by: J. M. S. Bartlett © Humana Press, Inc., Totowa, NJ

Fig. 1. Activation of caspase-3 (CPP32) protease in cDDP-treated apoptotic OVCAR-3 cells that can be prevented by caspase inhibitors. **A:** Apoptosis induced by cDDP treatment in OVCAR-3 cells. **B:** DEVD-cleaving activity in the cell lysates treated with 10 μg/mL of cDDP for 48 h in the absence or presence of 100 μg/mL of caspase inhibitor Z-Asp-CH₂DCB (Z-Asp). **C:** Processing of caspase-3 to active form p17 was determined by western blot analysis. **D:** Actin cleavage activity in apoptotic OVCAR-3 cell lysate which can be inhibited by Z-EVD-CH₂DCB (Z-EVD).

2.  Assay buffer. 20 m$M$ HEPES, pH 7.5, 2 m$M$ DTT, 10% (v/v) glycerol (*see* **Note 2**).
3.  Blocking buffer. TBST (10 m$M$ Tris-HCl, pH 7.5, 100 m$M$ NaCl, 0.1% (v/v)Tween-20) 5% (w/v) milk.
4.  Washing buffer. TBST (10 m$M$ Tris-HCl pH 7.5, 100 m$M$ NaCl, 0.1% (v/v) Tween-20).

Fig. 1C & D

## 3. Methods

### 3.1. Drug Treatment

1. Human ovarian carcinoma OVCAR-3 cells were maintained in RPMI-1640 medium (Nissui Co., Ltd. Tokyo, Japan) supplemented with 10% heat-inactivated fetal bovine serum and 100 μg/mL of kanamycin in a humidified atmosphere of 5% $CO_2$ and 95% air.

2. Logarithmically growing OVCAR-3 cells were harvested by trypsinization and seeded at an initial density of $2 \times 10^5$ cells in 10 mL of fresh medium in a 10-cm dish.

3. After overnight incubation, cDDP was added from 1000-fold concentrated stocks in dimethyl sulfoxide (DMSO) with a final concentration of 0.1% DMSO in medium in the presence or absence of Z-EVD-CH$_2$DCB or Z-Asp-CH$_2$DCB (Funakoshi, Tokyo, Japan) (*see* **Notes 3** and **4**).

4. After various periods of incubation, floating cells were collected and adhesive cells were trypsinized 5 min at 37°C, combined and sedimented at 800$g$ for 10 min, and then assays were performed.

5. The drug-treated cells were harvested, washed with ice-cold PBS once, and then resuspended in lysis buffer.

6. Cells were freeze-thawed four times at –80°C and 4°C and finally centrifuged for 20 min at 70,000$g$. The supernatant was taken as cell lysate.

## 3.2. Assay of DEVD-Cleaving Activity

1. The cDDP-treated cell lysate (10 µg of protein) was incubated with 1 m$M$ DEVD-MCA (Peptide Institute, Osaka, Japan) at 37°C for 30 min in the assay buffer (*see* **Note 5**).

2. The release of amino-4-methylcoumarin (AMC) was monitored by a spectrofluorometer (Hitachi F-2000), using an excitation wavelength of 380 nm and an emission wavelength of 460 nm. One unit was defined as the amount of enzyme required to release 1 pmol AMC per min at 37°C.

## 3.3. Detection of Caspase-3 Processing to Active Form p17

1. The cDDP-treated cell lysate 40 µg protein/lane was electrophoresed in 15/25% gradient polyacrylamide gel and then transferred to a nitrocellulose membrane (*see* Chapter 54 and **Note 6**).

2. After blocking 2 h at room temperature, the membrane was incubated for 2 h at 25°C with anti-CPP32 antibody (Transduction Laboratories, Lexington, KY), which was diluted 1:250 in blocking buffer.

3. Wash the membrane 10 min with washing buffer, three times.

4. Second antibody (antimouse IgG) was diluted to 1:250 with the blocking buffer, and the membrane was incubated for 1 h at room temperature.

5. After washing three times, immunodetection was performed using the enhanced chemiluminescence kit for Western blotting detection (Amersham, Arlington Heights, IL) (*see* **Note 7**).

## 3.4. Actin Cleavage Activity (ACA) Assay

1. Rabbit muscle actin was labeled with biotin by incubation with 100 µg/mL sulfosuccinimidyl-6-(biotinamido) hexanoate-biotin (Pierce, Rockfold, IL) at 25°C for 40 min in 1 $M$ HEPES (pH 8.0).

2. The biotinylated actin (0.2 µg/assay) was incubated with cell cytosolic fractions at 37°C for 3 h in the assay buffer.

3. The reaction mixtures were separated by 15/25% gradient polyacrylamide gel (Daiichi Chemical, Tokyo, Japan).

4. The electrophoresed proteins in the polyacrylamide gel were transblotted onto a nitrocellulose membrane.

5. After blocking, the blotted membrane was incubated with peroxidase-conjugated avidin (ABC kit, Vector Labs, Burkingame, CA) at 25°C for 1 h.

6. Wash three times with PBS –0.5% Tween-20.

7. Soak in an enhanced chemiluminescence (ECL) mixture (Amersham, Buckinghamshire, U.K.), and expose to Kodak X-Omat AR film.

## 4. Notes

1. Store at $-20°C$.
2. Make 5- or 10-fold concentrated solution, and store at $-20°C$.
3. Cisplatin should be stored at 4°C as powder, dissolved with DMSO to 1000-fold concentrated solution of final concentration just before use. Make fresh for every use.
4. Z-EVD-CH$_2$DCB and Z-Asp-CH$_2$DCB were dissolved in DMSO to 100 µg/µL, the final concentration was usually 100 µg/mL.
5. The amount of lysate (protein) or/and substrate DEVD-MCA and the incubation time can be changed according to the signal strength. Fluorogenic substrate DEVD-MCA is light-sensitive, should be dissolved in DMSO, and stored at $-20°C$ under light protection.
6. PVDF (polyvinylidene difluoride) membrane can also be used.
7. If the signal is weak, apply the lysate protein up to 100 µg/lane, and extend the exposure time to 1 h or even overnight.

## References

1. Kaufmann, S. H. (1989) Induction of endonucleolytic DNA cleavage in human acute myelogenous leukemia cells by etoposide, camptothecin, and other cytotoxic anti-cancer drugs: a cautionary note. *Cancer Res.* **49,** 5870–5878.
2. Meyn, R. E., Stephens, L. C., Hunter, N. R., and Milas, L. (1995) Apoptosis in murine tumors treated with chemotherapy agents. *Anticancer Drugs* **6,** 443–450.
3. Nicholson, D. W. and Thornberry, N. A. (1997) Caspase: killer proteases. *Trends Biochem. Sci.* **22,** 299–306.
4. Thornberry, N. A., Rosen, A., and Nicholson, D. W. (1997) Control of apoptosis by proteases. *Adv. Pharmacol.* **41,** 155–177.
5. Los, M., Van de Craen, M., Penning, L. C., Schenk, H., Westendorp, M., Baeuerle, P. A., et al. (1995) Requirement of an ICE/CED-3 protease for Fas/APO-1-mediated apoptosis. *Nature* **375,** 81–83.
6. Enari, M., Hug, H., and Nagata, S. (1995) Involvment of an ICE-like protease in Fas-mediated apoptosis. *Nature* **375,** 78–81.
7. Mashima, T., Naito, M., Kataoka, S., Kawai, H., and Tsuruo, T. (1995) Aspartate-based inhibitor of interleukin-1-β-converting enzyme prevents antitumor agent-induced apoptosis in human myeloid leukemia U937 cells. *Biochem. Biophys. Res. Commun.* **209,** 907–915.
8. Slee, E. A., Zhu, H., Chow, S. C., MacFarlane, M., Nicholson, D. W., and Cohen, G. M., (1996) Benzyloxycarbonyl-Val-Ala-Asp (OMe) fluoromethylketone (Z-VAD.FMK) inhibits apoptosis by blocking the processing of CPP32. *Biochem. J.* **315,** 21–24.
9. Nicholson, D. W., Ali, A., Thornberry, N. A., Vaillancourt, J. P., Ding, C. K., Gallant, M., et al. (1995) Identification and inhibition of the ICE/CED-3 protease necessary for mammalian apoptosis. *Nature* **376,** 37–43.
10. Dolle, R. E., Hoyer, D., Prasad, C. V., Schmidt, S. J., Helaszek, C. T., Miller, R. E., et al. (1994) P1 aspartate-based peptide a-((2,6-dichlorobenzoyl)oxy)methyl ketones as potent time-dependent inhibitors of interleukin-1-β-converting enzyme. *J. Med. Chem.* **37,** 563,564.
11. Rotonda, J., Nicholson, D. W., Fazil, K. M., Gallant, M., Gareau, Y., Labelle, M., et al. (1996) The three-dimensional structure of apopain/CPP32, a key mediator of apoptosis. *Nat. Struct. Biol.* **3,** 619–625.
12. Mashima, T., Naito, M., Fujita, N., Noguchi, K., and Tsuruo, T. (1995) Identification of actin as a substrate of ICE and an ICE-like protease and involvment of an ICE-like protease but not ICE in VP-16-induced U937 apoptosis. *Biochem. Biophys. Res. Commun.* **217,** 1185–1192.
13. Chen, Z., Naito, M., Mashima, T., and Tsuruo, T. (1996) Activation of actin-cleavable interleukin-1-β-converting enzyme (ICE) family protease CPP32 during chemotherapeutic agent-induced apoptosis in ovarian carcinoma cells. *Cancer Res.* **56,** 5224–5229.
14. Mashima, T., Naito, M., Noguchi, K., Miller, D. K., Nicholson, D. W., and Tsuruo, T. (1997) Actin cleavage by CPP32/apopain during the development of apoptosis. *Oncogene* **14,** 1007–1012.

# 79

# Differential Expression of Apoptosis-Associated Genes *bax* and *bcl*-2 in Ovarian Cancer

## Dagmar Marx and Harald Meden

## 1. Introduction

The deregulation of the balance between proliferation and programmed cell death is considered one of the most important features of malignant tumors. The search for new markers, which may reflect the tumor progress and response to various therapy regimens, has recently focused on alterations of genes involved in regulation of programmed cell death and apoptosis. The *bcl*-2-family is a still growing family of genes, which play a major role in regulation of cell suicide, acting either as inhibitors (e.g., *bcl*-2, *bcl*-$x_l$, *mcl*-1) or promoters (e.g., *bcl*-$x_s$, *bax*, *bak*, *bad*) of apoptosis *(1–3)*. The chromosomal translocation t(14;18), leading to overexpression of the *Bcl*-2 protein was first described in human B-cell lymphoma *(4)*. Later on, *Bcl*-2-overexpression without chromosomal translocations was also detected in various epithelial tumors *(5–12)*. It has been suggested that *Bcl*-2 as the major inhibitor of apoptosis plays a role in tumor development and progress by prolonging the survival of malignant cells. Unexpectedly, expression of *Bcl*-2 has been shown to be connected with parameters of favorable prognosis and prolonged survival in nonsmall-cell lung cancer *(6)*, breast *(7–9)*, and, recently, in ovarian cancer *(10–12)*. *Bax*-expression, in contrast, was associated with an unfavorable outcome, as well as negative histopathological features in breast *(13)* and ovarian cancer *(12)*. Moreover, the association of *Bax*-expression with predictors of poor clinical outcome was strongly connected with concomitant downregulation of *Bcl*-2-expression *(12,13)*. The unexpected effect of *Bcl*-2- and *Bax*-expression on prognosis of ovarian cancer patients is underlined by the survival curves of patients. Especially, patients with exclusively *Bax*-positive tumors had a statistically significantly reduced survival as compared to patients with exclusively *Bcl*-2-positive tumors *(12)*. This difference could be observed for patients with tumors of different stage and grade, as well as for patients with no evidence of disease or residual tumor after primary surgery *(12)*. One explanation for these observations is that the apoptosis inhibiting or promoting effect of these homologous proteins depends partly on protein–protein interactions. *Bax*, for example, the main antagonist of *Bcl*-2, heterodimerizes with *Bcl*-2 or *Bcl*-$X_1$ and homodimerizes with itself *(1–3)*. The ratio of *Bax*-heterodimers to *Bax*-homodimers seems to be the critical determinant for regulating cell death *(2,3)*. In cells in which 80% of *Bax* is found in homodimers, an apoptotic signal results in cell

From: *Methods in Molecular Medicine, Vol. 39: Ovarian Cancer: Methods and Protocols*
Edited by: J. M. S. Bartlett © Humana Press, Inc., Totowa, NJ

death *(2,3)*, suggesting a crucial role of the *Bax/Bcl*-2 balance for the regulation of proliferation or cell suicide.

From recent studies concerning breast and ovarian cancer, it may be suggested that during tumor development, expression of *Bcl*-2 is downregulated, whereas expression of *Bax* is unimpaired or activated *(12,13)*. Thus, deregulation of the *Bcl*-2/*Bax*-balance seems to be associated with malignant progression and may influence the clinical course by deregulation of programmed cell death and altered sensitivity to chemotherapy. Expression of *Bax* and *Bcl*-2 might therefore represent additional markers in predicting the prognosis of ovarian cancer patients. For this reason, easy and reproducible techniques, even successful for routinely formalin-fixed and paraffin-embedded material, have to be performed. Therefore, immunohistochemistry seems to be one method of choice.

## 2. Materials

1. Polyclonal rabbit anti-*Bax* antibody N-20 (Santa Cruz, CA; 100 µg/mL) in TBS.
2. Monoclonal mouse anti-*Bcl*-2 antibody (clone 124, Dako, Germany; 320 µg/mL) in TBS.
3. Rabbit antimouse antibody (Dako) diluted 1:50 in TBS/10% human serum.
4. Mouse antirabbit antibody (Dako) diluted 1:50 in TBS/10% human serum.
5. Mouse apaap-(alkaline phosphatase-antialkaline phosphatase-) complex (Dako)

**Note:** All undiluted antibodies are stable for at least 1 yr at 4°C; after dilution in TBS use within 2–3 d and store at 4°C.

6. Sodium citrate buffer (pH 6.0): Solution A: 21.00 g citric acid diluted to 1000 mL with aqua dest. Solution B: 29.41 g sodium citrate diluted to 1000 mL with aqua dest. Nine mL of solution A and 41 mL of solution B diluted to 500 mL with aqua dest.
7. Tris-buffered saline (TBS, pH 7.6): 6.01 g Tris-base, 8.50 g sodium chloride, diluted to 1000 mL with aqua dest.
8. Buffer solution for chromogen mixture: 8.70 g sodium chloride, 1.50 g Tris HCl, 4.90 g Tris base diluted to 1000 mL with aqua dest.

**Note:** Store all buffers at 4°C.

9. Chromogen mixture: Solution A:20 mg levamisole diluted in 35 mL chromogen-buffer mixed with 12.5 mL propandiol. Solution B: 10 mg sodium nitrite diluted in 250 µL aqua dest. mixed with 100 µL 5% new fuchsin (1 min reaction time). Solution C: 14 mg naphtol-as-biphosphate diluted in 300 µL dimethylformamide. After adjusting the prepared mixture (A+B+C) at pH 8.8, filter off and use immediately. **Note:** Chromogens are toxic.
10. Graded alcohol's (100%, 96%, and 75%).
11. Hematoxylin 0.1%: 2.0 g hematoxylin, 0.4 g sodium iodate, 100 g aluminium potassium sulphate diluted to 2000 mL with aqua dest. After incubation overnight, mix with 100g chloral hydrate and 2 g citric acid. **Note:** Useable after 4 wk incubation.

## 3. Methods

### 3.1. Immunohistochemistry on Paraffin Sections (see Chapter 51)

1. Immunostaining for *Bcl*-2 and *Bax* should be performed on 1–2 µm sections from formalin-fixed paraffin-embedded tumor tissue, which were air-dried overnight at 37°C (*see* **Notes 1** and **2**).
2. Slides are dewaxed in xylene (2 × 10 min) and rehydrated through graded alcohol's (100%, 100%, 96%, 96%, 75%; 2 min each).

3. Prior to immunohistochemical procedures, slides are heated in a microwave oven (720 W; 3 × 5 min) in excess sodium citrate buffer (pH 6.0).
4. After being heated, slides are washed (2 × 2 min) with TBS at pH 7.6.
5. Incubations are performed in a humidified chamber to avoid drying of the slides.

### 3.2. Immunohistochemical Staining of Bax-Expression

1. Incubation with the primary antibody is performed for 2 h in a solution of 1:200 in TBS (pH 7.6).
2. Slides are washed (2 × 2 min) in TBS (pH 7.6).
3. Incubation with mouse antirabbit antibody diluted 1:50 in TBS/10% human serum for 30 min.
4. Slides are washed (2 × 2 min) in TBS (pH 7.6).
5. Incubation with rabbit antimouse antibody diluted 1:50 in TBS/10% human serum for 30 min.
6. Slides are washed (2 × 2 min) in TBS (pH 7.6).
7. Incubation with the apaap-complex (1:100 in TBS) is performed for 50 min in the dark.
8. Slides are washed (2 × 2 minutes) in TBS (pH 7.6).

### 3.3. Immunohistochemical Staining of Bcl-2-Expression

1. Incubation with the primary antibody is performed for 2 h in a solution of 1:80 in TBS (pH 7.6, *see* **Note 3**).
2. Slides are washed (2 × 2 min) in TBS (pH 7.6).
3. Incubation with rabbit antimouse antibody diluted 1:50 in TBS/10% human serum for 30 min.
4. Slides are washed (2 × 2 min) in TBS (pH 7.6).
5. Incubation with the apaap-complex (1:100 in TBS) is performed for 50 min in the dark (*see* **Note 4**).
6. Slides are washed (2 × 2 min) in TBS (pH 7.6).

### 3.4. Chromogen-Reaction

1. After the immunohistochemical procedure slides are incubated with new fuchsin solution as chromogen for 30 min (shaking) at room temperature.
2. Slides are washed (2 × 2 min) in aqua dest.
3. Counterstaining of the nucleus is performed with hematoxylin for 5 min.
4. After rinsing in warm water, slides are covered with glycerin plates. The reaction products appear as red staining of the cytoplasm of the tumor cells with a homogenous staining pattern in most of the cases (*see* **Notes 5** and **6**).

## 4. Notes

Deregulation of the *Bcl-2/Bax*-balance may influence the clinical course of ovarian cancer patients by deregulation of programmed cell death and altered sensitivity to chemotherapy. Therefore, determination of *Bax*- and *Bcl*-2-expression might represent a useful additional marker in predicting the prognosis of ovarian cancer patients. There are different methods to evaluate the expression of these proteins, including immunohistochemistry, Western or Northern blots. Immunohistochemical evaluation of *Bax*- and *Bcl*-2-expression can be used for retrospective analyses on formalin-fixed paraffin-embedded material and is readily reproducible even for a routine laboratory. Quantitation of mRNA or protein expression might be assumed to provide a more accurate assessment of expression levels, however, immunohistochemical evaluation of *Bax* and especially *Bcl*-2 correlates directly with Northern blot RNA-analyses (Dr. Binder, personal communication). As it has been shown that *Bax* and *Bcl*-2 are expressed in normal tissue, too, immunohistochemically methods allow a specific association of positive immunoreaction especially to tumor cells. Nevertheless, there are some aspects to be mentioned for immunohistochemical analyses.

1. Formalin-fixed paraffin-embedded material may lead to loss of antigenity. To avoid false-positive or negative results external and internal controls are necessary. As external positive controls, use sections from lymph nodes, where *Bcl*-2 is located in the lymphocytes and *Bax* is expressed in the germ center of the lymph nodes confirming the lack of cross reactions, too.
2. Because staining intensity is influenced by section diameter, avoid semiquantitative evaluation without an internal control.
3. For *Bcl*-2 expression, the positivity of interspersed lymphocytes will be an additional internal positive control and allows a semiquantitative evaluation based on comparison of the color intensity of the stained tumor cells with the interspersed lymphocytes.
4. To enhance the primary signal the alkaline phosphatase-antialkaline phosphatase method (apaap) should be used.
5. All slides should be evaluated in blinded fashion by two investigators without knowledge of clinicopathological characteristics.
6. *Bax*- and *Bcl*-2-expression may be altered after cytostatic or radiological treatment caused by activation of the tumor suppressor gene *p53*, which has been shown to be a transcriptional activator of *Bax* and to repress *Bcl*-2 expression *(14,15)*. Therefore, avoid a different composition of the investigated cohorts especially in retrospective analyses.

## References

1. Oltvai, Z. N., Milliman, C. L., and Korsmeyer, S. J. (1993) Bcl-2 heterodimerizes in vivo with a conserved homolog, Bax, that accelerates programmed cell death. *Cell* **74,** 606–619.
2. Yang, E., Tha, J., Jockel, J., Boise, L. H., Thompsen, C. B., and Korsmeyer, S. J. (1995) Bad, a heterodimer partner for Bcl-Xl and Bcl-2, displaces Bax and promotes cell death. *Cell* **80,** 285–291.
3. Yang, E. and Korsmeyer, J. (1996) Molecular thanatopsis: a discourse on the Bcl-2 family and cell death. *Blood* **88,** 386–401.
4. Tsujimoto, Y., Gorham, J. J. C., Jaffe, E., and Croce, C. M. (1985) The t(14;18) chromosome translocations involved in B-cell neoplasm result from mistakes in VDJ joining. *Science* **299,** 1390–1393.
5. Hague, A., Moorghen, M., Hicks, D., Chapmen, M., and Paraskeva, C. (1994) Bcl-2 expression in human colorectal adenomas and carcinomas. *Oncogene* **9,** 3367–3370.
6. Pezella, F., Turley, H., Kuzu, L. I., Tungekar, M. F., Dunnill, M. S., Pierce, C. B., et al. (1993) Bcl-2 protein in non-small cell lung carcinoma. *N. Engl. J. Med.* **329,** 690–694.
7. Binder, C., Marx, D., Overhoff, R., Binder, L., Schauer, A., and Hiddemann, W. (1995) Bcl-2 protein expression in breast cancer in relation to established prognostic factors and other clinicopathological variables. *Ann. Oncol.* **6,** 1005–1010.
8. Joenssu, H., Pylkkänen, L., and Toikkanen, S. (1994) Bcl-2 protein expression and long-term-survival in breast cancer. *Am. J. Pathol.* **145,** 1191–1198.
9. Leek, R. D., Kaklamanis, L., Pezzella, F., Gatter, K. C., and Harris, A. L. (1994) Bcl-2 in normal human breast and carcinoma, association with estrogen receptor-positive, epidermal growth factor-receptor-negative tumors and in situ cancers. *Br. J. Cancer* **69,** 135–139.
10. Henriksen, R., Wilander, E., and Öberg, K. (1995) Expression and prognostic significance of Bcl-2 in ovarian tumors. *Br. J. Cancer* **72,** 1324–1329.
11. Diebold, J., Baretton, G., Felchner, M., Meier, W., Dopfer, K., Schmidt, M., et al. (1996) Bcl-2 expression, p53 accumulation, and apoptosis in ovarian cancer. *Am. J. Clin. Pathol.* **105,** 241–249.
12. Marx, D., Binder, C., Meden, H., Lenthe, T., Ziemek, T., Hiddemann, W., et al. (1997) Differential expression of apoptosis associated genes bax and bcl-2 in ovarian cancer; correlation to other predictive parameters and prognosis. *Anticancer Res.* **17,** 2233–2240.

13. Binder, C., Marx, D., Binder, L., Schauer, A., and Hiddemann, W. (1996) Expression of Bax in relation to Bcl-2 and other predictive parameters in breast cancer. *Ann. Oncol.* **7,** 129–133.
14. Miyashita, T., Harigai, M., Hanada, M., and Reed, J. C. (1994) Identification of a p53-dependent negative response element in the bcl-2 gene. *Cancer Res.* **54,** 5501–5507.
15. Miyashita, T. and Reed, J. (1995) Tumor suppressor p53 is a direct transcriptional activator of the human bax gene. *Cell* **80,** 293–299.

# 80

# DNA-Dependent Protein Kinase in Apoptosis

## John J. Turchi

## 1. Introduction

Programmed cell death or apoptosis can be induced by a variety of mechanisms including genotoxic stress *(1–3)*. The initiation of apoptosis involves the activation of a proteolytic cascade reminiscent of the blood-clotting pathway or activation of pancreatic proteases *(4)*. It has been suggested that a single DNA strand break or persistent DNA adduct is sufficient to induce apoptosis *(5)*. The protease cascade allows for the amplification of the initial signal and results in the degradation of cellular proteins and chromosomal DNA, which are packaged into apoptotic bodies and subsequently removed and recycled by phagocytic cells. The proteases involved in apoptosis employ active site cysteine residues, which catalyze the hydrolysis of the peptide bond following specific aspartic acid residues *(6)*. This class of proteases has been termed caspases for cysteinyl, aspartate-specific proteases. A current view of the caspase cascade is presented in **Fig. 1**. Genotoxic stress results in the generation of an as yet undefined signal that results in the release of cytochrome C from the intermembrane space of mitochondria into the cytoplasm. It is in the cytoplasm that cytochrome C can form a complex with apocaspase 9, apoptotic protease activating factor-1 (Apaf-1) and deoxyadenosine 5′triphosphate (dATP). This complex is competent for the autoproteolytic activation of caspase-9 *(7)*. Active caspase-9 then cleaves apocaspase-3 to generate an active caspase-3, which is responsible for cleaving specific target proteins, one of which is the catalytic subunit of DNA-dependent protein kinase (DNA-PKcs). The antiapoptotic factor *Bcl-x_L* can sequester cytochrome C and inhibit the formation of the caspase-9-Apaf-1 complex effectively blocking apoptosis *(8)*. The proapoptotic factor *Bcl-x_S* promotes apoptosis by binding to *Bcl-x_L* and thus blocking the inhibitory effect of this protein *(8)*.

DNA-dependent protein kinase (DNA-PK) is a trimeric protein consisting of two functional components, a 460-kDa kinase catalytic subunit and a heterodimeric DNA-binding component consisting of 70 and 80 kDa subunits, termed Ku70 and Ku80. Mutations in any of the DNA-PK subunits can result in hypersensitivity to ionizing radiation (IR), radiomimetic compounds, and an inability to catalyze *V(D)J* recombination *(9)*. DNA-PKcs is a member of the phosphatidylinositol 3-kinase family and inhibition of DNA-PK by wortmannin, a PI-3 kinase inhibitor, has revealed an

From: *Methods in Molecular Medicine, Vol. 39: Ovarian Cancer: Methods and Protocols*
Edited by: J. M. S. Bartlett © Humana Press, Inc., Totowa, NJ

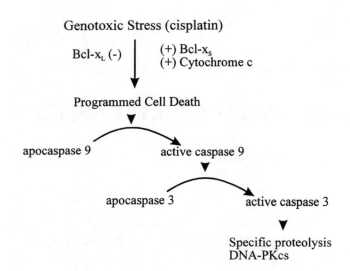

Fig. 1. Programmed cell death pathway in response to genotoxic stress.

increased sensitivity to ionizing radiation *(10,11)* indicating that DNA-PK may be a useful target for chemotherapeutic intervention in the treatment of cancer. The 460-kDa subunit is specifically cleaved by caspase-3 following the P1 aspartic acid of the DEVD sequence generating a 240-kDa inactive proteolytic fragment *(12)*. Both Ku70 and Ku80 subunits are unaffected by caspase-3.

More recently, cell lines deficient in DNA-PK as a result of mutation in either the Ku or DNA-PKcs genes, have been reported to have an increased sensitivity to DNA damaging agents that do not induce DSBs implicating a defect in nucleotide excision repair (NER) *(13)*. These results suggest a link between DNA-PK and sensitivity to DNA damage. Considering that the front-line treatment protocols for ovarian cancer include cisplatin, a DNA damaging agent, an important question is how DNA-PK is modulated by cisplatin. We have previously demonstrated that Ku70/Ku80 binds cisplatin damaged DNA in vitro, but is unable to activate DNA-PKcs *(14)*, and that the inhibitory effect was manifested as a decrease in catalytic efficiency of the enzyme *(15)*. We have also studied DNA-PK expression and activity in response to cisplatin using a series of ovarian cancer cell lines. Our results indicate that acquired cisplatin resistance does not result in a defective apoptotic process *(16)*. DNA-PK appears to be a central player in DNA metabolism and genetic maintenance. The degradation of DNA-PK is a hallmark of apoptosis and can be used to identify cells undergoing programmed cell death in response to external stimuli. In this chapter, we describe methods to measure DNA-PK activity and proteolytic degradation in cultured cell lines undergoing drug-induced apoptosis.

## 2. Materials

### 2.1. Cell Growth and Induction of Apoptosis

1. Cell culture media. Dulbecco's modified Eagle's medium (DMEM) supplemented with 10% fetal calf serum, 0.54 g/L l-glutamine, 100 U/mL penicillin, and 100 µg/mL streptomycin.
2. Cisplatin stock. Dissolve cisplatin (Sigma, St. Louis, MO) in water at a concentration of 1 m*M* and sonicate briefly to disperse the drug. Filter sterilize and store at –20°C (*see* **Note 1**).

3. PBS: 0.2 g/L KCl, 8 g/L NaCl, 1.15 g/L $Na_2HPO_4$, 2.16 g/L $NaH_2PO_4 \cdot 7H_2O$. Filter sterilize and store at room temperature.

## 2.2. Preparation of Cell Extracts

1. Wash buffer: 10 m$M$ HEPES-KOH (pH 7.5), 1.5 m$M$ $MgCl_2$, 10 m$M$ kCl, and 1 m$M$ β-mercaptoethanol. Make fresh prior to use.
2. Lysis buffer: 10 m$M$ Tris-Cl (pH7.5), 1 m$M$ $MgCl_2$, 1 m$M$ EGTA, 5 m$M$ β-mercaptoethanol, 10% glycerol, and 0.5% CHAPS. Make fresh prior to use.
3. High salt buffer: 50 m$M$ Tris-Cl (pH 7.5), 10 m$M$ $MgCl_2$, 2 m$M$ dithiothreitol (DTT), 25% sucrose, and 50% glycerol. Make fresh prior to use.
4. Dialysis buffer: 25 m$M$ HEPES (pH 7.8), 1 m$M$ EGTA, 0.01 % Nonidet P40, 10% glycerol, 1 m$M$ DTT, 0.1 m$M$ PMSF, 0.1 $M$ KCl. Make fresh prior to use.

## 2.3. Ku *DNA Binding Assay*

1. [γ-$^{32}$P]ATP (6000 Ci/mmol, 150 mCi/mL).
2. Duplex DNA substrate (*see* **Note 2**).
3. 10X binding buffer: 200 m$M$ HEPES-KOH (pH 7.5), 10 m$M$ DTT, 0.01% Nonidet P-40, 500 m$M$ NaCl, and acetylated BSA at 500 μg/mL.
4. 5X gel loading dye: 50% glycerol, 50 m$M$ ethylenediaminetetraacetic acid (EDTA) (pH 8.0), and 0.05% each bromophenol blue and xylene cyanole FF.

## 2.4. DNA-Dependent Protein Kinase Assay

1. [γ-$^{32}$P]ATP (30 Ci/mmol, 10 mCi/mL).
2. 10X kinase reaction buffer: 400 m$M$ HEPES (pH 7.5), 500 m$M$ KCl, 80 m$M$ $MgCl_2$, 2m$M$ EGTA, 10 mM DTT, and 25% glycerol.
3. Activated calf thymus DNA: 2 mg/mL in 10 m$M$ Tris-Cl (pH 8.0), and 1 m$M$ EDTA.

## 3. Methods

### 3.1. Cell Growth and Induction of Apoptosis

In this section, mammalian cells are plated and treated with a chemotherapeutic agent to induce apoptosis. The first part of the section describes the methods to determine the cytotoxicity for a given chemotherapeutic agent. The second part of the section describes large-scale drug treatment and the preparation of cellular extracts from both apoptotic and adherent cells in preparation for analysis of DNA-PK expression and activity. A flowchart outlining the experimental protocol is shown in **Fig. 2**.

1. Seed 500 cells in each of 20 100-mm dishes in cell medium plus supplements and incubate for 24 h at 37°C in a 5% $CO_2$ incubator.
2. Dilute cisplatin in complete medium to concentrations ranging from 0.1 μ$M$ to 200 μ$M$.
3. Treat plates in triplicate at each concentration for 4 h at 37°C.
4. Aspirate the drug containing medium and wash the cells three times with 10 mL of PBS.
5. Add 10 mL of complete medium and incubate for 7–14 d until colonies greater than 50 cells are observable by phase contrast microscopy.
6. Remove medium and wash cells once with 10 mL of PBS.
7. Add 5 mL of methylene blue staining solution (1% methylene blue in 70% ethanol) for 15 min at room temperature.
8. Remove the staining solution and wash the plates extensively with $H_2O$.
9. Count colonies with greater than 50 cells to determine percent survival by comparison with untreated controls. Determine the concentration of drug that results in 50 and 90% cell death, $IC_{50}$ and $IC_{90}$ values, respectively.

Fig. 2. Flowchart of experimental protocol to measure DNA-PK activity, expression, and degradation in response to chemotherapeutic treatment.

## 3.2. Large-Scale Cell Treatment and Preparation of Cell Extracts

Cells undergoing apoptosis release from the surface of the plate while cells that are resistant to apoptosis or are not as far along in the programmed cell death pathway remain adhered to the plate. Therefore, separate protein extracts are prepared from cells that have released from the plate and from cells that remain adhered to the plate.

1. Plate cells in complete growth media at subconfluent densities. Typically, $1–5 \times 10^6$ cells are plated in a 150-mm dish containing 30 mL of complete media. Cells are incubated at 37°C in a humidified 5% $CO_2$ atmosphere for 24 h.
2. Following incubation, apoptosis is induced by the addition of cisplatin. Typically, cells are treated for 4 h at 37°C in complete media at the previously determined $IC_{50}$ and $IC_{90}$ concentrations of drug.
3. Following incubation, the drug containing media is removed, and cell monolayers are washed three times with 10 mL of PBS and 20 mL of complete media is added and incubation continued for 24–96 h.
4. Remove media containing unadherent cells from the plate and collect the cells by sedimentation at 2000$g$ for 5 min.
5. Scrape the adherent cells from the plate in 2 mL of PBS and transfer to a 15-mL centrifuge tube also collect by sedimentation as above.
6. Wash both nonadherent and adherent cells separately in PBS, resuspend in 0.5 mL ice-cold wash buffer and transfer to a 1.5-mL microcentrifuge tube (*see* **Note 3**).
7. Collect the cells by sedimentation at 2000$g$ for 5 min and estimate the packed cell volume (PCV).
8. Resuspend the cell pellet in 4X PCV of ice-cold lysis buffer supplemented with protease inhibitors and incubate on ice for 30 min.
9. Slowly add 4X PCVs of high salt buffer and mix gently, but thoroughly.
10. Add saturated ammonium sulfate to a final concentration of 15% (1/2 PCV) from a saturated stock and incubation continued for an additional 30 min on ice.
11. Remove insoluble material by sedimentation at 14,000$g$ for 30 min at 4°C.
12. Dialyze the supernatant vs 500 mL of dialysis buffer using a multiwell microdialyzer (Gibco/Life Technologies, Gaithersburg, MD) at 4°C.
13. The cell extract is then frozen at –70°C in 50–100 μL aliquots.

### 3.3. Ku *DNA Binding Assay*

Extracts prepared from cells can be assayed directly for DNA-PK activity. The DNA binding activity is determined by an electrophoretic mobility shift assay (EMSA) and kinase activity is determined measuring phosphorylation of a synthetic peptide dependent on DNA in the reaction. The duplex DNA substrate is prepared by 5'-end labeling with $[^{32}P]$ATP.

1. Incubate duplex DNA (10 pmol) with 100 µCi of $[\gamma\text{-}^{32}P]$ATP (6000 Ci/mmol) and T4 polynucleotide kinase according to the manufacturers specifications in a volume of 45 µL.
2. Terminate the reaction by the addition of 5 µL of 0.5 $M$ EDTA. Determine the specific activity of the substrate by spotting 0.1 µL on a 1-sq cm piece of DE-81 filter paper (Whatman). Dry the filter and remove unincorporated ATP by washing three times with 10 mL of 0.5 $M$ NaPi (pH 7.0). Dry the filter and quantify the amount of radioactivity by liquid scintillation counting. The specific activity calculated is by dividing the CPM by 0.02 to obtain CPM/pmol.
3. Purify the remaining DNA from unincorporated ATP by Sephadex G-50 spin column chromatography. An aliquot of the purified DNA is used to determine the concentration and yield of DNA (*see* **Note 4**).
4. Mix 1–5 µg of protein from each extract with 50 fmol of duplex DNA substrate in 1X binding buffer on ice for 30 min in a volume of 20 µL.
5. Gently add 5 µL of gel loading dye and apply the samples immediately to the wells of an 8% native polyacrylamide gel prepared in 1X TBE using a 29:1 acrylamide to *bis*-acrylamide ratio (*see* **Note 5**).
6. Electrophorese the gel at 150 V for 1.5 h until the bromophenol blue dye has migrated about two-thirds of the distance of the gel (*see* **Note 6**).
7. Following electrophoresis, remove the gel and place on Whatman 3MM filter paper and cover with plastic wrap. Dry the gel with heat (85°C) under vacuum without pretreatment and detect radioactivity by autoradiography.
8. Quantification of the data is performed using a PhosphorImager and the fmol of DNA bound calculated (*see* **Note 7**).

### 3.4. *DNA-Dependent Protein Kinase Assay*

DNA-PK kinase activity is determined by the phosphorylation of a synthetic peptide dependent on the addition of DNA into the reactions. The cell extraction procedure employed minimizes the DNA contamination and thus assures DNA-PK activity can be accurately measured by the dependence on exogenously added DNA (*see* **Note 8**).

1. Assemble reactions on ice in triplicate in 1X kinase buffer containing 0.2 µCi $[\gamma^{32}P]$ATP (125 µ$M$) with and without activated calf thymus DNA in a final volume of 20 µL.
2. Initiate the reactions by the addition of protein (1–10 µg) and incubate at 30°C for 15 min.
3. During the incubation, cut a piece of Whatman P-11 filter paper and using a pencil draw a grid of 2.5 × 2.5-cm squares equal to the number of reactions performed.
4. Terminate the reactions by the addition 20 µL of 30% acetic acid.
5. Spot 35 µL of each reaction in a separate square of the P-11 filter.
6. Transfer the filter to a 9 × 9 Pyrex glass baking dish and dry the filter under a heat lamp for 15 min. Allow the filter to cool for 5 min.
7. Wash the filter five times each with 200 mL of 15% acetic acid for 5 min.
8. Aspirate the acetic acid and briefly rinse the filter in 100 mL of methanol.

9. Dry the filter, and spot 1 µL of one of the remaining samples and wrap the filter in plastic-wrap.
10. Expose the filter to a PhosphorImager screen for quantification of the radioactivity in each spot. The 1-µL control spot contains 125 pmol of ATP and can be used to calculate the amount of $[^{32}P]PO_4$ incorporated into the peptide.

### 3.5. Caspase-Catalyzed Degradation of DNA-PKcs

The catalytic subunit of DNA-PK is a specific substrate for caspase-3 and cleavage by caspase-3 generates a 240-kDa proteolytic fragment. Immunoblot analysis is an effective means to assess DNA-PKcs degradation by caspase-3. In addition, the Ku subunits are not substrates for caspase degradation and therefore serve as excellent controls. **Table 1** presents commercially available antibodies that can be employed to detect DNA-PKcs and the Ku subunits via immunoblot analysis. The procedures for SDS-PAGE separation of protein and immunoblotting are presented elsewhere in this volume (Chapter 54).

1. Separate protein by SDS-PAGE (*see* **Note 9**).
2. Transfer to PVDF membrane (*see* **Note 10**).
3. Block the membrane and probe with the primary antibody (*see* **Table 1** for recommended dilutions of the antibodies).
4. Wash the membrane and probe with a 1:1000 dilution of the appropriate secondary antibody (*see* **Note 11**).
5. Wash the membrane and detect the bound antibody using a commercially available chemiluminescent detection system.

## 4. Notes

1. Cisplatin is a yellowish solid and when dispersed at a concentration of 1 m*M* in water the solution should be clear. Although we employ cisplatin, any agent can be employed to induce cell death.
2. Almost any duplex DNA substrate can be employed in an EMSA for Ku. We routinely employ two complementary oligonucleotides which, when annealed, generate a duplex DNA 75-bp in length. The oligonucleotides can be 5′-end labeled with $^{32}P$ prior to annealing. Alternatively, a plasmid can be digested with a restriction enzyme and a duplex DNA fragment gel purified by agarose gel electrophoresis. Following elution from the gel the DNA can be quantified, labeled, and employed in the EMSA assay.
3. This step washes out the salt and places the cells in a hypotonic buffer, which makes cell lysis and protein extraction more efficient.
4. Alternatively, the DNA can be purified by electrophoresis on native polyacrylamide gel. The DNA can then be used in an EMSA following elution, precipitation, and quantification of the labeled DNA.
5. The percentage of gel employed will depend in part on the length of the DNA substrate used in the EMSA assay. For DNA substrates between 40 and 120 bp in length, an 8% gel should give excellent resolution between the free DNA and that bound by Ku.
6. In an 8% polyacrylamide gel run in 1X TBE, relative mobilities are calculated based on the migration of the bromophenol blue dye. The 75-bp duplex DNA has an R*f* of 0.85. Two Ku DNA complexes are often observed and represent one dimer bound to a DNA substrate, which migrates with an R*f* of 0.30. The slower migrating complex consists of two Ku dimers bound to a single DNA and exhibits an R*f* of 0.20.
7. The fmol of DNA bound is calculated by comparing the intensity of the protein-DNA complex with the intensity of the free control DNA obtained in the absence of added

**Table 1**
**DNA-PK Specific Antibodies**

| Subunit | Designation | Source | Type | Reference/supplier[a] | Dilution |
|---------|-------------|--------|------|----------------------|----------|
| DNA-PKcs | *DPK1 | rabbit | polyclonal | Lees-Miller (*3*) | 1:1000 |
| | 18-2 | mouse | monoclonal | Labvision | |
| | 25-4 | mouse | monoclonal | Labvision | |
| | 42-psc | mouse | monoclonal | Labvision | |
| | 4F10C5 | mouse | monoclonal | Pharmingen | |
| | C-19 | goat | polyclonal | Santa Cruz | |
| | N-20 | goat | polyclonal | Santa Cruz | |
| Ku 70 | *N3H10 | mouse | monoclonal | Labvision | 1:100 |
| | C-19 | goat | polyclonal | Santa Cruz | |
| | M-19 | goat | polyclonal | Santa Cruz | |
| | 1358 | rabbit | polyclonal | Chemicon | |
| Ku 80 | *111 | mouse | monoclonal | Labvision | 1:100 |
| | M20 | goat | polyclonal | Santa Cruz | |
| | C-20 | goat | polyclonal | Santa Cruz | |
| | 1357 | rabbit | polyclonal | Chemicon | |

[a]Information can be obtained at the following URL's: Labvision, www.labvision.com/; Pharmingen, www.pharmingen.com/; Santa Cruz, www.scbt.com/; Labvision, www.labvision.com/; Chemicon, www.chemicon.com/.

protein. Alternative methods can be employed to quantify the DNA bound. Scanning laser densitometry of autoradiographs or excising the bands from the gel and quantifying CPM by liquid scintillation counting are viable alternatives.

8. A synthetic peptide for DNA-PK (EPPLSQAEFADLWKK) is available from Promega (Madison, WI) or one can be purchased from any number of companies offering custom peptide synthesis. An additional control can be performed in reactions containing DNA, but with a peptide that cannot be phosphorylated by DNA-PK. The DNA-PK phosphorylation peptide where the LSQ sequence is rearranged to LQS is not phosphorylated by DNA-PK and can serve as an additional control.

9. We routinely use 10 × 10.5-cm minigels with a 4% stacking gel and an 8% resolving gel and electrophorese at a constant current of 30 mA.

10. A number of buffer systems are available for transferring protein to membranes. The large size of DNA-PKcs makes it a difficult protein to transfer out of SDS-gels. We routinely use 10 m*M* CAPS, pH 10.5 containing 10% methanol and transfer at 350 m*A* for 3 h at 4°C.

11. The secondary antibody needed will depend on the host of the primary antibody. Goat-antimouse IgG or goat-antirabbit IgG are the most common. We employ horseradish peroxidase conjugated secondary antibodies (Life Technologies, Bethesda, MD) and a 1:1000 dilution is sufficient for detection using chemiluminescence.

## Acknowledgments

The author thanks Karen M. Henkels, Steve Patrick, Ingrid Hermanson, and Elizabeth Smucker for their help and advice in preparing this manuscript. This research was supported by a grant from the National Institutes of Health (CA64374).

## References

1. Jeggo, P. A. (1997) DNAPK: at the cross-roads of biochemistry and genetics. *Mutat. Res.* **384,** 1–14.
2. Anderson, C. W. and Carter, T. H. (1996) The DNA-activated protein kinase DNA-PK. *Curr. Top. Microbiol. Immunol.* **217,** 91–111.

3. Lees-Miller, S. P. (1996) The DNA-dependent protein kinase, DNA-PK: 10 years and no ends in sight. *Biochem. Cell Biol.* **74,** 503–512.

4. Salvesen, G. S. and Dixit, V. M. (1997) Caspases: Intracellular Signaling by Proteolysis. *Cell.* **91,** 443–446.

5. Huang, L. C., Clarkin, K. C., and Wahl, G. M. (1996) Sensitivity and selectivity of the DNA damage sensor responsible for activating p53-dependent G1 arrest. *Proc. Natl. Acad. Sci. USA* **93,** 4827–4832.

6. Nicholson, D. W. and Thornberry, N. A. (1997) Caspases: killer proteases. *Trends in Biochem. Sci.* **22,** 299–306.

7. Li, P., Nijhawan, D., Budihardjo, I., Srinivasula, S. M., Ahmad, M., Alnemri, E. S., and Wang, X. (1997) Cytochrome c and dATP-dependent formation of Apaf-1/Caspase-9 complex initiaites an apoptotic protease cascade. *Cell.* **91,** 479–489.

8. Kharbanda, S., Pandey, P., Schofield, L., Israels, S., Roncinske, R., Yoshida, K., et al. (1997) Role for Bcl-xL as an inhibitor of cytosolic cytochrome C accumulation in DNA damageinduced apoptosis. *Proc. Natl. Acad. Sci. USA* **94,** 6939–6942.

9. Jackson, S. P. and Jeggo, P. A. (1995) DNA double-strand break repair and V(D)J recombination: involvement of DNA-PK. *Trends in Biochem. Sci.* **20,** 412–415.

10. Rosenzweig, K. E., Youmell, M. B., Palayoor, S. T., and Price, B. D. (1997) Radiosensitization of human tumor cells by the phosphatidylinositol 3-kinase inhibitors wortmannin and LY294002 correlates with inhibition of DNA-dependent protein kinase and prolonged G(2)-M delay. *Clinic. Cancer Res.* **3,** 1149–1156.

11. Okayasu, R., Suetomi, K., and Ullrich, R. L. (1998) Wortmannin inhibits repair of DNA doublestrand breaks in irradiated normal human cells. *Radiat. Res.* **149,** 440–445.

12. Song, Q., Lees-Miller, S. P., Kumar, S., Zhang, Z., Chan, D. W., Smith, G. C., et al. (1996) DNA-dependent protein kinase catalytic subunit: a target for an ICElike protease in apoptosis. *EMBO J.* **15,** 3238–3246.

13. Muller, C., Calsou, P., Frit, P., Cayrol, C., Carter, T., and Salles, B. (1998) UV sensitivity and impaired nucleotide excision repair in DNA-dependent protein kinase mutant cells. *Nucleic Acids Res.* **26,** 1382–1389.

14. Turchi, J. J. and Henkels, K. (1996) Human Ku autoantigen binds cisplatin-damaged DNA but fails to stimulate human DNA-activated protein kinase. *J. Biol. Chem.* **271,** 13,861–13,867.

15. Turchi, J. J., Patrick, S. M., and Henkels, K. M. (1997) Mechanism of DNA-dependent protein kinase inhibition by cis-diamminedichloroplatinum(II)-damaged DNA. *Biochemistry* **36,** 7586–7593.

16. Henkels, K. M. and Turchi, J. J. (1997) Induction of apoptosis in cisplatin-sensitive and -resistant human ovarian cancer cell lines. *Cancer Res.* **57,** 4488–4492.

# 81

## Detection of Telomerase Activity by PCR-Based Assay

### Satoru Kyo

## 1. Introduction

Telomeres are distal ends of human chromosomes composed of tandem repeats of the sequence TTAGGG. Possible functions of telomeres include prevention of chromosome degradation, end-to-end fusions, rearrangements, and chromosome loss. Human telomeres in somatic cells undergo progressive shortening with cell division, presumably caused by the inability of cells to fully replicate the ends of linear DNA templates *(1)*. When telomeres reach a critically short length with aging of cells, the cells exit from the cell cycle and stop dividing, so-called replicative senescence *(2,3)*.

Telomerase is a ribonucleotide protein enzyme, which functions as a DNA polymerase, and contains an integrated RNA with a short template element that directs synthesis of telomeric repeats (TTAGGG) at chromosome ends *(4,5)*. Telomerase activation is thus thought to be essential for prevention of telomere shortening with cell divisions and stabilization of telomeres, which may permit cells to escape from replicative senescence, leading to cellular immortality.

In 1994, Kim et al. developed a novel PCR-based method (Telomeric Repeat Amplification Protocol: TRAP) that can detect telomerase activity with a high degree of sensitivity *(6)*. Using the TRAP assay, a number of studies have revealed that telomerase is activated in most malignant tumors, irrespective of tumor type, but repressed in normal somatic tissues *(7–10)*. These findings suggest that telomerase activation may be a critical step in carcinogenesis. However, interestingly, subsequent studies have revealed that some types of normal somatic cells with high proliferative activity, such as human endometrial cells and trophoblasts in early pregnancy, can express telomerase activiy in a proliferation-dependent manner *(11,12)*. These findings suggested the hypothesis that special subsets of normal cells with stem-cell characteristics are capable of expressing telomerase activity, which is required for the stem cells to expand through the entire life of individuals.

The specific activation of telomerase in most malignant tumors has prompted researchers to utilize this activity for cancer diagnosis. A variety of materials including uterine cervical exfoliated cells, sedimented cells from urine, and fine needle aspirates from breast and lymph nodes have been used for the detection of telomerase activity with the TRAP assay *(13–15)*. The TRAP assay includes the two major steps,

From: *Methods in Molecular Medicine, Vol. 39: Ovarian Cancer: Methods and Protocols*
Edited by: J. M. S. Bartlett © Humana Press, Inc., Totowa, NJ

telomerase extension reaction and amplification of extended products (**Fig. 1**). The former step is based on the ability of telomerase to add telomeric repeat sequences to the ends of oligonucleotide primers (TS primer), which allows the oligonucleotides to be extended. The latter step is a PCR reaction to amplify the extended ologonucleotides with a special set of primers, TS and CX primers, the sequences of the latter are complementary to telomeric repeats. PCR products are heterogeneous in size, because template oligonucleotides extended to different lengths for each molecule and the primers used in the PCR reactions can anneal at random sites in internal teromeric repeat sequences of the templates. As a result, the PCR products generate DNA ladders in electrophoresis, which can be visualized with radioisotope labeling of the primers or simply by staining with special reagents that enable detection of small amounts of DNA in gels. We preferentially use a nonradioisotope method to visualize PCR procucts. The sensitivity of our nonradioisotope method with SYBR Green I staining has been proven to be similar to that of radioisotope method (*9*). In this chapter, techniques for nonradioisotope TRAP assay using SYBR Green I staining are described.

## 2. Materials

### 2.1. Reagents for TRAP Assay

1. Distilled water (DNase and RNase free).
2. Phosphate-buffered saline (PBS) pH 7.4, without $MgCl_2$ and $CaCl_2$.
3. Washing buffer (stored at –20°C) 10 m*M* HEPES-KOH, 1.5 m*M* $MgCl_2$, 10 m*M* KCl. Add 1 m*M* dithiothreitol (DTT) just before use.
4. Lysis buffer (stored at –20°C): 10 m*M* Tris-Hcl (pH 7.5), 1 m*M* $MgCl_2$, 1 m*M* EGTA, 0.5% 3-[(3-cholamidopropyl)dimethylamino]-1-propanesulfonate (CHAPS), 10% glycerol, 5 m*M* β-mercaptoethanol (add just before use), 0.1 m*M* phenylmethylsulfonyl fluoride (PMSF) (add just before use).
5. Ampliwax: PCR Gem 50 (Perkin Elmer, Norwalk, CT)
6. TS primer 5'-AATCCGTCGAGCAGAGTT-3'
7. CX primer 5'-CCCTT<u>A</u>CCCTT<u>A</u>CCCTT<u>A</u>CCCTAA-3' [CX primer is designed to be complementary to telomeric sequences. However, to avoid annealing of the CX primers to internal telomeric sequences of the templates in PCR reaction, the underlined bases are altered (A to T)]
8. 10X TRAP reaction buffer: 200 m*M* Tris-HCl (pH 8.3), 15 m*M* $MgCl_2$, 630 m*M* KCl, 0.05% Tween-20, 10 m*M* EGTA, 0.5 m*M* deoxynucleotide triphosphate, *Taq* polymerase (5 U/μL).
9. *T4* gene 32 protein (Boehringer-Mannheim, Germany)
10. Reagents for measuring protein concentration [Bio-Rad, Richmond, CA, Bio-Rad Protein Assay (#500-0006)].

### 2.2. Reagents for Polyacrylamide Gel Electrophoresis

1. 30% polyacrylamide/*bis*-acrylamide (19:1) stock solution.
2. 10% ammonium persulphate (APS). Prepare fresh on day of use.
3. *N,N,N'N'*-tetramethylethylenediamine (TEMED).
4. 10X TBE (for 1 L): 60.5 g tris base, 30 g boric acid, 4.12g EDTA.3Na.
5. 6X DNA dye: 0.25% bromophenol blue, 0.25% xylene cyanol, 50 m*M* EDTA, 50% glycerol.
6. SYBR Green 1 Nucleic Acid Gel Stain (FMC BioProducts, Rockland, ME).
7. SYBR Green I Photographic Filter (FMC BioProducts #50530).

Fig. 1. Principle of the TRAP assay.

## 2.3. Samples

1. Cultured cells: Approx $10^5$–$10^6$ cultured cells are collected by trypsynization and cell pellets are recovered by centrifugation. Pellets can be stored at –80°C until use.
2. Clinical samples
   a. Postoperative or biopsied tissue specimens. Small pieces of specimens (approx 50 to 500 mg) are collected with a sterile scalpel from postoperative or biopsied tissues and stored at –80°C until use.
   b. Exfoliated cells from tumors such as cervical cancer. Exfoliated cells are resuspended in ice-cold PBS and pellets are recovered by centrifugation and stored at –80°C until use.
   c. Sedimented cells from fluid samples such as urine, ascites, and pleural effusion. Cell fractions are collected by centrifugation and washed with PBS, and pellets are recovered by centrifugation and stored at –80°C until use. To isolate epithelial cells from several other types of contaminated materials such as blood cells and mucous, special treatments are sometimes required based on the source of materials.

## 3. Methods

### 3.1. Extraction of Telomerase

Subsequent steps should be performed on ice or at 4°C.

1. Cells ($10^4$–$10^6$) or tissue specimens (50 to 500 mg) are washed with 500 µL of washing buffer in 1.5- mL Eppendorf tubes (we can usually detect significant telomerase ladders in $10^2$ cells of C33A cervical cancer cell line, but not in 10 cells). After centrifugation (5000$g$) for 5 min, remove all the washing buffer carefully.
2. Add 200 µL of ice-cold lysis buffer and homogenize the cell pellets or tissues. For cultured cells, simply resuspend the pellets by repeated pipeting. For tissue specimens, several types of homogenizers can be used (Fisher, Pittsburgh, PA, PowerGen Model 35 Homoginizer, VWR: # KT749520-0000 or KT749540-0000).
3. Incubate homogenized cells or tissues on ice for 30 min and occasionally vortex the tubes.

Fig. 2. Single-tube arrangement in the TRAP assay.

4. Centrifuge at top speed (12,000*g*–15,000*g*) in a microfuge for 10 min.
5. Recover supernatants and transfer them to new Eppendorf tubes.
6. Measure protein concentration (Bradford assay). If concentration is higher than 10 µg/µL, dilute extracts with lysis buffer to 5 µg/µL.
7. Store supernatants at –80°C until use.

## 3.2. TRAP Assay

1. Prepare PCR tubes for 50 µL reaction volume (*see* **Note 1**).
2. Place the 2 µL of CX primers into the bottoms of tubes.
3. Layer AmpliWax onto CX primers and heat the tubes at 72°C for a few minitues in a thermal cycler. This step melts AmpliWax (**Fig. 2**).
4. Remove the PCR tubes from the thermal cycler, and place them on ice. Ampliwax will solidify and sequester the CX primers at the bottoms of tubes.
5. Prepare the following mixture for each sample: 5 µL 10X TRAP reaction buffer, 2 µL TS primer (100 ng/µL), 0.2 µL *T4* gene 32 protein, 0.4 µL *Taq* polymerase, 1–5 µL telomerase extracts (for 1–5 µg of protein) make up to 48 µL with ddH$_2$O.
6. Place the above mixtures onto the solidified Ampliwax in PCR tubes.
7. Place the tubes in a thermal cycler.
8. Start telomerase extension reaction at 23°C for 30 min.
9. Subsequently, start PCR reaction for amplification of telomerase extension products. 94°C 3 min/1 cycle (hot start), 94°C 45 s, 50°C 45 s, 72°C 60 s/30 cycles, 72°C 5 min/1 cycle. At 94°C in the first cycle, Ampliwax is melted and the wax barrier is destroyed, allowing CX primers to join PCR reaction mixtures and initiating PCR reaction with CX and TS primers.
10. After completion of PCR cycles, Ampliwax is located above the PCR reaction mixtures and solidifies at room temperature. Collect 17 µL of PCR reaction mixture with the tip penetrating into the Ampliwax.
11. Add 3 µL of 6X DNA dye to collected reaction mixtures and electrophorese on 12% polyacrylamide gel (200–300 V).

12. Stop electrophoresis when bromophenol blue is just out of the gel.
13. Dilute SYBR Green I 1:10000 in 1/2X TBE, which was used in electrophoresis, in a plastic polypropylene container.
14. Immerse gels in the above solutions and gently agitate at room temperature for 10–15 min. When protected from light, diluted SYBR Green I is stable for at least 24 h and can stain several gels (2 to 3) with progressive decrease in sensitivity. It is therefore better to cover the container with foil to protect against light.
15. Visualize PCR products on UV transilluminators using SYBR Green Stain Photographic Filter. If the samples have telomerase activity, DNA ladders composed of various sizes of PCR products can be observed (**Fig. 3**). Each ladder differs in size by 6 bp. The number of ladders and their staining intensities differ depending on the level of telomerase activity in extracts (*see* **Notes 2–4**).
16. Take a picture and measure the staining intensities of the ladders by picture analyzing software (*see* **Notes 5** and **6**).

## 4. Notes

1. The following control samples are required to evaluate the results of the TRAP assay.
   a. Heat-inactivation control: CHAPS extracts are preheated at 85°C for 10 min to inactivate telomerase activity. This control sample is used as a negative control.
   b. RNase I inactivation control (**Fig. 3**): Because telomerase is a ribonucleotide protein that includes integrated RNA with a short template for the synthesis of telomeric repeats, it is sensitive to RNase. Add 1 μg of RNase I to the CHAPS extract and preincubate at 37°C for 10 min before telomerase extension reaction. This control sample is used as a negative control.
   c. Positive control: Samples from cancer cell lines for which telomerase activity have been demonstrated can be used as positive controls. In general, samples from $10^4$ cells are sufficient for demonstration of telomerase signal (**Fig. 3**). However, because the intensity of telomerase activity varies among cell types, serially diluted cell extracts ($10^3$–$10^5$ cells) should be prepared and tested for each cell type.
2. Nonspecific signals are occasionally observed, which are caused by primer dimer formation. They can clearly be distinguished from specific telomerase signals as follows.
   a. The number of bands is no more than six.
   b. Several strong bands are usually found around 50–70 bp in size, and the interval separating the ladders is not regular and differs from that found in specific ladders.
3. PCR contamination is another difficulty we sometimes encounter. When telomerase ladders are observed in all the samples including negative controls, PCR contamination is a possibility. In case of contamination, all the reagents should be reprepared. To prevent contamination, it is recommended that aliquots of reagents be prepared.
4. A variety of reaction inhibitors are occasionally contained in the CHAPS extracts, such as *Taq* polymerase inhibitors. It sometimes happens that increasing amounts of extracts applied cause decrease in ladder intensity. This is probably caused by increasing effects of inhibitors. Because the TRAP assay is a one-tube reaction, such inhibitors may remain present following extension reaction and interfere with PCR reaction, generating false-negative samples. To identify samples that are false-negative because of reaction inhibitors, internal controls are generally used to monitor PCR efficiency.

   A 150-bp internal standard is prepared by synthesizing TS and CX oligonucleotides that contain an additional 15 bases at their 3′ ends that overlap with sequences encoding aa 97-132 of rat myogenin (*16*). (TS-overlap primer: 5′-AATCCGTCGAGCAGAG TT<u>GTGAATGAGGCCTTC</u>-3′, CX-overlap primer: 5′-CCCTTACCCTTACCCTTA CCCTTAA<u>TAGGCGCTCAATGTA</u>-3′). Myogenin sequences (15 bases each) are

Fig. 3. Representative results of nonradioisotope TRAP assay *(10)* using serially diluted extracts from C33A cells **(A)** and HEC 1 cells **(B)**. The numbers of C33A cells and amounts of protein extracts from HEC 1 cells applied per reaction are shown at the tops of the lanes. In control samples, lysis buffer was applied alone without addition of cell extracts. **(C)** TRAP assay to confirm specificity for telomerase activity. Extracts from HEC 1 and HEC 116 cells were pretreated with or without 1 µg of RNase A for 10 min. at 37°C. The extracts were then subjected to TRAP assay. **(D)** Representative results of TRAP assays using serially diluted extracts from tumor samples. C33A extracts were used as a positive control. The extracts from case 8 were mixed with those from C33A cells and subjected to TRAP assay, resulting in significant loss of the telomerase activity of C33A cells, suggesting the presence of reaction inhibitors in the extracts. To eliminate the inhibitors, the telomerase reaction mixture of case 8 was subjected to phenol/chloroform extractions followed by subsequent PCR. The signals were restored by this treatment.

underlined. TS- and CX-overlap primers are only used for the initial amplification, after which the 150-bp product is column purified for future use. Because the overlapping sequences of the primers recognize sequences of the *myo*-genin gene, PCR reaction with these primer sets using *myo*-genin cDNA as a template generates a 150-bp product. After purification of the products using the standard procedures to recover PCR products, they can be used as an internal control to monitor PCR efficacy, and are reamplified with the same TS and CX primers used to amplify the telomerase ladder in the standard TRAP assay. Fifteen attograms of internal standard products is usually used per reaction. False-negative samples can be identified by failure to amplify the internal standard.

The abundance of telomerase ladders sometimes increases with increasing amounts of *Taq* polymerase. This demonstrates that the molarity of these multiple amplification products causes *Taq* polymerase to become limiting. Thus, titration of *Taq* polymerase may also cause differences in PCR efficiency among samples, which can also be normalized with use of an internal standard. Commercially available research kits that include internal standard are available (TRAP-eze™, Oncor, Inc., Gaithersburg, MD).

Purification of telomerase extension products before PCR cycles can eliminate the effects of inhibitors (**Fig. 3**) *(10)*. After the extension reaction, reaction mixtures are purified by phenol/chloroform extractions followed by ethanol precipitation. Note that *Taq* polymerase is not required in the extension reaction. Dissolve the pellets in small amounts of distilled water or TE and add the PCR reaction mixture containing 10X TRAP reaction buffer, dNTPs, TS primer, CX primer, and *Taq* polymerase in 50-µL reaction volume, and start PCR reaction as described for the standard TRAP assay.

5. Telomerase activity can be semiquantified by a variety of methods. The most commonly used quantification method is measurement of the band intensity of telomerase ladders and normalization of it with that of the internal standard. In our SYBR Green I system, telomerase ladders are visualized on a UV transilluminator and photographed, and band intensities of the telomerase products and internal control are measured with picture analyzing software packages such as NIH Image. Normalization of telomerase ladders by internal control yields relative telomerase activities among samples.

An alternative method for estimation of telomerase activity is the dilution TRAP assay, in which serially diluted extracts (usually with 10-fold and 100-fold dilution) are examined. Because 5 µg protein extracts are used in the standard TRAP assay, 0.5 µg and 0.05 µg extracts are usually prepared simply by diluting the extracts with lysis buffer. Positive signals in diluted extracts suggest the presence of high-level telomerase activity in the samples. It occasionally happens that telomerase activity is positive with 0.05 µg extracts, but negative with 5 µg extracts (**Fig. 3**) *(10)*. This is also explained by the existence of reaction inhibitors, the effects of which decrease with dilution of extracts.

6. Another option to increase the capacity of quantification in the telomerase assay is use of specialized primers that contain unrelated tag sequences at their 5′ termini. PCR products in the TRAP assay progressively shorten with each cycle because the primers used are likely to anneal internal repeated sequences of the templates. Because the shorter templates are preferentially amplified in the PCR reaction, most of the PCR products in the TRAP assay are likely to be short and longer products are scarce. Thus, the processivity of telomerase is not accurately reflected by the TRAP assay. Stretch PCR assay is a powerful method for quantitation of telomerase activity *(17)*. This assay uses specialized primers that contain unrelated tag sequences at their 5′ termini (TAG-U primer: 5′-GTAAAACGACGGCCAGTTTGGGGTTGGGGTTGGGGTTG-3′, CTA-R primer: 5′-CAGGAAACAGCTATGACCCCTAACCCTAACCCTAACCCT-3′). Because the

primers contain tag sequences and the annealing temperature is extremely high (68°C), they tend to anneal the edge sequences of the templates which contain tag sequences, rather than the internal telomeric sequences, which do not contain tag sequences. Products obtained by stretch PCR are expected to be longer than those obtained by the TRAP assay and to much more accurately reflect the processivity of telomerase. Purification of telomerase extension products before PCR reaction is usually performed to increase capacity for quantitation. High annealing temperature (68°C) in stretch PCR will also reduce nonspecific signals. We developed a modified stretch PCR method, which is simpler than the original method and is therefore suitable for examination of numerous clinical samples *(18,19)*. Commercially available research kits that include internal standard are available for stretch PCR assay (TeloChaser, Toyobo Co., Ltd., Osaka, Japan).

## 4.1. Modified Stretch PCR

10X PCR buffer: 200 m$M$ Tris-Cl, 600 m$M$ KCl, 15 m$M$ MgCl$_2$, 0.05% Tween, 10 m$M$ EGTA.

1. Extension reaction 23°C 30 min. Reaction mixture: 5 µL 10X PCR buffer, 10 µL dNTPs (2.5 m$M$ each), 2 µL TAG-U primer (100 ng/µL), 31 µL H$_2$O, 2 µL CHAPS extract.
2. Add 150 µL of H$_2$O after completion of extension reaction
3. Two phenol/chloroform extractions followed by EtOH precipitation by the addition of 100 µL of 7.5 $M$ NH$_4$OAc (final concentration of NH$_4$OAc should be 2.5 $M$) and 750 µL of EtOH. It is recommended that carriers (carrier DNAs or glycogen) be used for easy recovery of pellets by ethanol precipitation.
4. Wash pellets with 1 mL of 70% EtOH and centrifuge at top speed.
5. Recover pellets and dry them in vacuum centrifugation at high temperature for a few minutes.
6. Add PCR mixture to the pellets and resuspend well (approx 20 times) by pipeting. PCR mixture: 5 µL 10X PCR buffer, 1 µL dNTPs, 1 µL CTA-R (100 ng/µL), 0.4 µL *Taq*, 42.6 µL H$_2$O.
7. Transfer above mixtures into PCR tubes.
8. PCR reaction: 93°C 3 min/1 cycle (hot start), 93°C 1 min, 68°C 1 min, 72°C 2 min/ 25 cycles, 72°C 10 min/1 cycle.
9. Electrophorese on 7% polyacrylamide gel (not 12% gel) and stain with SYBR Green for 10 min.

Longer products (ladders) than those observed in the TRAP assay can be observed. Because stretch PCR is performed under stringent conditions (high annealing temperature), the sensitivity of the assay is usually lower than that of the TRAP assay. Nonspecific signals are rarely observed and specificity is much higher than for the TRAP assay.

## References

1. Watson, J. D. (1972) Origin of concatameric T4 DNA. *Nature* **239,** 197–201.
2. Counter, C. M., Avilion, A. A., LeFeuvre, C. E., Stewart, N. G., Greider, C. W., and Harley, C. B. (1992) Telomere shortening associated with chromosome instability is arrested in immortal cells which express telomerase activity. *EMBO J.* **11,** 1921–1929.
3. Harley, C B., Futcher, B., and Greider, C. W. (1990) Telomeres shorten during ageing of human fibroblasts. *Nature (Lond.)* **345,** 458–460.
4. Greider, C. W. and Blackburn, E. H. (1989) A telomeric seqeunce in the RNA of *Tetrahymena* telomerase required for telomere repeat synthesis. *Nature* **337,** 331–337.
5. Yu, G. L., Bradley, J. D., Attardi, L. D., and Blackburn, E. H. (1990) In vivo alteration of telomerase sequences and senescence caused by mutated *Tetrahymena* telomerase RNAs. *Nature* **344,** 126–132.

6. Kim, N. W., Piatyszek, M. A., Prowse, K. R., Harley, C. B., West, M. D., Ho, P. L. C., et al. (1994) Specific association of human telomerase activity with immortal cells and cancer. *Science* **266,** 2011–2015.

7. Hiyama, K., Hiyama, E., Ishioka, S., Yamakido, M., Inai, K., Gazdar, A. F., et al. (1995) Telomerase activity in small-cell and non small-cell lung cancers. *J. Natl. Cancer Inst.* **87,** 895–901.

8. Hiyama, E., Gollahon, L., Kataoka, T., Kuroi, K., Yokoyama, T., Gazdar, A. F., et al. (1996) Telomerase activity in human breast tumors. *J. Natl. Cancer Inst.* **88,** 116.

9. Kyo, S., Ueno, H., Kanaya, T., and Inoue, M. (1996) Telomerase activity in gynecological tumors. *Clin. Cancer Res.* **2,** 2023–2028.

10. Kyo, S., Kunimi, K., Uchibayashi, T., Namiki, M., and Inoue, M. (1997) Telomerase activity in human urothelial tumors. *Am. J. Clin. Pathol.* **5,** 555–569.

11. Kyo, S., Takakura, M., Tanaka, M., Kanaya, T., Sagawa, T., Kohama, T., et al. (1997) Expression of telomerase activity in human chorion. *Biochem. Biophys. Res. Commun.* **241,** 498–503.

12. Kyo, S., Takakura, M., Kohama, T., and Inoue, M. (1997) Telomerase activity in human endometrium. *Cancer Res.* **57,** 610–614.

13. Kyo, S., Takakura, M., Ishikawa, H., Sasagawa, T., Satake, S., Tateno, M., and Inoue, M. (1997) Application of telomerase assay for the screening of cervical lesions. *Cancer Res.* **57,** 1863–1867.

14. Kinoshita, H., Ogawa, O., Kakehi, Y., Mishina, M., Mitsumori, K., Itoh, H., et al. (1997) Detection of telomerase activity in exfoliated cells in urine from patients with bladder cancer. *J. Natl. Cancer Inst.* **89,** 724–730.

15. Villa, R., Zaffaroni, N., Folini, M., Martelli, G., De Palo, G., Daidone, M. G., et al. (1998) Telomerase activity in benign and malignant breast lesions: a pilot prospective study on fine-needle aspirates. *J. Natl. Cancer Inst.* **90,** 537–539.

16. Wright, W. E., Shay, J. W., and Piatyszek, M. A. (1995) Modifications of a telomeric repeat amplification protocol (TRAP) result in increased reliabilty, linearity and sesitivity. *Necleic Acids Res.* **23,** 3794, 3795.

17. Tatematsu, K., Nakayama, J., Danbara, M., Shionoya, S., Sato, H., Omine, M., et al. (1996) A novel quantitative "stretch PCR assay", that detects a dramatic increase in telomerase activity during the progression of myeloid leukemias. *Oncogene* **13,** 2265–2274.

18. Kyo, S., Takakura, M., Tanaka, M., and Inoue, M. (1998) Telomerase activity in cervical cancer is quantitatively distinct from that in its precursor lesions. *Int. J. Cancer* **79,** 66–70.

19. Kyo, S., Takakura, M., Tanaka, M., Murakami, K., Saito, R, Hirano, H., et al. (1998) Quantitative differences in telomerase activity among malignant, premalignant, and benign ovarian lesions. *Clin. Cancer Res.* **4,** 399–405.

# X

## IMMUNO AND GENE THERAPY PROTOCOLS

# 82

## Immunological and Gene Therapy for Ovarian Cancer

*A Technical Overview*

### Charles Gourley and Hani Gabra

## 1. Introduction

Conventional medical approaches are limited in part on the prognosis of ovarian cancer. Although the advent of platinum- and taxane-based combination chemotherapy represents a significant advance in the treatment of ovarian carcinoma, the 5-yr survival of patients with intraperitoneal (ip) disseminated disease remains poor at only 30–40% *(1–3)*. The vast majority of patients present with disease that is advanced because of transcoelomic spread yet remains locoregionally contained, rather than truly metastatic to distant sites by blood or lymphatic spread.

Although 5-yr survival rates are poor owing to the late-presenting nature of ovarian cancer, the disease generally remains localized intraperitoneally throughout its natural history. Locoregional control, therefore, remains the primary objective of multimodal clinical management. These clinical realities should guide clinical research and the strategic objectives of translational and basic biological research, and afford a real opportunity for the locoregional testing of novel therapies by the ip route. The insertion of peritoneal catheters, such as those used for dialysis, allow safe delivery of agents to the peritoneum, and sampling of the effects of such interventions can also be made by peritoneal fluid washings at timed intervals.

Two innovative approaches being actively investigated are immunotherapy and gene therapy. Immunotherapy for cancer has, at its source, observations dating back several centuries, and has been actively investigated by workers over the last 50 yr. Rapid increases recently in our understanding of tumor immunology have stimulated a renaissance in this area of research.

Ten years of gene-therapy research have defined the criteria that are required to be met in order to evaluate such treatments rationally, and the limitations and difficulties of this modality have been defined. It is the objective of this chapter to outline progress for these modalities in ovarian cancer research and outline difficulties and pitfalls for those contemplating such translational and clinical research.

From: *Methods in Molecular Medicine, Vol. 39: Ovarian Cancer: Methods and Protocols*
Edited by: J. M. S. Bartlett © Humana Press, Inc., Totowa, NJ

## 2. Immunotherapy

Most of the scientific and clinical work on immunotherapy in human cancer has so far been conducted in malignant melanoma. This was a good tumor type to choose initially because of its documented response to immune-altering agents, such as interferon-γ (IFN-γ) and interleukin 2 (IL-2), as well as its well-characterized tumor-associated antigens (TAAs). Clinical trials have been conducted in melanoma using lymphokine-activated killer (LAK) cells ADDIN ENRfu *(4,5)*, tumor infiltrating lymphocytes (TILs) *(6)*, tumor lysate vaccines *(7)*, polyvalent melanoma cell vaccines *(8)*, peptide vaccines*(9)*, and pulsed dendritic cell vaccines *(10)*. Some of these strategies are currently being extended to ovarian cancer treatment.

There are several reasons why ovarian cancer is suitable for an immunotherapeutic approach for treatment. First, there are excellent severe combined immunodeficiency (SCID) mouse models in which human ovarian cancer cells can be injected intraperitoneally and whose subsequent growth is very similar to the pattern of tumor growth in humans *(11)*. These SCID mice also allow human T lymphocytes to be injected without rejection and, therefore, the opportunity arises to test immune strategies using human immune cells against human cancer cells in vivo. Second, ovarian cancer has been shown to respond intraperitoneally to cytokines such as IFN-γ and IL-2 *(12,13)* agents, which are also active in melanoma and renal cell carcinoma, the two tumor types considered the most immunogenic. Third, 90% of ovarian cancer patients present with disease confined to the peritoneum so the opportunity exists for ip administration of immunotherapeutic agents and for removal of peritoneal fluid via dialysis catheter to assess response of tumor cells or phenotype of immune cells.

Problems specific to ovarian cancer include its lack of immunological characterization, specifically a lack of defined cellular tumor antigens. Problems that have been encountered in immunotherapy in other tumor types and would have to be overcome in ovarian cancer include:

- The possibility that a conventional antibody response, no matter how vigorous, may not be useful in a therapeutic sense because it has not been shown to result in tumor cell death.
- The difficulty in activating T cells against a proposed tumor-associated antigen without inducing tolerance, anergy, or even apoptosis of the T cells.
- The possibility that not all tumor cells may express MHC class 1 and therefore present the tumor antigens in a context capable of priming T cells.
- The possibility of downregulation of a particular TAA or MHC molecule to allow immune escape from primed cytotoxic T cells.
- The lack of knowledge about the role of non-T-cell immunity in tumor rejection.

In the following section, we will consider ovarian cancer immunotherapy, first in terms of antibody-related approaches, then in terms of T-cell-related approaches, and finally, in terms of exogenous cytokine administration. Some techniques involve the use of both antibodies and T cells. Both of these approaches are considered further in **Subheading 2.3.**

### 2.1. Therapeutic Antibodies

#### 2.1.1. Membrane Folate Receptor

The membrane folate receptor (MFR), also known as the folate-binding protein (FBP), is one of the best-characterized ovarian tumor antigens and also has the advantage of being present on 90% of ovarian cancer cells. The murine monoclonal antibody (MAb) MOv18 attached to an Iodine 131 molecule has shown promising results in 16 ovarian cancer patients with minimal residual disease treated intraperitoneally (five had surgical complete response and six had stable disease at a third look operation) *(14)*.

Subsequently, chimeric MOv18 has been made to control the effector functions of the MAb and to reduce the immunogenicity of the murine MAb to allow for repeated administration in humans. The safety of intravenous infusion of such a construct has now been demonstrated in phase 1 clinical trials *(15)*. The most likely use for MAb MOv18 is as an immunoconjugate, either with β-emitters or chemotherapeutic moieties. Bispecific monoclonal antibodies have been used to retarget T lymphocytes against tumor cells. This is a means of overcoming the lack of known classical tumor-associated antigens as would be recognized by cytotoxic T cells. The most widely used construct (OC/TR) contains a specificity for the FBP molecule of ovarian carcinoma cells and a specificity for the CD 3 molecule of T lymphocytes. This antibody caused retargeting of in vitro-activated peripheral blood T lymphocytes from healthy donors and patients with ovarian carcinoma resulting in specific lysis of ovarian carcinoma cells in vitro *(16)* and increased survival in athymic mice xenotransplanted with ovarian carcinoma cells *(17)*. More recently, this form of bispecific MAb has been used in a phase-2 immunotherapy trial in patients with stage III or IV ovarian cancer *(18)*. A 27% overall response rate was obtained in 28 patients who received two cycles of five daily ip infusions of autologous in vitro-activated peripheral blood T lymphocytes retargeted with OC/TR plus recombinant IL-2 with or without a second daily infusion of OC/TR F (ab′) and IL-2. There was also evidence of disease response intraperitoneally with progression elsewhere, showing that this approach was locoregional in its effect with minimal systemic. The investigators then treated 13 patients with the same immunotherapeutic protocol and showed only low-serum concentrations of free, functional OC/TR and very weak coating of circulating T lymphocytes with OC/TR *(19)*. These peripheral blood T lymphocytes did not exert OC/TR-retargeted cytolytic activity. In this protocol, there is a requirement for in vitro activation of T lymphocytes prior to administration. An attempt has been made to improve the level of in vitro activation and simplify the protocol by using both monospecific anti-CD28 MAbs and bispecific anti-CD28/FBP MAbs. This increased the growth inhibition of tumor cells in vitro, but had no effect on the cytotoxicity of the T lymphocytes.

### 2.1.2. HMFG2

Monoclonal antibodies to human milk fat globule HMFG1 and HMFG2 identify surface antigens widely overexpressed on ovarian cancer cells. HMFG1 and HMFG2 have been extensively tested in ovarian cancer both as tools for imaging and therapy. Radio-labeled HMFG2 has been tested, particularly for ip radio-immunotherapy, and clear clinical responses have been obtained *(20,21)*. Future studies include discontinuing the radiotherapeutic component because cold antibody has been shown to have clinical efficacy in other scenarios, and thereby promoting its use to first-line adjuvant therapy during or immediately following chemotherapy.

### 2.1.3. c-erbB-2

Antibody to c-*erbB*-2 has been extensively evaluated as a treatment in breast cancer based on the observation that c-*erbB*-2 is overexpressed in one-third of cases, and that these patients have a worse prognosis. Herceptin, a humanized MAb, has been tested in patients with metastatic breast cancer in a randomized setting in combination with breast cancer. In 469 patients, addition of herceptin doubled the response rate from 36 to 62%. Additionally, survival time to disease progression increased from 5.5 to 8.6 mo. Both response and survival increases were statistically significant *(22)*.

c-*erbB*-2 is also elevated in one-third of ovarian cancer and is also an independent factor for poor prognosis *(23)*. It remains to be seen if this antibody provides similar efficacy in ovarian cancer.

### 2.1.4. Sialyl Tn-KLH

Sialyl Tn-KLH is a tumor-associated antigen generated by aberrant glycosylation of apomucin and correlates with poor prognosis. Its use as active specific immunotherapy in a randomized study for metastatic breast cancer has produced interesting results with improved survival in cancer vaccine arm, and these results have prompted its exploration in ovarian cancer *(24)*.

## 2.2. Therapeutic T Cells

### 2.2.1. Overview

It is considered that cell-mediated immunotherapy is more likely to be of therapeutic value than antibody approaches. However, cellular immunology is more complex and trials in humans have to be approached with more caution than antibody-related approaches. For this reason, it is useful to have good animal models. Recently, Walker and Gallagher *(11)* developed a model using SCID mice. When Ovan 4 ovarian carcinoma cells were transferred to the peritoneal cavity, the tumor distributed generally on the peritoneal wall and mesenteric membranes in a pattern similar to that seen in human ovarian cancer, rather than the ascitic pattern seen in previous models using athymic "nude" mice. SCID mice also do not reject human peripheral blood lymphocytes (PBLs ) and, therefore, the potential for infused immune cells to eradicate established tumors or protect against tumor cell challenge can be assessed. Indeed, it was shown that PBL-SCID mice all produced detectable levels of human immunoglobulin and that these mice survived significantly longer with the human ovarian tumor than nonreconstituted SCID mice. It is possible that the transfer of purified lymphocyte subpopulations may delineate which effector-cell populations are important in providing protection. This model can also be used to investigate immunization procedures, the protective effect of allogeneic vs autologous reconstituted lymphocytes and the use of ex vivo modified immune cells (whether genetically modified or immunologically primed).

Based on the assumption that TILs possess some degree of specific activity against the tumor which they infiltrate and following promising results in the melanoma setting, investigators infused TILs following a single small dose of cyclophosphamide (an *immunomodulating, not* a cytotoxic dose) in patients with advanced or recurrent disease and produced an overall response rate of 71.4% *(25)*. In a preliminary study, they also produced an improvement in the response rate to *cis*-platinum chemotherapy by using a combination of *cis*-platinum chemotherapy with TIL infusion, although the number of patients in the study were small. It is worth noting that regression of these tumors occurred at all sites, whether primary or metastatic.

### 2.2.2. Exogenous Cytokine Administration

There is concern that immunotherapy based on the principle of stimulation of a cytotoxic T-cell response could be hampered because tumor cells may not express or may actively downregulate the expression of MHC class 1 molecules. In this situation, combined immunotherapy with cytokines that have been shown to modulate MHC expression in other tumor types may be a useful therapeutic approach. Possible cytokines that could be employed include interferon α *(26,27)* interferon γ *(27–30)*, and retinoic acid *(29)*. One study *(31)*, conducted in metastatic pleural and peritoneal effusions in ovarian cancer patients showed that intrapleural or ip administration of IFN-α could produce a high local-response rate if the effusion contained a high ratio of tumor cells to mononuclear cells. If this ratio was low, the overall local response rate dropped from 100% (25% CR and 75% PR) to 17% (all PR).

## 2.3. Immunologically Based Gene Therapy

Unlike malignant melanoma, in ovarian and many other human cancers it is difficult to obtain tumor-specific T cells. To overcome this and broaden the applicability of cellular immunotherapy, T cells were transduced with a chimeric antibody/T-cell receptor gene consisting of the gene encoding the variable region of a MAb against a TAA (MOv-γ of the MAb MOv18 is classically used in ovarian carcinoma) linked to the Fc-receptor γ gene *(32–35)*. The construct was inserted into a retroviral transduction vector downstream of a human promoter, such as the human phosphoglycerate kinase (PGK) promoter. When T cells were transduced with these chimeric receptor genes, they recognized and lysed tumor cells and secreted cytokines when they encountered the appropriate mAb-defined antigen *(32,33)*. In a murine ovarian cancer model, the chimeric T-cell receptor gene was introduced into TILs, which were then administered intraperitoneally *(34)*. Mice treated with the MOv-γ transduced TILs had significantly increased survival compared to controls. Similarly, these TILs caused a decrease in 3-d pulmonary metastases from FBP-expressing tumor cells in C57BL/6 mice when administered intravenously *(34)*. Also, because the signaling motifs for the FcR and the TCR are highly related, it was felt that transduction of bone marrow cells with chimeric receptor genes may result in immune cells of several lineages (monocytes, NK cells, neutrophils, and T cells) all having antitumor activity. Therefore, Wang et al. *(35)* reconstituted lethally irradiated mice with murine bone marrow hemopoietic cells retrovirally transduced with the chimeric receptor gene directed against FBP on ovarian carcinoma cells. Successful transplants were conducted and all mice expressed the transgene, showing that the reconstituted stem cells were capable of maintaining long-term stability in vivo. When these mice were then challenged with sarcoma cells injected subcutaneously either expressing the FBP molecule or not, there was a reduction in size of the day-34 tumor by one-third in the sarcoma cells expressing the FBP molecule. FACS analysis showed that none of the remaining tumor cells expressed the FBP molecule demonstrating selection in the tumor-cell population of FBP negative cells. Most interestingly, when the mice were depleted of CD4 and CD8 cells, there was no decrease in the antitumor activity, suggesting that T cells may not be essential in this model. If this were the case, it would bypass many of the perceived problems with cellular immunotherapy such as requirement of costimulation for adequate activation of T cells.

A very different, but intriguing, approach has been taken by Hui et al. *(36)* who injected allogeneic MHC genes into cutaneous metastases in ovarian and cervical cancer patients and found that of the 10 patients in their phase 1 / 2 study, five exhibited a strong local response with shrinkage of the treated tumor lesion to less than 50% of the original size. Gene delivery was via DC-Chol/DOPE cationic liposomes. Although the number of patients was small, there was a suggestion that the immune response was somewhat dependent upon the immunizing MHC gene used with allogeneic HLA-A2 DNA being more effective than both allogeneic HLA-B13 DNA and xenogenic H-2K$^k$ DNA. In previous animal model studies, Hui et al. *(37)* showed that the introduction of allogeneic MHC genes into tumor cells generated vigorous CTL reactivities not only against the allogeneic MHC molecules, but also against the "wild-type" tumor cells. This has led them to ask whether the immune responses produced by introduction of allogeneic MHC genes would be strong enough to prevent or reduce the incidence of metastatic disease for ovarian or cervical carcinoma. The main problem of testing this would be how to design a safe trial that exposed allogeneic MHC molecules to the immune system in the context of a tumor cell in the adjuvant or low-volume disease setting.

Gene marking is also being used as an investigative tool to study immunotherapy. A neomycin resistance gene on a retroviral vector was transduced into purified ovarian TILs. Purified rIL-2 expanded CD3$^+$ CD8$^+$ neomarked TILs were administered ip. rIL-2 was also given ip as a bolus on days 2–4, 8–11, and 15–18. Laparoscopy was performed in patients with no clinical or radiological evidence of disease 1 mo after receiving the ip injected cells and serial sampling of cells was also conducted via a peritoneal catheter. The marked TILs were thereby used in ip adoptive immunotherapy of ovarian cancer patients to study TIL trafficking *(38,39)*.

## 3. Gene Therapy

Over the last 10 years, gene therapy has developed into a major cancer research discipline. Gene therapy is the alteration, using protocols that transfer nucleic acid to cells, of a somatic cell's genetic complement for therapeutic purposes. These alterations may be to knock out an abnormal gene product, to reconstitute the function of an inactivated gene, or to confer a new function on a cell to improve therapeutic outcome.

In order to engage in cancer gene therapy, first, the nucleic acid of interest should have functional activity in the cell of interest and proof of principle that the intervention is functional should be demonstrated in a preclinical model. Second, a method is required to deliver the nucleic acid of interest to the relevant somatic cell. Third, this method must be of sufficient efficiency of nucleic acid delivery to have the potential to demonstrate a clinical effect. Finally, the toxicities of the genetic therapy, just like any other medicine, must be tolerable.

### 3.1. Mechanisms of Gene Delivery

There are a large number of gene delivery systems that can be classified under two headings: viral and nonviral.

### 3.1.1. Nonviral Systems

Nonviral systems have the advantage of being nonbiohazards, which have relevance for issues of safety. Ex vivo manipulation of somatic cells can be achieved by transfection, electroporation, and lipofection. Nonviral systems have generally been regarded as less efficient than viral systems. However, newer nonviral systems are beginning to compete with viral-mediated gene delivery methods. New cationic liposomes enhanced with lipids promises great increases in transfection efficiency *(40–43)*. The use of transferrin-liposome systems *(44)*, also shows improved uptake efficiency promoted by lipofectin-DNA-transferrin complexes. The capacity of new lipid combinations to compact DNA *(42)* has provided a further efficiency increment. The use of receptor targeting *(44,45)* and the use of new peptides, such as protamine sulphate *(46)*, also hold promise for improving gene transfer efficiency.

Ovarian cancer gene therapy studies where gene delivery with nonviral systems is performed in vitro include lipofection of IL-2 into autologous ovarian tumor cells and their subsequent irradiation and reinfusion *(47)*; and expression of CEA by RNA transfer to autologous dendritic cells and their subsequent intravenous injection into ovarian cancer patients *(48)*. For ovarian-cancer in vivo gene therapy using nonviral systems, clinical protocols utilize lipofection of the DNA of interest. A study led by Hotobagyi is investigating the lipofection of the adenoviral *E1a* gene by ip injection in patients with ovarian cancer expressing *erbB*-2 *(49)*. This is based on the observation that *E1a* gene inhibits transcription at the *HER-2/neu* promoter *(50)* and murine studies that indicated suppression of tumor growth and improved survival in tumor-bearing mice treated with liposome/*E1a* gene complexes *(51,52)*. Another clinical study utilizing nonviral systems investigates the transfer of MHC DNA-liposome complexes using either HLA-A2, HLA-B13, or H-2K(k) gene complexed with DC-Chol/DOPE cationic liposomes injected intratumorally in patients with ovarian cancer who have either abdominal wall or lymph node metastases. This study was based on the observation that a previous phase I study in 19 advanced cancer patients demonstrated that the most common responding tumor type was ovarian cancer *(36)*.

### 3.1.2. Viral Delivery Systems

There is a growing list of viral vectors for gene delivery. In ovarian cancer trials, adenoviruses and retroviruses have been the main systems used, although there are also clinical trials using poxvirus vectors.

In general, retroviral vectors efficiently transduce replicating cells and animal studies have shown dramatic responses in experimental brain tumors, relying on the principle that these divide more rapidly than surrounding brain tissue *(53)*. Unfortunately, clinical studies with human gliomas were not clinically successful because of the much slower rate of division of naturally occurring human tumors.

Adenoviral vectors, in contrast, will transduce nondividing cells thereby being of more potential clinical utility. Unfortunately, one of the problems of adenoviral transduction in vivo is one of poor long-term expression of the transduced genes. This has been attributed to immune responses both humoral and cell-mediated against adenoviral antigens. In order to limit this problem, immunogenic antigens such as E2A and E4 have been deleted from the adenoviral construct. Furthermore, some workers have attempted to induce immunosuppression using drugs, cytokines, or T-cell depletion. A more sophisticated approach to the inhibition of T-cell activation is to interfere with the interaction between costimulatory molecules, specifically B7 on antigen-presenting cells and CTLA4 on T cells. Systemic injection of CTLA4Ig resulted in an improvement of transgene expression from the transduced adenoviral vectors *(54)*. Engineering of CTLA4Ig into an adenoviral vector followed by coinfection of this adenoviral construct with an adenoviral reporter construct carrying *LacZ* significantly prolonged the expression of the *lacZ* transgene. However, *LacZ* expression eventually faltered, and, after 5 mo, readministration of the *lacZ* reporter adenovirus resulted in re-expression suggesting that CTLA4Ig production continued and remained functionally suppressive for the humoral and cytotoxic response to adenoviral antigenicity *(55)*. This minimization of the immune response to adenoviral vectors is an important step forward in maintenance of long-term expression allowing effective multiple administration of gene therapy, which will almost certainly be required for cancer gene therapy.

Clinical ovarian cancer studies utilizing viral systems for in vitro manipulation include retroviral transduction of the *MDR-1* gene into autologous CD34 +ve bone marrow cells. The idea is to repopulate the marrow and confer resistance to chemotherapy agents thereby improving the patients tolerance to myelosuppression *(56)*.

Clinical studies utilizing in vivo viral systems for gene delivery to treat ovarian cancer have utilised the herpes simplex thymidine kinase (*HSV+K*) gene incorporated into either adenovirus *(57)* or retrovirus *(58)*.

## 3.2. Improving the Therapeutic Index of Cytotoxic Drugs

### 3.2.1. Prodrug Activation

The expression of a foreign gene in ovarian cancer cells that can specifically convert a nontoxic substrate to a toxic one is an attractive approach because a nontoxic compound (a prodrug) could be given to a patient that is selectively converted to the active drug in the cancer cells, which results in their selective destruction. The selective delivery of these genes to ovarian cancer cells is, however, problematic. A better approach is to place the prodrug activating gene under the control of a promoter, which is driven in ovarian cancer cells, but not in nonmalignant tissues. This principle underlies the concept of prodrug activation as a mechanism of improving the therapeutic index of the active drug. One method for employing relatively selective transduction of ovarian cancer cells is to use an adenovirus bearing the *HSVtk* gene. *HSVtk* converts the relatively nontoxic compound ganciclovir to toxic metabolites at high efficiency. Transfection of the Ad.RSVtk vector (where the *HSVtk* gene is under the control of the rous sarcoma virus promoter and is engineered into an adenoviral vector) to ovarian cancer cells in vitro followed by growth as murine xenografts and treatment of the mice subcutaneously or intraperitoneally with ganciclovir demonstrates the potential effectiveness of this system. Mice treated with ganciclovir had a 10- to 20-fold-lower tumor burden than control mice *(59)*. It was quickly noted that not all cells needed to be transfected and expressing for all cells to be killed. This so-called bystander effect was obvious when as few as 4% of cells were transfected in a mixed population. Treatment benefit appeared to be related to adenovirus dose and tumor burden *(60)*. Subsequently, it has been shown that the CMV promoter is more effective than the RSV promoter for *tk*-mediated ganciclovir cytotoxicity *(61)*. Animal studies have demonstrated clear survival advantage for tumor-bearing mice treated with this system *(62)*; and human studies are underway *(57)*.

Human umbilical vein endothelial cells (HUVECs) have been used to introduce *tk* activity intraperitoneally, and appear to have antitumor activity primarily caused by the bystander effect *(63)*. More recently, it has been shown that acyclovir could be more effective than ganciclovir as a prodrug *(64)*. Other bacterial prodrug-activating enzymes have been employed experimentally in ovarian cancer.

Bacterial carboxypeptidase G2 conferred approximately tenfold sensitivity for SKOV3 and approximately 100-fold sensitivity for A2780 with the mustard prodrug CMDA *(65)*. *Escherichia coli* nitroreductase expressing SKOV3 were approximately 200-fold more sensitive to the prodrug CB1954, and again, a significant bystander effect was in evidence *(66)*.

Control of the prodrug-activating enzyme using an ovarian-specific promoter would be an attractive approach, but has not been widely adopted in ovarian cancer. The CA125 and *Her2/neu* promoters would be obvious candidates, and secretory leucoprotease inhibitor gene has been suggested *(67)*, although in general downregulation of this marker seems to correlate with poor prognosis. As more differentially regulated genes are identified, so this approach will become more feasible.

### 3.2.2. Conferring Multidrug Resistance on Normal Tissues

Introduction of drug resistance genes into the normal hematopoietic tissue to confer resistance of these normal tissues to chemotherapy is an interesting idea that has actually been realized as a clinical trial in ovarian cancer *(56)*. The principle is that by conferring resistance to chemotherapy on the hematopoietic system (which is one of the main casualties of chemotherapy-induced toxicity), patients can be rendered more tolerant to the clinical toxicities associated with chemotherapy. In the Deisseroth study, analysis of MDR-1 transduced CFU-GM populations pre- and posttransplant showed that there was no difference in transduction efficiency pretransplant for two separate transfection protocols. However, posttransplant, transduction of adherent cells as opposed to transduction of suspension culture of CFU-GM populations appeared to predict for posttransplant MDR-1 positivity. However, the fact that these patients recover marrow function casts doubt on whether the CFU-GM population targeted has any contribution to play to repopulation of the bone marrow *(68)*. In another phase I study, retroviral transduction of CD34 positive cell populations in vitro prior to autologous transplantation resulted in a low level of MDR positivity in a population of transplant patients. This suggested normal untransduced CD34+ cells that were coinfused may have repopulated the marrow more extensively and competed out the transduced cells. Importantly, this study demonstrated that replication-competent retroviruses were not produced with this protocol, a critical issue for safety of this procedure *(69)*.

### 3.3. Manipulating the Flow of Cellular Information

#### 3.3.1. Antisense and Ovarian Cancer

It has been shown that deoxyoligonucleotides constructed in antisense to a particular mRNA can interfere with that mRNA's expression compared with sense or missense deoxyoligonucleotides. Furthermore, phosphorothioation of the oligonucleotide dramatically improves in vivo stability of the molecule. Laboratory research in ovarian cancer reveals an increasing range of targets in which antisense constructs appear to efficiently and specifically inhibit components of the malignant phenotype of ovarian cancer cell lines. IGF-1 *(70,71)*, IGF-2 *(72)*, IL6 *(73)*, c-*erb*B-2 *(74)*, EGFR *(75)*, uPA *(76)* cyclin-D1 *(77)*, and p53 *(78)* have all been successfully inhibited using antisense resulting in inhibition of a component of the malignant phenotype. Interesting antisense oligonucleotides to c-*raf*-kinase, developed by the ISIS corporation have shown potent broad-spectrum antitumor effects both in vitro and in murine xenograft models *(79)*, and these compounds have completed phase I clinical studies in which a dramatic CA125 marker response (97% reduction) was noted in a patient with ovarian cancer *(80)*.

### 3.3.2. Gene-Replacement/Correction in Ovarian Cancer

An observation that c-*erb*B-2 overexpression can be repressed by adenovirus E1A *(51,52)* has led to investigation of the clinical utility of this phenomenon within an ovarian and breast cancer phase I clinical trial *(49)*. The observation that *erb*B-2 modulation can have a clinical impact in breast cancer in several studies makes this a utilitarian approach as a starting point in clinical trials.

Gene replacement of wild-type *p53* inserted into an adenoviral vector and transfected into *p53*-mutant ovarian SKOV-3 cells reduced colony forming ability in vitro, and in a xenograft model, introduction of *p53* was associated with improved survival of the animals *(81)*. In vivo studies with SKOV-3 suggested a synergistic cytopathic effect between adenoviral *p53* construct and the microtubule disaggregation inhibitor paclitaxel. In vitro, it appears that paclitaxel concentrations too low for microtubule condensation and cytotoxicity may nevertheless promote adenoviral transduction *(82)*.

### 3.3.3. Manipulation of Intracellular Proteins

An approach has been developed whereby intracellular antibody to *erb*B-2 is delivered to tumor cells using an adenoviral vector resulting in cytotoxicity *(83)*. The cytotoxic mechanism was shown to be apoptosis *(84)*. In a phase I clinical trial of this gene therapy approach in ovarian cancer, expression of the c-*erb*B-2 sFv antibody mRNA could be detected by *in situ* hybridization in tumor tissue, and toxicities appeared to be minimal *(85,86)*. Further work is required to define the utility of this approach.

## 3.4. Technical Statements Regarding Clinical Gene Therapy

### 3.4.1. Phase I Trials

It has been argued that there has been an inappropriate and possibly unethical rush to clinically implement the limited molecular information available about ovarian cancer. However, clinical scientists working at the lab/clinic interface appreciate the formidable infrastructure required to connect molecular and clinical science. A major issue is the definition of the toxicity of these approaches, and it may be many years before we are able fully to appreciate potential risks to patients from this type of technology. This is of particular importance when incorporating gene therapy into the initial treatment package of patients, many of whom may survive for many years.

### 3.4.2. Toxicity

Issues of toxicity relate to both patient side effects of treatment, and wider safety issues relating to biohazards. Patient toxicities associated with the general modality of gene therapy are, in general, mild, restricted to mild fevers or allergic reactions, mild hematological toxicity, and the usual consequences of patient instrumentation. The toxicities relating to the specific moiety delivered will, of course, be specific to the active specific modification resulting from the genetic intervention. Hence, leaky prodrug activation strategies may produce milder forms of that active drug's toxicity profile; and specific inhibition of mRNA by antisense strategies affecting normal tissues may have unexpected clinical effects, such as coagulopathy and thrombocytopenia in association with c-*raf*-kinase antisense therapy. Viral infection may cause unwanted cytotoxicity, such as adenoviral transduction of glioma in vivo with consequent transduction and cytotoxicity of adjacent normal brain tissue. Each approach must enter proof-of-principle guided phase I studies in case of unexpected effects.

Safety issues have been a paramount concern of regulatory authorities monitoring gene therapy clinical trials. There is no doubt that tight regulation is required, particularly monitoring of viral vector studies with careful assessment of the capacity for apparently replication defective viruses to recombine and produce infectious titres from patients. In general, phase I studies have failed to detect such recombinant viruses. However, as we enter the next phase of viral vectorology, whereby researchers try to push ever higher the efficiency of in vivo gene transfer, it appears that the use of conditionally replicating viruses will become more common *(87)*. A recent clinical study *(88)*, not in ovarian cancer, using a replication-competent adenovirus that replicates preferentially in *p53* deficient cells has not shown toxicity, but this controversial approach remains in its infancy, currently limited by targeting strategies to tumor cells, avoiding normal tissues.

The pressing clinical need of future patients with ovarian cancer demands the creation of a gene therapy infrastructure now, and is a prerequisite for an approach based on the complete understanding of the molecular biology of ovarian cancer.

Phase I clinical trials commenced, primarily in the United States, have begun to lay down this infrastructure. The intraperitoneal (ip) route for gene therapy has been demonstrably successful in animal models, and phase I clinical trials, therefore, are predominantly using this route.

A website has been developed to keep track of the proliferating clinical trials database for gene therapy (The Wiley Gene Therapy Website at www.wiley.co.uk/genetherapy/). **Table I** shows the ovarian cancer trials available on this database as of October 20, 1998.

## 4. Conclusion

This review of technical activity in the fields of immuno- and gene therapy demonstrate the implementation of startling paradigm shifts, which have fuelled interest in these areas against the odds. It is hoped that the combination of a more-comprehensive understanding of the biology of ovarian cancer, and of cancer generally, and the implementation of many imperfectly selective methodologies in combined approaches will amplify the power of these approaches such that they acquire genuine clinical utility.

## Acknowledgement

The authors would like to thank the managing editor of Genetic Medicine, Wiley Europe for permission to reproduce the data from the Genetic Medicine website in **Table 1**.

**Table 1**
**Current Gene Therapy Protocols in Ovarian Cancer**

| Investigator | Disease | Country | Date Started | Gene | Vector | Patients |
|---|---|---|---|---|---|---|
| Alvarez | Ovarian Cancer | USA | 1/11/95 | TK | Adenovirus | 0 |
| Berchuck | Refractory metastatic Ovarian Cancer | USA | 30/9/95 | IL-2 | Lipofection | 0 |
| Curiel | Ovarian Cancer | USA | 15/5/96 | sFv against erbB-2 | Adenovirus | 0 |
| Deisseroth | Ovarian Cancer and Breast Cancer | USA | 1/12/93 | MDR-1 | Retrovirus | 20 |
| Freeman | Ovarian Cancer | USA | 1/2/93 | TK | Retroviral vector producing cells | 16 |
| Freeman | Ovarian Cancer | USA | 1/5/96 | TK | Retroviral vector producing cells | 0 |
| Hortobagyi | Metastatic Breast Cancer and Ovarian Cancer overexpressing her-2/neu | USA | N/C | E1A | Lipofection | 16 |
| Hwu | Advanced Ovarian Cancer | USA | 1/5/97 | Mov-gamma | Retrovirus | 2 |
| Link | Refractory or Recurrent Ovarian Cancer | USA | 1/6/95 | TK | Retroviral vector producing cells | 8 |
| Lyerly | Breast, Ovary | USA | 1/3/97 | CEA | RNA transfer | N/C |
| Hui | Ovarian and Cervical Cancer with Cutaneous Metastases | Singapore | 1/10/95 | HLA-A2 or HLA-B13 or H2K(k) | Lipofection | 10 |
| Freedman | Ovarian Cancer | USA | 15/8/97 | CD80(B7) and IL-12 | Poxvirus | N/C |
| Kieback | Ovarian Cancer | USA | 5/2/98 | TK | Adenovirus | N/C |

N/C = not communicated. Reproduced with permission from the Wiley Genetic Medicine website (http://www.wiley.co.uk/genetherapy).

## References

1. Venesmaa, P. (1994) Epithelial ovarian cancer : impact of surgery and chemotherapy on survival during 1977–1990. *Obstet. Gynecol.* **84,** 8–11.

2. Neijt, J. P., ten Bokkel Huinink, W. W., van der Burg, M. E., van Oosterom, A. T., Willemse, P. H., Vermorken, J. B., et al. (1991) Longterm survival in ovarian cancer. Mature data from the Netherlands Joint Study Group for Ovarian Cancer. *Eur. J. Cancer* **27,**

3. Di Saia, P. J. and Creasman, W. T. (1993) Epithelial ovarian cancer. *Clinic. Gynecolog. Oncol.* 333–425.

4. Rosenberg, S. A., Lotze, M. T., Muul, L. M., Chang, A. E., Avis, F. P., Leitman, S., et al. (1987) A progress report on the treatment of 157 patients with advanced cancer using lymphokine activated killer cells and interleukin-2 or high dose interleukin-2 alone. *N. Engl. J. Med.* **316,** 889–897.

5. Rosenberg, S. A., Lotze, M. T., Muul, L. M., Leitman, S., Chang, A. E., Ettinghausen, S. E., et al. (1985) Observations on the systemic administration of autologous lymphokine-activated killer cells and recombinant IL-2 to patients with metastatic cancer. *N. Engl. J. Med.* **313,** 1485–1492.

6. Rosenberg, S. A., Packard, B. S., and Aebersold, P. M. (1988) Use of tumor-infiltrating lymphocytes and IL-2 in the immunotherapy of patients with metastatic melanoma. *N. Engl. J. Med.* **319,** 1676–1680.

7. Mitchell, M. S., Harel, W., Kan-Mitchell, J., LeMay, L. G., Goedegebuure, P., Huang, X. Q., et al. (1993) Active specific immunotherapy of melanoma with allogeneic cell lysates. Rationale, results and possible mechanisms of action. *Ann. N.Y. Acad. Sci.* **690,** 153–166.

8. Morton, D. L., Hoon, D. S., Nizze, J. A., Foshag, L. J., Famatiga, E., Wanek, L. A., et al. (1993) Polyvalent melanoma vaccine improves survival of patients with metastatic melanoma. *Ann. N.Y. Acad. Sci.* **690,** 120–134.

9. Rosenberg, S. A., Yang, J. C., Schwartzentruber, D. J., Hwu, P., Marincola, F. M., Topalian, S. L., et al. (1998) Immunologic and therapeutic evaluation of a synthetic peptide vaccine for the treatment of patients with metastatic melanoma. *Nat. Med.* **4,** 321–327.

10. Nestle, F. O., Alijagic, S., Gilliet, M., Sun, Y., Grabbe, S., Dummer, R., et al. (1998) Vaccination of melanoma patients with peptide- or tumor lysate-pulsed dendritic cells. *Nat. Med.* **4,** 328–332.

11. Walker, W. and Gallacher, G. (1995) The development of a novel immunotherapy model of ovarian cancer in human PBL-severe combined immunodeficient (SCID) mice. *Clin. Exp. Immunol.* **101,** 494–501.

12. Berek, J. S., Hacker, N. F., Lichtenstein, A., Jung, T., Spina, C., Knox, R. M., et al. (1985) Intraperitoneal recombinant a interferon for salvage immunotherapy in stage 3 epithelial ovarian cancer: a Gynecologic Oncology Study Group. *Cancer Res.* **45,** 4447–4453.

13. Steis, R. G., Urba, W. J., VanderMolen, L. A., Bookman, M. A., Smith 2nd, J. W., Clark, J. W., et al. (1990) Intraperitoneal lymphokine activated killer cells and interleukin-2 therapy for malignancies limited to the peritoneal cavity. *J. Clin. Oncol.* **8,** 1618–1629.

14. Crippa, F., Bolis, G., Seregni, E., Gavoni, N., Scarfone, G., Ferraris, C., et al. (1995) Single dose intraperitoneal radioimmunotherapy with the murine monoclonal antibody I-131 MOv18: clinical results in patients with minimal residual disease of ovarian cancer. *Eur. J. Cancer* **31,** 686–690.

15. Molthoff, C. F. M., Prinssen, H. M., Kenemans, P., van Hof, A. C., den Hollander, W., and Verheijen, R. H. M. (1997) Escalating protein doses of chimeric monoclonal antibody MOv18 immunoglobulin G in ovarian carcinoma patients: a phase 1 study. *Cancer* **80,** 2712–2720.

16. Pupa, S. M., Canevari, S., Fontanelli, R., Menard, S., Mezzanzanica, D., Lanzavecchia, A., and Colnaghi, M. I. (1988) Activation of mononuclear cells to be used for hybrid monoclonal-antibody induced lysis of human ovarian carcinoma cells. *Int. J. Cancer* **42,** 455–459.

17. Mezzanzanica, D., Garrido, M. A., Neblock, D. S., Daddona, P. E., Andrew, S. M., Zurawski, V. R. J., et al. (1991) Human T-lymphocytes targeted against an established human ovarian carcinoma with a bispecific F (ab') antibody prolong host survival in a murine xenograft model. *Cancer Res.* **51,** 5716–5721.

18. Canevari, S., Stoter, G., Arienti, F., Bolis, G., Colnaghi, M. I., Di Re, E. M., et al. (1995) Regression of advanced ovarian carcinoma by intraperitoneal treatment with autologous T lymphocytes retargeted by a bispecific monoclonal antibody. *J. Natl. Cancer Inst.* **87,** 1463–1469.

19. Lamers, C. H. J., Bolhuis, R. L. H., Warnaar, S. O., Stoter, G., and Gratama, J. W. (1997) Local but no systemic immunomodulation by IP treatment of advanced ovarian cancer with autologous T lymphocytes retargeted by a bispecific monoclonal antibody. *Int. J. Cancer* **73,** 211–219.

20. Epenetos, A. A., Munro, A. J., Stewart, S., Rampling, R., Lambert, H. E., McKenzie, C. G., et al. (1987) Antibody-guided irradiation of advanced ovarian cancer with intraperitoneally administered radiolabeled monoclonal antibodies. *J. Clin. Oncol.* **5,** 1890–1899.

21. Riva, P., Marangolo, M., Lazzari, S., Agostini, M., Sarti, G., Moscatelli, G., et al. (1989) Locoregional immunotherapy of human ovarian cancer: preliminary results. *Int. J. Rad. Appl. Instrum. [B]* **16,** 659–666.

22. Slamon, D., Leyland-Jones, B., Shak, S., Paton, V., Bajamonde, A., Fleming, T., et al. (1998) Addition of Herceptin TM (humanized anti-Her2 antibody) to first line chemotherapy for Her2 overexpressing metastatic breast cancer (Her2+/mbc) markedly increases anticancer activity: a randomized, multinational controlled phase III trial. *Proc. ASCO* **17,** 98 (A377).

23. Berchuck, A., Kamel, A., Whitaker, R., Kerns, B., Olt, G., Kinney, R., et al. (1990) Overexpression of HER-2/neu is associated with poor survival in advanced epithelial ovarian cancer. *Cancer Res.* **50,** 4087–4091.

24. Freedman, R. S. K., Verschraegen, A. P., Edwards, C. F., Tomasovic, C. L., Kaplan, B., Bast, A., et al. (1998) Therapeutic anti-cancer vaccine: a randomized double blind dose comparison study of Sialyl TN-KLH with Detox-b se adjuvant for active specific immunotherapy of ovarian cancer (oc). *Proc. ASCO* **17,** 365 (A1409).

25. Aoki, Y., Takakuwa, K., Kodama, S., Tanaka, K., Takahashi, M., Tokunaga, A., and Takahashi, T. (1991) Use of adoptive transfer of tumor-infiltrating lymphocytes alone or in combination with cisplatin-containing chemotherapy in patients with epithelial ovarian cancer. *Cancer Res.* **51,** 1934–1939.

26. Boyer, C. M., Dawson, D. V., Neal, S. E., Winchell, L. F., Leslie, D. S., Ring, D., et al. (1989) Differential induction by interferons of major histocompatibility complex-encoded and non-major histocompatibility complex-encoded antigens in human breast and ovarian carcinoma cell lines. *Cancer Res.* **49,** 2928–2934.

27. Calvo, F., Jabrane, N., Faille, A., Gauville, C., de Cremoux, P., Lagier, G., et al. (1987) Quantitative modifications of major histocompatibility complex (MHC) antigens induced by recombinant gamma interferon in two human breast cancer lines. *Int. J. Immunopharmacol.* **9,** 459–468.

28. Marth, C. H., Zech, J., Bock, G., Mayer, I., and Daxenbichler, G. (1987) Effects of retinoids and interferon-gamma on cultured breast cancer cells in comparison with tumor necrosis factor alpha. *Int. J. Cancer* **40,** 840–845.

29. Jabrane-Ferrat, N., Faille, A., Loiseau, P., Poirier, O., Charron, D., and Calvo, F. (1990) Effect of gamma interferon on MHC class 1 and 2 transcription and protein expression in human breast adenocarcinoma cell lines. *Int. J. Cancer* **45,** 1169–1176.

30. Schwartz, R. H. (1992) Costimulation of T lymphocytes: the role of CD28, CTLA-4 and B7/BB1 in interleukin-2 production and immunotherapy. *Cell* **71,** 1065–1068.

31. Stathopoulos, G. P., Baxevanis, C. N., Papadopoulos, N. G., Zarkadis, I. K., Papacostas, P., Michailakis, E., et al. (1996) Local immunotherapy with interferon a in metastatic pleural and peritoneal effusions: correlation with immunologic parameters. *Anticancer Res.* **16,** 3855–3860.

32. Eshhar, Z. W., Gross, T., and Schindler, G. D. (1993) Specific activation and targeting of cytotoxic lymphocytes through chimeric single chains consisting of antibody-binding domains and the g or z subunits of the immunoglobulin and T cell receptors. *Proc. Natl. Acad. Sci. USA* **90,** 720–724.

33. Hwu, P., Shafer, G. E., Treisman, J., Schindler, D. G., Gross, G., Cowherd, R., et al. (1993) Lysis of ovarian cancer cells by human lymphocytes redirected with a chimeric gene composed of an antibody variable region and the Fc receptor g chain. *J. Exp. Med.* **178,** 361–366.

34. Hwu, P., Yang, J. C., Cowherd, R., Treisman, J., Shafer, G. E., Eshhar, Z., and Rosenberg, S. A. (1995) In vivo antitumor activity of T cells redirected with chimeric antibody/T cell receptor genes. *Cancer Res.* **55,** 3369–3373.

35. Wang, G. C., Royal, R. K., Yang, R. E., Rosenberg, J. C., et al. (1998) A T cell-independent antitumor response in mice with bone marrow cells retrovirally transduced with an antibody/Fc-g chain chimeric receptor gene recognising a human ovarian cancer antigen. *Nat. Med.* **4,** 168–172.

36. Hui, K. M. A., Huang, P. T., and Tay, L., (1997) Phase 1 study of immunotherapy of cutaneous metastases of human carcinoma using allogeneic and xenogeneic MHC DNA-liposome complexes. *Gene Ther.* **4,** 783–790.

37. Hui, K. S., Foo, T., and Oei, T. (1989) Tumor rejection mediated by transfection with allogeneic class 1 histocompatibility gene. *J. Immunol.* **143,** 3835–3843.

38. Freedman, R. S. P. and Deisseroth, C. D. (1996) Use of a retroviral vector to study the trafficking patterns of purified ovarian tumor infiltrating lymphocytes used in intraperitoneal adoptive immunotherapy of ovarian cancer patients. A pilot study. *Human Gene Ther.* **7,** 1351–1365.

39. Nash, M. A., Platsoucas, C. D., Wong, B. Y., Wong, P. M., Cottler-Fox, M., Otto, E., et al. (1995) Transduction of rIL-2 expanded CD4+ and CD8+ ovarian TIL-derived T cell lines with the G1Na (neoR ) replication-deficient retroviral vector. *Human Gene Ther.* **6,** 1379–1389.

40. Gorman, C. M., Aikawa, M., Fox, B., Fox, E., Lapuz, C., Michaud, B., et al. (1997) Efficient in vivo delivery of DNA to pulmonary cells using the novel lipid EDMPC. *Gene Ther.* **4,** 983–992.

41. Liu, Y., Mounkes, L. C., Liggitt, H. D., Brown, C. S., Solodin, I., Heath, T. D., and Debs, R. J. (1997) Factors influencing the efficiency of cationic liposome-mediated intravenous gene delivery. *Nat. Biotechnol.* **15,** 167–173.

42. Templeton, N. S., Lasic, D. D., Frederik, P. M., Strey, H. H., Roberts, D. D., and Pavlakis, G. N. (1997) Improved DNA: liposome complexes for increased systemic delivery and gene expression. *Nat. Biotechnol.* **15,** 647–652.

43. Wang, J., Guo, X., Xu, Y., Barron, L., and Szoka, F. C., Jr. (1998) Synthesis and characterization of long chain alkyl acyl carnitine esters. Potentially biodegradable cationic lipids for use in gene delivery. *J. Med. Chem.* **41,** 2207–2215.

44. Cheng, P. W. (1996) Receptor ligand-facilitated gene transfer: enhancement of liposome-mediated gene transfer and expression by transferrin. *Hum. Gene Ther.* **7,** 275–282.

45. Dachs, G. U., Dougherty, G. J., Stratford, I. J., and Chaplin, D. J. (1997) Targeting gene therapy to cancer: a review. *Oncol. Res.* **9,** 313–325.

46. Sorgi, F. L., Bhattacharya, S., and Huang, L. (1997) Protamine sulfate enhances lipid-mediated gene transfer. *Gene Ther.* **4,** 961–968.

47. Berchuck, A. and Lyerly, H. (1995) A phase I study of autologous human interleukin 2 (IL-2) gene modified tumor cells in patients with refractory metastatic ovarian cancer. *Human Gene Transfer Protocols*

48. Nair, S. K., Boczkowski, D., Morse, M., Cumming, R. I., Lyerly, H. K., and Gilboa, E. (1998) Induction of primary carcinoembryonic antigen (CEA)-specific cytotoxic T lymphocytes in vitro using human dendritic cells transfected with RNA. *Nat. Biotechnol.* **16,** 364–369.

49. Hortobagyi, G. N., Hung, M. C., and Lopez-Berestein, G. (1998) A Phase I multicenter study of E1A gene therapy for patients with metastatic breast cancer and epithelial ovarian cancer that overexpresses HER-2/neu or epithelial ovarian cancer. *Hum. Gene Ther.* **9,** 1775–1798.

50. Hung, M. C., Matin, A., Zhang, Y., Xing, X., Sorgi, F., Huang, L., et al. (1995) HER-2/neu-targeting gene therapy—a review. *Gene* **159,** 65–71.

51. Yu, D., Matin, A., Xia, W., Sorgi, F., Huang, L., and Hung, M. C. (1995) Liposome-mediated in vivo E1A gene transfer suppressed dissemination of ovarian cancer cells that overexpress HER-2/neu. *Oncogene* **11,** 1383–1388.

52. Zhang, Y., Yu, D., Xia, W., and Hung, M. C. (1995) HER-2/neu-targeting cancer therapy via adenovirus-mediated E1A delivery in an animal model. *Oncogene* **10,** 1947–1954.

53. Culver, K. W., Ram, Z., Wallbridge, S., Ishii, H., Oldfield, E. H., and Blaese, R. M. (1992) In vivo gene transfer with retroviral vector-producer cells for treatment of experimental brain tumors [see comments]. *Science* **256,** 1550–1552.

54. Kay, M. A., Meuse, L., Gown, A. M., Linsley, P., Hollenbaugh, D., Aruffo, A., et al. (1997) Transient immunomodulation with anti-CD40 ligand antibody and CTLA4Ig enhances persistence and secondary adenovirus-mediated gene transfer into mouse liver. *Proc. Natl. Acad. Sci. USA* **94,** 4686–4691.

55. Nakagawa, I., Murakami, M., Ijima, K., Chikuma, S., Saito, I., Kanegae, Y., et al. (1998) Persistent and secondary adenovirus-mediated hepatic gene expression using adenovirus vector containing CTLA4Ig. *Hum. Gene Ther.* **9,** 1739–1745.

56. Deisseroth, A. B., Kavanagh, J., and Champlin, R. (1994) Use of safety-modified retroviruses to introduce chemotherapy resistance sequences into normal hematopoietic cells for chemoprotection during the therapy of ovarian cancer: a pilot trial. *Hum. Gene Ther.* **5,** 1507–1522.

57. Alvarez, R. D. and Curiel, D. T. (1997) A phase I study of recombinant adenovirus vector-mediated intraperitoneal delivery of herpes simplex virus thymidine kinase (HSV- TK) gene and intravenous ganciclovir for previously treated ovarian and extraovarian cancer patients. *Hum. Gene Ther.* **8,** 597–613.

58. Link, C. J., Jr., Moorman, D., Seregina, T., Levy, J. P., and Schabold, K. J. (1996) A phase I trial of in vivo gene therapy with the herpes simplex thymidine kinase/ganciclovir system for the treatment of refractory or recurrent ovarian cancer. *Hum. Gene Ther.* **7,** 1161–1179.

59. Behbakht, K., Benjamin, I., Chiu, H. C., Eck, S. L., Van Deerlin, P. G., Rubin, S. C., and Boyd, J. (1996) Adenovirus-mediated gene therapy of ovarian cancer in a mouse model. *Am. J. Obstet. Gynecol.* **175,** 1260–1265.

60. Tong, X. W., Block, A., Chen, S. H., Contant, C. F., Agoulnik, I., Blankenburg, K., et al. (1996) In vivo gene therapy of ovarian cancer by adenovirus-mediated thymidine kinase gene transduction and ganciclovir administration. *Gynecol. Oncol.* **61,** 175–179.

61. Tong, X., Engehausen, D. G., Freund, C. T., Agoulnik, I., Guo, Z., Oehler, M. K., et al. (1998) The efficacy of adenovirus-mediated gene therapy of ovarian cancer is enhanced by using the cytomegalovirus promoter. *Anticancer Res.* **18,** 719–725.

62. Tong, X. W., Agoulnik, I., Blankenburg, K., Contant, C. F., Hasenburg, A., Runnebaum, L. B., et al. (1997) Human epithelial ovarian cancer xenotransplants into nude mice can be cured by adenovirus-mediated thymidine kinase gene therapy. *Anticancer Res.* **17,** 811–813.

63. Rancourt, C., Robertson, M. W., 3rd, Wang, M., Goldman, C. K., Kelly, J. F., Alvarez, R. D., et al. (1998) Endothelial cell vehicles for delivery of cytotoxic genes as a gene therapy approach for carcinoma of the ovary. *Clin. Cancer Res.* **4,** 265–270.

64. Tong, X. W., Engehausen, D. G., Kaufman, R. H., Agoulnik, I., Contant, C., Freund, C. T., et al. (1998) Improvement of gene therapy for ovarian cancer by using acyclovir instead of ganciclovir in adenovirus mediated thymidine kinase gene therapy. *Anticancer Res.* **18,** 713–718.

65. Marais, R., Spooner, R. A., Light, Y., Martin, J., and Springer, C. J. (1996) Gene-directed enzyme prodrug therapy with a mustard prodrug/carboxypeptidase G2 combination. *Cancer Res.* **56,** 4735–4742.

66. Friedlos, F., Court, S., Ford, M., Denny, W. A., and Springer, C. (1998) Gene-directed enzyme prodrug therapy: quantitative bystander cytotoxicity and DNA damage induced by CB1954 in cells expressing bacterial nitroreductase. *Gene Ther.* **5,** 105–112.

67. Garver, R. I., Jr., Goldsmith, K. T., Rodu, B., Hu, P. C., Sorscher, E. J., and Curiel, D. T. (1994) Strategy for achieving selective killing of carcinomas. *Gene Ther.* **1**, 46–50.

68. Hanania, E. G., Giles, R. E., Kavanagh, J., Fu, S. Q., Ellerson, D., Zu, Z., et al. (1996) Results of MDR-1 vector modification trial indicate that granulocyte/macrophage colony-forming unit cells do not contribute to posttransplant hematopoietic recovery following intensive systemic therapy. *Proc. Natl. Acad. Sci. USA* **93**, 15,346–15,351.

69. Hesdorffer, C., Ayello, J., Ward, M., Kaubisch, A., Vahdat, L., Balmaceda, C., et al. (1998) Phase I trial of retroviral-mediated transfer of the human MDR1 gene as marrow chemoprotection in patients undergoing high-dose chemotherapy and autologous stem-cell transplantation. *J. Clin. Oncol.* **16**, 165–172.

70. Resnicoff, M., Ambrose, D., Coppola, D., and Rubin, R. (1993) Insulin-like growth factor-1 and its receptor mediate the autocrine proliferation of human ovarian carcinoma cell lines. *Lab. Invest.* **69**, 756–760.

71. Muller, M., Dietel, M., Turzynski, A., and Wiechen, K. (1998) Antisense phosphorothioate oligodeoxynucleotide down-regulation of the insulin-like growth factor I receptor in ovarian cancer cells. *Int. J. Cancer* **77**, 567–571.

72. Yin, D. L., Pu, L., and Pei, G. (1998) Antisense oligonucleotide to insulin-like growth factor II induces apoptosis in human ovarian cancer AO cell line. *Cell Res.* **8**, 159–165.

73. Watson, J. M., Berek, J. S., and Martinez-Maza, O. (1993) Growth inhibition of ovarian cancer cells induced by antisense IL-6 oligonucleotides. *Gynecol. Oncol.* **49**, 8–15.

74. Wiechen, K. and Dietel, M. (1995) c-erbB-2 anti-sense phosphorothioate oligodeoxynucleotides inhibit growth and serum-induced cell spreading of P185c-erbB-2-overexpressing ovarian carcinoma cells. *Int. J. Cancer* **63**, 604–608.

75. Brader, K. R., Wolf, J. K., Chakrabarty, S., and Price, J. E. (1998) Epidermal growth factor receptor (EGFR) antisense transfection reduces the expression of EGFR and suppresses the malignant phenotype of a human ovarian cancer cell line. *Oncol. Rep.* **5**, 1269–1274.

76. Wilhelm, O., Schmitt, M., Hohl, S., Senekowitsch, R., and Graeff, H. (1995) Antisense inhibition of urokinase reduces spread of human ovarian cancer in mice. *Clin. Exp. Metastasis* **13**, 296–302.

77. Hung, W. C., Huang, J. S., and Chuang, L. Y. (1996) Antisense oligodeoxynucleotides targeted against different regions of cyclin D1 mRNA may exert different inhibitory effects on cell growth and gene expression. *Biochem. Biophys. Res. Commun.* **220**, 719–723.

78. Skilling, J. S., Squatrito, R. C., Connor, J. P., Niemann, T., and Buller, R. E. (1996) p53 gene mutation analysis and antisense-mediated growth inhibition of human ovarian carcinoma cell lines. *Gynecol. Oncol.* **60**, 72–80.

79. Monia, B. P. (1997) First- and second-generation antisense oligonucleotide inhibitors targeted against human c-raf kinase. *Ciba Found Symp.* **209**, 107–119.

80. Holmlund, J., Nemunaitis, J., Schiller, J., Dorr, A., and Kisner, D. (1998) Phase I trial of C-raf antisense oligonucleotide ISIS 5132 (CGP69846A) by 21-day continuous intravenous infusion (CIV) in patients with advanced cancer. *Proc. ASCO* **17**, 210 (A811).

81. Mujoo, K., Maneval, D. C., Anderson, S. C., and Gutterman, J. U. (1996) Adenoviral-mediated p53 tumor suppressor gene therapy of human ovarian carcinoma. *Oncogene* **12**, 1617–1623.

82. Nielsen, L. L., Lipari, P., Dell, J., Gurnani, M., and Hajian, G. (1998) Adenovirus-mediated p53 gene therapy and paclitaxel have synergistic efficacy in models of human head and neck, ovarian, prostate, and breast cancer. *Clin. Cancer Res.* **4**, 835–846.

83. Deshane, J., Siegal, G. P., Alvarez, R. D., Wang, M. H., Feng, M., Cabrera, G., et al. (1995) Targeted tumor killing via an intracellular antibody against erbB-2. *J. Clin. Invest.* **96**, 2980–2989.

84. Deshane, J., Grim, J., Loechel, S., Siegal, G. P., Alvarez, R. D., and Curiel, D. T. (1996) Intracellular antibody against erbB-2 mediates targeted tumor cell eradication by apoptosis. *Cancer Gene Ther.* **3**, 89–98.

85. Alvarez, R. D. and Curiel, D. T. (1997) A phase I study of recombinant adenovirus vector-mediated delivery of an anti-erbB-2 single-chain (sFv) antibody gene for previously treated ovarian and extraovarian cancer patients. *Hum. Gene Ther.* **8**, 229–242.

86. Deshane, J., Siegal, G. P., Wang, M., Wright, M., Bucy, R. P., Alvarez, R. D., and Curiel, D. T. (1997) Transductional efficacy and safety of an intraperitoneally delivered adenovirus encoding an anti-erbB-2 intracellular single-chain antibody for ovarian cancer gene therapy. *Gynecol. Oncol.* **64**, 378–385.

87. Russell, S. J. (1994) Replicating vectors for gene therapy of cancer. *Eur. J. Cancer* **30A**, 1165–1171.

88. Bischoff, J. R., Kirn, D. H., Williams, A., Heise, C., Horn, S., Muna, M., et al. (1996) An adenovirus mutant that replicates selectively in p53-deficient human tumor cells [see comments]. *Science* **274**, 373–376.

# 83

## Developing Anti-HER2/*neu* Single-Chain Fv Fragments from Phage Display Libraries

**Gregory P. Adams and Robert Schier**

## 1. Introduction

One of the major failures of conventional cancer therapy has been the inability to achieve a sufficient differential in toxicity between normal and neoplastic tissues. Since hybridoma technology was established *(1)*, monoclonal antibodies (MAbs) have been raised against a variety of tumor-associated antigens to overcome the lack of specificity. Unfortunately, MAbs have for the most part, failed to fulfill the expectations of being the desired "magic bullets" capable of directing cytotoxic effects strictly to malignant cells. The notable exception has been in the treatment of B-cell lymphomas that have exhibited an exciting response rate when treated with unconjugated *(2)* and radiolabeled *(3)* MAbs. However, similar progress has not been observed in the treatment of ovarian carcinoma and other solid malignancies. These tumors contain disordered vasculature and lack draining lymphatics, resulting in elevated interstitial pressure. In this environment, the diffusion of a relatively large, 150 kDa IgG molecule is limited to 1 mm in 2–3 d *(4)*. In contrast, smaller molecules such as 50 kDa Fab fragments exhibit faster movement through the tumor interstitium, on the order of 1 to 2 mm per day.

Single-chain Fv fragments (scFv) with their small size of approximately 25 kDa should exhibit an excellent penetration into solid tumors. These antibody fragments are comprised of the variable light ($V_L$) and variable heavy ($V_H$) chain domains of an Ig molecule linked by a short peptide spacer (typically 15 amino acids) *(5)*. These molecules present the functional monovalent antigen binding site of an antibody containing six antigen binding loops, or complementary determining regions (CDRs), flanked by the supporting framework regions. scFv derived from the antibody genes of hybridoma cells retain the tumor specificity of the original MAb with little or no decrement in binding affinity *(6)*. Furthermore, scFv consistently exhibit highly specific tumor retention and diffuse tumor penetration in their terminal distribution phase in immunodeficient mice bearing subcutaneous human tumor xenografts. However, the small size of these molecules also allows rapid elimination through the kidneys. These factors, coupled with the monovalent nature of the scFv's interaction with its target antigen lead to significantly lower quantitative tumor retention than is achievable with the

From: *Methods in Molecular Medicine, Vol. 39: Ovarian Cancer: Methods and Protocols*
Edited by: J. M. S. Bartlett © Humana Press, Inc., Totowa, NJ

parent MAbs. Typical results are in the order of 1% of the injected dose of radiolabeled scFv localizing per gram of tumor (% ID/g) compared with 20 % ID/g tumor for the parent IgG at 24 h postinjection.

Recent advances in phage display technology have simplified the process of generating scFv specific for a desired antigen. Large repertoires of human $V_H$ and $V_L$ genes were cloned and displayed as scFv on the surface of filamentous bacteriophage (7). Specific scFv can simply be isolated against any immobilized antigen using 2–5 cycles of phage rescue in *Escherichia coli*, phage preparation and phage selection. The selection strategy can be altered to increase the yield of scFv with desired characteristics. For example, selection against a biotinylated target in solution tends to result in a greater proportion of monomeric scFv recognizing the native antigen, while immobilizing the antigen on plastic (e.g., immunotubes or microtiter plates) often leads to the isolation of scFv binding to the denatured antigen with a propensity to spontaneously dimerize. The incubation time and amount of antigen employed are also important. Shortening the duration of the panning step can bias the selection in favor of scFv with rapid rates of association, while prolonging the duration of the panning step and decreasing the antigen concentration increases the likelihood of isolating scFv with slower rates of dissociation.

The scFv resulting from the selections described above can be further manipulated to address some of the obstacles encountered when scFv are used for in vivo tumor targeting. It is possible to selectively modify the affinity, size, and valence of scFv molecules. We have employed two distinct strategies, chain shuffling (8), and site-directed mutagenesis (9), to alter the affinity of an scFv for its target epitope. The affinities of scFv produced using these strategies can be in the picomolar range. Dimerization of scFv can also be used to enhance the "apparent affinity" (avidity) for the antigen without undertaking major modifications to the scFv. Although scFv dimers can be made by many different ways (10), two of these structures, the diabody and the gene-fused dimer, are referred to in this chapter. The decision as to which method will yield the best dimer is dependent upon the antigenic target and the planned application. The requirements of flexibility and the orientation of the targeted epitope on the antigen are likely to be critical determinants in the identification of the optimal structure.

In this chapter, we will describe the step-by-step methodology used for the isolation, characterization, and preparation for the in vitro evaluation and in vivo biodistributions of scFv molecules suitable for diagnosis and therapy. While we have employed these techniques to develop scFv-based agents specific for *HER2/neu*, these methods can be readily applied to other antigen systems.

## 2. Materials

### 2.1. Phage Display/scFv Manipulation

1. ELISA reader (405 n$M$).
2. Magnetic concentrator rack.
3. BIAcore (surface plasmon resonance inst.) (not necessary, but recommended).
4. Antibody library, antigen, phagemid vectors (e.g., Sheets Library; *see* **ref. 11**).
5. 2X TY: 16 g tryptone, 10 g yeast extract, and 5 g NaCl per 1 L distilled water (pH 7.4). Autoclave prior to use.
6. LB: 10 g tryptone, 5 g yeast extract, and 10 g NaCl per 1 L distilled water (pH 7.4). Autoclave prior to use.

7. 150 mm$^2$ agar plates: medium plus 15 g agar per 1 L distilled water. Autoclave prior to use.
8. 20% glucose (Glu).
9. 20% PEG (Polyethylenglycol 8000), 2.5 *M* NaCl.
10. Phosphate-buffered saline (PBS): 50 m*M* PBS pH 7.4 and 150 m*M* NaCl.
11. 2% Natriumazide stock (NaN$_3$) in.
12. Immunotubes and microtiter plates (Maxisorb, Nunc, Weisbaden-Biebrich, Germany).
13. Tween-20–10% stock solution.
14. Triethylamine (TEA)–100 m*M* stock solution.
15. 1 *M* Tris-HCl pH 7.4.
16. 5% MPBST: 5% low-fat milk powder, 0.05% Tween-20 in PBS.
17. Streptavidin magnetic beads (Dynal).
18. 50% sterile glycerol stock (Gly).
19. 1 *M* isopropyl-b-D-thiogalactopyranoside stock (IPTG) in H$_2$O.
20. 9E10 (anti-*myc*-tag) MAb (Santa Cruz Biotechnology, CA).
21. Antimouse IgG-HRP (horse radish peroxidase) (Sigma, St. Louis, MO).
22. ABTS solution (10 mg in 20 mL 50 m*M* citrate buffer pH 4.0 plus 20 μL 30% H$_2$O$_2$).
23. 50 m*M* citrate buffer pH 4.0.
24. 30% H$_2$O$_2$.
25. 3.2 mg/mL sodium fluoride (NaF) in distilled water.
26. PCR reagents : dNTPs, polymerase TAQ - VENT, buffer (all Promega, Madison, WI or Boehinger, Mannheim, Germany), primers (Genset).
27. Mineral oil.
28. Sterile double distilled H$_2$O.
29. LMB3 primer (CAG GAA ACA GCT ATG AC), fdSEQ1 primer (GAA TTT TCT GTA TGA GG).
30. Restriction enzymes : *Bst*NI, *Nco*I, *Not*I, *Xho*I (New England BioLabs, Beverly, MA).
31. PPB: 30 m*M* TRIS-HCl pH 8.0, 1 m*M* EDTA, 20% sucrose.
32. Primers of sequencing, PCR fingerprints and cloning (Genset).
33. 4 *M* MgCl$_2$.

## 2.2. scFv Expression

### 2.2.1. Equipment

1. HPLC system equipped with a Superdex 75 (Pharmacia, Uppsala, Sweden) or similar size exclusion column.
2. Two-liter glass shaker flasks with baffles.

### 2.2.2. Materials

1. pUC119mychis$_6$ plasmid.
2. 75 mm$^2$ LB/Amp/1% Glu agar plates.
3. 2X TY/Amp/1% Glu broth.
4. Miniprep kit (e.g., QIAprep Spin Miniprep Kit; Qiagen, Chatsworth, CA).
5. Restriction enzymes; *Nco*I and *Not*I.
6. Gel extraction kit (e.g., Qiagen).
7. T4 DNA ligase.
8. Competent TG1 *E. coli* (can be made or special ordered from Stratagene).
9. 75 mm$^2$ 2X TY/Amp/1%Gly agar plates.
10. 50% glycerol containing 5 m*M* MgCl$_2$.
11. LMB2 primer (GTA AAA CGA CGG CCA GT).
12. 2X TY plates (1.5% Agar/100 μg/mL Amp.).

13. 25 mL 2X TY broth with 75 μg/mL (w/v) carbenicillin and 1% (w/v) glucose.
14. 1 L 2X TY broth with 100 μg/mL Amp. and 0.1% (w/v) glucose.
15. 1 mL of 1 $M$ isopropyl-β-D-thiogalactopyranoside (IPTG) per liter of expression. Note: IPTG stocks can be made up in advance and stored in 1-mL aliquots at –10°C.
16. Periplasmic Extraction Buffer (PPB) –30 m$M$ Tris-HCl pH 8.0, 20% sucrose, 1 m$M$ EDTA.
17. Osmotic Shock Buffer (5 m$M$ $MgSO_4$).
18. IMAC loading buffer (20 m$M$ phosphate buffer pH 8.0 + 500 m$M$ NaCl + 20 m$M$ imidazole).
19. IMAC eluting buffer (20 m$M$ phosphate buffer pH 8.0 + 500 m$M$ NaCl + 250 m$M$ imidazole).
20. $Ni^{++}$ agarose resin (IMAC resin) (Qiagen).
21. 10% SDS-PAGE gels.
22. Proteins for specificity enzyme-linked immunosorbent assay (ELISA) [e.g., bovine serum albumin (BSA), lysozyme, avidin, streptavidin, ovalbumin].

## 2.3. In Vitro Assays

### 2.3.1. Materials

1. Sephadex G-50-80.
2. Biospin disposable chromatography columns (Bio-Rad, Richmond, CA).
3. 15-mL conical centrifuge tubes.
4. 1 mg/mL Chloramine T (CT) in $H_2O$.
5. Iodine-125.
6. 1 mg/mL sodium metabisulfite (SMB) in $H_2O$.
7. PBS.
8. HPLC molecular weight standards.
9. SK-BR-3 cell line (# HTB 30; American Type Culture Collection–ATCC).
10. SK-OV-3 cell line (# HTB 77; ATCC).
11. CEM cell line (# 119; ATCC).
12. 4 m$M$ EDTA in Hank's balanced salt solution (HBSS) without $Mg^{++}$ or $Ca^{++}$.
13. 0.5% Trypsin / 0.5 m$M$ EDTA in HBSS without $Mg^{++}$ or $Ca^{++}$.
14. 12 × 75 mm polypropylene tubes.

## 3. Methods

### 3.1. Phage Display

Here we describe the methods used to isolate, characterize, and affinity mature a scFv against HER2/*neu* from a human, naive scFv library (8,9,12–14). These methods are generally applicable to other antibody fragments and antibody libraries.

The first step into this technology involves the generation of an antibody fragment library. This could fill a whole chapter on its own and is described in detail elsewhere (7,12). Briefly, three types of antibody libraries (human, mouse, or synthetic) are commonly produced. Libraries can be generated using a commercial kit (e.g., Recombinant Phage Antibody System, Pharmacia Biotech) or access to a library can be acquired through academic collaborations (e.g., the "Sheets Library" from Dr. James Marks at the University of California San Francisco; see ref. **11**. Antibody fragments from human and synthetic libraries provide on average affinities between $10^{-6}$ and $10^{-9}$ $M$, which is sufficient for most applications. Antibody fragment libraries are generally stored as *E. coli* TG1 stocks. Each bacteria cell contains one unique *scFv* gene in a phagemid such as pHEN1 or pCANTAB5E (Pharmacia Biotech). Phage are retrieved or "rescued" by superinfecting an aliquot of the bacterial stock with a helper phage (VCSM13) to initiate phagemid replication, scFv expression and phage production. A protocol is presented below. Inoculation of culture medium (scaled up in **step 2**) with a tenfold excess of bacteria cell number over the library size should be sufficient to ensure that the whole library in the phage preparation is used for the selection process (*see* **Note 1**).

### 3.1.1. Rescue Phage from a Library Stock or from a Selection

1. Start at this step when performing phage rescue following selection (*see* **Subheading 3.1.3.**). After a selection round, 3 mL 2X TY/Amp/1% Glu/15% Gly is poured on each large selection plate and the bacterial colonies are scraped off and suspended in the broth. Remove an aliquot and store it at – 80°C.
2. Start at this step when rescuing phage from a library. 50 to 100 μL of the suspension (prepared in **step 1**, above) or of a phage library is used to inoculate 5 mL 2X TY/Amp/1% Glu ($OD_{600}$ of about 0.25).
3. Incubate bacterial culture for 30 to 60 min at 37°C in a shaker incubator to achieve an $OD_{600}$ of about 0.5.
4. Add approximately 5 to 10 μL of VCSM13 helper phage ($>1 \times 10^{10}$ phage/μL; the ratio to bacteria cells should be 10 to 1).
5. Incubate culture for 30 min at 37°C without shaking, then for another 30 min at 37°C in a shaker incubator (350 rpm) (*see* **Note 2**).
6. Check helper phage infection by plating 1 μL of the solution on an LB/Kan plate.
7. Spin down the bacteria at 4500$g$ for 5 min.
8. Resuspend the pellet in 25 mL × 2X TY/Amp/Kan (50 μg/mL) without glucose.
9. Incubate the culture at 30°C overnight in a shaker incubator (350 rpm).

### 3.1.2. Phage Preparation

1. Spin down bacteria from the overnight culture for 10 min at 4500$g$.
2. Remove the supernatant. Add 5 mL 20% PEG – 2.5 $M$ NaCl to supernatant, mix and incubate on ice for 30 min. Centrifuge the solution at 10,000$g$ for 10 min to isolate the phage pellet (*see* **Note 3**).
3. Resuspend the phage pellet in 2 mL PBS + 0.01% $NaN_3$ and transfer it to a 1.5-mL tube. Spin down bacterial debris at maximal $g$ force (typically > 13,000$g$) in a table-top microcentrifuge for 1 min.
4. Transfer the supernatant to a fresh tube (labeled "phage preparation") and store at 4°C for up to 2–4 wk. For longer storage, the supernatant is filtered through a 0.45-μm filter, glycerol should be added to a final concentration of 20% and the phage can be stored at –80°C.
5. Determine the titer of the phage preparation by making serial dilutions and infecting log phase *E. coli* TG1 for 30 min at 37°C. Plate the infected *E. coli* on 150 mm $^2$ LB/Amp plates (the phage titer should be on the order of $10^{12}$ to $10^{13}$ phage/mL) (*see* **Note 4**).

### 3.1.3. Phage Selection

The first round of phage selection can be started after phage are rescued from the library. The standard procedure is described below. Briefly, the antigen is immobilized on plastic and then incubated with the phage population. Nonspecifically adsorbed phage are washed off. Once the specific phage are eluted, *E. coli* TG1 cells are infected and plated on large agar plates. Two to five cycles of phage rescue, phage preparation and phage selection are usually required to enrich the phage population for specific binders. Although the standard procedure is presented below, it will likely be necessary to adjust it in response to both the individual target antigen and the phage library. Further adjustments are possible depending upon the specific desired properties of the resulting scFv molecules.

1. The night before the procedure: Coat antigen (e.g., HER2/*neu*) onto an Immunotube (Nunc) (*see* **Note 5**). Incubate 0.5 mL antigen solution in PBS overnight at 4°C in the Immunotube in which the selection will be performed. The concentration of the antigen employed should be in the range of 10 to 100 µg/mL.
2. In a 15-mL tube containing 2X TY broth, start an overnight culture of the TG1 cells. Use a single colony from an agar plate as the source of the bacteria.
3. The day of the procedure: Remove the antigen solution from the Immunotube and block with sufficient 5% low-fat milk powder - 0.05% Tween-20 - PBS (5% M-PBST) to fill the whole tube. Incubate for 1 h at 37°C.
4. Using a squeeze bottle of PBS, wash the Immunotube 1X.
5. Transfer approximately $10^{12}$ phage (~0.5 mL of the phage preparation) in 2.5% M-PBST into the blocked Immunotube.
6. Incubate the Immunotube with phage for 30 min at room temperature (RT) on a rotator.
7. Make a 1/100 dilution (1 mL into 100 mL 2X YT) of the overnight TG1 culture. Grow at 37°C in a shaker incubator to an $OD_{600}$ of 0.7 to 1.0.
8. Remove the Immunotube from the rotator and incubate it at RT for another 60 min without shaking.
9. Wash off nonspecific (unbound) phage (*see* **Note 6**). This process should be done very quickly using squeeze bottles and dumping the contents instead of aspirating them off. Alternate wash steps with PBST and PBS for a total of 10 washes with each buffer.
10. After removing all the wash solution, elute the specifically bound phage by adding 0.5 mL 100 m$M$ triethylamine (TEA) (*see* **Note 7**) and incubating the tube for 10 min at RT.
11. Transfer the eluted phage to a 2-mL tube containing 250 µL 1 M TRIS-HCl pH 7.4, mix and store on ice until the TGI *E. coli* culture reaches the proper $OD_{600}$.
12. Infect 5 mL TG1 $OD_{600}$ 0.7 to 1 by the addition of approximately 1/3 (250 µL) of the elutate. Mix gently by hand and incubate the mixture for 30 min at 37°C without shaking. Store the remaining elutate at 4°C. Take 1 to 10 µL of infected *E. coli* to check phage titer by plating on LB/Amp/1%Glu (as described above).
13. Spin down the infected bacteria for 5 min. at 4800$g$ (4°C) and resuspend in 500 µL 2X TY/Amp/1%Glu. Plate the cell suspension on 2 to 3 150 mm$^2$ LB/Amp/1% Glu agar plates and incubate overnight at 30°C.
14. Proceed with the phage rescue and preparation protocols presented above (in **Subheadings 3.1.1.** and **3.1.2.**). After several rounds of selection single colonies are picked and resuspended in 96-well plates containing media to produce a masterplate.

## 3.2. Initial Screening of Colonies

Purpose: Mini expressions and ELISA assays are performed to test single colonies from each round of selection for binding to the HER2/*neu* or other target antigen. First, a masterplate is made and clones are expressed in a 96-well format. Whole cell extracts are then directly employed in an scFv ELISA (*see* **Note 8**).

### 3.2.1. Miniexpression in a 96-Well Format

1. 96-well masterplate production. Using a new sterile toothpick each time, pick single colonies from the selection agar plate from the round to be analyzed. Resuspend each bacteria colony in a microtiter well containing 100 µL 2X TY/Amp/1% Glu.

2. Incubate the plate overnight at 37°C in a shaker incubator.

3. Add 100 μL 50% sterile glycerol to each well. Seal the microtiter plate and store at –80°C. This is the "masterplate." (Note: the following steps can be performed immediately, prior to freezing the plate, however, the "masterplate" should be stored frozen to serve as glycerol stocks for the individual colonies.)

4. Make a "working plate" using aliquots from the "masterplate." Being careful to maintain well positions, transfer 5–10 μL of the "masterplate" glycerol stocks to a fresh microtiter plate containing 100 μL 2X TY/Amp/0.1% Glu/well.

5. Grow bacteria to an $OD_{600}$ of 0.5 to 1.0 in a shaker incubator at 37°C (approximately 3–5 h).

6. Add 50 μL of 3 m$M$ IPTG diluted in 2X TY/Amp/well to induce protein expression. Incubate the plate overnight at 30°C in a shaker incubator.

7. The next day add 50 μL of 0.4% Tween 20/well and incubate the plate for 2 h at 37°C. Disrupt the cells using two freeze and thaw cycles (–80°C and 37°C) 5 min at each temperature.

8. Spin down bacteria debris for 15 min at 3000$g$ and remove 50 μL of the supernatant per well for assay in the ELISA described in **Subheading 3.2.2.**

## 3.2.2. Solid Phase scFv ELISA

1. The night before the procedure: Coat a sufficient number of wells in ELISA plates (Nunc Maxisorb) to assay all the glycerol stocks in the "masterplate(s)." Add 50 μL of HER2/*neu* (or other) antigen solution (1 to 10 μg/mL PBS) to each well, incubate overnight at 4°C (*see* **Notes 9** and **10**).

2. The day of the procedure: Remove the antigen solution by inverting the plate over a sink and shaking it out. Remove the remaining solution by gently tapping the plate onto paper towels.

3. Block the wells. Fill each well with 5% M-PBST and incubate for 1 h at 37°C.

4. Wash the plate one time with PBS. Empty the wash solution as in **step 1** above.

5. Transfer 50 μL of the *E. coli* supernatants from each well of the "working plate" to the corresponding well of the ELISA plate. If possible, add a mouse monoclonal antibody known to be reactive with the antigen to an extra well to serve as a positive control. Add 100 μL of 5% M-PBST to each well to dilute the stocks 1 : 3 and incubate for 1.5 h at RT.

6. Wash the ELISA plate twice with PBST and twice with PBS, by filling each well with buffer and removing each solution as in **step 1** above.

7. Add 50 μL of a 1 : 5000 dilution (in 5% M-PBST) of the anti*myc*-tag antibody 9E10 to each well (except the positive control well) and incubate for 1 h at RT (*see* **Note 11**).

8. Wash the ELISA plate two times with PBST and two times with PBS.

9. Add 50 μL antimouse IgG-HRP conjugate per well including the positive control well (Fc or whole molecule specific; diluted 1 : 5000 in 5% M-PBST) and incubate for 1 h at RT.

10. Wash ELISA plate three times with PBST and three times with PBS.

11. Add 100 μL of fresh ABTS solution (10 mg ABTS in 20 mL of 50 m$M$ citrate buffer pH 4 plus 20 μL 30% $H_2O_2$) and incubate for 20 to 30 min at RT.

12. Add 50 μL NaF solution (3.2 mg/mL water) to quench the enzymatic reaction; determine the absorbence at 405 nm in an ELISA reader. A clone is considered to be reactive with the target antigen if it is associated with an ELISA signal that is 2× background.

## 3.3. scFv Manipulation—Library Design and Construction for scFv Optimization

Strategies for in vitro affinity maturation are manifold and could easily be the subject of an entire chapter. In the interest of making the reader aware of the potential, the methods which we have found to be particularly effective are described in **Subheading 4.** The first two methods, chain shuffling and site-directed mutagenesis, are designed to increase the "intrinsic" affinity of the scFv for its target antigen. The final methods are designed to increase the "functional" affinity of the scFv by employing it in a dimeric structure such as a gene-fused (scFv)$_2$ or a diabody, which is capable of divalent association with target antigen. These methods are attractive as they do not require major modifications to the scFv molecule. Chain shuffling employs the natural occurring repertoire of *V* genes containing mutations in the frameworks and CDRs which were induced by somatic hypermutation of the germline genes *(8)* (*see* **Note 12**). The second method, randomization of CDRs or site-directed mutagenesis, is a synthetic approach by which new diversity is introduced *(9)* (*see* **Note 13**). The gene-fused dimer is produced by the addition of a flexible 15 amino acid peptide linker between two scFv molecules (*see* **Note 14**). Finally, the diabody is produced by decreasing the length of the peptide spacer between the scFv's light and heavy chains to prevent self-association. This leads to the formation of a noncovalent dimer with the variable heavy chain from one molecule paired with the variable light chain of the second and vice-versa *(16)* (*see* **Note 15**).

### 3.3.1. Affinity Phage Selection

Purpose: For many applications antibody fragments are required with subnanomolar affinities. Phage display can also be used for in vitro affinity maturation of a single binder by introducing additional diversity into the *scFv* gene. The scFv clones with the highest affinity can be discriminated from those with lower affinity by "affinity-driven selections." The method described here employs biotinylated antigen in solution. Antigens bound by scFv-phage are captured with streptavidin-coated magnetic beads, followed by the washing, elution, and infection procedures. An effective alternative to this method is "affinity discrimination by solid phase panning" using very long washing steps *(17,18)*.

1. The night before the procedure: In a 15-mL tube containing 2X TY broth, start an overnight culture of TG1 cells. Use a single colony from an agar plate as the source of the bacteria.
2. The day of the procedure: Block three $12 \times 75$ mm tubes (one empty and two containing 50 µL streptavidin [SA] magnetic beads) with 2 mL 5% M-PBST for 1 h at 37°C. Label the empty tube "E" and the SA-magnetic bead tubes SA-1 and SA-2.
3. Without emptying the tubes, transfer approximately $10^{12}$ phage in 2.5% M-PBST into the tube marked "SA-1." Incubate the phage with the SA-magnetic beads for 1 h at RT. Place the other two tubes aside at RT.
4. Remove the phage that contains scFv reactive with the SA-magnetic beads by placing the tube in a magnetic concentrator rack for 5 min at room temperature. While the tube is still in the concentrator rack, pour out the blocking solution from the tube labeled "E" (no SA-magnetic beads) and then pour the supernatant from tube "SA-1" into tube "E."
5. Add biotinylated antigen (*HER2/neu*) to tube "E." The concentration to be added should be decreased over successive rounds of selection (e.g., 1st round, 50 n*M*; 2nd round, 5 nM; 3rd round, 0.5 n*M*; 4th round, 0.05 n*M*) to increase the likelihood that high-affinity clones are selected (*see* **Note 16**).
6. Incubate the phage/antigen mixture for 1 h at RT on a clinical rotator.
7. Centrifuge the SA-magnetic beads in tube "SA-2" for 5 min at 2000*g*. Aspirate off the supernatant and resuspend the beads in 0.5 mL of 2.5% M-PBST. Transfer the bead solution into the phage/antigen mixture in tube "E." Incubate the suspension for 5 min at RT on a clinical rotator.

8. Collect the SA-magnetic beads by incubating tube "E" on a magnetic concentrator rack for 5 min.

9. Keeping the tube in the magnetic concentrator rack, wash off the nonspecific and weakly bound phage using quick washes with following scheme: three washes with PBST, two washes with 2.5% M-PBST, two washes with PBS, one wash with 2.5% M-PBS, and two washes with PBS. After the addition of buffer in each wash step, it is necessary to allow the magnetic beads to rebind to the magnet for 5 min before emptying the tube for the next wash cycle.

10. The elution, *E. coli* infection and plating steps are performed as described in **Subheading 3.1.3., steps 5, 8–12** presented above.

### 3.3.2. PCR Fingerprint Analysis

Purpose: While numerous colonies will result from a given selection, only a handful of distinct clones will actually be present. In the interest of reducing the number of colonies which will be expanded for further characterization, ELISA positive clones are analyzed by PCR fingerprint to identify unique full-length *scFv* genes. In this assay, the *scFv* gene from a single colony is amplified using primers [LMB3 and fdSEQ1 *(11)*] specific for the phage sequences that preceded and follow the inserted *scFv* gene. The PCR product is then digested with a 4-base pair cutting enzyme (*BstNI*) and run out on an agarose gel. Each distinct *scFv* clone will correlate with a unique restriction pattern.

PCR reaction mixture: 2 μL of 10X TAQ buffer (with 15 m$M$ MgC$_{12}$), 1 μL of 5 m$M$ dNTPs, 1 μL of primer LMB3 (10 pmol/μL), 1 μL of primer fdSEQ1 (10 pmol/μL) 0.1 μL of TAQ DNA Polymerase-Gibco (5 U/μL), 14.9 μL of H$_2$O.

1. Using a sterile toothpick, pick single colonies from the agar plate, and resuspended them in the reaction mixture. Add a few drops of mineral oil to the top of the reaction mixture if the thermocycler does not have a heated lid.

2. PCR cycles: 1×, 94°C / 3 min, 30×, 94°C / 1 min, 45°C / 1 min, 72°C / 1 min, 1×, 72°C / 10 min.

3. Load 5 μL of each tube or well (96-well format) on a 1.5% agarose gel using 6X gel loading buffer (0.25% bromophenol blue, 0.25% xylene cyanol, 40% w/v sucrose in H$_2$O) and a 100-bp DNA ladder (Gibco) as the molecular weight markers. (Determine % of full-length scFv clones in library or selection.)

4. Add 10 μL BstNI mixture to the remaining PCR reaction mixture and incubate at 60°C for 2 h.
   BstNI1 mixture: 1 μL of NEB2 buffer (NEB), 0.2 μL of BstNI (10 U/μL NEB), 8.8 μL of H$_2$O.

5. Load 15 to 20 μL on a 4% nusieve or FMC Metaphor agarose gel (FMC BioProducts).

6. Determine how many different restriction patterns are present. Each pattern will indicate the presence of a unique *scFv* clone.

7. A DNA preparation should be made from two to four clones representing each pattern. This should be used for sequencing of the clones to confirm the identities of distinct clones.

### 3.3.3 Expression and Sample Preparation for High Throughput Screening

Purpose: In this protocol, a small-scale expression and a periplasmic extraction of the scFv are performed to obtain material for off-rate ranking studies using surface plasmon resonance (SPR), specificity ELISA, and primary cell binding.

1. Inoculate 10 mL 2X TY / Amp/0.1% Glu with bacteria from a single colony and incubate bacterial culture in a shaker at 37°C until an $OD_{600}$ of 0.7 to 1.0 is achieved (usually 4 to 6 h).
2. Induce expression by adding 10 µL 1 $M$ IPTG (final conc. 1 m$M$). Incubate the culture over night at 25°C in shaker incubator.
3. Pellet the culture by centrifugation at 5000$g$ for 10 min at 4°C.
4. Remove the supernatant and resuspend the pellet in 0.5 mL precooled PPB (periplasmic extraction buffer). Transfer the suspension into a 1.5-mL microfuge tube and incubate the sample on ice for 30 min.
5. Spin down the bacteria for 5 min in a table top microcentrifuge at 13,000$g$ (supernatant = periplasmic preparation containing scFv).
6. Remove the supernatant and dilute it in PBS (or the HBS BIAcore buffer if the sample is to be analyzed by SPR) to a final volume of 2 mL. Dialyze the sample over night at 4°C against PBS (or HBS) containing 0.02% $NaN_3$. The samples are now ready to be used in most assays (e.g., specificity ELISA, cell binding). For BIAcore use, the samples should first be filtered (0.2 µm) and diluted 1:1 or 1:2 in running buffer.

### 3.3.4. Specificity ELISA

Purpose: Specificity ELISAs are performed using crude extracts of scFv (periplasmic fraction) to demonstrate that the expressed scFv are specific for the target antigen. The ELISA protocol is identical to the one described above with the exception that scFv are tested in triplicate against a panel of different antigens (e.g., BSA, lysozyme, avidin, streptavidin, ovalbumin) coated on the ELISA plate.

### 3.4. scFv Expression and Purification

### 3.4.1. Subcloning into Expression Vector

Purpose: This protocol is used to transfer the scFv gene from the phagemid vector to the expression vector pUC119mychis$_6$ *(13)*. The pUC119mychis$_6$ vector is useful as it adds a His$_6$ tag to the scFv's carboxy terminus. The His$_6$ tag facilitates rapid purification using an immobilized metal affinity chromatography (IMAC) column. While it is possible to perform the expressions with the scFv in the phagemid vector, the yields from large-scale expressions are typically very low owing to the toxicity of the phagemid gene III and the difficulty of purifying the scFv product.

1. Identify clones with the desired properties (e.g., specificity and affinity) from the results of the assays performed in **Subheading 3.3.**
2. Prepare overnight cultures of the desired clones. Using a sterile loop, streak the desired colonies from the "masterplate" onto LB/Amp/1% Glu agar plates and incubate at 37°C for up to 48 h.
3. Pick single colonies from the plates to inoculate 15-mL tubes containing 2X TY/Amp/1% Glu broth. Grow the cultures overnight in a 37°C shaker incubator (350 rpm).
4. Using a commercial miniprep kit isolate the phagemid DNA.
5. Digest the phagemid DNA with the *Nco*I and *Not*I restriction enzymes for 3 h at 37°C.
6. Purify the digested DNA on a 1% agarose gel alongside a 100-bp DNA ladder. The scFv DNA should run near the 400-bp marker. Isolate the scFv band using a gel extraction kit
7. Digest the vector pUC119mychis$_6$ with *Nco*I and *Not*I for 3 h at 37°C.
8. Ligate the *scFv* gene into the digested vector at a 10:1 molar ratio using T4 DNA ligase.
9. Add the entire ligation mixture to 20 µL 5X KCN, q.s. to 100 µL with sterile distilled $H_2O$.
10. Chill the solution on ice and then add to 0.1 mL of competent TG1 *E. coli*. Incubate for 20 min on ice and another 10 min at RT.

11. Add 1 mL of 2X TY broth and incubate at 37°C in a shaker incubator (350 rpm).
12. Plate increasing volumes on a series of 75 mm$^2$ 2X TY/Amp/Glu agar plates (e.g., 2 × 10 μL, 2 × 50 μL, and 2 × 200 μL).
13. Centrifuge the remaining cell suspension (5000$g$, 10 min), resuspend it in 200 μL of 2X TY broth and plate it out on a 150 mm$^2$ 2X TY/Amp/Glu agar plate.
14. Incubate the plates overnight at 37°C.
15. Identify colonies which contain the scFv insert. Choose 20 random colonies from the plates generated in **step 8** above. Stick the colonies with sterile toothpicks and swirl them in numbered individual PCR tubes containing 100 μL of the PCR reaction mix and then place each toothpick in an individual 15-mL centrifuge tube (matched numbers) containing 2 mL of 2X TY/Amp/1%Glu for the production of glycerol stocks.
16. Perform the PCR run as described below.
    PCR reaction mix: (amount per sample—prepare sufficient volume for 20 samples), 5 μL 10 *Taq* polymerase buffer, 2.5 μL 5 mm dNTP (mix), 2.5 μL LMB2 primer (10 pM/ μL), 2.5 μL LMB3 primer (10 pM/ μL), 35.5 μL H$_2$0, 1 μL *Taq* DNA polymerase (5 U/ μL) (add last).
    PCR cycles: 1× 94°C / 10 min., 30× 94°C / 30 s, 45°C / 30 s, 72°C / 1 min, 1× 72°C / 10 min.
17. Incubate the glycerol stock production tubes overnight at 37°C in a shaker incubator (350 rpm).
18. Pellet the bacteria at 5000$g$ (10 min).
19. Remove the supernatant and resuspend in 1 mL of 50 % glycerol containing 5 m$M$ MgCl$_2$ transfer to numbered cryotubes, freeze and store at –70°C.

### 3.4.2. Expression

This protocol describes larger scale expressions of scFv molecules in shake flasks (*see* **Note 17**). Maintain sterile technique throughout while growing the *E. coli* cultures.

1. Remove glycerol stock from the –70°C freezer and immediately transfer it to a prefrozen benchtop cooler to maintain the stock in a frozen state (*see* **Note 18**).
2. Using a small sterile loop, scrape the top of the frozen stock and streak it out on a 2X TY plate containing 1.5% agar and 100 μg/mL ampicillin. Incubate overnight at 37°C.
3. After the overnight incubation, numerous colonies should be visible on the plate. Late in the day select a single colony and aseptically transfer it to 20 mL of 2X TY/ 75 μg/mL carbenicillin/1.0% glucose. Grow the culture overnight (as short as possible) in a shaking incubator at 30°C (350 rpm).
4. Early the next day, the overnight culture should appear cloudy, indicating that the culture has aggressively multiplied. Inoculate 1 L of 2X TY / 100 μg/mL ampicillin /0.1% glucose with 10 mL of the overnight culture (*see* **Note 19**). Grow the bacteria in a shake flask at 37°C in a shaker incubator (250 rpm) until an OD$_{600}$ of 1.0 is achieved. Do not exceed an OD$_{600}$ of 1.0 (typically, it will take about 2 h if room temperature broth is used).
5. Move shaker flask containing the expression culture to a 30°C shaker incubator (*see* **Note 20**). Add 1 $M$ IPTG to a final concentration of 0.5 m$M$ (e.g., 0.5 mL of a 1-$M$ solution/L) to induce the expression of the scFv. Incubate the culture for 5 h at 28–30°C.
6. Place cultures on ice and swirl to cool. Keep everything at 4°C from this point.
7. Transfer the culture to 250-mL centrifuge buckets and spin at 4000$g$ for 20 minutes at 4°C to pellet the *E. coli*.
8. Discard the supernatants and resuspend the pellets in 10 mL of Periplasmic Extraction Buffer (PPB) (4°C) (*see* **Note 21**). Allow the suspension to sit on ice for 20 min.
9. Centrifuge the periplasmic extraction at 5000$g$ for 20 min at 4°C. Remove supernatant and store it on ice.

10. Resuspend bacterial pellet in 10 mL of osmotic shock buffer (5 m*M* MgSO₄) (4°C). Allow the suspension to sit on ice for 20 min.
11. Centrifuge the osmotic shock preparation at 7000*g* for 20 min at 4°C. Remove and save the supernatant (place on ice) and discard the cell pellets.
12. Combine the periplasmic and osmotic shock extractions and centrifuge them at 10,000*g* for 30 min at 4°C.
13. Transfer the supernatant to dialysis tubing (12,000–14,000 molecular weight cutoff) and dialyze overnight against PBS (*see* **Note 22**).

### 3.4.3. IMAC Purification

The six histidine residues at the carboxy terminus of the scFv have an affinity for $Ni^{++}$, which enables it to be purified on a $Ni^{++}$ agarose (Ni-NTA) column (*see* **Note 23**).

1. Equilibrate a 1-mL Ni-NTA column with 10 mL of PBS.
2. Imidozole is added to the scFv solution until a final concentration of 20 m*M* is achieved.
3. Load the scFv onto the equilibrated Ni-NTA column using a pump with a flow rate of 1 to 4 mL/min.
4. Wash column with 50-mL IMAC Loading Buffer.
5. Elute bound scFv with 4-mL IMAC Elution Buffer.
6. Check fractions for protein using absorbence at UV-280 nm or a Bradford assay.
7. Remove salt and imidazole using a desalting column or by overnight dialysis against PBS at 4°C.

### 3.4.4. Gel Filtration

Gel filtration is employed to separate monomeric scFv from the dimeric scFv, which is sometimes produced in the expression process (*see* **Note 24**).

1. Pool and concentrate IMAC fractions containing protein (scFv) in a centricon 10 concentrator (or a similar product) to a final volume of less than 1 mL.
2. Separate the dialyzed scFv on an HPLC or FPLC equipped with a Superdex 75 (or similar) size exclusion column (flow rate: 1 mL / min). Collect the fractions, which are predicted to be associated with 25 to 30 kDa proteins, and store them in separate tubes at 4°C for further characterization.
3. Determine the concentration of each fraction as described earlier.
4. Load a 5 μg aliquot of each fraction along with a series of molecular weight standards onto a 10% SDS-PAGE gel to determine the size and quality of the scFv eluted in each fraction. The monomeric fraction should be indicated by a single band of approximately 25 kDa.
5. The scFv can be stored at 4°C for 2–3 wk if sodium azide (0.02%) is included in the HPLC buffer to prevent bacterial growth. However, the sodium azide should be removed using a desalting column prior to using the scFv in the live cell or in vivo assays described below. It is usually possible to store the scFv for longer periods by freezing aliquots at –10 to –70°C in nonself-defrosting freezers.

## 3.5. In Vitro Assays

### 3.5.1. Radioiodination Methods for In Vitro and In Vivo Assays

Purpose: Trace labeled scFv is useful for determining in vitro and in vivo kinetics. However, it is important to note that producing useful radiolabeled scFv can be difficult. As the size of the protein to be labeled decreases, the probability increases that the attachment of a radioisotope to the protein will result in damage or steric hindrance, which can impair binding to the target antigen. Because the most facile radiolabeling methods involve the attachment of radioactive iodine (e.g., I-125, I-123, or I-131) to tyrosine residues, alternative methods such as radioiodine labeling of lysine residues or direct labeling with Tc-99m should be considered if the former methods interfere with antigen binding. Alternatively, site-directed mutagenesis can be employed to remove the targeted amino acid (e.g., tyrosine) from the scFv's CDR3 regions. Here, we will describe the chloramine T (CT) method for radioiodination of the tyrosine residues with iodine-125.

1. Prepare spin columns (one for every 250 µL of the reaction mixture) by adding Sephadex G-50-80 (preswelled overnight in PBS) to Biospin disposable chromatography columns (Bio-Rad; 732-6008). Let the resin settle in the column and add additional resin until the settled volume is 1.0–1.2 mL. Centrifuge the column for 2 min at 500*g*. The volume of the packed resin should be approx 0.7 mL. Cut the cap off of a 0.8-mL microfuge tube (one for each spin column) and place the capless tube in the bottom of a 15-mL conical centrifuge tube. Gently lower the spin column into the centrifuge tube such that the tip of the column fits into the mouth of the microfuge tube.

2. Suspend the desired amount of scFv in PBS at a concentration of 1.0–2.0 mg/mL in a capped 12 × 75 plastic tube (optimal total volumes range from 50 to 100 µL).

3. Add CT solution to the scFv to yield approximately a 1:10 CT : scFv molar ratio.

4. Add $^{125}$I to the scFv at an iodine to scFv molar ratio of 1:10 and allow the reaction to proceed at room temperature for 3 min.

5. At the conclusion of the incubation, quench the reaction by the addition of enough fresh SMB to yield a 1:10 SMB : scFv ratio.

6. Separate the unincorporated radioiodine from the labeled scFv by gel filtration using the spin columns prepared in **step 2.** above. Pipet the reaction mixture onto the resin in the spin column (maximum volume of 250 µL per column).

7. Seal the 15-mL centrifuge tube tightly with its cap prior to removing it from the hood. Spin the column for 2 min at 500*g*. Return the tube to the hood, uncap the tube and using forceps, remove the spin column, and place it in a radioactive waste bag.

8. Using forceps, remove the 0.8-mL microfuge tube from the centrifuge tube, cap the microfuge tube, and place it in a lead pig (store at 4°C). Place all radioactive waste in the waste bag and seal the bag to trap any volatile radioiodine. Dispose of the radioactive waste according to institutional guidelines.

9. Determine the purity of the radiolabeled scFv by HPLC analysis. Load 1 µL of the labeled scFv onto an HPLC equipped with a size exclusion column capable of distinguishing between monomeric scFv, dimerized scFv and unconjugated radioiodine (e.g., a Pharmacia Superdex 75 column). Run the HPLC at a flow rate of 1 mL per minute, collect 0.5-mL fractions and count the fractions in a gamma well counter. Compare the elution profile of the radiolabeled scFv to that of known molecular weight standards. The radioactivity should elute from the HPLC with the monomeric scFv peak (approx 25 kDa) and less than 1% of the activity should appear unconjugated.

10. Determine immunoreactivity of radioiodinated scFv.

### 3.6. Cell-Based Assays

Following the determination of affinity, it is critical that the reactivity with the target antigen be confirmed in the "native" setting, as all of the steps undertaken to this point depend upon an artificial presentation of the antigen. An example of the importance of this step is illustrated in the results of a selection we performed against a recombinant form of the extracellular domain (ECD) of the HER2/*neu* (c-*erbB*-2) protooncogene product, which is often overexpressed on the cell surface of a variety of cancers including carcinomas of the ovary and breast. Two distinct, promising scFv were isolated and expressed. Both exhibited an affinity for the HER2/*neu* ECD in ELISA assays and by surface plasmon resonance. However, only one of the scFv was capable of binding to HER2/*neu* in its native state on the surface of cancer cells in culture *(14)*. It is likely that the discrepancy between the results from the two assay systems was because of either conformational changes in the structure of the HER2/*neu* ECD molecule occurring when it was bound to the ELISA plate and BIAcore chip, or that the scFv, which was unable to bind to cell surface HER2/*neu*, targeted an epitope that was inaccessible because of a close proximity to the cell surface. This step is important when the antigen target will be encountered on the surface of a cell.

All of the cell-based assays, require cell lines that greatly overexpress the target antigen. In the case of our anti-HER2/*neu* scFv molecules, a number of appropriate cell lines are available from the American Type Culture Collection (ATCC, Rockville, MD). While we have found that the human breast carcinoma-derived SK-BR-3 line (ATCC # HTB 30), which expresses as many as $2 \times 10^6$ copies of HER2/*neu* per cell to be an excellent choice for the in vitro assays, however it is not tumorigenic in immuno-deficient mice. Accordingly, we typically employ the human ovarian carcinoma-derived SK-OV-3 line (ATCC # HTB 77), which expresses $1–1.5 \times 10^6$ copies of the antigen per cell and readily produces tumors in both nude and severe combined immu-nodeficient (SCID) mice.

### 3.6.1 Scatchard Analysis

This assay is performed to determine the affinity of an scFv for its target antigen (*see* **Notes 25** and **26**).

1. Harvest SK-OV-3 cells growing at log phase (if other than anti-HER2/*neu* scFv are being evaluated, substitute a cell line, which overexpresses the target antigen). Each confluent T-150 flask should contain approximately $1 \times 10^7$ cells.
2. Aspirate off the tissue culture media. Add 5 mL of 4-m$M$ EDTA in HBSS and let the cells sit for 5 min at rt.
3. Aspirate off the EDTA/HBSS solution and add 4 mL of Trypsin/EDTA to each flask of cells. Incubate flasks at 37°C for approx 5 min (until cells come free from the plastic when the flask is rapped with one hand).
4. Add 10 mL of tissue culture media containing 10% FCS to block further digestion by the trypsin. Pipet the cells up and down until all clumps are gone.
5. Transfer the cells into a 50-mL conical centrifuge tube and spin them for 5 min at 500*g*.
6. Resuspend the cells in fresh tissue culture media.
7. Remove a 100-µL aliquot and add 50-µL trypan blue dye to the aliquot. Determine cell viability and cell count in a hemocytometer.
8. Resuspend the cells in fresh tissue culture media at a final concentration of $1.67 \times 10^7$ cells per milliliter.
9. Prepare a stock solution containing 2.5 µg of $^{125}$I-scFv in 5 mL of tissue-culture media
10. Prepare solutions containing increasing concentrations (e.g., 0 ng, 20 ng, 40 ng, 200 ng, 2 µg, 4 µg, 20 µg, 40 µg, 80 µg, 200 µg, and 400 µg) of unlabeled scFv in a total volume of 400 µL of tissue-culture media.

11. In triplicate, add 100 µL of each of the solutions prepared in **step 3** to a 12 × 75 mm polyproplyene tube. Label the tubes with the concentrations added.
12. Add 100 µL (50 ng) of the stock solution prepared in **step 2** to each of the tubes prepared in **step 4**. Gently mix the tubes well.
13. Add 100 µL (50 µg) of the solution to three tubes labeled "total counts" and set these tubes aside until **step 19**.
14. Add 300 µL aliquots containing $5 \times 10^6$ cells (prepared in **step 1**) into each of the tubes prepared in **step 12**.
15. Mix each tube gently. Incubate at RT for 30 min.
16. Transfer the cells to ice. Add 3 mL of ice cold PBS to each tube.
17. Centrifuge for 5 min at 500*g* (4°C). Carefully aspirate off the supernatant.
18. Repeat **steps 16–17**.
19. Count the cell pellets and the tubes labeled "total counts" in a gamma counter.
20. Calculate the affinity and number of antigen binding sites. The reaction is described by a Scatchard plot *(18)*. The results of the assay are plotted with the bound over free (b/f) ratio of the scFv on the *y*-axis and the molar concentration of scFv bound to the cells on the *x*-axis. The affinity constant (*K*) of the scFv for the target antigen is determined from the slope of the line and the total concentration of antibody binding sites ($Ab_T$) in a hypo-thetical liter of cells is the concentration at the *x*-intercept.

### 3.6.3. Immunoreactivity Assay

Purpose: This assay is performed in a setting of antigen excess and antigen absence to determine if the antigen-binding properties of the scFv are altered following radioiodinations performed for in vivo biodistribution studies. The assay is performed similarly to the cell surface retention assay described above, except for the addition of negative control cells (e.g., CEM cells #119; ATCC) lacking the target antigen to assess nonspecific binding

1. Harvest SK-OV-3 and CEM (or other negative control) cells from tissue-culture flasks as described in **Subheading 3.6.1.** (if other than anti-HER2/*neu* scFv are being evaluated, substitute a cell line which overexpresses the target antigen). Resuspend the cells in fresh tissue culture media containing 10% FCS.
2. For each scFv to be evaluated, in triplicate, transfer $3 \times 10^6$ SK-OV-3 cells and $3 \times 10^6$ CEM cells into 15-mL polypropylene conical centrifuge tubes. Centrifuge the cells for 5 min at 500*g* and then carefully aspirate off the supernatant.
3. Dilute radiolabeled scFv in tissue-culture media containing 10% FCS to a final concentra-tion of 100 ng/mL.
4. Add 100 µL (10 ng) of the scFv solution to each tube and resuspend the cell pellet by gently pipetting up and down.
5. Incubate the tubes for 30 min at room temperature (*see* **Note 27**).
6. Add 2.0 mL of fresh tissue-culture medium to each tube and gently resuspend the cells as above.
7. Centrifuge the tubes for 5 min at 500*g*.
8. Transfer the supernatants to gamma counter tubes (labeled 1S, 2S, 3S, and so on), gently resuspend the cell pellets with 2.0 mL of PBS, and transfer them to gamma counter tubes (labeled 1C, 2C, 3C, and so on). Keep the supernatants and cell pellets from a single tube paired together. Count the tubes in a gamma counter along with an empty tube to deter-mine background counts.
9. Calculations: Subtract the background counts from each tube's counts. Determine the per-cent cell binding associated with each pair of tubes: cpm cell pellet/(cpm cell pellet + cpm

supernatant). Determine the average value for each group of three tubes representing the amount of specific binding and the amount of nonspecific binding. Typical live cell binding assays reveal >70% binding to the positive cells (SK-OV-3) and less than 3% binding to the negative control cells (CEM); However, the degree of binding to the positive control cells will be less when lower affinity scFv molecules (e.g., greater than $10^{-8}\,M$) are employed (*see* **Note 27**).

## 4. Notes

1. The culture volume has to be scaled up for rescuing the antibody fragment library to guarantee that the whole diversity of a library is present in the phage preparation. The number of bacteria cells in the library glycerol stock should be at least tenfold above the theoretical library size. The initial culture for phage rescue should be increased to a volume where the $OD_{600}$ ~0.25.

2. It is extremely important that the temperature during phage infection (helper phage, selected phage, titer determination) is 37°C and that the incubation step without shaking be allowed to proceed for at least 15 min. Failure to follow these instructions will lead to a poor efficiency of infection.

3. Precipitation during the phage preparation results in a white phage pellet that can be easily seen by eye. Darker pellets still contain bacteria cells and bacteria debris that should be removed. Filtration of redissolved phage usually results in a loss in phage titer and is only necessary for storage of phage preparations.

4. Phage titer can be calculated by serially diluting the phage and infecting *E. coli*. The number of "transducing units" or functional phage is determined by the number of antibiotic resistant bacteria colonies on the plate. The serial dilutions should be performed to bracket the likely titer. As $10^{12}$ to $10^{13}$ phage are usually present per mL of suspension, dilutions of $1/10^{11}$, $1/10^{12}$, $1/10^{13}$, and $1/10^{14}$ should be employed. Infect 1-mL aliquots of log phase TG1 *E. coli* ($OD_{600}$ approx 0.8) with 10 µL of diluted phage solution, plate out on a 150 mm$^2$ LB/Amp plate and incubate overnight at 37°C. Count the colonies and extrapolate back to determine the titer of the undiluted stock.

5. Nunc Maxisorb ELISA plates are an alternative to Immunotubes for phage selection.

6. Depending on the library used for selection, the antigen and the properties of scFv present in the library, the stringency of phage selection over multiple rounds should be increased to reduce the nonspecific background binding. This can be done by increasing the frequency and incubation time of washing. An effective alternative is to change the buffer composition (e.g., employing buffers with increased salt or detergent concentrations).

7. The most common eluents are solutions with high (TEA) or low pH (glycine buffer, HCl) or solutions containing chaotropic reagents (e.g., $MgCl_2$). Alternative elution strategies using free antigen or a specific peptide epitope of the antigen can be employed.

8. For the primary screening in an ELISA, a panel of clones must be expressed in an efficient manner. Miniexpression in 96-well microtiter plates is the method of choice. The supernatant of expression induced *E. coli* can be used directly in the ELISA. However, the concentrations of scFv in the supernatants are not always high enough to detect by ELISA. The logical alternative, the isolation of scFv from bacterial periplasm, is too time consuming. We have found that the easiest and fastest method to obtain sufficient crude scFv samples for the ELISA is to grow the cells in microtiter plates and produce bacterial extracts by adding Tween 20 and lysing the cells using freeze/thaw cycles. Finally, because it is true that a phage ELISA using crude scFv/phage preparations could be used in place of an scFv ELISA, the phage ELISA technique is often associated with nonspecific background binding to many antigens, and should be avoided.

9. There are many different ELISA formats available. The method of choice is usually the one that reflects the selection conditions. For example, a captured ELISA using

biotinylated antigen should be performed when selections were done with biotinylated antigen. Typically, the temperature and pH (buffer) used in the coating procedure can vary with the antigen. It may be necessary to try different conditions before successful coating has occurred. The potential for insufficient coating in this step makes the use of a positive control antibody very important.

10. To perform an scFv ELISA using biotinylated antigen, coat a plate as in **Subheading 3.2.2., step 1** with 50 µL avidin solution (5 µg/mL in PBS). Remove the avidin solution and block the plate as in **steps 2–4**. Add 50 µL of biotinylated antigen (1–10 µg/mL) to each well and incubate the plate for 30 min at room temperature. Dump out the antigen solution, blot dry on paper towels and wash the plate once with PBS. Proceed as described in **steps 5–12** of **Subheading 3.2.2.**

11. Different peptide-tags (e.g., *myc-*, *E-*, *his$_6$-tag*) can be used for the detection of scFv binding in the ELISA screening. Therefore the monoclonal antibodies, the enzyme conjugates and substrates have to be chosen depending on the requirements.

12. The primary requirement for the chain shuffling procedure is the availability (or generation) of $V_H$ and $V_L$ repertoire libraries. The $V_L$ shuffling for the anti-HER2 scFv C6.5 was made by cloning the VH gene of C6.5 via the restriction enzymes *Nco*I and *Xho*I into a light chain repertoire ($V_\kappa$ and $V_\lambda$). In a second step the optimized $V_L$ plus the C-terminal part of $V_H$ starting with the CDR3 to keep the specificity should be cloned into a $V_H$ fragment library (framework sections 1 to 3) using the restriction enzymes *Bss*HII and *Not*I.

13. For CDR3 randomization a library containing of $V_L$ or $V_H$ CDR3 mutants must be created. In order to accomplish this, an oligonucleotide is designed which randomizes, or partially randomizes the amino acids located in one of the CDR3 domains *(9)*. The mutations are generated by PCR amplification of the *scFv* gene under standard conditions followed by a second PCR to introduce the *Not*I restriction site. The gel purified DNA fragment is then digested with restriction enzymes and ligated into predigested pCANTAB5E (Pharmacia Biotech). Selections can then be performed against the target antigen and scFv with improved binding kinetics can be identified as aforementioned.

14. To create a gene-fused dimer, the *scFv* gene is ligated into the first and second positions of a bicistronic vector with an intervening spacer sequence. Although the $(G_4S)_3$ sequence, which is employed between the $V_L$ and $V_H$ chains of most scFv molecules is effective for this purpose because of its inherent flexibility, it is important to use different codon sequences to prevent difficulties in recombination. A major advantage of this technique is that it can be readily employed to create "bispecific" scFv molecules, which target two distinct antigens.

15. The creation of a diabody molecule employs a radically different approach from that used with the gene-fused dimer. Diabodies are noncovalent dimers, which result from shortening the intrachain peptide spacer from 15 aa's to 3-5 aa's, such that the $V_H$ chain and $V_L$ chain of a single molecule are prevented from associating. As these chains have a high affinity for each other, the $V_H$ chain from one scFv molecule will associate with the $V_L$ chain from a second molecule, and vice versa, resulting in the formation of a stable, rigid dimer with antigen-binding sites facing nearly 180° apart. To create a diabody, the $V_H$ and $V_L$ genes of an scFv are joined together by PCR splicing and overlap extension using an oligonucleotide which encodes a five amino acid linker ($G_4S$) between the C-terminus of the VH and the N-terminus of the *VL* gene. The resulting diabody gene product is digested with *Nco*I and *Not*I, gel purified and ligated into *Nco*I/*Not*I digested pUC119mychis$_6$. The ligation mixture is used to transform *E. coli* TG1, and clones containing the correct insert can be identified by PCR screening and DNA sequencing. The diabody is then expressed and purified in the same manner as the monomeric scFv molecule.

16. For in vitro affinity maturation the stringency of selection has to be increased for each round to separate the low-affinity binders from the high-affinity binders. The simplest

method is to decrease the antigen concentration. It has to be low enough to select only for scFv with the highest affinity, but sufficient antigen must remain to prevent a total loss of binding. Additional stringency can be build in by extending the incubation time for each washing step *(9)*. Finally, preelution or sequential elution with solutions having different pH or salt concentrations can be useful alternative methods to isolate rare binders with high affinity.

17. For large-scale expression of scFv the expression conditions regarding temperature, expression period, and IPTG induction must be optimized for each scFv. These parameters depend on the biophysical and biochemical properties of scFv. Also the location (cytoplasm, periplasm, culture supernatant) of the expressed material should be determined and the extraction method for scFv needs to be adjusted to the requirements.

18. It is important to maintain the stocks in a frozen state in order to prevent repeated freezing and thawing which will impair the viability of the transformed bacteria.

19. Larger or smaller expression volumes can be performed, however the ratio of the fresh broth to the overnight culture should be 100:1.

20. If a refrigerated shaking incubator is unavailable and the temperature is above 30°C, the temperature of a wet shaking incubator can be dropped to 30°C by the addition of ice directly into the water.

21. Although the culture supernatant usually contains functional scFv, we have found that higher quality preparations can be achieved (likely by avoiding proteolytic degradation) if only the scFv within the *E. coli* are harvested.

22. If the stability of the expressed scFv is poor (e.g., low yields or degraded scFv), add protease inhibitors to the extraction and dialysis buffers to prevent enzymatic digestion.

23. For IMAC purification the imidazole concentration in all the buffers can be varied. The optimal concentration may differ from construct to construct.

24. Whereas we typically employ an HPLC or FPLC system to simplify the process, it is possible to substitute a gravity-based column containing the appropriate sized Sephadex resin in a hand-filled column at 4°C.

25. In the Scatchard Assay, the quality of the scFv is very important in the generation of accurate results. Harsh radiolabeling conditions and the presence of dimeric species in the preparation can lead to erroneous affinity measurements.

26. If a BIAcore surface plasma resonance instrument is available, it can be used to simplify the process of affinity determination.

27. scFv molecules with an affinity lower than $10^{-8}$ $M$ have such a rapid dissociation from the antigen that they appear to have a lower immunoreactivity in this assay. Other than just accepting the fact that a low apparent immunoreactivity is normal for these molecules, it is possible to slow the dissociation by performing the entire assay at 4°C.

## Acknowledgments

We would like to thank Dr. Adrian McCall, Heidi Simmons, and Eva Horak of the Fox Chase Cancer Center for their critical reading of this manuscript. This work was supported by the Bernard A. and Rebecca S. Bernard Foundation and the Frank Strick Foundation.

## References

1. Kohler, G. and Milstein, C. (1975) Continuous clusters of fused cells secreting antibody of pre-defined specificity. *Nature* **256,** 495–497.
2. Brown, L., Miller, R. A., Horning, S. J., Czerwinski, D., Hart, S. M., Mcelderry, R., et al. (1989) Treatment of B-cell lymphomas with monoclonal anti-idiotype antibodies alone and in combination with alpha-interferon. *Blood* **73,** 651–661.

3. Kaminski, M. S., Zasady, K. R., Francis, I. R., Milik, A. W., Ross, C. W., Moon, S. D., et al. (1993) Radioimmunotherapy of B-cell lymphoma with 131I-anti-B1 (anti-CD20) antibody. *New Engl. J. Med.* **329,** 459–465.

4. Jain, R. K. (1989) Delivery of novel therapeutic agents in tumors: physiological barriers and strategies. *J. Natl. Cancer Inst.* **81,** 570–576.

5. Huston, J. S., Levinson, D., Mudgett-Hunter, M., Tai, M.-S., and Novotny, J. (1988) Protein engineering of antibody binding sites: recovery of specific activity in an anti-digoxin single-chain Fv analogue produced in *E coli*. *Proc. Natl. Acad. Sci. USA* **85,** 5879–5883.

6. Adams, G. P., McCartney, J. E., Tai, M-S, Oppermann, H., Huston, J. S., Stafford III, W. F., et al. (1993) Highly specific in vivo tumor targeting by monovalent and divalent forms of 741F8 anti-c-erbB-2 single-chain Fv. *Cancer Res.* **53,** 4026–4034.

7. Winter, G., Griffiths, A. D., Hawkins, R. E., and Hoogenboom, H. R. (1994) Making antibodies by phage display. *Annu. Rev. Immunol.* **12,** 433–455.

8. Schier, R., Bye, J., Apell, G., McCall, A., Adams, G. P., Malmqvist, M., et al. (1996) Isolation of high-affinity monomeric human anti-c-erbB-2 single chain Fv using affinity-driven selection. *J. Mol. Biol.* **255,** 28–43.

9. Schier, R., McCall, A., Adams, G. P., Marshall, K. W., Merritt, H., Yim, M., et al. (1996) Isolation of picomolar affinity anti-c-erbB-2 single-chain Fv by molecular evolution of the comllementarity determining regions in the center of the antibody binding site. *J. Mol. Biol.* **263,** 551–567.

10. Pluckthun, A. and Pack, P. (1997) New protein engineering approaches to multivalent and bispecific antibody fragments. *Immunotechnology* **3,** 83–105.

11. Sheets, M., et al. (1998) Sheets Library. *Proc. Natl. Acad. Sci.* **95,** 6157–6162.

12. Marks, J. D., Hoogenboom, H. R., Bonnert, T. P., McCafferty, J., Griffiths, A. D., and Winter, G. (1991) By-passing immunization. Human antibodies from V-gene libraries displayed on phage. *J. Mol. Biol.* **222,** 581–597.

13. Marks, J. D., Griffiths, A. D., Malmqvist, M., Clackson, T., Bye, J. M., and Winter, G. (1992) By-passing immunisation: building high affinity human antibodies by chain shuffling. *Bio/Technolo.* **10,** 779–783.

14. Schier, R., Marks, J. D., Wolf, E., Apell, G., Wong, C., McCartney, J., et al. (1995) In vitro and in vivo characterization of a human anti-c-erB2 single chain Fv isolated from a filamentous phage antibody library. *Immunotechnology* **1,** 73–81.

15. Adams, G. P., Schier, R., Marshall, K., Wolf, E. J., McCall, A. M., Marks, J. D., et al. (1998) Increased affinity leads to improved selective tumor delivery of single-chain Fv antibodies. *Cancer Res.* **58,** 485–490.

16. Holliger, P., Prospero, T., and Winter, G. (1993) 'Diabodies': small bivalent and bispecific antibody fragments. *Proc. Natl. Acad. Sci. USA* **90,** 6444–6448.

17. Barbas, C. F., Hu, D., Dunlop, N., Sawyer, L., Cabara, D., Hendry, R. M., et al. (1994) In vitro evolution of a neutralizing human antibody to human immunodeficiency virus type 1 to enhance affinity and broaden strain cross-reactivity. *Proc. Natl. Acad. Sci. USA* **91,** 3809–3813.

18. Yang, W.-P., Green, K., Pinz-Sweeney, S., Briones, A. T., Burton, D. R., and Barbas, C. F. (1995) CDR walking mutagenesis ffor the affinity maturation of a potent human anti-HIV-1 antibody into the picomolar range. *J. Mol. Biol.* **254,** 392–403.

19. Scatchard, G. (1949) The attractions of proteins for small molecules and ions. *Ann. NY Acad. Sci.* **51,** 660–672.

# 84

## Direction of the Recognition Specificity of Cytotoxic T Cells Toward Tumor Cells by Transduced, Chimeric T-Cell Receptor Genes

**Martina Maurer-Gebhard, Marc Azémar, Uwe Altenschmidt, Matjaz Humar, and Bernd Groner**

## 1. Introduction

Cellular transformation does not necessarily require the expression of proteins with neoantigenic properties, and for this reason, immunosurveillance does not register all tumor cells. They frequently express potentially immunogenic components, but are able to escape elimination by immune mechanisms. One explanation for this escape is poor antigen presentation by the tumor cells, resulting in little or no measurable antitumor immunity in immunocompetent hosts. T cells remain naive or even become anergic to the tumor cells. Reasons for the deficient antigen presentation by the tumor cells include the reduced or absent expression of major histocompatibility complex (MHC) molecules and the absence of tumor antigens in the groove of class I or class II MHC molecules as a consequence of defective protein processing. Other reasons are the absence or inadequate levels of expression of adhesion molecules, the absence or inadequate levels of costimulatory molecules or the expression of lymphocyte suppressive cytokines like transforming growth factor (TGF-β) or interleukin 10 (IL-10) by tumor cells (1–5).

Strategies are being developed to overcome the limitations for recognition of tumor cells by the immune system. Immunotherapy of solid tumors using autologous lymphocytes has been applied with only limited success in a few tumor types. Lymphokine-activated killer (LAK) cells (6) were initially expected to provide a basis for the generation of T-lymphocyte responses against tumors, but the clinical studies were disappointing (7). The tumor infiltrating lymphocytes (TILs) are 50 to 100 times more potent than LAK cells in the eradication of small metastases, but have no significant activity against large tumors (8). Their use is limited to a few malignancies from which TILs can be derived (9,10). Early studies have confirmed the safety of this approach and demonstrated the persistence and tumor localization of adoptively transferred TILs (11).

A general limitation in the use of lymphocytes for adoptive immunotherapy is the availability of sufficient numbers of lymphocytes specific for tumor cells. For this reason, efforts are aimed at enhancing the therapeutic efficacy of tumor immunotherapy. Large numbers of cytotoxic T lymphocytes with a predetermined recognition specificity for particular tumor cells can be generated through the genetic modification of T cells.

From: *Methods in Molecular Medicine, Vol. 39: Ovarian Cancer: Methods and Protocols*
Edited by: J. M. S. Bartlett © Humana Press, Inc., Totowa, NJ

The procedure is based on the derivation of monoclonal antibodies (MAbs) raised against antigens that are present specifically or preferentially on the surface of tumor cells *(12)*. The genetic information for these monoclonal antibodies expressed in clonal hybridoma cells can be used to modify the tumor cell recognition specificity of T cells.

To increase the number of tumors susceptible to adoptive T-cell therapy, chimeric receptors composed of single-chain antibodies (scFv) directed against tumor-associated antigens and fused to a signaling molecule, such as the Fc receptor (FcR)-$\gamma$ or TCR-$\zeta$ chain, have been constructed and introduced into T cells *(13–15)*. In early studies, fusion genes encoding Fv-z and Fv-g were stably introduced into hybridomas via protoplast fusion or electroporation. The transfectants showed expression of the chimeric receptors and were able to respond to antigen stimulation of these receptors by IL-2 production or target cell lysis *(13,14)*. Similar results were obtained with human TILs obtained from tumor biopsies. The cells were retrovirally transduced to enable them to express the Fv portion of an antibody specific for an ovarian carcinoma antigen *(16)*. Peripheral blood T lymphocytes, derived from different donors and retrovirally transduced to cause expression of a Fv-$\gamma$ receptor, showed lytic capacity of tumor cells and produced tumor necrosis factor-$\alpha$ and GM-CSF in vitro *(17)*.

Here we describe a method that shows how to isolate naive T lymphocytes from mice and redirect their target cell specificity toward tumor cells. This is achieved via the retroviral gene transfer of a chimeric T-cell receptor gene comprising a single-chain antibody domain coupled to the $\zeta$-chain of the TCR.

## 2. Materials

### 2.1. Preparation of Cell Suspensions from Spleen of Mice

1. Balb/c-mice (Balb/cAnNCrIBR) of 6 wk to 6 mo of age (Charles River, Deutschland), Haplotype: H-$2^d$.
2. Complete DMEM-medium supplemented with 10% heat-inactivated fetal calf serum (FCS), 2 m$M$ L-glutamine, 100 U/mL penicillin, 100 µg/mL streptomycin, 10 m$M$ HEPES, and 0.5 m$M$ β-mercaptoethanol.
3. 200 µm mesh screen (self-produced).
4. ACK-lysis buffer (0.15 $M$ NH$_4$Cl, 1 $M$ KHCO$_3$, 0.1 m$M$ Na$_2$EDTA, pH 7.2). Filter sterilize through a 0.2-µm filter and store at room temperature.
5. PBS (137 m$M$ NaCl, 2.7 m$M$ KCl, 4.3 m$M$ Na$_2$HPO$_4$, 1.4 m$M$ KH$_2$PO$_4$, pH 7.4).

### 2.2. Isolation of T Cells

#### 2.2.1. T-Cell Enrichment by Nonadherence to Nylon Wool Columns

1. Scrubbed nylon fiber wool (Type 200L, DuPont Biotechnology Systems Division, NEN Products).
2. 1% HCl (w/v) in double-distilled water (ddH$_2$O).
3. Canine grooming brushes.
4. 0.4% trypan blue solution.

#### 2.2.2. T-Cell Isolation by Magnetic Cell Sorting (MACS)

1. CD90 (Thy 1.2) MicroBeads (Miltenyi Biotec, Cologne) for isolation of mouse T cells.
2. MACS-column (Type LS$^+$, capacity $10^8$ marked cells, Miltenyi Biotec, Cologne, or other MACS-columns) comprising SuperMACS magnet and MACS-stand of high-grade steel.
3. Washing buffer (phosphate-buffered saline (PBS), 0.2 m$M$ EDTA, 0.5% FCS).

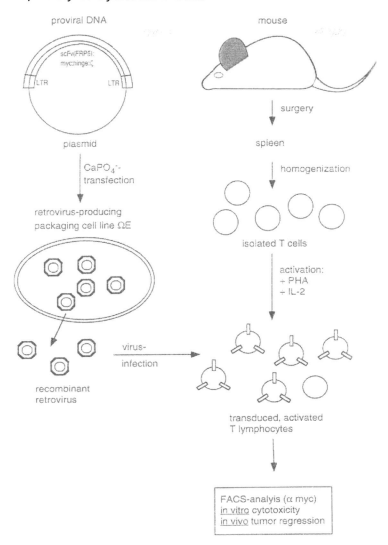

Fig. 1. Transduction of primary T cells. The retroviral vector encoding the ζ-chain construct was introduced into the packaging cell line ΩE by calcium phosphate transfection. Preactivated primary T cells isolated from mouse spleen were transduced by cocultivation with ΩE cells. Transduction efficacy was measured by FACS analysis. Activity of T cells was measured in vitro by standard LDH assays or chrome-release assays. In vivo effects were analyzed in tumor-bearing Balb/c mice.

## 2.3. Retroviral Transduction of T Cells

1. Ecotropic packaging cell line ΩE *(18)* transfected by calcium phosphate precipitation with pL[scFv(FRP5)/hinge/ζ]SN plasmid DNA *(19)*, cultivated in complete DMEM-medium.
2. Trypsin/EDTA (BioWhitticker, Walkersville, MD, 250 mg/L Versene (EDTA), 500 mg/L Trypsin 1:250).
3. 5 mg/mL phytohemagglutinin (PHA) (Sigma, St. Louis, MO).
4. 10 µg/mL recombinant mouse IL-2 (R & D Systems, Inc.) in PBS, 0.1% BSA.
5. 9 mg/mL polybrene (Sigma) in ddH$_2$O.

### 2.4. Detection of Transduced T Cells by FACS-Analysis

1. FACScan (Becton Dickinson, Rutherford, NJ).
2. FACS Flow (Becton Dickinson).
3. 0.1 mg/0.5 mL mouse antihuman c-*myc* antibody in 50 m*M* Tris-HCl, pH 8.0, 150 m*M* NaCl buffer containing 0.09% sodium azide (Pharmingen, San Diego, CA).
4. 0.5 mg/ml FITC-anti mouse IgG secondary antibody (Pharmingen).

### 2.5. Enrichment of Chimeric T Cells by MACS

1. Goat antimouse IgG Micro-Beads (Cat. No. 484-01, Miltenyi Biotec).

## 3. Methods

### 3.1. Preparation of Cell Suspensions from Spleen of Mice

Lymphocytes, mononuclear phagocytes, and related accessory cells are important constituents of the immune system. Of those, lymphocytes are the only immunocompetent cells, which are able to specifically recognize antigens on target cells. They consist of different subsets that perform different functions. They are concentrated in lymphoid tissue, e.g., in the spleen. The periarteriolar sheaths of the spleen contain many T lymphocytes, about two-thirds of which are of the $CD4^+$ T cells and one-third are $CD8^+$ cells.

1. Place freshly removed spleen on 200 μm mesh screen placed on a 100/20-mm petri dish. The subsequent procedure must be performed under sterile conditions at room temperature.
2. Using a circular motion, press the spleen against bottom of the mesh screen with the plunger of a 10-mL disposable plastic syringe until mostly fibrous tissue remains.
3. Remove cells from mesh screen with 5 mL of medium per spleen.
4. Centrifuge cells in a bench centrifuge for 10 min at 200*g* and discard supernatant.

### 3.2. Removal of Red Blood Cells from Spleen Cell Suspension

It is desirable to remove the red blood cells from spleen cell suspension because they are similar in size to the white blood cells and might interfere with experiments.

1. Resuspend pellet of spleen cells in ACK-lysis buffer, using 5 mL per spleen and incubate for 3 min at room temperature with occasional shaking or gentle pipeting (*see* **Note 1**).
2. Add 5 mL of PBS/spleen to stop lysis, spin 10 min at 200*g* in a bench centrifuge and discard supernatant.
3. Resuspend pellet in 5 mL of PBS/spleen, spin 10 min at 200*g* in a bench centrifuge and discard supernatant.
4. Determine cell number by trypan blue exclusion.

### 3.3. Isolation of T Cells

For many immunological experiments, it is necessary to prepare enriched populations of T cells. We describe two easy methods to isolate T cells from spleen of mice. With the help of these methods, up to $2 \times 10^7$ T cells can be prepared.

#### 3.3.1. T-Cell Enrichment by Nonadherence to Nylon Wool Columns

This protocol describes a commonly used method for the preparation of enriched T-cell populations from mouse spleen. The spleen cell suspension is passed through columns filled with nylon wool. B cells and macrophages preferentially adhere to nylon wool, whereas T cells do not. This method is easy to perform and the resulting T-cell population is about 80% pure.

### 3.3.1.1. PREPARATION OF STERILIZED NYLON WOOL COLUMNS

1. Place nylon wool in a 5-L beaker. Gloves must be used during the following procedure.
2. Saturate with an excess volume of 1% HCl.
3. Boil contents of beaker 5 to 10 min.
4. Allow to cool and pour off liquid.
5. Squeeze nylon wool to release trapped fluid and wash with distilled water.
6. Repeat washing until wash water is neutral (pH paper).
7. Dry nylon wool at room temperature by turning occasionally.
8. Fluff the nylon wool by combing between two canine grooming brushes until nylon is free of knots.
9. Remove the plunger from a 10-mL (or 20-mL) disposable syringe and use it to insert 1.2 g (or 2 g) of the fluffed nylon wool into the syringe.
10. Insert the plunger to compact the nylon wool then decompact.
11. Wrap the syringes in aluminium foil and autoclave in a baker (134°C, 10 min, 2 atm).

### 3.3.1.2. ENRICHMENT OF T CELLS BY NONADHERENCE TO NYLON *(22)* (*SEE* **NOTE 2**)

1. Place the column in an upright position and attach a three-way stopcock in an open position.
2. Equilibrate the column by running 50 mL of complete DMEM through the column at 37°C.
3. Remove trapped air bubbles by firmly tapping on the sides of the column until no dry areas are visible.
4. Close the stopcock and cover the nylon wool with 2 mL of medium to prevent drying of the wool.
5. Cover column with sterile aluminium foil and incubate it in a 37°C, 5% $CO_2$ humidified incubator for 45 min.
6. Open the stopcock and allow the medium to drain completely.
7. Add the cell suspension ($10^8$ cells/2 mL/10 mL syringe; $3 \times 10^8$/4 mL/20 mL syringe) and ensure that all cells penetrate the column.
8. Close the stopcock and add 2 mL medium to prevent drying and cover the column with aluminium foil to maintain sterility.
9. Incubate the column for at least 45 min at 37°C, 5% $CO_2$ in a humidified incubator.
10. Remove the column from the incubator and elute nonadherent cells with 15 mL (10-mL and 20-mL syringe) of complete DMEM.
11. Centrifuge the harvested cells 10 min at 200$g$ in a bench centrifuge.
12. Resuspend cells and determine viable cell yield using trypan blue exclusion.

### 3.3.2. T-Cell Isolation by MACS (see **Note 2**)

Mouse CD90 (Thy 1.2) microbeads are used for the positive selection of mouse T lymphocytes from lymphoid tissue. The Thy 1.2 antibody recognizes T cells of most common inbred mouse strains except AKR/J.

The magnetically labeled CD90$^+$ cells are passed through a separation column and retained in the magnetic field of a MACS separator. Unlabeled cells are depleted while CD90$^+$ cells can be eluted after removal of the column from the magnetic field. With the help of this method >95% purity can be achieved.

1. Isolate single cell suspension from spleen by standard preparation (**Subheading 3.1.**), and remove erythrocytes (*see* **Subheading 3.2.**).

2. Wash cells by adding 10 mL washing buffer (PBS, 0.2 m$M$ EDTA, 0.5% FCS) per $10^7$ total spleen cells.

3. Resuspend cell pellet in 900 µL of buffer per $10^8$ total cells. Add 100 µL of CD90 (Thy 1.2) Micro-Beads, mix well and incubate for 15 min at 6–12°C.

4. Place LS$^+$ column for positive selection into the magnetic field of a MACS-separator. Prepare the column by washing with 3 mL of washing buffer.

5. Apply cell suspension to the column and rinse column with 3 × 3 mL washing buffer to eliminate unlabeled cells.

6. Remove column from magnetic field, apply plunger, and firmly flush out the retained CD90$^+$ T cells.

7. Determine amount of isolated T cells by trypan blue exclusion.

## 3.4. Retroviral Transduction of T Cells

Retroviral gene transduction is used to introduce a nonviral gene into mitotic cells that cannot easily be transfected by conventional means, e.g., primary cells of various types. An infectious virus stock is made from cloned vectors. Plasmid DNA is transfected into packaging cell lines. These packaging cell lines are normally derived from stable mouse fibroblast lines and express the viral *gag*, *pol*, and *env* genes as a result of the introduction of these genes under the control of a cellular promoter. Although cellular RNAs are randomly encapsulated and bud with normal viral particles from these cell lines, the vector RNA is preferentially packaged because it contains the packaging sequence Ψ. The packaged retrovirus vectors enter the host cell via interaction of a viral envelope glycoprotein with a host-cell receptor. Postmitotic cells cannot be transduced because a cellular S phase seems to be a requirement for complete viral reverse transcription and integration.

1. Seed 5 × $10^4$ ΩE cells/well in 500 µL complete DMEM in a 12-well plate and let them adhere to the bottom of the dish for 3 h.

2. Add 2 × $10^6$ pretreated T cells in 500 µL of medium/well (activate with: 5 µg/mL phytohemagglutinin, 100 U rm IL-2, 9 µg/mL polybrene to increase the permeability of the cell membrane).

3. Cocultivate for 2 d at 37°C, 5% $CO_2$ in a humidified incubator (*see* **Note 3**).

4. Remove T cells from adherent packaging cell line. T cells that stick to the adherent packaging cells can be detached by gentle pipeting.

## 3.5. Detection of Transduced T Cells by FACS Analysis

T cells were transduced by pL[scFv(FRP5)/hinge/ζ]SN plasmid DNA encoding the chimeric TCR and a *myc*-tag for detection of infected cells. Analyze for the expression of the chimeric T-cell receptors by FACS analysis. Fluorescent staining was performed with a mouse antihuman c-*myc* antibody and subsequent incubation with a FITC-antimouse IgG secondary antibody.

## 3.6. Enrichment of Chimeric T Cells by MACS

1. Label transduced T cells with 4 µg mouse anti-*myc* antibody for $10^7$ T cells for 15 min at 6 to 12°C.

2. Resuspend pellet in 10 mL washing buffer per $10^7$ cells.

3. Discard supernatant, add 80 µL of washing buffer per $10^7$ total cells and 20 µL of MACS goat antimouse IgG Micro-Beads.

4. Mix well and incubate for 15 min at 6 to 12°C.

5. Proceed to magnetic separation (*see* **Subheading 3.3.2.**)

### *3.7. In Vivo Application of Genetically Modified T Cells in Balb/-Mice*

1. Suspend T cells after retroviral transduction in PBS.

2. Inject $10^7$ T cells in 100 µL PBS intratumorally or intravenously once per day for 5 d, in mice transplanted with tumor cells susceptible to the action of the transduced T cells. The efficacy of the transduced T cells is shown in in vitro killing assays.

## 4. Notes

1. A complete lysis of erythrocytes should be achieved to obtain very high purity of the isolated T-cell populations when using the nylon wool technique. Erythrocytes do not adhere to nylon wool and are flushed through the column together with the T-cell fraction. Lysis can be evaluated by the color of the pellet after centrifugation. Erythrocytes appear red in contrast to white blood cells. Incomplete lysis requires a second treatment with lysis buffer, but extensive lysis can also damage the T cells. That is why one should keep the procedure as short as possible.

2. Here we describe two different methods for enrichment of T cells from mouse spleen. Both techniques are very efficient for T-cell isolation, but if a high purity of T lymphocytes is required, we suggest the use of a MACS separator. We also could observe a higher yield of T cells by this method. The magnetic beads attached to the T cells had no adverse effects in our experiments. For preliminary studies we used the well-proven nylon wool column technique. Either methods yield in a high percentage (> 95%) of viable T cells as shown by propidium iodide staining in FACS analysis.

3. For the transduction of T cells, different procedures of retroviral gene transfer are described in the literature. We favor the coculture of T cells in the presence of the retrovirus producing packaging cell line as in our hands this method proved to be more efficient than the previously described transduction protocol using supernatant from those cell lines.

## References

1. Refisto, N. P., Kawakami, Y., Marincola, F., Shamamiau, P., Taggarse, A., Esquivel, F., et al. (1993) Molecular mechanisms used by tumors to escape immune recognition: immunogene therapy and the cell biology of major histocompatibility complex class I. *J. Immunother.* **14,** 182–190.
2. Allison, J. P., Hurwitz, A. A., and Leach D. R. (1995) Manipulation of costimulatory signals to enhance antitumor T cell responses. *Curr. Opinion Immunol.* **7,** 682–686.
3. Guinan, E. V., Gribben, J. G., Boussiotis, V. A., Freeman G. J., and Nadler, L. M. (1994) Pivotal role of B 7: CD 28 pathway in transplantation tolerance and tumor immunity. *Blood* **84,** 3261–3282.
4. Marrack, P. and Kappler, J. (1994) Subversion of the immune system by pathogens. *Cell* **76,** 323–332.
5. Moore, K. W., O'Garra, A., and de Waal Malefyt, R. (1993) Interleukin 10. *Annu Rev. Immunol.* **11,** 165–171.
6. Grimm, E. A., Muzumber, A., Zhang, H. Z., and Rosenberg, S. A. (1982) Lymphokine activated killer cell phenomenon. Lysis of natural killer resistant fresh solid tumor cells by interleukin 2 activated autologous human periferal blood lymphocytes. *J. Exp. Med.* **155,** 1823–1841.
7. Parmiani, G. (1990) An explanation of the variable clinical response to the interleukine 2 and LAK cells. *Immunol. Today* **11,** 113–115.
8. Rosenberg, S. A., Spiess, P. J., and Lafrenière, R. (1986) A new approach to the adoptive immunotherapy of cancer with tumor infiltrating lymphocytes. *Science* **233,** 1318–1321.
9. Rosenberg, S. A., Yannelli, J. R., Yang, J. C., Topolian, S. L., Schwarzentruber, D. J., Weber, J. S., et al. (1994) Treatment of patients with metastatic melanoma with autologous tumor infiltrating lymphocytes and interleukin 2. *J. Natl. Cancer Inst.* **86,** 1159–1166.
10. Rosenberg, S. A. (1992). The immunotherapy and gene therapy of cancer. *J. Clin. Oncol.* **10,** 180–199.

11. Fisher, B., Packard, B., and Read, E. (1989) Tumor localization of adoptively transfered indium 111 labeled tumor infiltrating lymphocytes in patients with metastatic melanoma. *J. Clin. Oncol.* **7,** 250–261.

12. Waldmann, T. A. (1991) Monoclonal antibodies in diagnosis and therapy. *Science* **253,** 1657–1662.

13. Brocker, T., Peter, A., Tannecker, A., and Karjalainen, K. (1993) New simplified molecular design for functional T cell receptor. *Eur. J. Immunol.* **23,** 1435–1439.

14. Eshar, Z., Waks, T., Gross, G., and Schindler, D. J. (1993) Specific activation and targeting of cytotoxic lymphocytes through chimeric single chains consisting of antibody-binding domains and the γ or ζ subunits of the immunoglobulin and T cell receptors. *Proc. Natl. Acad. Sci. USA* **90,** 720–724.

15. Moritz, D., Wels, W., Mattern, F., and Groner, B. (1994) Cytotoxic T lymphocytes with a grafted recognition specificity for erbB2 expressing tumor cells. *Proc. Natl. Acad. Sci. USA* **91,** 4318–4322.

16. Hwu, P., Schafer, G. E., Theisman, J., Schindler, D. G., Gross, G., Cowherd, R., et al. (1993) Lysis of ovarian cancer cells by human lymphocytes redirected with chimeric gene composed of antibody variable region and the Fc receptor γ chain. *J. Exp. Med.* **178,** 361–366.

17. Weijtens, M. E., Willemsen, R. A., Valerio, D., Stam, K., and Bolhuis, S. (1996) Single chain Ig/gammma gene-redirected human T lymphocytes produce cytokines, specifically lyse tumor cells and recycle lytic capacity. *J. Immunol.* **157,** 836–843.

18. Morgenstern, J. P. and Land, H. (1990) A series of mammalianexpression vectors and characterization of a reporter gene in stably and transiently transfected cells. *Nucleic Acid Res.* **18,** 3587–3596.

19. Moritz, D., et al. (1994) Cytotoxic T lymphocytes with a grafted recognition specificity for ERBB2-expressing tumor cells. *Proc. Natl. Acad. Sci. USA* **91,** 4318–4322.

# 85

# Eradication of c-erbB-2-Positive Ovarian Cancer Cells Mediated by Intracellular Expression of Anti-c-erbB-2 Antibody

## Jessy Deshane, Ronald D. Alvarez, and Gene P. Siegal

## 1. Introduction

Overexpression of *erbB*-2 is important in the pathogenesis of a variety of human neoplasms. Overexpression of the *erbB*-2 gene product has been associated with poor clinical prognosis with respect to malignancies originating in the ovary, breast, gastrointestinal tract, salivary gland, and lung *(1–4)* and has led to the development of several therapeutic strategies to target tumor cells exhibiting increased surface levels of *erbB*-2. Monoclonal antibodies that exhibit high-affinity binding to the extracellular domains of the *erbB*-2 protein have been developed *(5,6)*. Several studies have demonstrated that a subset of these antibodies can elicit growth inhibition of *erbB*-2 overexpressing cells both in vitro and in vivo *(5,6)*. Antitumor therapies directed at *erbB*-2 have also been developed utilizing targeted immunotoxins *(7)*. Gene-therapy strategies such as antisense technology has been widely used in these areas of research to achieve selected knockout of genes both at transcriptional or posttranscriptional levels *(8–10)*. Recombinant fusion proteins consisting of various bacterial toxins selectively targeted to the tumor by virtue of single-chain anti-*erbB*-2 antibody (sFv) moieties has also been utilized in this context *(7)*.

The rationale to develop new therapeutic modalities based on gene transfer has become increasingly compelling. The antineoplastic effect and cytotoxic effects of an intracellular single-chain antibody against *erbB*-2 have been demonstrated previously in the context of ovarian cancer *(11–16)* and breast cancer *(17)*. sFvs have also been used in the context of HIV disease for inhibition of human immunodeficiency virus replication *(18,19)*. Recently, modulation of *Bcl*-2 levels by an anti-*bcl*-2 sFv has been demonstrated to increase drug-induced cytotoxicity in the breast cancer cell line MCF-7 *(20)*.

Vectors have been developed for gene therapy for cancer based on mutation compensation associated with neoplastic transformation. For direct in vivo gene transfer, a variety of vector systems have been developed in a loco-regional context. These include viral vectors such as adenoviruses, retroviruses, HSV, and AAV-vectors. Recombinant adenoviral vectors have been shown to achieve the highest level of *in situ* gene transfer to airway epithelium *(21–25)*. This has led to the development of human

From: *Methods in Molecular Medicine, Vol. 39: Ovarian Cancer: Methods and Protocols*
Edited by: J. M. S. Bartlett © Humana Press, Inc., Totowa, NJ

clinical trials utilizing this approach. In the setting of in vivo gene transfer to the liver, the highest level of transduction of hepatocyte parenchymal cells after in vivo gene delivery have been observed with adenoviral vectors *(26–27)*. In the context of *in situ* transduction to a variety of nonneoplastic parenchymal cells and tumor cells, adenoviral vectors have shown the highest efficiency of in vivo gene delivery *(26–28)*. To study the utility of this novel strategy using an anti-*erbB*-2 sFv as applied to ovarian carcinoma cells, we and our colleagues constructed a replication incompetent recombinant adenoviral vector encoding an endoplasmic reticulum directed anti-*erbB*-2 sFv *(29)*.

## 2. Materials

### 2.1. Cytotoxicity Assay

1. XTT solution containing 1.0 mg/mL of XTT (2,3-*bis*(2-methoxy-4 nitro-5 sulfophenyl) 2-H tetrazolium-5-carboxanilide inner salt (XTT, sterile filtered; Sigma, St. Louis, MO), 0.0075 mg/mL of phenazine methasulfate in phenol red free RPMI medium.
2. Culture medium: RPMI medium (Mediatech, VA) with 10% fetal calf serum (FCS), (PAA Laboratories, Newport Beach, CA), 100 µg/mL penicillin, 300 µg/mL glutamine, 25 µg/mL streptomycin (Mediatech, VA).
3. Relevant plasmid constructs or recombinant adenoviruses pGT21 and Ad21.
4. Human ovarian carcinoma cell line overexpressing c-*erbB*-2 (SKOV3.ip1. cells) (Janet Price, Baylor University, Houston, TX).

### 2.2. Apoptotic Assay (Fluorescent Dye Uptake Method)

1. Dye containing 100 µg/mL acridine orange and 100 µg/mL ethidium bromide.
2. Cell suspension in complete RPMI medium at a density of $5 \times 10^5$ cells/mL.

### 2.3. Construction of a Recombinant Adenovirus (33)

1. Transfection reagent DOTAP (Boehringer-Mannheim Corporation, Indianapolis, IN).
2. 20 m*M* HEPES (cell culture grade, Life Technologies, Gaithersburg, MD), pH 7.4, sterile.
3. DNA constructs stored in storage buffer: 10 m*M* Tris-HCl, sterile.
4. Culture medium OPTI-MEM (Life Technologies).
5. Transformed primary human embryonal kidney cell line (ATCC, Rockville, MD).
6. Trypsin solution (Mediatech, VA).
7. DMEM/F12 media [complete and with 2% FCS (Mediatech, VA)].

### 2.4. Adenoviral Propagation (33)

1. 293 cells (ATCC, Rockville, MD).
2. DMEM + 2% FCS.
3. 5 m*M* HEPES, pH 7.8.
4. CsCl 1.33: 454.2 mg of CsCl/mL 5 m*M* HEPES, pH 7.8.
5. CsCl 1.45: 609.0 mg of CsCl/mL 5 m*M* HEPES, pH 7.8.
6. Viral preservation medium: For 100 mL–1 mL, 1 *M* Tris, pH 8.0, 2 mL, 5 *M* NaCl, 0.1 g BSA, bring up the volume to 50 mL with dH$_2$O. Add 50 mL glycerol, filter sterilize, and store at 4°C.
7. 3% Sucrose in 1X PBS for dialysis.
8. SW 28 tubes and SW41 tubes (Beckman, Palo Alto, CA).

### 2.5. Plaque Assay (33)

1. 1.35% of Noble Agar in water has to be kept at 44°C: For 500 mL 2X DMEM: DMEM 1 L Package (Mediatech, VA), 2X Pen-Strep, 2X glutamine, 3.7 g NaHCO$_3$, Add dH$_2$O to 500 mL. Adjust pH to 7.8, filter through 0.45 µm.

### 2.6. Chemical Linkage of Adenovirus and Polylysine

1. HBS (HEPES buffered saline)-5 m$M$ HEPES, pH 7.8; 150 m$M$ NaCl.
2. Poly-L-lysine (Sigma P-2636)-500 mg/50 mL HBS, adjust the pH to 7.8 and bring to a volume of 84 mL with HBS.
3. EDC (1-Ethyl-3-[3-Dimethylaminopropyl] carbodiimide Hydrochloride, Pierce #22980G)—1 gm in 4.0 mL dH$_2$O (prepared fresh before conjugation and discarded after use).

### 2.7. Preparation of Adenovirus-polylysine—DNA Complex

1. Poly-L-lysine (Sigma P-2636)- 1 mg/ml in HBS (20 mM HEPES, 150 m$M$ NaCl, pH 7.3).
2. EDC-linked AdpL (from **Subheading 3.7.**).

### 2.8. Flow Cytometric Analysis For the Determination of Optimum Vector For In Vivo Transduction

1. PCMVβ plasmid encoding the beta galactosidase reporter gene.
2. AdCMV*LacZ* (Recombinant adenovirus encoding the beta galactosidase reporter gene).
3. ACK Lysis buffer (0.15MNH$_4$Cl, 1.0 m$M$ KHCO$_3$, 0.1 m$M$ Na$_2$ EDTA, pH 7.4).
4. Biotinylated anti-*erbB*-2 antibody (3 µg/mL) (DAKO Corporation, Carpinteria, CA).
5. FACS buffer (10 m$M$ HEPES and 4% FCS in 1X PBS, pH 7.3, Store at 4°C).
6. 2 m$M$ fluorescein-di-galactoside (FDG) (Sigma).
7. Athymic nude mice.

### 2.9. Determination of In Vitro Efficacy of the Recombinant Adenovirus Encoding ER Directed Anti-erbB-2 sFv

1. HeLa (*erbB*-2 nonoverexpressing human cervical carcinoma cells).
2. Ad21 (Recombinant Adenovirus encoding ER-directed anti-*erbB*-2 sFv).

### 2.10. Analysis of Survival

1. CB-17 SCID mice (Jackson Labs).

## 3. Methods

### 3.1. Cytotoxicity Assay

The XTT assay is a colorimetric assay, which detects the ability of viable cells to convert tetrazolium salt to formazan.

1. A monolayer of cells is seeded (5000 cells/well) onto 96-well tissue-culture plates.
2. Transient transfection of target cells is carried out with plasmid constructs using the adenovirus polylysine (AdpL) method *(30)* or infection with recombinant adenoviruses *(14)*. Infections with recombinant adenoviruses are carried out at 37°C for 1 h in 2% FCS containing medium. The cells are infected at a multiplicity of infection (m.o.i.) of 100 PFU/cell in a volume of 100 µL standardized for 96-well plate, generally because for these specific viruses, a specific cytotoxic effect was achieved at those doses. After a 1-h incubation, the media was supplemented with complete medium. Transient transfection with AdpL was carried out as described in **Subheading 3.7.**
3. The plates are incubated for 0, 24, 48, 72, and 96 h. At each time-point, supernatants are removed and 50 µL of XTT solution are added to each well.
4. After 30 min, the A450 is determined spectophotometrically.
5. Percent viability is calculated from ODs by using the following formula: [(Infected cells—blank)/(uninfected cells—blank)] × 100.

### 3.2. Apoptotic Assay (Fluorescent Dye Uptake Method)

Fluorescent DNA binding dyes combined with fluorescence microscopy are used to visualize and count cells with aberrant chromatin organization *(31,32)*.

1. The cell suspension is prepared as noted above (*see* **Subheading 3.1., step 1**) and combined with 1 μL of dye.
2. Cells are stained with this mixture for 10 min at room temperature (25°C) and examined by fluorescent microscopy.
3. A total of 300 cells/slide are counted and the number of normal vs apoptotic nuclei are recorded using the following equation:

$$\% \text{ of apoptotic cells} = \frac{VA + NVA}{VN + VA + NVN + NVA} \times 100$$

where:

$VA$ = viable apoptotic (bright green chromatin that is highly condensed or fragmented) nuclei.

$NVA$ = nonviable apoptotic (bright orange chromatin that is highly condensed or fragmented) nuclei.

$NVN$ = nonviable normal (bright orange chromatin with organized structure) nuclei.

$VN$ = viable normal (bright green chromatin with organized structure) nuclei.

### 3.3. Construction of a Recombinant Adenovirus (33)

For best results only low passage 293 cells are used.

1. 293 cells are plated in 60-mm dishes 1–2 d prior to cotransfection in DMEM/F12 medium containing 10% FCS. At the time of cotransfection, the cells should be 50–70% confluent.
2. Preparing DOTAP/DNA complex: In a sterile polystyrene or glass tube mix: 2 μg of shuttle plasmid (*see* **Note 1**, Microbix Biosystems, Ontario, Canada), 3 μg of rescue plasmid (Microbix Biosystems), 15 μL of DOTAP, 20 m*M* HEPES, pH 7.4 to give a final volume of 100 μL.
3. Incubate the mixture at room temperature (25°C) for 10 min.
4. Remove the medium, wash the cells once with PBS and once with OPTI-MEM medium.
5. Add 1 mL of fresh OPTI-MEM per 60-mm dish.
6. Add DOTAP/DNA complex slowly to the medium (over a time period of 45 s).
7. Incubate under 5% $CO_2$ conditions at 37°C for 4–6 h and then replace the medium.
8. Change the medium again the day after transfection, and then every 2–3 d.
9. When monolayers of transfected cells are 100% confluent, remove the medium.
10. Wash the cells once with PBS, add 1 mL of trypsin solution per dish and incubate it for 1 min at room temperature (RT).
11. Remove the trypsin from the cells and incubate for an additional two minutes at RT.
12. Add 3–4 mL of fresh medium (containing 10% FCS) and resuspend trypsinized cells by pipeting up and down.
13. Split the cells into three 60-mm dishes and allow expansion until they are 60–70% confluent. Keep changing the medium every 3 d.
14. When monolayers become confluent, remove the medium and overlay the cells in each dish with 10 mL of DMEM/F12 containing 10% FCS and 0.8–1% low-melting-point agarose.
15. The day after overlaying with agarose, add 10 mL of DMEM/F12 medium containing 10% FCS per dish. Continue to incubate the dishes at 37°C in a humidified 5% $CO_2$ atmosphere. Count plaques appearing 2–4 wk after transfection.

## 3.4. Adenoviral Propagation (33)

1. Prepare 293 cells in 150-mm tissue-culture plates. (This protocol is for a 20–30 plate prep. Split the cells from three plates 1 : 10, and 5 d later they are ready to infect.)
2. When the cells are at approx 90% confluency, infect them with a $3 \times 10^{12}$ PFU/mL stock of the virus as follows: mix 20 µL of viral stock in 15 mL 2% FBS/DMEM + 1% Pen-Strep per dish.
3. Incubate at 37°C for 30–31 h (do not add complete media).
4. After 30–31 h infection, at the onset of visible cytopathic effect, harvest the virus by pipeting cells from plates.
5. Spin three plates per 50-mL tube at 3000$g$ force for 10 min at 4°C.
6. Resuspend pellets in a total volume of 10 mL of complete media (*see* **Note 2**).
7. Do three cycles of freeze (dry ice/ethanol; or –70°C) thaw (37°C) for 20 min each.
8. Spin at 3000$g$ force for 20 min and transfer supernatant to first gradient.
9. Prepare first gradient in SW28 tubes: 17 mL 1.33 CsCl, 9 mL 1.45 CsCl, 10 mL viral lysate.
10. Centrifuge at 30,000$g$ for 3 h at 18°C.
11. Remove cell debris from the gradient very carefully with a pipet, leaving approx 1 cm above the viral band.
12. Pull viral band in 2 mL or less and dilute in a reagent reservoir boat to 4 mL in 5 m$M$ HEPES (*see* **Note 3**).
13. Prepare the second gradient in SW 41 tubes: 4 mL 1.33 CsCl, 4 mL 1.45 CsCl, 4 mL viral band.
14. Centrifuge at 77,000$g$ force overnight at 18°C (at least 18 h).
15. Pull viral band in 1–11/2 mL only, again pull slowly and put into a reagent reservoir boat (easier to manipulate small volumes compared to a 15-mL tube).
16. Dilute 1 : 1 with viral preservation media, aliquot, and store at –70°C. Reserve 55 µL for OD reading and plaque assay.

## 3.5. Optional Dialysis Protocol

1. After removing viral band from second gradient, put directly into "slid-a-lyzer" dialysis chamber (Pierce, Rockford, IL) without diluting.
2. Dialyze against 3% sucrose in 1X PBS for 3 h, changing buffer every hour.
3. Remove virus from chamber, aliquot, and store at –70°C. Reserve approx 55 µL for OD reading and plaque assay.

## 3.6. Plaque Assay (33)

### 3.6.1. Infection: Day 1

1. Seed 6-well plates × 2 with 293 cells. Allow cells to reach 80–90% confluence.
2. Prepare several dilutions of the virus. Take 1 mL of 2% FCS containing DMEM/F12 media in three 1.5-mL Eppendorf tubes. Label the tubes as $10^{-3}$, $10^{-6}$, and $10^{-9}$. Take 1 µL from stock viral prep and add to the $10^{-3}$ tube. Take 1 µL from this dilution and add it to the $10^{-6}$ tube. Take 1 µL from this dilution and add it to the $10^{-9}$ tube.
3. To prepare cells for infection, aspirate media from cells. It is important at this step to be very careful. Tilt the plate and with a micropipet tip attached to suction, aspirate the medium without touching the cell monolayer.
4. Add 1 mL of 2% FCS containing DMEM/F12 media to all the wells.
5. Label the two 6-well plates as described below and infect the cells with the required volume of virus.

a. Plate 1: Well 1: $10^{-3}$ (1 µL of stock), Well 2: $10^{-7}$ (100 µL of $10^{-6}$), Well 3: $10^{-8}$ (10 µL of $10^{-6}$), Wells 4, 5, and 6: $10^{-9}$ (1 µL of $10^{-6}$).

b. Plate 2: Wells 1, 2, and 3: $10^{-10}$ (100 µL of $10^{-9}$), Wells 4, 5, and 6: $10^{-11}$ (10 µL of $10^{-9}$).

6. Incubate for 1 h and then add 2 mL of 10% FCS containing DMEM/F12 medium.
7. Incubate for 24 h at 37°C and then overlay the cells with Agar.

### 3.6.2. Overlay: Day 2

1. Aspirate the media from the cells.
2. Wash with PBS (pH 7.4) twice.
3. Add 1.5–2 mL of Agar, set for 30 min in the hood. As the plates dry, keep them upside down.

### 3.6.3. Count Plaques: Day 7

1. Wait 5 d and then count the plaques.

## 3.7. Chemical Linkage of Adenovirus and Polylysine

1. Prepare the virus as per the above protocol (**Subheading 3.4.**).
2. After the second spin, resuspend the virus in a final volume of 2.5 mL with 1.33 CsCl.
3. Load onto a PD10 column (Pharmacia, Piscataway, NJ) preequilibrated with HBS.
4. Elute with 2 mL HBS.
5. Resuspend to a final volume 3.6 mL with HBS.
6. Prepare final Reaction Mixture: 3.6 mL virus, 0.4 mL polylysine, 0.04 mL EDC.
7. Place Final Reaction Mixture on ice for 4 h.
8. Mix with 8 mL of 1.45 CsCl.
9. Centrifuge at 77,000$g$ for 18 h in SW41 tubes at 18°C.
10. Harvest the opalescent band, determine concentration.
11. Dilute with viral preservation medium to achieve a final concentration of $1 \times 10^{11}$ particles/mL. Aliquot and store at –70°C.

## 3.8. Preparation of Adenovirus-Polylysine-DNA Complex

Recipe for 6.0 µg DNA (transduction of approximately $1 \times 10^6$ cells may be scaled up or down accordingly.

1. Add 100 µL Adenovirus-polylysine (EDC-linked AdpL at $1 \times 10^{11}$ particles/mL) and 6.0 µg plasmid DNA in 100 µL HBS for 30 min at room temperature.
2. Then add 4.0 µL poly-L-lysine in 100 µL HBS and incubate at room temperature for 30 min.
3. Add this mixture to the cells which are in 1/2 total volume 2% FCS containing media.
4. Incubate for 60 min at 37°C.
5. Add the remaining volume of FCS containing media to bring the final concentration to maintenance level (*see* **Note 4**).

Plasmid DNA should be CsCl gradient purified for best results. Qiagen, Inc. (Valencia, CA) purification followed by endotoxin removal also provides the required purity of DNA for this process.

## 3.9. Flow Cytometric Analysis For the Determination of Optimum Vector For In Vivo Transduction

### 3.9.1. In Vivo Establishment of Tumor

1. SKOV3.ip1 cells are transplanted orthotopically into athymic nude mice via an intraperitoneal (ip) route.

2. Animals are challenged 48 h after tumor engraftment with different vectors encoding the *E.coli*-galactosidase reporter gene. These include: AdpL complexed with plasmid encoding *LacZ*, DOTAP complexed with the same plasmid and ADCMV*LacZ* delivered at 100 PFU/cell.

### 3.9.2. Recovery of Cells

The efficiency of gene transfer is assessed 48 h after gene delivery. Cells are retrieved by peritoneal lavage and flow cytometric analysis is used to calculate the percentage of cells with reporter gene transfer.

1. Tumor cells are harvested by intrainjecting cold phosphate-buffered saline (PBS), massaging the sides of the animals to ensure uniform distribution and removing tumor cells via the same needle.

### 3.9.3. Flow Cytometric Analysis

1. Pellet cells and add 5 mL ACK lysis buffer to lyse the red blood cells. Pipet up and down and incubate at room temperature for 5 min.
2. Lysis was terminated by the addition of 5 mL of complete media.
3. $10^6$ tumor cells are incubated with biotinylated polyclonal anti-*erbB*-2 antibody for 30 min at room temperature.
4. Cells are washed ($3 \times 20$ min) with PBS (pH 7.4) and incubated with streptavidin phycoerythrin.
5. Cells are washed again with PBS and resuspended in 100 µL FACS buffer in a 6-mL FACS tube.
6. Warm at 37°C for 10 min. Add 100 µL prewarmed 2 m*M* fluorescein-di-galactoside.
7. Incubate the cells at 37°C for exactly 1 min. Stop FDG loading by adding 1 mL FACS buffer.
8. Keep the cells on ice and in the dark until analysis is completed.
9. 10,000 cells can be easily size sorted first, and then sorted for *erbB*-2 and *Lac-Z* positivity.

## 3.10. Determination of In Vitro Efficacy of the Recombinant Adenovirus Encoding ER Directed Anti-erbB-2 sFv

1. Cells are plated at the required density for the XTT assay (*see* **Subheading 3.1.**).
2. Cells are then infected with the recombinant adenoviruses at 500 PFU/cell for 1.5 h.
3. This step is followed by the addition of complete medium.
4. 96 h after infection, the cells are assayed for cell viability using the XTT assay.

## 3.11. Determination of In Vivo Efficacy of Ad21

1. $2 \times 10^7$ SKOV3.ip1 cells are transplanted intraperitoneally into mice.
2. Recombinant adenoviruses Ad21 or AdCMV*LacZ* are administered intraperitoneally 2 d later at a dose of 500 PFU/cell.
3. Tumor cells are harvested by peritoneal lavage 48 h after viral administration.
4. XTT assays are performed to assay for cell viability.
5. Cells are also analyzed for apoptosis by the fluorescent dye uptake method as described above.

## 3.12. Analysis of Survival

1. $3 \times 10^7$ SKOV3. ip1. cells are injected intraperitoneally into CB-17 SCID mice.
2. Five days after tumor transplant, the recombinant adenoviruses (Ad21 or AdCMV*LacZ*) are administered at a dose of 500 PFU/cell. Control groups are of two types: those animals

that receive only the tumor inoculum and those animals which only received the vector (Ad21).

3. The animals are assayed for survival. Statistical analysis are performed at day 36. The log-rank test is used to calculate the statistical significance of difference. The proportional hazards model is used to estimate the relative risks of death comparing the control groups with the experimental group.

Here we have used a more efficient strategy of delivering an intracellular single-chain antibody directed to the endoplasmic reticulum of the target cells which overexpress the oncoprotein *erbB*-2. The gene is delivered via a recombinant adenoviral vector, which is capable of achieving the highest frequency of *in situ* transduction of tumor cells. The utility of recombinant adenoviral vectors in accomplishing gene delivery to human tumor xenografts that have been heterotopically transplanted into the peritoneum of nude mice has already been demonstrated *(34)*. In our studies a comparison of relative efficacy of the different vectors AdpL, lipid, and adenoviral vectors were carried out in vivo *(14)*. In this study, the recombinant adenoviral vectors accomplished transduction of >80% of the ascites tumor cell population. This transductional efficiency was significantly higher than that achieved with the other comparable vector systems.

The efficacy of the anti-*erbB*-2 sFv in achieving a cytotoxic effect was also studied both in vivo and in vitro. The recombinant adenoviral vector encoding the ER directed anti-*erbB*-2 sFv (Ad21) accomplished a marked reduction in the viability of SKOV3. ip1 cell. It is important to note that this cytotoxicity was not observed in the non-*erbB*-2 overexpressing HeLa cell line, which was used as a control in this experiment. It is also noteworthy that the control reporter gene encoding adenovirus was nontoxic when delivered at the same m.o.i., excluding the possibility of nonspecific vector-associated toxicity.

The adenoviral vector Ad21 also accomplished marked in vivo tumor cell cytotoxicity compared with the control vector AdCMV*LacZ* in *in situ* lavage-harvested tumor cells as evaluated by the XTT assay. Thus, in the context of mobile tumor cells in malignant ascites, the adenoviral vector was capable of achieving *in situ* transduction with selective tumor cell cytotoxicity. Experiments performed to look at phenotypic changes of the harvested tumor cells, also showed phenotypic changes indicative of apoptosis. Thus, the induced cytotoxicity appeared to be based on the selective induction of programmed cell death. Subsequent work in the laboratory has confirmed these observations.

The prolongation of survival of the animals following intraperitoneal administration of the Ad21 was also studied. This experiment was performed on SKOV3.ip1 tumor-bearing SCID animals. Significant differences in the survival of the treated mice were observed compared to the animals injected with the control virus ($p < 0.01$). The two control groups (cells only and the cells plus AdCMV*LacZ*) had an increased risk of death of 12.4 and 6.4 times, respectively.

One of the most interesting advantages of this approach is that although the adenoviral vectors are generally promiscuous as far as transduction of the host cells is concerned, this ER directed anti-*erbB*2 sFv encoding adenoviral vector is only cytotoxic for the *erbB*-2 overexpressing tumor cells. This is to say that ectopic expression of this sFv, even if it were to occur is not deleterious. Additionally, in ovarian cancer, where the containment of the intraperitoneally delivered vector is desired, ectopic expression of the therapeutic gene construct is not a major limitation. The disadvantage of this approach seems to be the fact that transduction of all neoplastic cells needs to be accomplished for efficient tumor eradication. Despite these problems, it has been shown by us that this strategy does provide tumor reduction at a level capable of giving a prolongation of survival.

Adenoviral vectors have also been limited by transient expression of the transgene and a markedly reduced rate of transduction following readministration. Neutralizing antibodies elicited by capsid proteins reduce the efficiency of vector administration whereas cytotoxic T lymphocytes (CTLs) directed against viral proteins and/or immunogenic transgene products expressed by transduced cells have the potential to limit persistence of expression. Several strategies have been proposed and used to circumvent this problem. Kolls et al. *(35)* have shown that administration of a depleting anti-CD4 antibody resulted in no antiadenoviral antibody response to the repeat administration of the vector and a second adenoviral transgene could be expressed in the animals treated with the antibody. Horowitz and coworkers *(36)* have demonstrated that insertion of the adenoviral E3 region into a recombinant viral vector prevents antiviral humoral and cellular immune responses and permits long-term gene expression. Transient administration of a novel immunosuppressant deoxyspergualin (DSG) has been shown to inhibit the development of both humoral and cell-mediated immune responses against Ad vector when delivered intranasally *(37)*.

Certain oncolytic agents such as etoposide and cyclophosphamide, which are commonly used for treatment of ovarian cancer patients, have also been demonstrated to suppress the immune response to adenoviral vectors and to enable repeated adenovirus-mediated cancer gene therapy. Scaria et al. *(38)* demonstrated in mice, a transient blockade of costimulation between activated T cells and B cells/antigen-presenting cells using a monoclonal antibody against the murine Cd40 ligand, which inhibits the development of neutralizing antibodies to adenoviral vector. This strategy also reduced the cellular immune response to Ad vector and allowed an increase in persistence of transgene expression. Furthermore, when administered with a second dose of Ad vector to mice preimmunized against vector, the monoclonal antibody was able to interfere with the development of a secondary antibody response and allowed for high levels of transgene expression upon administration of a third vector to the airway. TNF-alpha has been reported to play a central role in immune-mediated clearance of adenoviral vectors *(39)*. This is particularly important because the viral proteins that disable TNF-alpha function have been removed from most Ad vectors, rendering them highly susceptible to TNF-alpha mediated elimination. Wilson and coworkers *(40,41)* have reported a strategy that aims to inhibit CD4+ T-cell activation by transiently administering an inhibitor of the Cd28/B7 pathway, such as CTLAIg, at the time of administration of an E1- deleted adenovirus to the liver or lung. This appears to partially interfere with both arms of the immune response to adenovirus mediated gene transfer thus circumventing the need for chronic immune suppression *(41)*. Thus, with current efforts focused on developing an advanced vector system, this novel strategy can be translated into a clinical setting with therapeutic implications.

## 4. Notes

1. For our experiments, the shuttle vector used was not obtained from Microbix *(29)*. The shuttle vector was kindly provided by an investigator collaborating with Dr. David T. Curiel. Since then, efficient and comparable shuttle vectors with well-defined maps of the constructs available from Microbix have been successfully used for homologous recombination in the generation of recombinant adenoviral vectors.
2. Do not use more than 30 plates, which provide optimal conditions for the first gradient.
3. Pull the band very slowly to minimize the amount of CsCl pulled.
4. Poly-L-lysine (Sigma P-2636)-1 mg/mL in HBS stock stored in aliquots at –20°C.

## 5. Acknowledgment

The authors wish to thank Professor David T. Curiel for his careful review of the manuscript and his helpful suggestions.

## References

1. Slamon, D. J., Godolphin, W., and Jones, L. A. (1989) Studies of the HER-2/neu proto-oncogene in human breast and ovarian cancer. *Science* **244,** 707–712.
2. Semba, K., Kamata, N., Toyoshima, K., and Yamamoto, T. (1985) A v-erbB related protooncogene c-erbB-2, is distinct from the c-erbB-1/epidermal growth factor-receptor gene and is amplified in a human salivary gland adenocarcinoma. *Proc. Natl. Acad. Sci. USA* **82,** 6497–6501.
3. Fukushige, S. I., Matsubara, K. I., and Yoshida, M. (1986) Localization of a novel v-erbB-related gene, c-erbB-2, on human chromosome 17 and its amplification in a gastric cancer cell line. *Mol. Cell Biol.* **6,** 955–958.
4. Hynes, N. (1993) Amplification and overexpression of the erbB-2 gene in human tumors: its involvement in tumor development, significance as a prognostic factor and potential as a target for cancer therapy. *Cancer Biol.* **4,** 19–26.
5. Fendly, B. M., Winget, M., Hudziak, R. M., Lipari, M. T., Napier, M. A., and Ulrich, A. (1990) Characterization of murine monoclonal antibodies reactive to either the human epidermal growth factor receptor or HER2/neu gene product. *Cancer Res.* **50,** 1550–1558.
6. Drebin, J. A., Link, V. C., and Greene, M. I. (1988) Monoclonal antibodies specific for the neu oncogene product directly mediate antitumor effects in vivo. *Oncogene* **2,** 387–394.
7. Batra, J. K., Kasprzyk, P. G., Bird, R. E., Pastan, I., and King, C. R. (1992) Recombinant anti-erbB-2 immunotoxins containing Pseudomonas exotoxin. *Proc. Natl. Acad. Sci. USA* **89,** 5867–5871.
8. Ebbinghaus, S. W., Gee, J. E., Rodu, B., Mayfield, C. A., Sanders, S., and Miller, D. M. (1993) Triplex formation inhibits HER-2/neu transcription in vitro. *J. Clin. Invest.* **92,** 2433–2439.
9. Cooney, M., Czernuszewicz, G., Postel, E. H., Flint, S. J., and Hogan, M. E. (1988) Site-specific oligonucleotide binding represses transcription of the human c-myc gene in vitro. *Science* **241,** 456–459.
10. Mukhopadhyay, T., Tainsky, M., Cavendar, A. C., and Roth, J. A. (1991) Specific inhibition of K-ras expression and tumorigenicity of lung cancer cells by antisense RNA. *Cancer Res.* **51,** 1744–1748.
11. Deshane, J., Loechel, F., Conry, R. M., Siegal, G. P., King, C. R., and Curiel, D. T. (1994) Intracellular single-chain antibody directed against erbB-2 downregulates cell surface erbB-2 and exhibits a selective anti-proliferative effect in erbB-2 overexpressing cancer cell lines. *Gene Ther.* **1,** 332–337.
12. Deshane, J., Grim, J., Loechel, S., Siegal, G. P., Alvarez, R. D., and Curiel, D. T. (1996) Intracellular antibody against erbB-2 mediates targeted tumor cell eradication by apoptosis. *Cancer Gene Ther.* **3,** 89–98.
13. Deshane, J., Cabrera, G., Grim, J. E., Siegal, G. P., Pike, J., Alvarez, R. D., and Curiel, D. T. (1995) Targeted eradication of ovarian cancer mediated by intracellular exression of anti-erbB-2 single-chain antibody. *Gynecol Oncol.* **59,** 8–14.
14. Deshane, J., Siegal, G. P., Alvarez, R. D., Wang, M. H., Feng, M., Cabrera, G., et al. (1995) Targeted tumor killing via an intracellular antibody against erbB-2. *J. Clin. Invest.* **96,** 2980–2989.
15. Beerli, R. R., Wels, W., and Hynes, N. E. (1994) Intracellular expression of single chain antibodies reverts erbB-2 transformation. *J. Biol. Chem.* **269,** 23,931–23,936.
16. Graus-Porta, D., Beerli, R., and Hynes, N. E. (1995) Single-chain antibody-mediated intracellular retention of erbB-2 impairs Neu differentiation factor and epidermal growth factor signaling. *Mol. Cell Biol.* **15,** 1182–1191.

17. Wright, M., Grim, J., Deshane, J., Kim, M., Strong, T. V., Siegal, G. P., et al. (1997) An intracellular anti-erbB-2 single-chain antibody is specifically cytotoxic to human breast carcinoma cells overexpressing erbB-2. *Gene Ther.* **4,** 317–322.

18. Marasco, W. A., Haseltine, W. A., and Chen, S. Y. (1993) design, intracellular expression, and activity of a human anti-human immunodeficiency virus type 1 gp120 single-chain antibody. *Proc. Natl. Acad. Sci. USA* **90,** 7889–7893.

19. Pozansky, M. C., Foxall, R., Mhashilkar, A., Coker, R., Jones, S., Ramstedt, U., et al. (1998) Inhibition of human immunodeficiency virus replication and growth advantage of CD4+ T cells from HIV-infected individuals that express intracellular antibodies against HIV-1 gp120 or Tat. *Hum. Gene Ther.* **9,** 487–496.

20. Piche, A., Grim, J., Rancourt, C., Gomez-Navarro, J., Reed, J. C., and Curiel, D. T. (1998) Modulation of Bcl-2 protein levels by an intracellular anti-Bcl-2 single-chain antibody increases drug-induced cytotoxicity in the breast cancer cell line MCF-7. *Cancer Res.* **58,** 2134–2140.

21. Goldman, M. J., Yang, Y., and Wilson, J. M. (1995) Gene therapy in a xenograft model of cystic fibrosis lung corrects chloride transport more effectively that the sodium defect. *Nature Genet.* **9,** 126–131.

22. Engelhardt, J. F., Yang, Y., and Stratford-Perricaudet, L. D. (1993) Direct gene transfer of human CFTR into human bronchial epithelia of xenografts with E1-deleted adenoviruses. *Nature Genet.* **4,** 27–34.

23. Zsengeller, Z. K., Wert, S. E., and Hull, W. M. (1995) Persistence of replication deficient adenovirus-mediated gene transfer in lungs of immune-deficient(nu/nu) mice. *Hum. Gen. Ther.* **6,** 457–467.

24. Zabner, J., Couture, L. A., and Smith, A. E. (1994) Correction of cAMP-stimulated fluid secretion in cystic fibrosis air-way epithelia: efficiency of adenovirus-mediated gene transfer in vitro. *Hum. Gene Ther.* **5,** 585–593.

25. Johnson, L. G., Olsen, J. C., and Sarkadi, B. (1992) Efficiency of gene transfer for restoration of normal airway epithelial function in cystic fibrosis. *Nature Genet.* **2,** 21–25.

26. Kozarsky, K., Grossman, M., and Wilson, J. M. (1993) Adenovirus mediated correction of the genetic defect in hepatocytes from patients with familial hypercholesterolemia. *Somat. Cell. Mol. Genet.* **19,** 449–458.

27. Ye, X., Robinson, M. B., and Batshaw, M. L. (1996) Prolonged metabolic correction in adult ornithine transcarbamylase deficient mice with adenoviral vectors. *J. Biol. Chem.* **271,** 3639–3646.

28. Douglas, J. T. and Curiel, D. T. (1995) Adenoviruses as vectors for gene therapy. *Sci. Med.* **(1997),** 44–53.

29. Grim, J., Deshane, J., Feng, M., Lieber, A., Kay, M., and Curiel, D. T. (1996) erbB-2 knockout employing an intracellular single-chain antibody(sFv) accomplishes specific toxicity in erbB-2 expressing lung cancer cells. *Am. J. Respir. Cell Mol. Biol.* **15,** 348–354.

30. Curiel, D. T., Wagner, E., and Cotten, M., et al. (1992) High-efficiency gene transfer mediated by adenovirus coupled to DNA-polylysine complexes. *Human Gene Ther.* **3,** 147–154.

31. Mishell, B. B., Shiigi, S. M., and Henry, C. (1980) Preparation of mouse cell suspensions. *Select. Meth. Cell Immunol.* **1980,** 21,22.

32. Duke, R. C. and Cohen, J. J. (1992) Morphological and biochemical assays for apoptosis. *Cur. Protocol. Suppl.* **1992,** 3.

33. Graham, F. L. and Prevec, L. (1995) Methods for construction of adenovirus vectors. *Mol. Biotechnol.* **3,** 207–220.

34. (Sobol, R. E. and Scanlon, K. J. eds.), Clin Protocol. *Cancer Gene Ther.* (1995) **2,** 67–69.

35. Brody, S. L., Jaffe, A., Han, S. K., Wersto, R. P., and Crystal, R. G. (1994) Direct in vivo gene transfer and expression in malignant cells using adenoviral vectors. *Human Gene Ther.* **5,** 437–447.

36. Kolls, J. K., Lei, D., Odom, G., Nelson, S., Summer, W. R., Gerber, M. A., et al. (1996) Use of transient CD4 lymphocyte depletion to prolong transgene expression of E1-deleted adenoviral vectors. *Hum. Gene Ther.* **7,** 489–497.

37. Ilan, Y., Droguett, G., Chowdhury, N. R., Li, Y., Sengupta, K., Thummala, N. R., et al. (1997) Insertion of adenoviral E3 region into a recombinant viral vector prevents antiviral humoral and cellular immune responses and permits long-term expression. *Proc. Natl. Acad. Sci. USA* **94,** 2587–2592.

38. Kaplan, J. M. and Smith, A. E. (1997) Transient immunosuppression with deoxyspergualin improves longevity of transgene expression and ability to readminister adenoviral vector to the mouse lung. *Hum. Gene Ther.* **8,** 1095–1104.

39. Scaria, A., St. George, J. A., Gregory, R. J., Noelle, R. J., Wadsworth, S. C., Smith, A. E., et al. (1997) Antibody to CD40 Ligand inhibits both humoral and cellular immune responses to adenoviral vectors and facilitates repeated administration to mouse airway. *Gene Ther.* **4,** 611–617.

40. Elkon, K. B., Liu, C. C., Gall, J. G., Trevejo, J., Marino, M. W., Abrahamsen, K. A., et al. (1997) Tumor necrosis factor alpha plays a central role in immune-mediated clearance of adenoviral vectors. *Proc. Natl. Acad. Sci. USA* **94,** 9814–9819.

41. Schowalter, D. B., Meuse, L., Wilson, C. B., Linsley, P. S., and Kay, M. A. (1997) Constitutive expression of murine CTLA4Ig from a recombinant adenovirus vector results in prolonged gene expression. *Gene Ther.* **4,** 853–860.

42. Jooss, K., Turka, L. A., and Wilson J. M. (1998) Blunting of immune responses to adenoviral vectors in mouse liver and lung with CTLA4Ig. *Gene Ther.* **5,** 309–319.

# c-*erbB*-2 Antisense Oligonucleotides Inhibit Serum-Induced Cell Spreading of Ovarian Cancer Cells

## Kai Wiechen

## 1. Introduction

Amplification or overexpression of the c-*erbB*-2 oncogene (also known as *HER*-2, *neu*) is a frequent event in many types of human cancer including 20–30% of ovarian cancers where it characterizes a group of patients with poor prognosis *(1,2)*. The expression of *p185* (c-*erbB*-2) is in contrast quite restricted in normal adult tissues *(3)*. The c-*erbB*-2 oncogene product (*p185*$^{c\text{-}erbB\text{-}2}$) is a growth factor receptor (GFR) with extensive homology to the receptor for the epidermal growth factor (EGFR) and the c-*erbB*-3 and c-*erbB*-4 gene products *(4)*. According to the hypothesis that c-*erbB*-2 is involved in pathogenesis and progression of human cancer, the overexpression in fibroblasts leads to the appearance of a transformed phenotype, capable of forming colonies in soft agar and inducing tumors in mice *(5)*.

The clinical course of ovarian cancer is characterized by early abdominal spread and seeding of tumor cells rather than by generating distant metastases. Therefore, *p185*$^{c\text{-}erbB\text{-}2}$ may be important for cell spread and cell motility in ovarian cancer cells and may thus contribute to the early abdominal seeding of ovarian cancer. Carraway et al. *(6)* have shown that *p185*$^{c\text{-}erbB\text{-}2}$ is positioned in microvilli and pseudopodia of rat breast cancer cells. In addition in human breast cancer cells, *p185*$^{c\text{-}erbB\text{-}2}$ mediated spreading and motility could be observed *(7,8)*.

This chapter focuses on antisense approaches for the transient suppression of the c-*erbB*-2 oncogene product in human ovarian carcinoma cells to investigate the role of *p185*$^{c\text{-}erbB\text{-}2}$ in cellular motility. To transiently suppress the function of the c-*erbB*-2 oncogene in c-*erbB*-2-overexpressing SK-OV-3 ovarian cancer cells, nuclease-resistant phosphorothioate antisense oligodeoxynucleotides (sODNs) *(9)* were used. Problems using antisense sODNs may arise because many sites in a particular mRNA are probably not accessible for base pairing and accessible sites are not predictable. Therefore, optimal target sites for the antisense inhibition of c-*erbB*-2 have to be searched empirically *(10)*. The specificity and extent of the antisense effect was therefore measured by Western blotting. The influence of *p185*$^{c\text{-}erbB\text{-}2}$ on cellular motility

From: *Methods in Molecular Medicine, Vol. 39: Ovarian Cancer: Methods and Protocols*
Edited by: J. M. S. Bartlett © Humana Press, Inc., Totowa, NJ

**Table 1**
**Nucleotide Sequences**

|                    | sequence 5′ –> 3′        |
| ------------------ | ------------------------ |
| AS208              | GGG CAA GAG GGC GAG GAG   |
| AS631              | GAT CAA GAC CCC TCC       |
| Mismatch control   | CGC CTT ATC CGT AGC       |
| Sense control      | CTC CTC GCC CTC TTG CCC   |

was estimated qualitatively and semiquantitatively by measuring the spreading ability of the cells in serum-reduced media.

In the following, protocols are described for the detection of $p185^{c-erbB-2}$ and for measuring the influence of c-*erbB*-2 antisense sODNs on cellular proliferation and motility.

1. The inhibition of cellular proliferation by c-*erbB*-2 antisense sODNs is measured by a colorimetric XTT-assay.
2. The influence of $p185^{c-erbB-2}$ on cellular motility is estimated qualitatively and semiquantitatively by measuring the spreading ability of the cells in serum-reduced media.

## 2. Materials

### 2.1. Oligonucleotides

HPLC-purified or polyacrylamide gel-purified 18-mer phosphorothioate oligodeoxynucleotides (sODNs, Appligene, Heidelberg, Germany, or Eurogentec, Seraing, Belgium). Dissolve lyophilized sODNs in serum-free cell culture medium (DMEM) and store in aliquots for a single experiment at –20°C (**Table 1**).

### 2.2. Cell Culture

1. Dulbecco's modified Eagle's medium supplemented with 10% fetal bovine serum, 2 m*M* glutamine (DMEM/FBS).
2. 0.02 w/v trypsin, 50 m*M* ethylenediaminetetraacetic acid (EDTA) in PBS (pH 7.4).

### 2.3. XTT Proliferation Assay

1. XTT-kit (Boehringer Mannheim, Germany).
2. Microplate reader (Biokinetics Reader EL340, BioTek Instruments).

### 2.4. Cell-Spreading Assay

1. Laboratory equipment: 8-well chamber slides and 12-well culture plates (Nunc, Weisbaden-Biebrich, Germany).
2. Inverted photomicroscope (Olympus) with an ×20 objective.
3. Monoclonal antibody (MAb) 9G6 interfering with the extracellular domain of $p185$-$^{c-erbB-2}$ (Oncogene Science).
4. Mouse IgG with irrelevant specificity (Dianova, Hamburg, Germany).
5. Serum-free DMEM supplemented with 2 m*M* glutamine.

## 3. Methods

### 3.1. XTT Proliferation Assay (see Chapter 17)

1. Plate SK-OV-3 cells (American Type Culture Collection, HTB #77) growing in log phase in 96-well flat bottom microtiter plates in 100 μL DMEM, 10% FBS at a density of 500 cells per well (*see* **Note 1**).

2. After 48 h carefully remove medium using a Pasteur pipet and add 100 µL of DMEM supplemented with 2 m*M* glutamine and 1% FBS (*see* **Note 2**) with antisense sODNs or control sODNs (*see* **Note 5** for max. sODN concentration).
3. 72 h later add 50 µL XTT solution (mixed according to the manufacturers instructions) to each well. Mix by gentle agitation.
4. Measure formazan dye at 470 nm in the microplate reader.

### 3.2. Cell-Spreading Assay

The influence of *p185^(c-erbB-2)* on cellular motility was estimated qualitatively and semiquantitatively by measuring the spreading ability of the cells in serum-reduced media. To ensure that the spreading of SK-OV-3 ovarian cancer cells depends on *p185^(c-erbB-2)* the 9G6 c-*erbB*-2 monoclonal antibody that interferes with the extracellular domain of the receptor was additionally applied in a series of experiments.

1. Remove culture medium from stock cultures and wash once with phosphate-buffered saline (PBS) (*see* **Note 1**).
2. Detach SK-OV-3 cells from stock cultures with 1–2 mL trypsin/EDTA.
3. Pellet the cells by low-speed centrifugation at 1000*g* for 5 min, remove the supernatant and resuspend the pellet in serum-free DMEM.
4. Pellet the cells again, remove the supernatant and resuspend in serum-free medium.
5. Plate the cells in 8-well chamber slides or in 12-well culture plates at a density of 5000 cells per square centimeter (*see* **Note 1**) in serum-free DMEM supplemented with 2 m*M* glutamine. Under these conditions, the cells remain completely round and unattached on glass and plastic surfaces for at least 2 d.
6. After 4–24 h add sODNs (*see* **Note 3** for sODN concentration) or antibodies (MAb 9G6 and control IgG at 1–10 µg/mL) directly to the media. Do not change media because this will result in loss of the unattached SK-OV-3 cells. After addition gently agitate the wells.
7. After 16–24 h of incubation with sODNs, add FBS directly to the medium to produce a concentration of 1%. After addition gently agitate the wells. Do not change media at this step as this will result in loss of cells. After application of 1% FBS SK-OV-3 cells are completely spread within 2 h (*see* **Note 4**).
8. The effect can be assessed semiquantitatively by taking photographs 2 h after addition of FBS (objective ×20). We counted spread and round cells in at least 10 photomicrographs of each experiment (or at least 200 cells). Cells with a nuclear diameter larger than 9 µm and a total diameter more than 20 µm were scored in our experiments as spread (**Fig. 1**).

## 4. Notes

1. For the experiments SK-OV-3 cells with passage number 40–50 were used. The cells from stock cultures were trypsinized twice a week and diluted 1:5. It is important to use subconfluent SK-OV-3 cells in the experiments. The levels of *p185^(c-erbB-2)* are significantly higher in subconfluent cells than in confluent cells when the protein is detected by Western blot or flow cytometric analysis. In order to observe and to quantify cell spreading it is also necessary to use subconfluent SK-OV-3 cells.
2. A high concentration of FBS in the incubation medium (e.g., 10%) attenuates the antisense inhibition of c-*erbB*-2 with sODNs. This may be because of unspecific binding of sODNs to serum proteins. Therefore, FBS concentrations of 0–1% should be applied in the sODN incubation medium.
3. Phophorothioate oligodeoxynucleotides (sODNs) tend to inhibit protein synthesis and monolayer cell growth in an unspecific manner when applied in concentrations above 5 µ*M* in the culture medium. The interaction of sODNs with DNA and RNA polymerases

Fig. 1. Inhibition of serum-induced cell spreading of SK-OV-3 ovarian cancer cells by antisense sODNs. The cells were plated into chamberslides in serum-free DMEM with substance for 16 h. After this time, FBS was added to give a final concentration of 1%. Viable cells were photographed after 2 h (Olympus inverted microscope, objective x20). (Upper) untreated control, (middle) antisense sODN AS208 (5 μ*M*), (lower) sense sODN (5 μ*M*).

Fig. 2. Inhibition of serum-induced cell spreading of SK-OV-3 ovarian cancer cells. The cells were plated into chamberslides in serum-free DMEM with substance for 16 h. After this time FBS was added to give a final concentration of 1%. Viable cells were photographed after 2 h (Olympus inverted microscope, objective x20). Spread and round cells were counted in at least 10 microphotographs of each experiment (at least 200 cells). Cells with a nuclear diameter larger than 9 μm and a total diameter more than 20 μm were scored as spread. c-*erbB*-2 AS208 sODN (5 μ*M*), sense sODN (5 μ*M*), c-*erbB*-2 specific MAb 9G6 (10 μg/mL), IgG (10 μg/mL). Ordinate: percentage of round cells 2 h after addition of FBS.

and the forming of complexes with partially complementary sequences may account for nonspecific effects *(12)*. When using cationic lipids in conjunction with sODNs to enhance the antisense effects, the antisense concentration must be lowered to approximately 100 n*M* to avoid these nonantisense effects *(13)*.

4. Preincubation of SK-OV-3 cells with c-*erbB*-2 antisense sODNs completely inhibited cell spreading, whereas the control sODNs are not able to inhibit spreading (**Fig. 1**). The inhibition of cell spreading by the c-*erbB*-2 antisense sODN is dose-dependent with an $IC_{(50)}$ of approximately 1 μ*M*. Furthermore, the induction of cell spreading by FBS is strongly reduced by heat inactivation at 60°C for 2 h. The inhibition of cell spreading could be imitated by the monoclonal antibody 9G6 directed against the extracellular domain of $p185^{c-erbB-2}$ (**Fig. 2**).

## References

1. Berchuck, A., Kamel, A., Whitaker, R., Kerns, B., Olt, G., Kinney, R., et al. (1990) Overexpression of her-2/neu is associated with poor survival in advanced epithelial ovarian cancer. *Cancer Res.* **50**, 4087–4091.
2. Slamon, D. J., Godolphin, W., Jones, L. A., Holt, J. A., Wong, S. G., Keith, D. E., et al. (1989) Studies of the HER-2/neu proto-oncogene in human breast and ovarian cancer. *Science* **244**, 707–712.
3. de Potter, C. R., van Daele, S., van de Vijver, M. J., Pauwels, C., Maertens, G., de Boever, J., et al. (1989) The expression of the neu-oncogene product in normal fetal and adult human tissues. *Histopathology* **15**, 351–362.
4. Graus-Porta, D., Beerli, R. R., Daly, J. M., and Hynes, N. E. (1997) ErbB-2, the preferred heterodimerization partner of all ErbB receptors, is a mediator of lateral signaling. *EMBO J.* **16**, 1647–1655.

5. Hudziak, R. M., Schlessinger, J., and Ullrich, A. (1987) Increased expression of the putative growth factor receptor p185HER2 causes transformation and tumorigenesis of NIH 3T3 cells. *Proc. Natl. Acad. Sci. USA* **84,** 7159–7163.

6. Carraway, C. A. C., Carvajal, M. E., Li, Y., and Carraway, K. L. (1993) Association of p185neu with microfilaments via a large glycoprotein complex in mammary carcinoma microvilli. *J. Biol. Chem.* **268,** 5582–5587.

7. De Corte, V., De Potter, C., Vandenberghe, D., Van Laerebeke, N., Azam, M., Roels, H., et al. (1994) A 50 kDa protein present in conditioned medium of COLO-16 cells stimulates cell spreading and motility, and activates tyrosine phosphorylation of Neu/HER-2, in human SK-BR-3 mammary cancer cells. *J. Cell. Sci.* **107,** 405–416.

8. de Potter, C. R., Eeckhout, I., Schelfhout, A.-M., Geerts, M.-L., and Roels, H. J. (1994) Keratinocyte induced chemotaxis in the pathogenesis of paget's disease of the breast. *Histopathology* **24,** 349–356.

9. Stein, C. A. and Cheng, Y.-C. (1993) Antisense oligonucleotides as therapeutic agents—is the bullet really magical? *Science* **261,** 1004–1012.

10. Wagner, R. W., Matteucci, M. D., Lewis, J. G., Gutierrez, A. J., Moulds, C., and Froehler, B. C. (1993) Antisense gene inhibition by oligonucleotides containing C-5 propyne pyrimidines. *Science* **260,** 1510–1513.

11. Wiechen, K., Zimmer, C., and Dietel, M. (1998) Selection of a high activity c-erbB-2 ribozyme using a fusion gene of c-erbB-2 and the enhanced green flourescent protein. *Cancer Gene Ther.* **5,** 45–51.

12. Vlassov, V. V. and Yakubov, L. A. (1991) Oligonucleotides in cells and in organisms: Pharmacological considerations, in *Prospects for antisense nucleic acid therapy of cancer and AIDS* (Wickstrom, E., ed.), Wiley-Liss, New York, NY, pp. 243–266.

13. Müller, M., Dietel, M., Turzynski, A., and Wiechen, K. (1998) Antisense phosphorothioate oligodeoxynucleotide downregulation of the insulin-like growth factor I receptor in ovarian cancer cells. *Int. J. Cancer,* **77,** 567–571.

# 87

# *E1A*-Mediated Gene Therapy

## Mien-Chie Hung, Duen-Hwa Yan, and Su Zhang

## 1. Introduction

Ovarian carcinoma is the most lethal tumor of the female genital tract and continues to be a major cause of female cancer deaths, largely as a function of early abdominal seeding producing carcinomatosis. The high rate of mortality is mainly caused by the difficulties of early detection of this disease and the lack of effective treatment for advanced stages of ovarian cancers when they are detected. One of the common pathological features of many primary ovarian cancers is the amplification/overexpression of a transmembrane tyrosine kinase receptor, *HER*-2 (also known as *neu* or *ErbB2*) gene *(1)*. Although there are some discrepancies in the literature *(2)*, *HER*-2 overexpression in cancer cells correlates well with a greater resistance to chemotherapeutic agents in certain experimental systems *(3)*. In addition, *HER*-2 overexpression has been shown to enhance metastatic potential in many different model systems *(4)*. Therefore, the *HER*-2 gene has become an excellent target for developing therapeutic agents that could reverse malignant transformation of *HER*-2-overexpressing cancer cells *(5)*.

The choice of adenovirus 5 *E1A* as a therapeutic agent for the *HER*-2-overexpressing ovarian cancer cells was based on our previous findings that showed *E1A* not only is a transcription repressor of *HER*-2 gene *(6)*, but also is a potent inhibitor for the *HER*-2-mediated transformation, tumorigenicity, and metastasis in rodent cells *(7,8)* and in human ovarian cancer cells that overexpress *HER*-2 gene *(9)*. To test the efficiency and efficacy of the *E1A* gene therapy on ovarian cancer cells that overexpress *HER*-2 gene, we have developed an ovarian cancer animal model *(10)* that has been used to demonstrate an *E1A*-specific antitumor activity in vitro and in vivo using both liposome- *(10)* and adenovirus-mediated gene delivery systems. In this chapter, we will mainly focus on the *E1A*/liposome-mediated gene therapy protocol because this system has been shown to have a transfection efficiency with effective therapeutic efficacy and minimum toxicity *(11,12)*. A gene therapy protocol using adenovirus vector to carry *E1A* gene into cancer cells will also be described in **Note 6**. Compared with other virus delivery systems, such as retrovirus, the advantage of using adenovirus is the potentially ample supply of viruses and a higher expression efficiency. It has a broad host-cell range, and the virus can infect nonproliferative cells. Moreover, the adenovirus DNA does not integrate into the chromosomal DNA, but remains in an extrachromo-

From: *Methods in Molecular Medicine, Vol. 39: Ovarian Cancer: Methods and Protocols*
Edited by: J. M. S. Bartlett © Humana Press, Inc., Totowa, NJ

somal location and poses another advantage of maintaining genomic integrity of the infected cells. In the following sections, we will describe in detail how an orthotopic ovarian cancer mouse xenograft model is established and discuss how to use the liposome- and adenovirus-mediated *E1A* gene therapy in this animal model that bears human ovarian cancer cells overexpressing *HER*-2.

## 2. Materials

### 2.1. Tissue Culture

1. Dulbecco's modified Eagle's medium (DMEM-high glucose)/Ham's F12 (1:1) medium (incomplete medium) (Hyclone Laboratories, Inc., Logan, UT) with 10% (v/v) fetal bovine serum (FBS) (Gibco BRL, Grand Island, NY) and –1:100 100x antibiotics (penicillin, streptomycin, and fungizone, Gibco BRL), kept at 4°C.
2. 1X trypsin (Gibco BRL), kept at 4°C.
3. 10% dextrose (Baxter, Deerfield, IL), kept at 4°C.
4. 1X phosphate-buffered saline (PBS) (137m$M$ NaCl, 2.7 m$M$ KCl, 10 m$M$ Na$_2$HPO$_4$, 1.76 m$M$ KH$_2$PO$_4$, pH7.4).
5. 75% EtOH.
6. 20 m$M$ HEPES buffer (pH 7.8), kept at 4°C.
7. Sterile water (Baxter, Deerfield, IL), kept at 4°C.
8. *HER*-2 polyclonal antibody (Dako Corporation, Carpinteria, CA), kept at 4°C.

### 2.2. Plasmid DNA Preparation

1. LB medium: 1% Bacto-trypton (DIFCO Laboratories, Detroit, MI), 0.5% yeast extract (DIFCO Laboratories), and 1% NaCl. Autoclave and store at room temperature.
2. Antibiotics: 50 mg/mL ampicilin (Gibco BRL) and, 50 mg/mL kanamycin (Gibco BRL). Sterilize by filtration and store in aliquots at –20°C.
3. Resuspension buffer: 50 m$M$ Tris-Cl (pH 8.0), 10 m$M$ ethylenediaminetetraacetic acid (EDTA), 100 µg/mL RNase A, kept at 4°C.
4. Lysis buffer: 200 m$M$ NaOH, 1% sodium dodecyl sulfate (SDS).
5. Neutralization buffer: 3 $M$ potassium acetate (pH 5.5).
6. Equilibration buffer: 750 m$M$ NaCl 50 m$M$ MOPS (pH 7.0), 15% isopropanol, 0.15% Triton X-100.
7. Wash buffer: 1 $M$ NaCl, 50 m$M$ MOPS (pH 7.0), 15% isopropanol.
8. Elution buffer: 1.25 $M$ NaCl, 50 m$M$ MOPS (pH 8.5), 15% isopropanol.

### 2.3. Adenovirus Preparation

1. 1.5 g/mL CsCl: 30 g of CsCl dissolved in a final volume of 42.5 mL 1X PBS, filter sterilize.
2. 1.35 g/mL CsCl: 15 mL of 1.5 g/mL CsCl to a final volume of 21 mL with 1X PBS, filter sterilize.
3. 1.25 g/mL CsCl: 11 mL of 1.5 g/mL CsCl to a final volume of 20 mL with 1X PBS, filter sterilize.
4. Dialysis tubing (50,000 molecular weight cutoff, Spectrum®, Houston, TX, Spectro/Pro® 7), kept at 4°C.
5. Adenovirus dialysis buffer: 10 m$M$ Tris-HCl (pH 7.5), 1 m$M$ MgCl$_2$, 10% glycerol; autoclaved, kept at 4°C.
6. Glycerol: autoclaved.

## 3. Methods

### 3.1. Establishment of Ovarian Cancer Animal Model

1. SKOV3, a *HER-2/neu*-overexpressing human ovarian cancer cell line obtained from American Type Culture Collection (Cat.# ATCC HTB-77), or 2774, a human ovarian cancer cell line *(13,14)* with a basal level of *HER-2* expression, both cell lines are highly tumorigenic when ip-injected into nude mice. Cells are cultured in DMEM (high glucose)/ F12 medium (1 : 1) (incomplete medium) with 10% FBS and appropriate antibiotics (complete medium).

3. Harvest a fresh, rapidly growing cell culture by standard trypsinization and resuspend the cells in an appropriate volume of incomplete medium. Count the cell density using a hemocytometer (*see* **Note 1**).

4. Transfer the amount of cells necessary (with at least 10% more) for the injections to a sterile conical tube. Pellet the cells by low-speed centrifugation (200$g$) for 5 min at 4°C. Resuspend the cell pellet in 1x PBS so that the cell density is $2 \times 10^6$ cells/500 μL. Keep the cell suspension on ice and immediately proceed to the next step of ip injection.

5. Four- to six-wk-old athymic female homozygous *nu/nu* mice are used. The injection should be done in a sterile biohazard hood. Sterilize the lower region of the mouse abdomen with 75% EtOH. Inject 0.5 mL of cell suspension into the peritoneal cavity using a 25G5/8 needle with a 1-mL TB syringe containing $2 \times 10^6$ cells. Keep the injecting needle at a 45° angle into the abdominal cavity. Deliver the cells slowly to allow the cells to evenly spread in the abdominal cavity. At the end of injection, hold the syringe for another few seconds before withdrawing it quickly from the mouse (*see* **Note 1**).

Injection of these cells results in their dissemination into the peritoneal cavity which is a natural dissemination site of ovarian cancer cells. Typically, visible and palpable tumors will form in the abdominal cavity in 3–4 wk after injection. Tiny tumors (~0.5 mm in diameter) can be found on day 5 postinjection upon necropsy. To demonstrate these tumors are indeed originated from the injected cells, e.g., SKOV3, two assays can be used: (1) hematoxylin-eosin staining—the pathologic identity should be moderately differentiated adenocarcinomas; and (2) *HER-2* antibody staining—using a primary *HER-2* polyclonal antibody (1 : 300 dilution) specifically recognizes human *HER-2* encoded p185 protein. The p185 staining should be heavily stained in tumor sections obtained from both the mesentery and the inner side of the abdominal wall.

### 3.2. Liposome Delivery System

### 3.2.1. Preparation of Cationic Liposomes

1. To synthesize the cationic derivative of cholesterol (DC-Chol) *(12)*, 3β[N-(N′ N′-dimethylaminoethane)-carbamoyl] cholesterol, a solution of cholesteryl chloroformate (2.25 g, 5 mmol in 5 mL dry chloroform) was added dropwise to a solution of an excess N, N-dimethylethylendiamine (2 mL, 18.2 mmol in 3 mL dry chloroform) at 0°C. Cholesteryl chloroformate and N, N-dimethylethylenediamine can be purchased from Aldrich (Aldrich Chemical Co., Inc. Milwaukee, WI).

2. After the removal of solvent by evaporation, the residue was purified by recrystallization twice in absolute ethanol at 4°C and dried in vacuo, yielding 0.545 g of white powder of DC-Chol (21.8%).

3. A mixture of 1.2 μmol of DC-Chol and 0.8 μmol of Dioleoylphosphatidylethanolamine (DOPE) in chloroform (ratio 6:4) was dried, vacuum desiccated, and resuspended in

1 mL sterile 20 m*M* HEPES buffer (pH 7.8) in a sterile test tube. DOPE can be purchased from Avanti Polar Lipids.

4. After hydration for 24 h at 4°C, the suspension was sonicated for 5–10 min in a bath sonicator to form liposomes with 150–200 nm in average diameter.

### 3.2.2. Qiagen Maxi Plasmid DNA Preparation

1. Pick a single colony from a freshly streaked selective plate and inoculate a starter culture of 2–5 mL LB medium containing appropriate antibiotics (for pE1A-K2, use 50 µg/mL of kanamycin as final concentration; for pE1A-dl343, use 50 µg/mL of ampicillin as final concentration). Incubate for 8 h at 37°C with vigorous shaking (e.g., 300 rpm).
2. Dilute the starter culture 1/500 to 1/1000 into a 500 mL LB medium with a appropriate antibiotic. Shake for 12–16 h at 37°C.
3. Spin down the cells at 6000*g* for 15 min at 4°C. Resuspend the bacterial pellet in 10 mL of resuspension buffer.
4. Add 10 mL of lysis buffer, mix gently and thoroughly. Let sit at room temperature for 5 min.
5. Add 10 mL of neutralization buffer, mix gently and let sit on ice for 20 min.
6. Centrifuge at 20,000*g* for at 4°C for 30 min. Transfer the *clear* supernatant to a clean tube. It may be necessary to repeat this step to remove any residues that may clog the column in the next step.
7. Equilibrate a Qiagen-tip 500 by applying 10 mL of equilibration buffer onto the column and allow the buffer to flow through by gravity. Transfer the supernatant from **step 6** to the Qiagen-tip 500 and allow the supernatant to flow through the column by gravity.
8. Wash the Qiagen-tip twice with 30 mL of wash buffer.
9. Add 15 mL of elution buffer to the column and collect the eluent (about 15 mL).
10. Add 10.5 mL isopropanol to the eluent. Mix well and centrifuge at 15,000*g* at 4°C for 30 min. Carefully decant the supernatant.
11. Wash the DNA pellet with 5 mL of 70% ethanol and centrifuge at 15,000*g* for 10 min. Carefully decant the supernatant and air-dry the pellet for 10 min. Resuspend the DNA pellet in 0.5 mL sterile distilled water, kept at 4°C.

### 3.2.3. Adenovirus Preparation

To use adenovirus-mediated E1A gene therapy in vivo, one should first evaluate the virus infection efficiency using adenovirus ($10^9$ plaque forming unit [PFU]) carrying a reporter gene, e.g., Ad.RSV*LacZ*, an adenovirus type 5-based vector lacks *E1A*, *E1B*, and *E3* regions and contains a *LacZ* gene driven by Rous sarcoma virus-long terminal repeat. Three days after viral infection into the late-stage ip SKOV3 ovarian tumors in nude mice, we usually observed about 40–50% of malignant ascites and 30–70% of ip solid tumors that showed intracellular β-gal staining. In the therapeutic experiments, the tumor bearing mice can be divided into three groups: group 1 is the PBS control, only PBS is injected; group 2 is the negative control virus Ad.E1A(-), an adenovirus mutant (dl312), which lacks both *E1A* and *E3* regions, is injected; and group 3 is the therapeutic experiment virus Ad.E1A, an adenovirus (dl324) that contains *E1A*, but lacks *E1B* and *E3* regions, is injected. Our results indicated that all mice treated with either PBS or Ad.E1A(-) developed tumors and eventually died of intraabdominal tumors within 4.5 mo. In contrast, 80% of the Ad.E1A-treated mice remained tumor free for more than a year. Although the adenovirus vector has the higher transduction efficiency, the therapeutic effect of adenovirus-mediated *E1A* gene therapy is only slightly better than that of liposome-mediated therapy under the protocol described in the previous section.

1. Grow 293 cells (transformed primary human embryonal kidney cells, ATCC Cat.# CRL-1573) to 90% confluency on 150-mm dishes in DMEM/F12 (1:1) medium with 10% FBS and 1x antibiotics. Infect the cells with adenovirus in 5 mL of incomplete medium at a multiplicity of infection (MOI) of 10:1. Incubate the plates at 37°C for 1 h and occasionally rotate the plates for even distribution of the viral suspension.

2. Add 15 mL of complete medium to each plate and incubate the plates in a humidified incubator at 37°C with 5% $CO_2$ for 36–48 h.

3. After a complete cytopathic effect (CPE) appears, harvest the cells by centrifugation at 300$g$, 4°C for 15 min.

4. Lyse the cells by 3-time quick freeze-thaw cycles in a minimal volume of 1X PBS. Remove the cellular debris by centrifugation at 900$g$, 4°C for 10 min. Transfer and layer the supernatant onto the top of a CsCl step gradient (*see* **step 5**). In general, 4.5–5 mL supernatant obtained from 10 plates can be loaded in one centrifuge tube (Beckman, No. 344060, 14 × 95 mm) using an SW40Ti swing bucket rotor.

5. To make a CsCl step gradient, carefully layer the CsCl solutions from bottom to top of centrifuge tube in the following order:
   a. 0.5 mL of 1.5 g/mL CsCl
   b. 2.5 mL of 1.35 g/mL CsCl
   c. 2.5 mL of 1.25 g/mL CsCl

6. Centrifuge for 1 h at 10°C, 35,000 rpm (150,000$g$). Adenovirus will appear as a bluish-white band at the interface between the b. and c. layers. Carefully transfer the virus band (about 2–3 mL) into a new centrifuge tube and mix with 7–8 mL of 1.35 g/mL CsCl and centrifuge overnight (18 h) at 10°C, 35,000 rpm (150,000$g$).

7. Collect and transfer the virus band (bluish-white color) into a dialysis tubing and dialyzed in a cold, sterile adenovirus dialysis buffer at 4°C for 24 h with several changes of fresh dialysis buffer.

8. Add sterile glycerol to the virus preparation to a final concentration 10%. Aliquot the virus in appropriate volume and stored at –80°C.

9. Titrate the purified stock virus to determine the PFU: Take 25 μL of purified virus, mix with 465 μL of 1X PBS and 10 μL of 5% SDS in a 1.5 mL Eppendorf tube. Vortex for 1–2 min and brief centrifuge to remove any debris. Quantitate the viral DNA by measuring OD 260 nm absorption. One OD unit equals about $10^{12}$ viral particles per mL.

### 3.3. Gene Therapy for Mice Bearing Ovarian Tumors That Overexpress HER-2: E1A-*Mediated Gene Therapy by Liposome*

It is essential to determine the DNA:liposome ratio for the optimal transfection efficiency and the minimum animal toxicity (*see* **Note 2**). We generally use a *LacZ* gene expression vector encoding β-galactosidase to test the optimal DNA:liposome ratio. We have chosen 1:13 (e.g., 15 μg DNA : 200 nmol liposome) as our working condition in liposome/*E1A* gene therapy protocol because, under these conditions, we have consistently obtained high transfection efficiency with minimum toxicity. However, other DNA:liposome ratios, such as 1:1 (15 μg DNA : 15 nmol liposome), has been found as effective in animal model (*11*).

1. Dilute DNA stocks (pE1A-K2 and pE1A-dl343) with 5% dextrose to a concentration of 15 μg/100 μL in a clear plastic tube. pE1A-K2 is a plasmid expressing a wild-type *E1A* genomic clone. pE1Adl343 contains a 2 bp frame-shift deletion in the *E1A* coding region.

Both pE1A and pE1Adl343 DNA are prepared by a Qiagen Plasmid Kit (Qiagen Inc., Valencia, CA, Cat.# 12163) to ensure a high quality of plasmid DNA preparation.

2. Dilute DC-Chol:DOPE with 5% dextrose to the final concentration of 200 nmol/100 μL in a clear plastic tube.
3. Add the DNA solution dropwise into the liposome tube and mix gently.
4. Let the DNA/liposome mixture sit at room temperature for 10–15 min. (*see* **Note 5**).
5. Intraperitoneally inject the DNA/liposome complex into the tumor-bearing mice as described in the following section.

### 3.3.1. E1A *gene therapy*

Five days after ip injection of SKOV3 (or 2774) cells into nude mice, these tumor-bearing mice were randomly divided into five groups prepared for different treatments:

Group 1: the untreated control, mice will be injected with 5% dextrose.
Group 2: the *E1A* gene therapy treatment, each mouse will be injected with 15 mg pE1A-K2 DNA and 200 nmol liposome.
Group 3: the *E1A* frame-shift mutant (Efs) control, each mouse will be injected with 15 mg pE1A-dl343 DNA and 200 nmol liposome.
Group 4: E1A only control, each mouse will be injected with 15 mg pE1A-K2 DNA.
Group 5: liposome only control, each mouse will be injected with 200 nmol liposome.

All treatments are administered through ip injection with total volume of 200 μL per injection (*see* **Note 3**). Calculate the amount of material needed for injections and prepare at least 10% more to ensure a consistent injection volume. The treatment plan is designed as follows:

Day 6–8*: once a day injection for 3 d.
Day 13: starts 1×/wk injection for at least 20 wk (*see* **Note 4**).
* the number of days after SKOV3 (or 2774) cell inoculation.

All mice are observed once or twice a week for tumor development and then every other day when any or all of the following symptoms appear: abdominal bloating, significant weight loss, hunched posture, and decreased body movement.

### Notes

1. SKOV3 ovarian cancer model. SKOV3 cell line has been routinely used in the xenograft orthotopic ovarian cancer animal model for two reasons: (1) SKOV3 cells overexpress *HER*-2 at least 100-fold higher than other cancer cell lines derived from female genital tract; and (2) SKOV3 cells can readily form tumors when intraperitoneally-injected into nude mice. Because the number of cells for injection is critical in that it would affect the rate of tumor formation, death rate, and therapeutic outcome, caution should be given to ensure a reproducible cell counts. For example, we recommend that the estimated cell density in suspension should represent 50–200 cells per $0.1\text{-mm}^3$ cubic square on the hemocytometer. Four (two upper and two lower) cubic squares need to be counted to ensure the reproducibility of the cell counts. **Caution**: Immediate withdrawal of needle after ip cell inoculation may cause cell leakage from the site of injection and may also result in sc tumor growth later on.
2. *E1A*/liposome and animal toxicity. We have conducted a toxicity study concerning the effect of *E1A*/liposome on the injected mice. There were five mice in each group in the

single-dose acute toxicity experiments. Control mice were injected with 5% dextrose without DNA/liposome complex. The daily doses of *E1A* DNA used in this experiment were: 7.5, 15, 30, 60, 120, and 150 µg. The corresponding amounts (1:13) of liposome were: 100, 200, 400, 800, 1600, and 2000 nmol, respectively. The animals were observed for signs and symptoms of toxicity. After 2 wk, blood samples were drawn by orbital bleeding and assays of creatinine (renal function) and SGOT (liver function) were performed. No toxicity was observed at concentration levels of E1A DNA/liposome complex described above. At biopsy, there were no detectable abnormalities in any organ. In addition, we did another experiment in which E1A/liposome were injected daily for five consecutive days with doses of *E1A* DNA at 15, 30, 60, and 120 µg. The control group received no *E1A* DNA. All animals were monitored for 6 wk before sacrificed. There were minimal abnormalities detected at all doses. Also, another safety concern is integration of *E1A* DNA into chromosomes after transfection, which may alter the genetic integrity of the mice. To examine this possibility, we collected several major organs from *E1A*/liposome-treated tumor-bearing mice (which have survived for 1.5 yr after the last *E1A*/liposome injection) to analyze the existence of *E1A* in the genomic DNA obtained from these organs. PCRs were performed for these genomic DNA samples by using *E1A*-specific primers. There was no detectable *E1A* DNA signal found in any organs including ovaries, except for lung and kidney. This observation suggests that the germ cells may not transmit the *E1A* gene to the F1 offsprings in ovarian cancer mouse model by using our gene therapy protocol *(11)*.

3. The injection volume of *E1A*/liposome complex. In addition to the 200 µL ip injection volume that we have routinely used, we have also tried to use 1 mL injection volume of *E1A*/liposome complex. We did not observe any significant difference in terms of their transfection efficiency, toxicity, and therapeutic efficacy.

4. Duration of *E1A*/liposome treatment. Based on our experience, a longer *E1A*/liposome treatment usually results in a better survival rate.

5. DNA/liposome complex preparation. A well-prepared DNA/liposome complex will appear slightly milky in a clear plastic tube. If the milky appearance is absent in the DNA/liposome mixture or the presence of white precipitates in the tube, one should stop the current preparation. Check the DNA quality and concentration. Make sure the preparation procedure is carefully followed.

6. Adenovirus delivery system. In vitro experiments showed that infection of SKOV3 cells in culture with adenovirus vector encoding *E1A* led to a reduction of the growth rate of the cells, compared to control cells that were infected with adenovirus without *E1A*. A high quality of adenovirus preparation is essential for the success of adenovirus-mediated gene therapy.

## Acknowledgments

The authors are supported by NIH RO1 grants CA 58880 and CA 60856 (to M-C. Hung).

## References

1. Slamon, D. J., Godolphin, W., Jones, L. A., Holt, J. A., Wong, S. G., Keith, D. E., et al. (1989) Studies of the HER-2/neu proto-oncogene in human breast and ovarian cancer. *Science* **244**, 707–712.
2. Pergram, M. D., Finn, R. S., Arzoo, K., Beryt, M., Pietras, R. J., and Slamon, D. J. (1997) The effect of HER-2/neu overexpression on chemotherapeutic drug sensitivity in human breast and ovarian cancer cells. *Oncogene* **15**, 537–547.
3. Tsai, C.-M., Yu, D., Chang, K.-T., Wu, L.-H., Perng, P. R.-P., Ibrahim, N. K., and Hung, M.-C. (1995) Enhanced chemoresistance by elevation of the level of p185neu in HER-2/neu transfected human lung cancer cells. *J. Natl. Cancer Inst.* **87**, 682–684.

4. Yu, D. and Hung, M.-C. (1991) Expression of activated rat neu oncogene is sufficient to induce experimental metastasis in 3T3 cells. *Oncogene* **6,** 1991–1996.

5. Salomon, D. S., Brandt, R., Ciardiello, F., and Normanno, N. (1995) Epidermal growth factor-related peptides and their receptors in human malignancies. *Crit. Rev. Oncol.-Hematol.* **19,** 183–232.

6. Yu, D., Suen, T.-C., Yan, D.-H., Chang, L. S., and Hung, M.-C. (1990) Transcriptional repression of the *neu* protooncogene by the adenovirus 5 E1a gene products. *Proc. Natl. Acad. Sci. USA* **87,** 4499–4503.

7. Yu, D.-H., Scorsone, K., and Hung, M-C. (1991) The adenovirus-5 E1A gene products act as a transformation suppressor of HER-2/neu oncogene. *Mol. Cell. Biol.* **11,** 1745–1750.

8. Yu, D.-H., Hamada, J-I., Zhang, H., Nicolson, G. L., and Hung, M-C. (1992) Mechanisms of HER-2/neu oncogene-induced metastasis and repression of metastatic properties by adenovirus 5 E1A gene products. *Oncogene* **7,** 2263–2270.

9. Yu, D., Wolf, J. K., Scanlon, M., Price, J. E., and Hung, M.-C. (1993) Enhanced c-erbB-2/neu expression in human ovarian cancer cells correlates with more severe malignancy that can be suppressed by E1A. *Cancer Res.* **53,** 891–898.

10. Yu, D., Matin, A., Xia, W., Sorgi, F., Huang, L., and Hung, M.-C. (1995) Liposome-mediated in vivo E1A gene transfer suppressed dissemination of ovarian cancer cells that overexpress HER-2/neu. *Oncogene* **11,** 1383–1388.

11. Xing, X., Zhang, S., Chang, J., Tucker, S. D., Chen, H., Huang, L., et al. (1998) Safety study and characterization of E1A-liposome complex gene-delivery protocol in an ovarian cancer model. *Gene Ther.*, in press.

12. Gao, X. and Huang, L. (1991) A novel cationic liposome reagent for efficient transfection of mammalian cells. *Biochem. Biophys. Res. Commun.* **179,** 280–285.

13. Price, J. E., Wolf, J. K., and Pathak, S. (1998) Distinctive karyotypes and growth patterns in nude mice reveal cross-contamination in an established human cancer cell line. *Oncol. Rep.* **5,** 261–266.

14. Brader, K. R., Wolf, J. K., Chakrabarty, S., and Price, J. E. (1998) Epidermal growth factor receptor (EGFR) antisense transfection reduces the expression of EGFR and suppresses the malignant phenotype of a human ovarian cancer cell line. *Oncol. Rep.* **5,** 1269–1274.

# *p53* Adenovirus as Gene Therapy for Ovarian Cancer

**Jennifer L. Carroll, J. Michael Mathis, Maria C. Bell, and Joseph T. Santoso**

## 1. Introduction

Ovarian cancer arises from the accumulation of mutations in multiple combinations of genes *(1)*. The most extensively studied tumor suppressor gene in solid tumors is *p53*, a 53-kD nuclear phosphoprotein that binds DNA. The *p53* gene product plays a role in normal cellular proliferation by regulating gene transcription, cell cycle control, and apoptosis *(2)*. Mutations of *p53* are the most common molecular genetic abnormality to be described in human cancer, and have been identified in malignancies of the breast, colon, lung, esophagus, head and neck, and hematopoietic system *(3)*. Mutations of the *p53* gene have been identified in 30 to 79% of epithelial ovarian cancers *(4,5)*. Most of the mutations identified in *p53* are distributed throughout the open reading frame as missense mutations. We have identified a missense mutation in the *p53* gene in the 2774 ovarian cancer cell line that converts an arginine residue in the DNA binding region of the protein to a histidine residue *(6)*. The mutation in codon 273 we found in 2774 cells is one of the six major hotspots identified for *p53* missense mutations *(7)*.

### 1.1. Targeting p53

In spite of cancer's polygenic nature, there is strong evidence that correction of only one of the genetic defects in cancer cells in vitro can lead to the inhibition of cell growth and reversal of tumorigenicity *(6,8)*. The strategy of human gene therapy to alter the biology of human cancers is an area of investigation that shows significant potential for improving survival *(9)*. Functional impairment of *p53* resulting from gene deletion or mutation is associated with loss of cellular checkpoint signaling functions and inability to coordinate programmed cell death (apoptosis) in the presence of DNA damage *(10)*.

Our in vivo studies using the Balb/c athymic *nu/nu* mouse as a model for intraperitoneal (ip) cancer has demonstrated a survival advantage in animals treated with adenovirus-based *p53* gene therapy *(11,12)*. The mechanism of wild-type *p53* growth inhibition in tumor cells is complex and may involve cell cycle control through induction of target genes, may involve induction of apoptosis or programmed cell. Death of tumor cells modified with the wild-type *p53* gene may also lead to killing of uninfected

From: *Methods in Molecular Medicine, Vol. 39: Ovarian Cancer: Methods and Protocols*
Edited by: J. M. S. Bartlett © Humana Press, Inc., Totowa, NJ

neighboring tumor cells in a phenomenon termed the "bystander effect" *(13)*. Recently, we addressed the role of adenovirus-based *p53* gene therapy in the treatment of ovarian cancer *(12,13)*. Using an in vivo mouse model system, the ip route of administration of the adenovirus vector is a novel approach for the treatment of ovarian cancer metastasis, because iv administration is much less efficient *(14)*. The targeted role for adenovirus-based *p53* gene therapy in this study was treatment of advanced invasive ovarian carcinoma. Ovarian cancer remains confined to the peritoneal cavity for the majority of its course *(15)*. Therefore, therapeutic agents can be easily and effectively delivered to the tumor with pharmacokinetics that are often better than systemic administration.

## 2. Materials

### 2.1. Cell Culture

1. Dulbecco's modified Eagle medium/nutrient mixture F12 (DMEM/F12, Gibco BRL, Gaithersburg, MD).
2. Dulbecco's phosphate-buffered saline (PBS) without $CaCl_2$ or $MgCl_2$ (Gibco BRL).
3. Trypsin: ethylenediaminetetraacetic acid (EDTA) (Gibco BRL).

### 2.2. Adenovirus Preparation

1. 10 m*M* Tris-HCl pH 8.0.
2. 5% deoxycholate.
3. Saturated CsCl.

### 2.3. Plaque Formation Assay

1. Overlay solution: prepare 2X complete DMEM/F12 medium and 2% agarose, bring to 42°C and combine 1:1.

### 2.4. Western Analysis

1. RIPA buffer (100 mL): 1 mL NP40, 1 g sodium deoxycholate, 500 µL 20% SDS, 3 mL NaCl (5 *M*), 10 mL Tris-HCl (1.0 *M*, pH 7.5) 400 µL EDTA (0.5 *M*), and water.
2. Lysis buffer: 10 mL of RIPA buffer, 100 µL PMSF, 10 µL aprotinin, 10 µL pepstatin, and 10 µL macroglobulin.
3. 30% polyacrylamide/0.8% *bis*: 150 g of acrylamide, 4 g N,N′-methylene *bis*-acrylmide, water up to 500 mL, filter, and store at 4°C in the dark.
4. 4X Tris-HCl/SDS pH 6.8 (100 mL): 6.05 g Tris base, 40 mL water, adjust pH to 6.8 with 1 *M* HCl, bring volume to 100 mL with water, and filter. To filtered solution, add 0.4 g SDS and store at 4°C up to 1 mo.
5. 4X Tris-HCl/SDS pH 8.8 (500 mL): 91 g Tris base, 300 mL water, adjust pH to 8.8 with 1 *M* HCl, bring volume to 500 mL with water, and filter. To filtered solution, add 2 g SDS and store at 4°C up to 1 mo.
6. Resolving gel (10%): 5 mL 30% polyacrylamide, 3.75 mL Tris-HCl/SDS pH 8.8, 6.25 mL water, 50 µL 20% ammonium persulfate (APS), and 10 µL TEMED.
7. Stacking gel (3.9%): 1.3 ml 30% polyacrylamide, 2.5 mL Tris-HCl/SDS pH 6.8, 6.1 mL water, 50 µL 20% ammonium persulfate (APS), and 10 µL TEMED.
8. 5X SDS running buffer (dilute to 1X for use): 15.1 g Tris base, 72.0 g glycine, 5.0 g SDS, adjust volume to 1 L, and store at 4°C.
9. SDS sample buffer (6X): 7 mL Tris-HCl/SDS pH 6.8, 3.0 mL glycerol, 1 g SDS, 0.93 g DTT, 1.2 mg bromophenol blue, adjust volume to 10 mL, and store in 1-mL aliquots at –70°C.
10. Transfer buffer: 3.03 g Tris base, 14.4 g glycine, 600 mL water, 200 mL methanol, pH to 8.3–8.4, bring volume to 1 L with water, and store at 4°C.

11. Tris-buffered saline with Tween-20 (TTBS, 2 L): 18 mg NaCl, 24.2 g Tris base, pH to 7.5, and add 2 mL Tween-20.
12. Blocking buffer: 5% BSA in TTBS (filter).
13. Antibody diluent: 1% BSA in TTBS (filter).
14. ECL Western blotting system (Amersham, Arlington Hts., IL).

### 2.5. β-Galactosidase Assay

1. X-gal staining solution: 0.5 $M$ potassium ferrocyanide, 0.5 $M$ potassium ferricyanide, X-gal.

### 2.6. Growth Inhibition Assay

1. Staining solution: 1% crystal violet in methanol.
2. Destaining solution: 40 m$M$ HCl in 95% ethanol.

### 2.7. Cell Cycle Analysis

1. 70% ethanol.
2. 100X propidium iodine: prepare 10 mg/mL solution in water.
3. 100X RNase A: prepare 20 mg/mL solution in water and boil 10 min to inactivate DNase activity.

### 2.8. Apoptosis Assays

1. 3% $H_2O_2$.
2. 0.5% Triton X-100.
3. *In situ* cell death detection kit (Boehringer Mannheim Biochemicals, Indianapolis, IN).

### 2.9. Target Gene Expression (Immunohistochemistry)

1. For these studies, we use a variety of commercially available antibodies, such as mouse monoclonal antibodies *p53*, *p21*, cyclins (A, B, D, and E), and bax from Pharmingen, Inc., San Diego, CA.
2. A secondary antimouse IgG antibody with a horseradish peroxidase conjugated linker.
3. A 3-amino-9-ethlylcarbazole (AEC) detector chromogen kit (Biogenex, Inc., San Ramon, CA).

## 3. Methods
### 3.1. Virus Production and Analysis
#### 3.1.1. Adenovirus Preparation

The replication-defective human adenovirus (serotype 5-derived) vector containing a wild-type *p53* cDNA is produced by homologous recombination between two transfected plasmids containing adenovirus DNA fragments overlapped at the *E1a* flanking region *(8)*. The adenovirus stocks of Ad-CMV-*p53* and Ad-CMV-βgal are propagated in the human transformed embryonal kidney 293 cell line as described previously *(14)*. High titer adenovirus stocks are purified by cesium chloride gradient centrifugation *(16)*.

1. Subconfluent monolayers of 293 cells are infected in serum-free medium at a multiplicity of infection (MOI) of 10:1 for 4 h. After 4 h, cells are returned to serum-containing medium. The infection is allowed to proceed until the cells begin to lyse and are easily dislodged.
2. Infected cells are harvested, pelleted, and stored at –80°C.
3. Frozen cells are thawed on ice, and the cell pellets are resuspended in 10 vol of 10 m$M$ Tris-HCl and 0.1 vol of 5% deoxycholate.

4. Cellular DNA is sheared by sonication.
5. Crude lysates are centrifuged for 10 min at 150*g* at 4°C to remove cellular debris.
6. To each 3.1 mL of lysate is added 1.8 mL of saturated CsCl solution.
7. Crude CsCl lysates are centrifuged for 20 h at 35,000*g* at 4°C.
8. Banded virus is removed and is desalted by dialysis in PBS.
9. Glycerol is added to a final concentration of 10% and purified virus stocks are stored in small aliquots at –80°C.

### 3.1.2. Virus Titer

High-titer adenovirus stocks are purified and the titer of viral concentration is determined using a plaque-formation assay *(17)*.

1. Monolayers of 293 cells are grown in 60-mm dishes to near confluence and are infected with serial dilutions of viral stocks diluted in serum-free DME/F12.
2. After the cells are infected for 2 h, the medium is removed and replaced with 3 mL of overlay solution (1X DME/F12, 1% agarose).
3. After the agarose is hardened, the dishes are incubated and observed for the formation of plaques in 3–4 d, which are counted and used to calculate the viral concentration in plaque forming units/mL of viral stock (PfU/mL).

## 3.2. Gene Transfer and Expression

### 3.2.1. Ovarian Cancer Cell Lines

The characteristics of the human ovarian carcinoma cell lines we use are shown in **Table 1**. We obtained 2774, A2780, Caov-3, Caov-4, ES-2, HS 254.T, HS 38.T, HS 571.T, OV-1063, NIH:OVCAR-3, PA-1, SK-OV-3, and SW626 cell lines from the American Type Culture Collection. The cell lines are grown in DME/F12 media containing 10% fetal bovine serum (FBS), harvested with trypsin:EDTA, and pelleted by centrifugation at 150*g* for 5 min.

### 3.2.2. Gene Expression (Immunoblot) Analysis

To control for differences in *p53* expression, we determine *p53* levels by Western blot analysis in each cell line after infection with Ad-CMV-*p53* (*see* Chapter 54).

1. After solubilization in lysis buffer, samples are electrophoresed on a 10% SDS/polyacrylamide gel.
2. Proteins are transferred to nitrocellulose in a semidry electrophoretic blotting system (NovaBlot; Pharmacia, Uppsala, Sweden).
3. The nitrocellulose membranes are incubated for 1 h in blocking buffer, followed by incubation with buffer containing the mouse antihuman *p53* antibody (Oncogene Science).
4. Membranes are washed in PBS + 0.2% Tween-20 and incubated with HRP secondary antibody.
5. Finally, the membranes are washed and incubated for 1 min with ECL reagent and analyzed by autoradiography.

### 3.2.3. Gene Transfer (β-Galactosidase) Assays

It is possible that the differences in growth response to Ad-CMV-*p53* are nonspecific effects caused by differences in adenovirus infectivity or wild-type *p53* expression. To control for differences in adenovirus infectivity, we assay β-galactosidase activity *in situ* in each cell line after infection with increasing MOI of Ad-CMV-βgal,

**Table 1**
**Ovarian Cancer Cell Lines**

| Cell Line | Histology | Pt Age & Race | Source | *p53* Mutation |
|-----------|-----------|---------------|--------|----------------|
| 2774 | serous cystadenocarcinoma | 40; Caucasian | ATCC | mut R 287 H |
| A2780 | serous cystadenocarcinoma | unknown | ATCC | wild-type |
| Caov-3 | cystadenocarcinoma | 54; Caucasian | ATCC | mut Q 136 term |
| Caov-4 | cystadenocarcinoma | 45; Caucasian | ATCC | mut V 147 N |
| ES-2 | clear cell carcinoma | 47; Black | ATCC | unknown |
| HS 254.T | serous cystadenocarcinoma | 49; Caucasian | ATCC | unknown |
| HS 38.T | teratoma | unknown | ATCC | unknown |
| HS 571.T | cystadenocarcinoma | 65; Caucasian | ATCC | unknown |
| NIH:OVCAR-3 | cystadenocarcinoma | 60; Caucasian | ATCC | mut R 248 Q |
| OV-1063 | serous cystadenocarcinoma | 57; Caucasian | ATCC | unknown |
| PA-1 | teratocarcinoma | 12; Caucasian | ATCC | wild-type |
| SK-OV-3 | cystadenocarcinoma | 64; Caucasian | ATCC | del |
| SW626 | cystadenocarcinoma | 46; Caucasian | ATCC | mut G 262 V |

ranging from 0.1 : 1 to 100 : 1. The infected ovarian cancer cell lines are then analyzed for β-galactosidase activity.

1. Approximately $10^5$ cells are seeded into 60-mm$^2$ tissue-culture dishes. After 24 h, the cells are infected with Ad-CMV-βgal with an increasing MOI from 0.1 PFU per cell 100 PFU per cell in serum-free media for 4 h, and the cells are incubated for an additional 24–72 h in DME/F12 containing 10% FBS.
2. Infected cells are washed with PBS, fixed in formalin, and evaluated for β-galactosidase activity by incubation in X-gal staining solution.
3. To determine the efficiency of adenovirus vector to infect solid tumors, ovarian cancer cells are injected intraperitoneally into female athymic nude mice.
4. The animals then receive 1.0 mL ip injections of Ad-CMV-βgal.
5. At various times after injection (e.g., 24, 48, 72, 96, 120, 144, 168 h), the animals are culled.
6. Freshly resected ovarian tumor samples and peritoneal washings are analyzed histochemically for β-galactosidase activity.
7. The tumor samples are fixed in formalin, and stained with X-gal. Peritoneal washings are cytospun onto microscope slides, fixed in formalin, and stained with X-gal.
8. The tumor samples are subsequently embedded in paraffin or frozen in Tissue-Tek O.C.T. compound (Miles Laboratories Inc., Elkhart, IN) and sectioned.
9. Sections are counterstained with eosin.

### 3.2.4. Growth Inhibition Assays

The vast majority of *p53* mutations are missense mutations, resulting in a prolonged half-life and accumulation of the mutant protein. Because *p53* protein functions as a tetrameric complex, many *p53* mutations have a dominant-negative or inhibitory activity on wild-type protein. Thus, we hypothesize that cells with different *p53* mutations will respond with different sensitivities to Ad-CMV-*p53*. It is important then, to survey the effect of Ad-CMV-*p53* on the rates of cell growth in many ovarian cancer cell lines using the growth assay described below. As a control, changes in the rates of cell growth should be compared to uninfected cells or to cells infected with Ad-CMV-βgal.

1. On day 0, ovarian cancer cells are seeded into 96-well flat-bottom microtiter tissue-culture plates (Corning) at 3000 cells per well.
2. After adenovirus infection on day 1, and at subsequent time-points afterward, media from replicate wells are aspirated and the wells are washed with PBS.
3. The amount of viable adherent cells is determined by the method of Yamamoto et al. *(18)*.
4. Briefly, after aspiration of the PBS, the cells are stained with 1% crystal violet staining solution, washed with water, and dissolved in destaining solution.
5. The absorbence at 595 nm for each well is determined using a microplate reader.
6. Absorbance results are expressed as cell numbers by comparing the mean absorbance of six replicate wells to a standard curve prepared from known cell numbers.

## 3.3. Target Gene Expression Analysis

Induction of *p53* causes increased transcription of genes involved in cell cycle arrest (e.g., *p21*, *mdm2*, and *GADD45*) and apoptosis (e.g., *bak*, *bax*, and *bcl-X$_S$*). Thus, we determine the effect of Ad-CMV-*p53* infection on changes in cell cycle by flow cytometry and changes in apoptosis by an *in situ* (for terminal deoxynucleotidyl transferase-mediated dUTP nick end-labeling) (TUNEL) assay. Changes in *p21*, *GADD45*, *bak*, *bax*, and *bcl-X$_S$* after Ad-CMV-*p53* infection can also be determined by Western blot analysis (*see* Chapter 75 and *see* below). As a control, these changes should be compared to uninfected cells or to cells infected with Ad-CMV-βgal.

1. For these studies, ovarian cancer cells seeded onto tissue-culture slides and infected at 100:1 MOI Ad-CMV-*p53* or Ad-CMV-βgal.
2. After 48 h, the slides are harvested, fixed in ice-cold 95% ethanol/5% acetic acid, and stored at –20°C.
3. Rehydrate cells for 1 h in PBS.
4. Treat cells with 2% H$_2$O$_2$ in methanol.
5. Wash 3 × 5 min in PBS.
6. Block cells by incubating for 1 h in PBS with 1% FBS.
7. Incubate cells with primary antibody diluted 1:500 in PBS for 1 h.
8. Wash cells 3 × 5 min in PBS.
9. Incubate cells with horseradish peroxidase conjugated secondary antibody diluted 1:500 in PBS for 1 h.
10. Wash cells 3 × 5 min in PBS.
11. Visualize cells colorimetrically using a AEC detector chromogen kit (Biogenex, Inc.).
12. The cells are counterstained with hematoxylin.
13. The slides are analyzed at an Olympus BX-60 microscope equipped with X10, X20, X40, X60, and X100 Universal plan apochromatic objectives.
14. Two observers should independently score the slides for staining intensity.

## 3.4. Cell Cycle Analysis

1. Monolayers of cells are harvested with trypsin and washed in PBS.
2. Cell pellets (~1 × 10$^6$ cells) are resuspended in 750 µL of PBS, fixed by the dropwise addition of 2.0 mL of 70% ethanol (–20°C) while gently vortexing, and stored overnight at 4°C.
3. Fixed cells are pelleted, washed twice in PBS, and resuspended in 1X RNase A in PBS and incubated for 15 min at 37°C.
4. Propidium iodide is added to a concentration of 100 µg/mL.
5. The samples are stored at 4°C with EDTA (to prevent clumping) and are protected from light until analyzed.

6. DNA analysis is performed as described *(19)* using a FACScan flow cytometer (Becton Dickinson, San Jose, CA).
7. Aggregated nuclei and clumps are omitted from analysis, with pulse area vs pulse with gating.
8. Data from 20,000 nuclei is saved and displayed as a frequency distribution histogram of propidium iodide fluorescence at 575 nm.

### 3.5. Apoptosis Assays

To determine if the observed cell death involves apoptosis, an *in situ* TUNEL assay for nuclear fragmentation is performed. The TUNEL assay is acknowledged as the method of choice in the rapid identification and quantification of apoptosis. The TUNEL assay is based on the principle that terminal deoxynucleotidyl transferase catalyzes a template-independent addition of deoxynucleotides to free 3'-OH ends present in DNA breaks. This tailing is especially sensitive to the type of DNA fragmentation occurring in apoptotic, rather than necrotic cell death.

1. For studies on conventional paraffin-embedded sections from tumor tissues, slides are deparaffinized in xylene, rehydrated stepwise in graded ethanols (100, 95, 70, 50, and 0%), and pretreated with 20 mg/mL proteinase K for 15 min at room temperature.
2. The slides are then incubated in 3% $H_2O_2$ for 5 min to block endogenous peroxidase activity, permeabilized with 0.5% Triton X-100, and washed before TUNEL staining.
3. For TUNEL staining, the slides are treated with terminal deoxynucleotidyl transferase and biotinylated dUTP using reagents from an *in situ* cell death detection kit (Boehringer Mannheim Biochemicals).
4. Using this procedure, the 3'-OH ends of DNA are labeled with biotin-dUTP, which makes detection possible using an avidin-conjugated peroxidase.
5. After TUNEL staining and peroxidase detection, the slides are lightly counterstained with methyl green and mounted.
6. In each experiment, negative controls receive only the label solution without the terminal transferase, and positive controls are exposed to 1 mg/mL DNase I for 10 min at room temperature before the TUNEL reaction.
7. The degree of TUNEL staining in the sections is quantitated using a digital microscope to distinguish apoptosis-positive and apoptosis-negative tissues.

### 3.6. Preclinical Animal Models

Initially, we determine the course of disease by culling animals at days 3, 7, 10, 14, and 21 postinoculation of an $LD_{100}$ dose of ovarian cancer cells. We determine by gross and histologic examination the time-point that best approximates macroscopic residual disease. We then use this time as the starting point for evaluation of different treatment strategies of *p53* gene therapy.

### 3.6.1. In Vivo Adenovirus Distribution and Expression

Currently, few studies have addressed the in vivo pharmacokinetics of DNA when delivered to cells by viral vectors. Translational studies from in vitro cultured cells to whole animal studies, including those in humans, have been empirical and mainly designed to test the feasibility of the principle, rather than critical evaluation of the problems of optimal formation of a gene product. We evaluate the in vivo pharmacokinetics of adenovirus-based gene therapy administered intraperitoneally with Ad-CMV-βgal, including the distribution and extracellular elimination of adenovirus DNA after in vivo administration, as well as the half-life of gene product expression in tumor cells in vivo.

1. To determine adenovirus pharmacokinetics, 1.0-mL aliquots of the OVCAR-3 cell suspension are injected intraperitoneally into female athymic nude mice.
2. The animals then receive 1.0 mL ip injections of Ad-CMV-βgal at 14 d postinoculation.
3. At various times after adenovirus injection, the animals are culled and tumor samples are harvested, fixed in formalin, and stained with X-gal. Peritoneal washings are cytospun onto microscope slides, fixed in formalin, and stained with X-gal.
4. The tumor samples are subsequently embedded in paraffin or frozen in Tissue-Tek O.C.T. compound (Miles Laboratories Inc., Elkhart, IN) and sectioned.
5. Serial sections are counterstained with hematoxylin and eosin.
6. By directly visualizing transduced cells using X-gal staining, we systematically evaluate (1) the physical distribution of the viral vector delivered intrapraperitoneally, (2) the duration of reporter gene expression in tumor cells, (3) the efficiency of repetitive gene transfer in vivo on gene expression; and (4) the duration of adenovirus particles intraperitoneally in nude mice.

### 3.6.2. Tumor Inoculation In Vivo

Initial in vivo treatment arms should include Ad-CMV-*p53* administered intraperitoneally at escalating doses at days postinoculation of tumor cells. Appropriate controls with ip injections of normal saline and control virus (Ad-CMV-βgal) should be included in all experiments. Survival times for treatment groups are followed as described below. To assess the optimal treatment regimen of Ad-CMV-*p53* gene therapy, we perform gene transfer studies using adenovirus vectors carrying the *lacZ* gene (Ad-CMV-βgal).

1. Freshly harvested cells are washed and resuspended in PBS at $1 \times 10^7$ cells/mL.
2. To determine adenovirus efficacy and specificity on animal survival, 1.0 mL of the OVCAR-3 cell suspension is injected intraperitoneally into female athymic nude mice.
3. Importantly, ip transplantation of OVCAR-3 cells into athymic nude mice appears to produce two morphologically distinct tumor cell populations: ascites and solid tumors.

### 3.6.3. Tumor Analysis

1. The animals are monitored daily for changes in health, including overall appearance (i.e., weight changes, signs of inflammation, or ulceration) and activity.
2. Animals are monitored by gross examination and palpation for the presence of lesions that represented excessive size (>10% of body weight) or that impaired mobility.
3. Animals are euthanized at the designated times postimplantation of tumor cells by asphyxiation with methoxyflurane (Metofane).
4. A necropsy is performed on each animal to determine the gross extent and distribution of disease present, and tumor and ascites volumes are recorded.
5. Internal organs are removed and fixed in formalin, and paraffin sections are prepared, stained with hematoxylin and eosin, and examined by light microscopy.

### 3.6.4. Adenovirus Treatment In Vivo

1. The animals are divided into three treatment groups.
2. Each group receives 1.0 mL ip injections of the following treatments: Ad-CMV-*p53*, Ad-CMV-βgal (serving as a control adenovirus construct), or PBS (serving as a mock control treatment).

3. The adenoviral vectors are stored at −80° until immediately before use, and then thawed on ice.
4. The vectors are diluted to the appropriate titer with Dulbecco's PBS (GIBCO, pH 7.4), drawn into syringes, and administered to the animals within 15 min of dilution.

### 3.6.5. Chemotherapy Treatment

The *p53* tumor suppressor protein is involved in multiple central cellular processes, but is functionally inactivated in ovarian cancer by structural mutations and endogenous cellular mechanisms, such as overexpression of MDM2. This functional inactivation can, in some circumstances, produce resistance to DNA-damaging agents commonly used in cancer chemotherapy and radiotherapeutic approaches. These experiments are directed toward investigating the interaction between restoration of *p53* function through Ad-CMV-*p53* gene therapy and resensitization of chemoresistant ovarian cancer cell lines to chemotherapeutic agents, such as cisplatin and taxol. Preclinical knowledge of these potential interactions will lead to multimodal cancer therapies, in which clinical combination chemotherapeutic and gene-therapeutic strategies can be based. Chemotherapeutic agents that can be investigated initially include cisplatin (CDDP) and taxol, two agents that already have been shown to have some activity against ovarian adenocarcinoma.

1. The stock solutions of chemotherapeutic agents are diluted in medium to the desired concentration.
2. For determining the effect of CDDP in vivo, 0.1, 1.0, or 10 mg/kg CDDP is injected intraperitoneally at 3, 7, or 10 days postimplantation of $10^7$ OVCAR-3 cells in nude mice.
3. For determining the effect of CDDP and Ad-CMV-*p53* gene therapy, both treatments are injected simultaneously in the same procedure.
4. The synergistic, additive, less than additive, or protective effects of combinations of Ad-CMV-*p53* and chemotherapeutic agents are evaluated on cells using cell growth assays.
5. Statistical analysis for synergistic inhibition of cell growth is performed using isobolograms.

### 3.6.6. Survival Analysis

1. The effect of combinations of gene therapy and chemotherapeutic agents on human ovarian tumors growing in a nude mouse model is performed as described above.
2. Survival times are determined by the Kaplan-Meier method *(20)*, and comparisons between treatment arms are made by the log-rank test *(20)*.
3. Statistical significance is based on a *p* value of 0.05 or less. The isobologram and curve fitting analysis of Steel and Peckham as discussed in detail by Tsai et al. *(21)* is used to determine whether combinations of CDDP and Ad-CMV-*p53* have a synergistic cytotoxic effect against OVCAR-3 cells in vitro.

## 4. Notes

1. Repeated freeze/thaw cycles of the adenovirus stocks should be avoided and the viruses should be stored in small aliquots with 10% glycerol at −80°C.
2. For all experiments, in addition to treatment with Ad-CMV-*p53*, we use Ad-CMV-βgal as a control adenovirus treatment and PBS as a as a mock control treatment.
3. Because of the large number of data points that can be obtained from the cell growth assay described above, it is uniquely suited to generate three-dimensional isobolograms when exploring synergistic interactions between two agents.

4. In presenting the effects of various combinations of gene therapy and chemotherapeutic agents on cells, the data are reported in the following fashion: Synergistic (*S*)—the effects of a combination is statistically greater than the sum of each individual agent; Additive (*A*)—the effects of a combination is equal to the effects of the sum of each individual agent; Less than additive (*L*)—the effects of a combination is statistically less than the sum of the effects of each individual agent; Protective (*P*)—the effect of combination is less than either agent alone.

## References

1. Bast, R. C. Jr., Boyer, C. M., Jacobs, I., Xu, F. J., Wu, S., Wiener, J., et al. (1993) Cell growth regulation on epithelial ovarian cancer. *Cancer* **71,** 1597–1601.
2. Harris, C. C. and Hollstein M. (1993) Clinical implications of the p53 tumor-suppressor gene. *N. Engl. J. Med.* **329,** 1318–1327.
3. Crystal, R. G. (1995) Transfer of genes to humans: early lessons and obstacles to success. *Science* **270,** 404–410.
4. Kohler, M. F., Marks, J. R., Wiseman, R. W., Davidoff, A. M., Clarke-Pearson, D. L., Soper, J. T., et al. (1993) Spectrum of mutation and frequency of allelic deletion of the p53 gene in ovarian cancer. *J. Natl. Cancer Inst.* **85,** 1513–1519.
5. Kupryjnszyk, J., Thor, A., Beauchamp, R., Merrit, V., Edgerton, S. M., Bell, D. A., et al. (1993) P53 gene mutations and protein accumulation in human ovarian cancer. *Proc. Natl. Acad. Sci. USA* **90,** 4961–4965.
6. Santoso, J. T., Tang, D. C., Lane, S. B., Hung, J., Reed, D. S., Muller, C. Y., et al. (1995) Adenovirus-based p53 gene therapy in ovarian cancer. *Gynecolog. Oncol.* **69,** 197–204.
7. Levine, A. J., Perry, M. E., Chang, A., Silver, A., Dittmer, D., Wu, M., et al. (1994) The 1993 Walter Hubert Lecture: the role of the p53 tumorsuppressor gene in tumorigenesis. *Brit. J. Cancer* **69,** 409–416.
8. Fujiwara, T., Grimm, E. A., and Roth, J. A. (1994) Gene therapeutics and gene therapy for cancer. *Curr. Opin. Oncol.* **6,** 96–105.
9. Mulligan, R. C. (1993) The basic science of gene therapy. *Science* **260,** 926–932.
10. Harris, C. C. and Hollstein, M. (1993) Clinical implications of the p53 tumor-suppressor gene. *N. Engl. J Med.* **329,** 1318.
11. Von Greunigan, V. R., Santoso, J. T., Lane, S. B., Miller, D. S., and Mathis, J. M. (1998) Adenovirus-mediated p53 gene therapy for ovarian cancer. *Gynecolog. Oncol.,* in press.
12. Von Greunigan, V. R., O'Boyle, J. D., Coleman, R. A., Miller, D. S., and Mathis, J. M. (1999) Safety and efficacy of intraperitoneal adenovirus-mediated p53 gene therapy for ovarian cancer. *Int. J. Gynecolog. Cancer,* **9,** 365–372.
13. Cai, D. W., Mukhopadhyay, T., Liu, Y., Fujiwara, T., Roth, J. A. (1993) Stable expression of the wild-type p53 gene in human lung cancer cells after retrovirus-mediated gene transfer. *Hum. Gene Ther.* **4,** 617–624.
14. Tang, D. C., Johnston, S. A., and Carbone, D. P. (1994) Butyrate-inducible and tumor-restricted gene expression by adenovirus vectors. *Cancer Gene Ther.* **1,** 15–20.
15. Dvoretsky, P. M., Richards, K. A., Angel, C., Rabinowitz, L., Stoler, M. H., Beecham, J. B., et al. (1998) Distribution of disease at autopsy in 100 women with ovarian cancer. *Hum. Pathol.* **9,** 57–63.
16. Mittereder, N., March, K. L., and Trapnell, B. C. (1996) Evaluation of the concentration and bioactivity of adenovirus vectors for gene therapy. *J. Virol.* **70,** 7498–7509.
17. Graham, F. L. and Prevoc, L. (1991) Manipulation of adenovirus vectors, in Methods in Molecular Medicine Vol 7: Gene Transfer and Expression Protocols (Murray, E. J. ed.), Humana Press, Clifton, NJ, pp. 109–128.
18. Yamamoto, R. S., Kobayashi, M., Plunkett, J. M., Masunaka, I. K., Orr, S. L., and Granger, G. A. (1985) Production and detection of lymphotoxin in vitro: micro-assay for lymphotoxin, in *Investigation of Cell-Mediated Immunity* (Yoshido, T. ed.), Churchill Livingston, New York, pp. 126–134.
19. Gorman, A. M., Samali, A., McGowan, A. J., and Cotter, T. G. (1997) Use of flow cytometry techniques in studying mechanisms of apoptosis in leukemic cells. *Cytometry* **29,** 97–105.
20. Joseph, A., Ingelfinger, F., and Mosteller, J. H. (1993) *Biostatistics in Clinical Medicine,* 3rd Ed. McGraw-Hill, New York.
21. Tsai, C. M., Gazdar, A. F., Venzon, D. J., Steinberg, S. M., Dedrick, R. L., Mulshine, J. L., et al. (1989) Lack of in vitro synergy between etoposide and cis-diamminedichloroplatinum(II). *Cancer Res.* **49,** 2390–2397.

# 89

## Bispecific Antibody MDX-210 for Treatment of Advanced Ovarian and Breast Cancer

**Peter A. Kaufman, Paul K. Wallace, Frank H. Valone, Wendy A. Wells, Vincent A. Memoli, and Marc S. Ernstoff**

## 1. Introduction

A large number of monoclonal antibodies (MAbs) to various tumor cell lines have been developed *(1)*. However, MAbs have thus far had limited therapeutic impact in oncology, probably in part because many murine MAbs do not effectively recruit immune effector mechanisms, such as complement fixation and antibody-dependent cell-mediated cytotoxicity (ADCC) in humans. Additionally, although humanized MAbs are being developed, when used therapeutically their immunological effectiveness may be limited by high concentrations of nonspecific immunoglobulin (Ig) in patient serum. These nonspecific Ig will compete with conventional MAbs for binding to Type I Fc receptors (FcγRI) on immune effector cells, and may therefore limit conventional MAbs ability to recruit an immune response. Recently, however, clinical efficacy of a humanized MAb directed against *HER-2/neu* in patients with advanced breast cancer has been demonstrated *(2–4)*. Preclinical data suggests that mechanistically this activity may be as a consequence of modulation of important biologic properties of the *HER-2/neu* receptor itself, as opposed to through an immunologic mechanism of tumor cell destruction.

Bispecific antibodies (BsAb) are one approach to increasing the immunological effectiveness of therapy with MAbs *(5–8)*. BsAb are hybrid antibodies constructed from two parent MAbs, one specific for tumor cells and the other specific for immune effector cells. BsAb can direct the cytotoxic activities of T cells, natural killer (NK) cells, monocytes, macrophages, or activated granulocytes to destroy tumor targets. Tumor cells can be destroyed when certain "trigger molecules" are engaged during BsAb-mediated interaction of tumor and effector cells *(9–12)*.

For a BsAb to effectively target immunologic effector cells, it must bind to and activate a cell surface molecule capable of triggering cellular cytotoxicity. On monocytes, macrophages, and neutrophils (PMNs), the Fc receptors for IgG (FcγR), of which there are three structurally and functionally distinct classes, appear to be the only molecules capable of mediating ADCC of tumor cells *(5,13–15)*. FcγRI (CD 64) is a potent cytotoxic trigger molecule on monocytes, macrophages, and activated PMNs. FcγRII

From: *Methods in Molecular Medicine, Vol. 39: Ovarian Cancer: Methods and Protocols*
Edited by: J. M. S. Bartlett © Humana Press, Inc., Totowa, NJ

is a cytotoxic trigger molecule on monocytes, macrophages, PMNs, and eosinophils, but is also expressed by platelets and other cells. FcγRIII on macrophages and the NK cell/large granular lymphocyte population is a cytotoxic trigger molecule. On PMNs, FcγRIII is phosphatidylinositol glycan linked and does not mediate cytotoxicity. The primary trigger molecule on T cells is the αβ or γδ antigen receptor-CD3 complex. BsAb can react with this complex and redirect the T cell to mediate cytotoxicity that is not major histocompatibility complex (MHC) restricted.

Preliminary results with BsAb targeting of LGL/NK cells have been promising. Studies have suggested that these cells may be targeted with BsAb through FcγRIII for killing of tumor cells in vitro, and for preventing tumor growth in vivo *(16,17)*. A BsAb with specificity both for CD3 and human ovarian carcinoma antigens, when used in combination with human T cells, have been shown to induce significant inhibition of ovarian tumor growth in nude mice *(18)*. Another study reported significant activity with the use of interleukin-2 (IL-2) activated human PBL targeted with an anti-CD3 × mov18 (antiovarian carcinoma) BsAb, in a nude mouse model *(19)*. Others noted similarly encouraging results with another BsAb in studies of OKT3 targeting of colon carcinoma cells in nude mice *(20)*. More recently, apparent cure of established Hodgkin's lymphomas grown in SCID mice has been achieved by simultaneous targeting using anti-CD3 × antitumor plus anti-CD28 × antitumor BsAbs *(21)*. In another ovarian cancer model, targeting of NK cells via FcγRIII to tumor cells expressing *HER-2/neu* has been effective for increasing survival of SCID mice bearing human ovarian carcinoma xenografts that overexpress *HER-2/neu (9)*.

Studies of tumor cell killing by myeloid cells, mediated by BsAb targeted to FcγRI, have demonstrated killing of breast, ovarian, and colon cancers. In one study, for example, interferon-gamma (IFNγ) activated human macrophages, targeted through FcγRI against a human adenocarcinoma antigen, were cytotoxic against human colorectal adenocarcinoma cells in vitro and in a nude mouse model *(22)*. The precise mechanism(s) of BsAb-mediated tumor cell cytotoxicity have not been fully elucidated, and they may occur in part through release of cytokines, including tumor necrosis factor-alpha (TNFα) and IFNγ *(5,6,13)*. The signal for releasing such cytokines, the crosslinking of trigger molecules on immune effector cells, occurs when BsAb targeting is used. Thus, BsAbs, in addition to targeting direct tumor cell lysis by effector cells, may stimulate cytokine release at a tumor site in vivo. This then could impact on tumor cells sterically inaccessible to effector cells, or lacking the target antigen. In any case, there is accumulating in vitro and in vivo evidence demonstrating that BsAbs exhibit potent antitumor effects.

We have recently completed several Phase Ia/Ib trials of BsAb MDX-210 in patients with advanced breast and ovarian carcinomas, first evaluating toxicity of single-infusion therapy with MDX-210 in women with advanced breast or ovarian cancer refractory to standard therapy *(23)*, and more recently evaluating multiple dose therapy with MDX-210 *(24)*. MDX-210 is constructed from Fab fragments of murine MAb 22, that binds to FcγRI *(25,26)*, and murine MAb 520C9 that binds *HER-2/neu (27,28)*. A unique feature of MAb 22 is that it binds to FcγRI outside the normal ligand binding site for IgG *(25,26)*. Thus, immune effector mechanisms mediated via MAb 22 are not inhibited by saturating concentrations of human IgG, such as are found in vivo *(5,26)*. In vitro, MDX-210 mediates FcγRI-dependent functions including ADCC, phagocytosis, and superoxide generation *(5,25,26)*. Preclinical studies have demonstrated that MDX-210 effectively directs FcγRI positive effector cells to phagocytose tumor cells that overexpress *HER-2/neu (27,28)*.

## 2. Materials

### 2.1. Preparation of F(ab')$_2$

#### 2.1.1. Reagents

1. Pepsin (Sigma, St. Louis, MO, P-6887).
2. 1 *M* Tris[hydroxymethyl]aminomethane base (pH 8.0, Tris Base, Sigma).
3. AvidChrome F(ab')$_2$ kit (Unisyn Technologies, Hopkinton, MA, 1005-001).
4. Phosphate-buffered saline Ca$^{++}$ and Mg$^{++}$ free, pH 7.4 (PBS, 20 m*M* sodium phosphate, 0.15 *M* sodium chloride; or BioWhittaker, Walkersville, MD).

#### 2.1.2. Buffers

1. Dialysis buffer: 25 m*M* sodium acetate, pH 4.5.
2. Pepsin buffer: 70 m*M* sodium acetate containing 50 m*M* NaCl, pH to 3.8 with glacial acetic acid.
3. 100 m*M* phosphate buffer: Dissolve 16.3 g of sodium phosphate monobasic and 5.4 g of sodium phosphate dibasic (Sigma) in 1 L of distilled water, pH 7.0.

#### 2.1.3. Equipment

1. Dialysis cassettes: 10,000 molecular weight cutoff (Pierce, Rockford, IL, 0.5-3 mL: 66450ZZ; 3–15 mL: 66451ZZ).
2. Centriprep 10 (Millipore, Beverly, MA, 4304).
3. Amicon ultrafiltration stirred cell (Model 8010 catalog number 5121, has a 25-mm diameter and holds a maximum of 10 mL, model 8050 catalog number 5122, has a 43-mm diameter and holds a maximum of 50 mL) with a Diaflow 10,000 MW cutoff membrane filter (style PM 10, 25 mm catalog number 13112 and 43-mm catalog number 13122) using nitrogen pressure at 25 psi.
4. High-pressure liquid chromatography (HPLC). During digestion, antibody fragmentation is checked for completeness and purity on an HPLC sizing column. We use a system supplied by Waters Associates (Taunton, MA) consisting of a U6K universal injector, 510 solvent delivery system and 484 tunable absorbance detector. The fractionation is performed at 0.85 mL/min on a TSK-gel SW G3000 column (TASOhaas, Montgomeryville, PA, 05789) with TSK-gel-SW guard column (TASOhaas, 05371) equilibrated in 100 m*M* phosphate. A sample of undigested IgG should be run initially for comparisons during the digestion. A minimum of 10–25 µg of protein can be readily detected.

### 2.2. Bispecific Antibody Production

#### 2.2.1. Reagents

1. Mercaptoethylamine (MEA, Sigma), stock prepared as 500 m*M* MEA in PBS, pH 7.2.
3. *o*-phenylenedimaleimide (*o*-PDM, Sigma), use only freshly prepared reagent.
4. Dimethylformamide (DMF, Pierce).
5. Iodoacetamide (IAA, Sigma, I-6125), stock prepared as 500 m*M* IAA in PBS, pH 7.2.

#### 2.2.2. Buffers

1. 2 *M* Tris ethylenediaminetetraacetic acid (EDTA): Dissolve 242 g Tris Base, 37.2 g Na$_2$EDTA, 200 mL hydrochloric acid in 1 L of distilled water.

2. Working MEA: Prepare 10 m*M* MEA from a 500-m*M* stock as necessary.
3. SACE buffer: 50-m*M* anhydrous sodium acetate, 0.5 m*M* Na$_2$EDTA, pH to 5.3 with acetic acid.
4. 100-m*M* phosphate buffer: Dissolve 16.3 g of sodium hydrogen phosphate monobasic (Sigma, S-9638) and 5.4 g of sodium hydrogen phosphate dibasic (Sigma, S-9390) in 1 L of distilled water, pH 7.0.

### 2.2.3. Equipment

1. Two chromatography columns packed with Sephadex G-25 (Pharmacia, Piscataway, NJ, 17-0033-02) are required for small scale (2–30) mg of BsAb. These must be filled with two end flow adapters and water jacketed to allow chilling throughout the preparation (alternatively the chromatography procedures may be done in a 4°C cold room).
   Σ Column 1. (Pharmacia XK16/40) 1.6 cm in diameter, packed with 25 cm of gel and pumped at approximately 60 mL/h.
   Σ Column 2. (Pharmacia, XK26/40) 2.6 cm in diameter packed with 20 cm of gel and pumped at approx 200 mL/h.
2. Suitable UV monitor, chart recorder and fraction collector are required. We use a single path Pharmacia UV-1 280 nm UV optical unit with control unit, a Pharmacia P-1 peristaltic pump, and a Pharmacia FRAC-100 fraction collector.
3. HPLC. At each stage of construction, and for the final BsAb purification, antibody fragments and BsAb derivatives are checked for yield and purity on an HPLC sizing column. We use the Waters system described in **Subheading 2.1.3., item 4**. The fractionation is performed isocratically at 0.85 mL/min on a TSK-gel SW G3000 column (TASOhaas) equilibrated in 100 mM phosphate buffer. The final BsAb purification should be done using a column equilibrated with PBS.

## 2.3. Flow Cytometric Staining and Analysis

### 2.3.1. Reagents

1. Primary MAb or BsAb (*see* **Note 12**).
2. Second antibody, typically a goat antimouse IgG (H+L), F(ab')$_2$ FITC absorbed against human, bovine, and horse immunoglobulins (Jackson Immunoresearch, West Grove, PA, 115-096-062). For the detection of patient antitumor antibodies goat antihuman IgM, IgG and IgA (H+L), F(ab')$_2$ FITC (Jackson Immunoresearch, 109-096-064) was used.

### 2.3.2. Buffers

1. FCM buffer: To 1 L of PBS add 10 g BSA, 1 g sodium azide and 0.04 g Na$_2$EDTA, Stored at 4–8°C, this solution is stable for 6 mo.
2. 1% Formalin is prepared by diluting 10% stock in PBS (v/v).
3. HEPES-BSA: Add to RPMI-1640, 25 mM HEPES, 20 µg/mL gentamicin, 2 mg/mL BSA.
4. Block IgG is prepared by combining 6 mg/mL human IgG Cohn fraction II and III human globulins with HEPES-BSA. Stored frozen this material is stable for 1 yr.
5. RLF Lysing Solution (RLF-Lyse). Prepare one liter of RLF-Lyse by combining 8.3 g of dry ammonium chloride, 1 g potassium bicarbonate, and 10 mL of 10 m*M* Na$_2$EDTA. Bring the volume to 1 L with distilled water. Stored at 25°C (room temperature), this solution is stable for 6 mo. To make 10 m*M* disodium EDTA, dissolve 0.37 g of disodium EDTA in 100 mL water.

### 2.3.3. Equipment

1. Flow cytometer, we use a FACScan (Becton Dickinson, San Jose, CA). Linear forward scatter vs side scatter displays are used to set gates to define specific lymphocyte, mono-

cyte, and granulocyte populations and to eliminate small debris and large aggregates prior to collection of list mode data. Fluorescein fluorescence is detected using logarithmic amplification in the FL1 channel (530/30 bandpass filter). The data are collected on an HP 310 (Hewlett Packard, Palo Alto, CA) computer using FACScan Lysis II software. For each sample a minimum of 10,000 gated events is analyzed and the percent positive relative to an isotype control and the mean fluorescence intensity of each population are determined. The number of second antibody binding sites per cell can be determined by comparison to a standard curve generated with Rainbow microspheres (Sphereotech, Libertyville, IL) containing beads with six different levels of fluorochrome molecules per bead as previously described by the manufacturer *(25)*.

## 3. Methods

### 3.1. Preparation of F(ab')₂

The preparation of $F(ab')_2$ by limited proteolysis of mouse IgG has been described by many groups *(31,32)*. All the mouse IgG isotypes, with the exception of $IgG_2b$, can generally be cleaved to a $F(ab')_2$ product. Pepsin is the enzyme of choice for the preparation of murine $IgG_1$, and $IgG_2a$ $F(ab')_2$, although other reagents are available. Fragmentation of individual MAbs with pepsin is extremely pH variable, even within the same isotype. One $IgG_1$ may fragment rapidly at a pH of 3.8 or 4.0, whereas another $IgG_1$ may require a pH of 3.5. It is, therefore, best to pilot test small batches of antibody at different pH's and then scale up.

A commercial kit for pepsin digestions, which we have found reliable, is available from Unisyn Technologies. This kit is suitable for any user performing a limited number of digestions per year and is capable of digesting 100 mg of MAb. The above noted caution about pH is stressed with this kit, too. The buffers contained within the kit are at a pH of 4.0. During the digestion, which is monitored by HPLC, it may become necessary to drop the pH to 3.8 or lower. The user is advised to know how much glacial acetic acid that will be required to drop the volume in the digestion mixture down 0.1 U of pH. Otherwise, this is an excellent and easy alternative to the procedure described here.

1. Concentrate the pure mouse $IgG_1$ or $IgG_2a$ MAb to 5–10 mg/mL using a Centriprep 10 or Amicon concentrator under nitrogen pressure following the manufacturers recommendations.
2. Do a buffer exchange with dialysis buffer by placing the MAb into a dialysis cassette and placing this into 4 L of dialysis buffer at 4°C. Use a magnetic stirrer and stir bar to mix the buffer. After 18–24 h, harvest the MAb and place it in a 15-mL polypropylene tube.
3. Dissolve pepsin to 10 mg/mL in pepsin buffer and add to the MAb solution at a 3% ratio (w/w).
4. Incubate this mixture at 37°C in a water bath. At 1-h intervals remove 10 µg of digesting antibody and assay it by HPLC using a TSK3000 column to determine the extent of digestion. When less than 10% remains as IgG or when the $F(ab')_2$ peak is no longer increasing, stop the digestion by adjusting the pH back to 8.0 with 1 $M$ Tris base, pH 8.0. Under these conditions most $IgG_1$ and $IgG_2a$ MAbs will require 4–8 h for completion (*see* **Note 1**).
5. Samples from digestion are purified by HPLC using a TSK3000 column. Chromatography is performed isocratically at a 0.85 mL/min flow rate using 2 $M$ phosphate buffer or PBS. A maximum of 500 µg in 0.5 mL can be safely loaded onto this system.

### 3.2. Bispecific Antibody Production

Chemical linkage is the most straightforward procedure for making BsAb. It essentially involves purifying parent antibodies of two desired specificity's, or their Fab' or

F(ab')$_2$ fragments, coupling these antibodies together, and purifying the product from the reactants. Bifunctional reagents with ε-amino groups or with hinge region SH groups have been useful in preparing BsAb *(33,34)*. Although BsAb were originally made by coupling whole MAb and/or Fab' fragments with succinimidyl-3-(2-pyridyldithiol)-propionate (SPDP), this reagent causes random cross-linking and, while useful for preliminary preclinical studies, are too heterogeneous for clinical use *(35,36)*. Over the past few years, BsAb have been prepared in this laboratory using the chemical cross-linker *o*-PDM to activate thiols on Fab fragments of one of the MAb *(24)*. These Fab'-*o*-PDM derivatives are then combined with reduced Fab' fragments from the other MAb, yielding relatively homogeneous and functional BsAb. In this section, we outline the methodology for preparing these multivalent antibodies. For MDX-210, MAbA is MAb22 targeting CD64 *(25)* and MAbB is 520C9 targeting *HER*-2/*neu (26,27) (see* **Note 2**).

1. Prepare MAbA-Fab'-SH and MAbB-Fab'SH from their respective F(ab')$_2$ stocks by reducing them with 10 m*M* MEA for 30 min at 25°C. F(ab')$_2$ stocks, in PBS, should be at 5 mg/mL ± 1 mg/mL *(see* **Note 3**). The final Fab' must be free of F(ab')$_2$ species and may require a longer incubation with MEA. Monitor the reaction by HPLC (TSK3000) to determine when complete *(see* **Note 4**).
2. Remove free MEA by gel filtration through a G-25 column (number 1) equilibrated with SACE buffer.
3. Adjust protein concentrations to 5 mg/mL with Centriprep 10 following the manufacturers recommendations keeping these Fab'-SH solutions on ice *(see* **Note 5**).
4. Make 12 m*M o*-PDM solution (3.22 mg/mL) with DMF using glass tubes and pipets (not plastic) and keep this solution in a methanol ice bath (–20°C).
5. Swiftly add, with rapid mixing, one half volume of the 12 m*M o*-PDM solution in DMF to the chilled MAbA-Fab'-SH to a final concentration of 4 m*M o*-PDM. Incubate the reaction mixture for 30 min on ice.
6. Remove as rapidly as possible (less than 5 min) by using a pump, free *o*-PDM, and DMF from the MAbA-Fab'-S-*o*-PDM by gel filtration through a G-25 column (number 2) at 4°C, equilibrated with SACE buffer.
7. Collect the MAbA-Fab'-S-*o*-PDM coming off the column as the peak appears on the protein monitor into the tube containing the MAbB-Fab'-SH. A molar ratio of 1 : 1.2 (MAbA-Fab'-S-*o*-PDM:MAbB-Fab'-SH) is suggested *(see* **Note 6**).
8. At 4°C, concentrate the protein mixture to a concentration of 5 mg/mL (i.e., the original combined MAb-Fab' volumes) with an Amicon concentrator under nitrogen pressure.
9. Incubate the reaction mixture for 18 h at 4°C. This is optimally done by leaving the reaction mixture in the Amicon concentrator. The bulk of the reaction may well be completed in 2 h.
10. Monitor the process of conjugation formation by HPLC (TSK3000).
11. Take the reaction mixture out of the Amicon concentrator and rinse the chamber with 1 mL of 1 *M* Tris, pH 8.0, and combine this rinse with the reaction mixture whose pH will now be 8.0. If it is not, use an additional volume of 1 *M* Tris, pH 8.0 to bring the pH up to 8.0. All manipulations may now be done at room temperature.
12. Break any -S-S- bonds (i.e., MAbB-Fab'-S-S-Fab'-MAbB) formed during the incubation by treating the reaction mixture with 10 m*M* MEA for 30 min at 25°C.
13. Add IAA to a final concentration of 25 m*M* to alkylate free-SH groups on the proteins, if any, as well as the unreacted MEA, followed by a 10 minute incubation.
14. Purify the heterodimeric BsAb mixture (MAbA-Fab'-*o*-PDM-Fab'-MAbB) by gel filtration on a TSK3000 sizing gel using PBS *(see* **Note 7**).

15. Concentrate the protein mixture with an Amicon concentrator under nitrogen pressure to a concentration of approximately 1 mg/mL and then filter sterilize using a 0.2 μm filter.
16. Check the purity of the final product by SDS-PAGE and perform flow cytometric (or ELISA) binding studies (*see* **Note 8**).

### 3.3. Flow Cytometric Staining and Analysis

Immunofluorescence labeling was used to quantify the number of FcγRI sites per cell and the amount of BsAb bound to monocytes and granulocytes after BsAb therapy *(47,49)*. The procedure was performed on ice in 96-well, round bottom, polypropylene microtiter plates to prevent monocyte adherence using standard conditions defined below. A human IgG block was added to the cells prior to addition of murine MAb to block nonspecific binding of MAb to Fc receptor positive cells. All procedures should be done on ice with cold (4°C) reagents (*see* **Note 9**). A modification of this procedure described below in **Note 17** was used to measure patient antitumor antibodies in their serum.

1. Harvest cells and wash 1 time in FCM buffer, and perform a cell count and viability (*see* **Note 10**).
2. Resuspend cells to $5 \times 10^6$ cells/mL in FCM buffer (*see* **Note 11**).
3. Add 100 μL cells to each well (or $5 \times 10^5$ cells/well) (*see* **Notes 12** and **13**).
4. Spin the plate at 400*g* at 8°C for 5 min with no brake. Decant by smartly flicking the plate avoiding any loss of cells.
5. Resuspend the cells in each well with 50 μL of IgG block to block nonspecific binding especially with Fc-receptor positive cells. Incubate on ice for 10 min.
6. Add 50 μL of primary (test) antibody to the appropriate wells (*see* **Notes 14** and **15**). The ideal controls are MAb of the same species and isotype as the test MAb. In addition, it is advisable when trouble shooting becomes necessary to set up cells labeled with nothing (no primary or secondary MAb) and cells labeled only with the secondary goat antimouse.
7. Mix cells and MAb using eight-channel multipipet and incubate on ice for 30–60 min.
8. Wash three times with FCM buffer. Use 200 μL FCM buffer changes and centrifuge the plate at 400*g* at 8°C for 5 min. Decant each wash by smartly flicking the plate avoiding any loss of cells.
9. Add 50 μL goat antimouse F(ab′)₂ FITC to each well (except control well with cells only) and resuspend using eight-channel multipipet. Incubate on ice for 30–60 min avoiding direct exposure to light. Direct light will quench the fluorochrome, we cover the plate with aluminum foil (*see* **Note 16**).
10. Wash three times with FCM buffer. Use 200 μL FCM buffer changes and centrifuge the plate at 400*g* at 8°C for 5 min. Decant each wash by smartly flicking the plate avoiding any loss of cells (*see* **Note 17**).
11. At this point, the cells may be analyzed on the flow cytometer. If there will be a delay (greater than 4 h) resuspend the cells in each well with 175 μL of 1% formalin, wrap tightly in parafilm, and store covered at 4°C for up to 1 wk. It is advisable that once formalin is added the analysis by flow cytometry be delayed for 12 h to allow the fluorescence to equilibrate.

### 3.4. Analysis of HER-2/neu Overexpression (see Chapter 57)

*HER-2/neu* immunoreactivity was assessed with two different MAbs, CB-11 (Biogenix, San Ramon, CA) *(38)*, and 520C9 (the anti-*HER-2/neu* component of MDX-210) (Medarex, Annandale, NJ) *(27,28)*. Slides were scored both with regard to the percentage of positive tumor cells (<10%, 10–50%, or >50%) and the staining intensity (negative, moderate, or strong).

### 3.5. MDX-210 Clinical Trial Protocols

1. Patient Criteria: Eligibility for both clinical trials included: (1) Stage III or IV ovarian cancer resistant to at least one standard platinum-based chemotherapy regimen or stage IV breast carcinoma resistant to at least two standard chemotherapy regimens or to one hormonal and one chemotherapy regimen; (2) patients with primary or metastatic cancer that overexpressed *HER-2/neu* in >50% of tumor cells, with moderate to strong intensity; (3) Adequate hematologic (WBC >3000, ANC >1500, platelets >150,000); hepatic (bilirubin<1.5 mg/dL, SGPT and alkaline phosphatase <2X upper limits normal); and renal function (creatinine <1.5 mg/dL); and (4) ECOG performance status 0–2. These protocols were approved by the Norris Cotton Cancer Center Clinical Cancer Research Committee and the Dartmouth-Hitchcock Medical Center Committee for the Protection of Human Subjects, and all patients gave written informed consent. Toxicity was assessed using the NCI Common Clinical Trials Criteria. Exclusion criteria included a history of prior MAb immunotherapy or use of prior diagnostic MAbs, active immunological or inflammatory diseases, active infection, coexisting pregnancy or nursing, and a history of a psychiatric or addictive disorder that would prevent giving informed consent.

2. Administration of MDX-210: Secure venous access was established in each patient and IV fluids, typically normal saline, were administered throughout the treatment and posttreatment observation time. Patients were pretreated with acetaminophen 650 mg orally, diphenhydramine 25–50 mg orally or intravenously, and lorazepam 0.5–1.0 mg orally or intravenously, before administration of MDX-210. Posttreatment acetaminophen, diphenhydramine, and/or lorazepam was given as needed. A test dose of antibody (0.005–0.3 mg) was given intravenously in the single-dose trial. If the test dose was tolerated well, without evidence of allergic reaction, the remaining dose of BsAb was given within 30 min. MDX-210 was given intravenously at a rate of 6 mg/h with a maximum infusion duration of 2 h. Vital signs were monitored every 15 min for 2.5 h after the test dose, hourly for 6 h, and then every 4 h for 16 h. In the single-dose trial, patients were hospitalized overnight for observation to identify any delayed side effects. Follow-up evaluation occurred on days 2, 3, 4, 8, 15, 29, 57, and 85.

   In the multidose trial, two treatment schedules were employed: group A—therapy on day 1, 3, and 5; dose of 7 mg/m$^2$ (*n*=3); group B—therapy on day 1, 8, and 15; dose of 7 mg/m$^2$ (*n*=5), and 10 mg/m$^2$ (*n*=2). MDX-210 was administered via a 2-h iv infusion in this trial. Intravenous fluids were administered, and patients were pre- and posttreated with acetaminophen, diphenhydramine, and lorazepam as above. Vital signs were monitored every 15 min during BsAb infusion, and then hourly for 6 h.

3. Immunologic Monitoring: Serum cytokine levels including TNFα, interleukin-6 (IL-6), and granulocyte colony-stimulating factor (G-CSF) were quantified by ELISA (R & D Systems, Minneapolis, MN). For analysis of both peripheral blood monocyte and granulocyte bound MDX-210 by flow cytometry, 10 mL of heparinized whole blood was collected at baseline, at completion of the infusion of MDX-210, and at other selected time-points up to 48 h postinfusion. Buffy coat cells were isolated and flow cytometry was performed *(51)*. Total number of FcγRI expressed by circulating cells was determined (as described in **Subheading 3.3.**).

4. Plasma MDX-210 Pharmacokinetics: Venous blood aliquots (2 mL) were collected before and at the end of infusion and at various time-points up to 24 h after treatment. Plasma was separated and stored at –70°C for measurement of plasma MDX-210. Plasma concentrations of MDX-210 were estimated using a specific ELISA for murine immunoglobulin,

the limit of sensitivity of this assay is 0.02 µg/mL. Pharmacokinetic analyses were performed using the PC Nonlin version 4.2 pharmacokinetic program (SCI Software, Lexington, KT). The pharmacokinetic analysis performed was that for a constant rate intravenous infusion with a noncompartmental model (PC Nonlin model 202), the elimination constant ($\beta$) was estimated by linear regression of at least the terminal 3–6 plasma concentration time-points on the log plasma MDX-210 concentration vs time plot. $C_{max}$ and $T_{max}$ were the observed values on these plots. AUC was calculated using the linear trapezoidal rule with the extrapolated AUC from $C_{last}$ (last measurable plasma concentration) to infinity calculated from $C_{last}/k_\beta$. Clearance was calculated in the standard fashion, CL=Dose /AUC(0-infinity), and the volume of distribution ($Vd_{area}$) was subsequently calculated ($Vd_{area} = CL/k_\beta$).

5. Measurement of Serum Anti-Tumor Antibodies: Serum and/or plasma samples were obtained pretreatment and on days 30 and/or 60 postinfusion and frozen in 500 µL aliquots. Samples were analyzed for human antibodies reactive with SKBR3 (breast carcinoma) and SKOV3 (ovarian carcinoma) cell lines (as described in **Subheading 4.3.10.**).

## 3.6. Clinical Trials: Data Analyses

1. *HER-2/neu*: We have currently evaluated the overall incidence of *HER-2/neu* overexpression in 112 patients with either breast or ovarian cancer screened for MDX-210 clinical trials. In correlating between staining of tumor specimens by CB-11 and 520C9, data from the 105 patients reported below yielded comparable results with staining with both antibodies. Discordant immunohistochemical data were noted in the remaining patient specimens.

    *HER-2/neu* overexpression was determined for 40 patients with advanced ovarian cancer. Nine patients had essentially no detectable overexpression, and 10 were found to have overexpression in from 10%–50% of the tumor cell population, with nine of these demonstrating moderate staining intensity and one having strong staining intensity. Overexpression of *HER-2/neu* in greater than 50% of the tumor cell population was noted in 21 patients (53% of total), with 17 of these having strong staining intensity and four having moderate.

    *HER-2/neu* overexpression was similarly analyzed in the group of 65 patients with metastatic breast cancer. Six had essentially no detectable overexpression. Twelve patients were found to overexpress *HER-2/neu* in from 10%–50% of the tumor cell population. Overexpression of *HER-2/neu* in greater than 50% of the tumor cell population was noted in 47 patients, with 39 of these patients having strong staining intensity and eight having moderate staining. Thus, 72% of patients with metastatic breast cancer were found to have overexpression of *HER-2/neu* in greater than 50% of the tumor cell population.

2. Single-Dose Trial: In the single-dose trial, 15 patients were treated, nine had breast cancer, and six ovarian cancer. All were heavily pretreated, having received a median of four different prior chemotherapy or hormonal regimens. Treatment was generally well tolerated. Most patients developed low-grade fever, five patients had maximal temperatures of 38.0–39.0°C, which resolved rapidly. Most patients developed mild systolic hypotension. Two patients developed grade 3 hypotension, which resolved fully within 1–4 h, with iv fluids. Nine patients had nausea, one had emesis. Two patients who had significant pleural effusions and mild dyspnea before treatment developed increased dyspnea within 8 h of treatment. Dyspnea resolved spontaneously by hour 8 in one patient and after thoracentesis in the other.

    The number of peripheral blood monocytes decreased substantially within 1–2 h after starting the antibody infusion ($p<0.0001$) and then gradually returned to baseline by hour 24. These changes are considered evidence for immunological efficacy, and not a sign of hematological toxicity, as monocytes are the principal cells targeted by MDX-210. The median granulocyte count fell slightly 1–2 h after starting the infusion and then rebounded a few hours later, but the differences were not statistically significant. A slight decrease in lymphocytes occurred. There were no consistent changes in hemoglobin or platelets.

At doses $\geq 3.5$ mg/m$^2$ all monocytes demonstrated bound MDX-210 at the end of the infusion. Greater than 80% of monocytes continued to show bound BsAb 48 h after infusion, at the highest dose levels. MDX-210 saturated available monocyte Fc$\gamma$RI in a dose related manner with maximal saturation of 80–90% being achieved at doses $\geq 3.5$ mg/m$^2$ dose level. At the highest doses, 20–40% of monocyte receptors for Fc$\gamma$RI were occupied by BsAb 48 hours after antibody infusion.

Plasma concentrations of TNF$\alpha$, IL-6, G-CSF, and IFN$\gamma$ were determined at baseline and 1, 2, 3, 4, 6, 10, 24, and 48 h after BsAb. Treatment increased plasma concentrations of these cytokines in a complex manner. Increased plasma concentrations of TNF$\alpha$ were observed at hours 1–3 in some patients. Eight patients had increased plasma TNF$\alpha$, and there was no apparent dose response. Increased plasma concentrations of IL-6 and G-CSF were observed by hours 3–6. There appeared to be a threshold effect for stimulation of IL-6 and G-CSF in which low doses of MDX-210 did not stimulate release of these cytokines but once an active dose was reached there was no dose-response effect noted.

Two patients treated at the 10 mg/m$^2$ dose level underwent biopsies of cutaneous metastases 24–48 h after treatment. Immunohistochemical staining revealed in vivo binding of BsAb to tumor cells. In one patient, a mononuclear cell infiltrate and associated tumor cell necrosis were also observed. Two patients developed transient pain at sites of metastases within four hours of treatment.

3. Multidose Trial: Ten patients were treated in this trial, seven with breast cancer and three with ovarian cancer. Similar to the single-dose trial, flu-like symptoms, consisting of moderate fever and chills were common. Mild to moderate hypotension and mild gastrointestinal upset occurred occasionally as well. Overall, the clinical toxicity profile was mild, and similar to that noted with single-dose therapy. Of note, toxicities were manifest primarily on day 1 of therapy. One patient went off protocol after receiving one dose of BsAb (10 mg/m$^2$) because of transient grade 4 pulmonary toxicity. One patient went off protocol after receiving only one dose of BsAb (7 mg/m$^2$) because of progressive hepatic metastases.

No significant hematologic toxicity was seen. Monocyte counts in all patients decreased substantially on day 1, transiently, but diminished impact on monocyte counts was seen with successive doses of MDX-210.

Monocyte Fc$\gamma$RI saturation with BsAb was again evaluated, and approximately 75% saturation was noted in group A on both day 1 and day 5. Similarly, in group B, > 80% saturation of monocyte Fc$\gamma$RI was noted at the completion of the infusion on day 1, 8, and 15. In both groups of patients approximately 40% saturation of monocyte Fc$\gamma$RI was noted 24 h after therapy. Other immunologic parameters measured in this trial were similar overall to those noted above in patients treated on the single-dose trial.

An additional aspect of this therapy is that MDX-210, by directing macrophage phagocytosis of tumor cells, might result in enhanced presentation of tumor antigens and the induction of a humoral immune response. In 2/8 patients evaluated, increased serum immunoglobulins reactive with the *HER-2/neu* positive cell lines SKBR3 or SKOV3, on either day 30 or day 60 following treatment with MDX-210, were noted. One patient had breast cancer, and developed a twofold increase in antibodies reactive with SKBR3. Another patient had ovarian cancer, and developed a 1.4-fold increase in antibodies reactive with SKOV3, and additionally a 1.7-fold increase in antibodies reactive with SKBR3. These data suggest, therefore, that MDX-210 may in fact lead to enhanced tumor cell antigen presentation, and initiate more efficient development of an anti-tumor humoral immune response.

## 4. Notes

1. Because of the sensitivity of pepsin to pH, the period of digestion can be significantly extended or reduced by adjusting the pH by as little as 0.1 of a unit. Digestions which are not completed in a working day may be left overnight at 4°C and then continued the following day.

2. Mouse $IgG_1$ and $IgG_2a$ each possess two heavy-light chain and three heavy-heavy chain disulfide bonds (*S-S*). It follows, therefore, that the Fab'-SH from such molecules have five SH groups. It should be noted that under the conditions employed to reduce the $F(ab')_2$ that while all heavy chain *S-S* bonds are broken the heavy- and light-chain *S-S* bonds are not reduced. In this procedure, the SH groups on one parent Fab' (MAbA) are alkylated with a large molar excess of the cross-linker *o*-PDM. Immunochemical studies have shown that in this reaction *o*-PDM will usually cross-link adjacent SH groups intramolecularly. Thus, the two SH groups on the heavy chain probably become linked together through *o*-PDM, leaving a solitary SH group in the hinge region to react with just one end of the linker. The MAbA-Fab'-*o*-PDM is thus left with a single reactive maleimide group to react with the Fab'-SH from the selected partner (MAbB). Because this methodology relies on a single remaining SH after intramolecular crosslinking by *o*-PDM it is critical that the Fab' MAb chosen have an odd number of SH groups in the hinge region of the heavy chain. Among the mouse IgG subclasses $IgG_1$ and $IgG_2a$ (both with three bonds) and $IgG_3$ (one bond) qualify, whereas $IgG_2b$ (four bonds) does not.

3. The most common problem we encounter is starting off this procedure with an insufficient amount of antibody. Ideally, 10 mg of each $F(ab')_2$ should be used and 5 mg of each $F(ab')_2$ is a recommended minimum. Save a small amount of $F(ab')_2$ for use as an HPLC reference and for subsequent functional assays.

4. To most efficiently monitor the reduction, place the reaction mixture on ice to stop the reaction, and add 0.15 µL IAA to the sample you are running on HPLC. Proceed to **Subheading 3.1., step 2**, or warm the MAb mixture to 25°C to continue reduction.

5. MAb-SH from **Subheading 3.2., step 2** can be collected directly into the CentriPrep for concentration in **Subheading 3.2., step 3**.

6. We have found that a molar ratio of 1:1.2 or 1:1.3 MAbA:MAbB will give the greatest yield of BsAb. Other BsAbs using different MAb parents may differ slightly. If yields are low, adjusting this ratio may improve the yield. It is also important that all of the free *o*-PDM be removed in **Subheading 3.2., step 6**.

7. The conjugate yield should be over 50%, the first peak off the column is usually a small amount of trispecific antibody, followed by a large BsAb peak and then the uncoupled $F(ab')_2$ parents.

8. BsAb purity was assessed by nonreducing SDS-PAGE. The binding activity of each of the individual Fab' components of the bispecific antibody was checked using an indirect staining assay and FACS analysis *(39)*. For example, with MDX-210, the binding of the MAb 520C9 component was verified using the *HER-2/neu* expressing cell line SKBR3 *(40)* (ATCC, Rockville, MD), whereas the binding of the MAb22 component was checked with FcγRI expressing human monocytes and the U937 cell line *(41)* (ATCC, Rockville, MD). In addition, the bispecific nature of the molecule was verified by a bifunctional immunoassay to ascertain that both moieties were linked and functional. In this assay, BsAb was incubated with SKBR3 cells, then washed, and followed by addition of a soluble fusion protein consisting of the extracellular domain of human FcγRI (CD64) and human IgM heavy chain (sFcγRI-M) obtained from transiently transfected COS cells.

FITC-labeled goat-antihuman IgM was added and binding was assayed by flow-cytometry. Only BsAb bound to the SKBR3 cells and the sFcγRI-M would remain in the assay and be FITC positive. The parental antibodies (MAb22 and 520C9) should be negative in this assay.

9. Sodium azide is added to the FCM buffer to avoid bacterial contamination and importantly to also prevent capping and internalization of the fluorochrome (capping is an ATP-dependent process). Cells exposed to sodium azide at room temperature will be killed resulting in nonspecific antibody uptake. To avoid sodium azide induced death, all antibody labeling is done on ice with reagents at 4°C. Keeping the process cold also helps prevent capping. EDTA is added to the FCM buffer to facilitate the analysis of monocytes that would otherwise adhere to the plate.

10. In the clinical trials, both peripheral blood monocyte and granulocyte bound MDX-210 was quantified by flow cytometry. Ten milliliters of heparinized whole blood was collected at baseline, at completion of the infusion of MDX-210, and at other selected time points for up to 48 h after infusion completion. Buffy coat cells were isolated by spinning the heparinized blood at 400$g$ for 10 min. Red cells in the buffy coat were lysed by resuspending the buffy coat in 5 mL of RLF lyse at room temperature for 10 min. The cells were then centrifuged and washes once with FCM buffer.

11. Alternatively, resuspend the cells to $1 \times 10^7$ cells/mL in IgG block and add 50 uL of cells to each well ($5 \times 10^5$ cells per well). After the cells have been exposed to the block for 10 minutes proceed directly to **Subheading 3.3., step 6**.

12. We routinely add $5 \times 10^5$ cells/well, however $1 \times 10^5$ cells per well can be used when a minimum number of cells are available. No more than $1 \times 10^6$ cells per well should be used.

13. We routinely run our analysis in duplicate (i.e., two separate wells containing the same cells and MAb) this ensures that the results were reproducible. When a statistical treatments of the data is intended, we run each sample in triplicate.

14. The MAb dilution used will depend on the source and concentration of that MAb. In general primary MAb from a culture supernatant are usually saturating at 1X or 10X the supernatant concentration; a 1:1000 or greater dilution of ascites is typically saturating; purified MAb is saturating at 1 μg/mL final concentration. It should be stressed, however, that each MAb must be tested by titering to determine that a saturating concentration is being used.

15. In the clinical trials, the total number of FcγRI expressed by circulating cells was determined by incubating cells with a saturating dose of MAb32-FITC (Medarex, Inc., Annandale, NJ) another anti-FcγRI directed MAb, or MDX-210. The amount of BsAb bound in vivo to monocytes and granulocytes was determined by omitting **Subheading 3.3., steps 6–8**.

16. The dilution of secondary fluorochrome labeled goat anti-mouse antibody must be done by titering a stock to determine saturating conditions. In general we have found that 50 μL of a 1:40 dilution (v/v) of the goat antimouse F(ab')$_2$ FITC from Jackson Immunoresearch to be ideal.

17. Measurement of Patient Serum Anti-Tumor Antibodies: Serum and/or plasma samples were obtained pre-treatment and on days 30 and/or 60 postinfusion and frozen in 500-μL aliquots. Samples were analyzed for human antibodies reactive with SKBR3 and SKOV3 (ATCC) cell lines. Cells were counted and added to a 96-well plate as described in **Subheading 3.3., steps 1–4**. Cells are *not* resuspended in IgG block as described in **Subheading 3.3., step 5** because this reagent would cross-react with the goat antihuman detection reagent. A 1:10 dilution of serum or plasma was added as described in **Subheading 3.3., step 6**. The remainder of the procedure was performed as described except that unchanged,

except that a fluorescein conjugated goat antihuman Ig was used to detect human Ig bound to the tumor cells.

## References

1. Sparano, J. A. and O'Boyle, K. (1992) The potential role for biological therapy in the treatment of breast cancer. *Semin. Oncol.* **19,** 333–341.
2. Cobleigh, M. A., Vogel, C. L., Tripathy, D., Robert, N. J., Scholl, S., Fehrenbacher, L., et al. (1998) Efficacy and safety of Herceptin (humanized anti-HER2 antibody) as a single agent in 222 women with HER2 overexpression who relapsed following chemotherapy for metastatic breast cancer. *Proc. ASCO* **17,** 376A.
3. Slamon, D., Leyland-Jones, B., Shak, S., Paton, V., Bajamonde, A., Fleming, T., et al. (1998) Addition of Herceptin (humanized anti-HER2 antibody) to first line chemotherapy for HER2 overexpressing metastatic breast cancer markedly increases anticancer activity: a randomized, multinational controlled phase III trial. *Proc. ASCO* **17,** 377A.
4. Pegram, M. D., Lipton, A., Hayes, D. F., Weber, B. L., Baselga, J. M., Tripathy, D., et al. (1998) Phase II study of receptor-enhanced chemosensitivity using recombinant humanized anti-p185$^{HER2/neu}$ monoclonal antibody plus cisplatin in patients with HER2/*neu*-overexpressing metastatic breast cancer refractory to chemotherapy treatment. *J. Clin. Oncol.* **16,** 2659–2671.
5. Fanger, M. W., Morganelli, P. M., and Guyre, P. M. (1992) Bispecific antibodies. *Crit. Rev. Immunol.* **12,** 101–124.
6. Clark, M., Bolt, S., Tunnacliffe, A., and Waldman, H. (1991) *Bispecific Antibodies and Targeted Cellular Cytotoxicity* (Romet-Lemonne, J. L., Fanger, M. W., and Segal, D. M., eds.), Lienhart, pp. 243–247.
7. Fanger, M. W., Segal, D. M., and Romet-Lemonne, J. L. (1991) Bispecific antibodies and targeted cellular cytotoxicity. *Immunol. Today* **12,** 51–54.
8. Chokri, M., Girard, A., Borrelly, M. C., Oleron, C., Romet-Lemonne, J. L., and Bartholeyns, J. (1992) Adoptive immunotherapy with bispecific antibodies: targeting through macrophages. *Res. Immunol.* **143,** 95–99.
9. Weiner, L. M., Holmes, M., Adams, G. P., LaCreta, F., Watts, P., and Garcia de Palazzo, I. (1993) A human tumor xenograft model of therapy with a bispecific monoclonal antibody targeting c-erbB-2 and CD16. *Cancer Res.* **53,** 94–100.
10. Hsieh Ma, S. T., Eaton, A. M., Shi, T., and Ring, D. B. (1992) In vitro cytotoxic targeting by human mononuclear cells and bispecific antibody 2B1, recognizing c-erbB-2 protooncogene product and Fc gamma receptor III. *Cancer Res.* **52,** 6832–6839.
11. Barr, I. G., Miescher, S., von Fliedner, V., Buchegger, F., Barras, C., Lanzavecchia, A., et al. (1989) In vivo localization of a bispecific antibody which targets human T lymphocytes to lyse human colon cancer cells. *Int. J. Cancer* **43,** 501–507.
12. Ball, E. D., Guyre, P. M., Mills, L., Fisher, J., Dinces, N. B., and Fanger, M. W. (1992) Initial trial of bispecific antibody-mediated immunotherapy of CD15-bearing tumors: cytotoxicity of human tumor cells using a bispecific antibody comprised of anti-CD15 (MoAb PM81) and anti-CD64/Fc gamma RI (MoAb 32). *J. Hematother.* **1,** 85–94.
13. Fanger, M. W., Shen, L., Graziano, R. F., and Guyre, P. M. (1989) Cytotoxicity mediated by human Fc receptors for IgG. *Immunol. Today* **10,** 92–99.
14. van de Winkel, J. G. and Capel, P. A. (1993) Human IgG Fc receptor heterogeneity: molecular aspects and clinical implications. *Immunol. Today* **14,** 215–221.
15. Shen, L., Graziano, R. F., and Fanger, M. W. (1989) The functional properties of Fc gamma RI, II and III on myeloid cells: a comparative study of killing of erythrocytes and tumor cells mediated through the different Fc receptors. *Mol. Immunol.* **26,** 959–969.
16. de Palazzo, I. G., Gercel-Taylor, C., Kitson, J., and Weiner, L. M. (1990) Potentiation of tumor lysis by a bispecific antibody that binds to CA19-9 antigen and the Fc gamma receptor expressed by human large granular lymphocytes. *Cancer Res.* **50,** 7123–7128.
17. Weiner, L. M., Grecel-Taylor, C., Kitson, J., and Garcia de Palazzo, I. E. (1991) Properties of a bispecific monoclonal antibody binding CA19-9 tumor antigen and FcgRIII, in *Bispecific Antibodies and Targeted Cellular Cytotoxicity* (Romet-Lemonne J. L., Fanger, M. W., and Segal, D. M., eds), Lienhart, pp. 33–36.
18. Titus, J. A., Garrido, M. A., Hecht, T. T., Winkler, D. F., Wunderlich, J. R., and Segal, D. M. (1987) Human T cells targeted with anti-T3 cross-linked to antitumor antibody prevent tumor growth in nude mice. *J. Immunol.* **138,** 4018–4022.
19. Garrido, M. A., Valdayo, M. J., Winkler, D. F., Titus, J. A., Hecht, T. T., Perez, P., et al. (1990) Targeting human T-lymphocytes with bispecific antibodies to react against human ovarian carcinoma cells growing in nu/nu mice. *Cancer Res.* **50,** 4227–4232.

20. Nelson, H., Ramsey, P. S., Kerr, L. A., McKean, D. J., and Donohue, J. H. (1990) Regional and systemic distribution of anti-tumor x anti-CD3 heteroaggregate antibodies and cultured human peripheral blood lymphocytes in a human colon cancer xenograft. *J. Immunol.* **145,** 3507–3515.

21. Renner, C., Jung, W., Sahin, U., Denfeld, R., Pohl, C., Trumper, L., et al. (1994) Cure of xenografted human tumors by bispecific monoclonal antibodies and human T cells. *Science* **264,** 833–835.

22. Chokri, M., Girard, A., Deramoudt, F. X., Alonso, J. M., Bartholeyns, J., Jubault, C., et al. (1991) Experimental immunotherapy of colorectal tumors using cytotoxic macrophages and bispecific antibodies, in *Bispecific Antibodies and Targeted Cellular Cytotoxicity* (Romet-Lemonne, J. L., Fanger, M. W., and Segal, D. M., eds.), Lienhart, pp. 65–69.

23. Valone, F. H., Kaufman, P. A., Guyre, P. M., Lewis, L. D., Memoli, V., Deo, Y., et al. (1995) Phase Ia/Ib trial of bispecific antibody MDX-210 in patients with advanced breast or ovarian cancer that overexpresses the proto-oncogene HER-2/*neu*. *J. Clin. Oncol.* **13,** 2281–2292.

24. Kaufman, P. A., Guyre, P. M., Lewis, L. D., Valone, F. H., Memoli, V., Wells, W., et al. (1996) HER-2/*neu* targeted immunotherapy: A pilot study of multi-dose MDX-210 in patients with breast or ovarian cancers that overexpress HER-2/*neu* and a report of an increased incidence of HER-2/*neu* overexpression in metastatic breast cancer. *Tumor Targeting* **2,** 17–28.

25. Guyre, P. M., Graziano, R. F., Vance, B. A., Morganelli, P. M., and Fanger, M. W. (1989) Monoclonal antibodies that bind to distinct epitopes on Fc gamma RI are able to trigger receptor function. *J. Immunol.* **143,** 1650–1655.

26. Shen, L., Guyre, P. M., Anderson, C. L., and Fanger, M. W. (1986) Heteroantibody-mediated cytotoxicity: Antibody to the high-affinity Fc receptor for IgG mediates cytotoxicity by human monocytes which is enhanced by interferon-gamma and is not blocked by human IgG. *J. Immunol.* **137,** 3378–3382.

27. Ring, D. B., Clark, R., and Saxena, A. (1991) Identity of BCA200 and c-erbB-2 indicated by reactivity of monoclonal antibodies with recombinant c-erbB-2. *Mol. Immunol.* **28,** 915–917.

28. Ring, D. B., Kassel, J. A., Hsieh-Ma, S. T., Bjorn, M. J., Tringale, F., Eaton, A. M., et al. (1989) Distribution and physical properties of BCA200, a Mr 200,000 glycoprotein selectively associated with human breast cancer. *Cancer Res.* **49,** 3070–3080.

29. Fanger, M. W., Morganelli, P. M., and Guyre, P. M. (1993) Use of bispecific antibodies in the therapy of tumors. *Cancer Treat Res.* **68,** 181–194.

30. Fanger, M. W., Graziano, R. F., and Guyre, P. M. (1994) Production and use of anti-FcR bispecific antibodies. *Immunomethods* **4,** 72–81.

31. Mariani, M., Camagna, M., Tarditi, L., and Seccamani, E. (1991) A new enzymatic method to obtain high-yield F(ab)2 suitable for clinical use from mouse IgG1. *Mol. Immunol.* **28,** 69–77.

32. Parham, P. (1983) On the fragmentation of monoclonal IgG1, IgG2a, and IgG2b from BALB/c mice. *J. Immunol.* **131,** 2895–2902.

33. Graziano, R. F., Somasundaram, C., and Goldstein, J. (1995) The production of bispecific antibodies, in *Bispecific Antibodies* (Fanger, M. W., ed.), R. G. Landes Co., Austin, TX, pp. 1–26.

34. Hermanson, G. T. (1996) *Bioconjugate Techniques.* Academic, San Diego, CA.

35. Morganelli, P. M., Kitzmiller, T. J., Hemmer, R., and Fanger, M. W. (1992) Redirected targeting of LDL to human monocyte Fc gamma receptors with bispecific antibodies. *Arterioscler. Thromb.* **12,** 1131–1138.

36. Glennie, M. J., McBride, H. M., Worth, A. T., and Stevenson, G. T. (1987) Preparation and performance of bispecific F(ab'γ)2 antibody containing thioether-linked Fab'γ fragments. *J. Immunol.* **139,** 2367–2375.

37. Muirhead, K. A., Wallace, P. K., Schmitt, T. C., Frescatore, R. L., Franco, J. A., and Horan, P. K. (1986) Methodological considerations for implementation of lymphocyte subset analysis in a clinical reference laboratory. *Ann. NY Acad. Sci.* **468,** 113–127.

38. Corbett, I. P., Henry, J. A., Angus, B., Watchorn, C. J., Wilkinson, L., Hennessy, C., et al. (1990) NCL-CB11, a new monoclonal antibody recognizing the internal domain of the c-erbB-2 oncogene protein effective for use on formalin-fixed, paraffin-embedded tissue. *J. Pathol.* **161,** 15–25.

39. Guyre, P. M., Campbell, A. S., Kniffin, W. D., and Fanger, M. W. (1990) Monocytes and polymorphonuclear neutrophils of patients with streptococcal pharyngitis express increased numbers of type I IgG Fc receptors. *J. Clin. Invest.* **86,** 1892–1896.

40. Backman, K. A. and Guyre, P. M. (1994) Gamma-interferon inhibits Fc receptor II-mediated phagocytosis of tumor cells by human macrophages. *Cancer Res.* **54,** 2456–2461.

41. Looney, R. J., Abraham, G. N., and Anderson, C. L. (1986) Human monocytes and U937 cells bear two distinct Fc receptors for IgG. *J. Immunol.* **136,** 1641.

# Index